Taylor's
Clinical Nursing
Skills

Pamela Lynn, EdD, MSN, RN

Associate Professor
Gwynedd Mercy University
Frances M. Maguire School of Nursing
and Health Professions
Gwynedd Valley, Pennsylvania

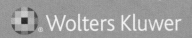

Wolters Kluwer

Philadelphia · Baltimore · New York · London
Buenos Aires · Hong Kong · Sydney · Tokyo

Vice President, Nursing Segment: Julie K. Stegman
Director, Nursing Education and Practice Content: Jamie Blum
Senior Product Manager: Betsy Gentzler
Senior Development Editor: Julie Vitale
Development Editor: Kelly Horvath
Editorial Coordinator: Erin Hernandez
Senior Content Editing Associate: Devika Kishore
Senior Production Project Manager: David Saltzberg
Marketing Manager: Greta Swanson
Manager, Graphic Arts & Design: Stephen Druding
Art Director, Illustration: Jennifer Clements
Manufacturing Coordinator: Margie Orzech-Zeranko
Prepress Vendor: Aptara, Inc.

6th Edition

9 8 7 6 5 4 3 2 1

Printed in Singapore

Library of Congress Cataloging-in-Publication Data

Names: Lynn, Pamela (Pamela Barbara), 1961- author.
Title: Taylor's clinical nursing skills : a nursing process approach /
    Pamela Lynn.
Other titles: Clinical nursing skills
Description: Sixth edition. | Philadelphia, PA : Wolters Kluwer Health,
    2023. | Includes bibliographical references and index.
Identifiers: LCCN 2022019841 (print) | LCCN 2022019842 (ebook) | ISBN
    9781975168704 (paperback) | ISBN 9781975168711 (ebook)
Subjects: MESH: Nursing Process | Nursing Care–methods | Case Reports |
    BISAC: MEDICAL / Nursing / Fundamentals & Skills | MEDICAL / Education &
    Training
Classification: LCC RT41 (print) | LCC RT41 (ebook) | NLM WY 100.1 | DDC
    610.73–dc23/eng/20220606
LC record available at https://lccn.loc.gov/2022019841
LC ebook record available at https://lccn.loc.gov/2022019842

shop.lww.com

In honor of nurses and nursing students everywhere
who continue to care with compassion and respect for the dignity and
individuality of each person—thank you, you are an inspiration!
—Pam Lynn

CONTRIBUTORS AND REVIEWERS

Contributor to this Edition

Heiddy DiGregorio, PhD, APRN, PCNS-BC, CHSE, CNE
Assistant Professor
Director of Simulation and Interprofessional Education
University of Delaware
College of Health Sciences, School of Nursing
Newark, Delaware
Chapter 5: Medications

Reviewers

Christie Cavallo, MSN, RN, EdD(c), CNE, CNEcl
Instructor
University of Tennessee Health Science Center
Memphis, Tennessee

Jennifer Delk, DNP, MSN, RN
Associate Professor and Chair of Undergraduate Programs
College of Nursing and Health Sciences
Union University
Jackson, Tennessee

Candice Entrekin
Pearl River Community College
Poplarville, Mississippi

Kathleen Fraley, ADN, BSN, MSN, RN
Professor of Nursing
St. Clair County Community College
Port Huron, Michigan

Carol Glaze, EdD(c), MSN, RN, CNE
Assistant Professor
University of Texas Medical Branch
School of Nursing
Galveston, Texas

Deanna Golden, DNP, MBA, RN
RN-BSN Program Faculty
School of Nursing & Health Sciences
Capella University
Minneapolis, Minnesota

Norlyn Hyde, RN, MSN
Professor of Nursing (Retired)
Skill Lab Instructor
Division of Nursing
Louisiana Tech University
Ruston, Louisiana

Gloria M. Loera, DNP, RN, NEA-BC
Assistant Professor
Program Director Graduate Studies
Gayle Greve Hunt School of Nursing
Texas Tech University Health Sciences Center El Paso
El Paso, Texas

Kristel Ray, DNP, MSN, BSN, RN, ANP-BC
Professor of Nursing and Simulation Coordinator
Mott Community College
Flint, Michigan

Robert Reynoso, MSN/Ed, BSN, AAAS, RN, CEN
Nursing Instructor
Shoreline Community College
Shoreline, Washington

Amy Roach, DNS, RN
Assistant Professor
Wellstar School of Nursing
Kennesaw State University
Kennesaw, Georgia

Christy Skinner
Gordon State College
Barnesville, Georgia

Shari Tenner-Hooban
Wesley College
Dover, Delaware

Stacy Thibodeau, DNP, MSN, RN
Assistant Professor of Nursing
University of Maine at Fort Kent
Fort Kent, Maine

Amy Witt, PhD, RN, CNE
Associate Professor
Bethel University
St. Paul, Minnesota

Taylor's Clinical Nursing Skills aims to help nursing students and graduate nurses incorporate cognitive, technical, interpersonal, and ethical/legal skills into safe, effective, thoughtful person-centered care. This book is written to meet the needs of novice to advanced nurses. Many of the skills shown in this book may not be encountered by the student while in school, but may be encountered once the graduate nurse has entered the workforce.

Because it emphasizes the basic principles of patient care, we believe this book can easily be used with any Fundamentals text. However, this Skills book was specifically designed to accompany *Fundamentals of Nursing: The Art and Science of Person-Centered Care,* Tenth Edition, by Taylor, Lynn, and Bartlett, to provide a seamless learning experience. Some of the Skills and Guidelines for Nursing Care from the Taylor *Fundamentals* book may also be found in this book, but its content has been embellished here to:

- Highlight the nursing process.
- Emphasize unexpected situations that the nurse may encounter, along with related interventions for how to respond to these unexpected situations.
- Draw attention to critical actions within skills.
- Illustrate specific actions within a skill through the use of nearly 1,000 four-color photographs and illustrations.
- Highlight available evidence for practice: best practice guidelines, research-based evidence, and support from appropriate professional literature.
- Reference appropriate case study or studies included at the end of the book, emphasizing which case studies utilize and enhance the content of each chapter.

In addition, this book contains several higher-level skills that are not addressed in the Taylor *Fundamentals* book.

Learning Experience

This text and the entire Taylor Suite have been created with the student's experience in mind. Care has been taken to appeal to all learning styles. The student-friendly writing style ensures that students will comprehend and retain information. The extensive art program enhances understanding of important actions. Accompanying skill videos clearly demonstrate and reinforce important skill steps; as students watch and listen to the videos, comprehension increases. In addition, each element of the Taylor Suite, which is described later in the preface, coordinates to provide a consistent and cohesive learning experience.

In Units I and II, the unexpected situations and special considerations content at the end of each skill challenges students to think critically, consider the context and multiple needs of patients, and prioritize care appropriately—supporting development of clinical judgment.

Organization

Taylor's Clinical Nursing Skills is organized into three units. Ideally, the text will be followed sequentially, but every effort has been made to respect the differing needs of diverse curricula and students. Thus, each chapter stands on its own merit and may be read independently of others.

Unit I: Actions Basic to Nursing Care

This unit introduces the foundational skills used by nurses: maintaining asepsis, measuring vital signs, assessing health, promoting safety, administering medication, and caring for surgical patients.

In Chapter 3, Health Assessment, physical assessment content reflects the practice needs of beginning and general nurses. Assessment procedures performed by advanced practice professionals are clearly identified. Assessments identified as advanced procedures and skills are available in the online resources for students.

Unit II: Promoting Healthy Physiologic Responses

This unit focuses on the physiologic needs of patients: hygiene; skin integrity and wound care; activity; comfort and pain management; nutrition; urinary elimination; bowel elimination; oxygenation; perfusion and cardiovascular care; fluid, electrolyte, and acid–base balance; neurologic care; and laboratory specimen collection.

Unit III: Integrated Case Studies

Although nursing skills textbooks generally present content in a linear fashion for ease of understanding, in reality, many nursing skills are performed in combination for patients with complicated health needs. The integrated case studies in this unit are designed to challenge the reader to think critically, consider the context and multiple needs of patients, and prioritize care appropriately—supporting development of clinical judgment, preparing the student and graduate nurse for complex situations that arise in everyday practice.

Teaching/Learning Package

To facilitate mastery of this text's content, a comprehensive teaching/learning package has been developed to assist faculty and students.

Resources for Instructors

Tools to assist you with teaching your course are available upon adoption of this text online at https://thepoint.lww.com/Lynn6e.

- The **Test Generator** has 450 NCLEX®-Style questions to help you put together exclusive new tests from a bank with questions spanning the book's topics, which will assist you in assessing your students' understanding of the material.
- **PowerPoint Presentations**, provided for each book chapter, enhance teaching by providing key visuals and reinforcing content. These provide an easy way for you to integrate the textbook with your students' learning experience, either via slide shows or handouts.
- **Skills Lab Teaching Plans** walk you through each chapter, objective by objective, and provide a lecture outline and teaching guidelines. In addition to one teaching plan for each chapter, there is one bonus teaching plan to assist with lab simulations.
- A **Master Checklist for Skills Competency** is provided to help you track your students' progress on all the skills in this book.
- **NEW! AACN Essentials Content Mapping**, which are competency-based and include expected competencies for entry-level nurses and advanced-level nurses.
- A **QSEN Competency Map** shows where in the text to find the Knowledge, Skills, and Attitudes (KSAs) that students will need to develop so they can ensure quality and safety in patient care.
- A sample **Syllabus** is provided to help you organize your course.
- **Journal Articles** offer access to current research available in Wolters Kluwer journals.
- The **Image Bank** provides free access to illustrations and photos from the textbook for use in PowerPoint presentations and handouts.

Resources for Students

Valuable learning tools for students are available online at https://thepoint.lww.com/Lynn6e, including:

- **Watch & Learn Videos**, **Practice & Learn Case Studies**, and **Concepts in Action Animations** demonstrate important concepts related to skills.
- **Journal Articles** offer access to current research available in Wolters Kluwer journals.
- A **Spanish–English Audio Glossary** provides helpful terms and phrases for communicating with patients who speak Spanish.

- **Dosage Calculation Quizzes** provide opportunities for students to practice math skills and calculate drug dosages.

Taylor Suite Resources

With expert authored content and engaging learning solutions, the Taylor Fundamentals/Skills suite is tailored to fit every learning style. This integrated suite of products offers students a seamless learning experience not found elsewhere. To learn more about any solution with the Taylor suite, please contact your local Wolters Kluwer representative.

- *Fundamentals of Nursing: The Art and Science of Person-Centered Care*, **10th Edition**, by Carol Taylor, Pamela Lynn, and Jennifer Bartlett. This Fundamentals text promotes nursing as an evolving art and science, directed to human health and well-being. It challenges students to cultivate the Quality and Safety Education for Nurses (QSEN) and blended competencies they will need to serve patients and the public well. The aim is to prepare nurses who combine the highest level of scientific knowledge and technologic skill with responsible, caring practice. The text challenges students to identify and master the cognitive and technical skills as well as the interpersonal and ethical/legal skills they will need to effectively nurse the patients in their care. The text includes engaging features to promote critical thinking, clinical reasoning, and clinical judgment.
- *Skill Checklists for Taylor's Clinical Nursing Skills*, **6th Edition**. This collection of checklists with convenient perforated pages is designed to accompany this Skills textbook and promote proper technique while increasing students' confidence.
- *Taylor's Video Guide to Clinical Nursing Skills*. With more than 12 hours of video footage and more than 170 videos, these videos—developed consistently with the written skill instructions—follow nursing students and their instructors as they perform a range of essential nursing procedures. Students can now access the full set of videos as part of Lippincott Skills for Nursing Education (see below.)

A Comprehensive, Digital, Integrated Skills Solution

Experience the content you love from this book in a new way in *Lippincott® Skills for Nursing Education*, an unparalleled nursing education skills solution to help student nurses develop skill competency and clinical judgment.

Available anytime, anywhere, *Lippincott Skills for Nursing Education* is designed specifically to empower nursing faculty and students to support teaching, learning, and reporting on nursing skills across the curriculum. Expert-authored skill instructions, evidence-based rationales, videos and case studies help the novice nursing student master new skills and confidently prepare for skills lab and clinical settings.

Used alone or integrated with *Lippincott® CoursePoint*, **Lippincott Skills for Nursing Education** offers an efficient learning experience backed with tools to monitor and motivate student preparedness and skill competency.

Taylor's Clinical Nursing Skills Collection, authored by Pamela Lynn, EdD, MSN, RN, delivers a robust set of essential skills for the undergraduate nurse and meets the needs of students throughout the curriculum.

Features include:

- A new **web-based user interface** goes beyond a traditional eBook, delivering essential pedagogy, nursing process approach and skill instruction optimized for online reading and on-the-go learning.
- **Trusted content** from *Taylor's Clinical Nursing Skills* and *Taylor's Video Guide to Clinical Nursing Skills* equips students with education-focused skill instructions and pedagogy.
- *Skill Overviews* use a consistent framework for each skill, with step-by-step implementation guidance and rationales.
- *Videos* bring skill instructions to life, with more than 170 videos showing nursing students and their instructors performing a range of essential nursing procedures, carefully matching written skill instructions.

- *Quizzes* for each skill assess students' understanding and preparedness for skills lab or clinical.
- *Case Studies* help students develop clinical judgment skills and apply their knowledge in the context of patient care, with two types of cases:
  - **Practice & Learn Interactive Case Studies** engage today's active learners in content review, case study practice application and assessment.
  - **Integrated Case Studies** reflect the complex combination of skills typically performed in nursing practice, challenging students to think critically and prioritize care.
- *Online Skill Checklists* allow instructors to customize student evaluation and easily track skill performance, enter comments, and save and share checklist records with students electronically.
- **Skill-based organization** of all resources ensures an efficient learning experience.
- **Enhanced reporting** provides in-depth dashboards with key data points to help instructors track student progress and identify strengths and weaknesses.

Pamela Lynn, EdD, MSN, RN

FOCUS ON PATIENT CARE!

Each chapter in Units I and II begins with a description of three real-world case scenarios that put the skills into context. These scenarios provide a framework for the chapter content to be covered.

GET READY TO LEARN!

Before reading the chapter content, read the **Learning Outcomes**. These roadmaps help you understand what is important and why. Create your own learning outline or use them for self-testing.

Review the **Nursing Concepts** list in the chapter opener that highlight connections to nursing concepts for ease of identification. **Key Terms** are bolded throughout the narrative; explanations to help you become familiar with new vocabulary are presented online at https://thepoint.lww.com/lynn6e.

15

Perfusion and Cardiovascular Care

Focusing on Patient Care

This chapter will help you develop some of the skills related to perfusion and cardiovascular care necessary to care for the following patients:

Coby Pruder, age 40, is to undergo an electrocardiogram as part of a physical examination. Although they report feeling healthy, they are also nervous.

Harry Stebbings, age 67, is admitted to the emergency department for chest pain and cardiac monitoring.

Ann Kribell, age 54, is a patient in the cardiac care unit. Ann has been diagnosed with heart failure and is receiving cardiac monitoring. The cardiac monitoring alarms are alarming very frequently, multiple times an hour.

Refer to Focusing on Patient Care: Developing Clinical Reasoning and Clinical Judgment at the end of the chapter to apply what you learn.

Learning Outcomes

After completing the chapter, you will be able to accomplish the following:

1. Perform cardiopulmonary resuscitation.
2. Perform emergency automated external defibrillation.
3. Perform emergency manual external defibrillation (asynchronous).
4. Obtain a 12-lead electrocardiogram.
5. Apply a cardiac monitor.
6. Apply and monitor a transcutaneous (external) pacemaker.
7. Remove a peripheral arterial catheter.

Nursing Concepts

- Assessment
- Clinical Decision Making/Clinical Judgment
- Perfusion
- Safety
- Tissue Integrity

957

DEVELOP CLINICAL REASONING AND CLINICAL JUDGMENT!

Fundamentals Review. Because of the breadth and depth of nursing knowledge that must be absorbed, nursing students and graduate nurses can easily become overwhelmed. Thus, this book is designed to eliminate excessive content and redundancy and to better focus the reader's attention. To this end, each chapter in Units I and II includes several boxes, tables, or figures that summarize important concepts that should be understood before performing a skill. For a more in-depth study of these concepts, readers are encouraged to refer to their Fundamentals textbook.

Enhance Your Understanding, located at the end of each chapter, gives readers an opportunity to further their understanding and apply what they have learned. It includes three sections:

Focusing on Patient Care: Developing Clinical Reasoning and Clinical Judgment asks readers to consider questions that reflect back to the opening scenarios for added cohesion throughout the chapters. Readers are challenged to apply the skills and use the new knowledge they have gained to "think through" learning exercises designed to show how critical thinking and clinical reasoning can result in a clinical judgment, leading to a possible change in outcomes and an impact on patient care.

Suggested Answers for Focusing on Patient Care: Developing Clinical Reasoning and Clinical Judgment represent possible nursing care solutions to the problems. The answers can be found after the bibliography section at the end of the chapter.

Integrated Case Study Connection refers readers to the appropriate case study or studies discussion in Unit III, emphasizing which case studies utilize and enhance the content of that chapter.

Fundamentals Review 14-1

FACTORS AFFECTING OXYGENATION AND PERFUSION

A variety of factors can affect cardiopulmonary functioning. This display reviews common factors.

LEVEL OF HEALTH

Acute and chronic illness can dramatically affect a person's cardiopulmonary function. Body systems (e.g., the cardiovascular system and respiratory system or the musculoskeletal system and the respiratory system) work together, so alterations in one may affect the other. For example, alterations in muscle function contribute to inadequate pulmonary **ventilation** and **respiration**, as well as to inadequate functioning of the heart.

DEVELOPMENTAL LEVEL

Respiratory function varies across the life span. The table below summarizes variations. Age-related variations in pulse rate and blood pressure can be found in Chapter 2, Fundamentals Review 2-1.

	Infant (Birth–1 year)	Early Childhood (1–5 years)	Late Childhood (6–12 years)	Adolescent and Adult (18+ years)
Respiratory rate	30–60 breaths/min	20–40 breaths/min	15–25 breaths/min	12–20 breaths/min
Respiratory pattern	Abdominal breathing, irregular in rate and depth	Abdominal breathing, irregular	Thoracic breathing, regular	Thoracic, regular
Shape of thorax	Round	Elliptical	Elliptical	Elliptical or barrel-shaped

MEDICATIONS

Many medications affect the function of the cardiopulmonary system. Patients receiving drugs that affect the central nervous system need to be monitored carefully for respiratory complications. The nurse should monitor rate and depth of respirations in patients who are taking certain medications, such as opioids or sedatives. Other medications decrease heart rate, with associated decreased cardiac output, and the potential to alter the flow of blood to body tissues.

(continued)

Enhance Your Understanding

Focusing on Patient Care: Developing Clinical Reasoning and Clinical Judgment

Consider the case scenarios at the beginning of the chapter as you answer the following questions to enhance your understanding and apply what you have learned.

QUESTIONS

1. Scott Mingus has a chest drain in place after thoracic surgery. The chest tube has been draining 20 to 30 mL of serosanguinous fluid every hour. Suddenly, the chest tube output is 110 mL/hr and the drainage is bright red. What should the nurse do?

2. Saranam Srivastava has a history of smoking and is scheduled for abdominal surgery. They need to learn how to use an incentive spirometer. What should the nurse include in patient education regarding the use of an incentive spirometer?

3. The nurse caring for Paula Cunningham determines that Ms. Cunningham needs to be suctioned via her endotracheal tube. What assessment findings might lead to this conclusion? How would the nurse determine if the suctioning of Ms. Cunningham's airway was effective?

You can find suggested answers after the Bibliography at the end of this chapter.

Integrated Case Study Connection

The case studies in the back of the book focus on integrating concepts. Refer to the following case studies to enhance your understanding of the concepts and skills in this chapter.

- Basic Case Studies: Kate Townsend, page 1205.
- Intermediate Case Studies: Olivia Greenbaum, page 1209; George Patel, page 1223.
- Advanced Case Studies: Cole McKean, page 1225; Damian Wallace, page 1227; George Patel, Gwen Galloway, Claudia Tran, and James White, page 1232.

Delegation Considerations assist students and graduate nurses in developing the critical decision-making skills necessary to transfer responsibility for the performance of an activity to another person and to ensure safe and effective nursing care. Delegation decision-making information is provided in each skill and Appendix A, using delegation guidelines based on American Nurses Association (ANA) and National Council of State Boards of Nursing (NCSBN) principles and recommendations.

DELEGATION CONSIDERATIONS The measurement of oxygen saturation using a pulse oximeter may be delegated to assistive personnel (AP) as well as to licensed practical/vocational nurses (LPN/LVNs). The decision to delegate must be based on careful analysis of the patient's needs and circumstances as well as the qualifications of the person to whom the task is being delegated. Refer to the Delegation Guidelines in Appendix A.

Skill 14-6	Caring for a Patient Receiving Noninvasive Continuous Positive Airway Pressure *(continued)*

allow to air dry. Reassemble the CPAP machine once components are fully dry. Inspect the components and replace as necessary; the mask and tube should be replaced as indicated by the manufacturer, usually every 3 to 12 months (ASA, 2021; Pinto & Sharma, 2021).
• Replace the CPAP machine filter every 4 weeks or according to the manufacturer's guidelines (ASA, 2021).

Evidence for Practice highlights available evidence for practice— best practice guidelines, research-based evidence, and support from appropriate professional literature.

EVIDENCE FOR PRACTICE ▶

IMPROVING ADHERENCE WITH CPAP

When used as prescribed, CPAP reduces daytime sleepiness, normalizes sleep architecture, and improves numerous health outcomes related to obstructive sleep apnea. Adherence to the prescribed use of CPAP is critical to achieve optimal effect of the therapy. However, a significant number of patients experience difficulties associated with use with resulting lack of adherence and compliance with the therapy (Pinto & Sharma, 2021). What can nurses do to help improve patient adherence to CPAP?

Related Research

López-López, L., Torres-Sánchez, I., Cabrera-Martos, I., Ortíz-Rubio, A., Granados-Santiago, M., & Valenza, M. C. (2020). Nursing interventions improve continuous positive airway pressure adherence in obstructive sleep apnea with excessive daytime sleepiness: A systematic review. *Rehabilitation Nursing, 45*(3), 140–146. https://doi.org/10.1097/rnj.000000000000190.

The purpose of this systematic review was to summarize the effectiveness of interventions in the literature to improve adherence to continuous positive airway pressure (CPAP) treatment in patients with excessive daytime sleepiness. Three data bases (MEDLINE, ScienceDirect, and Google Scholar) were systematically searched for randomized controlled trials published between January 2005 and May 2018 that included interventions to improve CPAP adherence in adult obstructive sleep apnea patients with high daytime sleepiness. Key words included *apnea, compliance, CPAP, adherence,* and *somnolence.* Eight trials were identified to meet the criteria. The methodologic quality of the included studies was classified according to the Jadad Scale (Jadad or Oxford score). Three trials had scores below 3 points, indicating lack of rigor; five trials had scores of 3, indicating rigor. The reviewed studies identified four categories of interventions to improve adherence to CPAP: educational (five studies), technological (one study), pharmacologic (one study) and multidimensional interventions, including patient education (one study). The majority of the trials reviewed examined the impact of patient education on CPAP adherence, and the results suggested that educational interventions are the most effective at improving adherence to CPAP. The researchers concluded that patient education strategies alone and in combination with other modalities, such as relaxation, improve patient adherence to CPAP.

Relevance to Nursing Practice

Nurses play a large role in designing interventions to positively impact patient outcomes. Nurses can support and encourage adherence to a prescribed CPAP intervention. Patient education can increase CPAP adherence. Nurses can also use therapeutic strategies to improve CPAP adherence and should consider multidimensional interventions to enhance compliance.

MASTER NURSING PROCESS!

The **nursing process** provides the organizational framework to integrate related nursing responsibilities for each of the five steps: Assessment, Diagnosis*, Outcome Identification and Planning, Implementation, and Evaluation.

The ANA's (2021). *Nursing Scope and Standards of Practice* highlights the continuing importance of nursing process,

> "Regardless of the theoretical knowledge base upon which nursing and its practice are derived, that knowledge fits within the multidimensional nursing process, the analytical, critical-thinking framework guiding professional thinking and activities." (p. 11)

Documentation Guidelines direct students and graduate nurses in accurate documentation related to implementation of the skill and related findings. **Sample Documentation** demonstrates proper documentation.

*The outcome of data interpretation related to a skill is presented as appropriate actual or potential health problems and needs identified in conjunction with diagnosing. This change reflects a balance between the educational value of teaching using the nursing process and the recognition that education needs to mirror clinical practice and the move away from the use of nursing diagnoses. Material related to identification of actual or potential health problems and needs is from the International Council of Nurses (ICN, 2019). *Nursing diagnosis and outcome statements. ICNP® is owned and copyrighted by the International Council of Nurses (ICN). Reproduced with permission of the copyright holder*. https://www.icn.ch/sites/default/files/inline-files/ICNP2019-DC.pdf; and *Problem-based care plans.* (2020). In *Lippincott Advisor*. Wolters Kluwer. https://advisor.lww.com/lna/home.do

Skill 14-9 — Suctioning an Endotracheal Tube: Open System (continued)

DELEGATION CONSIDERATIONS Suctioning an endotracheal tube is not delegated to assistive personnel (AP). Depending on the state's nurse practice act and the organization's policies and procedures, suctioning of an endotracheal tube in a stable situation, such as long-term care and other community-based care settings, may be delegated to licensed practical/vocational nurses (LPN/LVNs). The decision to delegate must be based on careful analysis of the patient's needs and circumstances as well as the qualifications of the person to whom the task is being delegated. Refer to the Delegation Guidelines in Appendix A.

EQUIPMENT
- Portable or wall suction unit with tubing
- A commercially prepared suction kit with an appropriate-size catheter (see General Considerations) or
- Sterile suction catheter with Y-port in the appropriate size
- Sterile, disposable container
- Sterile gloves
- Towel or waterproof pad
- Goggles and mask or face shield; N95 mask or equivalent, based on patient's health status
- Additional PPE, as indicated
- Disposable, clean gloves
- Resuscitation bag connected to 100% oxygen
- Assistant (optional)

ASSESSMENT Assess for indications for the need for suctioning: audible and/or visible secretions, reduced oxygen saturation, presence of coarse crackles over the trachea, deterioration of arterial blood gas values, reduced breath sounds, the patient's inability to generate an effective spontaneous cough, acute respiratory distress, or suspected aspiration of secretions (AARC, 2010; Patton, 2019; Sole et al., 2015). Assess lung sounds. Wheezes, coarse crackles, gurgling or diminished breath sounds may indicate the need for suctioning. Assess for the presence of visualized secretions in the artificial airway, audible secretions, and ineffective coughing (Morton & Fontaine, 2018; Sole et al., 2015). Assess the oxygen saturation level. Deterioration in oxygen desaturation may be an indication of the need for suctioning (AARC, 2010). Assess respiratory status, including respiratory rate and depth. Patients may become tachypneic when they need to be suctioned. Assess the patient for signs of respiratory distress, such as nasal flaring, retractions, or grunting. Assess for pain and the potential to cause pain during the intervention (Arroyo-Novoa et al., 2008; Chaseling et al., 2014; Wrona et al., 2021; Düzkaya & Kuğuoğlu, 2015). Anticipate the administration of pharmacologic (analgesic medication) and use of nonpharmacologic interventions for the patient before suctioning (Arroyo-Novoa et al., 2008; Düzkaya & Kuğuoğlu, 2015). Assess the appropriate suction catheter depth. Refer to Box 14-2. Assess the characteristics and amount of secretions while suctioning.

ACTUAL OR POTENTIAL HEALTH PROBLEMS AND NEEDS Many actual or potential health problems or issues may require the use of this skill as part of related interventions. An appropriate health problem or issue may include:
- Ineffective airway clearance
- Altered breathing pattern
- Impaired gas exchange

OUTCOME IDENTIFICATION AND PLANNING The expected outcome to achieve is that the patient will exhibit a clear, patent airway. Other outcomes that may be appropriate include that the patient will exhibit an oxygen saturation level within acceptable parameters, will demonstrate a respiratory rate and depth within acceptable parameters, and will remain free from any signs of respiratory distress and adverse effect.

IMPLEMENTATION

ACTION	RATIONALE
1. Gather equipment.	Assembling equipment provides for an organized approach to the task.
2. Perform hand hygiene and put on PPE, if indicated.	Hand hygiene and PPE prevent the spread of microorganisms. PPE is required based on transmission precautions.

Skill 14-9 — Suctioning an Endotracheal Tube: Open System (continued)

ACTION	RATIONALE
25. Turn off the suction. Remove the face shield or goggles and mask. Perform hand hygiene.	Removing the face shield or goggles and mask properly reduces the risk for infection transmission and contamination of other items. Hand hygiene prevents transmission of microorganisms.
26. Reassess the patient's respiratory status, including respiratory rate, effort, oxygen saturation, lung sounds, tracheal sounds, and the presence/absence of secretions in artificial airway, and the patient's response to the intervention.	These assess effectiveness of suctioning and the presence of complications.
27. Remove additional PPE, if used. Perform hand hygiene.	Proper removal of PPE reduces the risk for infection transmission and contamination of other items. Hand hygiene prevents the spread of microorganisms.

EVALUATION The expected outcomes have been met when the patient has exhibited a clear, patent airway; an oxygen saturation level within acceptable parameters; and a respiratory rate and depth within acceptable parameters; and the patient has remained free from any signs of respiratory distress and adverse effect.

DOCUMENTATION

Guidelines Document the time of suctioning, assessments before and after interventions, the reason for suctioning, oxygen saturation levels, and the characteristics and amount of secretions.

Sample Documentation

> 9/1/25 1850 Tan secretions noted in ET tube; coarse crackles noted to auscultation over trachea. Lung sounds coarse in lower lobes. Respirations 24 breaths/min, regular rhythm. Intercostal retractions noted. Endotracheal tube suctioning completed with 12-Fr catheter. Small amount of thin, tan secretions obtained. Specimen for culture collected and sent. After suctioning, no secretions noted in ET tube, auscultation over trachea clear, lung sounds clear, respirations 18 breaths/min, no intercostal retractions noted.
> —C. Bausler, RN

DEVELOPING CLINICAL REASONING AND CLINICAL JUDGMENT

UNEXPECTED SITUATIONS AND ASSOCIATED INTERVENTIONS
- *Catheter or sterile glove is contaminated:* Reconnect the patient to the ventilator or oxygen supply. Discard gloves and the suction catheter. Gather supplies and begin the procedure again.
- *When suctioning, your eye becomes contaminated with respiratory secretions:* After attending to the patient, perform hand hygiene and flush your eye with a large amount of sterile water. Contact employee health or your supervisor immediately for further treatment and complete adverse event documentation as per facility policy. Wear goggles or a face shield when suctioning to prevent exposure to body fluids.
- *Patient is extubated during suctioning:* Remain with the patient. Call for help to notify the health care team. Assess the patient's vital signs, ability to breathe without assistance, and oxygen saturation. Be ready to deliver assisted breaths with a bag-valve mask (see Skill 14-16) or administer oxygen. Anticipate the need for reintubation.
- *Oxygen saturation level decreases after suctioning:* Hyperoxygenate the patient. Auscultate lung sounds. If lung sounds are absent over one lobe, notify the health care team. Remain with the patient. The patient may have **pneumothorax** or a malplaced endotracheal tube. Anticipate a prescribed intervention for a stat chest x-ray and possible chest tube placement or reintubation.
- *Patient develops signs of intolerance to suctioning:* oxygen saturation level decreases and remains low after hyperoxygenation; patient becomes cyanotic; or patient becomes bradycardic: Stop

DEVELOP THE NECESSARY SKILLS!

Step-by-Step Skills. Each chapter presents numerous related step-by-step skills. The skills are presented in a concise, straightforward, and simplified two-column format to facilitate competent performance of nursing skills.

Scientific Rationales accompany each nursing action to promote a deeper understanding of the basic principles supporting nursing care.

Nursing Alerts draw attention to crucial information.

Photo Atlas Approach. When learning a new skill, it is often overwhelming to only *read* how to perform a skill. With nearly 1,000 photographs, this book offers a pictorial guide to performing each skill. The skill will not only be learned but also remembered through the use of text with pictures.

Skill 2-1 ▶ Assessing Body Temperature *(continued)*

ACTION	RATIONALE
37. Place the bed in the lowest position and elevate rails, as needed. Leave the patient clean and comfortable.	A low bed position and elevated side rails provide for patient safety.
38. Return the electronic thermometer to the charging unit.	The thermometer needs to be recharged for future use.
Measuring Rectal Temperature	
39. Adjust the bed to a comfortable working height (VHACEOSH, 2016). Put on nonsterile gloves.	Having the bed at the proper height prevents back and muscle strain. Gloves prevent contact with contaminants and body fluids.
40. Assist the patient to a side-lying position. Pull back the cover sufficiently to expose only the buttocks. Position a young infant supine with legs flexed (Kyle & Carmen, 2021).	The side-lying position allows the nurse to see the buttocks. Exposing only the buttocks keeps the patient warm and maintains their dignity. Rectal temperatures are not normally taken in newborns, infants, and young children (Jensen, 2019; Silbert-Flagg & Pillitteri, 2018) but may be indicated. Refer to the Special Considerations section at the end of the skill.
41. Remove the rectal probe from within the recording unit of the electronic thermometer. Cover the probe with a disposable probe cover, sliding it on until it snaps in place (Figure 14).	Using a cover prevents contamination of the thermometer.
42. **Lubricate about 1 inch of the probe with a water-soluble lubricant (Figure 15).**	Lubrication reduces friction and facilitates insertion, minimizing the risk of irritation or injury to the rectal mucous membranes.

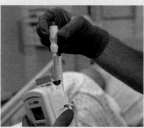 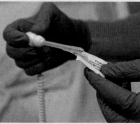

FIGURE 14. Removing appropriate probe and attaching disposable probe cover.

FIGURE 15. Lubricating thermometer tip.

ACTION	RATIONALE
43. Reassure the patient. Separate the buttocks until the anal sphincter is clearly visible.	If not placed directly into the anal opening, the thermometer probe may injure adjacent tissue or cause discomfort.
44. Insert the thermometer probe into the anus about 1.5 inches in an adult or no more than 1 inch in children (Figure 16) (Kyle & Carmen, 2021).	The depth of insertion must be adjusted based on the patient's age. Rectal temperatures are not normally taken in newborns, infants, and young children (Jensen, 2019; Silbert-Flagg & Pillitteri, 2018) but may be indicated. Refer to the Special Considerations section at the end of the skill.

Hand Hygiene icons alert you to this crucial step that is the best way to prevent the spread of microorganisms. Important information related to this icon is included inside the back cover.

Patient Identification icons alert you to this critical step ensuring the right patient receives the intervention, to help prevent errors. Important information related to this icon is included inside the back cover.

IMPLEMENTATION

ACTION	RATIONALE
1. Check the prescribed interventions or plan of care for frequency of measurement and route. More frequent temperature measurement may be appropriate based on nursing judgment.	Assessment and measurement of vital signs at appropriate intervals provide important data about the patient's health status.
2. Perform hand hygiene and put on PPE, if indicated.	Hand hygiene and PPE prevent the spread of microorganisms. PPE is required based on transmission precautions.
3. Identify the patient.	Identifying the patient ensures that the right patient receives the intervention and helps prevent errors.

Skill 2-2 ▶ Regulating Temperature Using an Overhead Radiant Warmer *(continued)*

IMPLEMENTATION

ACTION	RATIONALE
1. Check the prescribed interventions or plan of care for the use of a radiant warmer.	Provides for patient safety and appropriate care.
2. Perform hand hygiene and put on PPE, if indicated.	Hand hygiene and PPE prevent the spread of microorganisms. PPE is required based on transmission precautions.
3. Identify the patient.	Identifying the patient ensures the right patient receives the intervention and helps prevent errors.
4. Close curtains around the bed and close the door to the room, if possible. Discuss the procedure with the patient's family/caregivers.	This ensures the patient's privacy. Explanation reduces the family's/caregiver's apprehension and encourages cooperation.
5. Plug in the warmer. Turn the warmer to the manual setting. Allow the blankets to warm before placing the infant under the warmer.	By allowing the blankets to warm before placing the infant under the warmer, you are preventing heat loss through conduction. By placing the warmer on the manual setting, you are keeping the warmer at a set temperature no matter how warm the blankets become.
6. Insert probe securely into the heater unit. **Switch the warmer setting to automatic. Set the warmer to the**	The automatic setting ensures that the warmer will regulate the amount of radiant heat, depending on the temperature of

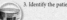

Skill 2-1 ▶ Assessing Body Temperature *(continued)*

Skill Variation **Assessing Body Temperature with a Temporal Artery Thermometer When the Temporal Artery and Behind the Ear Locations Are Not Accessible**

If the temporal artery and behind the ear locations are not accessible, the femoral artery, lateral thoracic artery, and axillary sites may be used to assess body temperature using a temporal artery thermometer (Exergen, n.d.b).

1. Assess the appropriateness and need for measurement at an alternate site using a temporal artery thermometer.
2. Refer to Steps 1–8 in Skill 2-1.
3. Refer to Steps 23–27 in Skill 2-1, with the following modifications for each specific alternate site: Femoral artery: Slide the probe across the groin.

Lateral thoracic artery: Scan side to side in the area, about midway between the axilla and nipple.
Axilla: Insert probe in the apex of the axilla for about 2 to 3 seconds.
4. Release the button and read the thermometer measurement.
5. Hold the thermometer over a waste receptacle. Gently push the probe cover with your thumb against the proximal edge to dispose of the probe cover.
6. The instrument will automatically turn off in 30 seconds, or press and release the power button.

EVIDENCE FOR PRACTICE ▶

FEVER AND ANTIPYRESIS

Temperature increase and fever are common clinical symptoms. Fever is an important part of a person's defense mechanisms against infection. Findings about antipyretic treatment have further challenged the need for routine or aggressive fever suppression. Unfortunately, many health care professionals continue to be "fever phobic," while their attitudes toward fever and antipyresis considerably affect antipyretic practice (Ludwig & McWhinnie, 2019). What are health care professionals' awareness of fever and antipyresis? Is nursing practice based on appropriate treatment for fever?

Related Evidence

Ludwig, J., & McWhinnie, H. (2019). Antipyretic drugs in patients with fever and infection: Literature review. *British Journal of Nursing, 28*(10), 610–618. https://doi.org/10.12968/bjon.2019.28.10.610

This literature review examined whether the administration of antipyretic drugs to adult patients with infection and fever, in secondary care, improves or worsens patient outcomes. Keywords, including fever, pyresis, infection, and antipyresis, were searched in the Cumulative Index to Nursing and Allied Health Literature (CINAHL) and Medline databases for the years 2010–2017. The target population for the review was hospitalized adult patients with fever and infection. Discussion of antipyretics in patients with infection and fever and/or discussion of the benefits/disadvantages of fever during infection were identified as criteria for inclusion in the review. Outcomes measured in the studies included patient mortality/morbidity, patient experiences and perceptions of fever/antipyretics, and professionals' attitudes toward fever/antipyretics. The database searches identified 1,523 articles; based on title and abstract review, 1,501 were excluded. Twenty-two articles were selected for full text review; after evaluation, 13 articles were chosen for inclusion in the final review. These final studies included randomized-controlled trials (3), cross-sectional survey/questionnaires (2), a qualitative interview (1), prospective observational studies (2), and retrospective observational studies (5). Each study was examined against the Critical Appraisal Skills Programme (CASP) quality checklists, and overall methodologic quality of the studies was deemed satisfactory. Two key themes identified included "antipyretics, fever and patient outcomes" and "professionals' and patients' experiences and perceptions of antipyretics and fever." Contrasting results were reported; two studies demonstrated improved patient outcomes following antipyretic administration, while several studies demonstrated increased mortality risk associate with antipyretics and/or demonstrated fever's benefits during infection. Results also demonstrated that health professionals continue to view fever as deleterious. The authors concluded the evidence does not support routine antipyretic administration. In addition, the researchers suggested health care providers should consider patients' comorbidities and symptoms of their underlying illness to promote safe, evidence-based, and appropriate administration of antipyretics.

Skill Variations, listed in the Table of Contents and the Skill title for ease of access, provide clear instructions for variations in equipment or technique.

Developing Clinical Reasoning and Clinical Judgment provides insight into prioritization and evidence-based practice and supports students' development of clinical reasoning and clinical judgment skills. This section includes:

Unexpected Situations are provided after the explanation of expected outcomes. Each situation is followed by an explanation of suggested possible intervention, with rationales. This feature serves as a starting point for group discussion.

DEVELOPING CLINICAL REASONING AND CLINICAL JUDGMENT
UNEXPECTED SITUATIONS AND ASSOCIATED INTERVENTIONS

- *Patient was previously fine on oxygen delivered by mask but is now short of breath, and the pulse oximeter reading is less than 93%:* Check to see that the oxygen tubing for the mask is still connected to the flow meter and the flow meter is still on the previous setting. Someone may have stepped on the tubing, pulling it from the flow meter, or the oxygen may have accidentally been turned off. Assess the patient's respiratory status, including respiratory rate, rhythm, effort, and lung sounds. Note any additional signs of respiratory distress. Collaborate with the health care team regarding any changes and assessment findings.
- *Areas over ear, face, or back of head are reddened:* Ensure that areas are adequately padded and that the elastic band for the mask is not pulled too tight. Consider consultation with the skin care team or wound nurse specialist.

Special Considerations, including **Infant, Child, Older Adult**, and **Community-Based Care Considerations** (e.g., modifications and home care), appear throughout to explain the varying needs of patients across the lifespan and in various care settings.

SPECIAL CONSIDERATIONS
General Considerations

- Different types of face masks are available for use (refer to Table 14-1 in Skill 14-4 for more information).
- It is important to ensure the mask fits snugly around the patient's face. If it is loose, it will not effectively deliver the right amount of oxygen.
- The mask may be removed for the patient to eat, drink, and take medications. If appropriate, consult with the health care team regarding the use of oxygen via nasal cannula for use during mealtimes and limit the number of times the mask is removed to maintain adequate oxygenation.

UNIT I

Actions Basic to Nursing Care

UNIT II   Promoting Healthy Physiologic Responses

Integrated Case Studies

Resources available on thePoint®

Appendix B: Equivalents

Appendix C: Adult Laboratory Values

ACKNOWLEDGMENTS

This updated edition is the work of many talented people. I would like to acknowledge the hard work of all who have contributed to the completion of this project. Thanks to Carol Taylor and Jennifer Bartlett for offering generous support and encouragement.

The work of this revision was skillfully coordinated by my dedicated team in the Nursing Education division of Wolters Kluwer. I am grateful to each of you for your patience, support, unending encouragement, and total commitment. My thanks to Julie Vitale, Senior Development Editor, and Kelly Horvath, Development Editor, for their insight and tireless work on this edition. My thanks to Betsy Gentzler, Senior Product Manager, for her hard work and guidance throughout the project; and to Erin Hernandez, Editorial Coordinator; Sadie Buckallew, Senior Production Project Manager; Stephen Druding, Manager, Graphic Arts & Design; and Jennifer Clements, Art Director, Illustration.

A special thanks to my colleagues at Gwynedd Mercy University who offer unending support and professional guidance.

Finally, I would like to gratefully acknowledge my family, for their love, understanding, and encouragement. Their support was essential during the long hours of research and writing.

—Pamela Lynn

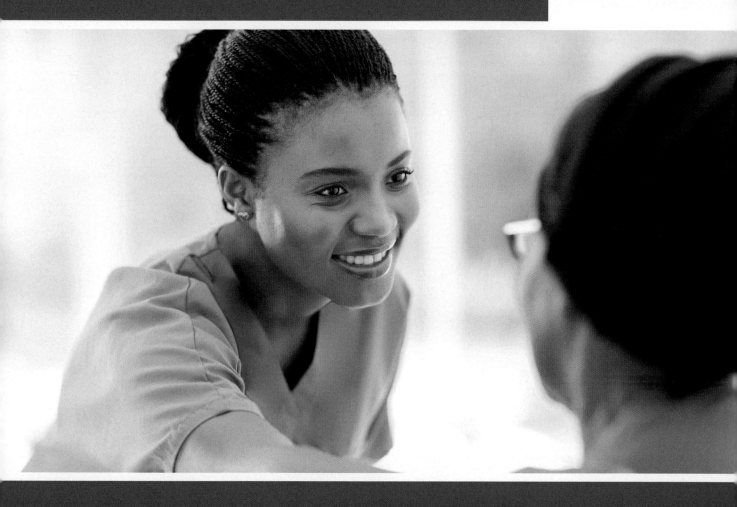

Actions Basic to Nursing Care

1

Asepsis and Infection Control

Focusing on Patient Care

This chapter will help you develop some of the skills related to asepsis and infection control necessary to care for the following patients:

Joe Wilson, age 64, is scheduled to undergo a cardiac catheterization later this morning.

Sheri Lawrence, age 28, has been ordered to have an indwelling urinary catheter inserted.

Edgar Barowski, age 78, is suspected of having tuberculosis and requires infection control precautions.

Refer to Focusing on Patient Care: Developing Clinical Reasoning and Clinical Judgment at the end of the chapter to apply what you learn.

Learning Outcomes

After completing the chapter, you will be able to accomplish the following:

1. Perform hand hygiene using an alcohol-based hand sanitizer.
2. Perform hand hygiene using soap and water (handwashing).
3. Put on and remove personal protective equipment safely.
4. Prepare a sterile field.
5. Add sterile items to a sterile field.
6. Put on sterile gloves and remove soiled gloves.

Nursing Concepts

- Clinical Decision Making/Clinical Judgment
- Infection
- Inflammation
- Safety

Nurses and other health care workers play a key role in preventing and controlling infection, minimizing complications, and reducing adverse outcomes for their patients. Prevention of **health care–associated infections (HAIs)** is a major challenge for health care providers. In the United States, more than a million HAIs occur every year, accounting for tens of thousands of deaths and billions of dollars in health care costs (Agency for Healthcare Research and Quality, 2019). Limiting the spread of microorganisms is accomplished by breaking the chain of infection. The practice of asepsis includes all activities to prevent infection or break the chain of infection. **Medical asepsis**, or clean technique, involves procedures and practices that reduce the number and transfer of **pathogens** (disease-producing microorganisms). Procedures incorporating medical asepsis include, for example, performing hand hygiene and wearing gloves. Refer to Fundamentals Review 1-1. **Surgical asepsis**, or sterile technique or aseptic technique, includes practices used to render and keep objects and areas free from microorganisms. Procedures incorporating surgical asepsis include, for example, inserting an indwelling urinary catheter or inserting an intravenous catheter. Refer to Fundamentals Review 1-2.

Hand hygiene is the most effective way to help reduce the spread of potentially infectious agents and reduce the risk of health care provider colonization or infection caused by germs from the patient (Centers for Disease Control and Prevention [CDC], 2019b). Hand hygiene means cleaning your hands by using either handwashing with soap and water, antiseptic hand wash, antiseptic handrub (alcohol-based hand sanitizer), or surgical hand antisepsis (CDC, 2019b). The Joint Commission has included a recommendation to use guidelines from the CDC or the World Health Organization (WHO) for hand hygiene as part of the 2020 Patient Safety Goal to "Prevent infection" (The Joint Commission, 2022). In addition, the WHO (2022) has identified the "My 5 Moments for Hand Hygiene" approach to define the key moments when health care workers should perform hand hygiene. These include:

- Moment 1: Before touching a patient
- Moment 2: Before a clean or aseptic procedure
- Moment 3: After body fluid exposure risk or risk of exposure
- Moment 4: After touching a patient
- Moment 5: After touching patient surroundings

Fundamentals Review 1-3 and 1-4 outline a summary of CDC-recommended practices for *Standard* and *Transmission-Based Precautions*, additional interventions that are an important part of protecting patients and health care providers and preventing the spread of infection.

This chapter focuses on nursing skills to assist in preventing the spread of infection. These skills include performing hand hygiene, using PPE, preparing a sterile field, adding sterile items to a sterile field, and putting on sterile gloves and removing after use.

Fundamentals Review 1-1

BASIC PRINCIPLES OF MEDICAL ASEPSIS IN PATIENT CARE

- Practice good hand hygiene techniques.
- Carry soiled items, including linens, equipment, and other used articles, away from the body to prevent them from touching the clothing.
- Do not place soiled bed linen or any other items on the floor, which is grossly contaminated. It increases contamination of both surfaces.
- Avoid allowing patients to cough, sneeze, or breathe directly on others. Provide patients with disposable tissues, and instruct them, as indicated, to cover their mouth and nose to prevent spread by airborne droplets.
- Move equipment away from you when brushing, dusting, or scrubbing articles. This helps prevent contaminated particles from settling on your hair, face, and uniform.
- Avoid raising dust. Use a specially treated or a dampened cloth. Dust and lint particles constitute a vehicle by which organisms can be transported from one area to another.

Fundamentals Review 1-1 continued

BASIC PRINCIPLES OF MEDICAL ASEPSIS IN PATIENT CARE

- Handle used textiles and fabrics, such as bed linens and patient garments, with minimum agitation to avoid contamination of air, surfaces, and people.
- Clean the least soiled areas first and then move to the more soiled ones. This helps prevent having the cleaner areas soiled by the dirtier areas.
- Dispose of soiled or used items directly into appropriate containers. Wrap items that are moist from body discharge or drainage in waterproof containers, such as plastic bags, before discarding into the refuse holder so that handlers will not come in contact with them.
- Pour liquids that are to be discarded, such as bath water, mouth rinse, and the like, directly into the drain to avoid splattering in the sink and onto you.

- Sterilize items that are suspected of containing pathogens. After sterilization, they can be managed as clean items if appropriate.
- Use personal grooming habits that help prevent spreading microorganisms. Shampoo your hair regularly, keep your fingernails short and free of broken cuticles and ragged edges, do not wear artificial fingernails if provision of care includes patient at high risk for infection and associated adverse outcomes; do not wear artificial fingernails or extenders if provision of care includes direct patient contact as identified by facility policy, and do not wear rings with grooves and stones that might harbor microorganisms.
- Follow guidelines conscientiously for infection control or barrier techniques as prescribed by your facility.

Source: Adapted from Centers for Disease Control and Prevention (CDC). (2007; updated 2019). *Guideline for isolation precautions: Preventing transmission of infectious agents in healthcare settings.* https://www.cdc.gov/infectioncontrol/guidelines/isolation/index.html.

Fundamentals Review 1-2

BASIC PRINCIPLES OF SURGICAL ASEPSIS IN PATIENT CARE

- Only a sterile object can touch another sterile object. Unsterile touching sterile means contamination has occurred.
- Open sterile packages so that the first edge of the wrapper is directed away from you to avoid the possibility of a sterile surface touching unsterile clothing. The outside of the sterile package is considered contaminated.
- Avoid spilling any solution on a cloth or paper used as a field for a sterile setup. The moisture penetrates the sterile cloth or paper and carries organisms by capillary action to contaminate the field. A wet field is considered contaminated if the surface immediately below it is not sterile.
- Hold sterile objects above waist level. This will ensure keeping the object within sight and preventing accidental contamination.

- Avoid talking, coughing, sneezing, or reaching over a sterile field or object. This helps to prevent contamination by droplets from the nose and the mouth or by particles dropping from your arm.
- Never walk away from or turn your back on a sterile field. This prevents possible contamination while the field is out of your view.
- All items brought into contact with broken skin, used to penetrate the skin to inject substances into the body, or used to enter normally sterile body cavities should be sterile. These items include dressings used to cover primary incisional wounds, needles for injection, and tubes (catheters) used to drain urine from the bladder.
- Consider the outer 1-inch edge of a sterile field to be contaminated.
- Consider an object contaminated if you have any doubt about its sterility.

Source: Adapted from Association of periOperative Registered Nurses (AORN). (2018). AORN guideline quick view: Sterile technique. *AORN Journal, 108*(6), 705–710. https://doi.org/10.1002/aorn.12458.

Fundamentals Review 1-3

STANDARD PRECAUTIONS

Standard Precautions are to be **used for all patients receiving health care in any setting** without regard to their diagnosis or presumed infection status. Standard Precautions apply to blood; all body fluids, secretions, and excretions except sweat, whether or not blood is present or visible; nonintact skin; and mucous membranes. Application is

(continued)

Fundamentals Review 1-3   continued

STANDARD PRECAUTIONS

determined by the nature of the health care provider–patient interaction and the extent of anticipated exposure. Standard Precautions reduce the risk of transmission of infectious agents among patients and health care personnel.

STANDARD PRECAUTIONS (TIER 1)

- Follow hand hygiene recommendations.
- Wear clean nonsterile gloves when touching (or when contact can be reasonably anticipated) blood, body fluids, excretions, secretions, contaminated items, mucous membranes, nonintact skin, and potentially contaminated skin. Change gloves between tasks on the same patient when moving from a contaminated body site to a clean body site, and remove gloves promptly after use.
- Wear personal protective equipment such as mask, eye protection (goggles), face shield, or fluid-repellent gown during procedures and care activities that involve touching blood, body fluids, excretions, secretions, contaminated items, mucous membranes, nonintact skin, and potentially contaminated skin or are likely to generate splashes or sprays of blood or body fluids. Use gown to protect skin and prevent soiling of clothing.
- Avoid recapping used needles. If you must recap, never use two hands. Use a needle-recapping device or the one-handed scoop technique. Place needles, sharps, and scalpels in appropriate puncture-resistant containers after use.
- Wear gloves to handle used patient care equipment that is soiled with blood or identified body fluids, secretions, and excretions to prevent transfer of microorganisms. Clean and reprocess items appropriately if used for another patient.
- Follow respiratory hygiene/cough etiquette. These strategies are targeted at patients and accompanying family members, caregivers and friends with undiagnosed transmissible respiratory infections. These strategies apply to any person entering a health care facility with signs of illness, including cough, congestion, rhinorrhea, or increased production of respiratory secretions. Educate patients and visitors to health care facilities to cover the mouth/nose with a tissue when coughing; to dispose of used tissues promptly; to use surgical masks on the coughing person when tolerated and appropriate; to use hand hygiene after contact with respiratory secretions; and to use spatial separation, ideally >3 ft, between people with respiratory infections in common waiting areas when possible. Health care personnel are advised to observe

Droplet Precautions (i.e., wear a mask) and perform hand hygiene when examining and caring for patients with signs and symptoms of a respiratory infection. Health care personnel who have a respiratory infection are advised to avoid direct patient contact, especially with high-risk patients. If this is not possible, then a mask should be worn while providing patient care.

- Use safe injection practices: Use basic principles of aseptic technique for the preparation and administration of parenteral medications, including the use of a sterile, single-use, disposable needle and syringe for each injection given and prevention of contamination of injection equipment and medication. Whenever possible, use of single-dose vials is preferred over multiple-dose vials, especially when medications will be administered to multiple patients.
- Wear a face mask for placement of a central venous catheter and for placement of a catheter or injecting material into the spinal or epidural space.

RESPIRATORY HYGIENE/COUGH ETIQUETTE

Standard Precautions generally apply to the recommended practices of health care providers during patient care. Respiratory Hygiene/Cough Etiquette applies broadly to all persons who enter a health care setting, **including health care personnel, patients, and visitors.**

- Provide *Respiratory Hygiene/Cough Etiquette* education for health care providers, patients, and visitors.
- Post signs, in language(s) appropriate to the population served, with *Respiratory Hygiene/Cough Etiquette* instructions for patients, family members, caregivers, friends, and visitors.
- Cover the mouth and nose with a tissue when coughing; promptly dispose of used tissues.
- Use surgical masks on a coughing person when tolerated and appropriate.
- Perform hand hygiene after contact with respiratory secretions.
- Provide spatial separation, ideally >3 ft, of persons with respiratory infections in common waiting areas when possible.
- Health care providers should observe Droplet Precautions when caring for patients with signs and symptoms of a respiratory infection.
- Health care providers who have a respiratory infection should avoid direct patient contact, especially with high-risk patients; if not possible, a mask should be worn while providing patient care.

Source: Adapted from the Centers for Disease Control and Prevention (CDC). (2007; updated 2019). *2007 Guideline for isolation precautions: Preventing transmission of infectious agents in healthcare settings.* https://www.cdc.gov/infectioncontrol/guidelines/isolation/index.html

Fundamentals Review 1-4

TRANSMISSION-BASED PRECAUTIONS

Transmission-Based Precautions are **used in addition** to Standard Precautions for patients with documented or suspected infection or colonization with pathogens that can be transmitted by airborne, droplet, or contact routes. Any of the three types can be used in combination with the others. Equipment required for patient care, such as a thermometer, sphygmomanometer, and stethoscope, should be disposable, kept in the patient's room, and not used for other patients. The 2007 Centers for Disease Control and Prevention (CDC, updated 2019) Guidelines include a directive to put on personal protective equipment (PPE) when entering the room of a patient with transmission-based precautions, and to remove the PPE only when leaving the room. Consult the 2007 CDC (2007; updated 2019) Guidelines—Appendix A—for information related to the type and duration of precautions recommended for specific infections and conditions. These categories recognize that a disease may have multiple routes of transmission and require more than one type of precaution (Taylor et al., 2023).

AIRBORNE PRECAUTIONS (TIER 2)

- Use *Airborne Precautions* for patients who have infections that spread through the air such as tuberculosis, varicella (chicken pox), rubeola (measles), and possibly severe acute respiratory syndrome (SARS) and patients with coronavirus (COVID-19) undergoing aerosol-generating procedures (CDC, 2020a).
- Place patient in a private room that has monitored negative air pressure in relation to surrounding areas, 6 to 12 air changes per hour, and appropriate discharge of air outside or monitored filtration if air is recirculated. Keep door closed and patient in room.
- Wear a mask or respirator, depending on the disease-specific recommendations that is put on prior to room entry. Whenever possible, nonimmune health care providers should not care for patient with vaccine-preventable airborne diseases (e.g., measles, chickenpox, smallpox).
- Transport patient out of room only when necessary and place a surgical mask on the patient if possible, and instruct the patient to observe Respiratory Hygiene/Cough Etiquette.

- Consult CDC Guidelines for additional prevention strategies for tuberculosis.

DROPLET PRECAUTIONS (TIER 2)

- Use *Droplet Precautions* for patients with an infection that is spread by large-particle droplets, that are generated when a patient coughs, sneezes, or talks (e.g., influenza, coronavirus, rubella, mumps, diphtheria, and the adenovirus infection in infants and young children.
- Use a private room, if available. Door may remain open.
- Wear PPE upon entry into the room for all interactions that may involve contact with the patient and potentially contaminated areas in the patient's environment.
- Transport patient out of the room only when necessary and place a surgical mask on the patient if possible.
- Keep visitors 3 ft away from the infected person.

CONTACT PRECAUTIONS (TIER 2)

- *Contact Precautions* are intended to prevent transmission of infectious agents that are spread by direct or indirect contact with the patient or the patient's environment (e.g., *Clostridioides difficile* [*C. difficile*], respiratory syncytial virus [RSV] [infants and young children], impetigo, norovirus).
- Use *Contact Precautions* for patients who are infected or colonized by multidrug-resistant organisms (MDROs).
- Observe *Contact Precautions* in the presence of excessive wound drainage, fecal incontinence, or other discharges from the body that suggest an increased potential for extensive environmental contamination and risk of transmission.
- Place patient in a private room if available.
- Wear a gown and gloves whenever you enter the room for all interactions that may involve contact with the patient or potentially contaminated areas in the patient's environment. Change gloves after having contact with infective material. Remove PPE before leaving the patient environment, and wash hands with an antimicrobial or waterless antiseptic agent.
- Limit movement of the patient out of the room.
- Avoid sharing patient care equipment.

Source: Adapted from Centers for Disease Control and Prevention (CDC). (2020a). *Coronavirus disease 2019 (COVID-19).* https://www.cdc.gov/coronavirus/2019-nCoV/hcp/; Centers for Disease Control and Prevention (CDC). (2007; updated 2019). *2007 Guideline for isolation precautions: Preventing transmission of infectious agents in healthcare settings.* https://www.cdc.gov/infectioncontrol/guidelines/isolation/index.html

Skill 1-1 ▶ Performing Hand Hygiene Using an Alcohol-Based Hand Sanitizer

Health care providers should use an alcohol-based hand sanitizer or wash with soap and water as part of routine hand hygiene interventions (Centers for Disease Control and Prevention [CDC], 2019b). Unless hands are soiled, alcohol-based hand sanitizers are the preferred method for cleaning of health care providers' hands in most clinical situations (CDC, 2019b). These products have an alcohol concentration between 60% and 95% and are available as foam, gel, or lotion. When using these products, check the product labeling for correct amount of product needed. During routine patient care, health care providers may use alcohol-based hand sanitizers (CDC, 2019b):

- If hands are not visibly soiled
- Before putting on gloves
- Before and after each patient contact
- Before performing a task requiring use of aseptic technique, such as inserting urinary catheters, peripheral vascular catheters, or invasive devices that do not require surgical placement or handling of medical devices
- Before donning sterile gloves prior to an invasive procedure (e.g., inserting a central intravascular catheter)
- Before moving from work on a soiled body site to a clean body site during patient care
- After contact with surfaces in the patient's environment immediately after removing gloves
- After contact with blood, body fluids or excretions, mucous membranes, nonintact skin, or contaminated surfaces

Alcohol-based hand sanitizers are fast-acting and cause less skin irritation and dryness than soap and water (CDC, 2019c).

Skill 1-2 provides guidelines for situations requiring handwashing, as opposed to hand hygiene with an alcohol-based hand sanitizer.

DELEGATION CONSIDERATIONS

The application and use of hand hygiene using alcohol-based hand sanitizers are appropriate for all health care providers.

EQUIPMENT

- Alcohol-based hand sanitizer
- Moisturizing hand lotion or cream approved by health care facility (optional)

ASSESSMENT

Assess hands for any visible soiling. If hands are visibly soiled, proceed with washing the hands with soap and water.

Assess for known or suspected exposure to certain microorganisms. Handwashing is required if known or suspected exposure to certain microorganisms, such as those causing anthrax, norovirus, or *Clostridioides difficile* (*C. difficile*). Alcohol-based hand sanitizers have poor activity against these organisms.

ACTUAL OR POTENTIAL HEALTH PROBLEMS AND NEEDS

Many actual or potential health problems or needs may require the use of this skill as part of related interventions. An appropriate health problem or need may include:
- Infection risk
- Knowledge deficiency
- Risk for Cross Infection

OUTCOME IDENTIFICATION AND PLANNING

The expected outcomes to achieve when performing hand hygiene with alcohol-based hand sanitizers are that transient microorganisms will be eliminated from the hands; the risk of transmission of microorganisms is reduced; the risk of health care worker colonization or infection caused by organisms acquired from the patient or environment is reduced; and morbidity, mortality, and costs associated with health care–associated infections (HAIs) are reduced. Other outcomes may be appropriate, depending on the specific diagnosis or patient problem.

IMPLEMENTATION

ACTION

1. Remove jewelry prior to patient contact, if possible, and secure in a safe place. A plain band may remain in place, based on facility policy.

2. Check the product labeling for correct amount of product needed.

3. Apply the product to the palm of one hand (Figure 1). Ensure use of the correct amount of product (Figure 2).

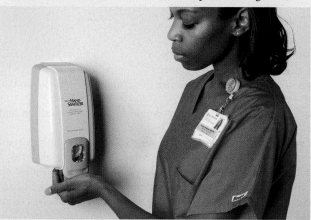

FIGURE 1. Applying the correct amount of product to the palm of one hand.

4. Rub hands together, **covering all surfaces of hands and fingers, between fingers, fingertips, and the area beneath the fingernails.**

5. Rub hands together until they are dry (approximately 20 seconds [CDC, 2019b]) (Figure 3).

6. Use moisturizing hand lotion or cream, as approved by facility policy.

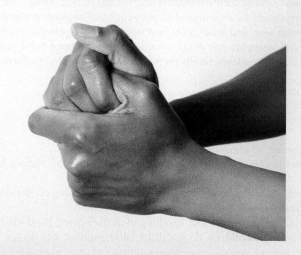

RATIONALE

Microorganisms may accumulate in settings of jewelry and underneath rings (CDC, 2019b), so it should not be worn during patient care. If jewelry was worn during patient care, it should be left on during handwashing.

Amount of product required to be effective varies from manufacturer to manufacturer.

Adequate amount of product is required to cover hand surfaces thoroughly.

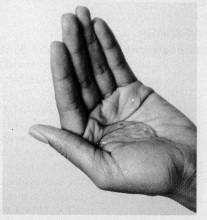

FIGURE 2. Ensuring use of the correct amount of product.

All surfaces must be treated to prevent disease transmission.

Drying ensures antiseptic effect.

Moisturizing hand lotion or cream helps to increase skin hydration to keep the skin soft and prevents dermatitis. It is best applied after patient care is complete, and from a small, personal container, according to facility policy. Avoid use of unapproved lotions or creams because they can cause deterioration of gloves or decrease the efficacy of some antiseptic agents. Follow facility policy.

FIGURE 3. Rubbing hands together until dry.

(continued on page 10)

Skill 1-1 ▶	**Performing Hand Hygiene Using an Alcohol-Based Hand Sanitizer** *(continued)*

EVALUATION

The expected outcomes have been met when transient microorganisms have been eliminated from the hands; the risk of transmission of microorganisms has been reduced; the risk of health care worker colonization or infection caused by organisms acquired from the patient has been reduced; and morbidity, mortality, and costs associated with HAIs has been reduced.

DOCUMENTATION

The performance of hand hygiene using an alcohol-based hand sanitizer is not generally documented.

DEVELOPING CLINICAL REASONING AND CLINICAL JUDGMENT

SPECIAL CONSIDERATIONS

General Considerations

- The use of gloves does not eliminate the need for hand hygiene.
- The use of hand hygiene does not eliminate the need for gloves.
- Ensure hands are dry before gloves are donned to decrease risk of dermatitis (Halm & Sandau, 2018).
- Hand hygiene performance by patients is an important intervention to reduce acquisition and transmission of HAIs (Srigley et al., 2020; Wong et al., 2020).
- Hand hygiene performance by family and nonfamily visitors to health care facilities is an important intervention to reduce acquisition and transmission of HAIs (Kim & Lee, 2019; Lary et al., 2020).
- Health care providers should educate patients, family, caregivers, and nonfamily visitors on the importance of hand hygiene. Informed patients, families, caregivers, and visitors are better engaged as members of the health care team and are better able to advocate for themselves (Kim & Lee, 2019; Lary et al., 2020).
- Health care consumers in all settings should be encouraged to "speak up for clean hands" and advocate for the use of hand hygiene by health care providers, family, and friends (CDC, 2016a; Gesser-Edelsburg et al., 2020).
- Germs can live under artificial fingernails before and after hand hygiene interventions. Health care providers should not wear artificial fingernails or extensions when having direct contact with patients at high risk (e.g., patients in intensive care units or operating rooms) (CDC, 2019b).
- Health care providers should keep natural nail tips less than ¼-in long (CDC, 2019b).

Infant and Child Considerations

- Children should only use alcohol-based hand sanitizer with adult supervision (U.S. Food and Drug Administration [FDA], 2020).

Community-Based Care Considerations

- Proper hand hygiene, including the use of alcohol-based hand sanitizers, is useful to reduce the risk of spread of microorganisms among family members and friends (CDC, 2016a). Patients, family members, and caregivers should be encouraged to perform hand hygiene, preferably by washing their hands; washing with soap and water is the best way to remove germs in most situations (CDC, 2020b). If soap and water are not readily available, alcohol-based hand sanitizer should be used (CDC, 2020b). Instruct patients, family members, and caregivers to perform hand hygiene (CDC, 2016a):
  - before preparing or eating food
  - before touching eyes, nose, or mouth
  - before and after changing wound dressings or bandages
  - after using the restroom
  - after blowing their nose, coughing, or sneezing
  - after touching hospital or other health care–setting surfaces such as doorknobs, phones, tables, and bed rails
- Instruct patients and family members on the importance of not wiping or rinsing off the alcohol-based hand sanitizer before it is dry (FDA, 2020).
- Teach patients, family members, and caregivers safe handling of alcohol-based hand sanitizers: Keep sanitizer out of reach of pets and children, do not drink hand sanitizer, and do not allow children or pets to ingest it. Ingestion of alcohol-based hand sanitizer can cause alcohol poisoning (FDA, 2020). However, eating with hands or licking hands after use is not of concern (FDA, 2020).

- Patients and their family members and caregivers should be cautioned to not attempt to make their own hand sanitizer, to avoid use of ineffective products and possible skin or eye irritation or burns (FDA, 2020).

EVIDENCE FOR PRACTICE ▶

IMPROVING THE USE OF HAND AND STETHOSCOPE HYGIENE

Health care workers have the potential to directly transmit organisms to susceptible people through touching. Indirect personal contact with an inanimate object (fomite), such as equipment or countertops, provides a potential means of transmission of microorganisms (Brunette & Nemhauser, 2019). Nurses use stethoscopes many times of the course of the day; stethoscopes, especially when unclean, have the potential to act as fomites of infection (Breen & Hessels, 2017). Stethoscope hygiene and proper hand hygiene can interrupt the transmission of dangerous microorganisms from nurses to patients (Breen & Hessels, 2017). Although best practice guidelines identify the importance of stethoscope and hand hygiene, health care professionals often fail to adhere to these guidelines (Holleck et al., 2020). How can we improve compliance with these important interventions?

Related Evidence

Holleck, J. L., Campbell, S., Alrawili, H., Frank, C., Merchant, N., Rodwin, B., Perez, M. F., Gupta, S., Federman, D. G., Chang, J. J., Vientos, W., & Dembry, L. (2020). Stethoscope hygiene: Using cultures and real-time feedback with bioluminescence-based adenosine triphosphate technology to change behavior. *American Journal of Infection Control, 48*(4), 380–385. https://doi.org/10.1016/j.ajic.2019.10.005

This quality improvement initiative utilized a preintervention-to-postintervention design. Medical students, house staff, and attending physicians at a Department of Veterans Affairs tertiary care teaching hospital participated in the project. Preintervention surveys exploring beliefs and barriers to stethoscope hygiene were administered prior to any intervention and postsurveys were administered 2 days after presentation of the results to participants. Participants cultured and swabbed their stethoscopes for bioluminescence-based adenosine triphosphate testing before and after use of several methods of stethoscope disinfection. Methods included disinfection with alcohol pads, alcohol-based handrub, and hydrogen peroxide disinfectant wipes. Data were collected at the start of clinical rotations and after presenting the culture images and bioluminescence results during the second and fourth weeks of the clinical rotations. This 4-week period was repeated for three cycles. Observations of hand and stethoscope hygiene were covertly recorded as well at the 1-, 2-, and 4-week intervals. Data included observed stethoscope and hand hygiene rates; bacteria identification and colony-forming units (CFU) from culture results; and bioluminescence scores, before and after the varying methods of disinfection. Survey responses exploring beliefs and barriers to stethoscope hygiene and self-reported disinfection rates were also reported. Observed hand hygiene opportunities showed that compliance improved ($p < .001$). Observed patient-provider encounters revealed no significant change in stethoscope hygiene rates ($p = .08$), although self-reported rates improved slightly. Perceptions regarding stethoscope hygiene importance improved ($p = .04$). Disinfection with alcohol pads, alcohol-based handrub, and hydrogen peroxide disinfectant wipes were equivalent in CFU reduction ($p = .21$). The top three barriers to stethoscope hygiene identified were forgetfulness, time constraints, and limited access to supplies. The researchers concluded that showing providers what is growing on their stethoscopes via cultures and bioluminescence technology before and after disinfection improved "buy in" regarding the importance of stethoscope hygiene, had an impact on cleaning behavior, and improved hand hygiene performance. The researchers identified that further research on the optimal methods to improve adherence with stethoscope hygiene is needed.

Relevance for Nursing Practice

Despite evidence of the importance of hand and stethoscope hygiene, adherence is a challenging issue. Nurses are positioned to advocate for and introduce ideas to increase compliance related to hand and stethoscope hygiene adherence, resulting in decreased HAIs and improved patient outcomes.

Refer to Skill 1-2 for additional evidence related to patient hand hygiene.

Skill 1-2 ▶ Performing Hand Hygiene Using Soap and Water (Handwashing)

Health care providers should wash with soap and water or use an alcohol-based hand sanitizer or as part of routine hand hygiene interventions (Centers for Disease Control and Prevention [CDC], 2019b).
Health care providers must wash with soap and water (CDC, 2019b):

- When hands are visibly soiled
- When caring for a patient with known or suspected infectious diarrhea
- After known or suspected exposure to spores (e.g., *Bacillus anthracis, Clostridioides difficile [C. difficile]* outbreaks)

During routine patient care, health care providers may wash hands with soap and water (CDC, 2019b):

- If hands are not visibly soiled
- Before and after each patient contact
- Before putting on gloves
- Before performing a task requiring use of aseptic technique, such as inserting urinary catheters, peripheral vascular catheters, or invasive devices that do not require surgical placement or handling of medical devices
- Before donning sterile gloves prior to an invasive procedure (e.g., inserting a central intravascular catheter)
- Before moving from work on a soiled body site to a clean body site during patient care
- After contact with surfaces in the patient's environment
- Immediately after removing gloves
- After contact with blood, body fluids or excretions, mucous membranes, nonintact skin, or contaminated surfaces

Using handwashing products that contain an antimicrobial (agent that kills microorganisms) or antibacterial ingredient is recommended in any setting where the risk for infection is high. When present in certain concentrations, these agents can kill bacteria or suppress their growth (Taylor et al., 2023).
Skill 1-1 provides guidelines for performing hand hygiene with alcohol-based hand sanitizer.

DELEGATION CONSIDERATIONS

The application and use of hand hygiene using soap and water is appropriate for all health care providers.

EQUIPMENT

- Antimicrobial or nonantimicrobial soap (if in bar form, soap must be placed on a soap rack)
- Paper towels
- Moisturizing hand lotion or cream approved by health care facility (optional)

ASSESSMENT

- Assess for any of the above requirements for handwashing. If no requirements are fulfilled, the health care provider has the option of performing hand hygiene with soap and water or using an alcohol-based hand sanitizer.
- Assess hands for any visible soiling. If hands are visibly soiled, proceed with washing the hands with soap and water.
- Assess for known or suspected exposure to certain microorganisms. Handwashing is required if known or suspected exposure to certain microorganisms, such as *C. difficile* and those causing anthrax or norovirus. Alcohol-based hand sanitizers have poor activity against these organisms.

ACTUAL OR POTENTIAL HEALTH PROBLEMS AND NEEDS

Many actual or potential health problems or needs may require the use of this skill as part of related interventions. An appropriate health problem or need may include:
- Infection risk
- Knowledge deficiency
- Risk for Cross Infection

OUTCOME
IDENTIFICATION
AND PLANNING

The expected outcomes to achieve when performing hand hygiene with soap and water are elimination of transient microorganisms from the hands; reduction in the risk of transmission of microorganisms; reduction in the risk of health care worker colonization or infection caused by organisms acquired from the patient or environment; and reduction in morbidity, mortality, and costs associated with HAIs. Other outcomes may be appropriate, depending on the specific diagnosis or patient problem identified.

IMPLEMENTATION

ACTION	RATIONALE
1. Gather the necessary supplies. Stand in front of the sink. Do not allow your clothing to touch the sink during the washing procedure (Figure 1).	The sink is considered contaminated. Clothing may carry organisms from place to place.
2. Remove jewelry prior to patient contact, if possible, and secure in a safe place. A plain band may remain in place, based on facility policy.	Microorganisms may accumulate in settings of jewelry and underneath rings (CDC, 2019b), so it should not be worn during patient care. If jewelry was worn during care, it should be left on during handwashing.
3. Turn on water and adjust force (Figure 2). Regulate the temperature until the water is warm.	Water splashed from the contaminated sink will contaminate clothing. Warm water is more comfortable and is less likely to open pores and remove oils from the skin. Organisms can lodge in roughened and broken areas of chapped skin.

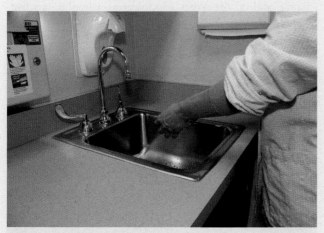

FIGURE 1. Standing in front of sink.

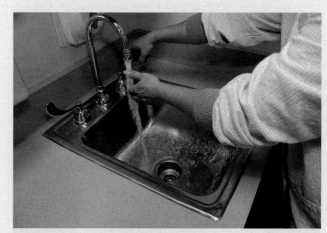

FIGURE 2. Turning on the water at the sink.

4. Wet the hands and wrist area. Keep hands lower than elbows to allow water to flow toward fingertips (Figure 3).	Water should flow from the cleaner area toward the more contaminated area. Hands are more contaminated than forearms.
5. Use about 1 teaspoon liquid soap from dispenser or rinse bar of soap and lather thoroughly, using a firm circular motion (Figure 4). Alternatively, use the amount of product recommended by the manufacturer. Cover all areas of hands with the soap product. If using bar soap, rinse soap bar again and return to soap rack without touching the rack.	Rinsing the soap before and after use removes the lather, which may contain microorganisms.

(continued on page 14)

Skill 1-2 ▶ Performing Hand Hygiene Using Soap and Water (Handwashing) *(continued)*

ACTION

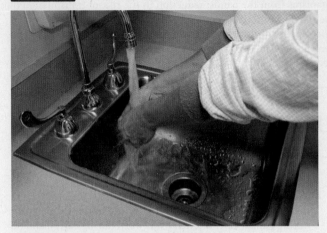

FIGURE 3. Wetting hands to the wrist.

6. Continuing with firm rubbing and circular motions. Wash the palms and backs of the hands; each finger; the areas between the fingers (Figure 5); and the knuckles, wrists, and forearms. **Wash at least 1 inch above area of contamination.** If hands are not visibly soiled, wash to 1 inch above the wrists (Figure 6).

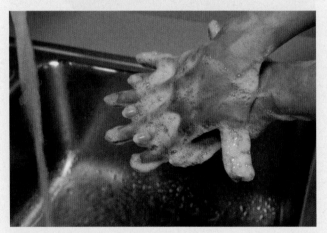

FIGURE 5. Washing areas between fingers.

7. Continue this friction motion for at least 15–20 seconds.

8. Use fingernails of the opposite hand to clean under fingernails (Figure 7).

9. Rinse hands thoroughly under running water with water flowing toward fingertips (Figure 8).

RATIONALE

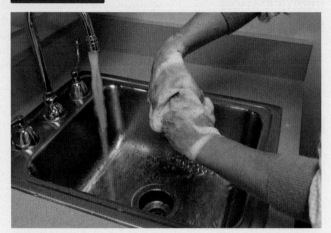

FIGURE 4. Lathering hands with soap and rubbing with firm circular motion.

Friction caused by firm rubbing and circular motions helps to loosen dirt and organisms that can lodge between the fingers, in skin crevices of knuckles, on the palms and backs of the hands, and on the wrists and forearms. Cleaning less contaminated areas (forearms and wrists) after hands are clean prevents spreading microorganisms from the hands to the forearms and wrists.

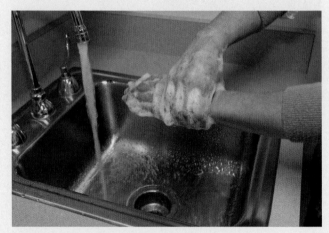

FIGURE 6. Washing to 1 inch above the wrist.

Effective handwashing requires at least a 15–20-second scrub with plain soap or disinfectant and warm water (CDC, 2019b). Hands that are visibly soiled need a longer scrub.

The area under nails has a high microorganism count, and organisms may remain under the nails, where they can grow and be spread to other people.

Running water rinses microorganisms and dirt into the sink.

ACTION

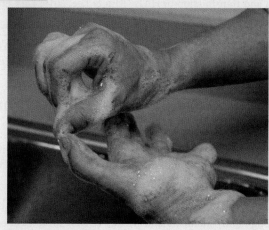

FIGURE 7. Using fingernails to clean under nails of opposite hand.

10. Pat hands dry with a paper towel, beginning with the fingers and moving upward toward forearms, and discard it immediately. Use another clean towel to turn off the faucet. Discard towel immediately without touching other clean hand.

11. Use moisturizing hand lotion or cream, as approved by facility policy.

RATIONALE

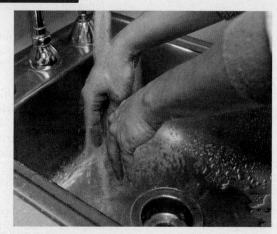

FIGURE 8. Rinsing hands under running water with water flowing toward fingertips.

Patting the skin dry prevents chapping. Dry hands first because they are considered the cleanest and least contaminated area. Turning the faucet off with a clean paper towel protects the clean hands from contact with a soiled surface.

Moisturizing hand lotion or cream helps to increase skin hydration to keep the skin soft and prevents dermatitis. It is best applied after patient care is complete, from a small, personal container, according to facility policy. Avoid use of unapproved lotions or creams because they can cause deterioration of gloves or decrease the efficacy of some antiseptic agents. Follow facility policy.

EVALUATION

The expected outcomes have been met when transient microorganisms have been eliminated from the hands; the risk of transmission of microorganisms has been reduced; the risk of health care worker colonization or infection caused by organisms acquired from the patient has been reduced; and morbidity, mortality, and costs associated with health care–associated infections (HAIs) has been reduced.

DOCUMENTATION

The performance of handwashing is not generally documented.

DEVELOPING CLINICAL REASONING AND CLINICAL JUDGMENT

SPECIAL CONSIDERATIONS

General Considerations

- The use of gloves does not eliminate the need for hand hygiene.
- The use of hand hygiene does not eliminate the need for gloves.
- Ensure hands are dry before gloves are donned to decrease risk of dermatitis (Halm & Sandau, 2018).
- Hand hygiene performance by patients is an important intervention to reduce acquisition and transmission of HAIs (Srigley et al., 2020; Wong et al., 2020).

(continued on page 16)

Skill 1-2 ▶ Performing Hand Hygiene Using Soap and Water (Handwashing) *(continued)*

- Hand hygiene performance by family and non-family visitors to health care facilities is an important intervention to reduce acquisition and transmission of HAIs (Kim & Lee, 2019; Lary et al., 2020).
- Health care providers should educate patients, family, and nonfamily visitors on the importance of hand hygiene. Informed patients, families, and visitors can be better engaged as members of the health care team and are better able to advocate for themselves (Kim & Lee, 2019; Lary et al., 2020).
- Health care consumers in all settings should be encouraged to "speak up for clean hands" and advocate for the use of hand hygiene by health care providers, family, and friends (CDC, 2016a; Gesser-Edelsburg et al., 2020).
- Germs can live under artificial fingernails before and after hand hygiene interventions. Health care providers should not wear artificial fingernails or extensions when having direct contact with patients at high risk (e.g., patients in intensive care units or operating rooms) (CDC, 2019b).
- Health care providers should keep natural nail tips less than ¼-in long (CDC, 2019b).

Community-Based Care Considerations

- Proper hand hygiene, including the use of alcohol-based hand sanitizers, is useful to reduce the risk of spread of microorganisms among family members and friends (CDC, 2016a). Patients, family members, and caregivers should be encouraged to perform hand hygiene, preferably by washing their hands; washing with soap and water is the best way to remove germs in most situations (CDC, 2020b). If soap and water are not readily available, alcohol-based hand sanitizer should be used (CDC, 2020b). Instruct patients, family members, and caregivers to perform hand hygiene (CDC, 2016a):
  - Before preparing or eating food
  - Before touching eyes, nose, or mouth
  - Before and after changing wound dressings or bandages
  - After using the restroom
  - After blowing their nose, coughing, or sneezing
  - After touching hospital or other health care–setting surfaces such as doorknobs, phones, tables, and bed rails

EVIDENCE FOR PRACTICE ▶

IMPROVING PATIENT HAND HYGIENE
Health care providers are the focus of many hand hygiene initiatives in health care facilities. Hand hygiene by patients is also an important means to prevent acquisition and dissemination of health care–associated pathogens.

Related Evidence
Knighton, S. C., Richmond, M., Zabarsky, T., Dolansky, M., Rai, H., & Donskey, C. J. (2020). Patients' capability, opportunity, motivation, and perception of inpatient hand hygiene. *American Journal of Infection Control, 48*(2), 157–161. https://doi.org/10.1016/j.ajic.2019.09.001

This study examined perceptions and behaviors of patients regarding patient hand hygiene behaviors relative to resources provided during admission to the hospital. A convenience sample of 107 participants attending a posthospital clinic visit completed a questionnaire that explored the capabilities, opportunities, and motivation for patient hand hygiene during the recent hospitalization. The researchers identified that content validity and reliability for the survey was established. Patients were asked whether they brought hand sanitizer to the hospital or used hospital resources to clean their hands as well as for their perspective on patient hand hygiene importance compared with hospital staff and their satisfaction or lack of satisfaction with hand hygiene independence. Responses to the questionnaire were collected using a structured interview. Most of the participants (60.7%) reported they were able to maintain cleaning their hands with little or no difficulty prior to hospital admission. During their hospital admission, only 19.6% of participants reported needing little or no assistance cleaning their hands. More than half of the participants reported mostly (31.8%) or completely (21.5%) agreeing that the hand hygiene of the health care staff was more important than that of the patients. Almost half (46.7%) of participants reported not being satisfied at all with their ability to maintain their hand hygiene in the hospital, whereas only 9.3% were very satisfied with their ability to maintain hand hygiene. The researchers concluded that clean hands are important to patients and interventions are needed to help patients achieve compliance and improved hand hygiene. The researchers concluded that increased efforts are needed to incorporate inpatient hand hygiene into existing infection control programs in inpatient settings.

Relevance for Nursing Practice
Effective hand hygiene is a critical means to help prevent the spread of microorganisms and infectious agents. Understanding patient perceptions related to barriers and facilitators of patient hand hygiene contributes to the development of approaches to improve patient hand hygiene. Nurses should consider undertaking studies related to improving hand hygiene compliance to ensure safe patient care. Such studies would also add to the body of knowledge to support evidence-based nursing practice.

Refer to Skill 1-1 for additional evidence related to hand and stethoscope hygiene.

Skill 1-3 ▶ Using Personal Protective Equipment

Personal protective equipment (PPE) refers to specialized clothing or equipment worn by an employee for protection against infectious materials. PPE is used in health care settings to improve personnel safety in the health care environment (Centers for Disease Control and Prevention [CDC], 2007, updated 2019). This equipment includes clean (nonsterile) and sterile gloves, impervious gowns/aprons, surgical and high-efficiency particulate air (HEPA) masks, N95 disposable masks, face shields, and protective eyewear/goggles.

Understanding the potential contamination hazards related to the patient's diagnosis and condition and the institutional policies governing PPE is very important. The type of PPE used will vary based on the type of exposure anticipated and category of precautions: **standard precautions** and **transmission-based precautions**, including contact, droplet, and airborne precautions. It is the nurse's responsibility to enforce the proper wearing of PPE during patient care for members of the health care team and patients or visitors, as appropriate. Refer to Fundamentals Review 1-3 and 1-4 for a summary of CDC-recommended practices for standard and transmission-based precautions. Box 1-1 provides Guidelines for Effective Use of PPE.

Box 1-1 Guidelines for Effective Use of PPE

- Put on PPE before contact with the patient, preferably before entering the patient's room. When using transmission-based precautions, put on PPE before entering the patient's room.
- Choose appropriate PPE based on the type of exposure anticipated and type of transmission-based precautions.
- When wearing gloves, work from "clean" areas to "dirty" areas.
- Change gloves between tasks on the same patient when moving from a contaminated body site to a clean body site, and remove gloves promptly after use.
- Touch as few surfaces and items with your PPE as possible.

- Avoid touching or adjusting PPE.
- Keep gloved hands away from your face.
- If gloves become torn or heavily soiled, remove and replace. Perform hand hygiene before putting on the new gloves.
- Personal glasses and contact lenses are not adequate eye protection and are not a substitute for goggles.
- As diseases/infections/conditions emerge or their prevalence increases, guidelines need to evolve. The CDC issued revised guidelines related to coronavirus disease (COVID-19), which are available at http://www.cdc.gov/vhf/ebola/healthcare-us/ppe/guidance.html.

Source: Adapted from Centers for Disease Control and Prevention (CDC). (2020a). *Coronavirus disease 2019 (COVID-19).* https://www.cdc.gov/coronavirus/2019-nCoV/hcp/; Centers for Disease Control and Prevention (CDC). (2007; updated 2019). *Guideline for isolation precautions: Preventing transmission of infectious agents in healthcare settings.* https://www.cdc.gov/infectioncontrol/guidelines/isolation/index.html

(continued on page 18)

Skill 1-3 ▶ Using Personal Protective Equipment *(continued)*

DELEGATION CONSIDERATIONS	The application and use of PPE are appropriate for all health care providers.

EQUIPMENT	• Gloves • Mask (surgical or particulate respirator) • Impervious gown • Goggles or face shield (protective eye wear; does not include eyeglasses) *Note: Equipment for PPE may vary depending on level of precautions required and facility policy.*

ASSESSMENT	• Assess the situation to determine the necessity for PPE. • Check the patient's medical record for information about a suspected or diagnosed infection or communicable disease. • Determine the possibility of exposure to blood and body fluids and identify the necessary equipment to prevent exposure; refer to the infection control manual provided by your facility. • Determine the need for Standard I or Transmission-based Precautions. Application is determined by the nature of the health care provider–patient interaction and the extent of anticipated exposure.

ACTUAL OR POTENTIAL HEALTH PROBLEMS AND NEEDS	Many actual or potential health problems or needs may require the use of this skill as part of related interventions. An appropriate health problem or need may include: • Infection risk • Knowledge deficiency • Risk for Cross Infection

OUTCOME IDENTIFICATION AND PLANNING	The expected outcome to achieve when using PPE is reduction in the risk of transmission of infectious agents among patients and health care personnel. Other outcomes that may be appropriate are that the patient and staff remain free from exposure to potentially infectious microorganisms and that the patient verbalizes information about the rationale for use of PPE.

IMPLEMENTATION

ACTION	**RATIONALE**
1. Check medical record and plan of care for type of precautions and review precautions in infection control manual.	Mode of transmission of organism determines type of precautions required.
2. Plan nursing activities before entering patient's room.	Organization facilitates performance of task and adherence to precautions.
3. Provide instruction about precautions and use of PPE to patient, family members, caregivers, and visitors.	Explanation encourages cooperation of patient, family, and caregivers and reduces apprehension about precaution procedures.
4. Perform hand hygiene.	Hand hygiene prevents the spread of microorganisms.
5. Put on gown, mask (surgical or particulate respirator), protective eyewear, and gloves based on the type of exposure anticipated and category of isolation precautions.	Use of PPE interrupts chain of infection and protects patient and nurse. Gown should protect all clothing and exposed skin on upper extremities. Gloves protect hands and wrists from microorganisms. Masks and particulate respirators protect wearer from direct contact with body fluids that may spray or splash; masks protect wearer from exposure to large-particle aerosols and particulate respirators protect wearer from inhalation of airborne droplet nuclei, and small-particle aerosols (Taylor et al., 2023). Eyewear protects mucous membranes in the eye from splashes.

ACTION

a. Put on the gown, with the opening in the back. Tie gown securely at neck and waist (Figure 1).

b. Put on the mask or respirator over your nose, mouth, and chin (Figure 2). Secure ties or elastic bands at the middle of the head and neck. Fit mask snug to face and below chin. Fit flexible band to nose bridge. If respirator is used, perform a fit check. Inhale: The respirator should collapse. Exhale: Air should not leak out.

c. Put on goggles (Figure 3). Place over the eyes and adjust to fit. Alternatively, a face shield could be used (Figure 4).

RATIONALE

The gown should fully cover the torso from the neck to knees, arms to the end of wrists, and wrap around the back.

Masks protect the nurse or patient from droplet nuclei and large-particle aerosols. A mask must fit securely to provide protection.

Eyewear protects mucous membranes in the eye from splashes; it must fit securely to provide protection.

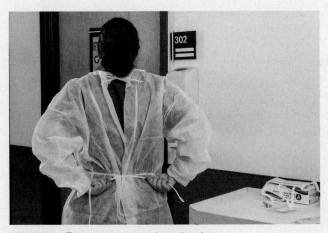

FIGURE 1. Tying gown at neck and waist.

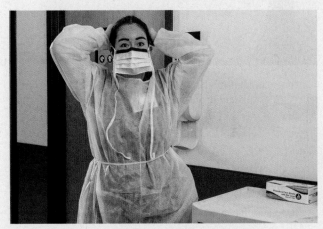

FIGURE 2. Applying mask over nose, mouth, and chin.

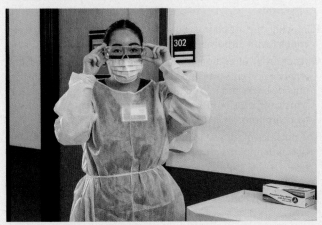

FIGURE 3. Putting on goggles.

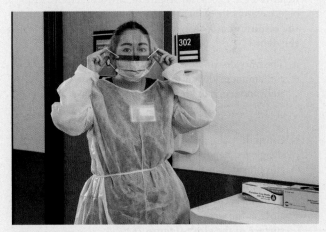

FIGURE 4. Putting on face shield.

(continued on page 20)

Skill 1-3 ▶ Using Personal Protective Equipment *(continued)*

ACTION

d. Put on clean disposable gloves. Extend gloves to cover the wrist of the gown (Figure 5).

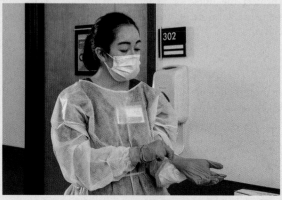

6. Identify the patient. Explain the procedure to the patient. Continue with patient care as appropriate.

Remove PPE

There are a variety of ways to remove PPE to achieve the goal of safe removal without contamination of clothes, skin, or mucous membranes (CDC, 2007; updated 2019). Two methods are outlined here, based on CDC recommendations.

Method A

7. Remove PPE: Except for respirator, if worn, remove PPE before exiting the patient room or in an anteroom. **Remove the respirator after leaving the patient's room and closing the door.**

   a. **The outsides of gloves are contaminated.** If hands are contaminated during gown or glove removal, immediately perform hand hygiene.

   b. Grasp the palm area of one gloved hand with the opposite gloved hand and peel off first glove, turning the glove inside out as you pull it off (Figure 6). Hold the removed glove in the remaining gloved hand.

   c. Slide fingers of the ungloved hand under the remaining glove at the wrist, **taking care not to touch the outer surface of the glove (Figure 7).**

   d. Peel off the second glove over the first glove, containing the first glove inside the other (Figure 8). Discard in appropriate container.

RATIONALE

Gloves protect hands and wrists from microorganisms.

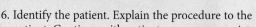
FIGURE 5. Putting on gloves, ensuring gloves cover gown cuffs.

Patient identification validates the correct patient and correct procedure. Discussion and explanation help allay anxiety and prepare the patient for what to expect.

Proper removal prevents contact with and the spread of microorganisms.

Removing the respirator outside the patient's room prevents contact with airborne microorganisms.

Outside front of equipment is considered contaminated. Hand hygiene prevents transmission of microorganisms. The inside, outside back, and ties on head and back are considered clean, which are areas of PPE that are not likely to have been in contact with infectious organisms.

The outsides of gloves are contaminated. This process contains the contaminated areas.

The ungloved hand is clean and should not touch contaminated areas.

This process contains the outside, contaminated areas of gloves. Proper disposal prevents transmission of microorganisms.

ACTION

e. To remove the goggles or face shield: **The outside of the goggles or face shield is contaminated—do not touch.** If hands are contaminated during goggle or face shield removal, immediately perform hand hygiene. Handle by the headband or earpieces and remove from the back (Figure 9). Lift away from the face. **Do not touch the front of the goggles or face shield.** Place in the designated receptacle for reprocessing or in an appropriate waste container.

RATIONALE

The outside of the goggles or face shield is contaminated; do not touch. Hand hygiene prevents transmission of microorganisms.

Handling by the headband or earpieces and lifting away from the face prevents transmission of microorganisms.

Proper disposal prevents transmission of microorganisms.

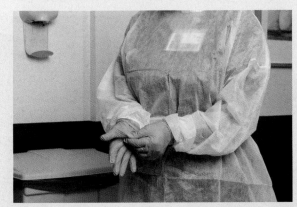

FIGURE 6. Grasping the palm area of one glove and peeling off.

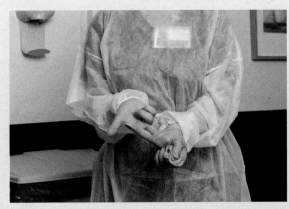

FIGURE 7. Sliding fingers of ungloved hand under the remaining glove at the wrist.

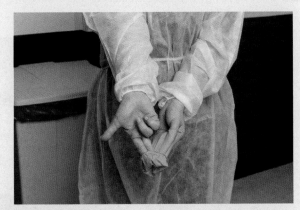

FIGURE 8. Peeling off the second glove, containing the first glove inside the other.

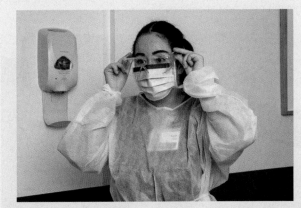

FIGURE 9. Removing goggles by grasping earpieces.

f. To remove the gown: **The gown front and sleeves are contaminated.** If hands are contaminated during gown removal, immediately perform hand hygiene. Unfasten ties, if at the neck and back, taking care that sleeves of gown do not contact the body. Allow the gown to fall away from shoulders. **Touching only the inside of the gown,** pull away from the neck and shoulders (Figure 10). Keeping hands on the inner surface of the gown, pull gown from arms (Figure 11). Turn gown inside out. Fold or roll into a bundle (Figure 12) and discard in an appropriate waste container.

The gown front and sleeves are contaminated. Hand hygiene prevents transmission of microorganisms.

Touching only the inside of the gown and pulling it away from the torso prevents transmission of microorganisms. This process contains the outside, contaminated areas of gown.

Proper disposal prevents transmission of microorganisms.

(continued on page 22)

Skill 1-3 ▶ Using Personal Protective Equipment *(continued)*

ACTION

g. To remove the mask or respirator: **The front of the mask/respirator is contaminated—do not touch.** If hands are contaminated during mask/respirator removal, immediately perform hand hygiene. Grasp the bottom ties or elastic of the mask/respirator, then top ties or elastic and remove. **Do not touch the front of mask or respirator** (Figure 13). Discard in an appropriate waste container. If using a reusable respirator, save for future use in the designated area.

RATIONALE

The front of the mask or respirator is contaminated; do not touch.

Not touching the front of the mask and proper disposal of the mask prevent transmission of microorganisms.

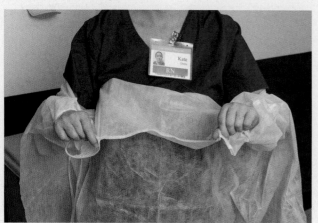

FIGURE 10. Touching only the inside of the gown, pull away from the neck and shoulders.

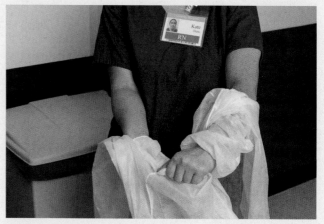

FIGURE 11. Keeping hands on the inner surface of the gown, pull gown from arms.

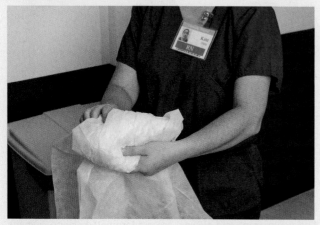

FIGURE 12. Turning gown inside out, rolling into a bundle.

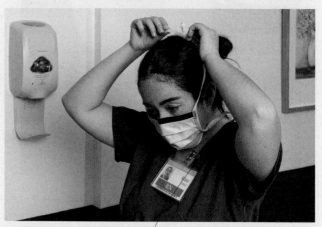

FIGURE 13. Removing mask or respirator, grasping the neck ties or elastic, taking care to avoid touching the front.

8. Perform hand hygiene immediately after removing all PPE.

Hand hygiene prevents spread of microorganisms.

Remove PPE

There are a variety of ways to remove PPE to achieve the goal of safe removal without contamination of clothes, skin, or mucous membranes (CDC, 2007; updated 2019).

ACTION

Method B

7. To remove the gown and gloves: **Gown front and sleeves and the outsides of gloves are contaminated.** If hands are contaminated during gown and glove removal, immediately perform hand hygiene. **Touching outside of the gown only with gloved hands,** grasp the gown in the front and pull away from the body, breaking the ties in the back (Figure 14). While removing the gown, fold or roll the gown inside-out into a bundle (Figure 15). As the gown is being removed, peel off gloves at the same time, **only touching the inside of the gloves and gown with bare hands (Figure 16).** Discard gown and gloves in an appropriate waste container.

8. To remove the goggles or face shield: **The outside of the goggles or face shield is contaminated—do not touch.** If hands are contaminated during goggle or face shield removal, immediately perform hand hygiene. Grasp the headband or earpieces and remove from the back (Figure 17). Lift away from the face. **Do not touch the front of goggles or face shield.** Place in designated receptacle for reprocessing or in an appropriate waste container.

RATIONALE

The front of the gown and sleeves, including waist strings, are contaminated. Hand hygiene prevents transmission of microorganisms.

The front of the gown and the outsides of gloves are contaminated.

This process contains the outside, contaminated areas of the gown.

Proper disposal prevents transmission of microorganisms.

The outside of the goggles or face shield is contaminated; do not touch. Hand hygiene prevents transmission of microorganisms.

Handling by the headband or earpieces and lifting away from face prevents transmission of microorganisms.

Proper disposal prevents transmission of microorganisms.

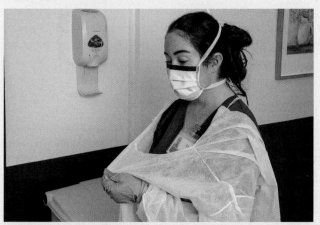

FIGURE 14. Grasping the outside of the front of gown and pulling away from the body.

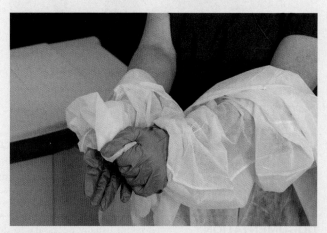

FIGURE 15. Rolling gown inside-out into a bundle.

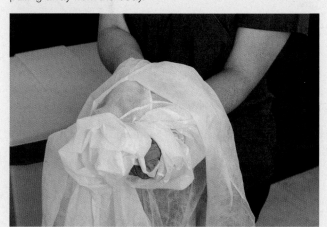

FIGURE 16. Peeling off gloves as gown is being removed, touching only the inside of the gloves and gown.

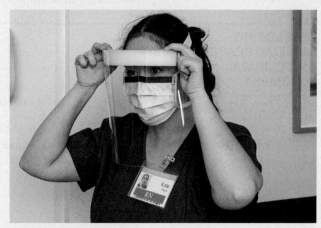

FIGURE 17. Removing the goggles or face shield, grasping the headband or earpieces.

(continued on page 24)

Skill 1-3 ▶ Using Personal Protective Equipment *(continued)*

ACTION

9. To remove mask or respirator: **Front of mask/respirator is contaminated—do not touch.** If hands are contaminated during mask/respirator removal, immediately perform hand hygiene. Grasp the bottom ties or elastic of the mask/respirator, then top ties or elastic, lift away from face, and remove (Figure 18). **Do not touch the front of mask or respirator.** Discard in an appropriate waste container. If using a reusable respirator, save for future use in the designated area.

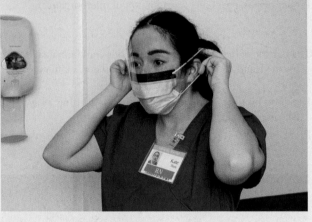

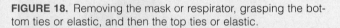

10. Perform hand hygiene immediately after removing all PPE.

RATIONALE

The front of mask or respirator is contaminated; do not touch.

Not touching the front of the mask and proper disposal of the mask prevent transmission of microorganisms.

Hand hygiene prevents spread of microorganisms.

FIGURE 18. Removing the mask or respirator, grasping the bottom ties or elastic, and then the top ties or elastic.

EVALUATION The expected outcomes have been met when the transmission of infectious agents among patients and health care providers has been prevented, patients and staff are free from exposure to potentially infectious microorganisms, and the patient verbalizes an understanding about the rationale for use of PPE.

DOCUMENTATION It is not usually necessary to document the use of specific articles of PPE or each application of PPE. However, document the implementation and continuation of specific transmission-based precautions as part of the patient's care.

DEVELOPING CLINICAL REASONING AND CLINICAL JUDGMENT

UNEXPECTED SITUATIONS AND ASSOCIATED INTERVENTIONS

- You did not realize the need for protective equipment at beginning of task: Stop task and obtain appropriate protective wear.
- You are accidentally exposed to blood and body fluids: Stop task and immediately follow facility protocol for exposure, including reporting the exposure.

- Standard Precautions are used for all patient care, based on risk assessment, and make use of common-sense practices and PPE to protect health care providers from infection and prevent the spread of infection from person to person (CDC, 2016b).
- Measures related to Respiratory Hygiene/Cough Etiquette should be implemented in community settings for any person with signs of illness including cough, congestion, rhinorrhea, or increased production of respiratory secretions (CDC, 2016b).

**EVIDENCE
FOR PRACTICE ▶**

PPE AND PREVENTION OF TRANSFER OF MICROORGANISMS

Prevention of health care–associated infections (HAIs) is a major challenge for health care providers. Infection-control guidelines recommend contact precautions for patients colonized or infected with specific multidrug-resistant organisms (MDROs) (CDC, 2007; updated 2019). These interventions include the use of nonsterile gloves during every interaction with patients to reduce the risk of transmission of microorganisms. Universal gloving has been suggested as an approach to reduce the transmission of MDROs (Chung et al., 2019). When universal gloving is implemented, health care providers wear gloves during every patient care activity for every patient. Does implementation of universal gloving prevent transmission of pathogens and decrease the incidence of HAIs?

Related Evidence

Chung, N. C. N., Kates, A. E., Ward, M. A., Kiscaden, E. J., Schacht Reisinger, H., Perencevich, E. N., Schweizer, M. L., & CDC Prevention Epicenters Program. (2019). Association between universal gloving and healthcare-associated infections: A systematic literature review and meta-analysis. *Infection Control & Hospital Epidemiology, 40*(7), 755–760. https://doi.org/10.1017/ice.2019.123

This systematic literature review and meta-analysis examined whether implementation of universal gloving is associated with decreased incidence of HAIs in clinical settings. A systematic literature search was conducted to identify relevant publications using search terms for universal gloving and HAIs. Pooled incidence rate ratios (IRRs) and 95% confidence intervals (CIs) were calculated using random effects models. Heterogeneity was evaluated using the Woolf test and the I^2 test. Eight heterogeneous ($I^2 = 59\%$) studies with varied results were included. Stratified analyses showed a nonsignificant association between universal gloving and incidence of methicillin-resistant *Staphylococcus aureus* (pooled IRR 0.94, 95% CI) and vancomycin-resistant enterococci (pooled IRR 0.94, 95% CI). Studies that implemented universal gloving alone showed a significant association with decreased incidence of HAIs (IRR 0.77, 95% CI), but studies implementing universal gloving as part of intervention bundles showed no significant association with incidence of HAIs (IRR 0.95, 95% CI). The researchers concluded universal gloving was associated with reduced incidence of HAIs and may be associated with a small protective effect against HAIs. The researchers suggested that, despite limited data, universal gloving may be considered in high-risk settings such as pediatric intensive care units and additional research is needed to determine the effects of universal gloving on a broader range of pathogens.

Relevance for Nursing Practice

Nurses should constantly strive to improve practice and be alert for interventions to help achieve better practice. As responsible practitioners, nurses and other health care personnel should continually review infection control standards and guidelines for best practice. It is important to examine and reflect on individual practice to ensure appropriate use of infection control measures, including use of PPE, to provide safe and responsible nursing care.

Skill 1-4 ▶ Preparing a Sterile Field Using a Packaged Sterile Drape

A sterile field is created to provide a surgically aseptic workspace. It should be considered a restricted area. A sterile drape may be used to establish a sterile field or to extend the sterile working area. The sterile drape should be waterproof on one side, with that side placed down on the work surface. After establishing the sterile field, add other sterile items, as needed, including solutions. Sterile items and sterile-gloved hands are the only objects allowed in the sterile field. Prepare the sterile field as close as possible to the time of use (AORN, 2018). Refer to Fundamentals Review 1-2 to review basic principles of surgical asepsis.

DELEGATION CONSIDERATIONS	Procedures requiring the use of a sterile field and other sterile items are not delegated to assistive personnel (AP). Depending on the state's nurse practice act and the organization's policies and procedures, these procedures may be delegated to licensed practical/vocational nurses (LPN/LVNs). The decision to delegate must be based on careful analysis of the patient's needs and circumstances as well as the qualifications of the person to whom the task is being delegated. Refer to the Delegation Guidelines in Appendix A.
EQUIPMENT	• Sterile-wrapped drape • Additional sterile supplies, such as dressings, containers, or solutions, as needed • PPE, as indicated
ASSESSMENT	Assess the situation to determine the necessity for creating a sterile field. Assess the area in which the sterile field is to be prepared. Move any unnecessary equipment out of the immediate vicinity. Assess that the sterile, packaged drape is dry and unopened. Assess the package expiration date, making sure that the date is still valid.
ACTUAL OR POTENTIAL HEALTH PROBLEMS AND NEEDS	Many actual or potential health problems or needs may require the use of this skill as part of related interventions. An appropriate health problem or need may include: • Infection risk • Risk for Cross Infection
OUTCOME IDENTIFICATION AND PLANNING	The expected outcomes to achieve when preparing a sterile field is that the sterile field is created without contamination, and the patient remains free of exposure to pathogens.

IMPLEMENTATION

ACTION	**RATIONALE**
1. Perform hand hygiene and put on PPE, if indicated.	Hand hygiene and PPE prevent the spread of microorganisms. PPE is required based on transmission precautions.
2. Identify the patient. Explain the procedure to the patient.	Patient identification validates the correct patient and correct procedure. Discussion and explanation help allay anxiety and prepare the patient for what to expect.
3. Check that the packaged sterile drape is dry and unopened. Also note expiration date, making sure that the date is still valid.	Moisture contaminates a sterile package. Expiration date indicates period that package remains sterile.
4. Select a work area that is waist level or higher.	Work area is within sight. Bacteria tend to settle, so there is less contamination above the waist.

ACTION

5. Open the outer covering of the drape. Remove sterile drape, lifting it carefully by its corners. Hold away from body and above the waist and work surface.
6. Continue to hold only by the corners. Allow the drape to unfold, away from your body and any other surface (Figure 1).
7. Position the drape on the work surface with the moisture-proof side down (Figure 2). This would be the shiny or blue side. Avoid touching any other surface or object with the drape. If any portion of the drape hangs off the work surface, that part of the drape is considered contaminated.

RATIONALE

The outer 1 inch (2.5 cm) of drape is considered contaminated. Any item touching this area is also considered contaminated.

Touching the outer side of the wrapper maintains the sterile field. Contact with any surface would contaminate the field.

Moisture-proof side prevents contamination of the field if it becomes wet. The moisture penetrates the sterile cloth or paper and carries organisms by capillary action to contaminate the field. A wet field is considered contaminated if the surface immediately below it is not sterile.

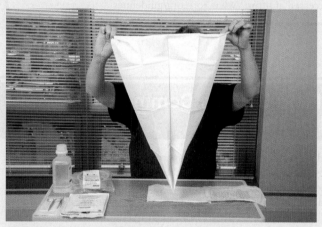

FIGURE 1. Holding drape by corners and allowing it to unfold away from body and surfaces.

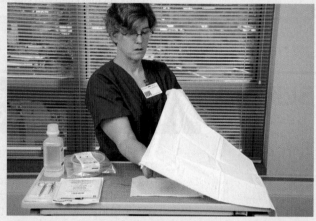

FIGURE 2. Positioning drape on work surface with the moisture-proof side down.

8. Place additional sterile items on field as needed. Refer to Skill 1-6. Continue with the procedure as indicated.

9. When procedure is completed, remove PPE, if used. Perform hand hygiene.

Sterility of the field is maintained.

Proper removal of PPE reduces the risk for infection transmission and contamination of other items. Hand hygiene prevents the spread of microorganisms.

EVALUATION

The expected outcomes have been met when the sterile field has been prepared without contamination, and the patient has remained free of exposure to pathogens.

DOCUMENTATION

It is not usually necessary to document the preparation of a sterile field. However, document the use of sterile technique for any procedure performed using sterile technique.

DEVELOPING CLINICAL REASONING AND CLINICAL JUDGMENT

UNEXPECTED SITUATIONS AND ASSOCIATED INTERVENTIONS

- *A part of the sterile field becomes contaminated:* When any portion of the sterile field becomes contaminated, discard the sterile field and any items on the field, and start over.
- *You realize a supply is missing after setting up the sterile field:* Call for help. Do not leave the sterile field unattended. If the nurse is not able to directly see the sterile field at all times, it is considered contaminated.

(*continued on page 28*)

Skill 1-4 ▶ Preparing a Sterile Field Using a Packaged Sterile Drape *(continued)*

- *The patient touches the sterile field:* If the patient touches the sterile field, discard the supplies and prepare a new sterile field. If the patient is confused, have someone assist by holding the patient's hands and/or provide reassurance and explanation of the procedure.

EVIDENCE FOR PRACTICE ▶	**AORN GUIDELINE QUICK VIEW: STERILE TECHNIQUE** Association of periOperative Registered Nurses (AORN). (2018). AORN guideline quick view: Sterile technique. *AORN Journal, 108*(6), 705–710. https://doi.org/10.1002/aorn.12458 This AORN guideline Quick View provides key points for implementation of sterile technique from the *AORN Guideline Essentials.* These guidelines provide evidence-based recommendations to guide implementation of sterile technique to promote safety and optimal outcomes for patients. Access to the full set of *Guidelines for Perioperative Practice* is included with AORN membership and can be accessed at https://www.aorn.org/guidelines

Skill 1-5 ▶ Preparing a Sterile Field Using a Commercially Prepared Sterile Kit or Tray

A sterile field is created to provide a surgically aseptic workspace. Consider it a restricted area. Commercially prepared sterile kits and trays are wrapped in a sterile wrapper that, once opened, becomes the sterile field. Sterile items and sterile-gloved hands are the only objects allowed in the sterile field. If the area is breached, the entire sterile field is considered contaminated. Prepare the sterile field as close as possible to the time of use (AORN, 2018). Refer to Fundamentals Review 1-2 to review basic principles of surgical asepsis.

DELEGATION CONSIDERATIONS	Procedures requiring the use of a sterile field and other sterile items are not delegated to assistive personnel (AP). Depending on the state's nurse practice act and the organization's policies and procedures, these procedures may be delegated to licensed practical/vocational nurses (LPN/LVNs). The decision to delegate must be based on careful analysis of the patient's needs and circumstances as well as the qualifications of the person to whom the task is being delegated. Refer to the Delegation Guidelines in Appendix A.
EQUIPMENT	• Commercially prepared sterile package • Additional sterile supplies, such as dressings, containers, or solutions, as needed • PPE, as indicated
ASSESSMENT	Assess the situation to determine the necessity for creating a sterile field. Assess the area in which the sterile field is to be prepared. Move any unnecessary equipment out of the immediate vicinity. Assess that the commercially prepared package is dry and unopened. Assess the package expiration date, making sure that the date is still valid.
ACTUAL OR POTENTIAL HEALTH PROBLEMS AND NEEDS	Many actual or potential health problems or needs may require the use of this skill as part of related interventions. An appropriate health problem or need may include: • Infection risk • Risk for Cross Infection
OUTCOME IDENTIFICATION AND PLANNING	The expected outcomes to achieve when opening a commercially packaged sterile kit or tray is that a sterile field is created without contamination, the contents of the package remain sterile, and the patient remains free of exposure to pathogens.

IMPLEMENTATION

ACTION	RATIONALE

 1. Perform hand hygiene and put on PPE, if indicated.

Hand hygiene and PPE prevent the spread of microorganisms. PPE is required based on transmission precautions.

 2. Identify the patient. Explain the procedure to the patient.

Patient identification validates the correct patient and correct procedure. Discussion and explanation help allay anxiety and prepare the patient for what to expect.

3. Check that the packaged kit or tray is dry and unopened. Also note expiration date, making sure that the date is still valid.

Moisture contaminates a sterile package. Expiration date indicates period that package remains sterile.

4. Select a work area that is waist level or higher.

Work area is within sight. Bacteria tend to settle, so there is less contamination above the waist.

5. Open the outside cover of the package (Figure 1) and remove the kit or tray. Place in the center of the work surface, with the topmost flap positioned on the far side of the package. Discard outside cover.

This allows sufficient room for sterile field.

6. Reach around the package and grasp the outer surface of the end of the topmost flap, holding no more than 1 inch from the border of the flap. Pull open away from the body, keeping the arm outstretched and away from the inside of the wrapper (Figure 2). Allow the wrapper to lie flat on the work surface.

This maintains sterility of inside of wrapper, which is to become the sterile field. The outer surface of the wrapper is considered unsterile. The outer 1-inch border of the wrapper is considered contaminated.

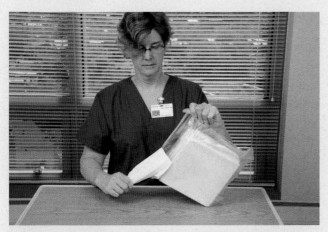

FIGURE 1. Opening outside cover of package.

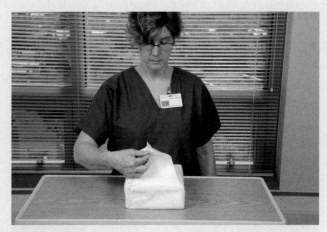

FIGURE 2. Pulling top flap open, away from body.

7. Reach around the package and grasp the outer surface of the first side flap, holding no more than 1 inch from the border of the flap. Pull open to the side of the package, keeping the arm outstretched and away from the inside of the wrapper (Figure 3). Allow the wrapper to lie flat on the work surface.

This maintains sterility of the inside of the wrapper, which is to become the sterile field. The outer surface of the wrapper is considered unsterile. The outer 1-inch border of the wrapper is considered contaminated.

8. Reach around the package and grasp the outer surface of the remaining side flap, holding no more than 1 inch from the border of the flap. Pull open to the side of the package, keeping the arm outstretched and away from the inside of the wrapper (Figure 4). Allow the wrapper to lie flat on the work surface.

This maintains sterility of the inside of the wrapper, which is to become the sterile field. The outer surface of the wrapper is considered unsterile. The outer 1-inch border of the wrapper is considered contaminated.

(continued on page 30)

Skill 1-5 ▶ Preparing a Sterile Field Using a Commercially Prepared Sterile Kit or Tray *(continued)*

ACTION

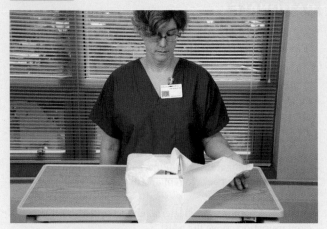

FIGURE 3. Pulling open the first side flap.

9. Stand away from the package and work surface. Grasp the outer surface of the remaining flap closest to the body, holding not more than 1 inch from the border of the flap. Pull the flap back toward the body, keeping arm outstretched and away from the inside of the wrapper (Figure 5). Keep this hand in place. Use other hand to grasp the wrapper on the underside (the side that is down to the work surface). Position the wrapper so that when flat, edges are on the work surface, and do not hang down over sides of work surface (Figure 6). Allow the wrapper to lie flat on the work surface.

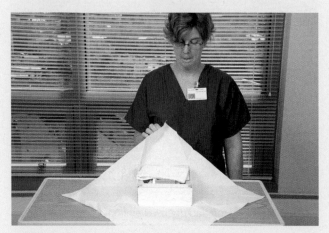

FIGURE 5. Pulling open flap closest to body.

10. The outer wrapper of the package has become a sterile field with the packaged supplies in the center (Figure 7). Do not touch or reach over the sterile field. Place additional sterile items on field as needed. Refer to Skill 1-6. Continue with the procedure as indicated.

RATIONALE

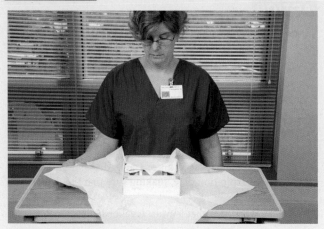

FIGURE 4. Pulling open the remaining side flap.

This maintains sterility of the inside of the wrapper, which is to become the sterile field. The outer surface of the wrapper is considered unsterile. The outer 1-inch border of the wrapper is considered contaminated.

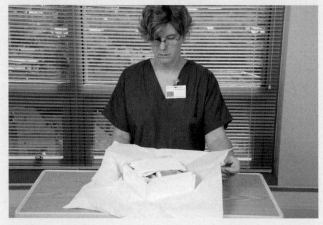

FIGURE 6. Positioning wrapper on work surface.

Sterility of the field and contents are maintained.

| ACTION | RATIONALE |

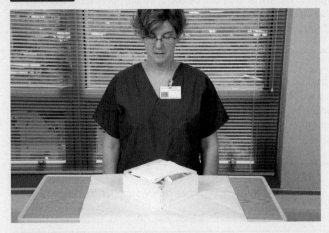

FIGURE 7. Outside wrapper of package is now sterile field.

11. When procedure is completed, remove PPE, if used. Perform hand hygiene.

Proper removal of PPE reduces the risk for infection transmission and contamination of other items. Hand hygiene prevents the spread of microorganisms.

EVALUATION

The expected outcomes have been met when the sterile field has been prepared without contamination, the contents of the package remained sterile, and the patient has remained free of exposure to pathogens.

DOCUMENTATION

It is not usually necessary to document the preparation of a sterile field. However, do document the use of sterile technique for any procedure performed using sterile technique.

DEVELOPING CLINICAL REASONING AND CLINICAL JUDGMENT

UNEXPECTED SITUATIONS AND ASSOCIATED INTERVENTIONS

- *A part of the sterile field becomes contaminated:* When any portion of the sterile field becomes contaminated, discard the sterile field and any items on the field and start over.
- *You realize a supply is missing after setting up the sterile field:* Call for help. Do not leave the sterile field unattended. If you are unable to directly see the sterile field at all times, it is considered contaminated.
- *The patient touches the sterile field:* If the patient touches the sterile field, discard the supplies and prepare a new sterile field. If the patient is confused, have someone assist by holding the patient's hands and/or provide reassurance and explanation of the procedure.

EVIDENCE FOR PRACTICE ▶

AORN GUIDELINE QUICK VIEW: STERILE TECHNIQUE
Association of periOperative Registered Nurses (AORN). (2018). AORN guideline quick view: Sterile technique. *AORN Journal, 108*(6), 705–710. https://doi.org/10.1002/aorn.12458
Refer to details in Skill 1-4, Evidence for Practice.

Skill 1-6 ▶ Adding Sterile Items to a Sterile Field

A sterile field is created to provide a surgically aseptic workspace. It should be considered a restricted area. After establishing the sterile field, add other sterile items, including solutions, as needed. Items can be wrapped and sterilized within the facility, or they can be commercially prepared. Take care to ensure that nothing unsterile touches the field or other items in the field, including hands or clothes. Refer to Fundamentals Review 1-2 to review basic principles of surgical asepsis.

DELEGATION CONSIDERATIONS

Procedures requiring the use of a sterile field and other sterile items are not delegated to assistive personnel (AP). Depending on the state's nurse practice act and the organization's policies and procedures, these procedures may be delegated to licensed practical/vocational nurses (LPN/LVNs). The decision to delegate must be based on careful analysis of the patient's needs and circumstances as well as the qualifications of the person to whom the task is being delegated. Refer to the Delegation Guidelines in Appendix A.

EQUIPMENT

- Sterile field
- Sterile gauze, forceps, dressings, containers, solutions, or other sterile supplies, as needed
- PPE, as indicated

ASSESSMENT

Assess the situation to determine the necessity for creating a sterile field. Assess the area in which the sterile field is to be prepared. Move any unnecessary equipment out of the immediate vicinity. Identify additional supplies needed for the procedure.

Assess that the sterile, packaged supplies are dry and unopened. Assess the package expiration date, making sure that the date is still valid.

ACTUAL OR POTENTIAL HEALTH PROBLEMS AND NEEDS

Many actual or potential health problems or needs may require the use of this skill as part of related interventions. An appropriate health problem or need may include:
- Infection risk
- Risk for Cross Infection

OUTCOME IDENTIFICATION AND PLANNING

The expected outcomes to achieve when adding items to a sterile field are that the sterile field is created without contamination, the sterile supplies are added to the sterile field and are not contaminated, and the patient remains free from exposure to pathogens.

IMPLEMENTATION

ACTION	RATIONALE
1. Perform hand hygiene and put on PPE, if indicated.	Hand hygiene and PPE prevent the spread of microorganisms. PPE is required based on transmission precautions.
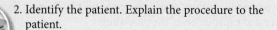 2. Identify the patient. Explain the procedure to the patient.	Patient identification validates the correct patient and correct procedure. Discussion and explanation help allay anxiety and prepare the patient for what to expect.
3. Check that the sterile, packaged drape and supplies are dry and unopened. Also note expiration date, making sure that the date is still valid.	Moisture contaminates a sterile package. An expiration date indicates period that package remains sterile.
4. Select a work area that is waist level or higher.	Work area is within sight. Bacteria tend to settle, so there is less contamination above the waist.
5. Prepare sterile field as described in Skill 1-4 or Skill 1-5.	Proper technique maintains sterility.

ACTION	**RATIONALE**

6. Add sterile item:

To Add a Facility-Wrapped and Sterilized Item

a. Hold facility-wrapped item in the dominant hand, with top flap opening away from the body. With other hand, reach around the package and unfold top flap and both sides.

Only sterile surface and item are exposed before dropping onto sterile field.

b. Keep a secure hold on the item through the wrapper with the dominant hand. Grasp the remaining flap of the wrapper closest to the body, taking care not to touch the inner surface of the wrapper or the item. Pull the flap back toward the wrist, so the wrapper covers the hand and wrist.

Only sterile surface and item are exposed before dropping onto sterile field.

c. Grasp all the corners of the wrapper together with the nondominant hand and pull back toward wrist, covering hand and wrist. Hold in place.

Only sterile surface and item are exposed before dropping onto sterile field.

d. Hold the item 6 inches above the surface of the sterile field and drop onto the field. **Be careful to avoid touching the surface or other items or dropping any item onto the 1-inch border.**

This prevents contamination of the field and inadvertent dropping of the sterile item too close to the edge or off the field. Any items landing on the 1-inch border are considered contaminated.

To Add a Commercially Wrapped and Sterilized Item

a. Depending on the type of package, hold package in one hand. Pull back top cover with other hand. Alternatively, carefully peel the edges apart using both hands (Figure 1).

This allows contents to remain uncontaminated by hands.

b. After top cover or edges are partially separated, hold the item 6 inches above the surface of the sterile field. Continue opening the package and drop the item onto the field (Figure 2). **Be careful to avoid touching the surface or other items or dropping an item onto the 1-inch border.**

This prevents contamination of the field and inadvertent dropping of the sterile item too close to the edge or off the field. Any items landing on the 1-inch border are considered contaminated.

c. Discard wrapper.

A neat work area promotes proper technique and avoids inadvertent contamination of the field.

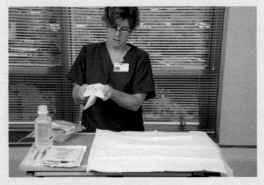

FIGURE 1. Carefully peeling edges apart.

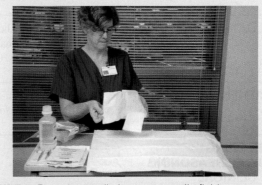

FIGURE 2. Dropping sterile item onto sterile field.

To Add a Sterile Solution

a. Obtain appropriate solution and check expiration date.

Once opened, label any bottles with date and time. Solution may be kept for use for 24 hours once opened.

b. Open solution container according to directions and **place cap on table away from the field with edges up (Figure 3).**

Sterility of the inside of the cap is maintained.

(continued on page 34)

Skill 1-6 ▶ Adding Sterile Items to a Sterile Field *(continued)*

ACTION

c. Hold bottle outside the edge of the sterile field with the label side facing the palm of your hand and prepare to pour from a height of 4 to 6 inches (10 to 15 cm). **Do not touch the tip of the bottle to the sterile container or field.**

d. Pour required amount of solution steadily into sterile container previously added to the sterile field and positioned at side of sterile field or onto dressings (Figure 4). **Avoid splashing any liquid.**

e. Touch only the outside of the lid when recapping. Label solution with date and time of opening.

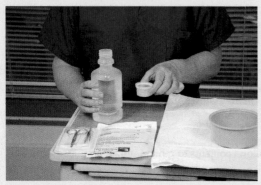

FIGURE 3. Opening bottle of sterile solution and placing cap on table with edges up.

7. Continue with procedure as indicated.

 8. When procedure is completed, remove PPE, if used. Perform hand hygiene.

RATIONALE

The label remains dry, and solution may be poured without reaching across sterile field. Minimal splashing occurs from that height.

Accidentally touching the tip of the bottle to a container or dressing contaminates them both.

A steady stream minimizes the risk of splashing; moisture contaminates sterile field.

The solution remains uncontaminated and available for future use.

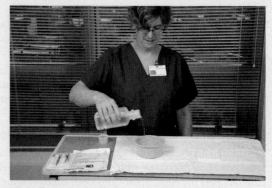

FIGURE 4. Pouring solution into sterile container.

Proper removal of PPE reduces the risk for infection transmission and contamination of other items. Hand hygiene prevents the spread of microorganisms.

EVALUATION

The expected outcomes have been met when the sterile field has been created without contamination, the sterile supplies have not been contaminated, and the patient has remained free of exposure to pathogens.

DOCUMENTATION

It is not usually necessary to document the addition of sterile items to a sterile field. However, document the use of performing sterile technique for any procedure.

DEVELOPING CLINICAL REASONING AND CLINICAL JUDGMENT

UNEXPECTED SITUATIONS AND ASSOCIATED INTERVENTIONS

- *The item being added falls close to or on the edge of the field:* Consider the outer 1-inch edge of a sterile field to be contaminated. Any item within the outer 1-inch is considered contaminated.
- *A part of the sterile field becomes contaminated:* When any portion of the sterile field becomes contaminated, discard the sterile field and any items on the field and start over.
- *You realize a supply is missing after setting up the sterile field:* Call for help. Do not leave the sterile field unattended. If you are unable to see the sterile field at all times, it is considered contaminated.
- *The patient touches the sterile field:* If the patient touches the sterile field, discard the supplies and prepare a new sterile field. If the patient is confused, have someone assist by holding the patient's hands and/or reinforcing what is happening.

EVIDENCE
FOR PRACTICE ▶

AORN GUIDELINE QUICK VIEW: STERILE TECHNIQUE
Association of periOperative Registered Nurses (AORN). (2018). AORN guideline quick view: Sterile technique. *AORN Journal, 108*(6), 705–710. https://doi.org/10.1002/aorn.12458
Refer to details in Skill 1-4, Evidence for Practice.

Skill 1-7 ▶ Putting on Sterile Gloves and Removing Soiled Gloves

When applying and wearing sterile gloves, keep hands above waist level and away from nonsterile surfaces. Replace gloves if they develop an opening or tear; the integrity of the material becomes compromised; or the gloves come in contact with any nonsterile surface or nonsterile item. Refer to Fundamentals Review 1-2 for additional guidelines related to working with sterile gloves. It may be a good idea to bring an extra pair of gloves with you when gathering supplies, according to facility policy. That way, if the first pair is contaminated in some way and needs to be replaced, you will not have to leave the procedure to get a new pair.

DELEGATION CONSIDERATIONS

Procedures requiring the use of sterile gloves and other sterile items are not delegated to assistive personnel (AP). Depending on the state's nurse practice act and the organization's policies and procedures, these procedures may be delegated to licensed practical/vocational nurses (LPN/LVNs). The decision to delegate must be based on careful analysis of the patient's needs and circumstances as well as the qualifications of the person to whom the task is being delegated. Refer to the Delegation Guidelines in Appendix A.

EQUIPMENT

• Sterile gloves of the appropriate size
• PPE, as indicated

ASSESSMENT

Assess the situation to determine the necessity for sterile gloves. In addition, check the patient's medical record for information about a possible latex allergy. Also, question the patient about any history of allergy, including latex allergy, or sensitivity and signs and symptoms that have occurred. If the patient has a latex allergy, anticipate the need for latex-free gloves. Assess that the sterile glove package is dry and unopened. Assess the package expiration date, making sure that the date is still valid.

ACTUAL OR POTENTIAL HEALTH PROBLEMS AND NEEDS

Many actual or potential health problems or needs may require the use of this skill as part of related interventions. An appropriate health problem or need may include:
• Infection risk
• Risk for Cross Infection

OUTCOME IDENTIFICATION AND PLANNING

The expected outcomes to achieve when putting on sterile gloves and removing soiled gloves is that the gloves are applied without contamination, gloves are removed without transmission of infectious agents, and the patient remains free from exposure to infectious microorganisms.

(*continued on page 36*)

Skill 1-7 ▶ Putting on Sterile Gloves and Removing Soiled Gloves *(continued)*

IMPLEMENTATION

ACTION

1. Perform hand hygiene and put on PPE, if indicated.

2. Identify the patient. Explain the procedure to the patient.

3. Check that the sterile glove package is dry and unopened. Also note expiration date, making sure that the date is still valid.

4. Place sterile glove package on clean, dry surface at or above your waist.

5. Open the outside wrapper by carefully peeling the top layer back (Figure 1). Remove inner package, handling only the outside of it.

6. Place the inner package on the work surface with the side labeled "cuff end" closest to the body.

7. Carefully open the inner package. Fold open the top flap, then the bottom and sides (Figure 2). **Do not touch the inner surface of the package or the gloves.**

RATIONALE

Hand hygiene and PPE prevent the spread of microorganisms. PPE is required based on transmission precautions.

Patient identification validates the correct patient and correct procedure. Discussion and explanation help allay anxiety and prepare the patient for what to expect.

Moisture contaminates a sterile package. Expiration date indicates the period that the package remains sterile.

Moisture could contaminate the sterile gloves. Any sterile object held below the waist is considered contaminated.

This maintains sterility of gloves in inner packet.

This allows for ease of glove application.

The inner surface of the package is considered sterile. The outer 1-inch border of the inner package is considered contaminated. The sterile gloves are exposed with the cuff end closest to the nurse.

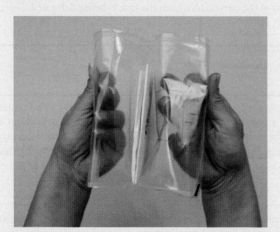

FIGURE 1. Pulling top layer of outside wrapper back.

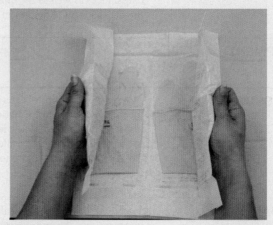

FIGURE 2. Folding back side flaps.

8. With the thumb and forefinger of the nondominant hand, grasp the folded cuff of the glove for the dominant hand, touching only the exposed inside of the glove (Figure 3).

9. Keeping the hands above the waistline, lift and hold the glove up and off the inner package with fingers down (Figure 4). **Do not let it touch any unsterile object.**

The unsterile hand touches only the inside of the glove. The outside remains sterile.

The glove is contaminated if it touches any unsterile objects.

ACTION

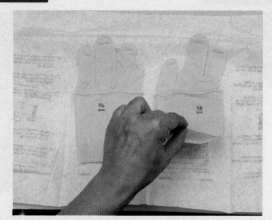

FIGURE 3. Grasping cuff of glove for dominant hand.

10. Carefully insert dominant hand palm up into glove (Figure 5) and pull glove on. Leave the cuff folded until the opposite hand is gloved.
11. Hold the thumb of the gloved hand outward. Place the fingers of the gloved hand inside the cuff of the remaining glove (Figure 6). Lift it from the wrapper, taking care not to touch anything with the gloves or hands.

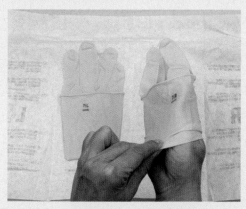

FIGURE 5. Inserting dominant hand into glove.

12. Carefully insert nondominant hand into glove. Pull the glove on, taking care that the skin does not touch any of the outer surfaces of the gloves.
13. Slide the fingers of one hand under the cuff of the other and fully extend the cuff down the arm, **touching only the sterile outside of the glove (Figure 7).** Repeat for the remaining hand.
14. Adjust gloves on both hands, if necessary, **touching only sterile areas with other sterile areas (Figure 8).**

RATIONALE

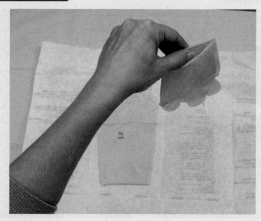

FIGURE 4. Lifting glove from package.

Attempting to turn upward with unsterile hand may result in contamination of a sterile glove.

The thumb is less likely to become contaminated if held outward. Sterile surface touching sterile surface prevents contamination.

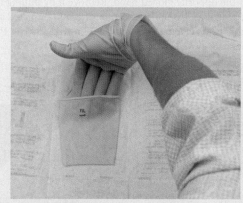

FIGURE 6. Sliding fingers under cuff of glove for nondominant hand.

Sterile surface touching sterile surface prevents contamination.

Sterile surface touching sterile surface prevents contamination.

Sterile surface touching sterile surface prevents contamination.

(continued on page 38)

Skill 1-7 ▶ Putting on Sterile Gloves and Removing Soiled Gloves *(continued)*

ACTION	RATIONALE

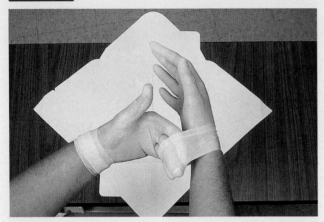

FIGURE 7. Sliding fingers of one hand under cuff of other hand and extending cuff down the arm.

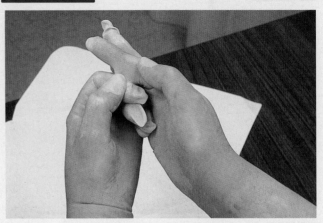

FIGURE 8. Adjusting gloves as necessary.

15. Continue with the procedure as indicated.

Removing Soiled Gloves

16. **Outside of gloves is contaminated.** If hands are contaminated during gown or glove removal, immediately perform hand hygiene. Grasp the palm area of one gloved hand with the opposite gloved hand. Remove it by pulling it off, inverting it as it is pulled, keeping the contaminated area on the inside (Figure 9). Hold the removed glove in the remaining gloved hand.

Hand hygiene prevents the spread of microorganisms.

The contaminated area does not come in contact with hands or wrists.

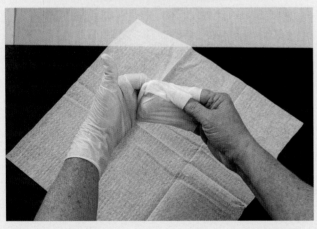

FIGURE 9. Inverting glove as it is removed.

17. Slide fingers of the ungloved hand between the remaining glove and the wrist (Figure 10). **Take care to avoid touching the outside surface of the glove.** Remove it by pulling second glove over the first glove, inverting it as it is pulled, keeping the contaminated area on the inside, and securing the first glove inside the second (Figure 11).

The contaminated area does not come in contact with hands or wrists.

18. Discard gloves in appropriate container. Remove additional PPE, if used. Perform hand hygiene.

Proper removal and disposal of PPE reduces the risk for infection transmission and contamination of other items. Hand hygiene prevents the spread of microorganisms.

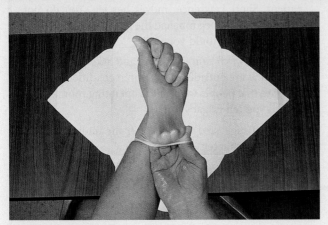

FIGURE 10. Sliding fingers of ungloved hand inside remaining glove.

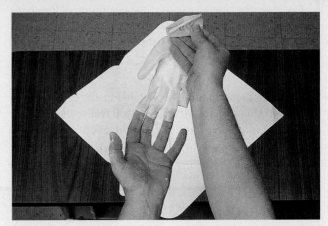

FIGURE 11. Inverting glove as it is removed, securing first glove inside it.

EVALUATION	The expected outcomes have been met when gloves have been applied without contamination, gloves have been removed without transmission of infectious agents, and the patient remained free from exposure to infectious microorganisms.

DOCUMENTATION	It is not usually necessary to document the application of sterile gloves and removal. However, document the use of sterile technique for any procedure performed using sterile technique.

DEVELOPING CLINICAL REASONING AND CLINICAL JUDGMENT

UNEXPECTED SITUATIONS AND ASSOCIATED INTERVENTIONS

- Contamination occurs during application of the sterile gloves: Discard gloves and open new package of sterile gloves.
- A hole or tear is noticed in one of the gloves: Discard gloves and open a new package of sterile gloves.
- A hole or tear is noticed in one of the gloves during the procedure: Stop procedure. Remove damaged gloves. Perform hand hygiene and put on new sterile gloves.
- The patient touches the nurse's hand: If the patient touches your hands and nothing else, you may remove the contaminated gloves and put on new sterile gloves. It may be a good idea to bring two pairs of sterile gloves into the room, depending on facility policy, so that you will not have to leave the procedure to get a new pair.
- If the patient touches the sterile field, discard the supplies and prepare a new sterile field. If the patient is confused, have someone assist you by holding the patient's hands or reinforcing what is happening.
- Patient has a latex allergy: Obtain latex-free sterile gloves.

EVIDENCE FOR PRACTICE ▶

AORN GUIDELINE QUICK VIEW: STERILE TECHNIQUE
Association of periOperative Registered Nurses (AORN). (2018). AORN guideline quick view: Sterile technique. *AORN Journal, 108*(6), 705–710. https://doi.org/10.1002/aorn.12458
    Refer to details in Skill 1-4, Evidence for Practice.

Enhance Your Understanding

Focusing on Patient Care: Developing Clinical Reasoning and Clinical Judgment

Consider the case scenarios at the beginning of the chapter as you answer the following questions to enhance your understanding and apply what you have learned.

QUESTIONS

1. While preparing the sterile table in the cardiac catheterization lab for Mr. Wilson, you realize that a sterile bowl is missing. How can you obtain a sterile bowl?

2. While you are putting on sterile gloves in preparation for an indwelling urinary catheter insertion, your patient, Sheri Lawrence, moves her leg. You do not think that Sheri's leg touched the glove, but you are not positive. What should you do?

3. Edgar Barowski's son is visiting and asks you why the masks that are outside Edgar's room are different from the ones that people wear in the operating room. What should you tell Edgar's son?

You can find suggested answers after the Bibliography at the end of this chapter.

Integrated Case Study Connection

The case studies in the back of the book focus on integrating concepts. Refer to the following case studies to enhance your understanding of the concepts and skills in this chapter.

- Basic Case Studies: Tiffany Jones, page 1195; John Willis, page 1199.
- Intermediate Case Studies: Tula Stillwater, page 1213; Gwen Galloway, page 1221; George Patel, page 1223.

Bibliography

Agency for Healthcare Research and Quality (AHRQ). (2019). AHRQ's healthcare-associated infections program. https://www.ahrq.gov/hai/index.html

Alzyood, M., Jackson, D., Brooke, J., & Aveyard, H. (2018). An integrative review exploring the perceptions of patients and healthcare professionals towards patient involvement in promoting hand hygiene compliance in the hospital setting. *Journal of Clinical Nursing, 27*(7–8), 1329–1345. https://doi.org/10.1111/jocn.14305

Association for Professionals in Infection Control and Epidemiology (APIC). (2015). *Guide to hand hygiene programs for infection prevention.* http://apic.org/Professional-Practice/Implementation-guides#HandHygiene

Association of periOperative Registered Nurses (AORN). (2018). AORN guideline quick view: Sterile technique. *AORN Journal, 108*(6), 705–710. https://doi.org/10.1002/aorn.12458

Association of periOperative Registered Nurses (AORN). (2020). *Guidelines for Perioperative Practice.* https://www.aorn.org/guidelines

Atif, S., Lorcy, A., & Dubé, E. (2019). Healthcare workers' attitudes toward hand hygiene practices: Results of a multicentre qualitative study in Quebec. *Canadian Journal of Infection Control, 34*(1), 41–48.

Azor-Martinez, E., Yui-Hifume, R., Muñoz-Vico, F. J., Jimenez-Noguera, E., Strizzi, J. M., Martinez-Martinez, I., Garcia-Fernandez, L., Seijas-Vasquez, M. L., Torres-Alegre, P., Fernández-Campos, M. A., & Gimenez-Sanchez, F. (2018). Effectiveness of a hand hygiene program at child care centers: A cluster randomized trial. *Pediatrics, 142*(5), e20181245. https://doi.org/10.1542/peds.2018-1245

Baloh, J., Thom, K. A., Perencevich, E., Rock, C., Robinson, G., Ward, M., Herwaldt, L., & Schacht Reisinger, H. (2019). Hand hygiene before donning nonsterile gloves: Healthcare workers' beliefs and practices. *American Journal of Infection Control, 47*(5), 492–497. https://doi.org/10.1016/j.ajic.2018.11.015

Boyce, J. M., Laughman, J. A., Ader, M. H., Wagner, P. T., Parker, A. E., & Arbogast, J. W. (2019). Impact of an automated hand hygiene monitoring system and additional promotional activities on hand hygiene performance rates, and healthcare–associated infections. *Infection Control & Hospital Epidemiology, 40*(7), 741–747. https://doi.org/10.1017/ice.2019.77

Breen, A., & Hessels, A. (2017). Stethoscopes: Friend or fomite? *Nursing Management, 48*(12), 9–11. https://doi.org/10.1097/01.NUMA.0000526917.85088.eb

Brunette, G. W., & Nemhauset, J. B. (Eds.) (2019). *CDC yellow book 2020: Health information for international travel.* Oxford University Press.

Calfee, D. P., Salgado, C. D., Milstone, A. M., Harris, A. D., Kuhar, D. T., Moody, J., Aureden, K., Huang, S. S., Maragakis, L. L., Yokoe, D. S., & Society for Healthcare Epidemiology of America. (2014). Strategies to prevent methicillin-resistant Staphylococcus aureus transmission and infection in acute care hospitals: 2014 update. *Infection Control and Hospital Epidemiology, 35*(7), 772–796. https://doi.org/10.1086/676534

Centers for Disease Control and Prevention (CDC). (n.d.). *Sequence for putting on personal protective equipment and how to safely remove personal protective equipment* [Poster]. https://www.cdc.gov/hai/pdfs/ppe/PPE-Sequence.pdf

Centers for Disease Control and Prevention (CDC). (2002). Guidelines for hand hygiene in health-care settings. *Morbidity and Mortality Weekly Report, 51*(RR-16), 1–45. http://www.cdc.gov/mmwr/PDF/rr/rr5116.pdf

Centers for Disease Control and Prevention (CDC). (2007; updated 2019). *Guideline for isolation precautions: Preventing transmission of infectious agents in healthcare settings.* https://www.cdc.gov/infectioncontrol/guidelines/isolation/index.html

Centers for Disease Control and Prevention (CDC). (2016a). *Hand hygiene in healthcare settings. Patients. Clean hands count for patients.* https://www.cdc.gov/handhygiene/patients/index.html

Centers for Disease Control and Prevention (CDC). (2016b). *Healthcare-associated infections. Outpatient settings. Guide to infection prevention in outpatient settings: Minimum expectations for safe care.* https://www.cdc.gov/hai/settings/outpatient/outpatient-settings.html

Centers for Disease Control and Prevention (CDC). (2017). *Healthcare Infection Control Practices Advisory Committee (HICPAC). Core infection prevention and control practices for safe healthcare delivery in all settings.* https://www.cdc.gov/hicpac/recommendations/core-practices.html

Centers for Disease Control and Prevention (CDC). (2018). *Ebola (Ebola virus disease). Personal protective equipment (PPE).* https://www.cdc.gov/vhf/ebola/healthcare-us/ppe/index.html

Centers for Disease Control and Prevention (CDC). (2019a). *Hand hygiene in healthcare settings.* https://www.cdc.gov/handhygiene/index.html

Centers for Disease Control and Prevention (CDC). (2019b). *Hand hygiene in healthcare settings. Healthcare providers. Clean hands count for healthcare providers.* https://www.cdc.gov/handhygiene/providers/index.html

Centers for Disease Control and Prevention (CDC). (2019c). *Hand hygiene in healthcare settings. Show me the science.* https://www.cdc.gov/handhygiene/science/index.html

Centers for Disease Control and Prevention (CDC). (2020a). *Coronavirus disease 2019 (COVID-19).* https://www.cdc.gov/coronavirus/2019-nCoV/hcp/

Centers for Disease Control and Prevention (CDC). (2020b). *Handwashing: Clean hands save lives. When and How to wash your hands.* https://www.cdc.gov/handwashing/when-how-handwashing.html

Chung, N. C. N., Kates, A. E., Ward, M. A., Kiscaden, E. J., Schacht Reisinger, H., Perencevich, E. N., Schweizer, M. L., & CDC Prevention Epicenters Program. (2019). Association between universal gloving and healthcare-associated infections: A systematic literature review and meta-analysis. *Infection Control & Hospital Epidemiology, 40*(7), 755–760. https://doi.org/10.1017/ice.2019.123

Cobb, A., & Lazar, B. (2020). Mobile device usage contributes to nosocomial infections. *Radiologic Technology, 91*(3), 303–307.

Ford, C., & Park, L. J. (2018). Hand hygiene and handwashing: Key to preventing the transfer of pathogens. *British Journal of Nursing, 27*(20), 1164–1166. https://doi.org/10.12968/bjon.2018.27.20.1164

Gesser-Edelsburg, A., Cohen, R., Zemach, M., & Halavi, A. M. (2020). Discourse on hygiene between hospitalized patients and health care workers as an accepted norm: Making it legitimate to remind health care workers about hand hygiene. *American Journal of Infection Control, 48*(1), 61–67. https://doi.org/10.1016/j.ajic.2018.10.026

Halm, M., & Sandau, K. (2018). Skin impact of alcohol-based hand rubs vs handwashing. *American Journal of Critical Care, 27*(4), 334–337. https://doi.org/10.4037/ajcc2018727

Hauk, L. (2018). Guideline for sterile technique. *AORN Journal, 108*(4), P10–P12. https://doi.org/10.1002/aorn.12409

Healthy People 2020. (n.d.; updated April 2020). *Healthcare-associated infections.* Office of Disease Prevention and Health Promotion. https://www.healthy-people.gov/2020/topics-objectives/topic/healthcare-associated-infections

Healthy People 2030. (n.d.). *Health care-associated infections.* https://health.gov/healthypeople/objectives-and-data/browse-objectives/health-care-associated-infections

Hinkle, J. L., & Cheever, K. H. (2018). *Brunner & Suddarth's textbook of medical-surgical nursing* (14th ed.). Wolters Kluwer Health.

Holleck, J. L., Campbell, S., Alrawili, H., Frank, C., Merchant, N., Rodwin, B., Perez, M. F., Gupta, S., Federman, D. G., Chang, J. J., Vientos, W., & Dembry, L. (2020). Stethoscope hygiene: Using cultures and real-time feedback with bioluminescence-based adenosine triphosphate technology to change behavior. *American Journal of Infection Control, 48*(4), 380–385. https://doi.org/10.1016/j.ajic.2019.10.005

Iversen, A. M., Kavalaris, C. P., Hansen, R., Hansen, M. B., Alexander, R., Kostadinov, K., Holt, J., Kristensen, B., Knudsen, J. D., Møller, J. K., & Ellermann-Eriksen, S. (2020). Clinical experiences with a new system for automated hand hygiene monitoring: A prospective observational study. *American Journal of Infection Control, 48*(5), 527–533. https://doi.org/10.1016/j.ajic.2019.09.003

Jain, S., Clezy, K., & McLaws, M. L. (2018). Safe removal of gloves from contact precautions: The role of hand hygiene. *American Journal of Infection Control, 46*(7), 764–767. https://doi.org/10.1016/j.ajic.2018.01.013

The Joint Commission. (2022). *National patient safety goals. Hospital: 2022 National patient safety goals.*

https://www.jointcommission.org/standards/national-patient-safety-goals/hospital-national-patient-safety-goals/

Jordan, V. (2020). Coronavirus (COVID-19): Infection control and prevention measures. *Journal of Primary Health Care, 12*(1), 96–97. https://doi.org/10.1071/HC15950

Kim, D., & Lee, O. (2019). Effects of audio-visual stimulation on hand hygiene compliance among family and non-family visitors of pediatric wards: A quasi-experimental pre-post intervention study. *Journal of Pediatric Nursing, 46*, e92–e97. https://doi.org/10.1016/j.pedn.2019.03.017

Knighton, S. C., Richmond, M., Zabarsky, T., Dolansky, M., Rai, H., & Donskey, C. J. (2020). Patients' capability, opportunity, motivation, and perception of inpatient hand hygiene. *American Journal of Infection Control, 48*(2), 157–161. https://doi.org/10.1016/j.ajic.2019.09.001

Lary, D., Calvert, A., Nerlich, B., Segal, J., Vaughan, N., Randle, J., & Hardie, K. R. (2020). Improving children's and their visitors' hand hygiene compliance. *Journal of Infection Prevention, 21*(2), 60–67. https://doi.org/10.1177/1757177419892065

Link, T. (2019). Guideline implementation: Sterile technique. *AORN Journal, 110*(4), 415–422. https://doi.org/10.1002/aorn.12803

Mills, J. P., Zhu, Z., Mantey, J., Hatt, S., Patel, P., Kaye, K. S., Gibson, K., Cassone, M., Lansing, B., & Mody, L. (2019). The devil is in the details: Factors influencing hand hygiene adherence and contamination with antibiotic-resistant organisms among healthcare providers in nursing facilities. *Infection Control & Hospital Epidemiology, 40*(12), 1394–1399. https://doi.org/10.1017/ice.2019.292

Norris, T. L. (2019). *Porth's essentials of pathophysiology* (5th ed.). Wolters Kluwer.

Office of Disease Prevention and Health Promotion. (n.d.). *Health care-associated infections (HAIs).* U.S. Department of Health and Human Services. https://health.gov/our-work/health-care-quality/health-care-associated-infections

Osei-Bonsu, K., Masroor, N., Cooper, K., Doern, C., Jefferson, K. K., Major, Y., Adamson, S., Thomas, J., Lovern, I., Albert, H., Stevens, M. P., Archer, G., Beraman, G., & Doll, M. (2019). Alternative doffing strategies of personal protective equipment to prevent self-contamination in the health care setting. *American Journal of Infection Control, 47*(5), 534–539. https://doi.org/10.1016/j.ajic.2018.11.003

Rai, H., Saldana, C., Gonzalez-Orta, M. I., Knighton, S., Cadnum, J. L., & Donskey, C. J. (2019). A pilot study to assess the impact of an educational patient hand hygiene intervention on acquisition of colonization

with health care-associated pathogens. *American Journal of Infection Control, 47*(3), 334–336. https://doi.org/10.1016/j.ajic.2018.09.004

Srigley, J. A., Cho, S. M., O'Neill, C., Bialachowski, A., Ali, R. A., Lee, C., & Mertz, D. (2020). Hand hygiene knowledge, attitudes, and practices among hospital inpatients: A descriptive study. *American Journal of Infection Control, 48*(5), 507–510. https://doi.org/10.1016/j.ajic.2019.11.020

Suen, L. K. P., Wong, J. W. S., Lo, K. Y. K., & Lai, T. K. H. (2019). The use of hand scanner to enhance hand hygiene practice among nursing students: A single-blinded feasibility study. *Nurse Education Today, 76*, 137–147. https://doi.org/10.1016/j.nedt.2019.01.013

Taylor, C., Lynn, P., & Bartlett, J. (2023). *Fundamentals of nursing: The art and science of person-centered care* (10th ed.). Wolters Kluwer.

U.S. Food & Drug Administration (FDA). (2020). *Consumer updates. Safely using hand sanitizer.* https://www.fda.gov/consumers/consumer-updates/safely-using-hand-sanitizer

Wong, M. W. H., Xu, Y. Z., Bone, J., & Srigley, J. A. (2020). Impact of patient and visitor hand hygiene interventions at a pediatric hospital: A stepped wedge cluster randomized controlled trial. *American Journal of Infection Control, 48*(5), 511–516. https://doi.org/10.1016/j.ajic.2019.09.026

Woodard, J. A., Leekha, S., Jackson, S. S., & Thom, K. A. (2019). Beyond entry and exit: Hand hygiene at the bedside. *American Journal of Infection Control, 47*(5), 487–491. https://doi.org/10.1016/j.ajic.2018.10.026

World Health Organization. (2020). *Infection prevention and control.* https://www.who.int/infection-prevention/en/

World Health Organization (WHO). (2017, May 5). *Evidence of hand hygiene as the building block for infection prevention and control.* https://www.who.int/publications/i/item/WHO-HIS-SDS-2017.7

World Health Organization (WHO). (2022). *SAVE LIVES—Clean your hands.* https://www.who.int/campaigns/world-hand-hygiene-day

Wound, Ostomy and Continence Nurses Society (WOCN®). (2016). *Core curriculum wound management.* Wolters Kluwer.

Yousef, R. H. A., Salem, M. R., & Mahmoud, A. T. (2020). Impact of implementation of a modified World Health Organization multimodal hand hygiene strategy in a university teaching hospital. *American Journal of Infection Control, 48*(3), 249–254. https://doi.org/10.1016/j.ajic.2019.07.019

SUGGESTED ANSWERS FOR FOCUSING ON PATIENT CARE: DEVELOPING CLINICAL REASONING AND CLINICAL JUDGMENT

1. You should call for or ask another staff member to obtain the bowl. Never walk away from or turn your back on a sterile field. This prevents possible contamination while the field is out of your view.

2. You should change gloves. Only a sterile object can touch another sterile object. Nonsterile touching sterile means contamination has occurred. Consider an object contaminated if you have any doubt about its sterility.

3. You should explain the rationale for transmission-based precautions, including specific information about airborne precautions. Airborne precautions are used for patients who have infections that spread through the air, such as tuberculosis, varicella (chicken pox), rubeola (measles), and possibly SARS. Place patient in a private room that has monitored negative air pressure in relation to surrounding areas, 6 to 12 air changes per hour, and appropriate discharge of air outside or monitored filtration if air is recirculated. Keep door closed and patient in room.

2

Vital Signs

Focusing on Patient Care

This chapter will explain some of the skills related to vital signs necessary to care for the following patients:

Tyrone Jeffries, age 5, is in the emergency department with a temperature of 101.3°F (38.9°C).

Toby White, age 26, has a history of asthma and is now breathing 32 times per minute.

Carl Glatz, age 58, has recently started taking medications to control his hypertension (high blood pressure).

Refer to Focusing on Patient Care: Developing Clinical Reasoning and Clinical Judgment at the end of the chapter to apply what you learn.

Learning Outcomes

After completing the chapter, you will be able to accomplish the following:

1. Assess body temperature via the oral, tympanic, temporal, axillary, and rectal routes.
2. Regulate an infant's temperature using an overhead radiant warmer.
3. Regulate temperature using a hypothermia blanket.
4. Assess peripheral pulses by palpation.
5. Assess an apical pulse by auscultation.
6. Assess peripheral pulses using Doppler ultrasound.
7. Assess respiration.
8. Assess blood pressure using an automated, electronic oscillometric device.
9. Assess blood pressure by auscultation.
10. Assess systolic blood pressure using Doppler ultrasound.

Nursing Concepts

- Assessment
- Clinical Decision Making/Clinical Judgment
- Oxygenation
- Perfusion
- Safety
- Thermoregulation

V

ital signs are indicators of physiologic functioning and include a person's temperature, pulse, respiration, and blood pressure, abbreviated as T, P, R, and BP. The health status of a person is reflected in these indicators of body function. Identification of a change in data related to assessment of vital signs is a crucial part of determining and recognizing deterioration in the status of a patient (Dalton et al., 2018). Pain assessment is often included along with measurement of vital signs and is discussed in Chapter 10. Pulse oximetry, the noninvasive measurement of arterial oxyhemoglobin saturation, is also often included with the measurement of vital signs and is discussed in Chapter 14.

Vital signs are assessed and compared with accepted normal values and the patient's usual patterns in a wide variety of instances. Consideration is given to potential variations in vital signs related to specific health conditions, illnesses and complications, medications, environmental factors, and therapies. Monitoring and analysis of the significance vital signs are important nursing responsibilities and are crucial to identifying changes in patient status (Dalton et al., 2018). Monitoring and evaluation of trends in intermittently measured vital signs is an important part of early identification of risk for a serious adverse event, contributing to timely intervention and improved patient outcomes (Brekke et al., 2019; Churpek et al., 2016).

Examples of appropriate times to measure vital signs include, but are not limited to, screenings at health fairs and clinics, in the home, upon admission to a health care setting, when medications are given that may affect one of the vital signs, before and after invasive diagnostic and surgical procedures, and in emergency situations. Nurses take vital signs as often as the condition of a patient requires such assessment, prioritizing and adapting assessment of vital signs to address the patient's unique situation. The nurse should consider the patient's medical diagnosis, comorbidities, types of treatments and medications received, the patient's level of acuity and risk for complications, trends in the patient's vital signs, prescribed interventions, and facility policies to help guide the frequency of assessment for an individual patient (Burchill et al., 2015; Jarvis & Eckhardt, 2020).

Although vital sign measurement may be delegated to other health care personnel when the condition of the patient is stable, it is the nurse's responsibility to ensure the accuracy of the data, interpret vital sign findings, and communicate abnormal findings. Principles of delegation should be followed (see Appendix A). If a patient has abnormal or unusual physical signs or symptoms (e.g., chest pain or dizziness) or has unexpected changes in vital signs, the nurse should validate the findings and further assess the patient. Techniques for measuring each of the vital signs are presented in this chapter. Fundamentals Review 2-1 outlines age-related variations in normal vital signs. Fundamentals Review 2-2 provides guidelines for obtaining vital signs for infants and children.

Fundamentals Review 2-1

AGE-RELATED VARIATIONS IN NORMAL VITAL SIGNS

Age	Temperature °C °F	Pulse beats/min	Respirations breaths/min	Blood Pressure mm Hg
Newborns	36.2–37.7 97.2–99.9	95–170	30–60	60–70/40
Infants	35.6–37.6 96–99.7	85–170	30–50	85/37
Toddler	35.6–37.2 96–99	70–150	20–40	88/42
Child	35.6–37.2 96–99	65–130	15–25	95/57
Adolescent	35.8–37.5 96.4–99.5	60–115	12–20	102/60
Adult	35.8–37.5 96.4–99.5	60–100	12–20	<120/80

Source: Adapted from Chiocca, E. M. (2019). *Advanced pediatric assessment* (3rd ed.). Springer Publishing Company; Hogan-Quigley, B., Palm, M. L., & Bickley, L. S. (2017). *Bates' nursing guide to physical examination and history taking* (2nd ed.). Wolters Kluwer; and Kyle, T., & Carman, S. (2021). *Essentials of pediatric nursing* (4th ed.). Wolters Kluwer.

Fundamentals Review 2-2

TECHNIQUES FOR OBTAINING VITAL SIGNS OF INFANTS AND CHILDREN

- Due to the "fear factor" of blood pressure measurement, save the blood pressure measurement for last. Children and infants often begin to cry during blood pressure assessment, and this may affect the respiration and pulse rate assessment.
- Perform as many tasks as possible while the child is sitting on the parent's lap or in a chair next to the parent.
- Let the child see and touch the equipment before you begin to use it.

- Make measuring vital signs a game. For instance, if you are using a tympanic thermometer that makes a chirping sound, tell the child you are looking for "birdies" in the ear. While auscultating the pulse, tell the child you are listening for another type of animal.
- If the child has a doll or stuffed animal, pretend to take the doll's vital signs first.

Skill 2-1 ▶ Assessing Body Temperature

Skill Variation: *Assessing Body Temperature Using a Noncontact Infrared Thermometer*

Skill Variation: *Assessing Body Temperature with a Temporal Artery Thermometer When the Temporal Artery and Behind the Ear Locations Are Not Accessible*

Body **temperature** is the difference between the amount of heat produced by the body and the amount of heat lost to the environment, measured in degrees. Heat is generated by metabolic processes in the core tissues of the body, transferred to the skin surface by the circulating blood, and then dissipated to the environment. Core body temperature (intracranial, intrathoracic, and intra-abdominal) is higher than surface body temperature. Normal body temperature is 35.9° to 38°C (96.7° to 100.5°F), depending on the route used for measurement (Jensen, 2019). There are individual variations of these temperatures as well as variations related to age, sex assigned at birth, physical activity, state of health, and environmental temperatures. Body temperature also varies during the day, with temperatures being lowest in the early morning and highest in the late afternoon (Boron & Boulpaep, 2016, as cited in Norris, 2019).

The nurse is expected to choose an appropriate site, and the correct equipment for temperature measurement based on the patient's condition, facility policy, and prescribed interventions. Factors affecting site selection include the patient's age, state of consciousness, amount of pain, and other care or treatments (such as oxygen administration) being provided. Health facility policies and procedures may provide guidance related to the site to be used for assessing patients' temperatures.

Several types of equipment and different procedures might be used to measure body temperature. Different types of thermometers are illustrated in Figure 1. To obtain an accurate measurement, choose an appropriate site, the correct equipment, and the appropriate tool based on the patient's condition. If a temperature reading is obtained from a site other than the oral route, document the site used along with the measurement. If no site is listed with the documentation, it is generally assumed to be the oral route.

The procedures for assessing body temperature at the oral, tympanic, temporal artery, axillary, and rectal sites are outlined below. See the accompanying Skill Variation on page 55 for a description of the procedure for assessing body temperature using a noncontact infrared thermometer.

Refer to Box 2-1 for normal temperature ranges based on measurement site.

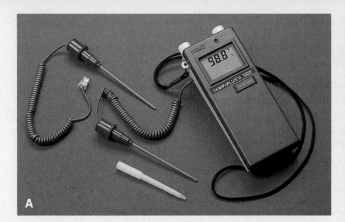
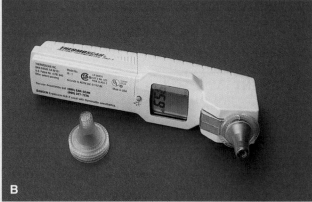
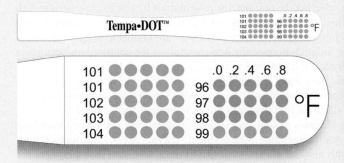
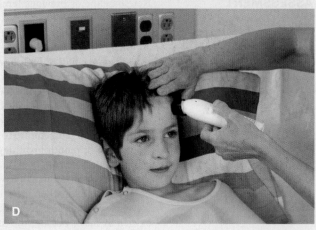
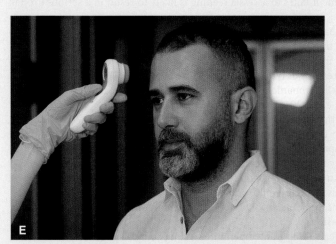

FIGURE 1. Types of thermometers. **A.** Electronic thermometer. **B.** Tympanic membrane thermometer. **C.** Disposable thermometer for measuring oral temperature; the dots change color to indicate temperature. **D.** Temporal artery thermometer. **E.** Noncontact infrared thermometer. (*Source:* Used with permission. Part **C.** Medical Indicators, Inc. Part **E.** iStock. *Photo by ozgurdonmaz.*)

Box 2-1   Normal Temperature Variations Based on Measurement Site

Measurement Site	Normal Temperature Range
Oral temperature	35.9° to 37.5°C (96.6° to 99.5°F)
Tympanic temperature	36.8° to 38.3°C (98.2° to 100.9°F)
Temporal artery	36.3° to 38.1°C (98.7° to 100.5°F)
Axillary	35.4° to 36.9°C (95.6° to 98.5°F)
Rectal	36.3° to 38.1°C (97.4° to 100.5°F)

Source: Adapted from Jensen, S. (2019). *Nursing health assessment. A best practice approach* (3rd ed.). Wolters Kluwer; Weber, J. R., & Kelley, J. H. (2018). *Health assessment in nursing* (6th ed.). Wolters Kluwer.

(*continued on page 46*)

Skill 2-1 ▶ Assessing Body Temperature *(continued)*

DELEGATION CONSIDERATIONS	Measurement of body temperature may be delegated to assistive personnel (AP) as well as to licensed practical/vocational nurses (LPN/LVNs). The decision to delegate must be based on careful analysis of the patient's needs and circumstances as well as the qualifications of the person to whom the task is being delegated. Refer to the Delegation Guidelines in Appendix A.

EQUIPMENT

- Digital or electronic thermometer, appropriate for site to be used
- Disposable probe covers
- Water-soluble lubricant for rectal temperature measurement
- Nonsterile gloves, if appropriate
- Additional personal protective equipment (PPE), as indicated
- Toilet tissue, if needed
- Electronic record or pen and paper or flow sheet

ASSESSMENT

Note baseline or previous temperature measurements. Assess the patient for the presence of the following:

Cognitive functioning: When selecting the oral site, the patient must be able to close their mouth around the probe. Therefore, this site is not suitable for use in children younger than 6 years old, in some children with developmental delay, in patients who are unable to follow directions, with patients with changes in or inflammation of the oral mucosa, or for confused and comatose patients (Jensen, 2019; Mason et al., 2017; Opersteny et al., 2017).

Consumption of food or drink: If a patient has had either hot or cold food or fluids or has been smoking or chewing gum, the general recommendation is to wait 15 to 30 minutes before measurement of an oral temperature to allow the oral tissues to return to normal temperature.

Presence of mouth breathing, diseases of oral cavity, facial surgery, seizures: Mouth breathing can influence the results of an oral temperature measurement (Jensen, 2019). Oral temperatures should not be taken in people with diseases of the oral cavity, in those who have had surgery of the nose or mouth, or when there is a risk of seizures (Sund-Levander & Grodzinsky, 2013).

Delivery of oxygen by mask: Oral temperatures should not be assessed in patients receiving oxygen by mask, because the time it takes to assess a reading is likely to result in a serious drop in the patient's blood oxygen level.

Ear pain or ache: If a patient has an earache, do not use the affected ear to take a tympanic temperature. The movement of the tragus may cause severe discomfort.

Presence of ear drainage, ear infection or a scarred tympanic membrane: These conditions can contribute to inaccurate measurement of tympanic temperature (Jensen, 2019).

Presence of cerumen (earwax): Tympanic temperature readings may be negatively impacted by the presence of cerumen (Oguz et al., 2018; Robertson & Hill, 2019).

Patient positioning: If the patient has been sleeping or lying with the head turned to one side, take a tympanic temperature in the other ear. Measure only the side of the head exposed to the environment when using a temporal artery thermometer. Heat may be increased on the side that was against the pillow, especially if it is a plastic-covered pillow.

Presence of head coverings: Anything covering the area, such as a hat, hair, wigs, or bandages will insulate the area, resulting in falsely high temporal artery temperature readings.

Presence of scars, open lesions, or abrasions: Do not measure temporal artery temperature over scar tissue, open lesions, or abrasions.

Presence of diaphoresis or sweat: Temporal temperature readings may be negatively impacted in the presence of diaphoresis or sweat (Jensen, 2019).

Patient's ability to hold arm tightly against the body: Axillary readings are affected by ambient temperature, local blood flow, appropriate placement of the probe, and closure of the axillary cavity (Oguz et al., 2018; Sund-Levander & Grodzinsky, 2013).

Recent rectal, anal, vaginal, or prostate surgery: The rectal site should not be used in patients who have undergone recent rectal, anal, vaginal, or prostate surgeries or have a disease of the rectum to avoid trauma and injury (Jensen, 2019; Weber & Kelley, 2018).

Presence of heart disease or recent cardiac surgery: Because the insertion of the thermometer into the rectum can slow the heart rate by stimulating the vagus nerve, assessing a rectal temperature for patients with heart disease or after cardiac surgery should be avoided (Jensen, 2019).

Presence of neutropenia: Assessing a rectal temperature is contraindicated in patients who are neutropenic (have low white blood cell counts, such as in leukemia) due to the increased risk of infection (Jensen, 2019).

Presence of thrombocytopenia: Do not insert a rectal thermometer into a patient who has thrombocytopenia (low platelet count). The rectum is very vascular, and a thermometer could cause rectal bleeding.

ACTUAL OR POTENTIAL HEALTH PROBLEMS AND NEEDS	Many actual or potential health problems or needs may require the use of this skill as part of related interventions. An appropriate health problem or need may include: • Hyperthermia • Impaired comfort • Impaired Thermoregulation
OUTCOME IDENTIFICATION AND PLANNING	The expected outcomes to achieve when performing temperature assessment are that the patient's temperature is assessed accurately without injury, and the patient experiences minimal discomfort. Other outcomes may be appropriate, depending on the specific diagnosis or patient problem.

IMPLEMENTATION

ACTION	**RATIONALE**
1. Check the prescribed interventions or plan of care for frequency of measurement and route. More frequent temperature measurement may be appropriate based on nursing judgment.	Assessment and measurement of vital signs at appropriate intervals provide important data about the patient's health status.
2. Perform hand hygiene and put on PPE, if indicated.	Hand hygiene and PPE prevent the spread of microorganisms. PPE is required based on transmission precautions.
3. Identify the patient.	Identifying the patient ensures that the right patient receives the intervention and helps prevent errors.
4. Close the curtains around the bed and close the door to the room, if possible. Discuss the procedure with the patient and assess the patient's ability to assist with the procedure.	This ensures the patient's privacy. Explanation relieves anxiety and facilitates cooperation. Dialogue encourages patient participation and allows for individualized nursing care.
5. Assemble equipment on the overbed table within reach.	Organization facilitates task performance.
6. Ensure that the electronic or digital thermometer is in working condition.	Improperly functioning thermometer may not give an accurate reading.
7. Put on gloves, if indicated.	Gloves prevent contact with blood and body fluids. Gloves are usually not required for an oral, axillary, or tympanic temperature measurement, unless contact with blood or body fluids is anticipated. Gloves should be worn for rectal temperature measurement.
8. Select the appropriate site based on assessment data.	This ensures safety and accuracy of measurement.
9. Follow the steps as outlined below for the appropriate type of thermometer.	
10. When measurement is completed, remove gloves, if worn. Remove additional PPE, if used. Perform hand hygiene.	Proper removal of PPE reduces the risk for infection transmission and contamination of other items. Hand hygiene prevents the spread of microorganisms.

Measuring an Oral Temperature

11. Remove the electronic unit from the charging unit and remove the probe from within the recording unit.	The electronic unit must be taken into the patient's room to assess the patient's temperature. On some models, the machine is turned on when the probe is removed.
12. Cover thermometer probe with disposable probe cover, sliding it on until it snaps into place (Figure 2).	Using a cover prevents contamination of the thermometer probe.

(continued on page 48)

Skill 2-1 ▶ Assessing Body Temperature *(continued)*

ACTION	**RATIONALE**

13. Place the probe beneath the patient's tongue in the posterior sublingual pocket (Figure 3). Ask the patient to close their lips around the probe.

When the probe rests deep in the posterior sublingual pocket, it is in contact with blood vessels lying close to the surface.

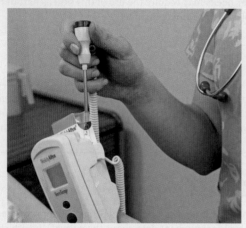

FIGURE 2. Putting probe cover on the thermometer.

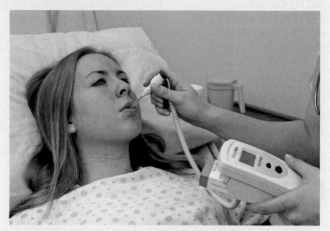

FIGURE 3. Placing thermometer under the tongue in the posterior sublingual pocket.

14. Continue to hold the probe until you hear a beep (Figure 4). Note the temperature reading.

If left unsupported, the weight of the probe tends to pull it away from the correct location. The probe must remain in the sublingual pocket for the full period of measurement to ensure accurate measurement. The signal indicates that the measurement is completed. The electronic thermometer provides a digital display of the measured temperature.

15. Remove the probe from the patient's mouth. Dispose of the probe cover by holding the probe over an appropriate receptacle and pressing the probe-release button (Figure 5).

Disposing of the probe cover ensures that it will not be reused accidentally on another patient. Proper disposal prevents spread of microorganisms.

16. Return the thermometer probe to the storage place within the unit. Return the electronic unit to the charging unit, if appropriate.

The thermometer needs to be recharged for future use. If necessary, the thermometer should stay on the charger so that it is ready to use at all times.

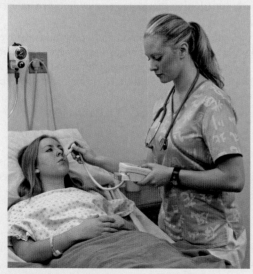

FIGURE 4. Holding probe in the patient's mouth.

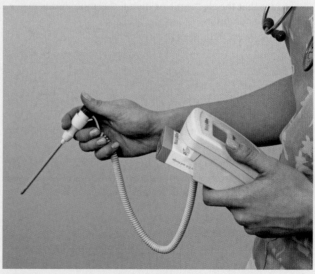

FIGURE 5. Pushing button to dispose of cover.

ACTION

Measuring a Tympanic Membrane Temperature

17. If necessary, push the "ON" button and wait for the "ready" signal on the unit.

18. Attach the disposable cover onto the tympanic probe (Figure 6).

19. **Insert the probe snugly into the external ear using gentle but firm pressure, angling the thermometer toward the patient's jaw line. Pull the pinna up and back to straighten the ear canal in an adult (Figure 7).**

RATIONALE

For proper function, the thermometer must be turned on and warmed up.

Use of a disposable cover deters the spread of microorganisms.

If the probe is not inserted correctly, the patient's temperature may be noted as lower than normal.

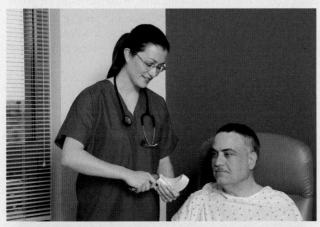

FIGURE 6. Attaching the disposable cover onto the tympanic probe.

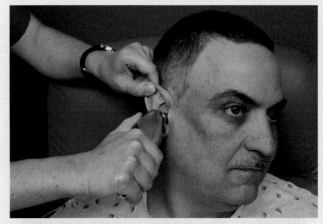

FIGURE 7. Thermometer in patient's ear canal with pinna pulled up and back.

20. Activate the unit by pushing the trigger button. The reading is immediate (usually within 2 seconds). Note the reading.

21. Discard the probe cover in an appropriate receptacle by pushing the probe-release button or use the rim of cover to remove it from the probe (Figure 8). Replace the thermometer in its charger, if necessary.

The digital thermometer must be activated to record the temperature.

Discarding the probe cover ensures that it will not be reused accidentally on another patient. Proper disposal prevents the spread of microorganisms. If necessary, the thermometer should stay on the charger so that it is always ready to use.

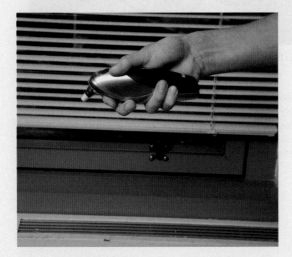

FIGURE 8. Disposing of probe cover.

(continued on page 50)

Skill 2-1 ▶ Assessing Body Temperature *(continued)*

ACTION	**RATIONALE**
Measuring Temporal Artery Temperature	If the temporal artery and behind the ear locations are not accessible, the femoral artery, lateral thoracic artery, and axillary sites may be used to assess body temperature using a temporal artery thermometer (Exergen, n.d.b). Refer to the Skill Variation on page 55.
22. Brush the patient's hair aside if it is covering the temporal artery area.	Anything covering the area—such as a hat, hair, wigs, or bandages—would insulate the area, resulting in falsely high readings. Measure only the side of the head exposed to the environment.
23. Apply a probe cover.	Using a cover prevents contamination of the thermometer probe.
24. Hold the thermometer like a remote control device, with your thumb on the red "ON" button. Place the probe flush on the center of the forehead, with the body of the instrument sideways (not straight up and down) so that it is not in the patient's face (Figure 9).	This allows for easy use of the device and reading of the display. Holding the instrument straight up and down could be intimidating for the patient, particularly young patients and/or those with alterations in mental status.
25. Depress the "ON" button. Keep the button depressed throughout the measurement.	
26. **Slowly slide the probe straight across the forehead, midline, to the hairline, maintaining contact with the skin (Figure 10). Do not move the probe down the side of the face.**	Midline on the forehead, the temporal artery is <2 mm below the skin, whereas at the side of the face, the temporal artery is much deeper. Measuring there would result in falsely low readings. Slow movement and continuous contact with the skin are necessary to ensure accurate results.

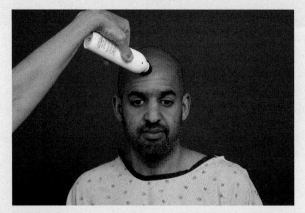

FIGURE 9. Placing the thermometer probe on the center of the forehead.

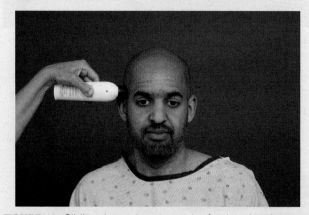

FIGURE 10. Sliding the probe across the forehead to the hairline.

27. If required, based on specific thermometer in use, brush hair aside if it is covering the ear, exposing the area of the neck under the ear lobe. Keeping the button depressed, lift the probe from the forehead and touch on the neck just behind the ear lobe, in the depression just below the mastoid (Figure 11).	Sweat causes evaporative cooling of the skin on the forehead, possibly leading to a falsely low reading. During diaphoresis, the area on the head behind the ear lobe exhibits high blood flow necessary for the arterial measurement; it is a double check for the thermometer (Exergen, n.d.a).

ACTION

RATIONALE

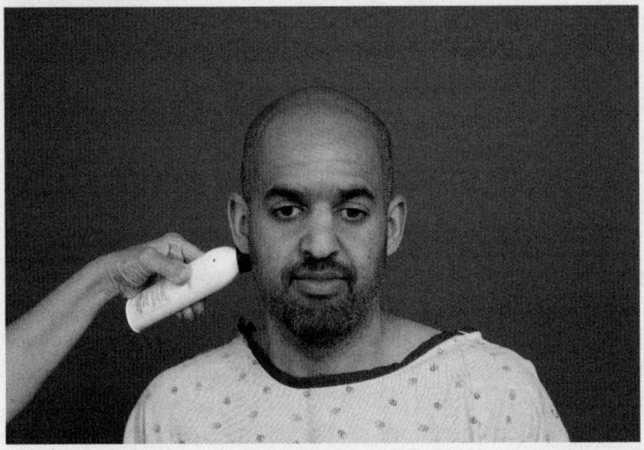

FIGURE 11. Touching the probe behind the ear.

28. Release the button and read the thermometer measurement.
29. Hold the thermometer over a waste receptacle. Gently push the probe cover with your thumb against the proximal edge to dispose of the probe cover.

Discarding the probe cover ensures that it will not be reused accidentally on another patient.

30. The instrument will automatically turn off in 30 seconds, or press and release the power button.

This turns the thermometer off.

Measuring Axillary Temperature

31. Remove the probe from the recording unit of the electronic thermometer. Place a disposable probe cover on by sliding it on and snapping it securely.

Using a cover prevents contamination of the thermometer probe.

32. Move the patient's clothing to expose only the axilla (Figure 12).

The axilla must be exposed for placement of the thermometer. Exposing only the axilla keeps the patient warm and maintains their dignity.

33. **Place the end of the probe in the center of the axilla (Figure 13). Have the patient bring the arm down and close to the body.** Hold the patient's arm by the patient's side until the measurement is complete.

The deepest area of the axilla provides the most accurate measurement; surrounding the bulb with skin surface provides a more reliable measurement.

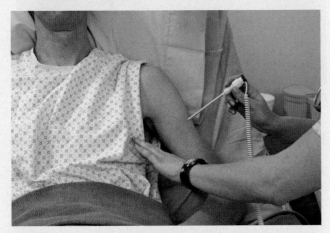

FIGURE 12. Exposing axilla to assess temperature.

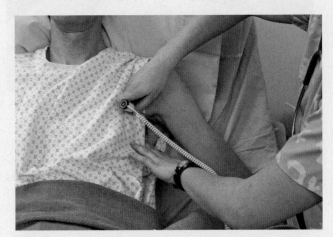

FIGURE 13. Placing thermometer in the center of the axilla.

34. Hold the probe in place until you hear a beep, and then carefully remove the probe. Note the temperature reading.

Axillary thermometers must be held in place to obtain an accurate temperature.

35. Cover the patient and help them to a position of comfort.

This ensures patient comfort.

36. Dispose of the probe cover by holding the probe over an appropriate waste receptacle and pushing the release button.

Discarding the probe cover ensures that it will not be reused accidentally on another patient.

(continued on page 52)

Skill 2-1 ▶ Assessing Body Temperature *(continued)*

ACTION	**RATIONALE**
37. Place the bed in the lowest position and elevate rails, as needed. Leave the patient clean and comfortable.	A low bed position and elevated side rails provide for patient safety.
38. Return the electronic thermometer to the charging unit.	The thermometer needs to be recharged for future use.

Measuring Rectal Temperature

ACTION	**RATIONALE**
39. Adjust the bed to a comfortable working height (VHACEOSH, 2016). Put on nonsterile gloves.	Having the bed at the proper height prevents back and muscle strain. Gloves prevent contact with contaminants and body fluids.
40. Assist the patient to a side-lying position. Pull back the covers sufficiently to expose only the buttocks. Position a young infant supine with legs flexed (Kyle & Carmen, 2021).	The side-lying position allows the nurse to see the buttocks. Exposing only the buttocks keeps the patient warm and maintains their dignity. Rectal temperatures are not normally taken in newborns, infants, and young children (Jensen, 2019; Silbert-Flagg & Pillitteri, 2018) but may be indicated. Refer to the Special Considerations section at the end of the skill.
41. Remove the rectal probe from within the recording unit of the electronic thermometer. Cover the probe with a disposable probe cover, sliding it on until it snaps in place (Figure 14).	Using a cover prevents contamination of the thermometer.
42. **Lubricate about 1 inch of the probe with a water-soluble lubricant (Figure 15).**	Lubrication reduces friction and facilitates insertion, minimizing the risk of irritation or injury to the rectal mucous membranes.

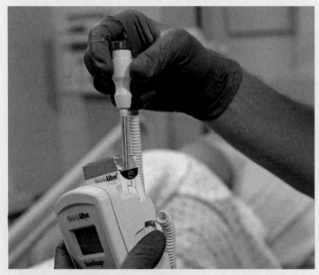

FIGURE 14. Removing appropriate probe and attaching disposable probe cover.

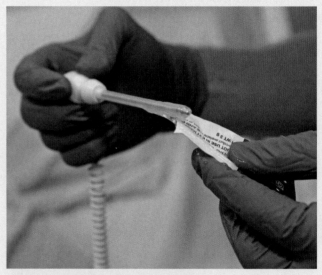

FIGURE 15. Lubricating thermometer tip.

ACTION	**RATIONALE**
43. Reassure the patient. Separate the buttocks until the anal sphincter is clearly visible.	If not placed directly into the anal opening, the thermometer probe may injure adjacent tissue or cause discomfort.
44. **Insert the thermometer probe into the anus about 1.5 inches in an adult or no more than 1 inch in children (Figure 16)** (Kyle & Carmen, 2021).	The depth of insertion must be adjusted based on the patient's age. Rectal temperatures are not normally taken in newborns, infants, and young children (Jensen, 2019; Silbert-Flagg & Pillitteri, 2018) but may be indicated. Refer to the Special Considerations section at the end of the skill.

ACTION

RATIONALE

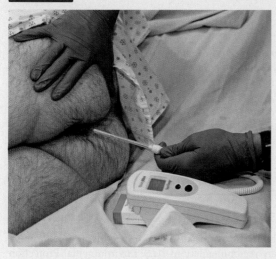

FIGURE 16. Inserting thermometer into the anus.

45. Hold the probe in place until you hear a beep, then carefully remove the probe. Note the temperature reading on the display.

If left unsupported, movement of the probe in the rectum could cause injury and/or discomfort. The signal indicates that the measurement is completed. The electronic thermometer provides a digital display of the measured temperature.

46. Dispose of the probe cover by holding the probe over an appropriate waste receptacle and pressing the release button.

Proper probe cover disposal reduces risk of microorganism transmission.

47. Using toilet tissue, wipe the anus of any feces or excess lubricant. Dispose of the toilet tissue. Remove gloves and discard them. Perform hand hygiene.

Wiping promotes cleanliness. Disposing of the toilet tissue avoids transmission of microorganisms.

48. Cover the patient and help them a position of comfort.

This ensures patient comfort.

49. Place the bed in the lowest position; elevate rails as needed.

These actions provide for the patient's safety.

50. Perform hand hygiene.

Hand hygiene prevents the spread of microorganisms.

51. Return the thermometer to the charging unit.

The thermometer needs to be recharged for future use.

EVALUATION

The expected outcomes have been met when the patient's temperature has been assessed accurately without injury, and the patient has experienced minimal discomfort.

DOCUMENTATION

Guidelines

Record temperature in the electronic record or flow sheet. Communicate abnormal findings to the appropriate person. Identify the site of assessment used if other than oral.

Sample Documentation

Lippincott
DocuCare

Practice documenting body temperature and other vital signs in *Lippincott DocuCare*

10/20/25 Tympanic temperature assessed. Temperature 102.5°F. Patient states she has "a pounding" headache; denies chills, malaise. Physician notified. Received order to give 650 mg PO acetaminophen now. Incentive spirometer × 10 q 2 hours.
—M. Evans, RN

(continued on page 54)

Skill 2-1 ▶ Assessing Body Temperature *(continued)*

DEVELOPING CLINICAL REASONING AND CLINICAL JUDGMENT

UNEXPECTED SITUATIONS AND ASSOCIATED INTERVENTIONS

- *Temperature reading is higher or lower than expected based on your assessment:* Reassess temperature with a different thermometer. The thermometer may not be calibrated correctly. If using a tympanic thermometer, improper positioning of the probe can contribute to errors (Jensen, 2019).
- *During rectal temperature assessment, the patient reports feeling light-headed or passes out:* Remove the thermometer immediately. Quickly assess the patient's blood pressure and heart rate. Vagal stimulation during insertion of the probe may cause reduction in the patient's heart rate (Jensen, 2019). Notify the health care provider. Do not attempt to take another rectal temperature on this patient.

SPECIAL CONSIDERATIONS

General Considerations

- Glass thermometers with mercury-filled bulbs are not used in health care institutions to measure body temperature due to federal safety recommendations (U.S. Environmental Protection Agency [EPA], n.d.).
- If the patient smoked, chewed gum, or consumed hot or cold food or fluids recently, wait 15 minutes before taking an oral temperature to allow the oral tissues to return to baseline temperature (Mayo Clinic, 2020a).
- Nasal oxygen is not thought to affect oral temperature readings. Do not assess oral temperatures in patients receiving oxygen by mask. Removal of the mask for the time required for assessment could result in a serious drop in the patient's blood oxygen level.
- When using a tympanic thermometer, make sure to insert the probe into the ear canal sufficiently tightly to seal the opening to ensure an accurate reading.
- A dirty probe lens and cone on the temporal artery thermometer can cause a falsely low reading. If the lens is not shiny in appearance, clean the lens with an alcohol swab or gauze moistened in alcohol (Exergen, n.d.b).
- If the temporal artery and behind the ear locations are not accessible, the femoral artery, lateral thoracic artery, and axilla sites may be used to assess body temperature using a temporal artery thermometer (Exergen, n.d.b). Refer to the Skill Variation on page 55.
- If the patient's axilla has been washed recently, wait 15 to 30 minutes before taking an axillary temperature to allow the skin to return to baseline temperature.

Infant and Child Considerations

- Pull the pinna back and down when measuring tympanic temperature on a child younger than 3 years of age. For children older than 3 years of age, there is no need to manipulate the pinna (Kyle & Carman, 2021).
- Small children have a limited attention span and difficulty keeping their lips closed long enough to obtain an accurate oral temperature reading. Based on an assessment of the child's ability to cooperate, it may be more appropriate to use the temporal or tympanic site.
- For children under 3 months (90 days) old, the axillary method is safest and is good for screening (Seattle Children's, 2022). If the axillary temperature is above 99 F, recheck with a rectal measurement. The rectal or temporal method should be used for children 3 months to 4 years old; the tympanic method can be used after 6 months of age (Seattle Children's, 2022). In children age 4 years or older, it is safe to measure temperature orally, in addition to tympanic and axillary methods (Seattle Children's, 2022).

Community-Based Care Considerations

- Teach patients who use electronic or digital thermometers to clean the probe after use to prevent transmission of microorganisms among family members. Clean according to the manufacturer's directions.
- Patients may still be using glass mercury thermometers at home. Encourage patients to use alternative devices, such as digital thermometers.

- Teach patients using nonmercury glass thermometers to clean the thermometer after use in luke-warm soapy water and rinse in cool water. Store it in an appropriate place to prevent breakage and injury from the glass. Encourage patients to use alternative devices, such as digital thermometers.
- Teach patients that glass thermometers should never be used to take a temperature for a person who is unconscious or for infants and young children.
- Pacifier thermometers, which use the supralingual area, are available to screen for fever, but are not recommended for newborns. Leave this thermometer in place for 3 to 5 minutes, based on the manufacturer's recommendations (Mayo Clinic, 2020).

Skill Variation Assessing Body Temperature Using a Noncontact Infrared Thermometer

Noncontact infrared (IFR) thermometers measure body temperature by capturing the heat emitted by the skin over body surfaces at various locations. Comparisons of noncontact IFR thermometer measurements with tympanic, temporal artery, and axillary body temperature measurement have resulted in inconsistent findings related to accuracy of measurements (Aw, 2020; Berksoy et al., 2018; Franconi et al., 2018; Wang et al., 2013). As a result, this method of temperature measurement has been suggested for possible use as screening for fever, not for ongoing monitoring of body temperature (Aw, 2020; Bayhan et al., 2014; Berksoy et al., 2018; Canadian Agency for Drugs and Technologies in Health, 2014). Locations recommended for use for measurement include over the forehead (temporal artery), the neck (carotid artery), umbilicus, axilla, and the nape of the neck (Berksoy et al., 2018; U.S. Food and Drug Administration [FDA], 2020; Wang et al., 2013). **Proper use of the noncontact thermometer is essential to achieve as accurate measurement as possible and prevent inaccurate measurement (FDA, 2020).**

1. Ensure the noncontact IFR thermometer has been exposed to the testing environment or room for 10 to 30 minutes prior to use to allow the thermometer to adjust to the environment.
2. Refer to Steps 1–8 in Skill 2-1.
3. Follow specific manufacturer instructions for use.
4. Use in a draft-free space that is out of direct sun and away from radiant heat sources (FDA, 2020).
5. The patient's forehead should not be blocked or covered during measurement.
6. Clean and dry the patient's forehead.
7. Power the thermometer on.
8. Change mode setting, if necessary, based on thermometer features, to "Body."

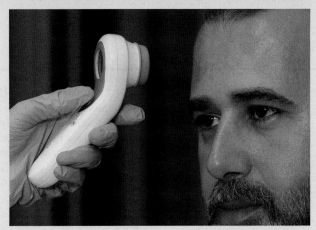

FIGURE A. Holding the device perpendicular from the patient's forehead. (*Source:* Used with permission from iStock. *Photo by ozgurdonmaz.*)

9. Hold the device perpendicular and 1 to 2 inches from the patient's forehead, or the distance recommended by the manufacturer (Figure A).
10. Press the "Scan" button. Measurement is almost instantaneous; note temperature measurement.
11. If a repeat measurement is necessary, follow the manufacturer's directions for the appropriate time interval between readings.

12. When measurement is completed, remove gloves, if worn. Remove additional PPE, if used. Perform hand hygiene.

(*continued on page 56*)

Skill 2-1 ▶ Assessing Body Temperature *(continued)*

Skill Variation Assessing Body Temperature with a Temporal Artery Thermometer When the Temporal Artery and Behind the Ear Locations Are Not Accessible

If the temporal artery and behind the ear locations are not accessible, the femoral artery, lateral thoracic artery, and axillary sites may be used to assess body temperature using a temporal artery thermometer (Exergen, n.d.b).

1. Assess the appropriateness and need for measurement at an alternate site using a temporal artery thermometer.
2. Refer to Steps 1–8 in Skill 2-1.
3. Refer to Steps 23–27 in Skill 2-1, with the following modifications for each specific alternate site: Femoral artery: Slide the probe across the groin.

Lateral thoracic artery: Scan side to side in the area, about midway between the axilla and nipple.
Axilla: Insert probe in the apex of the axilla for about 2 to 3 seconds.

4. Release the button and read the thermometer measurement.
5. Hold the thermometer over a waste receptacle. Gently push the probe cover with your thumb against the proximal edge to dispose of the probe cover.
6. The instrument will automatically turn off in 30 seconds, or press and release the power button.

EVIDENCE FOR PRACTICE ▶

FEVER AND ANTIPYRESIS

Temperature increase and fever are common clinical symptoms. Fever is an important part of a person's defense mechanisms against infection. Findings about antipyretic treatment have further challenged the need for routine or aggressive fever suppression. Unfortunately, many health care professionals continue to be "fever phobic," while their attitudes toward fever and antipyresis considerably affect antipyretic practice (Ludwig & McWhinnie, 2019). What are health care professionals' awareness of fever and antipyresis? Is nursing practice based on appropriate treatment for fever?

Related Evidence

Ludwig, J., & McWhinnie, H. (2019). Antipyretic drugs in patients with fever and infection: Literature review. *British Journal of Nursing, 28*(10), 610–618. https://doi.org/10.12968/bjon.2019.28.10.610

This literature review examined whether the administration of antipyretic drugs to adult patients with infection and fever, in secondary care, improves or worsen patient outcomes. Keywords, including fever, pyresis, infection, and antipyresis, were searched in the Cumulative Index to Nursing and Allied Health Literature (CINAHL) and Medline databases for the years 2010–2017. The target population for the review was hospitalized adult patients with fever and infection. Discussion of antipyretics in patients with infection and fever and/or discussion of the benefits/disadvantages of fever during infection were identified as criteria for inclusion in the review. Outcomes measured in the studies included patient mortality/morbidity, patient experiences and perceptions of fever/antipyretics, and professionals' attitudes toward fever/antipyretics. The database searches identified 1,523 articles; based on title and abstract review, 1,501 were excluded. Twenty-two articles were selected for full text review; after evaluation, 13 articles were chosen for inclusion in the final review. These final studies included randomized-controlled trials (3), cross-sectional survey/questionnaires (2), a qualitative interview (1), prospective observational studies (2), and retrospective observational studies (5). Each study was examined against the Critical Appraisal Skills Programme (CASP) quality checklists, and overall methodologic quality of the studies was deemed satisfactory. Two key themes identified included "antipyretics, fever and patient outcomes" and "professionals' and patients' experiences and perceptions of antipyretics and fever." Contrasting results were reported; two studies demonstrated improved patient outcomes following antipyretic administration, while several studies demonstrated increased mortality risk associate with antipyretics and/or demonstrated fever's benefits during infection. Results also demonstrated that health professionals continue to view fever as deleterious. The authors concluded the evidence does not support routine antipyretic administration. In addition, the researchers suggested health care providers should consider patients' comorbidities and symptoms of their underlying illness to promote safe, evidence-based, and appropriate administration of antipyretics.

Relevance to Nursing Practice

Nurses must engage in lifelong education to engage in evidence-based practice. There is a need for continuing education of nursing professionals in relation to fever and antipyresis that includes knowledge, clinical skills, attitudes, and barriers to change in practice. Advancing nurses' knowledge will contribute to the elimination of "fever phobia" and promote implementation of evidence-based nursing care, resulting in improved patient outcomes and patient safety (Ludwig & McWhinnie, 2019).

Skill 2-2 ▶ Regulating Temperature Using an Overhead Radiant Warmer

Neonates, infants who are exposed to stressors or chilling (e.g., from undergoing numerous procedures), and infants who have an underlying condition that interferes with thermoregulation (e.g., prematurity) are highly susceptible to heat loss. Therefore, radiant warmers are used for infants who have trouble maintaining body temperature. In addition, use of a radiant warmer minimizes the oxygen and calories that the infant would expend to maintain body temperature, thereby minimizing the effects of body temperature changes on metabolic activity.

An overhead radiant warmer uses infrared light to warm the infant. The infant's skin is warmed, causing an increase in blood flow, which heats both the underlying blood and tissue surfaces. The warmer is adjusted to maintain an anterior abdominal skin temperature of 95.9° to 97.7°F (35.5° to 36.5°C) using an automatic thermostat (Bell, n.d.; Silbert-Flagg & Pillitteri, 2018).

DELEGATION CONSIDERATIONS

Measurement of body temperature for an infant in a radiant warmer is not delegated to assistive personnel (AP). Depending on the state's nurse practice act and the organization's policies and procedures, the measurement of body temperature for an infant in a radiant warmer may be delegated to a licensed practical/vocational nurse (LPN/LVN). The decision to delegate must be based on careful analysis of the patient's needs and circumstances as well as the qualifications of the person to whom the task is being delegated. Refer to the Delegation Guidelines in Appendix A.

EQUIPMENT

- Overhead warmer
- Temperature probe
- Aluminum foil probe cover
- Axillary or rectal thermometer, based on facility policy
- PPE, as indicated

ASSESSMENT

Assess the patient's temperature using the route specified in facility policy, and assess the patient's fluid intake and output.

ACTUAL OR POTENTIAL HEALTH PROBLEMS AND NEEDS

Many actual or potential health problems or needs may require the use of this skill as part of related interventions. An appropriate health problem or need may include:
- Hyperthermia
- Hypothermia
- Impaired Thermoregulation

OUTCOME IDENTIFICATION AND PLANNING

The expected outcome to achieve when using an overhead warmer is that the infant's temperature is maintained within normal limits without injury. Other outcomes may be appropriate, depending on the specific diagnosis or patient problem identified for the patient.

(continued on page 58)

Skill 2-2 ▶ Regulating Temperature Using an Overhead Radiant Warmer *(continued)*

IMPLEMENTATION

ACTION	**RATIONALE**
1. Check the prescribed interventions or plan of care for the use of a radiant warmer.	Provides for patient safety and appropriate care.
2. Perform hand hygiene and put on PPE, if indicated.	Hand hygiene and PPE prevent the spread of microorganisms. PPE is required based on transmission precautions.
3. Identify the patient.	Identifying the patient ensures the right patient receives the intervention and helps prevent errors.
4. Close curtains around the bed and close the door to the room, if possible. Discuss the procedure with the patient's family/caregivers.	This ensures the patient's privacy. Explanation reduces the family's/caregiver's apprehension and encourages cooperation.
5. Plug in the warmer. Turn the warmer to the manual setting. Allow the blankets to warm before placing the infant under the warmer.	By allowing the blankets to warm before placing the infant under the warmer, you are preventing heat loss through conduction. By placing the warmer on the manual setting, you are keeping the warmer at a set temperature no matter how warm the blankets become.
6. Insert probe securely into the heater unit. **Switch the warmer setting to automatic. Set the warmer to the desired abdominal skin temperature, usually 95.9° to 97.7°F (35.5° to 36.5°C)** (Bell, n.d.; Silbert-Flagg & Pillitteri, 2018).	The automatic setting ensures that the warmer will regulate the amount of radiant heat, depending on the temperature of the infant's skin. The temperature should be adjusted so that the infant does not become too warm or too cold.
7. Place the infant under the warmer. Attach the probe to the infant's abdominal skin at mid-epigastrium, halfway between the xiphoid and the umbilicus. Cover with a foil-backed shield (Figure 1). If the infant is prone, attach the probe to the skin over either flank (not between the scapulae) (Bell, n.d.; Silbert-Flagg & Pillitteri, 2018).	The foil-backed shield prevents direct warming of the probe, allowing the probe to read only the infant's temperature.
8. When the abdominal skin temperature reaches the desired set point, check the patient's temperature using the route specified in facility policy to be sure it is within the normal range (Figure 2).	By monitoring the infant's temperature, you are watching for signs of **hyperthermia** or **hypothermia**.

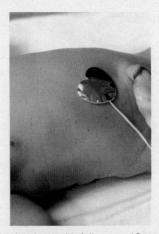

FIGURE 1. Probe in place with foil cover. (*Source:* Used with permission from Shutterstock. *Photo by Joe Mitchell.*)

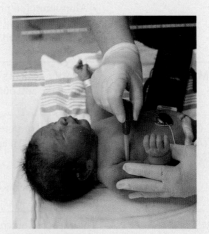

FIGURE 2. Taking infant's axillary temperature. (*Source:* Used with permission from Shutterstock. *Photo by Joe Mitchell.*)

ACTION	RATIONALE
9. Adjust the warmer's set point slightly, as needed, if the patient's temperature is abnormal. Do not change the set point if the temperature is normal.	By monitoring the infant's temperature, you are watching for signs of hyperthermia or hypothermia. This prevents the infant from becoming too warm or too cool.
10. Remove additional PPE, if used. Perform hand hygiene.	Proper removal of PPE reduces the risk for infection transmission and contamination of other items. Hand hygiene deters the spread of microorganisms.
11. Check the position of the probe frequently to ensure the probe maintains contact with the patient's skin. Continue to monitor temperature measurement and other vital signs.	Poor contact will cause overheating. Entrapment of the probe under the arm or between the infant and mattress will cause a falsely high reading and underheating (Bell, n.d.; Silbert-Flagg & Pillitteri, 2018). Poor contact with skin will cause overheating (Bell, n.d.). Monitoring of vital signs assesses patient status.

EVALUATION

The expected outcomes have been met when the infant has been placed under the radiant warmer, the infant's temperature was well controlled, and the infant experienced no injury.

DOCUMENTATION

Guidelines

Document initial assessment of the infant, including body temperature; the placement of the infant under the radiant warmer; and the settings of the radiant warmer. Document infant's skin and axillary (or rectal) temperatures, and other vital sign measurements.

Sample Documentation

> 10/13/25 1110 Infant placed under radiant warmer. Warmer on automatic setting 36.7°C (98°F), baby's skin temperature 36.8°C (98.2°F), rectal temperature 37°C (98.6°F).
>
> —M. Evans, RN

DEVELOPING CLINICAL REASONING AND CLINICAL JUDGMENT

UNEXPECTED SITUATIONS AND ASSOCIATED INTERVENTIONS

- *The infant becomes **febrile** under the radiant warmer:* Do not turn the warmer off and leave the infant naked. This could cause cold stress and even death. Leave the warmer on automatic and lower the set temperature. Notify the primary care provider.
- *The warmer's temperature is fluctuating constantly or is inaccurate:* Change the probe cover. If this does not improve the temperature variations, change the probe as well.

SPECIAL CONSIDERATIONS

Infant and Child Considerations

- Radiant warmers result in increased insensible water loss. This water loss needs to be taken into account when daily fluid requirements are calculated.

Skill 2-3 ▶ Regulating Temperature Using a Hypothermia Blanket

A hypothermia blanket, or cooling pad, is a blanket-sized aquathermia pad that conducts a cooled solution, usually distilled water, through coils in a plastic blanket or pad (Figure 1). Placing a patient on a hypothermia blanket or pad helps to lower body temperature. The nurse monitors the patient's body temperature and can reset the blanket setting accordingly. The blanket also can be preset to maintain a specific body temperature; the device continually monitors the patient's body temperature using a temperature probe (which is inserted rectally or in the esophagus or placed on the skin) and adjusts the temperature of the circulating liquid accordingly.

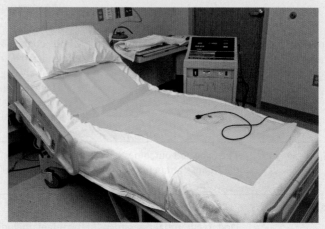

FIGURE 1. Hypothermia blanket.

DELEGATION CONSIDERATIONS	The application of a hypothermia pad is not delegated to assistive personnel (AP). The measurement of a patient's body temperature while a hypothermia pad is in use may be delegated to AP. Depending on the state's nurse practice act and the organization's policies and procedures, the application of a hypothermia pad may be delegated to a licensed practical/vocational nurse (LPN/LVN). The decision to delegate must be based on careful analysis of the patient's needs and circumstances as well as the qualifications of the person to whom the task is being delegated. Refer to the Delegation Guidelines in Appendix A.
EQUIPMENT	• Disposable hypothermia blanket or pad • Electronic control panel • Distilled water to fill the device, if necessary • Thermometer, if needed to monitor the patient's temperature • Sphygmomanometer • Stethoscope • Temperature probe, if needed • Thin blanket or sheet • Towels • Clean gloves • Additional PPE, as indicated
ASSESSMENT	Assess the patient's condition, including current body temperature, to determine the need for the hypothermia blanket. Consider alternative measures to help lower the patient's body temperature before implementing the cooling blanket. Also verify the prescribed interventions for the application of a hypothermia blanket. Assess the patient's vital signs, neurologic status, peripheral circulation, and skin integrity. Assess the equipment to be used, including the condition of cords, plugs, and cooling elements. Look for fluid leaks. Once the equipment is turned on, make sure there is a consistent distribution of cooling.

ACTUAL OR POTENTIAL HEALTH PROBLEMS AND NEEDS	Many actual or potential health problems or needs may require the use of this skill as part of related interventions. An appropriate health problem or need may include: • Hyperthermia • Injury risk • Altered skin integrity risk
OUTCOME IDENTIFICATION AND PLANNING	The expected outcome to achieve when using a hypothermia blanket is that the patient maintains the desired body temperature. Other outcomes that may be appropriate include: the patient does not experience shivering; the patient's vital signs are within normal limits; and the patient does not experience alterations in skin integrity, neurologic status, peripheral circulation, or fluid and electrolyte balance. Other outcomes may be appropriate, depending on the specific diagnosis or patient problem identified for the patient.

IMPLEMENTATION

ACTION	**RATIONALE**
1. Review the prescribed interventions for the application of the hypothermia blanket. Obtain consent for the therapy per facility policy.	Reviewing the order validates the correct patient and correct procedure.
2. Perform hand hygiene and put on PPE, if indicated.	Hand hygiene and PPE prevent the spread of microorganisms. PPE is required based on transmission precautions.
3. Identify the patient. Determine if the patient has had any previous adverse reaction to hypothermia therapy.	Identifying the patient ensures the right patient receives the intervention and helps prevent errors. Individual differences exist in tolerating specific therapies.
4. Assemble equipment on the overbed table within reach.	Organization facilitates task performance.
5. Close curtains around the bed and close the door to the room, if possible. Explain what you are going to do and why you are going to do it to the patient.	This ensures the patient's privacy. Explanation relieves anxiety and facilitates cooperation.
6. Check that the water in the electronic unit is at the appropriate level. Fill the unit two thirds with distilled water, or to the fill mark, if necessary. Check the temperature setting on the unit to ensure it is within the safe range.	Sufficient water in the unit is necessary to ensure proper function of the unit. Tap water leaves mineral deposits in the unit. Checking the temperature setting helps to prevent skin or tissue damage.
7. Assess the patient's vital signs, neurologic status, peripheral circulation, and skin integrity.	Assessment supplies baseline data for comparison during therapy and identifies conditions that may contraindicate the application.
8. Adjust the bed to comfortable working height, usually elbow height of the caregiver (VHACEOSH, 2016).	Having the bed at the proper height prevents back and muscle strain.
9. Make sure the patient's gown has cloth ties, not snaps or pins.	Cloth ties minimize the risk of cold injury.
10. Apply lanolin or a mixture of lanolin and cold cream to the patient's skin where it will be in contact with the blanket.	These agents help protect the skin from cold.
11. Turn on the blanket and make sure the cooling light is on. **Verify that the temperature limits are set within the desired safety range (Figure 2).**	Turning on the blanket prepares it for use. Keeping temperature within the safety range prevents excessive cooling.
12. Cover the hypothermia blanket with a thin sheet or bath blanket.	A sheet or blanket protects the patient's skin from direct contact with the cooling surface, reducing the risk for injury.
13. Position the blanket under the patient so that the top edge of the pad is aligned with the patient's neck (Figure 3).	The blanket's rigid surface may be uncomfortable. The cold may lead to tissue breakdown.

(continued on page 62)

Skill 2-3 ▶ Regulating Temperature Using a Hypothermia Blanket *(continued)*

ACTION	RATIONALE

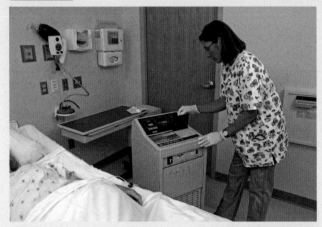

FIGURE 2. Turning the hypothermia blanket control unit on and checking the settings.

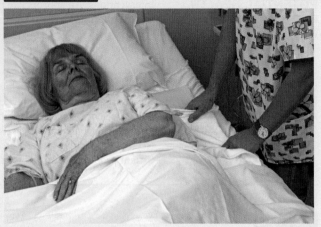

FIGURE 3. Positioning the hypothermia blanket under the patient.

 14. Put on gloves. Lubricate the rectal probe and insert it into the patient's rectum unless contraindicated. Or tuck the skin probe deep into the patient's axilla and tape it in place. For patients who are comatose or anesthetized, use an esophageal probe. Remove gloves. Perform hand hygiene. Attach the probe to the control panel for the blanket.

The probe allows continuous monitoring of the patient's core body temperature. Rectal insertion may be contraindicated in patients with a low white blood cell or platelet count.

15. Wrap the patient's hands and feet in gauze if ordered, or if the patient desires. For male patients, elevate the scrotum off the hypothermia blanket with towels.

These actions minimize chilling, promote comfort, and protect sensitive tissues from direct contact with cold.

16. Place the patient in a comfortable position. Lower the bed. Dispose of any other supplies appropriately.

Repositioning promotes patient comfort and safety.

17. Recheck the thermometer and settings on the control panel.

Rechecking verifies that the blanket temperature is maintained at a safe level.

 18. Remove any additional PPE, if used. Perform hand hygiene.

Proper removal of PPE reduces the risk for infection transmission and contamination of other items. Hand hygiene prevents the spread of microorganisms.

19. **Turn and position the patient regularly (every 30 minutes to 1 hour).** Keep linens free from condensation. Reapply cream, as needed. Observe the patient's skin for change in color, changes in lips and nail beds, edema, pain, and sensory impairment.

Turning and repositioning prevent alterations in skin integrity and provide for assessment of potential skin injuries.

20. **Monitor vital signs and perform a neurologic assessment, per facility policy, usually every 15 minutes, until the body temperature is stable.** In addition, monitor the patient's skin integrity, peripheral circulation and fluid and electrolyte status, as per facility policy.

Continuous monitoring provides evaluation of the patient's response to the therapy and permits early identification and intervention if adverse effects occur.

21. Avoid cooling to the point of shivering (Morton & Fontaine, 2018). Observe for signs of shivering, including verbalized sensations, facial muscle twitching, hyperventilation, or twitching of extremities.

Shivering increases heat production and is often controlled with medications.

22. Assess the patient's level of comfort.

Hypothermia therapy can cause discomfort. Prompt assessment and action can prevent injuries.

ACTION	**RATIONALE**
23. Turn off the blanket according to facility policy, usually when the patient's body temperature reaches 1 degree above the desired temperature. **Continue to monitor the patient's temperature until it stabilizes.**	Body temperature can continue to fall after this therapy.

EVALUATION

The expected outcome has been met when the patient has maintained the desired body temperature and other vital signs within acceptable parameters. In addition, the patient remained free from shivering and did not experience alterations in skin integrity, neurologic status, peripheral circulation, or fluid and electrolyte balance.

DOCUMENTATION

Guidelines

Document assessments, such as vital signs, neurologic, peripheral circulation, and skin integrity status prior to use of the hypothermia blanket. Record verification of prescribed interventions and that the procedure was explained to the patient. Document the control settings, time of application and removal, and the route of the temperature monitoring. Include the application of lanolin cream to the skin as well as the frequency of position changes. Document the patient's response to the therapy, especially noting a decrease in temperature and level of discomfort. Record the use of medication to reduce shivering or other discomforts, if implemented. Include any pertinent patient and family teaching.

Sample Documentation

11/10/25 1800 Patient's temperature 106°F (41°C), pulse 122, respirations 24, BP 118/72. Dr. Fenter notified. Order received for application of hypothermia blanket. Procedure explained to patient. Lanolin applied to skin, bath sheet applied between blanket and patient, axillary probe applied, hypothermia blanket setting 99°F (37.2°C) per order. Vital signs, neurologic, neurovascular, and skin assessment every 30 minutes; see electronic flow sheets. Patient without evidence of shivering.

—*J. Lee, RN*

11/10/25 1930 Patient reports chills and shivering. Temperature 100°F (37.8°C), pulse 104, respirations 20, BP 114/68. Dr. Fenter notified. Hypothermia blanket discontinued per order.

—*J. Lee, RN*

DEVELOPING CLINICAL REASONING AND CLINICAL JUDGMENT

UNEXPECTED SITUATIONS AND ASSOCIATED INTERVENTIONS

- *The patient is cold and has chills. You observe shivering of the extremities:* Obtain vital signs. Assess for other symptoms. Increase the blanket temperature to a more comfortable range. If shivering persists or is excessive, discontinue the therapy. Notify the primary care provider of the findings and document the event in the patient's record.
- *When performing a skin assessment during therapy, you note increased pallor on pressure points and sluggish capillary refill. The patient reports alterations in sensation on these points:* Discontinue therapy, obtain vital signs, assess for other symptoms, notify the primary care provider, and document the event in the patient's record.

SPECIAL CONSIDERATIONS

Older Adult Considerations

- Older adults are more at risk for skin and tissue damage because of their thin skin, loss of cold sensation, decreased subcutaneous tissue, and changes in the body's ability to regulate temperature. Check these patients more frequently during therapy.

Skill 2-4 ▶ Assessing a Peripheral Pulse by Palpation

Skill Variation: *Assessing Peripheral Pulse Using a Portable Doppler Ultrasound*

The peripheral **pulse** is a throbbing sensation that can be palpated (felt) over a peripheral artery, such as the radial artery or the carotid artery. Peripheral pulses result from a wave of blood being pumped into the arterial circulation by the contraction of the left ventricle. Each time the left ventricle contracts to eject blood into an already full aorta, the arterial walls in the cardiovascular system expand to compensate for the increase in pressure of the blood. The peripheral pulses may be felt wherever an artery passes over a solid structure, such as bone or cartilage. Characteristics of the peripheral pulse include rate, rhythm, strength (amplitude), and elasticity. These characteristics are indicators of the effectiveness of the heart as a pump, the volume of blood ejected with each heartbeat (stroke volume), and the adequacy of peripheral blood flow.

Pulse rates are measured in beats per minute. The normal pulse rate for adolescents and adults ranges from 60 to 100 beats per minute. Pulse strength (amplitude) refers to and describes the quality of the pulse in terms of its fullness, indicates the volume of blood flowing through the vessel, and reflects the strength of left ventricular contraction. It is assessed by the feel of the blood flow through the vessel and may be described as full and bounding when it is forceful or weak, and thready when it is decreased in quality. Pulse rhythm is the pattern of the pulsations and the intervals between them. Pulse rhythm is normally regular; the pulsations and the pauses between occur at evenly spaced intervals. An irregular pulse rhythm occurs when the pulsations and pauses between beats occur at unequal, varied intervals. Pulse elasticity is assessed by the feel of the blood vessel upon palpation. The normal artery feels smooth, straight, and resilient (springy) (Jensen, 2019; Weber & Kelley, 2018). Blood vessels may feel more rigid, less resilient, and crooked from loss of elasticity, such as occurs with aging, for example.

Assess the pulse by palpating peripheral arteries (refer to the steps outlined below), by auscultating the apical pulse with a stethoscope (see Skill 2-5), or by using a portable Doppler ultrasound (see the accompanying Skill Variation on page 68). To assess the pulse accurately, you need to know which site to choose and what method is most appropriate for the patient.

The most commonly used sites to palpate peripheral pulses and one example of a scale used to describe pulse amplitude are illustrated in Box 2-2. Place your fingers over the artery so that the ends of your fingers are flat against the patient's skin when palpating peripheral pulses. Do not press with the tip of the fingers only (refer to Figure 1, Step 8).

See the accompanying Skill Variation on page 68 for a description of the procedure for assessing a peripheral pulse using a portable Doppler ultrasound.

DELEGATION CONSIDERATIONS	The measurement of the radial and brachial peripheral pulses may be delegated to assistive personnel (AP). The measurement of peripheral pulses may be delegated to licensed practical/vocational nurses (LPN/LVNs). The decision to delegate must be based on careful analysis of the patient's needs and circumstances as well as the qualifications of the person to whom the task is being delegated. Refer to the Delegation Guidelines in Appendix A.
EQUIPMENT	• Watch with second hand or digital readout • Electronic record or pen and paper or flow sheet • Nonsterile gloves, if appropriate; additional PPE, as indicated
ASSESSMENT	Choose a site to assess the pulse. For an adult patients and children, the most common site for obtaining a peripheral pulse is the radial pulse. Apical pulse measurement is the preferred method of pulse assessment for infants and children less than 2 years of age (Jarvis & Eckhardt, 2020; Kyle & Carmen, 2021). (Refer to Skill 2-5.) Assess for factors that could affect pulse characteristics, such as the patient's age, physical activity, fluid balance, medications, body temperature, and presence of disease and/or health conditions. Note baseline or previous pulse measurements.
ACTUAL OR POTENTIAL HEALTH PROBLEMS AND NEEDS	Many actual or potential health problems or needs may require the use of this skill as part of related interventions. An appropriate health problem or need may include: • Altered tissue perfusion • Impaired Cardiac Output • Impaired comfort

Box 2-2 | Pulse Sites and Pulse Amplitude

Pulse Sites

Arteries commonly used for assessing the pulse include the temporal, carotid, brachial, radial, femoral, popliteal, posterior tibial, and dorsalis pedis.

Pulse Amplitude

- 0: Absent, unable to palpate
- +1: Diminished, weaker than expected
- +2: Normal; brisk, expected
- +3: Bounding

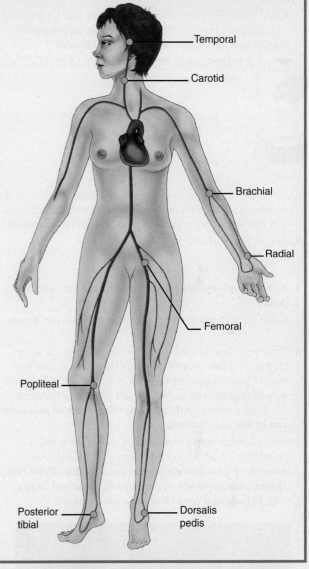

Temporal

Carotid

Brachial

Radial

Femoral

Popliteal

Posterior tibial

Dorsalis pedis

Source: Adapted from Writing Committee Members; Gerhard-Herman, M. D., Gornik, H. L., Barrett, C., Barshes, N. R., Corriere, M. A., Drachman, D. E., Fleisher, L. A., Fowkes, F. G. R., Hamburg, N. M., Kinlay, S., Lookstein, R., Misra, S., Mureebe, L., Olin, J. W., Patel, R. A. G., Regensteiner, J. G., Schanzer, A., Shishehbor, M. H., . . . Wijeysundera, D. N. (2017). 2016 AHA/ACC Guideline on the management of patients with lower extremity peripheral artery disease: Executive Summary. *Vascular Medicine, 22*(3), NPI–NP43. https://doi.org/10.1177/1358863X17701592

OUTCOME IDENTIFICATION AND PLANNING

The expected outcomes to achieve when measuring a pulse rate are that the patient's pulse is assessed accurately without injury, and that the patient experiences minimal discomfort. Other outcomes may be appropriate, depending on the specific diagnosis or patient problem identified for the patient.

(*continued on page 66*)

Skill 2-4 ▶ Assessing a Peripheral Pulse by Palpation *(continued)*

IMPLEMENTATION

ACTION	RATIONALE
1. Check prescribed interventions or plan of care for frequency of pulse assessment. More frequent pulse measurement may be appropriate based on nursing judgment.	Assessment and measurement of vital signs at appropriate intervals provide important data about the patient's health status.

ACTION	RATIONALE
2. Perform hand hygiene and put on PPE, if indicated.	Hand hygiene and PPE prevent the spread of microorganisms. PPE is required based on transmission precautions.

ACTION	RATIONALE
3. Identify the patient.	Identifying the patient ensures the right patient receives the intervention and helps prevent errors.
4. Close the curtains around the bed and close the door to the room, if possible. Discuss the procedure with the patient and assess the patient's ability to assist with the procedure.	This ensures the patient's privacy. Explanation relieves anxiety and facilitates cooperation.
5. Put on gloves, if indicated.	Gloves are not usually worn to obtain a pulse measurement unless contact with blood or body fluids is anticipated. Gloves prevent contact with blood and body fluids.
6. Select the appropriate peripheral site based on assessment data.	Ensures safety and accuracy of measurement.
7. Move the patient's clothing to expose only the site chosen.	The site must be exposed for pulse assessment. Exposing only the site keeps the patient warm and maintains their dignity.
8. Place your first, second, and third fingers over the artery (Figure 1). Place your fingers over the artery so that the ends of your fingers are flat against the patient's skin when palpating peripheral pulses. Do not press with the tip of the fingers only. **Lightly compress the artery so pulsations can be felt and counted.**	The sensitive fingertips can feel the pulsation of the artery.
9. Using a watch with a second hand, count the number of pulsations felt for 30 seconds (Figure 2). Multiply this number by 2 to calculate the rate for 1 minute. **If the rate, rhythm, or amplitude of the pulse is abnormal in any way, palpate and count the pulse for 1 minute.**	Ensures accuracy of measurement and assessment.

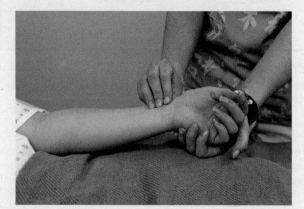

FIGURE 1. Placing fingers over the artery.

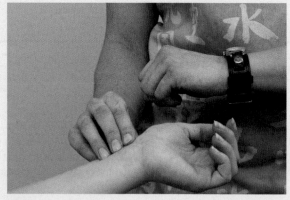

FIGURE 2. Counting the pulse.

ACTION	**RATIONALE**
10. Note the rhythm and amplitude of the pulse, as well as the elasticity of the blood vessel.	Provides additional assessment data regarding the patient's cardiovascular status.
11. When measurement is completed, remove gloves, if worn. Perform hand hygiene. Cover the patient and help them to a position of comfort.	Proper removal of gloves reduces the risk for infection transmission and contamination of other items. Hand hygiene prevents the spread of microorganisms. Covering and positioning the patient ensures patient comfort.
12. Remove additional PPE, if used. Perform hand hygiene.	Proper removal of PPE reduces the risk for infection transmission and contamination of other items. Hand hygiene prevents the spread of microorganisms.

EVALUATION

The expected outcomes have been met when the patient's pulse has been assessed accurately without injury, and the patient experienced minimal discomfort.

DOCUMENTATION

Guidelines

Record pulse rate, strength, rhythm, and elasticity in the electronic record or flow sheet. Identify site of assessment. Communicate abnormal findings to the primary care provider.

Sample Documentation

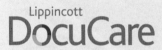

Practice documenting pulse and other vital signs in *Lippincott DocuCare*.

> <u>2/6/125</u> 1000 Pulses 84, regular, 2+, normal elasticity; equal bilaterally in radial, popliteal, and dorsalis pedis sites.
>
> —*M. Evans, RN*

DEVELOPING CLINICAL REASONING AND CLINICAL JUDGMENT

UNEXPECTED SITUATIONS AND ASSOCIATED INTERVENTIONS

- *The pulse is irregular:* Monitor the pulse for a full minute. If the pulse is difficult to assess, validate pulse measurement by taking the apical pulse for 1 minute. If this is a change for the patient, notify the primary care provider.
- *The pulse is palpated easily, but then disappears:* Apply only moderate pressure to the pulse. Applying too much pressure may obliterate the pulse.
- *You cannot palpate a pulse:* Use a portable Doppler ultrasound to assess the pulse. If this is a change in assessment or if you cannot find the pulse using a Doppler ultrasound, notify the primary care provider. If you can find the pulse using a Doppler ultrasound, place a small X over the spot where the pulse is located, based on facility policy. This can make palpating the pulse easier because the exact location of the pulse is known.

SPECIAL CONSIDERATIONS

General Considerations

- The normal heart rate varies by age. Refer to Fundamentals Review 2-1 on page 43.
- The carotid pulse should be palpated only in the lower third of the neck to avoid stimulation of the carotid sinus (Jensen, 2019, p. 95). When palpating a carotid pulse, lightly press only one side of the neck at a time. Never attempt to palpate both carotid arteries at the same time. Bilateral palpation could result in reduced cerebral blood flow and cause the patient to lose consciousness (Jensen, 2019).
- If a peripheral pulse is difficult to assess accurately because it is irregular, feeble, or extremely rapid, assess the apical rate.

(continued on page 68)

Skill 2-4 ▶ Assessing a Peripheral Pulse by Palpation *(continued)*

Infant and Child Considerations

- In children younger than 2 years of age, auscultate an apical pulse rate (see Skill 2-5) (Jarvis & Eckhardt, 2020; Kyle & Carmen, 2021).
- In children older than age 2 years, use the radial site for pulse assessment and count for 1 minute (Jarvis & Eckhardt, 2020; Kyle & Carmen, 2021).
- Measure the apical rate if the child has a cardiac problem or congenital heart defect (see Skill 2-5).

Community-Based Care Considerations

- Teach the patient and family members/caregivers how to take the patient's pulse, if appropriate.
- Inform the patient and family/caregivers about digital pulse monitoring devices.
- Teach family members/caregivers how to locate and monitor peripheral pulse sites, if appropriate.

Skill Variation ▶ Assessing Peripheral Pulse Using a Portable Doppler Ultrasound

A Doppler ultrasound device may be used to assess pulses that are difficult to palpate or auscultate. The device has an audio unit with an ultrasound transducer that amplifies changes in sound frequency as the blood flows through the blood vessel at a pulse site (Jarvis & Eckhardt, 2020; Jensen, 2019). The amplified sounds, whooshing pulsatile beats, can be measured to assess a peripheral pulse (Jarvis & Eckhardt, 2020).

1. Refer to Steps 1–7 in Skill 2-4.
2. Remove Doppler from charger and turn it on. Make sure that volume is set at low.
3. Apply conducting gel to the site where you expect to auscultate the pulse.
4. Hold the Doppler base in your nondominant hand. With your dominant hand, touch the probe lightly to the skin with the probe tip in the gel. Adjust the volume, as needed. Hold the probe perpendicular to the skin. Slowly move the Doppler tip around until the pulse is heard (Figure A).
5. **Using a watch with a second hand, count the heartbeat for 1 minute. Note the rhythm of the pulse.**
6. Remove the Doppler tip and turn the Doppler off. Wipe excess gel off the patient's skin with a tissue.
7. Place a small X over the spot where the pulse is located with an indelible pen, based on facility policy. Marking the site allows for easier future assessment. It can also make palpating the pulse easier because the exact location of the pulse is known.

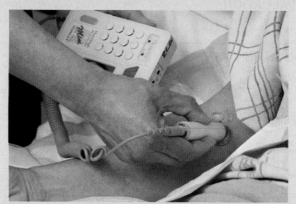

FIGURE A. Moving the Doppler tip until pulse is heard.

8. Cover the patient and help them to a position of comfort.
9. Wipe any gel remaining on the Doppler probe off with a tissue. Clean the Doppler probe per facility policy or manufacturer's recommendations.

10. Remove PPE, if used. Perform hand hygiene.

11. Return the Doppler ultrasound device to the charge base.
12. Record pulse rate, rhythm, and site, and that it was obtained with a Doppler ultrasound.

Skill 2-5 ▶ Assessing the Apical Pulse by Auscultation

Skill Variation: *Assessing the Apical–Radial Pulse Deficit*

An apical pulse is auscultated (listened to) over the apex of the heart, as the heart beats. Heart sounds, which are produced by closure of the valves of the heart, are characterized as "lub-dub." The apical pulse is the result of closure of the mitral and tricuspid valves ("lub") and the aortic and pulmonic valves ("dub"). The combination of the two sounds is counted as one beat. Pulse rates are measured in beats per minute. The normal pulse rate for adolescents and adults ranges from 60 to 100 beats per minute. Pulse rhythm is also assessed. Pulse rhythm is the pattern of the beats and the intervals between them. Pulse rhythm is normally regular; the "lub-dubs" and the pauses between occur at evenly spaced intervals. An irregular rhythm occurs when the beats and pauses between beats occur at unequal, varied intervals.

An apical pulse should be assessed when a peripheral pulse is difficult to assess accurately because it is irregular, weak, or very rapid. An apical pulse is also assessed when administering medications that alter heart rate and rhythm. In adults, the apical pulse is counted for 1 full minute. Apical pulse measurement is the preferred method of pulse assessment in children less than 2 years of age (Jarvis & Eckhardt, 2020; Kyle & Carmen, 2021).

Patients with irregularities in pulse rhythm may have a resulting **pulse deficit**. Assessment of the apical–radial pulse may be indicated. See the accompanying Skill Variation on page 72 for a description of the procedure for assessing the apical–radial pulse to identify a pulse deficit.

DELEGATION CONSIDERATIONS	The assessment of an apical pulse is not delegated to assistive personnel (AP). The measurement of an apical pulse may be delegated to a licensed practical/vocational nurse (LPN/LVN). The decision to delegate must be based on careful analysis of the patient's needs and circumstances as well as the qualifications of the person to whom the task is being delegated. Refer to the Delegation Guidelines in Appendix A.
EQUIPMENT	• Watch with second hand or digital readout • Stethoscope • Alcohol swab • Electronic record or pen and paper or flow sheet • Nonsterile gloves, if appropriate; additional PPE, as indicated
ASSESSMENT	Assess for factors that could affect pulse characteristics, such as the patient's age, physical activity, fluid balance, medications, body temperature, and presence of disease and/or health conditions. Note baseline or previous pulse measurements.
ACTUAL OR POTENTIAL HEALTH PROBLEMS AND NEEDS	Many actual or potential health problems or needs may require the use of this skill as part of related interventions. An appropriate health problem or need may include: • Altered tissue perfusion • Impaired Cardiac Output • Fluid Imbalance
OUTCOME IDENTIFICATION AND PLANNING	The expected outcomes to achieve when measuring an apical pulse rate are that the patient's pulse is assessed accurately without injury, and the patient experiences minimal discomfort. Other outcomes may be appropriate, depending on the specific diagnosis or patient problem identified for the patient.

IMPLEMENTATION

ACTION	RATIONALE
1. Check prescribed interventions or plan of care for frequency of pulse assessment. More frequent pulse measurement may be appropriate based on nursing judgment. Identify the need to obtain an apical pulse measurement.	Provides for patient safety and appropriate care.
2. Perform hand hygiene and put on PPE, if indicated.	Hand hygiene and PPE prevent the spread of microorganisms. PPE is required based on transmission precautions.

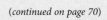

(continued on page 70)

Skill 2-5   ▶ Assessing the Apical Pulse by Auscultation   *(continued)*

ACTION	RATIONALE

3. Identify the patient.

Identifying the patient ensures the right patient receives the intervention and helps prevent errors.

4. Close curtains around the bed and close the door to the room, if possible. Discuss the procedure with the patient and assess the patient's ability to assist with the procedure.

This ensures the patient's privacy. Explanation relieves anxiety and facilitates cooperation.

5. Put on gloves, if indicated.

Gloves are not usually worn to obtain a pulse measurement unless contact with blood or body fluids is anticipated. Gloves prevent contact with blood and body fluids.

6. Use an alcohol swab to clean the **diaphragm** of the stethoscope. Use another swab to clean the earpieces, if necessary.

Cleaning with alcohol deters transmission of microorganisms.

7. Assist the patient to a sitting or reclining position and expose the chest area.

This position facilitates identification of the site for stethoscope placement.

8. Move the patient's clothing to expose only the apical site.

The site must be exposed for pulse assessment. Exposing only the apical site keeps the patient warm and maintains their dignity.

9. Hold the stethoscope diaphragm against the palm of your hand for a few seconds.

Warming the diaphragm promotes patient comfort.

10. **Palpate the space between the fifth and sixth ribs (fifth intercostal space), and move to the left midclavicular line.** Place the stethoscope diaphragm over the apex of the heart (Figures 1 and 2).

Position the stethoscope over the apex of the heart, where the heartbeat is best heard.

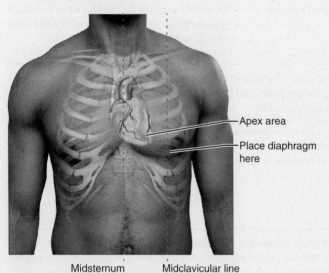

FIGURE 1. Locating the apical pulse: apex area.

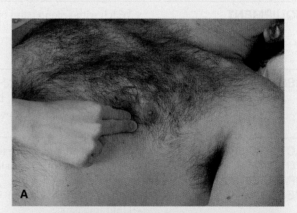

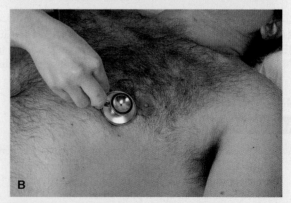

FIGURE 2. The apical pulse is usually found at (**A**) the fifth intercostal space just inside the midclavicular line and can be heard (**B**) over the apex of the heart.

ACTION	**RATIONALE**
11. Listen for heart sounds ("lub-dub"). Each "lub-dub" counts as one beat.	These sounds occur as the heart valves close.
12. Using a watch with a second hand, count the heartbeat for 1 minute.	Counting for a full minute increases the accuracy of assessment.
13. Note the rhythm of the beats.	Provides additional assessment data regarding the patient's cardiovascular status.
14. Clean the diaphragm of the stethoscope with an alcohol swab. Remove gloves. Perform hand hygiene.	Cleaning deters transmission of microorganisms.
15. Cover the patient and help them to a position of comfort.	Covering and positioning the patient ensures patient comfort.
16. Remove additional PPE, if used. Perform hand hygiene.	Proper removal of PPE reduces the risk for infection transmission and contamination of other items. Hand hygiene prevents the spread of microorganisms.

EVALUATION

The expected outcomes have been met when the patient's apical pulse has been assessed accurately without injury, and the patient experienced minimal discomfort.

DOCUMENTATION

Guidelines

Record pulse rate and rhythm in the electronic record or flow sheet. Communicate abnormal findings to the appropriate person. Identify site of assessment.

Sample Documentation

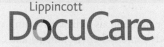

Practice documenting the apical pulse and other vital signs in *Lippincott DocuCare*.

2/6/25 1000 Apical pulse 82 and regular. Digoxin 0.125 mg administered orally as prescribed. Patient verbalized understanding of actions and untoward effects of medication.

—B. Clapp, RN

DEVELOPING CLINICAL REASONING AND CLINICAL JUDGMENT

UNEXPECTED SITUATIONS AND ASSOCIATED INTERVENTIONS

- If the apical rate is irregular, assess the patient for other symptoms, such as lightheadedness, dizziness, shortness of breath, or palpitations. Communicate findings to the appropriate health care provider.

SPECIAL CONSIDERATIONS

Infant and Child Considerations

- Assess the apical pulse just above and outside the left nipple of the infant at the third or fourth intercostal space. As the child ages, the location for assessment moves to a more medial and slightly lower area until 7 years of age. In children 7 years of age or older, assess the apical pulse at the fourth or fifth intercostal space at the midclavicular line (Jensen, 2019).
- The apical pulse rate is most reliable for infants and children younger than 2 years of age. Count the rate for 1 full minute in infants and children (Jensen, 2019; Silbert-Flagg & Pillitteri, 2018).
- Allow the young child to examine or handle the stethoscope to become familiar with the equipment.
- Assess the apical rate if the child has a cardiac problem or congenital heart defect.

(continued on page 72)

Skill 2-5 ▶ Assessing the Apical Pulse by Auscultation *(continued)*

Skill Variation ▶ Assessing the Apical–Radial Pulse Deficit

Measurement of the apical–radial pulse deficit may be utilized to assess the effectiveness of the contractions of the heart, specifically the left ventricle. Counting of the pulse at the apex of the heart and at the radial artery simultaneously is used to assess the apical–radial pulse deficit. Comparison of these two pulse rates provides an indirect evaluation of the ability of each heart contraction to eject enough blood into the peripheral circulation to create a pulse (Jensen, 2019). A difference between the apical and radial pulse rates is called the pulse deficit and indicates that not all the heartbeats are reaching the peripheral arteries or are too weak to be palpated (Taylor et al., 2023). Two nurses are required to perform this skill; one listens with a stethoscope over the apex of the heart for the apical heart rate and the other counts the pulse rate at the radial artery.

1. Refer to Steps 1–10 in Skill 2-5.

2. One watch with a sweep second hand is placed so that both nurses can read it simultaneously.
3. The nurses determine where they can best hear and feel the pulse and decide on a time to start counting, such as when the second hand on the watch is at a specified place (e.g., the number 12).
4. Both nurses count for 1 full minute and record their counts. The difference between the apical and radial pulse rates is the pulse deficit.

5. Clean the diaphragm of the stethoscope with an alcohol swab. Remove gloves, if used. Perform hand hygiene.

6. Cover the patient and help them to a position of comfort.

7. Remove additional PPE, if used. Perform hand hygiene.

Skill 2-6 ▶ Assessing Respiration

Measuring respirations allows for baseline assessment of respiratory function, as well as providing insight into the status of the patient's homeostatic control (the body's internal environment) and presence of physiologic conditions, such as hypoxia (Rolfe, 2019). Respiratory rate abnormalities are important predictors of deteriorating patient conditions and serious events, including cardiac arrest and intensive care admission (Malyca et al., 2019; Tessorolo Souza et al., 2019). Accurate assessment and interpretation of respirations as part of vital sign measurement are important parts of clinical assessment (Rolfe, 2019).

Ventilation (or breathing) is movement of gases in and out of the lungs; inspiration (or inhalation) is the act of breathing in, and expiration (or exhalation) is the act of breathing out. The cycle of **inspiration** and **expiration** is counted as one breath. Respiratory rates are measured in breaths per minute. Under normal conditions, healthy adults breathe about 12 to 20 times per minute (**respirations** per minute); infants and children breathe more rapidly (Hess et al., 2021). Fundamentals Review 2-1 outlines respiratory rate ranges for different age groups. The depth of respirations varies normally from shallow to deep. Respiratory rhythm is the pattern of the breaths and the intervals between them. Respiratory rhythm is normally regular; the breaths and the pauses between occur at evenly spaced intervals. An irregular respiratory rhythm occurs when the breaths and pauses between beats occur at unequal, varied intervals. Table 2-1 outlines various respiratory patterns.

Assess respiratory rate, depth, and rhythm by inspection (observing and listening) or by listening with the stethoscope. Determine the rate by counting the number of breaths per minute.

Move immediately from the pulse assessment to counting the respiratory rate to avoid letting the patient know you are counting respirations. Patients should be unaware of the respiratory assessment because awareness of measurement by observation can alter breathing patterns or rate (Hill et al., 2018).

DELEGATION CONSIDERATIONS

The measurement of respirations may be delegated to assistive personnel (AP) as well as to licensed practical/vocational nurses (LPN/LVNs). The decision to delegate must be based on careful analysis of the patient's needs and circumstances as well as the qualifications of the person to whom the task is being delegated. Refer to the Delegation Guidelines in Appendix A.

Table 2-1 | Patterns of Respiration

	DESCRIPTION	PATTERN	ASSOCIATED FEATURES
Normal	12–20 breaths/min; Regular		Normal pattern
Tachypnea	>24 breaths/min; Shallow		Fever, anxiety, exercise, respiratory disorders
Bradypnea	<10 breaths/min; Regular		Depression of the respiratory center by medications, brain damage
Hyperventilation	Increased rate and depth		Extreme exercise, fear, diabetic ketoacidosis (Kussmaul's respirations), overdose of aspirin
Hypoventilation	Decreased rate and depth; irregular		Overdose of narcotics or anesthetics
Cheyne–Stokes respirations	Alternating periods of deep, rapid breathing followed by periods of **apnea**; regular		Drug overdose, heart failure, increased intracranial pressure, renal failure
Biot's respirations	Varying depth and rate of breathing, followed by periods of apnea; irregular		Meningitis, severe brain damage

EQUIPMENT	• Watch with second hand or digital readout • Electronic record or pen and paper or flow sheet • PPE, as indicated
ASSESSMENT	Assess the patient for factors that could affect respirations, such as physical activity, medications, body temperature, smoking, anxiety, pain, and presence of disease and/or health conditions. Note baseline or previous respiratory measurements. Assess patient for any signs of respiratory distress, which include retractions, nasal flaring, grunting, **dyspnea**, **orthopnea**, or **tachypnea**.
ACTUAL OR POTENTIAL HEALTH PROBLEMS AND NEEDS	Many actual or potential health problems or needs may require the use of this skill as part of related interventions. An appropriate health problem or need may include: • Altered breathing pattern • Impaired gas exchange • Ineffective airway clearance
OUTCOME IDENTIFICATION AND PLANNING	The expected outcomes to achieve when assessing respirations are that the patient's respirations are assessed accurately without injury, and the patient experiences minimal discomfort. Other outcomes may be appropriate, depending on the specific diagnosis or patient problem identified for the patient.

(continued on page 74)

Skill 2-6 ▶ Assessing Respiration *(continued)*

IMPLEMENTATION

ACTION	RATIONALE
1. **While your fingers are still in place for the pulse measurement, after counting the pulse rate, observe the patient's respirations (Figure 1).**	The patient may alter the rate of respirations if aware they are being counted (Hill et al., 2018).

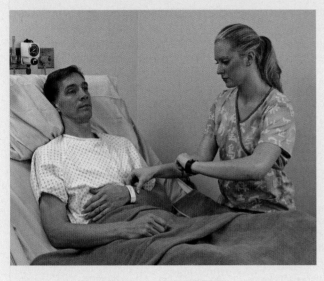

FIGURE 1. Assessing respirations.

2. Note the rise and fall of the patient's chest.	A complete cycle of an inspiration and an expiration composes one respiration.
3. Using a watch with a second hand, count the number of respirations for 30 seconds. Multiply this number by 2 to calculate the respiratory rate per minute. **Avoid counting for a 15-second interval.**	Sufficient time is necessary to observe the rate, depth, and other characteristics (Hill et al., 2018; Jarvis & Eckhardt, 2020). Use of a 15-second interval and multiplying by 4 can result in a respiratory count that is significantly incorrect (Hill et al., 2018; Jarvis & Eckhardt, 2020). Some literature suggests 60-second counts should be implemented whenever possible to ensure accuracy (Kallioinen et al., 2017).
4. **If respirations are abnormal in any way, count the respirations for at least 1 full minute** (Jarvis & Eckhardt, 2020).	Increased time allows the detection of unequal timing between respirations.
5. Note the depth and rhythm of the respirations.	This provides additional assessment data regarding the patient's respiratory status (Jarvis & Eckhardt, 2020).
6. When measurement is completed, remove gloves, if worn. Perform hand hygiene. Cover the patient and help them to a position of comfort.	Proper removal of gloves reduces the risk for infection transmission and contamination of other items. Hand hygiene prevents the spread of microorganisms. Covering and positioning the patient ensures patient comfort.
7. Remove additional PPE, if used. Perform hand hygiene.	Proper removal of PPE reduces the risk for infection transmission and contamination of other items. Hand hygiene deters the spread of microorganisms.

EVALUATION

The expected outcome has been met when the patient's respirations have been assessed accurately without injury, and the patient experienced minimal discomfort.

DOCUMENTATION

Guidelines   Document respiratory rate, depth, and rhythm on electronic record or flow sheet. Communicate any abnormal findings to the appropriate person.

Sample Documentation

Lippincott
DocuCare

Practice documenting respiration and other vital signs in *Lippincott DocuCare*.

10/23/25 0830 Patient breathing at a rate of 16 respirations per minute. Respirations regular and unlabored.

—M. Evans, RN

DEVELOPING CLINICAL REASONING AND CLINICAL JUDGMENT

UNEXPECTED SITUATIONS AND ASSOCIATED INTERVENTIONS

- *The patient is breathing with such shallow respirations that you cannot count the rate:* Sometimes it is easier to count respirations by auscultating the lung sounds. Auscultate lung sounds and count respirations for 30 seconds. Multiply by 2 to calculate the respiratory rate per minute. If the respiratory rate is irregular, count for a full minute. Notify the primary health care provider of the respiratory rate and the shallowness and irregularity of the respirations.

SPECIAL CONSIDERATIONS

General Considerations

- If respiratory rate or depth is irregular, count respirations for 1 minute.
- If respirations are very shallow and difficult to detect, observe the sternal notch, where respiration is more apparent.
- If respirations are difficult to detect, such as with patients who are obese or with children, place a hand on the upper chest or abdomen to feel the respiratory rate (Jarvis & Eckhardt, 2020). Alternatively place a hand on the patient's shoulder to feel the respiratory rate (Jensen, 2019).

Infant and Child Considerations

- For infants and children, count respirations for 1 full minute to ensure accuracy (Kyle & Carmen, 2021).
- Infants' respirations are primarily diaphragmatic; count abdominal movements to assess respiratory rate for infants (Jensen, 2019; Kyle & Carmen, 2021).
- Count thoracic movements to assess respiratory rate for infants and children older than 1 year of age (Kyle & Carmen, 2021).
- Assess respirations before taking the temperature so that the child is not crying, which would alter the respiratory status.
- Assess respirations in infants and children when the child is resting or sitting quietly, because respiratory rate often changes when infants or young children cry, feed, or become more active. The most accurate respiratory rate is obtained when the infant or child is at rest (Jensen, 2019; Kyle & Carmen, 2021).

EVIDENCE FOR PRACTICE ▶

ACCURATE RESPIRATION MEASUREMENT

Measurement of respirations is part of a baseline assessment of respiratory function and provides insight into the status of the patient. Respiratory rate abnormalities are important predictors of deteriorating patient conditions and serious events, including cardiac arrest and intensive care admission (Malyca et al., 2019; Tessorolo Souza et al., 2019). Accurate assessment and interpretation of respirations as part of vital sign measurement are important parts of clinical assessment (Rolfe, 2019).

Related Research

Kallioinen, N., Hill, A., Christofidis, M. J., Horswill, M. S., & Watson, M. O. (2021). Quantitative systematic review: Sources of inaccuracy in manually measured adult respiratory rate data. *Journal of Advanced Nursing, 77*(1), 98–124. https://doi.org/10.1111/jan.14584

(continued on page 76)

Skill 2-6 ▶ Assessing Respiration *(continued)*

The purpose of this systematic review was to identify potential sources of inaccuracy in manually measured adult respiratory rate data and quantify their effects. A search of Medline, CINAHL, and Cochrane library databases was performed (from databased inception to July 31, 2019). Quantitative studies were included that investigated manual measurement of adult patients' respiratory rate (RR) in clinical settings; identified at least one specific potential source of inaccuracy in the observation or documentation of RR; and, in relation to each source of inaccuracy identified, quantified the prevalence or independent effect on documented RR values. Evidence quality was evaluated by using the Standard Quality Assessment Criteria for Evaluating Primary Research Papers from a Variety of Fields (Kmet et al., 2004, as cited in Kallioinen et al., 2021, p. 100). Studies presenting data on individual sources of inaccuracy in the manual measurement of adult RR were analyzed, assessed for quality, and grouped according to the source of inaccuracy investigated. Quantitative data were extracted and synthesized, and meta-analyses performed where appropriate. Identified studies ($n = 49$) identified five sources of inaccuracy: (1) the *awareness effect* creates an artefactual reduction in actual RR; (2) *observation methods* involving shorter counts cause systematic underscoring of RR; (3) *inter-* or *intraobserver variability* causes substantial differences between individual RR measurement observations; (4) *value bias* in which particular RRs are overrepresented, suggesting estimation; and (5) *recording omission*, resulting in higher average rates in inpatient versus triage/admission contexts. The researchers concluded manually measured RR data are subject to several potential sources of inaccuracy and a single measurement may be affected by several factors. The researchers suggested health care providers should interpret recorded RR data cautiously unless systems are in place to ensure its accuracy. According to the authors, nurses should count rather than estimate RR, and 60-second counts should be implemented whenever possible to ensure accuracy. Nurses should ensure patients are unaware that their RR is being measured and take care to accurately document the resulting RR value.

Relevance to Nursing Practice

Measurement of respirations provides insight into the status of the patient and is an important predictor of changes and declines in a patient's status. Assessing vital signs as part of a nursing assessment is an important component of care in all health care settings. The usefulness of respiratory rate data depends on the accuracy of the observations and documentation. Nurses have a responsibility to obtain and record accurate measurements of respiratory rate to contribute to accurate and appropriate identification of and changes in patient status.

Skill 2-7 ▶ Assessing Blood Pressure Using an Automated, Electronic Oscillometric Device

Measurement of blood pressure is an important part of vital sign measurement, identification of a patient's baseline status, and identification of changes in a patient's status (Taylor et al., 2023). Normal blood pressure is defined as a systolic pressure <120 mm Hg and 80 mm Hg (Whelton et al., 2018). Table 2-2 identifies the categories for blood pressure levels in adults.

Automated, electronic oscillometric blood pressure devices determine blood pressure by analyzing the sounds of blood flow or measuring the amplitude of the oscillations (fluctuations) in blood flow upon deflation or inflation of the cuff (Figure 1). These devices can be set to take and record blood pressure readings at preset intervals. There has been a shift away from manual auscultatory blood pressure measurement to the use of oscillometric measurement method, supported by improved device technology, as well as the recommendation to obtain multiple blood pressure readings to increase accuracy (Muntner et al., 2019). The measurement of blood pressure using the manual auscultatory method is described in Skill 2-8 on page 85. Systolic blood pressure can also be estimated by palpation or using a Doppler ultrasound device (refer to the Skill Variation in Skill 2-8 on page 93).

Table 2-2	Categories for Blood Pressure Levels in Adults (Ages 18 and Older)

	BLOOD PRESSURE LEVEL (mm Hg)		
CATEGORY	Systolic		Diastolic
Normal	<120	*and*	<80
Elevated	120–129	*and*	<80
Hypertension Stage 1	130–139	*or*	80–89
Hypertension Stage 2	≥140	*or*	≥90
Hypertensive crisis	>180	*and/or*	>120

Source: Whelton, P. K., Carey, R. M., Aronow, W. S., Casey, D. E., Collins, K. J., Himmelfarb, C. D., DePalma, S. M., Gidding, S., Jamerson, K. A., Jones, D. W., MacLaughlin, E. J., Muntner, P., Ovbiagele, B., Smith, S. C., Spencer, C. C., Stafford, R. S., Taler, S. J., Thomas, R. J., Williams, Sr., K. A., ... Wright, J. T., Jr. (2018). 2017 ACC/AHA/AAPA/ABC/ACPM/AGS/APhA/ASH/ASPC/NMA/PCNA Guideline for the prevention, detection, evaluation, and management of high blood pressure in adults. *Hypertension, 71*(4), 1269–1324. https://doi.org/10.1161/HYP.0000000000000066

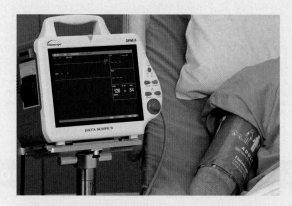

FIGURE 1. The electronic oscillometric blood pressure monitor reports systolic and diastolic blood pressure as well as mean blood pressure. (*Source:* Used with permission from Shutterstock. *Photo by B. Proud.*)

The nurse must know the appropriate equipment to use, including choosing the appropriate blood pressure cuff (Table 2-3), how to accurately obtain the measurement, and which site to choose to accurately assess blood pressure. Refer to Box 2-3 for important considerations related to accurate blood pressure measurement.

Oscillometric devices are commonly used to measure blood pressure in a variety of settings, including clinics, ambulatory, home, and acute care (Muntner et al., 2019). Many of these devices have additional integrated equipment, such as a thermometer and pulse oximetry, to perform multiple vital sign measurements.

Regardless of the method used to measure blood pressure, health care providers must ensure the use of careful, accurate technique to avoid errors in blood pressure measurement (Muntner et al., 2019; Pickering et al., 2005; Whelton et al., 2018). Box 2-4 identifies potential sources of blood pressure measurement error.

Various sites can be used to assess blood pressure. The brachial artery and the popliteal artery are used most commonly. This skill discusses using the brachial artery site to obtain a blood pressure measurement.

At times, it is necessary to assess a patient for orthostatic hypotension (postural hypotension). Assessment for orthostatic hypotension may be accomplished using either an automated, electronic oscillometric blood pressure device or the auscultatory method of measuring blood pressure. Box 2-5 outlines the procedure to assess for orthostatic hypotension.

(*continued on page 78*)

Skill 2-7 ▶ Assessing Blood Pressure Using an Automated, Electronic Oscillometric Device *(continued)*

Table 2-3 Recommended Blood Pressure Cuff Sizes

CUFF SIZE	CUFF BLADDER DIMENSIONS (cm)	ARM CIRCUMFERENCE[a] (cm)
Neonates, infants, children	Cuff bladder length should encircle 80–100% of arm Cuff bladder width-to-arm circumference ratio 0.45–0.55	
Small adult size	12 × 22	22–26
Adult size	16 × 30	27–34
Large adult size	16 × 36	35–44
Adult thigh size	16 × 42	45–52

[a]Select a blood pressure cuff that has a bladder length 75% to 100% of the arm circumference and a width that is 37% to 50% of the arm circumference.

Source: Adapted from Flynn, J. T., Kaelber, D. C., Baker-Smith, C. M., Blowey, D., Carroll, A. E., Daniels, S. R., de Ferranti, S. D., Dionne, J. M., Falkner, B., Flinn, S. K., Gidding, S. S., Goodwin, C., Leu, M. G., Powers, M. E., Rea, C., Samuels, J., Simasek, M., Thaker, V. V., Urbina, E. M., . . . Subcommittee on Screening and Management of High Blood Pressure in Children. (2017). Clinical practice guideline for screening and management of high blood pressure in children and adolescents. *Pediatrics, 140*(3), e20171904. https://doi.org/10.1542/peds.2017-1904; Muntner, P., Shimbo, D., Carey, R. M., Charleston, J. B., Gaillard, T., Misra, S., Myers, M. G., Ogedegbe, G., Schwartz, J. E., Townsend, R. R., Urbina, E. M., Viera, A., J., White, W. B., & Wright, J. T. Jr. (2019). Measurement of blood pressure in humans. A scientific statement from the American Heart Association. *Hypertension, 73*(5), e35–e66. https://doi.org/10.1161/HYP.0000000000000087; and Pickering, T. G., Hall, J. E., Appel, L. J., Falkner, B. E., Graves, J., Hill, M. N., Jones, D. W., Kurtz, T., Sheps, S. G., & Roccella, E. J. (2005). Recommendations for blood pressure measurement in humans and experimental animals. Part 1: Blood pressure measurement in humans: A statement for professionals from the subcommittee of professional and public education of the American Heart Association Council on High Blood Pressure Research. *Circulation, 111*(5), 697–716. http://circ.ahajournals.org/content/111/5/697.abstract.

Box 2-3 Considerations Related to Measurement of Blood Pressure

Blood Pressure
- Blood pressure (BP) refers to the force of the blood against arterial walls.
- **Systolic pressure** is the highest point of pressure on arterial walls when the ventricles contract and push blood through the arteries at the beginning of systole. When the heart rests between beats during diastole, the pressure drops. The lowest pressure present on arterial walls during diastole is the **diastolic pressure** (Taylor et al., 2023).
- BP is measured in millimeters of mercury (mm Hg) and recorded as a fraction. The numerator is the systolic pressure; the denominator is the diastolic pressure.
- The difference between the systolic and diastolic pressures is called the **pulse pressure**.
- BP readings can be within a wide range and still be normal. It is important to know the normal blood pressure range of a particular person. A rise or fall of 20 to 30 mm Hg in a person's blood pressure is significant, even if it is within the generally accepted normal range.

Accurate Assessment of Blood Pressure
- Ensure use of validated and calibrated devices

- Obtain BP measurements
  - In a quiet environment, the patient should not talk or move during measurement
  - After the patient relaxes
  - After the patient has not consumed caffeine, exercised, or smoked for 30 minutes
  - With the patient in a supine or sitting position
  - (Sitting) with the patient's arm supported on a table at heart level or held up by the health care provider (midpoint of the sternum). The patient's feet and back should be supported as well (Whelton et al., 2018).
  - (Supine) with the patient's arm supported with a pillow at heart level (Muntner et al., 2019).
  - With the patient's legs uncrossed (Liu et al., 2016, as cited in Muntner et al., 2019).

Measuring BP Related to the Diagnosis/ Management of Hypertension
- BP measurements should be obtained ≥2 readings on ≥2 occasions and the measurements averaged to estimate the person's level of blood pressure (Whelton et al., 2018).

Box 2-4 | Sources of Error in Blood Pressure Measurement

- Use of noncalibrated, nonvalidated, nonmaintained device
- Use of a cuff of incorrect size
- Patient movement during measurement
- Patient talking during the measurement
- Incorrect placement and/or orientation of the cuff
- Incorrect positioning of the patient
- Use of inaccurate measurement technique
  - Incorrect positioning of the limb used for measurement
- Inflation of cuff that is too rapid
- Deflation of cuff that is too rapid (faster than 2 to 3 mm Hg per second)
- Environmental noise
- Failure to allow for a rest period prior to measurement
- Incorrect interpretation
- Reliance on blood pressures measured at a single occasion

Source: Adapted from Muntner, P., Shimbo, D., Carey, R. M., Charleston, J. B., Gaillard, T., Misra, S., Myers, M. G., Ogedegbe, G., Schwartz, J. E., Townsend, R. R., Urbina, E. M., Viera, A. J., White, W. B., & Wright, J. T. Jr. (2019). Measurement of blood pressure in humans. A scientific statement from the American Heart Association. *Hypertension, 73*(5), e35–e66. https://doi.org/10.1161/HYP.0000000000000087; Whelton, P. K., Carey, R. M., Aronow, W. S., Casey, D. E. Jr., Collins, K. J., Dennison Himmelfarb, C., DePalma, S. M., Gidding, S., Jamerson, K. A., Jones, D. W., MacLaughlin, E. J., Muntner, P., Ovbiagele, B., Smith, S. C. Jr., Spencer, C. C., Stafford, R. S., Taler, S. J., Thomas, R. J., Williams, K. A. Sr., ... Wright, J, T. Jr. (2018). 2017 ACC/AHA/AAPA/ABC/ACPM/AGS/APhA/ASH/ASPC/NMA/PCNA Guideline for the prevention, detection, evaluation, and management of high blood pressure in adults. *Hypertension, 71*(6), e13–e115. https://doi.org/10.1161/HYP.0000000000000065

Box 2-5 | Assessing for Orthostatic Hypotension

Assess for signs and symptoms of hypotension, such as dizziness, lightheadedness, pallor, diaphoresis, or syncope throughout the procedure. If the patient is attached to a cardiac monitor, assess for arrhythmias. Immediately return the patient to a supine position if symptoms appear during the procedure. Do not have the patient stand if symptoms of hypotension occur when the patient is sitting. Use the following guidelines to assess for orthostatic hypotension:

- Lower the head of the bed. Place the bed in a low position.
- Ask the patient to lie in a supine position for 3 to 10 minutes. At the end of this time, take initial blood pressure and pulse measurements.

- Assist the patient to a sitting position on the side of the bed with the legs dangling. After 1 to 3 minutes, take the blood pressure and pulse measurements.
- Assist the patient to stand, unless standing is contraindicated. Wait 2 to 3 minutes, then take blood pressure and pulse measurements.
- Record the measurements for each position, noting the position with the readings. A decrease in systolic blood pressure of ≥20 mm Hg or a decrease in diastolic blood pressure of ≥10 mm Hg within 3 minutes of standing when compared with blood pressure from the sitting or supine position is significant for orthostatic hypotension (Angelousi et al., 2014).

Source: Adapted from Angelousi, A., Gererd, N., Benetos, A., Frimat, L., Gautier, S., Weryha, G., & Boivin, J. M. (2014). Association between orthostatic hypotension and cardiovascular risk, cerebrovascular risk, cognitive decline and falls as well as overall mortality: A systematic review and meta-analysis. *Journal of Hypertension, 32*(8), 1562–1571; discussion 1571. https://doi.org/10.1097/HJH.0000000000000235; Lanier, J. B., Mote, M. B., & Clay, E. C. (2011). Evaluation and management of orthostatic hypotension. *American Family Physician, 84*(5), 527–536; and Pickering, T. G., Hall, J. E., & Appel, L. J. (2005). American Heart Association Scientific Statement. Recommendations for blood pressure measurement in humans and experimental animals. Part 1: Blood pressure measurement in humans: A statement for professionals from the subcommittee of professional and public education of the American Heart Association Council on High Blood Pressure Research. *Circulation, 111*(5), 697–716. http://circ.ahajournals.org/content/111/5/697.abstract

DELEGATION CONSIDERATIONS	The measurement of brachial artery blood pressure may be delegated to assistive personnel (AP) as well as to licensed practical/vocational nurses (LPN/LVNs). The decision to delegate must be based on careful analysis of the patient's needs and circumstances as well as the qualifications of the person to whom the task is being delegated. Refer to the Delegation Guidelines in Appendix A.
EQUIPMENT	<ul><li>Blood pressure cuff of appropriate size</li><li>Automated, electronic oscillometric blood pressure device</li><li>Electronic record or pen and paper or flow sheet</li><li>PPE, as indicated</li></ul>

(continued on page 80)

Skill 2-7 ▶ Assessing Blood Pressure Using an Automated, Electronic Oscillometric Device *(continued)*

ASSESSMENT	Assess the brachial pulse, or the pulse appropriate for the site being used. Assess for an intravenous infusion or breast or axilla surgery on the side of the body corresponding to the arm used. Assess for the presence of a cast, arteriovenous shunt, or injured or diseased limb. If any of these conditions are present, do not use the affected arm to monitor blood pressure. Assess the size of the limb so that the appropriate-sized blood pressure cuff can be used (see Table 2-3). Assess for factors that could affect blood pressure reading, such as the patient's age, physical activity, weight, fluid balance, medications, and presence of disease and/or health conditions. Note baseline or previous blood pressure measurements. Assess the patient for pain. If the patient reports pain, give pain medication as ordered before assessing blood pressure. If the blood pressure is taken while the patient is in pain, make a notation concerning the pain if the blood pressure is elevated.
ACTUAL OR POTENTIAL HEALTH PROBLEMS AND NEEDS	Many actual or potential health problems or needs may require the use of this skill as part of related interventions. An appropriate health problem or need may include: • Impaired Cardiac Output • Hypertension risk • Hypotension risk
OUTCOME IDENTIFICATION AND PLANNING	The expected outcome to achieve when measuring blood pressure is that the patient's blood pressure is measured accurately without injury. Other outcomes may be appropriate depending on the patient's health problems or issues.

IMPLEMENTATION

ACTION	**RATIONALE**
1. Check the prescribed interventions or plan of care for frequency of blood pressure measurement. More frequent measurement may be appropriate based on nursing judgment.	Provides for patient safety.
2. Perform hand hygiene and put on PPE, if indicated.	Hand hygiene and PPE prevent the spread of microorganisms. PPE is required based on transmission precautions.
3. Identify the patient.	Identifying the patient ensures the right patient receives the intervention and helps prevent errors.
4. Close the curtains around the bed and close the door to the room, if possible. Discuss the procedure with the patient and assess patient's ability to assist with the procedure. Validate that the patient has relaxed for several minutes.	This ensures the patient's privacy. Explanation relieves anxiety and facilitates cooperation. Activity immediately before measurement can result in inaccurate results.
5. Put on gloves, if indicated.	Gloves prevent contact with blood and body fluids. Gloves are usually not required for measurement of blood pressure, unless contact with blood or body fluids is anticipated.
6. Select the appropriate arm (or alternate site) for measurement and blood pressure cuff (refer to Table 2-3).	Decision on measurement site and cuff size is based on the nurse's assessment of individual patient circumstances. Incorrect cuff size contributes to the most frequent error in measurement in nonacute care settings (Muntner et al., 2019).

ACTION

7. Have the patient assume a comfortable lying or sitting position with the forearm supported at the level of the heart and the palm of the hand upward (Figure 2). If the measurement is taken in the supine position, support the arm with a pillow. In the sitting position, support the arm yourself or by using the bedside table. If the patient is sitting, have the patient sit back in the chair so that the chair supports their back. In addition, make sure the patient keeps the legs uncrossed.

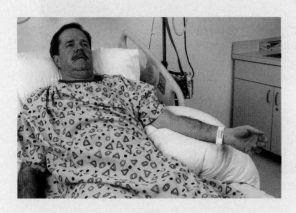

FIGURE 2. Proper positioning for blood pressure assessment using brachial artery.

8. Expose the brachial artery by removing garments or move a sleeve if it is not too tight, above the area where the cuff will be placed.

9. Palpate the location of the brachial artery. Center the bladder of the cuff over the brachial artery, about midway on the upper arm, so that the lower edge of the cuff is about 2.5 to 5 cm (1 to 2 inches) above the inner aspect of the elbow (Figure 3). **Line up the artery marking on the cuff with the patient's brachial artery.** The tubing should extend from the edge of the cuff nearer the patient's elbow (Figure 4).

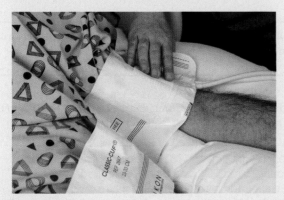

FIGURE 3. Centering the bladder of the cuff over the brachial artery.

RATIONALE

The position of the arm can have a major influence when the blood pressure is measured; if the upper arm is below the level of the right atrium, the readings will be too high. If the arm is above the level of the heart, the readings will be too low (Muntner et al., 2019; Pickering et al., 2005). This position places the brachial artery on the inner aspect of the elbow so that the bell or diaphragm of the stethoscope can rest on it easily. Support for the patient's arm prevents isometric exercise that will affect the blood pressure level (Muntner et al., 2019). If the back is not supported, the diastolic pressure may be elevated falsely; if the legs are crossed, the systolic pressure may be elevated falsely (Muntner et al., 2019; Pickering et al., 2005).

Clothing over the artery interferes with the ability to hear sounds and can cause inaccurate blood pressure readings. A tight sleeve would cause congestion of blood and possibly inaccurate readings (Muntner et al., 2019).

Pressure in the cuff applied directly to the artery provides the most accurate readings. If the cuff gets in the way of the stethoscope, readings are likely to be inaccurate. A cuff placed upside down with the tubing toward the patient's head may give a false reading.

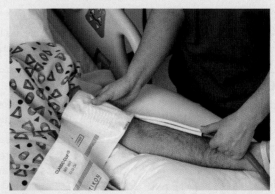

FIGURE 4. Cuff tubing extending from the edge of the cuff nearer the patient's elbow.

(*continued on page 82*)

Skill 2-7 ▶ Assessing Blood Pressure Using an Automated, Electronic Oscillometric Device (continued)

ACTION	RATIONALE
10. Wrap the cuff around the arm smoothly and snugly, and fasten it (Figure 5). Do not allow any clothing to interfere with the proper placement of the cuff.	A smooth cuff and snug wrapping produce equal pressure and help promote an accurate measurement. A cuff wrapped too loosely results in an inaccurate reading.
11. Turn on the machine. **If the machine has different settings for infants, children, and adults, select the appropriate setting.** Push the start button. Instruct the patient to hold the limb still and refrain from speaking.	Keeping the limb still and refraining from talking provide for accurate measurement of blood pressure levels (Muntner et al., 2019).
12. Wait until the machine beeps and the blood pressure reading appears. Note the reading (Figure 6).	A beep signals the completion of reading.

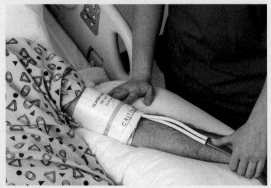

FIGURE 5. Wrapping the cuff around the arm smoothly and snugly.

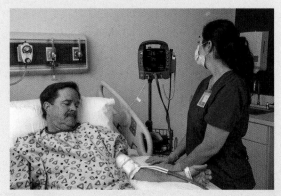

FIGURE 6. Noting the blood pressure reading.

ACTION	RATIONALE
13. Remove the cuff from the patient's limb and clean and store the equipment.	Cleaning of equipment prevents transmission of microorganisms and prepares equipment for future use.
14. Remove gloves, if worn. Perform hand hygiene. Cover the patient and help them to a position of comfort.	Removing gloves properly reduces the risk for infection transmission and contamination of other items. Hand hygiene prevents the spread of microorganisms. Covering and positioning the patient ensures patient comfort.
15. Remove additional PPE, if used. Perform hand hygiene.	Proper removal of PPE reduces the risk for infection transmission and contamination of other items. Hand hygiene deters the spread of microorganisms.

EVALUATION

The expected outcome has been met when the blood pressure has been measured accurately without injury and minimal patient discomfort.

DOCUMENTATION

Guidelines

Record the findings on the electronic record or flow sheet. Communicate abnormal findings to the primary health care provider. Identify arm used or site of assessment if other than brachial.

Sample Documentation

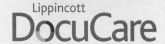

Practice documenting blood pressure and other vital signs in *Lippincott DocuCare*.

> 10/18/25 0945 Blood pressure taken in right arm 180/88. Dr. Brown notified. Patient denies dizziness, headache. Captopril 25 mg PO twice a day prescribed. Blood pressure to be repeated 30 minutes after administering medication.
> —M. Evans, RN

DEVELOPING CLINICAL REASONING AND CLINICAL JUDGMENT

SPECIAL CONSIDERATIONS

General Considerations

- Blood pressure measurements should be checked in both arms at the first examination (Muntner et al., 2019; Pickering et al., 2005). Most people have differences in blood pressure readings between arms. When there is a consistent interarm difference, use the arm with the higher pressure (Muntner et al., 2019; Pickering et al., 2005).
- Separate repeated blood pressure measurements in the same arm by 1 to 2 minutes to avoid inaccurate results (Muntner et al., 2019).
- Blood pressure can be assessed by auscultation with a sphygmomanometer and stethoscope (see Skill 2-8); systolic blood pressure can be assessed using Doppler ultrasound (see the accompanying Skill Variation).
- Incorrect cuff size contributes to the most frequent error in measurement in nonacute care settings (Muntner et al., 2019). *If the cuff is too narrow*, the reading could be erroneously high because the pressure is not evenly transmitted to the artery. *If a cuff is too wide,* the reading may be erroneously low because pressure is dispersed over a disproportionately large surface area.
- Diastolic blood pressure measured while the patient is supine is approximately 1 to 5 mm Hg higher than when measured while the patient is sitting; systolic blood pressure measured while the patient is supine is approximately 3 to 10 mm Hg higher than when measured while the patient is sitting (Muntner et al., 2019).
- Automated electronic oscillometric wrist monitors have been developed that measure blood pressure in the forearm using the radial artery. Forearm measurements tend to be higher than the upper arm measurements (Halm, 2014). The accuracy of readings with forearm monitors is affected by the position of the wrist relative to the heart. This can be avoided if the wrist is always at heart level when the reading is taken (Pickering et al., 2005).
- The wrist site for measurement has been suggested as an alternative for obtaining blood pressure readings in people who are obese. It is often difficult to obtain the appropriately sized cuff for the upper arm, given arm circumference and conical-shaped upper arms common in obesity. The conical shape of the upper arm makes it difficult to fit the cuff to the arm, increasing the likelihood of inaccurate blood pressure measurement (Halm, 2014). Thus, measurement in the forearm can be a possible solution to this problem (Muntner et al., 2019; Palatini, 2018).
- When the patient's brachial artery is inaccessible or use of the upper arm is contraindicated, assess blood pressure using the popliteal artery in the leg. The systolic blood pressure is at least 15 to 20 mm Hg higher at this site than the arm, although the diastolic pressure is the same (Muntner et al., 2019; Sheppard et al., 2019).

Infant and Child Considerations

- Use oscillometric devices that have been validated for use with children and adolescents (Muntner et al., 2019).
- In children, if elevated blood pressure is present when measure with an oscillometric device, auscultation should be performed to define blood pressure levels (Muntner et al., 2019).
- The use of wrist monitors is not recommended for pediatric patients (Muntner et al., 2019).
- Blood pressure should be taken in the right arm for children to align with normative data (Muntner et al., 2019).
- In infants and small children, the lower extremities are commonly used for blood pressure monitoring at the popliteal, dorsalis pedis, and posterior tibial sites. In children older than 1 year of age, the systolic pressure in the thigh tends to be 10 to 40 mm Hg higher than in the arm; the diastolic pressure remains the same (Kyle & Carman, 2021).
- Infants and children presenting with cardiac complaints may have blood pressures assessed in all four extremities. Large differences among blood pressure readings between the upper and lower extremities can indicate heart defects, such as coarctation of the aorta (Kyle & Carman, 2021).

Community-Based Care Considerations

- Patient and family/caregiver education related to home blood pressure monitoring (HBPM) should include information about hypertension, selection of equipment, appropriate procedures, and interpretation of results (Whelton et al., 2018).

(continued on page 84)

Skill 2-7 ▶ Assessing Blood Pressure Using an Automated, Electronic Oscillometric Device *(continued)*

- Automated blood pressure devices in public locations are generally inaccurate and inconsistent. In addition, the cuffs on these devices are inadequate for people with large arms (Pickering et al., 2005).
- Explain to the patient that it is important to use a cuff size appropriate for limb circumference. Inform the patient that cuff sizes range from a pediatric cuff to a large thigh cuff and that a poorly fitting cuff can result in an inaccurate measurement.
- Use of an automated validated digital monitoring device is suggested as best practice for HBPM (Whelton et al., 2018). Inform the patient about digital blood pressure monitoring equipment. Although more costly than manual cuffs, most provide an easy-to-read recording of systolic and diastolic measurements. Use of auscultatory devices is not recommended for HBPM because patients, family, and caregivers rarely master the technique required for accurate use of these devices (Whelton et al., 2018).
- Optimally, patients should measure and record blood pressure daily. Explain that two readings, at least 1 minute apart, should be taken in the morning before taking medications and in the evening (Muntner et al., 2019; Whelton et al., 2018). Measurement should occur following the guidelines detailed in Skill 2-7. Ideally, patients should measure weekly blood pressure readings beginning 2 weeks after a change in the treatment regimen and during the week before a follow-up visit (Whelton et al., 2018). The readings should be recorded to show to the health care provider. If possible, monitor with built-in memory should be brought to all health care visits.
- Explain that home monitoring devices should be checked for accuracy every 1 to 2 years. Readings should be compared with auscultated measurement by a health care provider to ensure accuracy.

EVIDENCE FOR PRACTICE ▶

MEASUREMENT OF BLOOD PRESSURE IN HUMANS

Muntner, P., Shimbo, D., Carey, R. M., Charleston, J. B., Gaillard, T., Misra, S., Myers, M. G., Ogedegbe, G., Schwartz, J. E., Townsend, R. R., Urbina, E. M., Viera, A., J., White, W. B., & Wright, J. T. Jr. (2019). Measurement of blood pressure in humans. A scientific statement from the American Heart Association. *Hypertension*, *73*(5), e35–e66. https://doi.org/10.1161/HYP.0000000000000087

This scientific statement and guideline provide evidence-based recommendations to guide measurement of blood pressure.

Refer to details in the Evidence for Practice in Skill 2-8.

EVIDENCE FOR PRACTICE ▶

PREVENTION, DETECTION, EVALUATION, AND MANAGEMENT OF HIGH BLOOD PRESSURE IN ADULTS

Whelton, P. K., Carey, R. M., Aronow, W. S., Casey, D. E., Collins, K. J., Himmelfarb, C. D., DePalma, S. M., Gidding, S., Jamerson, K. A., Jones, D. W., MacLaughlin, E. J., Muntner, P., Ovbiagele, B., Smith, S. C., Spencer, C. C., Stafford, R. S., Taler, S. J., Thomas, R. J., Williams, Sr., K. A., … Wright, J. T., Jr. (2018). 2017 ACC/AHA/AAPA/ABC/ACPM/AGS/APhA/ASH/ASPC/NMA/PCNA Guideline for the prevention, detection, evaluation, and management of high blood pressure in adults. *Hypertension*, *71*(4), 1269–1324. https://doi.org/10.1161/HYP.0000000000000065

This scientific statement and guideline provide evidence-based recommendations to guide measurement of blood pressure.

Refer to details in the Evidence for Practice in Skill 2-8.

Skill 2-8 ▶ Assessing Blood Pressure by Auscultation

Skill Variation: *Assessing Systolic Blood Pressure Using Doppler Ultrasound*

Measurement of blood pressure is an important part of vital sign measurement, identification of a patient's baseline status, and identification of changes in a patient's status (Taylor et al., 2023). Normal blood pressure is defined as a systolic pressure <120 mm Hg and <80 mm Hg (Whelton et al., 2018). Table 2-2 on page 77 identifies the categories for blood pressure levels in adults.

The auscultatory method has been the traditional approach to measurement of systolic and diastolic blood pressure and remains an acceptable method for measuring blood pressure (Muntner et al., 2019). This method is described below.

However, this method is being replaced more and more by oscillometric devices in clinical practice (Muntner et al., 2019). The use of an automated, electronic oscillometric blood pressure device to measure blood pressure is outlined in Skill 2-7 on page 76. Systolic blood pressure can also be estimated by palpation or using a Doppler ultrasound device (refer to the Skill Variation on page 93).

The nurse must know the appropriate equipment to use, including choosing the appropriate blood pressure cuff (see Table 2-3), how to accurately obtain the measurement, how to describe the sounds that are heard during the auscultatory method of measurement, and which site to choose to accurately assess blood pressure. Refer to Box 2-3 on page 78 for important considerations related to accurate blood pressure measurement.

A sphygmomanometer, along with a stethoscope, is used to assess blood pressure in the auscultatory method of blood pressure measurement. The sphygmomanometer consists of a cuff (with an air compartment), a pump, and the manometer (pressure dial) (Figure 1). The series of sounds for which to listen when assessing blood pressure using the auscultatory method are called **Korotkoff sounds**. Table 2-4 on page 86 describes and illustrates these sounds.

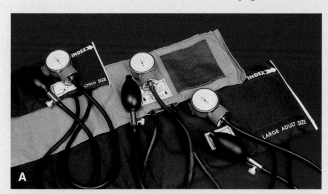
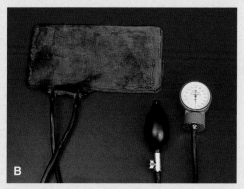

FIGURE 1. Sphygmomanometer. **A.** Three cuff sizes: a small cuff for a child or a small or frail adult, a normal-sized cuff, and a large adult cuff. A cuff sized for use on the thigh is also available. **B.** Parts of a sphygmomanometer. (Part **B** used with permission from Weber, J. R., & Kelley, J. H. (2018). *Health assessment in nursing* (6th ed.). Wolters Kluwer, p. 135.)

Regardless of the method used to measure blood pressure, health care providers must ensure the use of careful, accurate technique to avoid errors in BP measurement (Muntner et al., 2019; Pickering et al., 2005; Whelton et al., 2018). Box 2-4 on page 79 identifies potential sources of blood pressure measurement error.

Various sites can be used to assess blood pressure. The brachial artery and the popliteal artery are used most commonly. This skill discusses using the brachial artery site to obtain a blood pressure measurement. The skill begins with the procedure for estimating systolic pressure. Estimation of systolic pressure prevents inaccurate readings in the presence of an auscultatory gap (a pause in the auscultated sounds). To identify the first Korotkoff sound accurately, the cuff must be inflated 20 to 30 mm Hg above the point at which the pulse can no longer be felt (Muntner et al., 2019).

At times, it is necessary to assess a patient for orthostatic hypotension (postural hypotension). Assessment for orthostatic hypotension may be accomplished using either an automated, electronic oscillometric blood pressure device or the auscultatory method of measuring blood pressure. Box 2-5 on page 79 outlines the procedure to assess for orthostatic hypotension.

(*continued on page 86*)

Skill 2-8 ▶ Assessing Blood Pressure by Auscultation *(continued)*

Table 2-4 Korotkoff Sounds

PHASE	DESCRIPTION	ILLUSTRATION
Phase I	Characterized by the first appearance of faint, but clear tapping sounds that gradually increase in intensity; the first tapping sound is the systolic pressure.	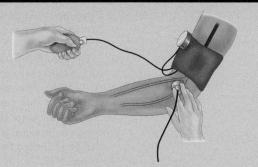 **FIGURE A.** Blood flow interrupted by inflated cuff.
Phase II	Characterized by muffled or swishing sounds; these sounds may temporarily disappear, especially in hypertensive people; the disappearance of the sound during the latter part of phase I and during phase II is called the *auscultatory gap* and may cover a range of as much as 40 mm Hg; failing to recognize this gap may cause serious errors of underestimating systolic pressure or overestimating diastolic pressure.	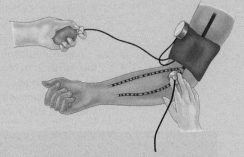 **FIGURE B.** As the pressure in the cuff is released, blood starts flowing again and Korotkoff sounds are audible.
Phase III	Characterized by distinct, loud sounds as the blood flows relatively freely through an increasingly open artery.	
Phase IV	Characterized by a distinct, abrupt, muffling sound with a soft, blowing quality; in adults, the onset of this phase is considered the first diastolic pressure.	
Phase V	The last sound heard before a period of continuous silence; the pressure at which the last sound is heard is the second diastolic pressure.	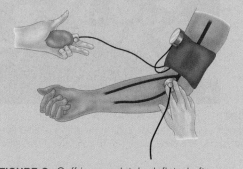 **FIGURE C.** Cuff is completely deflated after Phase V, restoring complete blood flow.

DELEGATION CONSIDERATIONS	The measurement of brachial artery blood pressure may be delegated to assistive personnel (AP) as well as to licensed practical/vocational nurses (LPN/LVNs). The decision to delegate must be based on careful analysis of the patient's needs and circumstances as well as the qualifications of the person to whom the task is being delegated. Refer to the Delegation Guidelines in Appendix A.

EQUIPMENT	• Stethoscope • Sphygmomanometer • Blood pressure cuff of appropriate size • Electronic record or pen and paper or flow sheet • Alcohol swab • PPE, as indicated

ASSESSMENT

Assess the brachial pulse, or the pulse appropriate for the site being used. Assess for an intravenous infusion or breast or axilla surgery on the side of the body corresponding to the arm used. Assess for the presence of a cast, arteriovenous shunt, or injured or diseased limb. If any of these conditions are present, do not use the affected arm to monitor blood pressure. Assess the size of the limb so that the appropriate-sized blood pressure cuff can be used (refer to Table 2-3). Assess for factors that could affect blood pressure reading, such as the patient's age, physical activity, weight, fluid balance, medications, and presence of disease and/or health conditions. Note baseline or previous blood pressure measurements. Assess the patient for pain. If the patient reports pain, give pain medication as ordered before assessing blood pressure. If the blood pressure is taken while the patient is in pain, make a notation concerning the pain if the blood pressure is elevated.

ACTUAL OR POTENTIAL HEALTH PROBLEMS AND NEEDS

Many actual or potential health problems or needs may require the use of this skill as part of related interventions. An appropriate health problem or need may include:
- Impaired Cardiac Output
- Hypertension risk
- Hypotension risk

OUTCOME IDENTIFICATION AND PLANNING

The expected outcome to achieve when measuring blood pressure is that the patient's blood pressure is measured accurately without injury. Other outcomes may be appropriate, depending on the specific diagnosis or patient problem identified for the patient.

IMPLEMENTATION

ACTION

RATIONALE

1. Check the prescribed interventions or plan of care for frequency of blood pressure measurement. More frequent measurement may be appropriate based on nursing judgment.

Provides for patient safety.

2. Perform hand hygiene and put on PPE, if indicated.

Hand hygiene and PPE prevent the spread of microorganisms. PPE is required based on transmission precautions.

3. Identify the patient.

Identifying the patient ensures the right patient receives the intervention and helps prevent errors.

4. Close the curtains around the bed and close the door to the room, if possible. Discuss the procedure with the patient and assess patient's ability to assist with the procedure. Instruct the patient to hold the limb still and refrain from speaking during the measurement. Validate that the patient has relaxed for several minutes.

This ensures the patient's privacy. Explanation relieves anxiety and facilitates cooperation. Keeping the limb still and refraining from talking provide for accurate measurement of BP levels (Muntner et al., 2019). Activity immediately before measurement can result in inaccurate results.

5. Put on gloves, if indicated.

Gloves prevent contact with blood and body fluids. Gloves are usually not required for measurement of blood pressure, unless contact with blood or body fluids is anticipated.

6. Select the appropriate arm (or alternate site) for measurement and blood pressure cuff (refer to Table 2-3).

Decision on measurement site and cuff size is based on nurse's assessment of individual patient circumstances. Incorrect cuff size contributes to the most frequent error in measurement in nonacute care settings (Muntner et al., 2019).

(continued on page 88)

Skill 2-8 ▶ Assessing Blood Pressure by Auscultation *(continued)*

ACTION

7. Have the patient assume a comfortable lying or sitting position with the forearm supported at the level of the heart and the palm of the hand upward (Figure 2). If the measurement is taken in the supine position, support the arm with a pillow. In the sitting position, support the arm yourself or by using the bedside table. If the patient is sitting, have the patient sit back in the chair so that the chair supports their back. In addition, make sure the patient keeps the legs uncrossed.

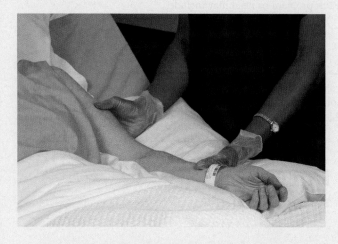

8. Expose the brachial artery by removing garments or move a sleeve if it is not too tight, above the area where the cuff will be placed.

9. Palpate the location of the brachial artery. Center the bladder of the cuff over the brachial artery, about midway on the upper arm, so that the lower edge of the cuff is about 2.5 to 5 cm (1 to 2 inches) above the inner aspect of the elbow. **Line up the artery marking on the cuff with the patient's brachial artery.** The tubing should extend from the edge of the cuff nearer the patient's elbow (Figure 3).

10. Wrap the cuff around the arm smoothly and snugly, and fasten it. Do not allow any clothing to interfere with the proper placement of the cuff.

RATIONALE

The position of the arm can have a major influence when the blood pressure is measured; if the upper arm is below the level of the right atrium, the readings will be too high. If the arm is above the level of the heart, the readings will be too low (Muntner et al., 2019; Pickering et al., 2005). This position places the brachial artery on the inner aspect of the elbow so that the bell or diaphragm of the stethoscope can rest on it easily. Support for the patient's arm prevents isometric exercise that will affect the BP level (Muntner et al., 2019). If the back is not supported, the diastolic pressure may be elevated falsely; if the legs are crossed, the systolic pressure may be elevated falsely (Muntner et al., 2019; Pickering et al., 2005).

FIGURE 2. Positioning for blood pressure assessment using brachial artery. (*Source:* Used with permission from Shutterstock. *Photo by B. Proud.*)

Clothing over the artery interferes with the ability to hear sounds and can cause inaccurate blood pressure readings. A tight sleeve would cause congestion of blood and possibly inaccurate readings (Muntner et al., 2019).

Pressure in the cuff applied directly to the artery provides the most accurate readings. If the cuff gets in the way of the stethoscope, readings are likely to be inaccurate. A cuff placed upside down with the tubing toward the patient's head may give a false reading.

A smooth cuff and snug wrapping produce equal pressure and help promote an accurate measurement. A cuff wrapped too loosely results in an inaccurate reading.

ACTION	RATIONALE

11. Check that the needle on the aneroid gauge is within the zero mark (Figure 4).

If the needle is not in the zero area, the blood pressure reading may not be accurate.

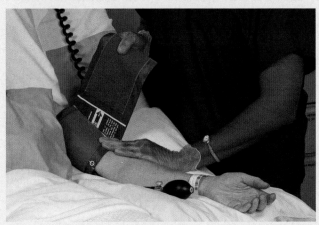

FIGURE 3. Placing the blood pressure cuff on the upper arm. (*Source:* Used with permission from Shutterstock. *Photo by B. Proud.*)

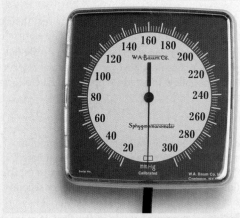

FIGURE 4. Ensuring gauge starts at zero. (*Source:* Used with permission from Shutterstock. *Photo by B. Proud.*)

Estimating Systolic Pressure

12. Palpate the pulse at the brachial or radial artery by pressing gently with the fingertips (Figure 5).

To identify the first Korotkoff sound accurately, the cuff must be inflated 20 to 30 mm Hg above the point at which the pulse can no longer be felt (Muntner et al., 2019).

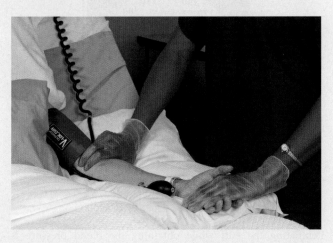

FIGURE 5. Palpating the brachial pulse. (*Source:* Used with permission from Shutterstock. *Photo by B. Proud.*)

13. Tighten the screw valve on the air pump.

The bladder within the cuff will not inflate with the valve open.

14. **Inflate the cuff while continuing to palpate the artery. Note the point on the gauge where the pulse disappears.**

The point where the pulse disappears provides an estimate of the systolic pressure. To identify the first Korotkoff sound accurately, the cuff must be inflated to a pressure above the point at which the pulse can no longer be felt.

15. Deflate the cuff and wait 1 minute.

Allowing a brief pause before continuing permits the blood to refill and circulate through the arm.

(*continued on page 90*)

Skill 2-8 ▶ Assessing Blood Pressure by Auscultation *(continued)*

ACTION

Obtaining Blood Pressure Measurement

16. Assume a position that is no more than 3 ft away from the gauge.

17. Place the stethoscope earpieces in your ears. Direct the earpieces forward into the canal and not against the ear itself.

18. Place the bell or diaphragm of the stethoscope firmly but with as little pressure as possible over the brachial artery (Figure 6). Do not allow the stethoscope to touch clothing or the cuff.

19. Pump the pressure 20 to 30 mm Hg above the point at which the systolic pressure was palpated and estimated. Open the valve on the manometer and allow air to escape slowly (allowing the gauge to drop 2 mm Hg per second) (Muntner et al., 2019).

20. **Note the point on the gauge at which the first of at least two consecutive beats appears (Figure 7). Read the pressure to the closest 2 mm Hg. Note this number as the systolic pressure.**

RATIONALE

A distance of more than about 3 ft can interfere with accurate reading of the numbers on the gauge.

Proper placement blocks extraneous noise and allows sound to travel more clearly.

Having the bell or diaphragm directly over the artery allows more accurate readings. Heavy pressure on the brachial artery distorts the shape of the artery and the sound. Placing the bell or diaphragm away from clothing and the cuff prevents noise, which would distract from the sounds made by blood flowing through the artery.

Increasing the pressure above the point where the pulse disappeared ensures a period before hearing the first sound that corresponds with the systolic pressure. It prevents misinterpreting phase II sounds as phase I sounds.

Systolic pressure is the point at which the blood in the artery is first able to force its way through the vessel at a similar pressure exerted by the air bladder in the cuff. The first sound is phase I of Korotkoff sounds.

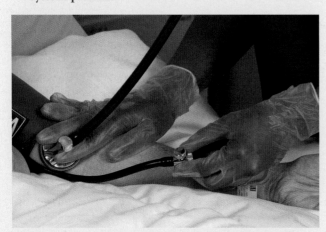

FIGURE 6. Placement of diaphragm of stethoscope. (*Source:* Used with permission from Shutterstock. *Photo by B. Proud.*)

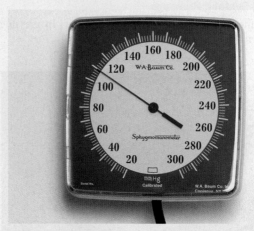

FIGURE 7. Noting the point on the gauge at which the first of at least two consecutive beats appears. (*Source:* Used with permission from Shutterstock. *Photo by B. Proud.*)

21. Do not reinflate the cuff once the air is being released to recheck the systolic pressure reading.

Reinflating the cuff while obtaining the blood pressure is uncomfortable for the patient and can cause an inaccurate reading. Reinflating the cuff causes congestion of blood in the lower arm, which lessens the loudness of Korotkoff sounds.

ACTION

RATIONALE

22. **Note the point at which the sound completely disappears (Figure 8). Read the pressure to the closest 2 mm Hg. Note this number as the diastolic pressure.**

The point at which the sound disappears corresponds to the beginning of phase V Korotkoff sounds and is generally considered the diastolic pressure reading (Muntner et al., 2019; Pickering et al., 2005).

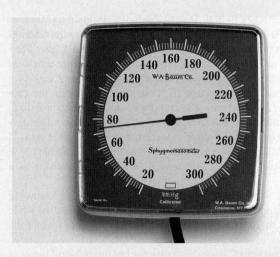

FIGURE 8. Noting the point at which the sound completely disappears. (*Source:* Used with permission from Shutterstock. *Photo by B. Proud.*)

23. Allow the remaining air to escape quickly. Repeat any suspicious reading, but wait at least 1 to 2 minutes. Deflate the cuff completely between attempts to check the blood pressure.

False readings are likely to occur if there is congestion of blood in the limb while obtaining repeated readings.

24. When measurement is completed, remove the cuff. Remove gloves, if worn. Perform hand hygiene. Cover the patient and help them to a position of comfort.

Removing gloves properly reduces the risk for infection transmission and contamination of other items. Hand hygiene prevents the spread of microorganisms. Covering and positioning the patient ensures patient comfort.

25. Clean the bell or diaphragm of the stethoscope with the alcohol wipe. Clean and store the sphygmomanometer, according to facility policy.

Appropriate cleaning deters the spread of microorganisms. Equipment should be left ready for use.

26. Remove additional PPE, if used. Perform hand hygiene.

Proper removal of PPE reduces the risk for infection transmission and contamination of other items. Hand hygiene deters the spread of microorganisms.

EVALUATION

The expected outcome has been met when the blood pressure has been measured accurately without injury and with minimal patient discomfort.

DOCUMENTATION

Guidelines

Record the findings on the electronic record or flow sheet. Communicate abnormal findings to the primary health care provider. Identify arm used and site of assessment if other than brachial.

Sample Documentation

Lippincott
DocuCare

Practice documenting blood pressure and other vital signs in *Lippincott DocuCare.*

10/18/25 0945 Blood pressure taken in right arm 180/88. Patient denies headache, dizziness. Dr. Brown notified. Captopril 25 mg PO twice per day prescribed. Blood pressure to be repeated 30 minutes after administering medication.

—M. Evans, RN

(continued on page 92)

Skill 2-8 ▶ Assessing Blood Pressure by Auscultation *(continued)*

DEVELOPING CLINICAL REASONING AND CLINICAL JUDGMENT

SPECIAL CONSIDERATIONS

General Considerations

- Blood pressure measurements should be checked in both arms at the first examination (Muntner et al., 2019; Pickering et al., 2005). Most people have differences in blood pressure readings between arms. When there is a consistent interarm difference, use the arm with the higher pressure (Muntner et al., 2019; Pickering et al., 2005). Separate repeated blood pressure measurements in the same arm by 1 to 2 minutes to avoid inaccurate results (Muntner et al., 2019).
- Incorrect cuff size contributes to the most frequent error in measurement in nonacute care settings (Muntner et al., 2019). *If the cuff is too narrow,* the reading could be erroneously high because the pressure is not evenly transmitted to the artery. *If a cuff is too wide,* the reading may be erroneously low because pressure is dispersed over a disproportionately large surface area.
- Blood pressure can be assessed using an automatic electronic blood pressure monitor (see Skill 2-7); systolic blood pressure can be assessed using Doppler ultrasound (see the accompanying Skill Variation).
- Diastolic blood pressure measured while the patient is supine is approximately 1 to 5 mm Hg higher than when measured while the patient is sitting; systolic blood pressure measured while the patient is supine is approximately 3 to 10 mm Hg higher than when measured while the patient is sitting (Muntner et al., 2019).
- The wrist site for measurement has been suggested as an alternative for obtaining blood pressure readings in people who are obese. It is often difficult to obtain the appropriately sized cuff for the upper arm, given arm circumference and conical-shaped upper arms common in obesity. The conical shape of the upper arm makes it difficult to fit the cuff to the arm, increasing the likelihood of inaccurate blood pressure measurement (Halm, 2014). Thus, measurement in the forearm can be a possible solution to this problem (Muntner et al., 2019; Palatini, 2018).
- When the patient's brachial artery is inaccessible and/or the use of the upper arm is contraindicated, you can assess the blood pressure using the popliteal artery in the leg. The systolic blood pressure is at least 15 to 20 mm Hg higher at this site than the arm, although the diastolic pressure is the same (Muntner et al., 2019; Sheppard et al., 2019).

Infant and Child Considerations

- In children, if elevated blood pressure is present when measuring with an oscillometric device, auscultation should be performed to define blood pressure levels (Muntner et al., 2019).
  - Blood pressure should be taken in the right arm for children to align with normative data (Muntner et al., 2019).
  - In infants and small children, the lower extremities are commonly used for blood pressure monitoring at the popliteal, dorsalis pedis, and posterior tibial sites. In children older than 1 year of age, the systolic pressure in the thigh tends to be 10 to 40 mm Hg higher than in the arm; the diastolic pressure remains the same (Kyle & Carman, 2021).
- Infants and children presenting with cardiac complaints may have blood pressures assessed in all four extremities. Large differences among blood pressure readings between the upper and lower extremities can indicate heart defects, such as coarctation of the aorta (Kyle & Carman, 2021).

Community-Based Care Considerations

- Patient and family/caregiver education related to home blood pressure monitoring (HBPM) should include information about hypertension; selection of equipment; appropriate procedures; and interpretation of results (Whelton et al., 2018).
- Automated blood pressure devices in public locations are generally inaccurate and inconsistent. In addition, the cuffs on these devices are inadequate for people with large arms (Pickering et al., 2005).
- Use of an automated validated digital monitoring device is suggested as best practice (Whelton et al., 2018). Use of auscultatory devices is not recommended for HBPM because patients, family, and/or caregivers rarely master the technique required for accurate use of these devices (Whelton et al., 2018). Refer to information in Skill 2-7.

Skill Variation ▶ Assessing Systolic Blood Pressure Using Doppler Ultrasound

An indirect blood pressure measurement may be obtained a Doppler ultrasound device, which amplifies sound, and a sphygmomanometer. It is especially useful if the sounds are indistinct or inaudible with a regular stethoscope. This method provides only an estimate of systolic blood pressure.

1. Determine the need to use a Doppler ultrasound device for measurement of systolic blood pressure.

2. Perform hand hygiene and put on PPE, if indicated.

3. Identify the patient.

4. Explain the procedure to the patient.
5. Close the curtains around the bed and close the door to the room, if possible.
6. Select the appropriate limb for application of cuff.
7. Have the patient assume a comfortable lying or sitting position with the appropriate limb exposed.
8. Center the bladder of the cuff over the artery, lining up the artery marker on the cuff with the artery.
9. Wrap the cuff around the limb smoothly and snugly, and fasten it. Do not allow any clothing to interfere with proper placement of the cuff.
10. Check that the needle on the aneroid gauge is within the zero mark, if using a sphygmomanometer.
11. Place a small amount of conducting gel to the site where you expect to auscultate the pulse.
12. Hold the Doppler device in your nondominant hand. Using your dominant hand, touch the probe lightly to the skin with the probe tip in the gel. Adjust the volume, as needed. Hold the probe perpendicular to the skin. Slowly move the Doppler tip around until you hear the pulse.
13. Once the pulse is found using the Doppler device, close the valve to the sphygmomanometer. Tighten the screw valve on the air pump.
14. Inflate the cuff while continuing to use the Doppler device on the artery. Note the point on the gauge where the pulse disappears (Figure A).

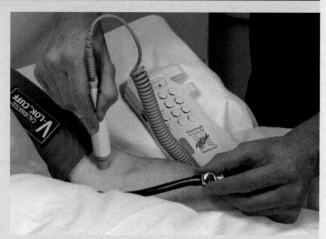

FIGURE A. Inflating cuff while listening to artery pulsations. (*Source:* Used with permission from Shutterstock. *Photo by B. Proud.*)

15. Open the valve on the manometer and allow air to escape quickly. Repeat the measurement if a suspicious reading is obtained, but wait at least 1 minute between readings to allow normal circulation to return in the limb. Deflate the cuff completely between attempts to check the blood pressure.
16. Remove the Doppler tip and turn off the Doppler device. Wipe excess gel off the patient's skin with tissue. Remove the cuff.
17. Wipe any gel remaining on the Doppler probe off with a tissue. Clean the Doppler device according to facility policy or manufacturer's recommendations.
18. Return the Doppler device to the charge base.

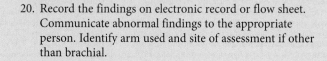

19. Remove PPE, if used. Perform hand hygiene.

20. Record the findings on electronic record or flow sheet. Communicate abnormal findings to the appropriate person. Identify arm used and site of assessment if other than brachial.

EVIDENCE FOR PRACTICE ▶

SCREENING AND MANAGEMENT OF HIGH BLOOD PRESSURE IN CHILDREN AND ADOLESCENTS

Flynn, J. T., Kaelber, D. C., Baker-Smith, C. M., Blowey, D., Carroll, A. F., Daniels, S. R., de Ferranti, S. D., Dionne, J. M., Falkner, B., Flinn, S. K., Gidding, S. S., Goodwin, C., Leu, M. G., Powers, M. E., Rea, C., Samuels, J., Simasek, M., Thaker, V. V., & Urbina, E. M. (2017). Clinical practice guideline for screening and management of high blood pressure in children and adolescents. *Pediatrics, 140*(3), e2 0171904. https://doi.org/10.1542/peds.2017-1904

This guideline provides evidence-based recommendations to guide measurement of blood pressure in children and adolescents.

Refer to details in the Evidence for Practice in Skill 2-7.

Enhance Your Understanding

Focusing on Patient Care: Developing Clinical Reasoning and Clinical Judgment

Consider the case scenarios at the beginning of the chapter as you answer the following questions to enhance your understanding and apply what you have learned.

QUESTIONS

1. Tyrone Jeffries, who is 5 years old with a fever of 101.3°F (38.5°C), is suspected of having a middle-ear infection. You need to obtain another set of vital signs for him. As you approach with the electronic thermometer, Tyrone begins to scream, saying, "Go away. I don't want it!" How would you respond?

2. Toby White, who is 26 years old with a history of asthma, has a respiratory rate of 32 breaths per minute. What other assessments would be most important to make?

3. Carl Glatz, the 58-year-old man receiving medications for hypertension, asks you about how he should monitor his blood pressure at home. What information would you suggest?

You can find suggested answers after the Bibliography at the end of this chapter.

Integrated Case Study Connection

The case studies in the back of the book focus on integrating concepts. Refer to the following case studies to enhance your understanding of the concepts and skills in this chapter.

- Basic Case Studies: Abigail Cantonelli, page 1193; James White, page 1196; Naomi Bell, page 1198; Joe LeRoy, page 1203.

- Intermediate Case Studies: Olivia Greenbaum, page 1209; Victoria Holly, page 1211; Jason Brown, page 1215; Lucille Howard, page 1219; Janice Romero, page 1220; Gwen Galloway, page 1221.
- Advanced Case Studies: Cole McKean, page 1225.

Bibliography

Allan, J., & Sheppard, K. (2018). Monitoring a pulse in adults. *British Journal of Nursing, 27*(21), 1237–1239. https://doi.org/10.12968/bjon.2018.27.21.1237

Alne, T. (2020). Therapeutic hypothermia. Comparing surface vs intravascular cooling. *Dimensions of Critical Care Nursing, 39*(1), 12–22. https://doi.org/10.1097/DCC.0000000000000398

American Academy of Pediatrics (AAP). (2020). *AAP pediatric hypertension guidelines.* https://www.mdcalc.com/aap-pediatric-hypertension-guidelines

American Heart Association. (2017). *Understanding blood pressure readings.* http://www.heart.org/HEARTORG/Conditions/HighBloodPressure/KnowYourNumbers/Understanding-Blood-Pressure-Readings_UCM_301764_Article.jsp#.WrZcg4jwaUl

Angelousi, A., Gererd, N., Benetos, A., et al. (2014). Association between orthostatic hypotension and cardiovascular risk, cerebrovascular risk, cognitive decline and falls as well as overall mortality: A systematic review and meta-analysis. *Journal of Hypertension, 32*(8), 1562–1571.

Arnold, A., & McNaughton, A. (2018). Accuracy of non-invasive blood pressure measurements in obese patients. *British Journal of Nursing, 27*(1), 35–40. https://doi.org/10.12968/bjon.2018.27.1.35

Asher, C., & Northington, L. (2008). Society of Pediatric Nurses. Position statement for measurement of temperature/fever in children. *Journal of Pediatric Nursing, 23*(3), 234–326. https://doi.org/10.1016/j.pedn.2008.03.005

Aw, J. (2020). The non-contact handheld cutaneous infra-red thermometer for fever screening during the COVID-19 global emergency. *Journal of Hospital Infection, 104*(4), 451. https://doi.org/10.1016/j.jhin.2020.02.010

Backer Mogensen, C., Wittenhoff, L., Fruerhøj, G., & Hansen, S. (2018). Forehead or ear temperature measurement cannot replace rectal measurements, except for screening purposes. *BMC Pediatrics, 18*(1), 15. https://doi.org/10.1186/s12887-018-0994-1

Bayhan, C., Özsürekçi, Y., Tekçam, N., Güloğlu, A., Ehliz, G., Ceyhan, M., & Kara, A. (2014). Comparison of infrared tympanic thermometer with non-contact infra-red thermometer. *Journal of Pediatric Infectious Diseases, 8*, 52–55. DOI:10.5152/ced.2014.1698

Bell, E. (n.d.). *Iowa neonatology handbook. Servocontrol: Incubator and radiant warmer.* University of Iowa Stead Family Children's Hospital. https://uichildrens.org/health-library/servocontrol-incubator-and-radiant-warmer?id=234214

Berksoy, E. A., Bağ, Ö, Yazici, S., & Çelik, T. (2018). Use of noncontact infrared thermography to measure temperature in children in a triage room. *Medicine, 97*(5), e9737. https://doi.org/10.1097/MD.0000000000009737

Bickley, L. S. (2021). *Bates' guide to physical examination and history taking* (13th ed.). Wolters Kluwer.

Brekke, I. J., Puntervoll, L. H., Pedersen, P. B., Kellett, J., & Brabrand, M. (2019). The value of vital sign trends in predicting and monitoring clinical deterioration: A systematic review. *PloS One, 14*(1), e0210875. https://doi.org/10.1371/journal.pone.0210875

Broskinski, C., Valdez, S., Riddell, A., & Riffenburgh, R. H. (2018). Comparison of temporal artery versus rectal temperature in emergency department patients who are unable to participate in oral temperature assessment. *Journal of Emergency Nursing, 44*(1), 57–63. https://doi.org/10.1016/j.jen.2017.04.015

Burchill, C., Anderson, B., & O'Connor, P. (2015). Exploration of nurse practices and attitudes related to postoperative vital signs. *Medsurg Nursing, 24*(4), 249–255.

Burns, S. M., & Delgado, S. A. (2019). *AACN Essentials of critical care nursing* (4th ed.). McGraw-Hill Education.

Canadian Agency for Drugs and Technologies in Health. (2014). *Non-contact thermometers for detecting fever: A review of clinical effectiveness.* https://www.ncbi.nlm.nih.gov/books/NBK263237/pdf/Bookshelf_NBK263237.pdf

Centers for Disease Control and Prevention (CDC). (n.d.). *Sequence for putting on personal protective equipment and how to safely remove personal protective equipment* [Poster]. https://www.cdc.gov/hai/pdfs/ppe/PPE-Sequence.pdf

Centers for Disease Control and Prevention (CDC). (2007; updated 2019). *Guideline for isolation precautions: Preventing transmission of infectious agents in healthcare settings.* https://www.cdc.gov/infectioncontrol/guidelines/isolation/index.html

Centers for Disease Control and Prevention (CDC). (2019). *Hand hygiene in healthcare settings.* https://www.cdc.gov/handhygiene/index.html

Cheng, R. Z., Bhalla, V., & Chang, T. I. (2019). Comparison of routine and automated office blood pressure measurement. *Blood Pressure Monitoring, 24*(4), 174–178. https://doi.org/10.1097/MBP.0000000000000392

Churpek, M. M., Adhikari, R., & Edelson, D. P. (2016). The value of vital sign trends for detecting clinical deterioration on the wards. *Resuscitation, 102*, 1–5. https://doi.org/10.1016/j.resuscitation.2016.02.005

Dalton, M., Harrison, J., Malin, A., & Leavey, C. (2018). Factors that influence nurses' assessment of patient acuity and response to acute deterioration. *British Journal of Nursing, 27*(4), 212–218. https://doi.org/10.12968/bjon.2018.27.4.212

Eliopoulos, C. (2018). *Gerontological nursing* (9th ed.). Wolters Kluwer.

Elliott, M., & Baird, J. (2019). Pulse oximetry and the enduring neglect of respiratory rate assessment: A commentary on patient surveillance. *British Journal of Nursing, 28*(19), 1256–1259. https://doi.org/10.12968/bjon.2019.28.19.1256

Exergen. (n.d.a). *Temporal artery thermometry.* https://www.exergen.com/tathermometry/index.htm

Exergen. (n.d.b). *Temporal artery temperature measurement. Training handout for nursing staff.*

https://www.exergen.com/wp-content/uploads/2018/05/TAT-5000-Training-Trifold.pdf

Fitzwater, J., Johnstone, C., Schuppers, M., Cordoza, M., & Norman, B. (2019). A comparison of oral, axillary, and temporal artery temperature measuring devices in adult acute care. *Medsurg Nursing, 28*(1), 35–41.

Flynn, J. T., Kaelber, D. C., Baker-Smith, C. M., Blowey, D., Carroll, A. F., Daniels, S. R., de Ferranti, S. D., Dionne, J. M., Falkner, B., Flinn, S. K., Gidding, S. S., Goodwin, C., Leu, M. G., Powers, M. E., Rea, C., Samuels, J., Simasek, M., Thaker, V. V., & Urbina, E. M. (2017). Clinical practice guideline for screening and management of high blood pressure in children and adolescents. *Pediatrics, 140*(3), e2 0171904. https://doi.org/10.1542/peds.2017-1904

Franconi, I., La Cerra, C., Marucci, A. R., Petrucci, C., & Lancia, L. (2018). Digital axillary and non-contact infrared thermometers for children. *Clinical Nursing Research, 27*(2), 180–190. https://doi.org/10.1177/1054773816676538

Freeman, R., Abuzinadah, A. R., Gibbons, C., Jones, P., Miglis, M. G., & Sinn, D. I. (2018). Orthostatic hypotension. JACC State-of-the-art review. *Journal of the American College of Cardiology, 72*(11), 1294–1309. https://doi.org/10.1016/j.jacc.2018.05.079

Gates, D., Horner, V., Bradley, L., Fogle Sheperd, T., John, O., & Higgins, M. (2018). Temperature measurements. Comparison of different thermometer types for patients with cancer. *Clinical Journal of Oncology Nursing, 22*(6), 611–617. https://doi.org/10.1188/18.CJON.611-617

Godbole, G. P., & Aggarwal, B. (2018). Review of management strategies for orthostatic hypotension in older people. *Journal of Pharmacy Practice and Research, 48*(5), 483–491. https://doi.org/10.1002/jppr.1484

Halm, M. A. (2014). Arm circumference, shape, and length: How interplaying variables affect blood pressure measurement in obese persons. *American Journal of Critical Care, 23*(2), 166–170. https://doi.org/10.4037/ajcc2014364

Harvard Medical School. (2019). *Reading the new blood pressure guidelines.* Harvard Health Publishing. https://www.health.harvard.edu/heart-health/reading-the-new-blood-pressure-guidelines

Hayward, G., Verbakel, J. Y., Ismail, F. A., Edwards, G., Wang, K., Fleming, S., Holtman, G. A., Glogowska, M., Morris, E., Curtis, K., & van den Bruel, A. (2020). Non-contact infrared versus axillary and tympanic thermometers in children attending primary care: A mixed-methods study of accuracy and acceptability. *British Journal of General Practice, 70*(693), e236–e244. https://doi.org/10.3399/bjgp20X708845

Hess, D. R., MacIntyre, N. R., Galvin, W. F., & Mishoe, S. C. (2021). *Respiratory care. Principles and practice* (4th ed.). Jones & Bartlett Learning.

Hill, A., Kelly, E., Horseill, M. S., & Watson, M. O. (2018). The effects of awareness and count duration on adult respiratory rate measurements: An experimental study. *Journal of Clinical Nursing, 27*(3-4), 546–554. https://doi.org/10.1111/jocn.13861

Hinkle, J. L., & Cheever, K. H. (2018). *Brunner & Suddarth's textbook of medical-surgical nursing* (14th ed.). Wolters Kluwer.

Hogan-Quigley, B., Palm, M. L., & Bickley, L. S. (2017). *Bates' nursing guide to physical examination and history taking* (2nd ed.). Wolters Kluwer.

Jarvis, C., & Echkardt, A. (2020). *Physical examination & health assessment* (8th ed.). Elsevier.

Jensen, S. (2019.) *Nursing health assessment: A best practice approach* (3rd ed.). Wolters Kluwer.

Joseph, R. A., Derstine, S., & Killian, M. (2017). Ideal site for skin temperature probe placement on infants in the NICU. *Advances in Neonatal Care, 17*(2), 114–122. https://doi.org/10.1097/ANC.0000000000000369

Kallioinen, N., Hill, A., Horswill, M. S., Ward, H. E., & Watson, M. O. (2017). Sources of inaccuracy in the measurement of adult patients' resting blood pressure in clinical settings: A systematic review. *Journal of Hypertension, 35*(3), 421–441. https://doi.org/10.1097/HJH.0000000000001197

Kersey-Matusiak, G. (2019). *Delivering culturally competent nursing care. Working with diverse and vulnerable populations* (2nd ed.). Springer Publishing Company.

Kiekkas, P., Aretha, D., Almpani, E., & Stefanopoulos, N. (2019). Temporal artery thermometry in pediatric patients: Systematic review and meta-analysis. *Journal of Pediatric Nursing, 46*, 89–99. https://doi.org/10.1016/j.pedn.2019.03.004

Kurnat-Thoma, E., Edwards, V., & Emery, K. (2018). Axillary, tympanic and temporal thermometry comparison in a community hospital pediatric unit. *Pediatric Nursing, 44*(5), 235–246.

Kyle, T., & Carman, S. (2021). *Essentials of pediatric nursing* (4th ed.). Wolters Kluwer.

Lipsitz, L. A. (2017). Orthostatic hypotension and falls. *Journal of the American Geriatrics Society, 65*(3), 470–471. https://doi-org.libproxy.gmercyu.edu/10.1111/jgs.14745

Ludwig, J., & McWhinnie, H. (2019). Antipyretic drugs in patients with fever and infection: Literature review. *British Journal of Nursing, 28*(10), 610–618. https://doi.org/10.12968/bjon.2019.28.10.610

Mason, T. M., Boubekri, A., Lalau, J., Patterson, A., Hartranft, S. R., & Sutton, S. K. (2017). Equivalence study of two temperature-measurement methods in febrile adult patients with cancer. *Oncology Nursing Forum, 44*(2), E82–E87. https://doi.org/10.1188/17.ONF.E82-E87

Mayo Clinic. (2020a). *Thermometer basics: Taking your child's temperature.* https://www.mayoclinic.org/healthy-lifestyle/infant-and-toddler-health/in-depth/thermometer/art-20047410

Mayo Clinic. (2020b). *Get the most out of home blood pressure monitoring.* https://www.mayoclinic.org/diseases-conditions/high-blood-pressure/in-depth/high-blood-pressure/art-20047889

Morton, P. G., & Fontaine, D. K. (2018). *Critical care nursing. A holistic approach* (11th ed.). Wolters Kluwer.

Muntner, P., Shimbo, D., Carey, R. M., Charleston, J. B., Gaillard, T., Misra, S., Myers, M. G., Ogedegbe, G., Schwartz, J. E., Townsend, R. R., Urbina, E. M., Viera, A., J., White, W. B., & Wright, J. T. (2019). Measurement of blood pressure in humans. A scientific statement from the American Heart Association. *Hypertension, 73*(5), e35–e66. https://doi.org/10.1161/HYP.0000000000000087

Myers, M. G., Asmar, R., & Staessen, J. A. (2018). Office blood pressure measurement in the 21st century. *Journal of Clinical Hypertension, 20*(7), 1104–1107. https://doi.org/10.1111/jch.13276

National Heart, Lung, and Blood Institute (NHLBI). (n.d.). *Low blood pressure. Also known as hypotension.* Retrieved February 28, 2021, from http://www.nhlbi.nih.gov/health/health-topics/topics/hyp

Norris, T. L. (2019). *Porth's essentials of pathophysiology* (5th ed.). Wolters Kluwer.

Oguz, F., Yildiz, I., Varkal, M. A., Hizli, Z., Toprak, S., Kaymakci, K., Saygili, S. K., Kilic, A., & Unuvar, E. (2018). Axillary and tympanic temperature measurement in children and normal values for ages. *Pediatric Emergency Care, 34*(3), 169–173. https://doi.org/10.1097/PEC.0000000000000693

Opersteny, E., Anderson, H., Bates, J., Davenport, K., Husby, J., Myking, K., & Oron, A. P. (2017). Precision, sensitivity and patient preference of non-invasive thermometers in a pediatric surgical acute care setting. *Journal of Pediatric Nursing, 35*, 36–41. https://doi.org/10.1016/j.pedn.2017.02.003

Palatini, P. (2018, August 15). Blood pressure measurement in the obese: Still a challenging problem. *E-Journal of Cardiology Practice, 16*(21). https://www.escardio.org/Journals/E-Journal-of-Cardiology-Practice/Volume-16/Blood-pressure-measurement-in-the-obese-still-a-challenging-problem

Pickering, T. G., Hall, J. E., Appel, L. J., Falkner, B. E., Graves, J., Hill, M.N., Jones, D. W., Kurtz, T., Sheps, S. G., & Roccella, E. J. (2005). Recommendations for blood pressure measurement in humans and experimental animals. Part 1: Blood pressure measurement in humans: A statement for professionals from the subcommittee of professional and public education of the American Heart Association Council on High Blood Pressure Research. *Circulation, 111*, 697–716. http://circ.ahajournals.org/content/111/5/697.abstract

Pouy, S., & Chehrzad, M. M. (2019). Identification of the best skin temperature probe attachment place in premature neonates nursed under radiant warmers in NICU: A diagnostic clinical trial study. *Journal of Neonatal Nursing, 25*(2), 69–73. https://doi.org/10.1016/j.jnn.2018.10.001

Robertson, M., & Hill, B. (2019). Monitoring temperature. *British Journal of Nursing, 28*(6), 344–347.

Rolfe, S. (2019). The importance of respiratory rate monitoring. *British Journal of Nursing, 28*(8), 504–508. https://doi.org/10.12968/bjon.2019.28.8.504

Ryan-Wenger, N. A., Sims, M. A., Patton, R. A., & Williamson, J. (2018). Selection of the most accurate thermometer devices for clinical practice: Part 1: Meta-analysis of the accuracy of non-core thermometer devices compared to core body temperature. *Pediatric Nursing, 44*(3), 116–133.

Seattle Children's. (2022, April 6). Fever—How to take the temperature. https://www.seattlechildrens.org/conditions/a-z/fever-how-to-take-the-temperature/

Sheppard, J. P., Albasri, A., Franssen, M., Fletcher, B., Pealing, L., Roberts, N., Obeid, A., Pucci, M., McManus, R. J., & Martin, U. (2019). Defining the relationship between arm and leg blood pressure readings: A systematic review and meta-analysis. *Journal of Hypertension, 37*(4), 660–670. https://doi.org/10.1097/HJH.0000000000001958

Silbert-Flagg, J., & Pillitteri, A. (2018). *Maternal & child health nursing* (8th ed.). Wolters Kluwer.

Stergiou, G. S., Dolan, E., Kollias, A., Poulter, N. R., Shennan, A., Staessen, J. A., Ahang, Z. Y., & Weber, M. A. (2018). Blood pressure measurement in special populations and circumstances. *Journal of Clinical Hypertension (Greenwich), 20*(7), 1122–1127. https://doi.org/10.1111/jch.13296

Stergiou, G. S., Kario, K., Kollias, A., McManus, R. J., Ohkubo, T., Parati, G., & Imai, Y. (2018). Home blood pressure monitoring in the 21st century. *Journal of Clinical Hypertension, 20*(7), 1116–1121. https://doi.org/10.1111/jch.13284

Sund-Levander, M., & Grodzinsky, E. (2013). Assessment of body temperature measurement options. *British Journal of Nursing, 22*(16), 942, 944–950.

Taylor, C., Lynn, P., & Bartlett, J. (2023). *Fundamentals of nursing: The art and science of person-centered care* (10th ed.). Wolters Kluwer.

Tessorolo Souza, B., Teixeira Lopes, M. C. B., Okuno, M. F. P., Batista, R. E. A., Teixeira de Góis, A. F., & Campanharo, C. R. V. (2019). Identification of warning signs for prevention of in-hospital cardiorespiratory arrest. *Revista Latino-Americana de Enfermagem, 27*, e3072. DOI: 10.1590/1518-8345.2853.3072

Toughy, T. A., & Jett, K. (2018). *Ebersol and Hess' Gerontological nursing & healthy aging* (5th ed.). Elsevier.

U.S. Environmental Protection Agency (EPA). (n.d.). *Mercury thermometers.* Retrieved February 28, 2021, from https://www.epa.gov/mercury/mercury-thermometers

U.S. Food and Drug Administration (FDA). (2020). *Non-contact infrared thermometers.* https://www.fda.gov/medical-devices/general-hospital-devices-and-supplies/non-contact-infrared-thermometers

U.S. National Library of Medicine. (2020, February 25). *Low blood pressure.* MedlinePlus. https://medlineplus.gov/ency/article/007278.htm

VHA Center for Engineering & Occupational Safety and Health (CEOSH) (VHACEOSH). (2016). Safe patient handling and mobility guidebook. http://www.tnpatientsafety.com/pubfiles/Initiatives/workplace-violence/sphm-pdf.pdf

Wang, K., Gill, P., Wolstenholme, J., Heneghan, C., Thompson, M., Price, C. P., Van den Bruel, A., & Plüddemann, A. (2013). *Non-contact infrared thermometers.* National Institute for Health Research. https://www.community.healthcare.mic.nihr.ac.uk/reports-and-resources/horizon-scanning-reports/hs-report-0025

Weber, J. R., & Kelley, J. H. (2018). *Health assessment in nursing* (6th ed.). Wolters Kluwer.

Whelton, P. K., Carey, R. M., Aronow, W. S., Casey, D. E., Collins, K. J., Himmelfarb, C. D., DePalma, S. M., Gidding, S., Jamerson, K. A., Jones, D. W., MacLaughlin, E. J., Muntner, P., Ovbiagele, B., Smith, S. C., Spencer, C. C., Stafford, R. S., Taler, S. J., Thomas, R. J., Williams, Sr., K. A.,... Wright, J. T., Jr. (2018). 2017 ACC/AHA/AAPA/ABC/ACPM/AGS/APhA/ASH/ASPC/NMA/PCNA Guideline for the prevention, detection, evaluation, and management of high blood pressure in adults. *Hypertension, 71*(4), 1269–1324. https://doi.org/10.1161/HYP.0000000000000065

World Health Organization (WHO). (2019, September 13). *Hypertension.* https://www.who.int/news-room/fact-sheets/detail/hypertension

Writing Committee Members; Gerhard-Herman, M. D., Gornik, H. L., Barrett, C., Barshes, N. R., Corriere, M. A., Drachman, D. E., Fleisher, L. A., Fowkes, F. G. R., Hamburg, N. M., Kinlay, S., Lookstein, R., Misra, S., Mureebe, L., Olin, J. W., Patel, R. A. G., Regensteiner, J. G., Schanzer, A., Shishehbor, M. H.,… Wijeysundera, D. N. (2017). 2016 AHA/ACC Guideline on the management of patients with lower extremity peripheral artery disease: Executive Summary. *Vascular Medicine, 22*(3), NPI–NP43. https://doi.org/10.1177/1358863X17701592

SUGGESTED ANSWERS FOR FOCUSING ON PATIENT CARE: DEVELOPING CLINICAL REASONING AND CLINICAL JUDGMENT

1. First, assess the problem, talking with Tyrone and his mother, using age-appropriate communication with Tyrone. Because potentially he is thought to have an ear infection, he may be having pain in one or both ears. Assess his status and ability to cooperate and consider another route for temperature measurement. Temporal artery or axillary measurement may be indicated, based on your assessment and facility policy.

2. In addition to the respiratory rate, note the depth and rhythm of the respirations. Auscultate lung sounds. Measure the patient's oxygen saturation level with pulse oximetry. Ask the patient about recent activity and the presence of factors that may have caused an acute asthma attack, and for factors that could affect respirations, such as exercise, medications, smoking, chronic illness or conditions, neurologic injury, pain, and anxiety. Note baseline or previous respiratory measurements. Assess patient for any signs of respiratory distress, which include retractions, nasal flaring, grunting, and orthopnea (breathing more easily in an upright position).

3. Home monitoring of blood pressure for patients with hypertension is strongly recommended. Advise Mr. Glatz that automated blood pressure devices in public areas are generally inaccurate and inconsistent. Use a cuff size appropriate for limb circumference. Inform him that cuff sizes range from a pediatric cuff to a large thigh cuff and that a poorly fitting cuff can result in an inaccurate measurement. Discuss digital blood pressure monitoring equipment. Use of an automated validated digital monitoring device is suggested as best practice for HBPM (Whelton et al., 2018). Although more costly than manual cuffs, most provide an easy-to-read recording of systolic and diastolic measurements.

3

Health Assessment

Focusing on Patient Care

This chapter will help you develop some of the assessment skills related to health assessment necessary to care for the following patients:

William Lincoln, age 54, comes to the clinic for a routine checkup.

Lois Felker, age 30, has a history of type 1 diabetes. She is a patient in the hospital.

Bobby Williams, age 14, has been brought to the emergency department by his parents and is suspected of having appendicitis.

Refer to Focusing on Patient Care: Developing Clinical Reasoning and Clinical Judgment at the end of the chapter to apply what you learn.

Learning Outcomes

After completing the chapter, you will be able to accomplish the following:

1. Describe the components of a health assessment.
2. Describe and perform the components of a general survey.
3. Weigh a patient using a bed scale.
4. Describe and conduct a health history and physical assessment.
5. Use appropriate equipment while performing health assessment.
6. Position the patient correctly to perform a systematic physical assessment.
7. Verbalize the appropriate rationales for performing the specific systematic assessment techniques.
8. Assess the skin, hair, and nails.
9. Assess the head and neck.
10. Assess the thorax, lungs, and breasts.
11. Assess the cardiovascular system.
12. Assess the abdomen.
13. Assess female genitalia.
14. Assess male genitalia.
15. Assess the neurologic, musculoskeletal, and peripheral vascular systems.

Nursing Concepts

- Assessment
- Clinical Decision Making/Clinical Judgment
- Communication
- Therapeutic communication

97

Health assessment involves gathering information about the health status of the patient, the overall level of physical, psychological, sociocultural, developmental, functional, and spiritual health of a patient. A nursing health assessment is a holistic collection of information about how a person's health status is affecting activity levels and abilities to perform tasks. A nursing health assessment also explores how patients are coping with their health issues and any related loss of function or change in ability to function (Jensen, 2019). The nurse gathers, evaluates, and synthesizes information (**data**). The type and amount of information obtained vary and are determined based on the patient's needs, health care setting, and circumstances. The nurse identifies actual or potential health problems and/or needs that require nursing care based on evaluation of the gathered data. Assessment data are used to plan and implement nursing interventions and evaluate patient care outcomes to deliver the best possible care for each patient. A health assessment includes a health history and a physical assessment.

A **health history** is a collection of subjective data that provides information about the patient's health status. Information is ideally collected during an interview with the patient. However, the patient's family members and/or caregivers may also be an important source of data. If available, the health records of the patient can be a source of additional information. Components of the health history include biographical data, the reason the patient is seeking health care, present health concerns or history of those health concerns, past health history, family health history, functional health, and a review of systems. Questions should be adapted to the individual patient, based on the setting, situation, and ongoing information as the health assessment proceeds. Be sure to use language the patient can understand; avoid using medical terms and jargon. Nurses use therapeutic communication skills, including interviewing techniques, during the health history to gather data to identify actual and potential health problems as well as sources of patient strength. In addition, during the health history, the nurse begins to establish an effective nurse–patient relationship. Fundamentals Review 3-1 summarizes major components of a health history.

Physical assessment is a collection of objective data that provides information about changes in the patient's body systems. These data are obtained through direct observation or elicited through examination techniques, such as **inspection**, **palpation**, **percussion**, and **auscultation** (Fundamentals Review 3-2). The use of percussion and deep palpation are advanced physical assessment skills, usually performed by advanced practice professionals, health care providers with advanced education. *Percussion and deep palpation will not be discussed as part of physical assessment in this chapter. Refer to information on a health assessment text for details of these advanced assessment skills.* To perform a physical examination, the nurse requires knowledge of anatomy and physiology, the equipment used for assessing body systems, and proper patient positioning and draping.

Nurses should be familiar with the general health beliefs of various cultural and ethnic groups to improve the effectiveness of health care services and provide care within a cultural context. Nurses should know risk factors for alterations in health that are based on racial inheritance and ethnic backgrounds. They should also be aware of the normal variations that occur within races, and should understand how cultural characteristics, such as religion and spirituality, may impact health. When working with a patient from an unfamiliar culture, inquire about preferences and practices before beginning the examination (Jensen, 2019).

Laboratory tests and diagnostic procedures provide crucial information about a patient's health. These results become a part of the total health assessment. Nurses assist before, during, and after some diagnostic tests, and complete other testing as prescribed. Refer to Chapter 18 for information related to laboratory specimen collection for commonly prescribed laboratory testing.

For a comprehensive assessment, the nurse integrates individual assessments following a systematic head-to-toe format. *However, not all assessments included in a comprehensive physical assessment are covered in this chapter.* Advanced practice professionals (health care providers with advanced education) typically perform some of the assessments included in a comprehensive or focused exam, such as an internal eye examination, a vaginal examination, or a rectal examination. *Refer to information on a health assessment text for details of these advanced assessment skills.*

It is often not necessary to perform a comprehensive assessment during each patient encounter. Assessment focused on the circumstances and the needs of a particular patient can help to prioritize care. A short, focused general assessment can be used to establish a baseline to prioritize nursing care. This basic assessment is based on the patient's diagnosis, health problems, individual circumstances, and potential complications helps to quickly identify changes in the patent's clinical status (Henley Haugh, 2015). Nursing knowledge, expertise, and clinical reasoning and judgment guide the nurse in decisions about which assessments are a priority for an individual patient. This prioritized initial assessment may also identify specific findings to follow up on later. Fundamentals Review 3-3 provides an example of a brief, general assessment to gather pertinent data to provide a basis for prioritizing nursing care. Nurses should use clinical judgment to adapt this generic assessment to the individual circumstances of an individual patient and to monitor for changes that might require further intervention (Henley Haugh, 2015).

Fundamentals Review 3-1

COMPONENTS OF A HEALTH HISTORY

BIOGRAPHIC DATA

Biographic information is often collected during admission to a health care facility or agency and documented on a specific form; it helps to identify the patient. Depending on the health care setting, some biographic data may be collected by people other than the nurse.

Biographic data include the patient's name, address, billing, and insurance information. Additional biographical information may include sex assigned at birth, sexual orientation, gender identity, age and birth date, marital status, occupation, race, ethnic origin, religious preference, presence of an advance directive/living will, and the patient's primary health care provider.

The source of the information is also recorded. Differences in language and culture may have an effect on the quality and safety of health care. Language has been identified as contributing to health disparities, as a significant barrier to access to health care, and a barrier to quality health care and appears to increase the risks to patient safety (Ali & Watson, 2018; Chung et al., 2020; Kersey-Matusiak, 2019; Ku & Jewers, 2013). It is important to note the patient's preferred language for discussing health care as well as any sensory or communication needs.

REASON FOR SEEKING HEALTH CARE

The reason for seeking care is a statement in the patient's own words that describes the patient's reason for seeking care. This can help to focus the rest of the assessment. Ask an open-ended question, such as, "Tell me why you are here today." Record whatever it is the person says, their description in exact words. Avoid paraphrasing or interpreting.

HISTORY OF PRESENT HEALTH CONCERN

When taking the patient's history of present health concern, be sure to explore the symptoms thoroughly. Encourage the patient to describe and explain any symptoms. The description should include information regarding the onset of the problem; location; duration; intensity; quality/description; relieving/exacerbating factors; associated factors; past occurrences; any treatments; and how the problem has affected the patient.

PAST HEALTH HISTORY

A patient's past health history may provide insight into causes of current symptoms. It also alerts the nurse to certain risk factors. A past health history includes childhood and adult illnesses, chronic health problems and treatment, and previous surgeries or hospitalizations. This history should also include accidents or injuries, obstetric history, allergies, and the date of most recent immunizations. Vaccine recommendations are updated each year by the Centers for Disease Control and Prevention (CDC). Current guidelines for different age groups can be found on the CDC's website at www.cdc.gov (CDC, n.d.). Ask the patient about health maintenance screenings, such as routine mammograms and colorectal tests, including dates and results, as well as the use of safety measures. Ask the patient about prescribed and over-the-counter medications, including vitamins, supplements, and any home or herbal remedies. Include the name, dose, route, frequency, and purpose for each medication.

FAMILY HEALTH HISTORY

A person's family history will provide insight into diseases and conditions for which a patient may be at increased risk. Certain disorders have genetic links. Information regarding contact with family members with communicable diseases or environmental hazards can provide clues to the patient's current health or risk factors for health issues. This information can also identify important topics for health teaching and counseling.

(continued)

Fundamentals Review 3-1 continued

COMPONENTS OF A HEALTH HISTORY

FUNCTIONAL HEALTH

Information about a patient's functional health helps to identify the effects of health or illness on a patient's self-care abilities and quality of life including the strengths of the patient and areas that need to improve (Jarvis & Eckhardt, 2020; Jensen, 2019). Psychosocial factors and lifestyle and health practices can contribute to and influence a patient's overall health and well-being. Social determinants of health, the conditions (social, economic, and physical) in the environments in which people live their lives, affect a wide range of health, functioning and quality-of-life outcomes and risks (USDHHS & ODPHP, 2020).

Obtain information about the patient's social support, interpersonal relationships, available care givers, resources, and supporters that are available to help the patient cope with alterations in health and related alterations in functioning and quality of life. Obtain information about the patient's values, beliefs, and spiritual resources; self-esteem and self-concept; and coping and stress management.

Question the patient regarding personal habits, including use of alcohol, illicit drugs, and/or tobacco; environmental and occupational hazards; and intimate partner and family/caregiver (domestic) violence.

Assess the patient's level of activity, ask about the patient's level of activity and exercise; sleep and rest; and nutrition. Ask about the patient's ability to perform **activities of daily living (ADLs)**. Eating, bathing, dressing, and toileting are examples of ADLs. Assess the patient's ability to perform **instrumental activities of daily living (IADLs)**. Housekeeping, meal preparation, management of finances, and transportation are examples of IADLs. Functional health may be further assessed using a formal tool, such as the Katz Index of Independence in Activities of Daily Living, which is used with older adults (Figure 3-1).

Obtain information about the patient's mental health. Regular screenings in primary care and other health care settings enable earlier identification of mental health and substance use disorders, leading to earlier treatment and care. Screenings should be provided to people of all ages, even the young and older adults (American Mental Health Counselors Association, 2017). There are many assessment tools available to assist with screening for mental health disorders. Specific tools are available to screen for depression or suicide, for example, and to be used with specific populations, such as adolescents or older adults. The Patient Health Questionnaire-9 (PHQ-9), the most common screening tool to identify depression, is one example of a mental health assessment tool (Figure 3-2).

ACTIVITIES POINTS (1 OR 0)	INDEPENDENCE: (1 POINT) **NO** supervision, direction, or personal assistance	DEPENDENCE: (0 POINTS) **WITH** supervision, direction, personal assistance, or total care
BATHING POINTS:_____	**(1 POINT)** Bathes self completely or needs help in bathing only a single part of the body such as the back, genital area, or disabled extremity.	**(0 POINTS)** Needs help with bathing more than one part of the body, getting in or out of the tub or shower. Requires total bathing.
DRESSING POINTS:_____	**(1 POINT)** Gets clothes from closets and drawers and puts on clothes and outer garments complete with fasteners. May have help tying shoes.	**(0 POINTS)** Needs help with dressing self or needs to be completely dressed.
TOILETING POINTS:_____	**(1 POINT)** Goes to toilet, gets on and off, arranges clothes, cleans genital area without help.	**(0 POINTS)** Needs help transferring to the toilet, cleaning self, or uses bedpan or commode.
TRANSFERRING POINTS:_____	**(1 POINT)** Moves in and out of bed or chair unassisted. Mechanical transferring aides are acceptable.	**(0 POINTS)** Needs help in moving from bed to chair or requires a complete transfer.
CONTINENCE POINTS:_____	**(1 POINT)** Exercises complete self-control over urination and defecation.	**(0 POINTS)** Is partially or totally incontinent of bowel or bladder.
FEEDING POINTS:_____	**(1 POINT)** Gets food from plate into mouth without help. Preparation of food may be done by another person.	**(0 POINTS)** Needs partial or total help with feeding or requires parenteral feeding.

TOTAL POINTS = _____ 6 = High (*patient independent*) 0 = Low (*patient very dependent*)

FIGURE 3-1. Katz Index of Independence in Activities of Daily Living. (*Source:* Slightly adapted from Katz, S., Down, T. D., Cash, H. R., & Grotz, R. C. [1970]. Progress in the development of the index of ADL. *The Gerontologist, 10*[1], 20–30. Copyright © The Gerontological Society of America. Reproduced [Adapted] by permission of the publisher.)

Fundamentals Review 3-1   continued

COMPONENTS OF A HEALTH HISTORY

Over the last 2 weeks, how often have you been bothered by any of the following problems? *(Use "✓" to indicate your answer)*	Not At All	Several Days	More Than Half the Days	Nearly Every Day
1. Little interest or pleasure in doing things	0	1	2	3
2. Feeling down, depressed, or hopeless	0	1	2	3
3. Trouble falling or staying asleep, or sleeping too much	0	1	2	3
4. Feeling tired or having little energy	0	1	2	3
5. Poor appetite or overeating	0	1	2	3
6. Feeling bad about yourself—or that you are a failure or have let yourself or your family down	0	1	2	3
7. Trouble concentrating on things, such as reading the newspaper or watching television	0	1	2	3
8. Moving or speaking so slowly that other people could have noticed. Or the opposite—being so fidgety or restless that you have been moving around a lot more than usual	0	1	2	3
9. Thoughts that you would be better off dead or of hurting yourself in some way	0	1	2	3

FOR OFFICE CODING 0 + _____ + _____ + _____

= Total Score: _____

If you checked off any problems, how difficult have these problems made it for you to do your work, take care of things at home, or get along with other people?

Not difficult at all	Somewhat difficult	Very difficult	Extremely difficult
☐	☐	☐	☐

How to Score PHQ-9

Major Depressive Syndrome is suggested if:

- Of the 9 items, 5 or more are checked as at least "More than half the days"
- Either item #1 or #2 is positive, that is, at least "More than half the days"

Other Depressive Syndrome is suggested if:

- Of the 9 items, 2, 3, or 4 are check as at least "More than half the days"
- Either item #1 or #2 is positive, that is, at least "More than half the days"

FIGURE 3-2. From Patient Health Questionnaire (PHQ) Screeners. Developed by Dr. Robert L. Spitzer, Dr. Janet B. W. Williams, Dr. Kurt Kroenke, and colleagues, with an educational grant from Pfizer Inc. No permission required to reproduce, translate, display, or distribute. http://www.phqscreeners.com.

Use neutral and inclusive terms (e.g., partner) and a nonjudgmental manner to obtain information about the patient's sexual history, sexual activity, gender identity, and sexual orientation. This information will help identify the needs of individual patients and provide patient-centered, culturally considerate care (Altarum Institute, 2019; Cahill et al., 2020). Some suggested strategies and essential health questions related to assessment of sexual health are included here (Altarum Institute, 2019; Cahill et al., 2020).

- In a matter-of-fact manner, inform the patient that sexual health is important to overall health and these questions are asked of everyone.
- Allow the patient the opportunity to ask questions or voice concerns.

- Assure the patient that all information is confidential.
- Ask the following questions using neutral and inclusive terms:
  - Have you been sexually active in the last year? If yes, what types of sex do you have? With men, women, or both? How many partners have you had?
  - If no, have you ever been sexually active?
  - How do you think of yourself? Lesbian, gay, heterosexual/straight, bisexual; something else (specify); don't know
  - What is your current gender identity? Male, female, female-to-male/transgender male/transgender man, male-to-female/transgender female/transgender woman, nonbinary or nonconforming, genderqueer, additional category (specify), decline to answer

(continued)

Fundamentals Review 3-1   continued

COMPONENTS OF A HEALTH HISTORY

- What sex were you assigned at birth, as shown on your birth certificate? Male, female, decline to answer
- What are your pronouns? He/him, she/her, they/their; something else (specify)
- What do you do to protect yourself from STIs?
- Have you been vaccinated against human papillomavirus? Hepatitis A? Hepatitis B?
- What questions do you have about your body and/or sex?

Additional points related to assessment of sexual and reproductive health are included in Skills 3-8 and 3-9.

REVIEW OF SYSTEMS

A review of systems is a series of questions about all body systems that helps to reveal concerns or problems as part of the health history. Questions should be adapted to the individual patient, omitting questions that do not apply and adding questions that seem pertinent, based on the setting, situation, and ongoing information as the health assessment proceeds. The nurse should avoid using medical terms and jargon and use language the patient can understand. Examples of health history questions related to each body system (review of systems) are included in the discussion of each region of the physical examination discussed in this chapter.

Fundamentals Review 3-2

PHYSICAL ASSESSMENT TECHNIQUES

Inspection is the process of performing deliberate, purposeful observations in a systematic manner. The nurse closely observes visually, but also uses hearing and smell to gather data throughout the assessment. The nurse assesses details of the patient's appearance, behavior, and movement. Inspection begins with the initial patient contact and continues through the entire assessment. Adequate natural or artificial lighting is essential for distinguishing the color, texture, and moisture of body surfaces. The nurse inspects each area of the body for size, color, shape, position, movement, and symmetry, noting normal findings and any deviations from normal.

Palpation uses the sense of touch. The hands and fingers are sensitive tools that can assess skin temperature, turgor, texture, and moisture as well as vibrations within the body (e.g., the heart) and shape or structures within the body (e.g., the bones). Specific parts of the hand are more effective at assessing different qualities. The dorsum (back) surfaces of the hand and fingers are used for gross measure of temperature. The palmar (front) surfaces of the fingers and fingerpads are used to assess firmness, contour, shape, tenderness, and consistency. The fingerpads are best at fine discrimination. Use fingerpads to locate pulses, lymph nodes, and other small lumps, and to assess skin texture and edema. Vibration is palpated best with the ulnar, or outside, surface of the hand. For light palpation, apply pressure with the fingers together and lightly depressing the skin and underlying structures about 1 to 2 cm (0.5 to 0.75 inch). Light palpation is used to feel for pulses, tenderness, surface skin texture, temperature, moisture, and muscular resistance (Jarvis & Eckhardt, 2020; Jensen, 2019; Weber & Kelley,

2018). Advanced health care providers usually perform deep palpation. Deep palpation is used to assess organs, masses, structures that are covered by thick muscle, and tenderness (Jensen, 2019; Weber & Kelley, 2018). Refer to information on a health assessment text for details of this advanced assessment skill.

Percussion is the act of striking one object against another to produce sound. The fingertips are used to tap the body over body tissues to produce vibrations and sound waves. The characteristics of the sounds produced are used to assess the location, shape, size, and density of tissues. Abnormal sounds suggest alteration of tissues, such as an emphysematous lung, or the presence of a mass, such as an abdominal tumor. A quiet environment allows sounds to be heard. Advanced health care providers usually perform percussion. Refer to information on a health assessment text for details of this advanced assessment skill.

Auscultation is the act of listening with a stethoscope to sounds produced within the body. This technique is used to listen for blood pressure, and heart, lung, and bowel sounds. Four characteristics of sound are assessed by auscultation: (1) pitch (ranging from high to low); (2) loudness (ranging from soft to loud); (3) quality (e.g., gurgling or swishing); and (4) duration (short, medium, or long). When auscultating, use the proper part of the stethoscope (diaphragm or bell) for specific sounds. Use the bell of the stethoscope to detect low-pitched sounds (such as some heart murmurs). Hold the bell lightly against the body part being auscultated. Use the diaphragm of the stethoscope to detect high-pitched sounds (such as normal heart sounds, breath sounds, and bowel sounds). Hold the diaphragm firmly against the body part being auscultated.

Fundamentals Review 3-3

BRIEF GENERAL PHYSICAL ASSESSMENT

ASSESSMENT	COMPONENTS
Safety	Assess: bed position, call bell location, appropriate emergency equipment, assistive devices, fall risk/hazards
Vital signs	Assess: temperature, pulse, respirations, blood pressure, oxygen saturation, pain assessment
Mental status	Assess: level of consciousness; orientation to person, place, and time; speech
Psychosocial	Assess: behavior and affect
Head, eyes, ears, nose, throat, neck	Assess: eyes, pupils, mouth, carotid arteries, swallowing, facial color, moisture, lesions, wounds, glasses, hearing aid, ability to hear conversation, ability to see
Chest	Assess: chest color, moisture, lesions, wounds, quality of respirations, heart sounds, lung sounds, cough, sputum
Abdomen	Assess: abdomen color, moisture, lesions, wounds, bowel sounds, tenderness, distention, pain/discomfort, ability to eat, urine elimination pattern and urine characteristics, bowel elimination pattern and stool characteristics
Upper and lower extremities	Assess: skin, color, pulses, temperature, tenderness, edema, capillary refill, strength, sensation, range of motion, lesions, wounds
Activity	Assess: movement and ambulation, ability to move in bed, ability to get out of bed, ability to walk and distance, gait
Therapeutic devices	Assess: peripheral and central venous access devices, supplemental oxygen setting, pacemaker, cardiac monitor, urinary catheters, gastric tubes, chest tubes, dressings, braces, slings

Nurses should use clinical judgment to adapt this generic assessment to the individual circumstances of an individual patient and to monitor for changes that might require further intervention (Henley Haugh, 2015).

Source: Adapted from Henley Haugh, K. (2015). Head-to-toe: Organizing your baseline patient physical assessment. *Nursing, 45*(12), 58–61. Used with permission; Anderson, B., Nix, E., Norman, B., & McPike, H. D. (2014). An evidence based approach to undergraduate physical assessment practicum course development. *Nurse Education in Practice, 14*(3), 242–246.

Skill 3-1 ▶ Performing a General Survey

The **general survey** is the first component of the physical assessment, beginning with the first moment of patient contact and continuing throughout the nurse–patient relationship. The general survey helps to develop an overall impression of the patient. It includes observing the patient's overall appearance and behavior; taking vital signs; measuring height, weight, and waist circumference; head circumference (infants and children) and calculating the **body mass index (BMI)**. BMI and waist circumference are indicators of risk for developing obesity-associated diseases or conditions, such as cardiovascular disease, high blood pressure, and type 2 diabetes (National Heart, Lung, and Blood Institute, n.d.).

DELEGATION CONSIDERATIONS

Measurement of the patient's weight and height, and vital signs may be delegated to assistive personnel (AP). Depending on the state's nurse practice act and the organization's policies and procedures, the licensed practical/vocational nurses (LPN/LVNs) may perform some or all the parts of the general survey. The decision to delegate must be based on careful analysis of the patient's needs and circumstances as well as the qualifications of the person to whom the task is being delegated. Refer to the Delegation Guidelines in Appendix A.

(continued on page 104)

Skill 3-1 ▶ Performing a General Survey (continued)

EQUIPMENT	• Adequate lighting • Tape measure • A scale with height attachment; chair scale; or bed scale • PPE, as indicated
ASSESSMENT	Develop an overall impression of the patient, focusing on appearance and behavior, vital signs, height, and weight. Ask the patient about any changes in weight, pain or discomfort, sleeping patterns, and any difficulty sleeping.
ACTUAL OR POTENTIAL HEALTH PROBLEMS AND NEEDS	Many actual or potential health problems or needs may require the use of this skill as part of related interventions. An appropriate health problem or need may include: • Bathing/hygiene ADL deficit • Impaired comfort • Coping impairment
OUTCOME IDENTIFICATION AND PLANNING	The expected outcome to achieve in performing a general survey is that the assessment is completed without the patient experiencing anxiety or discomfort, an overall impression of the patient is formulated, the findings are documented, and the appropriate referral is made to other health care professionals, as needed, for further evaluation. Other outcomes may be appropriate, depending on the specific diagnosis or patient problem identified for the patient.

IMPLEMENTATION

ACTION	**RATIONALE**
1. Perform hand hygiene and put on PPE, if indicated.	Hand hygiene and PPE prevent the spread of microorganisms. PPE is required based on transmission precautions.
2. Identify the patient.	Identifying the patient ensures the right patient receives the intervention and helps prevent errors.
3. Close curtains around the bed and the door to the room, if possible. Explain the purpose of the health examination and what you are going to do. Answer any questions.	This ensures the patient's privacy. Explanation relieves anxiety and facilitates cooperation.
4. Assess the patient's overall appearance and behavior. Observe if the patient appears to be their stated age. Note the patient's mental status. Is the person alert and oriented, responsive to questions, and responding appropriately? Are the facial features symmetric? Note any signs of acute distress, such as shortness of breath, pain, or anxiousness.	Appearance provides information about various aspects of the patient's health. Changes in cognitive processes, asymmetry, and signs of distress can be indicators of health abnormalities.
5. Assess the patient's body structure. Does the person's height appear within normal range for stated age and genetic heritage? Does the person's weight appear within normal range for height and body build? Note if body fat is evenly distributed. Do body parts appear equal bilaterally and relatively proportionate? Is the patient's posture erect and appropriate for age?	Height that is excessively short or tall, asymmetry, one-sided atrophy or hypertrophy, abnormal posture, and abnormal body proportion can be indicators of health problems.
6. Assess the patient's mobility. Is the patient's gait smooth, even, well balanced, and coordinated? Is joint mobility smooth and coordinated with a general full range of motion (ROM)? Are involuntary movements evident?	Abnormalities in gait and ROM can indicate health concerns.

ACTION

7. Assess the patient's behavior. Are facial expressions appropriate for the situation? Does the patient maintain eye contact, based on cultural norms? Does the person appear comfortable and relaxed with you? Is the patient's speech clear and understandable? Observe the person's hygiene and grooming. Is the clothing appropriate for climate, fit well, appear clean, and appropriate for the person's culture and age group? Does the person appear clean and well groomed, appropriate for age and culture?

8. Assess for pain. (Refer to Chapter 10.)

9. Have the patient remove shoes and heavy outer clothing. Weigh the patient using a scale (Figure 1). Compare the measurement with previous weight measurements and recommended range for height.

10. With shoes off, and standing erect, measure the patient's height using a wall-mounted measuring device or measuring pole (Figure 2).

RATIONALE

Facial expressions, speech, eye contact, and other behaviors provide clues to mood and mental health. Deficits in hygiene and grooming may indicate alterations in health.

Pain can indicate alterations in physical and psychological health.

Weight loss or gain may indicate health problems.

Ratio of height and weight is a general assessment of overall health, hydration, and nutrition.

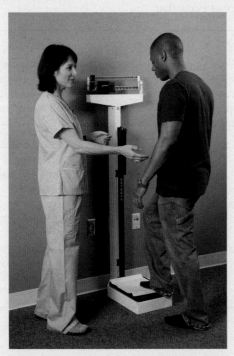

FIGURE 1. Weighing patient using scale. (*Source:* Used with permission from Shutterstock. *Photo by B. Proud.*)

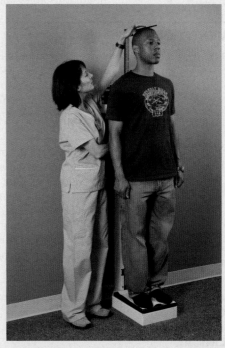

FIGURE 2. Measuring patient's height. (*Source:* Used with permission from Shutterstock. *Photo by B. Proud.*)

11. Use the patient's weight and height measurements to calculate the patient's BMI.

$$\text{Body mass index} = \frac{\text{weight in kilograms}}{\text{height in meters}^2}$$

BMI, an indicator of total body fat stores in the general population, provides a more accurate weight calculation than weight measurement alone. In addition, it provides an estimation of risk for diseases, such as heart disease, type 2 diabetes, and hypertension (National Heart, Lung, and Blood Institute, n.d.).

(*continued on page 106*)

Skill 3-1 ▶ Performing a General Survey *(continued)*

ACTION	RATIONALE
12. Using the tape measure, measure the patient's waist circumference. Place the tape measure snugly around the patient's waist at the level of the umbilicus.	Waist circumference is a good indicator of abdominal fat. It is thought to be an important and reliable indicator of risk for obesity-associated diseases or conditions (National Heart, Lung, and Blood Institute, n.d.).
13. Measure the patient's temperature, pulse, respirations, blood pressure, and oxygen saturation. (Refer to Chapter 2 and Chapter 14 for specific techniques.)	Vital signs and oxygen saturation are measured to establish a baseline for the database and to detect actual or potential health problems.
14. Remove PPE, if used. Clean the equipment, based on facility policy. Perform hand hygiene. Continue with assessments of specific body systems as appropriate or indicated. Initiate appropriate referral to other health care providers for further evaluation as indicated.	Proper removal of PPE reduces the risk for infection transmission and contamination of other items. Cleaning of equipment prevents transmission of microorganisms. Hand hygiene prevents the spread of microorganisms. Additional assessments should be completed, as indicated, to evaluate the patient's health status. Intervention by other health care providers may be indicated to evaluate and treat the patient's health status.

EVALUATION

The expected outcomes have been met when the assessment has been completed without the patient experiencing anxiety or discomfort; an overall impression of the patient has been formulated; the findings have been documented; and the appropriate referrals have been made to other health care professionals, as needed, for further evaluation.

DOCUMENTATION

Guidelines

Document findings related to assessment of the patient's physical appearance, body structure, mobility, and behavior. Document the patient's height, weight, BMI, and waist circumference. Document the presence or absence of pain as well as an initial pain assessment if present. Record the patient's temperature (T), pulse (P), respiration (R), and blood pressure (BP) measurements as well as the oxygen saturation measurement. Note any referrals.

Sample Documentation

Lippincott
DocuCare

Practice documenting assessment techniques and findings in *Lippincott DocuCare*.

1/26/25 1015 Patient admitted to room 432. Patient is a 23-year-old Asian female graduate student at a local university, living in an apartment with three other female students. Appears well nourished, disheveled, clothing appropriate for age and season, and tired. Oriented, cooperative, with no signs of acute distress; patient denies pain at present. T 98.9°F, P 78, R 16, BP 114/58 mm Hg (left arm), sitting O_2 sat 96% on room air. Height 144 cm (5 ft). Weight 55 kg (121 lb). BMI 26.5. Waist circumference 32 inches. Information provided regarding use of call bell, lights, and phone, and location of bathroom. Patient verbalizes an understanding of information.
—R. Robinson, RN

DEVELOPING CLINICAL REASONING AND CLINICAL JUDGMENT

UNEXPECTED SITUATIONS AND ASSOCIATED INTERVENTIONS

- *Patient is unable to tolerate standing for height or weight measurement:* Obtain a chair scale or bed scale to measure weight (refer to Skill 3-2). Obtain a measuring stick to measure height. Alternatively, use tape to mark the patient's length in the bed with the patient supine, the head in the midline position, and the legs extended flat on the bed. Measure the resulting length.

**SPECIAL
CONSIDERATIONS**

General Considerations

- BMI may not be accurate for people, such as athletes, with a large muscle mass; people with **edema** or dehydration; older adults and others who have lost muscle mass (Dudek, 2018; National Institutes of Health [NIH], n.d.).
- According to the guidelines published by the National Heart, Lung, and Blood Institute, an adult with a BMI below 18.5 is underweight, a BMI of 25 to 29.9 indicates that a person is overweight, and a BMI of 30 or greater indicates obesity (National Heart, Lung, and Blood Institute, n.d.).
- Disease risk increases with a waist measurement of more than 40 inches in men and 35 inches in women (National Heart, Lung, and Blood Institute, n.d.).

*Infant and Child
Considerations*

- Measure height (length) in children up to age 2 years in the recumbent position with legs fully extended (Kyle & Carman, 2021).
- Measure head circumference at birth and each physical examination for infants and children up to age 2 years to track the pattern of head growth (Bright Futures/American Academy of Pediatrics, 2021; Weber & Kelley, 2018). Circle the tape measure around the infant or child's head (not including the ears), beginning at the forehead just above the eyebrows, bringing the tape around the head just above the occipital prominence at the back of the head, using the widest span (Jarvis & Eckhardt, 2020; Kyle & Carmen, 2021).
- Weigh infants without clothing.
- Weigh children in their underwear.
- BMIs for children and teens use weight and height, and add sex assigned at birth and age into the calculation, listed as a percent. This percentage indicates a child's BMI in relation to the BMIs of other children of the same sex assigned at birth and age (NIH, n.d.).
- Children ages 2 years and older are considered at a healthy weight if their BMI falls between the 5th and 85th percentiles, overweight if their BMI is between the 85th and 95th percentiles, and obese if their BMI is at or higher than the 95th percentile (NIH, n.d.).
- Information about BMI-for-age and growth charts for children can be found at the Centers for Disease Control and Prevention (CDC)'s BMI-for-age calculator (CDC, 2018).

Skill 3-2 ▶ Using a Portable Bed Scale

Obtaining a patient's weight is an important component of assessment. In addition to providing baseline information of the patient's overall status, weight is a valuable indicator of nutritional status and fluid balance. Changes in a patient's weight can provide clues to underlying problems, such as nutritional deficiencies or fluid excess or deficiency, or it can indicate the development of new problems, such as fluid overload.

Typically, the nurse will measure weight by having the patient stand on an upright scale. However, doing so requires that the patient is mobile and can maintain their balance. Chair scales are available for patients who are unable to stand. For patients who are confined to the bed, have limited mobility, or cannot maintain a balanced upright or standing position for a short period of time, a bed scale can be used. With a bed scale, the nurse places the patient in a sling and raises the patient above the bed. To ensure safety, a second nurse should be on hand to assist with weighing the patient. Many facilities provide beds with built-in scales. The following procedure explains how to weigh the patient with a portable bed scale.

**DELEGATION
CONSIDERATIONS**

Measurement of body weight may be delegated to assistive personnel (AP) as well as to licensed practical/vocational nurses (LPN/LVNs). The decision to delegate must be based on careful analysis of the patient's needs and circumstances as well as the qualifications of the person to whom the task is being delegated. Refer to the Delegation Guidelines in Appendix A.

EQUIPMENT

- Bed scale with sling
- Cover for sling
- Sheet or bath blanket
- PPE, as indicated

(continued on page 108)

Skill 3-2 ▶ Using a Portable Bed Scale *(continued)*

ASSESSMENT

Assess the patient's ability to stand for a weight measurement. If the patient cannot stand, assess the patient's ability to sit in a chair or to lie still for a weight measurement. Assess the patient for pain. If necessary, give medication for pain or sedation before placing the patient on a bed scale. Assess for the presence of any material, such as tubes, drains, or (intravenous) IV tubing, which could become entangled in the scale or pulled during the weighing procedure.

ACTUAL OR POTENTIAL HEALTH PROBLEMS AND NEEDS

Many actual or potential health problems or needs may require the use of this skill as part of related interventions. An appropriate health problem or need may include:
- Impaired Mobility
- Impaired Nutritional Status
- Overweight

OUTCOME IDENTIFICATION AND PLANNING

The expected outcomes to achieve when weighing a patient using a portable bed scale are that the patient's weight is measured accurately without injury to the patient, and the patient experiences minimal discomfort. Other outcomes may be appropriate, depending on the specific diagnosis or patient problem identified for the patient.

IMPLEMENTATION

ACTION	**RATIONALE**
1. Check the prescribed interventions or plan of care for frequency of weight measurement. More frequent measurement of the patient's weight may be appropriate based on nursing judgment. Obtain the assistance of a second caregiver, based on the patient's mobility and ability to cooperate with the procedure.	This provides for patient safety and appropriate care.
2. Perform hand hygiene and put on PPE, if indicated.	Hand hygiene and PPE prevent the spread of microorganisms. PPE is required based on transmission precautions.
3. Identify the patient.	Identifying the patient ensures that the right patient receives the intervention and helps prevent errors.
4. Close the curtains around the bed and close the door to the room if possible. Discuss the procedure with the patient and assess the patient's ability to assist with the procedure.	This ensures the patient's privacy. Explanation relieves anxiety and facilitates cooperation.
5. Place a cover over the sling of the bed scale.	Using a cover deters the spread of microorganisms.
6. Attach the sling to the bed scale. Lay the sheet or bath blanket in the sling. Turn on the scale. **Balance the scale so that weight reads 0.0.**	Scale will add the sling, blanket, and cover into the weight unless it is zeroed with the sling, blanket, and cover.
7. Adjust the bed to a comfortable working position (VHACEOSH, 2016). Position one caregiver on each side of the bed, if two caregivers are present. Raise side rail on the opposite side of the bed from where the scale is located, if not already in place. Cover the patient with the sheet or bath blanket. Remove other covers and any pillows.	Having the bed at the proper height prevents back and muscle strain. Having one caregiver on each side of the bed provides for patient safety and appropriate care. Side rail assists patient with movement. Blanket maintains patient's dignity and provides warmth.
8. Turn the patient onto their side facing the side rail, keeping their body covered with the sheet or blanket. Remove the sling from the scale. Place the cover on the sling. Roll cover and sling lengthwise. Place rolled sling under the patient, making sure the patient is centered in the sling.	Rolling the patient onto their side facilitates placing the patient onto the sling. Blanket maintains patient's dignity and provides warmth.

ACTION

RATIONALE

9. Roll the patient back over the sling and onto the other side. Pull the sling through, as if placing sheet under patient, unrolling the sling as it is pulled through.

This facilitates placing the patient onto the sling.

10. Roll the scale over the bed so that the arms of the scale are directly over the patient. **Spread the base of the scale.** Lower the arms of the scale and place the arm hooks into the holes on the sling.

By spreading the base, you are giving the scale a wider base, thus preventing the scale from toppling over with the patient. Hooking sling to scale provides secure attachment to the scale and prevents injury.

11. Once the scale arms are hooked onto the sling, gradually elevate the sling so that the patient is lifted up off the bed (Figure 1). **Assess all tubes and drains, making sure that none have tension placed on them as the scale is lifted. Once the sling is no longer touching the bed, ensure that nothing else is hanging onto the sling (e.g., ventilator or IV tubing). If any tubing is connected to the patient, raise it up so that it is not adding any weight to the patient.**

The scale must be hanging free to obtain an accurate weight. Any tubing that is hanging off the scale will add weight to the patient.

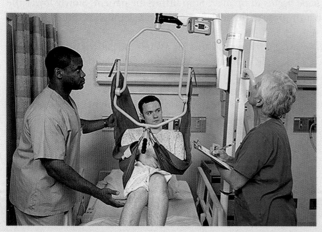

FIGURE 1. Using a bed scale.

12. Note the weight reading on the scale. Slowly and gently, lower the patient back onto the bed. Disconnect the scale arms from the sling. Close the base of the scale and pull it away from the bed.

Lowering the patient slowly does not alarm the patient. Closing the base of the scale facilitates moving the scale.

13. Raise the side rail. Turn the patient to the side rail. Roll the sling up against the patient's backside.

Raising the side rail is a safety measure.

14. Raise the other side rail. Roll the patient back over the sling and up facing the other side rail. Remove the sling from the bed. Remove gloves, if used. Raise the remaining side rail. Perform hand hygiene.

The patient needs to be removed from the sling before it can be removed from the bed. Hand hygiene deters the spread of microorganisms.

15. Cover the patient and help them to a position of comfort. Place the bed in the lowest position.

Ensures patient comfort and safety.

16. Remove the disposable cover from the sling and discard in the appropriate receptacle.

Using a cover deters the spread of microorganisms.

17. Remove additional PPE, if used. Clean equipment based on facility policy. Perform hand hygiene.

Proper removal of PPE reduces the risk for infection transmission and contamination of other items. Cleaning equipment prevents transmission of microorganisms. Hand hygiene deters the spread of microorganisms.

18. Replace the scale and sling in the appropriate spot. Plug the scale into the electrical outlet.

Scale should be ready for use at any time.

(continued on page 110)

Skill 3-2 ▶ Using a Portable Bed Scale *(continued)*

EVALUATION

The expected outcome has been met when the patient has been weighed accurately without injury, and the patient has experienced minimal discomfort.

DOCUMENTATION

Guidelines

Document weight, unit of measurement, and scale used.

Sample Documentation

10/15/25 0230 Patient reports pain in legs 5/10. Premedicated with oxycodone 5 mg and acetaminophen 325 mg 2 tabs PO before obtaining weight per order. Patient weighed using bed scale, 75.2 kg.

—M. Evans, RN

DEVELOPING CLINICAL REASONING AND CLINICAL JUDGMENT

UNEXPECTED SITUATIONS AND ASSOCIATED INTERVENTIONS

- *As the patient is being lifted, the scale begins to tip over:* Stop lifting the patient. Slowly lower the patient back to the bed. Ensure that the base of the scale is spread wide enough before attempting to weigh the patient.
- *Weight differs from the previous day's weight by more than 1 kg:* Weigh the patient using the same scale at the same time each day. Check scale calibration. Make sure that the patient is wearing the same clothing. Make sure that no tubes or containers are hanging on the scale. If the patient is incontinent, make sure undergarments are clean and dry.
- *Patient becomes agitated as the sling is raised into the air:* Stop lifting the patient and reassure them. If the patient continues to be agitated, lower them back to the bed. Reevaluate necessity of obtaining weight at that exact time.

Skill 3-3 ▶ Assessing the Skin, Hair, and Nails

The integumentary system includes the skin, hair, nails, sweat glands, and sebaceous glands. Assessment of the skin, hair, and nails provides information about the nutritional and hydration status and overall health of the patient. This assessment can provide information associated with certain systemic diseases, infection, immobility, excessive sun exposure, and allergic reactions. It also provides information about self-care activities related to personal hygiene. Assessment often begins with an overall inspection of the skin's condition and skin assessment is integrated throughout the entire health assessment. Assessment of specific regions is usually integrated into specific body system assessments. Skin assessment is presented separately in this text for learning purposes.

DELEGATION CONSIDERATIONS

The assessment of the patient's skin, hair, and nails should not be delegated to assistive personnel (AP). However, the AP may notice some items while providing care. The nurse must then validate, analyze, document, communicate, and act on these findings, as appropriate. Depending on the state's nurse practice act and the organization's policies and procedures, the licensed practical/vocational nurses (LPN/LVNs) may perform some or all the parts of assessment of the patient's skin, hair, and nails. The decision to delegate must be based on careful analysis of the patient's needs and circumstances as well as the qualifications of the person to whom the task is being delegated. Refer to the Delegation Guidelines in Appendix A.

EQUIPMENT

- Gloves
- Additional PPE, as indicated
- Bath blanket or other drape
- Measuring tape or ruler
- Adequate light source

ASSESSMENT

Complete a health history, focusing on the integumentary system. Identify risk factors for altered health by asking about the following:

- History of rashes, lesions, change in color, or itching
- History of bruising or bleeding in the skin
- History of allergies to medications, plants, foods, or other substances
- History of bathing routines and products
- Exposure to the sun and sunburn history
- Presence of lesions (wounds, bruises, abrasions, or burns)
- Presence of body piercings and/or tattoos
- Change in the color, size, or shape of a mole
- Exposure to chemicals that may be harmful to the skin, hair, or nails
- Degree of mobility
- Types of food eaten and liquids consumed each day
- Cultural practices related to skin

ACTUAL OR POTENTIAL HEALTH PROBLEMS AND NEEDS

Many actual or potential health problems or needs may require the use of this skill as part of related interventions. An appropriate health problem or need may include:

- Altered skin integrity
- Altered body image perception
- Altered skin integrity risk

OUTCOME IDENTIFICATION AND PLANNING

The expected outcome to achieve in performing assessment of the skin, hair, and nails is that the assessment is completed without the patient experiencing anxiety or discomfort, the findings are documented, and the appropriate referral is made to the other health care professionals, as needed, for further evaluation. Other outcomes may be appropriate, depending on the specific diagnosis or patient problem identified for the patient.

IMPLEMENTATION

ACTION	RATIONALE
1. Perform hand hygiene and put on PPE, if indicated.	Hand hygiene and PPE prevent the spread of microorganisms. PPE is required based on transmission precautions.
2. Identify the patient.	Identifying the patient ensures the right patient receives the intervention and helps prevent errors.
3. Close curtains around the bed and the door to room, if possible. Explain the purpose of the integumentary examination and what you are going to do. Answer any questions.	This ensures the patient's privacy. Explanation relieves anxiety and facilitates cooperation.
4. Ask the patient to remove all clothing and put on an examination gown (if appropriate). The patient remains in the sitting position for most of the examination but will need to stand or lie on the side when the posterior part of the body is examined, exposing only the body part being examined.	Exposing only the body part being examined provides privacy for the patient. During the initial part of the examination, assess the skin areas that are exposed (e.g., face, arms, and hands). As the different assessments are completed, incorporate skin examination within these systems.
5. Use the bath blanket or drape to cover any exposed area other than the one being assessed. Inspect the overall skin coloration (Figure 1).	Use of a bath blanket or drape provides for comfort and warmth. Overall coloration is a good indication of health status. Skin color varies among races and people; individual skin color should be relatively consistent across the body. Abnormal findings include **cyanosis**, **pallor**, **jaundice**, and **erythema**.
6. Inspect skin for vascularity, bleeding, or **ecchymosis**.	These signs may relate to injury or cardiovascular, hematologic, or liver dysfunction.

(continued on page 112)

Skill 3-3 ▶ Assessing the Skin, Hair, and Nails *(continued)*

ACTION	RATIONALE
7. Inspect the skin for lesions. Note bruises, scratches, cuts, insect bites, and wounds. (Refer to General Wound Assessment [Fundamentals Review 8-1] in Chapter 8.) If present, note size, shape, color, exudates, and distribution/pattern, and presence of drainage or odor. Assess the location and condition of body piercings and/or tattoos.	Lesions can be normal variations, such as a macule or freckle, or an abnormal lesion, such as a melanoma.
8. Palpate skin using the back of your hands to assess temperature. Wear gloves when palpating any potentially open area of the skin (Figure 2).	The back of the hand is more sensitive to temperature. Increase in skin temperature may indicate elevated body temperature.

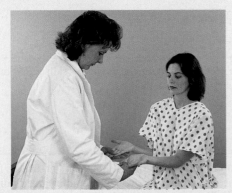

FIGURE 1. Inspecting overall skin coloration. (*Source:* Used with permission from Shutterstock. *Photo by B. Proud.*)

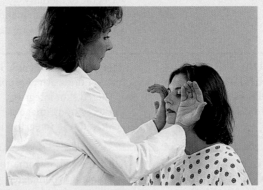

FIGURE 2. Assessing skin temperature. (*Source:* Used with permission from Shutterstock. *Photo by B. Proud.*)

9. Palpate for texture and moisture.	In a dehydrated patient, skin is dry, loose, and wrinkled. Elevated body temperature may result in increased perspiration.
10. Assess skin **turgor** by gently pinching the skin under the clavicle (Figure 3).	Provides information about the patient's hydration status as well as skin mobility and elasticity. Decreased elasticity may be present in dehydrated patients.

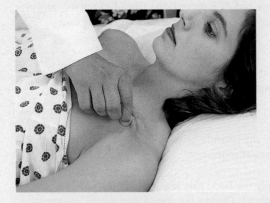

FIGURE 3. Assessing skin turgor. (*Source:* Used with permission from Shutterstock. *Photo by B. Proud.*)

11. Palpate for edema, which is characterized by swelling, with taut and shiny skin over the edematous area.	Edema may be the result of overhydration, heart failure, kidney dysfunction, or peripheral vascular disease.
12. If lesions are present, put on gloves and palpate the lesion.	Palpation of lesions may result in drainage, which provides clues to the type or cause of the lesion. Gloves prevent contact with blood and body fluids.
13. Inspect the nail condition, including the shape, texture, and color as well as the nail angle; note if any clubbing is present.	Nail condition provides information about underlying illness and oxygenation status. Nails are normally convex, and the cuticle is pink and intact. The angle of nail attachment is 160 degrees. Clubbing is present when the nail angle base exceeds 180 degrees.

ACTION

14. Palpate nails for texture and capillary refill.

15. Inspect the hair and scalp for color, texture, and distribution (Figure 4). Wear gloves if lesions or infestation is suspected or if hygiene is poor.

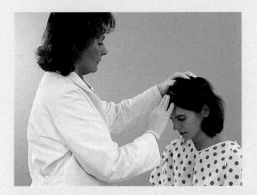

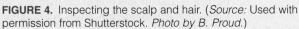
FIGURE 4. Inspecting the scalp and hair. (*Source:* Used with permission from Shutterstock. *Photo by B. Proud.*)

16. Remove gloves and any additional PPE, if used. Perform hand hygiene. Continue with assessments of specific body systems, as appropriate or indicated. Initiate appropriate referral to other health care providers for further evaluation, as indicated.

RATIONALE

Normally, nails are firm and smooth and capillary refill should be brisk, less than 3 seconds.

Hair condition provides information about nutritional and oxygenation status. Hair should be evenly distributed over the scalp. There are variations in hair color.

Proper removal of PPE reduces the risk for infection transmission and contamination of other items. Hand hygiene prevents the spread of microorganisms. Additional assessments should be completed, as indicated, to evaluate the patient's health status. Intervention by other health care providers may be indicated to evaluate and treat the patient's health status.

EVALUATION

The expected outcomes have been met when the patient has participated in the integumentary assessment; the assessment has been completed without the patient experiencing anxiety or discomfort; the findings are documented; and the appropriate referrals have been made to the other health care professionals, as needed, for further evaluation.

DOCUMENTATION

Guidelines

Describe specific findings, including coloration, texture, moisture, temperature, turgor, capillary refill, and edema. Note hair distribution and texture. Describe the condition of nails, including any abnormal findings. If lesions are present, document specifics, describing type, size, shape (use tape measure if necessary), elevation, coloring, location, drainage, distribution, and patterns.

Sample Documentation

> <u>5/2/25</u> 1030 Skin assessment performed. Patient reports history of atopic dermatitis. Uniform skin coloring (tan) with pink undertones. Skin on all areas, but the hands, is soft and warm. Skin returns to position when pinched. Multiple lesions, consistent with dermatitis, observed on the hands. Lesions are red, scaly, and dry. Brown hair, shiny and evenly distributed. Nails are firm and the cuticle is pink and intact and without ridging or pitting.
> —B. Gentzler, RN

DEVELOPING CLINICAL REASONING AND CLINICAL JUDGMENT

UNEXPECTED SITUATIONS AND ASSOCIATED INTERVENTIONS

- *While assessing the skin of a patient with dark skin tone, you are unsure if the change in coloration in a particular area of the body is normal or abnormal:* It is especially important when assessing people with dark skin tones to conduct the assessment with natural light rather than artificial lighting. When an abnormal condition is present, first examining an area of the skin that is not

(continued on page 114)

Skill 3-3 ▶ Assessing the Skin, Hair, and Nails *(continued)*

affected by the dermatologic disorder provides a comparison for identifying abnormal color conditions. Skin temperature becomes important to detect erythema in people with dark skin tones; areas of erythema will feel warm compared with surrounding skin. Pallor in patients with dark skin tones is seen as an ashen gray or yellow tinge. Also, lesions that look red or brown on light skin may present as black or purple on dark skin.

SPECIAL CONSIDERATIONS

Older Adult Considerations
- In the older adult patient expect to find overall thinning of the skin, reduced sweating and oil, and reduced skin turgor.

Cultural Considerations
- Pallor in people with dark skin tones appears as ashen gray or yellow tinged. Brown-toned skin appears more yellowish brown, dull; darker skin looks ashen, gray, dull. Assess areas with least pigmentation, such as conjunctivae and mucous membranes (Jarvis & Eckhardt, 2020).
- Assess cyanosis in people with darker skin tones by examining the oral mucosa, nail beds, and the conjunctivae (Jarvis & Eckhardt, 2020).
- Assess jaundice in people with darker skin tones by observing the sclera of the eyes, the palms of the hands, and the junction of the hard and soft palate (Jarvis & Eckhardt, 2020).
- Congenital dermal melanocytosis is a common variation of hyperpigmentation in newborns of African American, Asian, Native American, Latino heritage. It is a blue black to purple macular area of hyperpigmentation that is usually located at the sacrum or buttocks, but sometimes occurs on the abdomen, thighs, shoulders, or arms. Mongolian spot gradually fades during the first year of life. It is important not to confuse these areas of hyperpigmentation with bruises (Jarvis & Eckhardt, 2020; Jensen, 2019; Weber & Kelly, 2018).
- Patients of Southeast Asian heritage may have a common variation of diminished body and facial hair (Jarvis & Eckhardt, 2020; Jensen, 2019).
- African American individuals and other people with curly hair may experience pseudofolliculitis barbae. This is a common condition in which tightly curved hairs grow back into the skin, causing a foreign-body reaction with inflammation (Jensen, 2019).

Skill 3-4 ▶ Assessing the Head and Neck

Examination of the head and neck region includes the assessment of multiple structures and body systems. The eyes, ears, nose, mouth, and throat are located within the facial structures. Anterior neck structures include the trachea, esophagus, and the thyroid gland as well as the arteries, veins, and lymph nodes. Posterior neck areas involve the upper portion of the spine. Assessment of the size and consistency of the thyroid gland is performed by advanced practice professionals. Refer to information on a health assessment text for details.

DELEGATION CONSIDERATIONS

Assessment of the patient's head and neck should not be delegated to assistive personnel (AP). However, the AP may notice some items while providing care. The nurse must then validate, analyze, document, communicate, and act on these findings, as appropriate. Depending on the state's nurse practice act and the organization's policies and procedures, the licensed practical/vocational nurses (LPN/LVNs) may perform some or all the parts of assessment of the patient's head and neck. The decision to delegate must be based on careful analysis of the patient's needs and circumstances as well as the qualifications of the person to whom the task is being delegated. Refer to the Delegation Guidelines in Appendix A.

EQUIPMENT

- Stethoscope
- Gloves
- Additional PPE, as indicated
- Bath blanket or other drape
- Lighting, including a penlight
- Tongue blades
- Visual acuity chart

ASSESSMENT

Complete a health history, focusing on the head and neck. Identify risk factors for altered health by asking about the following:
- Changes with aging in vision or hearing
- History of use of corrective lenses or hearing aids
- History of allergies
- History of disturbances in vision or hearing
- History of chronic illnesses, such as hypertension, diabetes mellitus, or thyroid disease
- Exposure to harmful substances or loud noises
- History of smoking, chewing tobacco, or cocaine use
- History of eye or ear infections
- Presence of body piercings and/or tattoos
- Oral and dental care practices

ACTUAL OR POTENTIAL HEALTH PROBLEMS AND NEEDS

Many actual or potential health problems or needs may require the use of this skill as part of related interventions. An appropriate health problem or need may include:
- Impaired Swallowing
- Impaired Dentition
- Impaired Hearing

OUTCOME IDENTIFICATION AND PLANNING

The expected outcome to achieve in performing an examination of the structures in the head and neck region is that the assessment is completed without the patient experiencing anxiety or discomfort, the findings are documented, and the appropriate referral is made to the other health care professionals, as needed, for further evaluation. Other outcomes may be appropriate, depending on the specific diagnosis or patient problem identified for the patient.

IMPLEMENTATION

ACTION	**RATIONALE**
1. Perform hand hygiene and put on PPE, if indicated.	Hand hygiene and PPE prevent the spread of microorganisms. PPE is required based on transmission precautions.
2. Identify the patient.	Identifying the patient ensures the right patient receives the intervention and helps prevent errors.
3. Close the curtains around the bed and close the door to the room, if possible. Explain the purpose of the head and neck examination and what you are going to do. Answer any questions.	This ensures the patient's privacy. Explanation relieves anxiety and facilitates cooperation.
4. Inspect the head for size and shape. Inspect the face for color, symmetry, lesions, and distribution of facial hair. Note facial expression. Palpate the skull.	In general, the shape of the head is normocephalic and symmetric. Abnormal findings include a lack of symmetry or unusual size or contour of the head, which may be a result of trauma or disease. Facial expression is appropriate. The skull should be mobile and nontender.
5. Inspect the external eye structures (eyelids, eyelashes, eyeball, and eyebrows), cornea, conjunctiva, and sclera. Note color, edema, symmetry, and alignment.	Inspection detects abnormalities, such as ptosis, styes, conjunctivitis, or scleral color. Some abnormalities are associated with systemic disorders.

(continued on page 116)

Skill 3-4 ▶ Assessing the Head and Neck *(continued)*

| ACTION | RATIONALE |

ACTION

6. Examine the pupils for equality of size and shape (Figure 1). Examine the pupillary reaction to light:

   a. Darken the room.

   b. Ask the patient to look straight ahead.

   c. Bring the penlight from the side of the patient's face and briefly shine the light on the pupil (Figure 2).

   d. Observe the pupil's reaction; it normally constricts rapidly (direct response). Note pupil size.

   e. Repeat the procedure and observe the other eye; it too normally will constrict (consensual reflex).

   f. Repeat the procedure with the other eye.

RATIONALE

Testing pupillary response to light and accommodation assesses cranial nerve III, the oculomotor nerve. The pupils are normally black, equal in size, round, and smooth. The normal and consensual pupillary response is constriction.

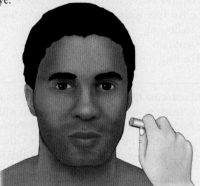

FIGURE 1. Pupillary gauge measures pupils in millimeters (mm).

1 2 3 4 5 6 7

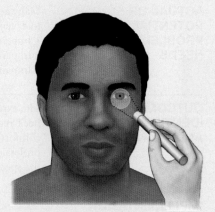

FIGURE 2. Assessing pupillary reaction to light.

7. Test for pupillary accommodation:

   a. Hold the forefinger, a pencil, or other straight object about 10 to 15 cm (4 to 6 inches) from the bridge of the patient's nose.

   b. Ask the patient to first look at the object, then at a distant object, and then back to the object being held. The pupil normally constricts when looking at a near object (Figure 3A) and dilates when looking at a distant object (Figure 3B).

Testing pupillary response to light and accommodation assesses cranial nerve III, the oculomotor nerve. The normal pupillary response is constriction when focusing on a near object.

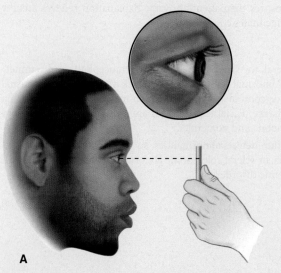

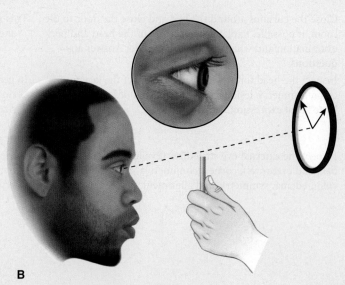

A   **B**

FIGURE 3. Assessing pupillary accommodation.

ACTION

8. Assess extraocular movements.

   a. Ask the patient to hold the head still and follow the movement of your forefinger or a penlight with the eyes as you move the patient's eyes through the six cardinal positions of gaze.

   b. Keeping your finger or penlight about 1 ft from the patient's face, move it slowly through the cardinal positions: up and down, right and left, diagonally up and down to the left (Figure 4A), diagonally up and down to the right (Figure 4B).

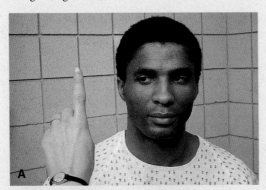

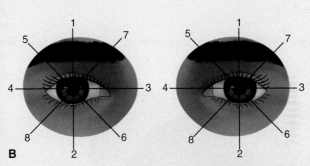

FIGURE 4. Assessing extraocular movements.

9. Test convergence:

   a. Hold your finger about 6 to 8 inches from the bridge of the patient's nose.

   b. Move your finger toward the patient's nose (Figure 5). The patient's eyes should normally converge (assume a cross-eyed appearance).

10. Test the patient's visual acuity with a Snellen chart. Have the patient stand 20 ft from the chart and ask the patient to read the smallest line of letters possible, first with both eyes and then with one eye at a time (with the opposite eye covered). Note whether the patient's vision is being tested with or without corrective lenses (Figure 6).

RATIONALE

This evaluates the function of each of the six extraocular eye muscles (EOMs) and tests cranial nerves III, IV, and VI (oculomotor, trochlear, and abducens nerves). Normally, both eyes move together, are coordinated, and are parallel.

The patient's eyes should normally converge; converging eyes normally follow the object to within 5 cm of the nose (assume a cross-eyed appearance).

Evaluates the patient's distance vision and function of cranial nerve II (optic nerve). Additional tools are used to test for color perception.

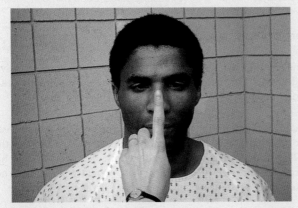

FIGURE 5. Assessing convergence.

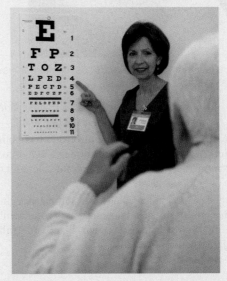

FIGURE 6. Testing visual acuity with a Snellen chart.

(continued on page 118)

Skill 3-4 ▶ Assessing the Head and Neck *(continued)*

ACTION	RATIONALE
11. Inspect the external ear bilaterally for shape, size, and lesions. Palpate the ear and mastoid process. Inspect the visible portion of the ear canal. Note cerumen (wax), edema, discharge, or foreign bodies.	Inspection may reveal abnormalities, such as uneven color, size, drainage, or lesions; inflammation (edema) or infection; nodules, lesions, or tenderness. Cerumen may normally be dark orange, brown, yellow, gray, or black and soft, moist, dry, or hard.
12. Use a whispered voice as a general hearing screening test. Stand about 1 to 2 ft away from the patient out of the patient's line of vision. Ask the patient to cover the ear not being tested. Determine whether the patient can hear a whispered sentence or group of numbers from 1 to 2 ft. away. Perform the test on each ear.	Provides a gross assessment of cranial nerve VIII (acoustic nerve) and provide clues to the need for further evaluation. The patient should repeat what has been said.
13. Put on gloves. Inspect and palpate the external nose (Figure 7).	Gloves prevent contact with blood and body fluids. These actions assess for the color, shape, consistency, and tenderness of the nose.
14. Palpate over the frontal and maxillary sinuses (Figure 8).	Sinus palpation is used to elicit tenderness, which may indicate sinus congestion or infection. Normally, the sinuses are not painful when palpated.

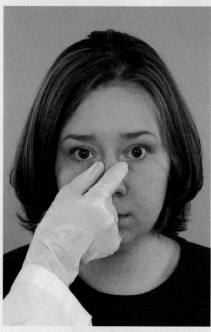

FIGURE 7. Palpating the nose. (*Source:* Used with permission from Shutterstock. *Photo by B. Proud.*)

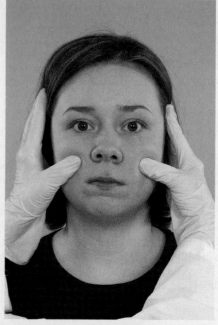

FIGURE 8. Palpating the sinuses. (*Source:* Used with permission from Shutterstock. *Photo by B. Proud.*)

15. Occlude one nostril externally with a finger while patient breathes through the other; repeat for the other side.	This technique checks the patency of the nasal passages.
16. Inspect each anterior naris and the turbinates by tipping the patient's head back slightly and shining a light into the nares. Examine the mucous membranes for color and the presence of lesions, exudate, or growths.	This technique can detect edema, inflammation, and excessive drainage. The nasal mucosa is moist and darker red than the oral mucosa.
17. Inspect the lips, oral mucosa, hard and soft palates, gingivae, teeth, and salivary gland openings. Ask the patient to open the mouth wide and use a tongue blade and penlight to visualize structures.	Evaluates the condition of the oral structures and hydration level of the patient. The lips should be pink, moist, and smooth. The gums should be pink and smooth. The teeth should be regular and free of cavities or have dental restoration. The tonsils, if present, are small, pink, and symmetric in size.

ACTION

18. Inspect the tongue. Ask the patient to stick out the tongue. Place a tongue blade at the side of the tongue while patient pushes it to the left and right with the tongue. Inspect the uvula by asking the patient to say "ahh" while sticking out the tongue (Figure 9). Palpate the tongue for muscle tone and tenderness. Remove gloves. Sticking out the tongue evaluates the function of cranial nerve XII (hypoglossal nerve). Saying "ahh" checks for movement of the uvula and soft palate.

RATIONALE

The tongue and mucous membranes are normally pink, moist, and free of swelling or lesions. The uvula is normally centered and freely movable. The tongue should feel soft with positive muscle tone and be nontender.

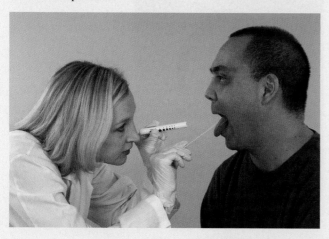

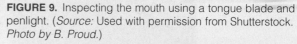

FIGURE 9. Inspecting the mouth using a tongue blade and penlight. (*Source:* Used with permission from Shutterstock. *Photo by B. Proud.*)

19. Inspect and palpate the lymph nodes (Figure 10) for enlargement, tenderness, and mobility, using the fingerpads in a slow, circular motion (Figure 11).

Palpation can determine size, shape, mobility, consistency, and/or tenderness of enlarged lymph nodes.

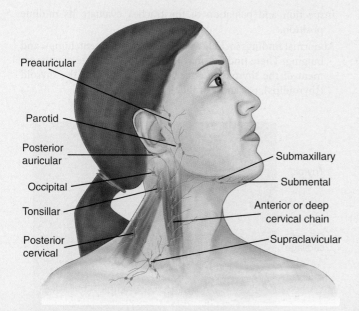

Preauricular

Parotid

Posterior auricular

Occipital

Tonsillar

Posterior cervical

Submaxillary

Submental

Anterior or deep cervical chain

Supraclavicular

FIGURE 10. Location of lymph nodes in neck.

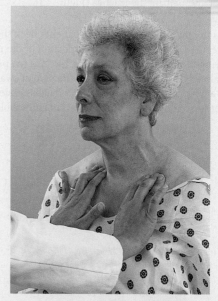

FIGURE 11. Palpating lymph nodes. (*Source:* Used with permission from Shutterstock. *Photo by B. Proud.*)

(*continued on page 120*)

Skill 3-4 ▶ Assessing the Head and Neck *(continued)*

ACTION	**RATIONALE**

20. Inspect and palpate (Figure 12A) the left and then the right carotid arteries. **Palpate only one carotid artery at a time.** Note the strength of the pulse and grade it as with peripheral pulses. Use the bell of the stethoscope to auscultate the carotid arteries (Figure 12B).

This is part of the assessment of the peripheral vascular system in Skill 3-10. However, some health care providers include this assessment here for organizational convenience and time management. Palpation of this area assesses flow of blood through the arteries. Palpating both arteries at once can reduce blood flow to the brain, potentially causing dizziness or loss of consciousness (Jensen, 2019). Auscultation can detect a **bruit**.

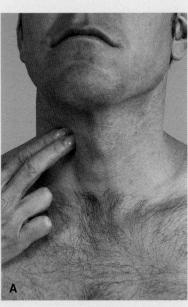
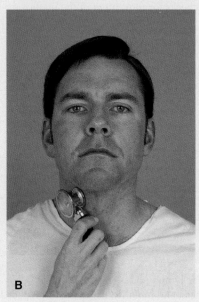

FIGURE 12. Palpating (**A**) and auscultating (**B**) the carotid arteries. (*Source:* Used with permission from Shutterstock. *Photos by B. Proud.*)

21. Inspect and palpate the trachea (Figure 13).

Inspection and palpation of the trachea evaluate its midline position.

22. Assess the thyroid gland with the patient's neck slightly hyperextended. Observe the lower portion of the neck overlying the thyroid gland (Figure 14). Ask the patient to swallow. Observe the area while the patient swallows. Offer a glass of water, if necessary, to make it easier for the patient to swallow. Assess for symmetry and visible masses.

Abnormal findings include asymmetry, enlargement, lumps, and bulging. These findings may indicate the presence of enlargement of the thyroid (a goiter), inflammation of the thyroid (thyroiditis), or cancer of the thyroid.

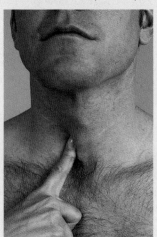

FIGURE 13. Palpating to determine position of trachea. (*Source:* Used with permission from Shutterstock. *Photo by B. Proud.*)

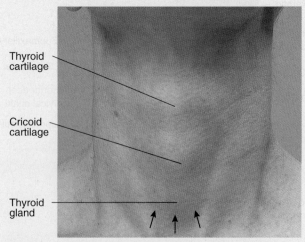

Thyroid cartilage

Cricoid cartilage

Thyroid gland

FIGURE 14. Assessing the thyroid gland. (*Source:* From Hogan-Quigley et al. [2017]. *Bates' nursing guide to physical examination and history taking* [2nd ed., p. 223]. Wolters Kluwer.)

ACTION

23. Inspect the ability of the patient to move the neck. Ask the patient to touch chin to chest and to each shoulder, each ear to the corresponding shoulder, and then tip the head back as far as possible.

 24. Remove any additional PPE, if used. Perform hand hygiene. Continue with assessments of specific body systems, as appropriate or indicated. Initiate appropriate referral to other health care providers for further evaluation, as indicated.

RATIONALE

These actions assess neck ROM, which is normally smooth and controlled.

Proper removal of PPE reduces the risk for infection transmission and contamination of other items. Hand hygiene prevents the spread of microorganisms. Additional assessments should be completed, as indicated, to evaluate the patient's health status. Intervention by other health care providers may be indicated to evaluate and treat the patient's health status.

EVALUATION

The expected outcomes have been met when the patient has participated in head and neck assessment; the assessment has been completed without the patient experiencing anxiety or discomfort; the findings have been documented; and the appropriate referrals have been made to the other health care professionals, as needed, for further evaluation.

DOCUMENTATION

Guidelines

Describe specific findings. For the head and face, document symmetry, coloration, and presence of lesions or edema. Note visual acuity, pupillary reaction, and condition of the external eye. Document results of tests for accommodation, convergence, and extraocular muscles. Describe condition of the ear, noting any lesions or discharge. Document results of any hearing tests. Note condition of the nose and sinuses. Describe condition of lips, gums, tongue, and buccal mucosa. Document quality of carotid pulse. Note position of trachea and any enlargement of the thyroid. Describe quality of any lymph nodes palpable. Note ROM of the neck. Document presence of pain or discomfort.

Sample Documentation

6/10/25 1545 Head and neck examination completed. Patient denies history of any sensory changes or sensory difficulties, but states, "I have some sores in my mouth." Overall skin coloring consistent, with pink undertones. Head symmetric and normal in size. Eyes are symmetric. No lesions or redness noted. Pupils equal and reactive to light; positive accommodation and convergence. Visual acuity 20/20 in both eyes. Eyes move smoothly through six fields of gaze. External ears and canal free of discharge, lesions, or tenderness. Whisper test negative for hearing loss. Nose and sinuses nontender. Minimal clear discharge present in the nostrils; nostrils patent. Lips free of lesions. Multiple white lesions approximately 1 cm in diameter noted on buccal mucosa and tongue. Uvula rise normal. No palpable lymph nodes. Carotid pulse strong bilaterally. Trachea midline. Thyroid does not appear enlarged.

—B. Gentzler, RN

DEVELOPING CLINICAL REASONING AND CLINICAL JUDGMENT

UNEXPECTED SITUATIONS AND ASSOCIATED INTERVENTIONS

- *While you are testing a patient's visual acuity, the patient states that he can't see anything without his glasses:* Stop the test. Instruct the patient to put on his glasses, and then resume testing.
- *While performing an examination of the regional lymph nodes in the neck area, you palpate a lymph node that feels hard and fixed:* Ask the patient if he has felt this node before and, if so, for how long it has been present and if it is painful. Refer the patient to a primary health care provider for follow-up care.

(continued on page 122)

Skill 3-4 ▶ Assessing the Head and Neck *(continued)*

SPECIAL CONSIDERATIONS

General Considerations

- A patient who wears corrective lenses should have them on when visual acuity is being tested.
- A Snellen picture chart or Snellen E-chart can be used to test vision in children and in patients who are unable to read English. The E-chart uses the capital letter E in varying sizes pointing in different directions. The patient points their fingers in the direction the legs of the E are pointing.
- Near vision is tested with a handheld vision screen with varying sizes of print. A Jaeger card can be used for this measurement. The patient holds the card 14 inches from the eyes. Ask the patient to read the smallest line of letters possible, with one eye at a time (with the opposite eye covered), and corrective lenses in place, if used. The results are recorded as a fraction and written as 14 over the smallest line read by the patient. A normal result is 14/14.

Infant and Child Considerations

- When examining the neck of an infant or child, the preferred approach to assess ROM of the neck is to assess one movement at a time, rather than a full rotation of the neck, to avoid dizziness on movement.
- When examining the head of an infant, inspect and gently palpate the fontanels and sutures.
- Keep in mind that an infant's nose is usually slightly flattened.
- For a child younger than age 8 years, do not assess the frontal sinuses; they are usually too small to assess.
- Be aware that lymph nodes may be palpable in children younger than age 12 years, which is considered a normal variation.
- Note the number of teeth in a child; a child may have up to 20 temporary teeth.

Older Adult Considerations

- Look for a thin, grayish ring in the cornea (arcus senilis). This may be a normal finding in an older adult.
- When evaluating the older adult patient, expect to find normal age-related changes, such as a decrease in vision, hearing, smell, and taste.
- If the patient wears dentures, ask them to remove them for inspection of the gums and roof of the mouth.

Cultural Considerations

- Exophthalmos, protrusion of the eyeball, can be a normal finding in patients of African American heritage.

EVIDENCE FOR PRACTICE ▶

SCREENING FOR HEARING AND VISUAL IMPAIRMENT

Hearing impairment (hearing loss) is a common age-associated change in older adults. Despite being considered part of the normal aging process, age-related sensory impairment can have significant impact on the quality of life and functional status of older adults. These impacts are exacerbated when hearing impairment co-occurs with other conditions, such as visual or cognitive impairment (Meyer & Hickson, 2020). How can nurses best support older adults with hearing impairments and improve patient outcomes?

Related Evidence

Meyer, C., & Hickson, L. (2020). Evidence-based practice guideline. Nursing management of hearing impairment in nursing facility residents. *Journal of Gerontological Nursing*, 46(7), 15–25. DOI: 10.3928/00989134-20200605-04

This guideline provides a summary of the evidence about the impacts of hearing impairment and the factors that are associated with increased risk of hearing impairment. The guideline also offers evidence-based assessment criteria for measuring impairment as well as evidence-based nursing interventions for the management of hearing impairment in older adults.

Relevance to Nursing Practice

Sensory impairment can have negative effects on communication and the functional abilities of older adults. Nurses and caregivers play a key role in recognizing sensory impairment in older adults and implementing interventions to support and improve their quality of life.

Skill 3-5 ▶ Assessing the Thorax, Lungs, and Breasts

The thorax is composed of the lungs, rib cage, cartilage, and intercostal muscles. A thorough examination of the respiratory system is essential because the primary purpose of this system is to supply oxygen to, and remove carbon dioxide from, the body. Recognizing and identifying normal and abnormal breath sounds, a crucial component of lung assessment, takes practice (Tables 3-1 and 3-2). Assessment of the breasts and axillae is also included in this assessment. Regular clinical breast exam and breast self-exam are not recommended; however, women should be familiar with how their breasts normally look and feel from everyday self-care and promptly report changes to a health care provider (American Cancer Society [ACS], 2020; U.S. Preventive Services Task Force and the American Congress of Obstetricians and Gynecologists, as cited in Johns Hopkins Medicine, n.d.).

Table 3-1 Normal Breath Sounds

TYPE, DESCRIPTION, AND LOCATION	RATIO OF INSPIRATION TO EXPIRATION
Bronchial or Tubular	
Blowing, hollow sounds; auscultated over the larynx and trachea	Sound on expiration is longer, lower, and higher-pitched than inspiration
Bronchovesicular	
Medium-pitched, medium intensity, blowing sounds; auscultated over the first and second intercostal spaces anteriorly and the scapula posteriorly	Inspiration and expiration sounds have similar pitch and duration
Vesicular	
Soft, low-pitched, whispering sounds; heard over most of the lung fields	Sound on inspiration is longer, louder, and higher-pitched than expiration

Table 3-2 Adventitious Breath Sounds

TYPE AND CHARACTERISTICS	ILLUSTRATION
Wheeze (Sibilant) • Musical or squeaking • High-pitched, continuous sounds • Auscultated during inspiration and expiration • Air passing through narrowed airways	
Rhonchi (Sonorous Wheeze) • Sonorous or coarse; snoring quality • Low-pitched, continuous sounds • Auscultated during inspiration and expiration • Coughing may somewhat clear the sound • Air passing through or around secretions	
Crackles • Bubbling, crackling, popping • Low- to high-pitched, discontinuous sounds • Auscultated during inspiration and expiration • Opening of deflated small airways and alveoli; air passing through fluid in the airways	
Stridor • Harsh, loud, high-pitched • Auscultated on inspiration • Narrowing of upper airway (larynx or trachea); presence of foreign body in airway	
Friction Rub • Rubbing or grating • Loudest over lower lateral anterior surface • Auscultated during inspiration and expiration • Inflamed pleura rubbing against chest wall	

(continued on page 124)

Skill 3-5 ▶ Assessing the Thorax, Lungs, and Breasts *(continued)*

DELEGATION CONSIDERATIONS	Assessment of the patient's thorax, breasts, axillae, and lungs should not be delegated to assistive personnel (AP). However, the AP may notice some items while providing care. The nurse must then validate, analyze, document, communicate, and act on these findings, as appropriate. Depending on the state's nurse practice act and the organization's policies and procedures, the licensed practical/vocational nurses (LPN/LVNs) may perform some or all the parts of assessment of the patient's thorax, breasts, axillae, and lungs. The decision to delegate must be based on careful analysis of the patient's needs and circumstances as well as the qualifications of the person to whom the task is being delegated. Refer to the Delegation Guidelines in Appendix A.
EQUIPMENT	• Bath blanket or other drape • Examination gown • Light source • Stethoscope • PPE, as indicated
ASSESSMENT	Complete a health history, focusing on the thorax and lungs. Identify risk factors for altered health by asking about the following: • History of trauma to the ribs or history of lung surgery • Number of pillows used when sleeping • History of persistent cough with or without producing sputum • History of allergies • Environmental exposure to chemicals, asbestos, or smoke • History of smoking (including pack-years) • History of lung disease in family members or self • History of frequent or chronic respiratory infections • Breast discomfort, masses, or lumps, nipple discharge • History of breast disease, biopsy, or surgeries • Menstrual and pregnancy history, breastfeeding
ACTUAL OR POTENTIAL HEALTH PROBLEMS AND NEEDS	Many actual or potential health problems or needs may require the use of this skill as part of related interventions. An appropriate health problem or need may include: • Ineffective airway clearance • Impaired gas exchange • Altered health maintenance
OUTCOME IDENTIFICATION AND PLANNING	The expected outcome to achieve in performing an examination of the thorax, lungs, breasts, and axillae is that the assessment is completed without the patient experiencing anxiety or discomfort, the findings are documented, and the appropriate referral is made to the other health care professionals, as needed, for further evaluation. Other outcomes may be appropriate, depending on the specific diagnosis or patient problem identified for the patient.

IMPLEMENTATION

ACTION	RATIONALE
1. Perform hand hygiene and put on PPE, if indicated.	Hand hygiene and PPE prevent the spread of microorganisms. PPE is required based on transmission precautions.
2. Identify the patient.	Identifying the patient ensures the right patient receives the intervention and helps prevent errors.

ACTION

3. Close the curtains around the bed and close the door to the room, if possible. Explain the purpose of the thorax, lung, breast, and axillae examination and what you are going to do. Answer any questions.

4. Help the patient undress, if needed, and provide a patient gown. Assist the patient to a sitting position and expose the posterior thorax.

5. Use the bath blanket to cover any exposed area other than the one being assessed.

6. Inspect the posterior thorax. Examine the skin (Figure 1), bones, and muscles of the spine, shoulder blades, and back as well as symmetry of expansion and accessory muscle use during respirations.

7. Assess the anteroposterior (AP) and lateral diameters of the thorax.

8. Palpate over the spine and posterior thorax. Use the dorsal surface of the hand to palpate for temperature. Use the palmar surface of the hand to palpate in a sequential pattern for tenderness, muscle development, and masses (Figure 2).

RATIONALE

This ensures the patient's privacy. Explanation relieves anxiety and facilitates cooperation.

Having the patient wear a gown facilitates examination of the thorax while maintaining the patient's privacy.

Use of a bath blanket provides for comfort and warmth.

Examination provides information about lung expansion and accessory muscle use during respiration. Inspection of skin reveals color, presence of lesions, rashes, or masses.

This assessment helps to detect deformities, such as a barrel chest. Normally, the AP is less than the transverse diameter (1:2 ratio).

Palpation may reveal abnormal findings, such as excessively dry or moist skin, muscle asymmetry, masses, tenderness, or vibrations.

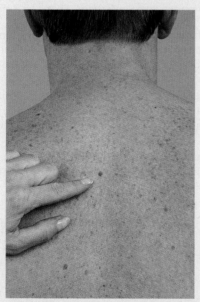

FIGURE 1. Inspecting the skin for abnormalities and variations. (*Source:* Used with permission from Shutterstock. *Photo by B. Proud.*)

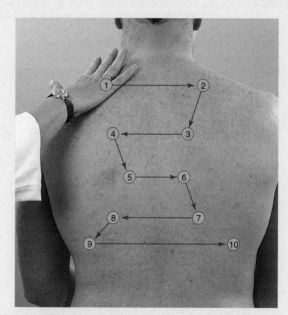

FIGURE 2. Palpating the posterior thorax.

9. Assess thoracic expansion by standing behind the patient and placing both thumbs on either side of the patient's spine at the level of T9 or T10 (Figure 3A). Ask the patient to take a deep breath and note movement of your hands (Figure 3B).

Movement should be symmetric bilaterally.

(*continued on page 126*)

Skill 3-5 ▶ Assessing the Thorax, Lungs, and Breasts *(continued)*

ACTION

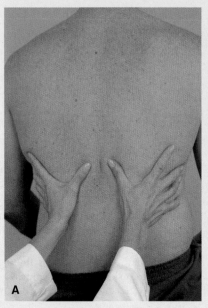 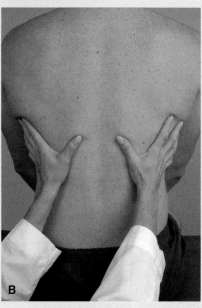

FIGURE 3. Palpating posterior thoracic excursion. **A.** The nurse's hands are placed symmetrically on the patient's back. **B.** As the patient inhales, the nurse's hands should move apart symmetrically. (*Source:* Used with permission from Shutterstock. *Photos by B. Proud.*)

10. As the patient breathes slowly and deeply through the mouth, auscultate the lungs across and down the posterior thorax to the bases of lungs in a sequential pattern, comparing sides (Figure 4).

11. Inspect the anterior thorax. With the patient sitting, rearrange the gown so the anterior chest is exposed. Inspect the skin, bones, and muscles as well as symmetry of lung expansion and accessory muscle use.

12. Palpate the anterior thorax across and down the anterior thorax to the bases of lungs in a sequential pattern (Figure 5). Use the palmar surface of the hand to palpate for temperature, tenderness, muscle development, and masses.

RATIONALE

Lung auscultation assesses for normal breath sounds and for **adventitious breath sounds**. Abnormal breath sounds indicate respiratory compromise or diseases, such as asthma or bronchitis.

Examination of the anterior thorax provides information about lung expansion and accessory muscle use during respiration. Inspection of skin reveals color, presence of lesions, rashes, or masses.

Palpation may reveal abnormal findings, such as excessively dry or moist skin, muscle asymmetry, masses, tenderness, or vibrations.

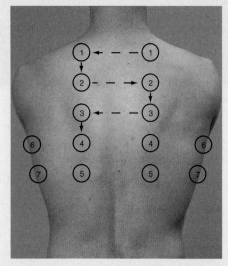 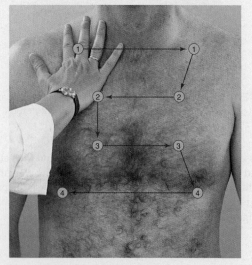

FIGURE 4. Auscultating the posterior thorax. (*Source:* From Hogan-Quigley et al. [2017]. *Bates' nursing guide to physical examination and history taking* [2nd ed., p. 344]. Wolters Kluwer.)

FIGURE 5. Palpating the anterior thorax.

ACTION

13. As the patient breathes slowly and deeply through the mouth, auscultate the lungs across and down the anterior thorax to the bases of lungs in a sequential pattern, comparing sides (Figure 6).

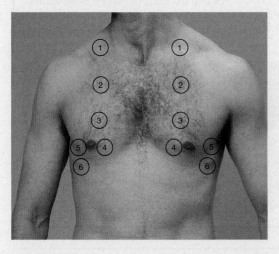

FIGURE 6. Auscultating the anterior thorax. (*Source:* From Hogan-Quigley et al. [2017]. *Bates' nursing guide to physical examination and history taking* [2nd ed., p. 351]. Wolters Kluwer.)

14. If assessment of the breasts is required, inspect the breasts. Ask the patient to rest hands on both sides of the body, then on the hips and finally above the head. With the patient holding each position, inspect the breasts for size, shape, symmetry, color, texture, and skin lesions. Inspect the areola and nipples for size and shape and the nipples for discharge, crusting, and inversion.

15. Palpate the axillae with the patient's arms resting against the side of the body. If any nodes are palpable, assess their location, size, shape, consistency, tenderness, and mobility.

16. Assist the patient into a supine position. Place a small pillow or towel under the patient's back and ask the patient to place a hand on the side being examined under the head, if possible.

17. Wear gloves if there is any discharge from the nipples or if a lesion is present. Palpate each quadrant of each breast in a systematic method, using either the circular, wedge, or vertical strip technique (see Box 3-1). Palpate the nipple and areola and gently compress the nipple between the thumb and forefinger to assess for discharge. Remove gloves, if worn, and perform hand hygiene.

18. Assist the patient into a comfortable position and in replacing the gown. Remove gloves and any additional PPE, if used. Perform hand hygiene. Continue with assessments of specific body systems, as appropriate or indicated. Initiate appropriate referral to other health care providers for further evaluation, as indicated.

RATIONALE

Lung auscultation assesses for normal breath and abnormal (adventitious) breath sounds. Abnormal breath sounds indicate respiratory compromise or diseases, such as asthma or bronchitis.

This technique evaluates the general condition of the breasts and helps to identify any abnormalities.

Palpating the axillae helps to detect nodular enlargement, tenderness, and other abnormalities.

Positioning facilitates the exam.

Gloves prevent contact with blood and body fluids. Palpating the breasts evaluates the consistency and elasticity of breast tissue and nipples and for presence of lumps, masses, or discharge. Proper removal of gloves reduces the risk for infection transmission and contamination of other items. Hand hygiene prevents the spread of microorganisms.

Replacing the gown ensures patient comfort. Proper removal of PPE reduces the risk for infection transmission and contamination of other items. Hand hygiene prevents the spread of microorganisms. Additional assessments should be completed, as indicated, to evaluate the patient's health status. Intervention by other health care providers may be indicated to evaluate and treat the patient's health status.

(*continued on page 128*)

Skill 3-5 ▶ Assessing the Thorax, Lungs, and Breasts (continued)

Box 3-1 | Methods for Palpating the Breasts

Wedge Method
- Work in a clockwise direction and palpate from the periphery toward the areola.
- Use the pads of the first three fingers to gently compress the breast tissue against the chest wall.

Circular Method
- Start at the tail of Spence and move in increasing smaller circles, moving in toward areola.
- Use the pads of the first three fingers to gently compress the breast tissue against the chest wall.

Vertical Strip Method
- Start at the outer edge of the breast and palpate up and down the breast.
- Use the pads of the first three fingers to gently compress the breast tissue against the chest wall.

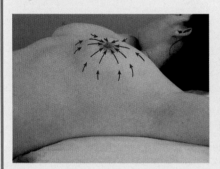 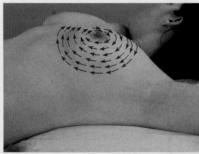 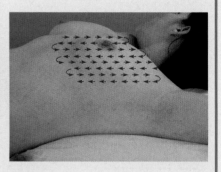

EVALUATION

The expected outcomes have been met when the patient has participated in the assessment of the thorax, lungs, breasts, and axillae; the patient has verbalized understanding of these assessment techniques as appropriate; the assessment has been completed without the patient experiencing anxiety or discomfort; the findings have been documented; and the appropriate referrals have been made to the other health care professionals, as needed, for further evaluation.

DOCUMENTATION

Guidelines

Describe specific findings. Include specific findings for all assessment techniques performed. Note the location of elicited abnormalities. For breast assessment, clock position (using the positioning of the hands of an analog clock) is often used to describe the location of findings.

Sample Documentation

Lippincott DocuCare

Practice documenting assessment techniques and findings in *Lippincott DocuCare.*

6/10/25 2025 Patient states that she "has had a dry cough for the past week and feels weak." Skin pale. RR 30. Breathing effort moderately labored; right-sided intercostal retraction noted. Barrel-shaped chest. Vibrations palpated on right anterior and posterior chest. Rhonchi (sonorous wheezes) auscultated in RUL, RML, and RLL of lung fields. Breasts symmetric, skin smooth with even tone. Breasts and axillae without lumps, masses, dimpling, or discharge.

—B. Gentzler, RN

DEVELOPING CLINICAL REASONING AND CLINICAL JUDGMENT

UNEXPECTED SITUATIONS AND ASSOCIATED INTERVENTIONS

- *When assessing a patient's lungs, you hear short, high-pitched popping sounds on inspiration:* Ask the patient to cough and auscultate again. If the sounds remain, suspect fine crackles and ask the patient if they are experiencing any difficulty in breathing or shortness of breath. Crackles may indicate disease, such as pneumonia or heart failure. Document the findings. Continue to assess the patient and notify the appropriate health care providers, as indicated.

SPECIAL CONSIDERATIONS

General Considerations

- Warm equipment, such as a stethoscope, before using it to prevent chilling the patient.
- Warm hands before palpating thorax and breasts to prevent chilling the patient and causing any discomfort.
- Attempt to reduce the noise level in the room while auscultating for breath sounds to ensure accuracy in listening. Also, note that the presence of chest hair may mimic the sound of crackles and bumping the stethoscope against clothing may distort the sound.

Infant and Child Considerations

- Auscultate a child's lungs before performing other assessment techniques that may cause crying.
- Expect to hear breath sounds that are harsher or more bronchial than those of an adult.
- Expect use of abdominal muscles during respiration (infants and young children up to school-age).

Older Adult Considerations

- Expect to find a reduction in respiratory effort due to age-related changes.
- A common finding in the older adult is kyphosis, an exaggerated posterior curvature of the spine causing bowing out of the upper spine (Eliopoulos, 2018; Jensen, 2019).

Skill 3-6 ▶ Assessing the Cardiovascular System

The cardiovascular system transports oxygen, nutrients, and other substances to the body tissues and removes metabolic waste products to the kidneys and lungs. Careful assessment of this vital system is essential. In this skill, assessment data associated with the heart will be presented. The peripheral vascular system assessment is included in Skill 3-10, because peripheral vascular, neurologic, and musculoskeletal systems are usually combined when performing a head-to-toe assessment. Assessment of the carotid pulses is included in Skill 3-4, because this assessment is commonly included while assessing the neck as part of a head-to-toe assessment.

While assessing the heart, careful auscultation is important. Identifying heart sounds takes practice. Table 3-3 provides a review of normal heart sounds in relation to the cardiac cycle and information about abnormal heart sounds.

DELEGATION CONSIDERATIONS

Assessment of the patient's cardiovascular system should not be delegated to assistive personnel (AP). However, the AP may notice some items while providing care. The nurse must then validate, analyze, document, communicate, and act on these findings, as appropriate. Depending on the state's nurse practice act and the organization's policies and procedures, the licensed practical/vocational nurses (LPN/LVNs) may perform some or all the parts of assessment of the patient's cardiovascular system. The decision to delegate must be based on careful analysis of the patient's needs and circumstances as well as the qualifications of the person to whom the task is being delegated. Refer to the Delegation Guidelines in Appendix A.

EQUIPMENT

- Bath blanket or other drape
- Examination gown
- Stethoscope
- Centimeter ruler
- PPE, as indicated

ASSESSMENT

Complete a health history, focusing on the heart. Identify risk factors for altered health by asking about the following:
- History of chest pain, tightness, palpitations, dizziness, or fatigue
- Swelling in the ankles and feet
- Number of pillows used to sleep
- Type and amount of medications taken daily

(continued on page 130)

Skill 3-6 ▶ Assessing the Cardiovascular System   *(continued)*

Table 3-3 │ Heart Sounds

Normal Heart Sounds

During auscultation, the first heart sound, S_1, is heard as the "lub" of "lub-dub." This sound occurs when the mitral and tricuspid valves close, and it corresponds to the onset of ventricular contraction. The sound, low-pitched and dull, is heard best at the apical area. The second heart sound, S_2, occurs at the termination of systole and corresponds to the onset of ventricular diastole. The "dub" of "lub-dub," it represents the closure of the aortic and pulmonic valves. The sound of S_2 is higher-pitched and shorter than S_1. The two sounds occur within 1 second or less, depending on the heart rate. Normal findings include S_1 that is louder at the tricuspid and apical areas, with S_2 louder at the aortic and pulmonic areas.

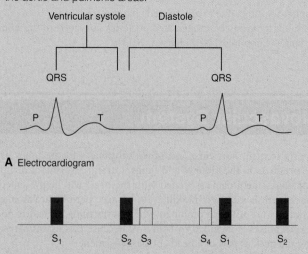

A Electrocardiogram

B Heart sounds

Heart sounds in relation to the cardiac cycle and an electro-cardiogram.

Abnormal Heart Sounds

Abnormal findings include extra heart sounds at any of the cardiac landmarks and abnormal rate or rhythm. A wide variety of conditions may alter the normal heart rate or rhythm, including serious infections, anemia, diseases of the heart muscle or conducting system, dehydration or overhydration, endocrine disorders, respiratory disorders, and head trauma. Extra heart sounds may be S_3, S_4, or murmurs.

- S_3, known as the third heart sound, follows S_2, and is often represented by a "lub-dub-dee" pattern ("dee" being S_3). This sound is best heard with the stethoscope bell at the mitral area, with the patient lying on the left side. S_3 is considered normal in children and young adults and abnormal in middle-aged and older adults.
- S_4 is the fourth heart sound, occurring right before S_1, and is often represented by a "dee-lub-dub" pattern ("dee" being S_4). S_4 is considered normal in older adults but abnormal in children and adults.
- Heart murmurs are extra heart sounds caused by some disruption of blood flow through the heart. The characteristics of a murmur and grading depend on the adequacy of valve function, rate of blood flow, and size of the valve opening. Usually, nurses are more concerned with recognizing changes in murmurs rather than in diagnosing and labeling them (Jensen, 2019, p. 467). Refer to information on a health assessment text for grading details and additional information related to assessment of heart sounds.

- History of heart defect, rheumatic fever, or chest or heart surgery
- Personal or family history of hypertension (high blood pressure), myocardial infarction (heart attack), coronary artery disease, high blood cholesterol levels, or diabetes mellitus
- History of smoking (including pack-years)
- Alcohol use
- Type and amount of exercise
- Usual foods eaten each day

ACTUAL OR POTENTIAL HEALTH PROBLEMS AND NEEDS	Many actual or potential health problems or needs may require the use of this skill as part of related interventions. An appropriate health problem or need may include: • Impaired Cardiac Output • Activity Intolerance • Risk for Impaired Cardiac Function
OUTCOME IDENTIFICATION AND PLANNING	The expected outcome to achieve in performing an examination of the cardiovascular structures is that the assessment is completed without causing the patient to experience anxiety or discomfort, the findings are documented, and the appropriate referral is made to other health care professionals, as needed, for further evaluation. Other outcomes may be appropriate, depending on the specific diagnosis or patient problem identified for the patient.

IMPLEMENTATION

ACTION

 1. Perform hand hygiene and put on PPE, if indicated.

 2. Identify the patient.

3. Close the curtains around the bed and close the door to the room, if possible. Explain the purpose of the cardiovascular examination and what you are going to do. Answer any questions.

4. Help the patient undress, if needed, and provide a patient gown. Assist the patient to a supine position with the head elevated about 30 to 45 degrees, if possible, and expose the anterior chest. Use the bath blanket to cover any exposed area other than the one being assessed.

5. If not performed previously with the assessment of the head and neck, inspect and palpate the left and then the right carotid arteries. **Palpate only one carotid artery at a time.** Note the strength of the pulse and grade it as with peripheral pulses.

6. Inspect the neck for distention of the jugular veins.

7. Inspect the **precordium** for contour, pulsations, and heaves (Figure 1). Observe for the apical impulse at the fourth to fifth intercostal space (ICS) at the left midclavicular line.

8. Using the palmar surface, with the four fingers held together, gently palpate the precordium for pulsations. Remember that hands should be warm. Palpation proceeds in a systematic manner, with assessment of specific cardiac landmarks—the aortic, pulmonic, tricuspid, and mitral areas and Erb's point (see Figure 1). Palpate the apical impulse in the mitral area (Figure 2). Note size, duration, force, and location in relationship to the midclavicular line.

RATIONALE

Hand hygiene and PPE prevent the spread of microorganisms. PPE is required based on transmission precautions.

Identifying the patient ensures the right patient receives the intervention and helps prevent errors.

This ensures the patient's privacy. Explanation relieves anxiety and facilitates cooperation.

Having the patient wear a gown facilitates examination of the cardiovascular system. Use of a bath blanket provides for comfort and warmth.

Palpation of this area evaluates circulation through the arteries. Palpating both arteries at once can reduce blood flow to the brain, potentially causing dizziness or loss of consciousness (Jensen, 2019).

Jugular venous distention (fullness) is associated with heart failure and fluid volume overload.

Precordium inspection helps detect pulsations. There are normally no pulsations, except for the apical impulse.

Normal findings include no pulsation palpable over the aortic and pulmonic areas, with a palpable apical impulse. Abnormal findings include precordial thrills, which are fine, palpable, rushing vibrations over the right or left second ICS, and any lifts or heaves, which involve a rise along the border of the sternum with each heartbeat.

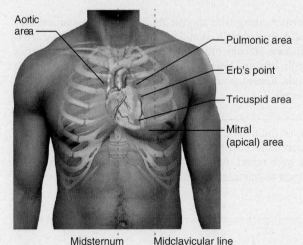

Aortic area
Pulmonic area
Erb's point
Tricuspid area
Mitral (apical) area
Midsternum   Midclavicular line

FIGURE 1. Precordium cardiac landmarks.

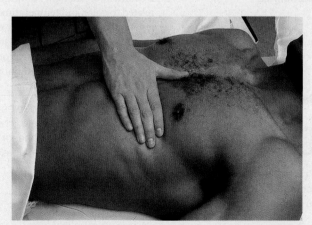

FIGURE 2. Palpating the apical impulse in the mitral area.

(continued on page 132)

Skill 3-6 ▶ Assessing the Cardiovascular System *(continued)*

ACTION

9. Auscultate heart sounds at the cardiac landmarks (Figure 1). Ask the patient to breathe normally. Use the diaphragm of the stethoscope first to listen to high-pitched sounds. Then use the bell to listen to low-pitched sounds. Focus on the overall rate and rhythm of the heart and the normal heart sounds (Table 3-3). Begin at the aortic area, move to the pulmonic area, then to Erb's point, then the tricuspid area, and finally listen at the mitral area (Figure 3).

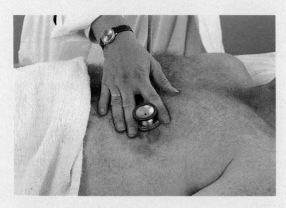

RATIONALE

Auscultation evaluates heart rate and rhythm and assesses for normal sounds (the lub, S_1; the dub, S_2) and abnormal heart sounds. The normal heart sounds (S_1 and S_2) are generated by the closing of the valves (the aortic, pulmonic, tricuspid, mitral). Extra heart sounds are often heard when the patient has anemia or heart disease. A wide variety of conditions may alter the normal heart rate or rhythm, including serious infections, diseases of the heart muscle or conducting system, dehydration or overhydration, endocrine disorders, respiratory disorders, and head trauma. Extra heart sounds may be S_3, S_4, or murmurs.

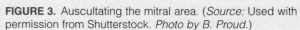

FIGURE 3. Auscultating the mitral area. (*Source:* Used with permission from Shutterstock. *Photo by B. Proud.*)

10. Assist the patient in replacing the gown. Remove PPE, if used. Perform hand hygiene. Continue with assessments of specific body systems as appropriate or indicated. Initiate appropriate referral to other health care providers for further evaluation, as indicated.

Replacing the gown ensures patient comfort. Proper removal of PPE reduces the risk for infection transmission and contamination of other items. Hand hygiene prevents the spread of microorganisms. Additional assessments should be completed as indicated to evaluate the patient's health status. Intervention by other health care providers may be indicated to evaluate and treat the patient's health status.

EVALUATION

The expected outcomes have been met when the patient has participated in the assessment of the cardiovascular system; the patient has verbalized understanding of these assessment techniques as appropriate; the assessment has been completed without the patient experiencing anxiety or discomfort; the findings have been documented; and the appropriate referrals have been made to the other health care professionals, as needed, for further evaluation.

DOCUMENTATION

Guidelines

Document assessment techniques performed, along with specific findings. Note assessment data related to color and temperature of the skin. Record inspection findings related to the carotid arteries, jugular veins, and anterior chest wall area. Document findings related to palpation of anterior chest wall for presence of pulsations, thrills, lifts, and heaves. Note auscultation findings, including rate, rhythm, pitch, and location of sounds. Record the normal heart sounds (S_1 and S_2) as well as the presence of any extra (abnormal) sounds.

Sample Documentation

Lippincott DocuCare

Practice documenting assessment techniques and findings in *Lippincott DocuCare*.

5/10/25 1015 Patient denies chest pain but states, "I have palpitations occurring about once a week." Skin pale, cool to touch, brisk capillary refill. Inspection and palpation of chest: no lifts, pulsations, or heaves were noted. Auscultation: S_1 loudest at the apex; S_2 loudest at the base; no extra sounds auscultated. Carotid pulse 88, regular rhythm, +2, equal bilaterally.

—S. Moses, RN

DEVELOPING CLINICAL REASONING AND CLINICAL JUDGMENT

SPECIAL CONSIDERATIONS

General Considerations

- Warm equipment, such as a stethoscope, before using it to prevent chilling the patient.

Infant and Child Considerations

- The presence of abnormal heart sound S_3 is considered normal in children and young adults.
- The presence of abnormal heart sound S_4 is considered abnormal in children.

Older Adult Considerations

- The presence of abnormal heart sound S_3 is considered abnormal in middle-aged and older adults.
- The presence of abnormal heart sound S_4 is considered normal in older adults.

Skill 3-7 ▶ Assessing the Abdomen

The abdominal cavity, the largest cavity in the body, contains the stomach, small intestine, large intestine, liver, gallbladder, pancreas, spleen, kidneys, urinary bladder, adrenal gland, and major blood vessels. In women, the uterus, fallopian tubes, and ovaries are also located in the abdomen. Not all of these organs can be assessed. For identification and documentation purposes, the abdomen can be divided into four quadrants (Figure 1).

The order of the techniques differs for the abdominal assessment from the other systems. Assessment of the abdomen starts with inspection, then auscultation, percussion, and palpation. The order of assessment differs for this system because palpation and percussion before auscultation may alter the sounds heard on auscultation. Advanced practice professionals perform percussion and deep palpation of the abdomen. Therefore, these techniques will not be discussed here. Before beginning the abdominal assessment, ask the patient to empty their bladder because a full bladder may cause discomfort during the examination.

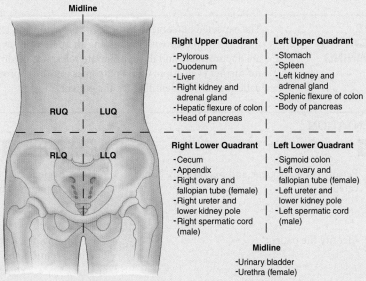

Right Upper Quadrant
- Pylorous
- Duodenum
- Liver
- Right kidney and adrenal gland
- Hepatic flexure of colon
- Head of pancreas

Left Upper Quadrant
- Stomach
- Spleen
- Left kidney and adrenal gland
- Splenic flexure of colon
- Body of pancreas

Right Lower Quadrant
- Cecum
- Appendix
- Right ovary and fallopian tube (female)
- Right ureter and lower kidney pole
- Right spermatic cord (male)

Left Lower Quadrant
- Sigmoid colon
- Left ovary and fallopian tube (female)
- Left ureter and lower kidney pole
- Left spermatic cord (male)

Midline
- Urinary bladder
- Urethra (female)

FIGURE 1. Abdominal quadrants and underlying organs.

(continued on page 134)

Skill 3-7 ▶ Assessing the Abdomen *(continued)*

DELEGATION CONSIDERATIONS

Assessment of the patient's abdomen should not be delegated to assistive personnel (AP). However, the AP may notice some items while providing care. The nurse must then validate, analyze, document, communicate, and act on these findings, as appropriate. Depending on the state's nurse practice act and the organization's policies and procedures, the licensed practical/vocational nurses (LPN/LVNs) may perform some or all the parts of assessment of the patient's abdomen. The decision to delegate must be based on careful analysis of the patient's needs and circumstances as well as the qualifications of the person to whom the task is being delegated. Refer to the Delegation Guidelines in Appendix A.

EQUIPMENT

- PPE, as indicated
- Bath blanket or other drape
- Examination gown
- Stethoscope

ASSESSMENT

Complete a health history, focusing on the abdomen. Identify risk factors for altered health by asking about the following:
- History of abdominal pain
- History of indigestion, nausea or vomiting, constipation or diarrhea
- History of food allergies or lactose intolerance
- Appetite and usual food and fluid intake
- Usual bowel and bladder elimination patterns
- History of gastrointestinal disorders
- History of urinary tract disorders
- History of abdominal surgery or trauma
- Amount and type of alcohol ingestion
- For women, menstrual history

ACTUAL OR POTENTIAL HEALTH PROBLEMS AND NEEDS

Many actual or potential health problems or needs may require the use of this skill as part of related interventions. An appropriate health problem or need may include:
- Constipation
- Acute pain
- Diarrhea

OUTCOME IDENTIFICATION AND PLANNING

The expected outcome to achieve in performing an examination of the abdomen is that the assessment is completed without causing the patient to experience anxiety or discomfort, the findings are documented, and the appropriate referral is made to other health care professionals, as needed, for further evaluation. Other outcomes may be appropriate, depending on the specific diagnosis or patient problem identified for the patient.

IMPLEMENTATION

ACTION	RATIONALE
1. Perform hand hygiene and put on PPE, if indicated.	Hand hygiene and PPE prevent the spread of microorganisms. PPE is required based on transmission precautions.
2. Identify the patient.	Identifying the patient ensures the right patient receives the intervention and helps prevent errors.
3. Close the curtains around bed and close the door to the room, if possible. Explain the purpose of the abdominal examination and what you are going to do. Answer any questions.	This ensures the patient's privacy. Explanation relieves anxiety and facilitates cooperation.

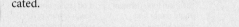

ACTION

4. Help the patient undress, if needed, and provide a patient gown. Assist the patient to a supine position, if possible, and expose the abdomen. Use the bath blanket to cover any exposed area other than the one being assessed.

5. Inspect the abdomen for skin color, contour, pulsations, the umbilicus, and other surface characteristics (rashes, lesions, masses, scars).

6. Auscultate all four quadrants of the abdomen (Figure 1) for bowel sounds. Warm the stethoscope and, using light pressure, place the flat diaphragm on the right lower quadrant of the abdomen, then move to the right upper quadrant (Figure 2), left upper quadrant, and finally left lower quadrant. Listen carefully for bowel sounds (gurgles and clicks), and note their frequency and character.

7. Auscultate the abdomen for vascular sounds. Using the bell of the stethoscope, auscultate over the abdominal aorta, femoral arteries, and iliac arteries for **bruits** (Figure 3).

RATIONALE

Having the patient wear a gown facilitates examination of the abdomen. Use of a bath blanket provides for comfort and warmth.

The umbilicus should be centrally located and may be flat, rounded, or concave. The abdomen should be evenly rounded or symmetric, without visible peristalsis. In thin people, an upper midline pulsation may normally be visible. Abnormal findings include asymmetry (possibly from an enlarged organ or mass), distention (possibly indicating retained gas or air; obesity), swelling of the abdomen (possibly indicating **ascites**) and abdominal masses, or unusual pulsations.

Performing auscultation before percussion or palpation prevents percussion and palpation techniques from interfering with findings. Traditionally, bowel sounds are assessed in all four quadrants. Bowel sounds usually occur every 5 to 15 seconds. Before documenting bowel sounds as absent, listen for 1 minute or longer in each abdominal quadrant (Jensen, 2019; Weber & Kelley, 2018). Abnormal findings include increased bowel sounds (often heard with diarrhea or in early bowel obstruction), decreased bowel sounds (heard after abdominal surgery or late bowel obstruction), or absent bowel sounds (indicating peritonitis or paralytic ileus). Bowel sounds of high-pitched tinkling or rushes of high-pitched sounds indicate a partial bowel obstruction.

A bruit may be heard in the presence of stenosis (narrowing) or occlusion of an artery. Bruits may also be caused by abnormal dilation of a vessel.

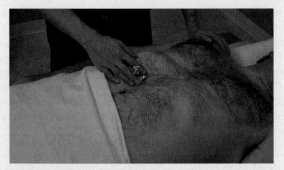

FIGURE 2. Auscultating the abdomen. (*Source:* From Jensen, S. [2019]. *Nursing health assessment* [3rd ed., p. 558]. Wolters Kluwer.)

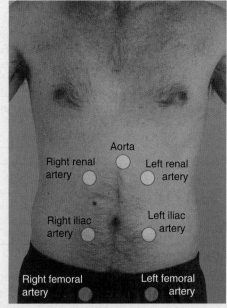

FIGURE 3. Locations to auscultate for vascular sounds. (*Source:* Used with permission from Shutterstock. *Photo by B. Proud.*)

(continued on page 136)

Skill 3-7 ▶ Assessing the Abdomen *(continued)*

ACTION

8. Palpate the abdomen lightly in all four quadrants. The pads of the fingers are used to apply pressure with the fingers together and lightly depressing the skin and underlying structures about 1 to 2 cm (0.5 to 0.75 inch) (Jarvis & Eckhardt, 2020; Jensen, 2019; Weber & Kelley, 2018). Watch the patient's face for nonverbal signs of pain during palpation. Palpate each quadrant in a systematic manner, noting muscular resistance, tenderness, enlargement of the organs, or masses (Figure 4). **If the patient reports pain or discomfort in a particular area of the abdomen, palpate that area last.**

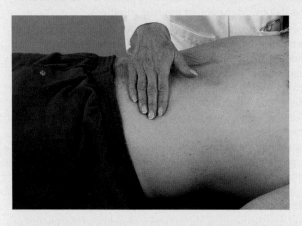

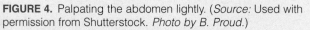

FIGURE 4. Palpating the abdomen lightly. (*Source:* Used with permission from Shutterstock. *Photo by B. Proud.*)

RATIONALE

Palpation provides information about the location, size, tenderness, and condition of the underlying structures. The abdomen should normally be soft, relaxed, and free of tenderness. Abnormal findings include involuntary rigidity, spasm, masses, and pain (which may indicate trauma, peritonitis, infection, tumors, or enlarged or diseased abdominal organs, such as appendicitis).

9. Palpate and then auscultate the femoral pulses in the groin. Note the strength of the pulse and grade it as with peripheral pulses (see Skill 3-10). Use the bell of the stethoscope to auscultate the arteries.

10. Assist the patient into a comfortable position and in replacing the gown. Remove PPE, if used. Perform hand hygiene. Continue with assessments of specific body systems, as appropriate, or indicated. Initiate appropriate referral to other health care providers for further evaluation, as indicated.

This is part of the assessment of the peripheral vascular system in Skill 3-10. However, some health care providers include this assessment here for organizational convenience and time management. This technique assesses flow of blood through the arteries. Auscultation can detect a bruit.

Replacing the gown ensures patient comfort. Proper removal of PPE reduces the risk for infection transmission and contamination of other items. Hand hygiene prevents the spread of microorganisms. Additional assessments should be completed, as indicated, to evaluate the patient's health status. Intervention by other health care providers may be indicated to evaluate and treat the patient's health status.

EVALUATION

The expected outcomes have been met when the patient participated in the assessment of the abdomen; the patient verbalized understanding of the assessment techniques as appropriate; the assessment has been completed without the patient experiencing anxiety or discomfort; the findings have been documented; and the appropriate referrals have been made to the other health care professionals, as needed, for further evaluation.

DOCUMENTATION

Guidelines

Document assessment techniques performed, along with specific findings. Note assessment data related to color of the skin, presence of symmetry/asymmetry, distention, swelling, lesions, rashes, scars, or masses. Note the character of the bowel sounds and if any bruits are present. Note the overall softness or hardness of the abdomen, presence of palpable masses, the presence of pain or tenderness, and unusual pulsations.

Sample Documentation

Lippincott
DocuCare

Practice documenting assessment techniques and findings in *Lippincott DocuCare*.

> 3/30/25 0930 Patient states, "I have been feeling sick to my stomach for the last 24 hours." Denies any abdominal pain. Abdomen symmetric; soft, slightly distended, umbilicus midline, no scars or pulsations, bowel sounds present in all four quadrants, but decreased.
>
> —B. Gentzler, RN

DEVELOPING CLINICAL REASONING AND CLINICAL JUDGMENT

SPECIAL CONSIDERATIONS

General Considerations

- Warm equipment, such as a stethoscope, before using it to prevent chilling the patient.
- Some sources suggest bowel sounds radiate widely over the abdomen, and listening in all four quadrants is not necessary; assessment of presence and hypoactivity (decreased)/hyperactivity (increased) is sufficient (Jarvis & Eckhardt, 2020; McGee, 2018).

Infant and Child Considerations

- Umbilical cord in newborns; dries and falls off within the first few weeks of life.
- In infants, expect a large abdomen in relation to the pelvis.
- The abdomen of a child is normally protuberant.

Older Adult Considerations

- Decreased bowel sounds are a normal finding in the older adult.
- Decreased abdominal tone is a normal finding in the older adult.
- Fat accumulation on the abdomen and hips is a common finding in the older adult.

Skill 3-8 ▶ Assessing the Female Genitalia

The external female genitalia consist of the mons pubis, labia majora and minora, clitoris, vestibular glands, vaginal vestibule, vaginal orifice, and urethral opening (Figure 1). During the physical assessment, examine the external genitalia by inspection and palpation. The internal pelvic examination is a skill most often performed by an advanced practice professional. Women from some cultures or those who practice certain religions may agree to a physical examination of the genitalia only if it is performed by a female nurse or female practitioner.

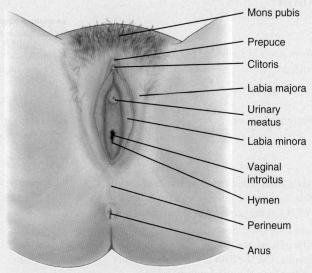

Mons pubis
Prepuce
Clitoris
Labia majora
Urinary meatus
Labia minora
Vaginal introitus
Hymen
Perineum
Anus

FIGURE 1. External female genitalia.

(continued on page 138)

Skill 3-8 ▶ Assessing the Female Genitalia *(continued)*

DELEGATION CONSIDERATIONS	Assessment of the patient's genitalia should not be delegated to assistive personnel (AP). However, the AP may notice some items while providing care. The nurse must then validate, analyze, document, communicate, and act on these findings, as appropriate. Depending on the state's nurse practice act and the organization's policies and procedures, the licensed practical/vocational nurses (LPN/LVNs) may perform some or all the parts of assessment of the patient's genitalia. The decision to delegate must be based on careful analysis of the patient's needs and circumstances as well as the qualifications of the person to whom the task is being delegated. Refer to the Delegation Guidelines in Appendix A.

EQUIPMENT	• PPE, as indicated • Examination gown • Bath blanket or other drape • Gloves

ASSESSMENT	Complete a health history, focusing on the female genital system. Identify risk factors for altered health by asking about the following: • Menstrual history (age of first and last period, length of flow, type of flow, pain) • Sexual history (age at which sexual activity began, number and sex of partners assigned at birth, practices) • Pain with intercourse, difficulty achieving orgasm • Number of pregnancies and live births • History of sexually transmitted infection (STI) • Use of contraceptives/protection from STIs • Frequency of pelvic examinations and Pap smears • History of vaginal discharge, itching, or pain on urination • Use of hormones and tobacco (how long, how much, how many packs/day)

ACTUAL OR POTENTIAL HEALTH PROBLEMS AND NEEDS	Many actual or potential health problems or needs may require the use of this skill as part of related interventions. An appropriate health problem or need may include: • Altered health maintenance • Infection risk • Impaired Sexual Functioning

OUTCOME IDENTIFICATION AND PLANNING	The expected outcome to achieve in performing an examination of the female genitalia is that the assessments are completed without causing the patient to experience anxiety or discomfort, the findings are documented, and the appropriate referral is made to other health care professionals, as needed, for further evaluation. Other outcomes may be appropriate, depending on the specific diagnosis or patient problem identified for the patient.

IMPLEMENTATION

ACTION	**RATIONALE**
1. Perform hand hygiene and put on PPE, if indicated.	Hand hygiene and PPE prevent the spread of microorganisms. PPE is required based on transmission precautions.
2. Identify the patient.	Identifying the patient ensures the right patient receives the intervention and helps prevent errors.
3. Close the curtains around bed and close the door to the room, if possible. Explain the purpose of the examination of genitalia and what you are going to do. Answer any questions.	This ensures the patient's privacy. Explanation relieves anxiety and facilitates cooperation.
4. Help the patient undress, if needed, and provide a patient gown. Assist the patient to a supine position, or lying on her side, if possible. Use the bath blanket to cover any exposed area other than the one being assessed.	Having the patient wear a gown facilitates examination of the genitalia. Use of a bath blanket provides for comfort and warmth.

ACTION

5. Put on gloves. Inspect the external genitalia for color, size of the labia majora and vaginal opening, lesions, and discharge.

6. Palpate the labia for masses. Remove gloves and perform hand hygiene.

7. Assist the patient to a comfortable position.

8. Remove additional PPE, if used. Perform hand hygiene. Continue with assessments of specific body systems, as appropriate, or indicated. Initiate appropriate referral to other health care providers for further evaluation, as indicated.

RATIONALE

Gloves prevent contact with blood and body fluids. The vulva normally has more pigmentation than other skin areas, and the mucous membranes are dark pink and moist. The skin and mucosa should be smooth, without lesions or swelling. The labia should be symmetric without lesions or swelling. Lesions may be the result of infections (e.g., herpes or syphilis). There may normally be a small amount of clear or whitish vaginal discharge.

The vulva should be without lumps or masses. Removal of gloves reduces the risk for infection transmission and contamination of other items. Hand hygiene prevents the spread of microorganisms.

This ensures the patient's comfort.

Proper removal of PPE reduces the risk for infection transmission and contamination of other items. Hand hygiene prevents the spread of microorganisms. Additional assessments should be completed, as indicated, to evaluate the patient's health status. Intervention by other health care providers may be indicated to evaluate and treat the patient's health status.

EVALUATION

The expected outcomes have been met when the patient has participated in the assessment of the genitalia; the patient has verbalized an understanding of the assessment techniques as appropriate; the assessment has been completed without the patient experiencing anxiety or discomfort; the findings have been documented; and the appropriate referrals have been made to the other health care professionals, as needed, for further evaluation.

DOCUMENTATION

Guidelines

Document assessment techniques performed, along with specific findings. Note and record the color, size of the labia majora and vaginal opening, lesions, and presence of any discharge. Document any patient statements of pain and risk factors.

Sample Documentation

> <u>1/12/25</u> 1645 Patient denies vaginal itching, pain, lumps, or discharge. Vulva with darker pigmentation than surrounding skin tone; mucous membranes are dark pink and moist. Skin and mucosa smooth, without lesions or swelling. Labia are symmetric without lesions or swelling. No discharge noted. Vulva is without lumps or masses.
> —B. Holmes, RN

DEVELOPING CLINICAL REASONING AND CLINICAL JUDGMENT

SPECIAL CONSIDERATIONS

Infant and Child Considerations

- In newborns, enlargement of the labia and clitoris and breast enlargement occur, resulting from exposure to maternal hormones in utero and normally seen in the first week after birth, subsiding by the second week after birth.
- Pubic hair and breast development occur at puberty and follow a regular sequence of development.
- Menstruation begins about 2.5 years after puberty begins.
- Irregular menstrual cycle is common for first 2 years.

Older Adult Considerations

- Decreased size of labia is a common finding in older adults.
- Decreased amount of pubic hair is a normal finding in older adults.
- Decreased vaginal secretion is a common finding in older adults.

(continued on page 140)

Skill 3-9 ▶ Assessing the Male Genitalia

The external male genitalia (Figure 1) include the penis and scrotum. In addition, the inguinal area may be assessed as part of this assessment. During the physical assessment, the nurse examines the external genitalia by inspection and palpation, and the inguinal area by inspection. Examination of the prostate gland is a skill performed by an advanced practice professional.

The American Cancer Society (ACS, 2018) advises men to be aware of testicular cancer and to see a health care provider right away if they find a lump in a testicle. Routine testicular self-exams can give a patient greater awareness of the condition of their testicles and help detect changes (Mayo Clinic, 2018).

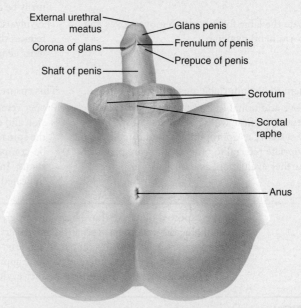

FIGURE 1. External male genitalia. (*Source:* From Pansky, B., & Gest, T. R. [2013]. *Lippincott's concise illustrated anatomy: Thorax, abdomen & pelvis* [p. 205]. Wolters Kluwer; Figure 3.1F.)

DELEGATION CONSIDERATIONS	The assessment of the patient's genitalia should not be delegated to assistive personnel (AP). However, the AP may notice some items while providing care. The nurse must then validate, analyze, document, communicate, and act on these findings, as appropriate. Depending on the state's nurse practice act and the organization's policies and procedures, the licensed practical/vocational nurses (LPN/LVNs) may perform some or all the parts of assessment of the patient's genitalia. The decision to delegate must be based on careful analysis of the patient's needs and circumstances as well as the qualifications of the person to whom the task is being delegated. Refer to the Delegation Guidelines in Appendix A.
EQUIPMENT	• PPE, as indicated • Bath blanket or other drape • Examination gown • Gloves
ASSESSMENT	Complete a health history, focusing on the male genitalia. Identify risk factors for altered health by asking about the following: • Frequency of digital rectal examinations • Frequency of testicular self-examination • Use of contraceptives/protection from sexually transmitted infections (STIs) • Occupational exposure to chemicals (tire and rubber manufacturing, farming, mechanics) • Sexual history (age at which sexual activity began, number and sex of partners assigned at birth, practices) • History of STI • History of discharge from the penis • Difficulty with urination (incontinence, hesitancy, frequency, voiding at night) • History of erectile dysfunction, pain with intercourse

ACTUAL OR POTENTIAL HEALTH PROBLEMS AND NEEDS	Many actual or potential health problems or needs may require the use of this skill as part of related interventions. An appropriate health problem or need may include: • Altered health maintenance • Infection risk • Impaired Sexual Functioning
OUTCOME IDENTIFICATION AND PLANNING	The expected outcome to achieve in performing an examination of the male genitalia is that the assessments are completed without causing the patient to experience anxiety or discomfort, the findings are documented, and the appropriate referral is made to other health care professionals, as needed, for further evaluation. Other outcomes may be appropriate, depending on the specific diagnosis or patient problem identified for the patient.

IMPLEMENTATION

ACTION

RATIONALE

1. Perform hand hygiene and put on PPE, if indicated.

Hand hygiene and PPE prevent the spread of microorganisms. PPE is required based on transmission precautions.

2. Identify the patient.

Identifying the patient ensures the right patient receives the intervention and helps prevent errors.

3. Close the curtains around the bed and close the door to the room, if possible. Explain the purpose of the examination of genitalia and what you are going to do. Answer any questions.

This ensures the patient's privacy. Explanation relieves anxiety and facilitates cooperation.

4. Help the patient undress, if needed, and provide a patient gown. Assist the patient to a supine or sitting position, if possible. Use a bath blanket to cover any exposed area other than the one being assessed.

Having the patient wear a gown facilitates examination of the genitalia. Use of a bath blanket provides for comfort and warmth.

5. Put on gloves. Inspect the external genitalia for size, placement, contour, appearance of the skin, redness, edema, and discharge. If the patient is uncircumcised, retract the foreskin for inspection of the glans penis and return foreskin back over the glans penis after inspection. Assess the location of the urinary meatus. Inspect the scrotum for symmetry.

Gloves prevent contact with blood and body fluids. The size and shape of the scrotum should be similar bilaterally. It is not unusual for the left testicle to lie lower in the scrotal sac than the right testicle. Normal findings include skin that is free of lesions, and a foreskin (if present) that is intact, uniform in color, and easily retracted. The urinary meatus is normally located in the center of the glans penis and is free of discharge. If the foreskin is left retracted, it may cause venous congestion in the glans of the penis, leading to edema. Abnormal findings include lesions, redness, edema, discharge, and displacement of the urinary meatus or difficulties with voiding. Lesions may be the result of infections (e.g., herpes or syphilis). Edema, redness, or discharge may indicate an infection. Voiding difficulties may result from scarring caused by infections or prostate enlargement.

6. Palpate the scrotum for consistency, nodules, masses, and tenderness.

The consistency of the scrotal contents (i.e., testes) should be similar bilaterally. The scrotum and testes should be free of masses and nontender. Pain may indicate an infection.

7. Inspect the inguinal area. Ask the patient to bear down and look for bulging of the area. Remove gloves and perform hand hygiene.

Normally, the inguinal area is free of bulges. Removal of gloves reduces the risk for infection transmission and contamination of other items. Hand hygiene prevents the spread of microorganisms.

(continued on page 142)

Skill 3-9 ▶ Assessing the Male Genitalia *(continued)*

ACTION

8. Assist the patient to a comfortable position.

9. Remove additional PPE, if used. Perform hand hygiene. Continue with assessments of specific body systems, as appropriate, or indicated. Initiate appropriate referral to other health care providers for further evaluation, as indicated.

RATIONALE

This ensures the patient's comfort.

Proper removal of PPE reduces the risk for infection transmission and contamination of other items. Hand hygiene prevents the spread of microorganisms. Additional assessments should be completed, as indicated, to evaluate the patient's health status. Intervention by other health care providers may be indicated to evaluate and treat the patient's health status.

EVALUATION

The expected outcomes have been met when the patient has participated in the assessment of the genitalia; the patient has verbalized understanding of the assessment techniques as appropriate; the assessment has been completed without the patient experiencing anxiety or discomfort; the findings have been documented; and the appropriate referrals have been made to the other health care professionals, as needed, for further evaluation.

DOCUMENTATION

Guidelines

Document assessment techniques performed, along with specific findings. Note and record the size, placement, contour, appearance of the skin, presence of foreskin, redness, edema, location of urinary meatus, and discharge. Document any patient statements of pain and risk factors.

Sample Documentation

> 09/23/25 1730 Patient denies pain and discharge from penis; denies lumps or changes in scrotum. Patient reports no difficulty with urination. Scrotum of equal size and shape. Skin without lesions, edema, redness; foreskin present and intact, uniform in color, and easily retracted. Urinary meatus located in the center of the glans penis and is free of discharge. Scrotum and testes free of masses and nontender. Inguinal area is free of bulges.
>
> —B. Holmes, RN

DEVELOPING CLINICAL REASONING AND CLINICAL JUDGMENT

SPECIAL CONSIDERATIONS

Infant and Child Considerations

- In newborns, breast enlargement occurs, resulting from exposure to maternal hormones in utero and normally seen in the first week after birth, subsiding by the second week after birth.
- Development of pubic hair and enlargement of the scrotum, testes, and penis occur at puberty and follow a regular sequence to adult configuration.
- Spontaneous nocturnal emission of seminal fluid occurs at puberty.

Older Adult Considerations

- Decreased penis size is a normal finding in older adults.
- Decreased pubic hair is a common finding in older adults.
- Decreased size and firmness of testes is a normal finding in older adults.

Skill 3-10 ▶ Assessing the Neurologic, Musculoskeletal, and Peripheral Vascular Systems

The following assessment integrates the findings from the neurologic, musculoskeletal, and peripheral vascular systems. These systems are usually combined when performing a head-to-toe assessment. In assessing the neurologic system, ask the patient to respond to a series of questions that will enable you to obtain data related to overall cognitive function. In addition, evaluate sensation in different areas of the body as well as selected cranial nerves. Musculoskeletal examination will provide information concerning the condition and functioning of certain muscles and joints throughout the body. The peripheral vascular system assessment will identify the condition of the arteries and veins in the extremities as gained through inspection and palpation of the skin and peripheral pulses.

Musculoskeletal trauma, crush injuries, orthopedic surgery, and external pressure from a cast or tight-fitting bandage can cause damage to blood vessels and nerves. This damage causes localized inflammation and tissue edema, which can lead to significantly diminished perfusion and severe ischemia, with resulting severe and permanent dysfunction of the affected area and/or loss of a limb. Assessment of neurovascular status is focused assessment and is an important nursing intervention leading to early identification of neurovascular impairment and timely intervention (Agency for Clinical Innovation, 2018; Johnston-Walker & Hardcastle, 2011; Turney et al., 2013). A neurovascular assessment includes assessing for changes in circulation, motor function, and sensation. Box 3-2 outlines the components of a neurovascular assessment.

Box 3-2 Components of a Neurovascular Assessment

- Pain: Extreme pain, especially on passive motion, is a significant sign of probable neurovascular impairment in an extremity. Subjective and objective assessments should be included. Opioid analgesia is unlikely to relieve the pain.
- Pallor (perfusion): Comparison between affected and unaffected limb is important. Color and temperature of the extremity: Pale skin, decreased tone, or white color may indicate poor arterial perfusion. Cyanosis may indicate venous stasis. Coolness or decreased temperature may indicate decreased arterial supply. Compare distal to proximal temperature variation in affected limb. Assess capillary refill. Using your thumb and forefinger, squeeze the patient's fingernail or toenail until it appears white. Release the pressure and observe the time it takes for normal color to return. Normally, color returns immediately, in less than 2 to 3 seconds.
- Peripheral pulses: Comparison between affected and unaffected limb is important. Assess the consistency of arterial blood flow (pulse presence, rate, quality) up to

and past the affected area. Assess capillary refill, especially in patients whose pulses cannot be palpated due to casts or bandages and in nonverbal patients.
- Paresthesia (sensation): May be first symptom of changes in sensory nerves to appear. Compare sensation to touch between affected and unaffected limb. Numbness, tingling, or "pins and needles" sensations may be reported. Evaluate the areas above and below the affected area.
- Paralysis (movement): The ability of the patient to move the extremity distal to the injury. Paralysis of an extremity may be the result of prolonged nerve compression or irreversible muscle damage.
- Pressure: Comparison between affected and unaffected limb is important. Swelling occurs as a physiologic response to injury. Affected area may become taut and firm to the touch, with surrounding skin appearing shiny. The feeling of tightness or pressure may be present.
- Blood loss/ooze: Assess blood loss on dressings, casting materials, and any surgical drains.

Source: Adapted from Hinkle, J. L., & Cheever, K. H. (2018). *Brunner & Suddarth's textbook of medical–surgical nursing* (14th ed.). Wolters Kluwer; Johnston-Walker, E., & Hardcastle, J. (2011). Neurovascular assessment in the critically ill patient. *Nursing in Critical Care, 16*(4), 170–177.

DELEGATION CONSIDERATIONS

The assessment of the patient's neurologic, musculoskeletal, and peripheral vascular systems should not be delegated to assistive personnel (AP). Some items may be noticed while providing care and noted by the AP. The nurse must then validate, analyze, document, communicate, and act on these findings, as appropriate. Depending on the state's nurse practice act and the organization's policies and procedures, the licensed practical/vocational nurses (LPN/LVNs) may perform some or all the parts of assessment of the patient's neurologic, musculoskeletal, and peripheral vascular systems. The decision to delegate must be based on careful analysis of the patient's needs and circumstances as well as the qualifications of the person to whom the task is being delegated. Refer to the Delegation Guidelines in Appendix A.

(continued on page 144)

Skill 3-10 ▶ Assessing the Neurologic, Musculoskeletal, and Peripheral Vascular Systems *(continued)*

EQUIPMENT
- PPE, as indicated
- Bath blanket or other drape
- Tongue depressor
- Examination gown
- Gloves
- Containers of odorous materials (e.g., coffee or chocolate), as indicated
- Miscellaneous items (e.g., pin, cotton, paper clip)
- Cotton-tipped applicators

ASSESSMENT

Complete a health history, focusing on the neurologic, musculoskeletal, and peripheral vascular systems. Identify risk factors for altered health by asking about the following:
- History of numbness, tingling, or tremors
- History of seizures
- History of headaches or dizziness
- History of trauma to the head or spine
- History of high blood pressure or stroke
- Changes in the ability to hear, see, taste, or smell
- Loss of ability to control bladder and bowel
- History of smoking
- History of chronic alcohol use
- History of diabetes mellitus or cardiovascular disease
- Use of prescription and over-the-counter medications
- Frequency of blood cholesterol tests and results
- History of trauma, arthritis, or neurologic disorder
- History of pain or swelling in the joints or muscles
- Frequency and type of usual exercise
- Dietary intake of calcium
- Changes in color or temperature of the extremities
- History of pain in the legs when sleeping or pain that worsens by walking
- History of blood clots or sores on the legs that do not heal

ACTUAL OR POTENTIAL HEALTH PROBLEMS AND NEEDS

Many actual or potential health problems or needs may require the use of this skill as part of related interventions. An appropriate health problem or need may include:
- Fall risk
- Impaired Verbal Communication
- Risk for Impaired Peripheral Neurovascular Function

OUTCOME IDENTIFICATION AND PLANNING

The expected outcome to achieve in performing an examination of the neurologic, musculoskeletal, and peripheral vascular systems is that the assessments are completed without causing the patient to experience anxiety or discomfort, the findings are documented, and the appropriate referral is made to other health care professionals, as needed, for further evaluation. Other outcomes may be appropriate, depending on the specific diagnosis or patient problem identified for the patient.

IMPLEMENTATION

ACTION	RATIONALE
1. Perform hand hygiene and put on PPE, if indicated.	Hand hygiene and PPE prevent the spread of microorganisms. PPE is required based on transmission precautions.
2. Identify the patient.	Identifying the patient ensures the right patient receives the intervention and helps prevent errors.

ACTION

3. Close the curtains around the bed and close the door to the room, if possible. Explain the purpose of the neurologic, musculoskeletal, and peripheral vascular examinations and what you are going to do. Answer any questions.

4. Help the patient undress, if needed, and provide a patient gown. Assist the patient to a supine position, if possible. Use the bath blanket to cover any exposed area other than the one being assessed.

5. Begin with a survey of the patient's overall hygiene and physical appearance.

6. Assess the patient's mental status.
   a. Evaluate level of consciousness. Refer to Chapter 17 for standardized assessment tools to assess level of consciousness.

   b. Evaluate the patient's orientation to person, place, and time.

   c. Assess memory (immediate recall and past memory).

   d. Evaluate the patient's ability to understand spoken and written word.

7. Test cranial nerve (CN) function, as indicated.

   a. Ask the patient to close the eyes, occlude one nostril, and then identify the smell of different substances, such as coffee, chocolate, or alcohol. Repeat with the other nostril.

   b. Test visual acuity and pupillary constriction. Refer to previous discussion in the assessment of the head and neck.

   c. Move the patient's eyes through the six cardinal positions of gaze. Refer to previous discussion in the assessment of the head and neck.

   d. Ask the patient to smile, frown, wrinkle the forehead, and puff out cheeks (Figure 1).

RATIONALE

This ensures the patient's privacy. Explanation relieves anxiety and facilitates cooperation.

Having the patient wear a gown facilitates examination of the neurologic, musculoskeletal, and peripheral vascular systems. Use of a bath blanket provides for comfort and warmth.

This provides initial impressions of the patient. Hygiene and appearance can provide clues about the patient's mental state and comfort level.

This helps identify the patient's level of awareness.

The patient should be awake and alert. Patients with altered level of consciousness may be lethargic, stuporous, or comatose.

Memory problems may indicate neurologic impairment.

Evaluation of the patient's ability to understand spoken and written word helps assess for aphasia.

It is not necessary to assess every cranial nerve for every patient. Assessment should be individualized based on the patient's needs and health care setting and circumstances (Jensen, 2019).

This action tests the function of CN I (olfactory nerve).

This tests function of CN II and CN III (optic and oculomotor nerves).

This testing evaluates the function of tests CN III, CN IV, and CN VI (oculomotor, trochlear, and abducens nerves).

This maneuver evaluates the motor function of CN VII (facial nerve).

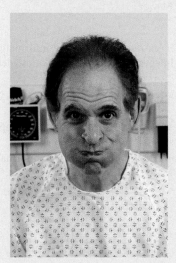

FIGURE 1. Puffing out cheeks.

(continued on page 146)

Skill 3-10 ▶ Assessing the Neurologic, Musculoskeletal, and Peripheral Vascular Systems *(continued)*

ACTION	RATIONALE
e. Ask the patient to protrude tongue and push against the cheek with the tongue.	This evaluates function of CN XII (hypoglossal nerve).
f. Palpate the jaw muscles. Ask the patient to open and clench jaws. Stroke the patient's face with a cotton ball.	This evaluates function of CN V (trigeminal nerve).
g. Test hearing with the whispered voice test. Refer to previous discussion in the assessment of the head and neck.	This evaluates function of CN VIII (acoustic nerve).
h. Put on gloves. Ask patient to open mouth. While observing soft palate, ask patient to say "ah"; observe upward movement of the soft palate. Test the gag reflex by touching the posterior pharynx with the tongue depressor. Explain to patient that this may be uncomfortable. Ask the patient to swallow. Remove gloves.	Gloves prevent contact with blood and body fluids. An intact gag reflex and swallowing indicate normal functioning of CNs IX and X (glossopharyngeal and vagus nerves).
i. Place your hands on the patient's shoulders (Figure 2) while they shrug against resistance. Then place your hand on the patient's left cheek, then the right cheek, and have the patient push against it.	These actions check CN XI (spinal accessory nerve) function and trapezius and sternocleidomastoid muscle strength.
8. Check the patient's ability to move their neck. Ask the patient to touch their chin to the chest and to each shoulder, then move each ear to the corresponding shoulder (Figure 3), and then tip the head back as far as possible.	These actions assess neck ROM, which is normally smooth and controlled.

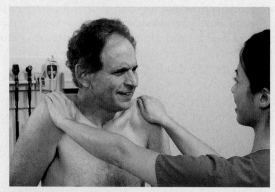

FIGURE 2. Assessing function of the spinal accessory nerve (CN XI) and muscular strength. (*Source:* From Weber, J. R., & Kelley, J. H. [2018]. *Health assessment in nursing* [6th ed., p. 585]. Wolters Kluwer.)

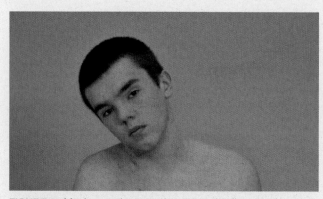

FIGURE 3. Moving each ear to the corresponding shoulder. (*Source:* From Jensen, S. [2019]. *Nursing health assessment* [3rd ed., p. 601]. Wolters Kluwer.)

9. Inspect the upper extremities. Observe for skin color, presence of lesions, rashes, and muscle mass. Palpate for skin temperature, texture, and presence of masses.	Examination of the upper extremities provides information about the circulatory, integumentary, and musculoskeletal systems.
10. Ask the patient to extend arms forward and then rapidly turn palms up and down.	This maneuver tests proprioception and cerebellar function.
11. Ask the patient to flex upper arm and to resist examiner's opposing force (Figure 4).	This technique assesses the muscle strength of the upper extremities.
12. Inspect and palpate the hands, fingers, wrists (Figure 5), and elbow joints.	Inspection and palpation provide information about abnormalities, tenderness, and ROM.

ACTION

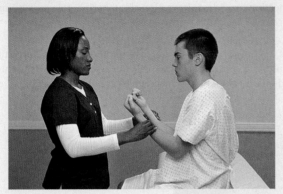

FIGURE 4. Assessing muscle strength of the upper extremities. (*Source:* From Jensen, S. [2019]. *Nursing health assessment* [3rd ed., p. 604]. Wolters Kluwer.)

13. Ask the patient to bend and straighten the elbow, and flex and extend the wrists and hands.

14. Palpate the skin and the radial and brachial pulses. Assess the pulse rate, quality or amplitude, and rhythm. Test capillary refill (Refer to "Pallor" in Box 3-2).

15. Cross your index and middle fingers. Have the patient squeeze your index and middle fingers (Figure 6).

16. Assist the patient to a supine position. Palpate (Figure 7A) and then use the bell of the stethoscope to auscultate the femoral pulses in the groin (Figure 7B), if not done during assessment of the abdomen. Note the strength of the pulse and grade it as with peripheral pulses.

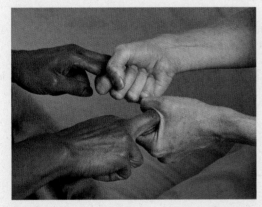

FIGURE 6. Testing grip. Patient squeezes nurse's crossed index and middle fingers. (*Source:* Used with permission from Shutterstock. *Photo by B. Proud.*)

RATIONALE

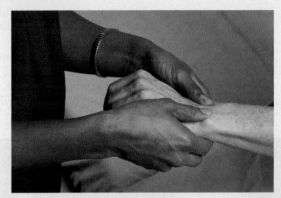

FIGURE 5. Palpating the wrist. (*Source:* Used with permission from Shutterstock. *Photo by B. Proud.*)

Tests ROM of elbow joint and wrists.

Pulse palpation and capillary refill evaluate the peripheral vascular status of the upper extremities.

This maneuver tests the muscle strength of the hands.

This technique assesses flow of blood through the arteries. Auscultation can detect a bruit.

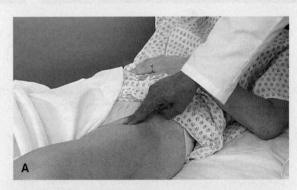

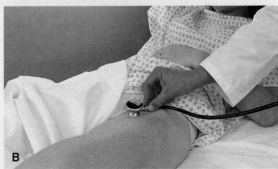

FIGURE 7. Palpating (**A**) and auscultating (**B**) the femoral pulses. (*Source:* Used with permission from Shutterstock. *Photos by B. Proud.*)

(*continued on page 148*)

Skill 3-10 ▶ Assessing the Neurologic, Musculoskeletal, and Peripheral Vascular Systems *(continued)*

ACTION	**RATIONALE**
17. Examine the lower extremities. Inspect the legs and feet for color, lesions, varicosities, hair growth, nail growth, edema, and muscle mass.	Inspection provides information about peripheral vascular function.
18. Assess for pitting edema in the lower extremities by pressing fingers into the skin at the pretibial area and dorsum of the foot (Figure 8A). If an indentation remains in the skin after the fingers have been lifted, pitting edema is present (Figure 8B).	This technique reveals information about excess interstitial fluid. Refer to an edema scale in assessing the amount of edema: 1+ about 2 mm deep to 4+ about 8 mm deep.

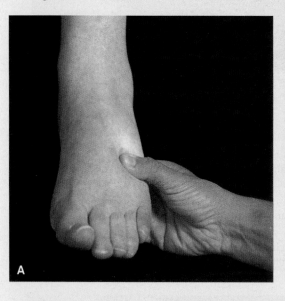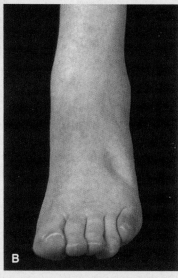

FIGURE 8. Assessing for pitting edema in lower extremities. (*Source:* From Hogan-Quigley et al. [2017]. *Bates' nursing guide to physical examination and history taking* [2nd ed., p. 453]. Wolters Kluwer.)

19. Palpate for pulses and skin temperature at the posterior tibial, dorsalis pedis, and popliteal areas. Assess the pulse rate, quality or amplitude, and rhythm. Test capillary refill (Refer to "Pallor" in Box 3-2).	Pulses, skin temperature, and capillary refill provide information about the patient's peripheral vascular status.
20. Ask the patient to move one leg laterally with the knee straight to test abduction of the hip. Keeping knee straight, move leg medially to test adduction of the hip. Repeat with other leg.	This maneuver assesses ROM and provides information about joint problems.
21. Ask the patient to raise the thigh against the resistance of your hand (Figure 9); next have the patient push outward against the resistance of your hand; then have the patient pull backward against the resistance of your hand. Repeat on the opposite side.	These measures assess motor strength of the upper and lower legs.

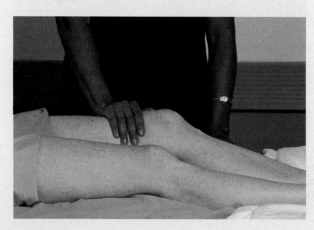

FIGURE 9. Testing motor strength of upper leg. Patient attempts to raise thigh against nurse's resistance. (*Source:* Used with permission from Shutterstock. *Photo by B. Proud.*)

ACTION

RATIONALE

22. Ask the patient to dorsiflex and then plantarflex both feet against opposing resistance (Figure 10).

These measure ankle flexion and dorsiflexion.

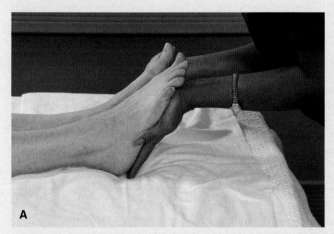

A

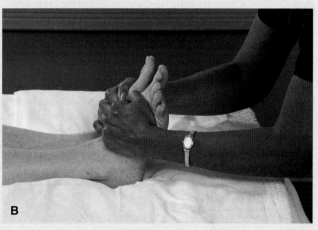

B

FIGURE 10. A. Testing ankle flexion and dorsiflexion. The patient first pushes the balls of the feet against resistance of the nurse's hands. **B.** Then attempts to pull against nurse's resistance. (*Source:* Used with permission from Shutterstock. *Photos by B. Proud.*)

23. As needed, assist the patient to a standing position. Observe the patient as they walk with a regular gait, on the toes, on the heels, and then heel to toe (Figure 11).

This procedure evaluates cerebellar and motor function.

24. Perform the Romberg's test; ask the patient to stand straight with feet together, both eyes closed with arms at side (Figure 12). Wait 20 seconds and observe for patient swaying and ability to maintain balance. Be alert to prevent a patient fall or injury related to losing balance during this assessment.

This test checks cerebellar functioning and evaluates balance, equilibrium, and coordination. Slight swaying is normal, but patient should be able to maintain balance.

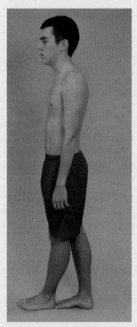

FIGURE 11. Testing heel to toe walking. (*Source:* From Jensen, S. [2019]. *Nursing health assessment* [3rd ed., p. 652]. Wolters Kluwer.)

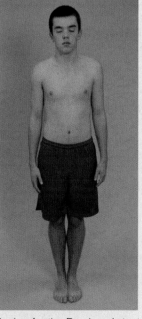

FIGURE 12. Positioning for the Romberg's test. (*Source:* From Jensen, S. [2019]. *Nursing health assessment* [3rd ed., p. 653]. Wolters Kluwer.)

(*continued on page 150*)

Skill 3-10 ▶ Assessing the Neurologic, Musculoskeletal, and Peripheral Vascular Systems *(continued)*

ACTION	**RATIONALE**
25. Assist the patient to a comfortable position.	This ensures the patient's comfort.
26. Remove PPE, if used. Perform hand hygiene. Continue with assessments of specific body systems, as appropriate, or indicated. Initiate appropriate referral to other health care providers for further evaluation, as indicated.	Proper removal of PPE reduces the risk for infection transmission and contamination of other items. Hand hygiene prevents the spread of microorganisms. Additional assessments should be completed, as indicated, to evaluate the patient's health status. Intervention by other health care providers may be indicated to evaluate and treat the patient's health status.

EVALUATION

The expected outcomes have been met when the patient has participated in the assessment of the neurologic, musculoskeletal, and peripheral vascular systems; the patient has verbalized understanding of the assessment techniques as appropriate; the assessment has been completed without the patient experiencing anxiety or discomfort; the findings have been documented; and the appropriate referrals have been made to the other health care professionals, as needed, for further evaluation.

DOCUMENTATION

Guidelines

Document assessment techniques performed, along with specific findings. Note the cognitive responses of the patient, the tested cranial nerves, and sensation and motor responses. Document any patient statements of pain, muscle weakness, or joint abnormality. Record findings, including color, turgor, temperature, pulses, and capillary refill.

Sample Documentation

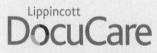

Practice documenting assessment techniques and findings in *Lippincott DocuCare*.

> 4/4/25 Patient alert, oriented, cognitively appropriate. Full ROM of all joints. Muscles soft, firm, nontender, no atrophy. Patient states pain in right calf. Right calf skin paler tone and slightly cooler compared with left calf. Peripheral pulses 72, +2, regular rhythm, equal bilaterally; exception—right posterior tibial and dorsalis pedis pulses +1. Capillary refill right lower extremity sluggish, >3 seconds, +sensation in feet, equal bilaterally.
>
> —S. Moses, RN

DEVELOPING CLINICAL REASONING AND CLINICAL JUDGMENT

SPECIAL CONSIDERATIONS

General Considerations

- Before performing the mental status examination, inform the patient that some of the questions may seem unusual, but that you are attempting to evaluate overall cognitive function.

Infant and Child Considerations

- In an infant, jerky and brief twitching of the extremities may be noted and considered a normal finding.
- The Babinski sign is a normal finding in children ages 24 months and younger (Jensen, 2019).
- The infant's extremities move symmetrically through ROM but lack full extension.
- Motor control develops in head, neck, trunk, and extremities in sequence.
- Coordination of movement varies according to the developmental level of the young child.

Older Adult Considerations

- Be aware that short-term memory, such as recall of recent events, may diminish with age. Older adults may also experience slowed reaction time as well.
- In the older adult patient, expect to find decreased musculoskeletal function, such as loss of muscle strength.
- Slower gait, with a wider base and flexed hips and knees.
- Keep in mind that older adults may take longer to perform certain actions, such as completing activities for testing coordination.

Enhance Your Understanding

Focusing on Patient Care: Developing Clinical Reasoning and Clinical Judgment

Consider the case scenarios at the beginning of the chapter as you answer the following questions to enhance your understanding and apply what you have learned.

QUESTIONS

1. When obtaining the history from Mr. Lincoln, he reports having a stuffed-up nose, postnasal drip, and a cough that sometimes produces mucus. He has smoked about one and a half packs of cigarettes a day for the past 20 years. Which areas of his physical examination would be most important?

2. Lois Felker, who has a history of type 1 diabetes mellitus, has arrived for her appointment with the health care provider. What systems will be most important to include in the physical assessment portion of the routine checkup related to this health problem?

3. Bobby Williams is suspected of having appendicitis. Which aspects of the health assessment are significant in relation to this health problem?

You can find suggested answers after the Bibliography at the end of this chapter.

Integrated Case Study Connection

The case studies in the back of the book focus on integrating concepts. Refer to the following case studies to enhance your understanding of the concepts and skills in this chapter.
- Basic Case Studies: James White, page 1196; Naomi Bell, page 1198; Joe LeRoy, page 1203; Kate Townsend, page 1205.
- Intermediate Case Studies: Olivia Greenbaum, page 1209; Victoria Holly, page 1211; Jason Brown, page 1215; Kent Clark, page 1217; Lucille Howard, page 1219; George Patel, page 1223.
- Advanced Case Studies: Cole McKean, page 1225; Damian Wallace, page 1227; Robert Espinoza, page 1230.

Bibliography

Agency for Clinical Innovation (ACI). ACI Musculoskeletal Network. (2018). *Neurovascular assessment*. New South Wales Government. https://aci.health.nsw.gov.au/__data/assets/pdf_file/0004/458185/ACI_0147-MSK-compartment-guide_V4.pdf

Ali, P. A., & Watson, R. (2018). Language barriers and their impact on provision of care to patients with limited English proficiency: Nurses' perspectives. *Journal of Clinical Nursing, 27*(5–6), e1152–e1160. https://doi.org/10.1111/jocn.14204

Altarum Institute. (2019). *Sexual health and your patients: A provider's guide*. National Coalition for Sexual Health. https://nationalcoalitionforsexualhealth.org/tools/for-healthcare-providers

American Cancer Society (ACS). (2018). *Testicular cancer early detection, diagnosis, and staging*. https://www.cancer.org/content/dam/CRC/PDF/Public/8845.00.pdf

American Cancer Society (ACS). (2020). *Breast cancer. American Cancer Society recommendations for early detection of breast cancer*. https://www.cancer.org/cancer/breast-cancer/screening-tests-and-early-detection/american-cancer-society-recommendations-for-the-early-detection-of-breast-cancer.html

American Mental Health Counselors Association. (2017, January 27). *AMHCA Clinical practice briefs. The need for early mental health screening and intervention across the lifespan*. https://www.amhca.org/viewdocument/the-need-for-early-mental-health-sc-2?LibraryFolderKey=&DefaultView=folder

American Speech-Language Hearing Association. (n.d.). *Adult hearing screening*. Screening for disability (activities and participation). Self-assessment tools. https://www.asha.org/PRPSpecificTopic.aspx?folderid=8589942721&section=Key_Issues

Anderson, B., Nix, E., Norman, B., & McPike, H. D. (2014). An evidence based approach to undergraduate physical assessment practicum course development. *Nurse Education in Practice, 14*(3), 242–246.

Andrews, M., Boyle, J. S., & Collins, J. (2020). *Transcultural concepts in nursing care* (8th ed.). Wolters Kluwer.

Bright Futures/American Academy of Pediatrics. (2021). Recommendations for preventive pediatric health care. https://downloads.aap.org/AAP/PDF/periodicity_schedule.pdf

Cahill, S., Baker, K., & Makadon, H. (2020). *Do ask, do tell: A toolkit for collecting sexual orientation and gender identify information in clinical settings*. The Fenway Institute and the Center for American Progress. https://doaskdotell.org/

Centers for Disease Control and Prevention (CDC). (n.d.). *Immunization schedules*. https://www.cdc.gov/vaccines/schedules/

Centers for Disease Control and Prevention. (2018). *Healthy weight. About child & teen BMI. What is BMI?* https://www.cdc.gov/healthyweight/assessing/bmi/childrens_bmi/about_childrens_bmi.html

Chung, S., Huang, Q., LaMori, J., Doshi, D., & Romanelli, R. J. (2020). Patient-reported experiences in discussing prescribed medications with a health care provider: Evidence for racial/ethnic disparities in a large health care delivery system. *Population Health Management, 23*(1), 78–84. DOI: 10.1089/pop.2018.0206

Dalton, M., Harrison, J., Malin, A., & Leavey, C. (2018). Factors that influence nurses' assessment of patient acuity and response to acute deterioration. *British Journal of Nursing, 27*(4), 212–218.

Derbyshire, J., & Hill, B. (2018). Performing neurological observations. *British Journal of Nursing, 27*(19), 1110–1114.

Dudek, S. (2018). *Nutrition essentials for nursing practice* (8th ed.). Wolters Kluwer.

Eliopoulos, C. (2018). *Gerontological nursing* (9th ed.). Wolters Kluwer.

Greenshields, S. (2019). Neurological assessment in children and young people. *British Journal of Nursing, 28*(16), 1056–1059.

Hall, A. (2018). Heart sounds: Auscultation for valvular heart disease. *British Journal of Cardiac Nursing, 13*(1), 12–18.

Hess, D. R., MacIntyre, N. R., Galvin, W. F., & Mishoe, S. C. (2021). *Respiratory care. Principles and practice* (4th ed.). Jones & Bartlett Learning.

Hickey, J. V. (2019). *The clinical practice of neurological and neurosurgical nursing* (8th ed.). Wolters Kluwer.

Hinkle, J. L., & Cheever, K. H. (2018). *Brunner & Suddarth's textbook of medical-surgical nursing* (14th ed.). Wolters Kluwer.

Hogan-Quigley, B., Palm, M. L., & Bickley, L. (2017). *Bates' nursing guide to physical examination and history taking* (2nd ed.). Wolters Kluwer.

Holleck, J. L., Campbell, S., Alrawili, H., Frank, C., Merchant, N., Rodwin, B., Perez, M. F., Gupta, S., Federman, D. G., Chang, J. J., Vientos, W., & Dembry, L. (2020). Stethoscope hygiene: Using cultures and real-time feedback with bioluminescence adenosine triphosphate technology to change behavior. *American Journal of Infection Control, 48*(4), 380–385. https://doi.org/10.1016/j.ajic.2019.10.005

Jarvis, C., & Eckhardt, A. (2020). *Physical examination & health assessment* (8th ed.). Elsevier.

Jensen, S. (2019). *Nursing health assessment: A best practice approach* (3rd ed.). Wolters Kluwer Health.

Johns Hopkins Medicine. (n.d.). *Health. Wellness and prevention. Breast self-awareness*. https://www.hopkinsmedicine.org/health/wellness-and-prevention/breast-self-awareness

Johnston-Walker, E., & Hardcastle, J. (2011). Neurovascular assessment in the critically ill patient. *Nursing in Critical Care, 16*(4), 170–177.

Keltner, N. L., & Steele, D. (2019). *Psychiatric nursing* (8th ed.). Elsevier.

Kersey-Matusiak, G. (2019). Delivering culturally competent nursing care. *Working with diverse and vulnerable populations* (2nd ed.). Springer Publishing Company.

Ku, L., & Jewers, M. (2013). *Health care for immigrant families: Current policies and issues.* Migration Policy Institute. https://www.migrationpolicy.org/research/health-care-immigrant-families-current-policies-and-issues

Kyle, T., & Carman, S. (2021). *Essentials of pediatric nursing* (4th ed.). Wolters Kluwer Health.

Mayo Clinic. (2018). *Testicular exam.* https://www.mayoclinic.org/tests-procedures/testicular-exam/about/pac-20385252

McCormick, R., Robin, A. T., Gluch, J., & Lipman, T. H. (2019). Oral health assessment in acute care pediatric nursing. *Pediatric Nursing, 45*(6), 299–309.

McGee, S. R. (2018). Chapter 53. Auscultation of the abdomen. *Evidence-based physical diagnosis* (4th ed.). Elsevier.

Meyer, C., & Hickson, L. (2020). Evidence-based practice guideline. Nursing management of hearing impairment in nursing facility residents. *Journal of Gerontological Nursing, 46*(7), 15–25. DOI: 10.3928/00989134-20200605-04

Mitchell, A., & Elbourne, S. (2020). Lower limb assessment. *British Journal of Nursing, 29*(1), 18–21.

National Heart, Lung, and Blood Institute. (n.d.). *Aim for a health weight. Assessing your weight and health risk.* https://www.nhlbi.nih.gov/health/educational/lose_wt/risk.htm

National Institutes of Health (NIH). (n.d.). *How are overweight and obesity diagnosed?* Eunice Kennedy Shriver National Institute of Child Health and Human Development. https://www.nichd.nih.gov/health/topics/obesity/conditioninfo/diagnosed

Norris, T. L. (2019). *Porth's essentials of pathophysiology* (5th ed.). Wolters Kluwer.

Ohns, M. J., Walsh, E., & Douglas, Z. (2020). Acute compartment syndrome in children: Don't miss this elusive diagnosis. *The Journal for Nurse Practitioners, 16*, 19–22. https://doi.org/10.1016/j.nurpra.2019.07.012

SAMHSA-HRSA Center for Integrated Health Solutions (CIHS). (2020). *Resources for screening, brief intervention, and referral to treatment (SBIRT).* Substance Abuse and Mental Health Services Administration (SAMHSA), U. S. Department of Health and Human Services, and Health Resources and Services Administration (HRSA). https://www.samhsa.gov/integrated-health-solutions

Senger, B. A., & Smith, D. W. (2020). Augmenting a focused bedside history for prelicensure nursing students. *Journal of Nursing Education, 59*(3), 178. https://doi.org/10.3928/01484834-20200220-14

Silbert-Flagg, J., & Pillitteri, A. (2018). *Maternal and child health nursing* (8th ed.). Wolters Kluwer.

Taylor, C., Lynn, P., & Bartlett, J. (2023). *Fundamentals of nursing: The art and science of person-centered care* (10th ed.). Wolters Kluwer.

Taylor, E. J. (2020). Initial spiritual screening and assessment: Five things to remember. *Korean Journal of Hospice & Palliative Care, 23*(1), 1–4. https://doi.org/10.14475/kjhpc.2020.23.1.1

Turney, J., Raley Noble, D., & Chae Kim, S. (2013). Orthopaedic nurses' knowledge and interrater reliability of neurovascular assessments with 2-point discrimination test. *Orthopaedic Nursing, 32*(3), 167–172. https://doi.org/10.1097/NOR.0b013e3182920abb

U. S. Department of Health and Human Services (USDHHS). Office of Disease Prevention and Health Promotion (ODPHP). (2020). Healthy People 2030. *Social determinants of health.* https://health.gov/healthypeople/objectives-and-data/social-determinants-health

VHA Center for Engineering & Occupational Safety and Health (CEOSH). (2016). Safe patient handling and mobility guidebook. http://www.tnpatientsafety.com/pubfiles/Initiatives/workplace-violence/sphm-pdf.pdf

Videbeck, S. L. (2020). *Psychiatric mental health nursing* (8th ed.). Wolters Kluwer.

Waterhouse, C. (2005). The Glasgow Coma Scale and other neurological observations. *Nursing Standard, 19*(33), 56–64; quiz 66–67.

Weber, J. R., & Kelley, J. H. (2018). *Health assessment in nursing* (6th ed.). Wolters Kluwer.

Wijdicks, E. F., Bamlet, W. R., Maramattom, B. V., Manno, E. M., & McClelland, R. L. (2005). Validation of a new coma scale: The FOUR Score. *Annals of Neurology, 58*(4), 585–593. https://doi.org/10.1002/ana.20611

Zappa, S., Fagoni, N., Bertoni, M., Selleri, C., Venturini, M. A., Finazzi, P., Metelli, M., Rasulo, F., Piva, S., Latronico, N., & Imminent Brain Death (IBD) Network Investigators. (2020). Determination of imminent brain death using the Full Outline of Unresponsiveness Score and the Glasgow Coma Scale: A prospective, multicenter, pilot feasibility study. *Journal of Intensive Care Medicine, 35*(2), 203–207. https://doi.org/10.1177/0885066617738714

SUGGESTED ANSWERS FOR FOCUSING ON PATIENT CARE: DEVELOPING CLINICAL REASONING AND CLINICAL JUDGMENT

1. Assessment of the patient's head and neck, as well as his thorax and lungs, would be most important. Examination of his head and neck will provide additional information related to his nasal symptoms as well as his cough. Assessment of his thorax and lungs will provide additional information related to his cough and possible effects of smoking.

2. Assessment of integumentary, neurologic, and peripheral vascular systems would be important to include when caring for a patient with diabetes. Major complications of diabetes include retinopathy, nephropathy, and neuropathy. Assessment of these systems would aid in identifying possible complications from diabetes that should be addressed.

3. Assessment of the patient's abdomen would be important to aid in confirming concerns related to appendicitis. In particular, you should assess for tenderness and pain, which can indicate peritoneal irritation, such as from appendicitis. Other symptoms may include nausea, vomiting, and lack of appetite.

4

Safety

Focusing on Patient Care

This chapter will help you develop some of the skills related to safety issues that may be necessary to care for the following patients:

Megan Lewis, an 18-month-old who has an IV access in her left forearm.

Kevin Mallory, a 35-year-old professional body builder admitted with a severe closed head injury. He is intubated and is constantly reaching for his endotracheal tube.

John Frawley, a 72-year-old diagnosed with Alzheimer disease who continues to try to get out of bed after falling and breaking a hip.

Refer to Focusing on Patient Care: Developing Clinical Reasoning and Clinical Judgment at the end of the chapter to apply what you learn.

Learning Outcomes

After completing the chapter, you will be able to accomplish the following:

1. Perform a situational assessment.
2. Implement nursing interventions related to reducing fall risk and risk of fall-related injury.
3. Implement nursing interventions to be used as alternatives to restraints.
4. Identify guidelines for the use of physical restraints.
5. Apply an extremity restraint correctly and safely.
6. Apply a waist restraint correctly and safely.
7. Apply an elbow restraint correctly and safely.
8. Apply a mummy restraint correctly and safely.

Nursing Concepts

- Assessment
- Clinical Decision Making/Clinical Judgment
- Safety

Safety and security are basic human needs. Safety is a paramount concern that underlies all nursing care, and patient safety is a responsibility of all health care providers. It is a focus in all health care facilities as well as in the home, workplace, and community. Nursing strategies that identify potential hazards and promote wellness from a person-centered perspective evolve from an awareness of individual factors that affect a patient's safety. Fundamentals Review 4-1 outlines patient safety risks related to developmental stage, as well as patient teaching to promote patient safety. Guidelines to promote patient safety are provided by health care accrediting, professional, and governmental organizations and agencies. For example, the Joint Commission identifies National Patient Safety Goals (NPSGs). The purpose of the NPSGs is to improve patient safety, focusing on problems in health care safety and how to solve them. These NPSGs are identified for a range of patient care settings, including ambulatory care, home care, hospitals, behavioral care, and office-based surgery. They are updated yearly and can be found on the Joint Commission website at https://www.jointcommission.org/en/standards/national-patient-safety-goals/.

The American Nurses Association (ANA) is a professional organization that also provides guidance to promote patient safety. A position statement from the ANA defines the nurses' role in reducing **restraint** use in health care. These recommendations are presented in Box 4-2 in Skill 4-3.

This chapter covers skills nurses will need when working with patients to monitor for safety, prevent injury, and to intervene when safety issues arise. The first skill addresses the use of a general patient and environmental survey to identify immediate patient concerns, as well as safety concerns. The next two skills address prevention of injury and discuss reduction of fall risk and utilizing alternatives to the use of restraints. The remaining skills address how to use several types of physical restraints safely and correctly. A physical restraint is any manual method, physical or mechanical device, material, or equipment that the person cannot remove easily, which immobilizes or reduces the person's freedom of movement or normal access to one's body (CMS, 2006). **Physical restraints should be considered as a last resort after other care alternatives have been unsuccessful.**

Whether or not a specific device is considered a restraint is determined by several factors:

- Intended use of a device, such as physical restriction
- Its involuntary application
- Identified patient need

For example, if a bed rail is used to facilitate a patient's mobility in and out of bed, it is not a restraint. If side rails could potentially restrict a patient's freedom to leave the bed, the rails would be a restraint. If a patient can release or remove a device, it is not a restraint. Side rails that are raised with the *intent* to prevent the patient from voluntarily attempting or actually getting out of bed, would be considered a restraint; if the *intent* of raising the side rails is to prevent a patient from inadvertently falling out of bed, or if the patient lacks the physical ability to even attempt to get out of bed, side rails would not be considered a restraint (The Joint Commission, 2017).

When it is necessary to apply a restraint, the nurse should use the least restrictive method and should remove it at the earliest possible time. Consider the laws regulating the use of restraints and facility regulations and policies. Ensure compliance with ordering, assessment, and maintenance procedures. Fundamentals Review 4-2 provides general guidelines for restraint use. Always treat patients with respect and protect their dignity.

Fundamentals Review 4-1

PREVENTING ACCIDENTS AND PROMOTING SAFETY AT VARYING DEVELOPMENTAL STAGES

Developmental Stage/Safety Risks	Teaching Tip	Why Is This Important
Fetus Abnormal growth and development	• Abstain from alcohol and caffeine while pregnant. • Stop smoking or reduce the number of cigarettes smoked per day. • Avoid all drugs, including OTC drugs, unless prescribed by the health care provider. • Avoid exposure to pesticides and certain environmental chemicals. • Avoid exposure to radiation.	Any factors, chemical or physical, can adversely affect the fertilized ovum, embryo, and developing fetus. A fetus is extremely vulnerable to environmental hazards.
Neonate (first 28 days of life) Infection Falls SIDS	• Wash hands frequently. • Never leave an infant unsupervised on a raised surface without side rails. • Use the appropriate infant car seat that is secured in the backseat facing the rear of the car. • Handle the infant securely while supporting the head. • Place infant on the back to sleep.	Physical care for the newborn includes maintaining a patent airway, protecting the baby from infection and injury, and providing optimal nutrition.
Infant Falls Injuries from toys Burns Suffocation or drowning Inhalation or ingestion of foreign bodies	• Supervise the child closely to prevent injury. • Select toys appropriate for developmental level. • Use appropriate safety equipment in the home (e.g., locks for cabinets, gates, electrical outlet covers). • Never leave the child alone in the bathtub. • Childproof the entire house.	Infants progress from rolling over to sitting, crawling, and pulling up to stand. They are very curious and will explore everything in their environment that they can.
Toddler Falls Cuts from sharp objects Burns Suffocation or drowning Inhalation or ingestion of foreign bodies/poisons	• Have poison control center phone number in readily accessible location. • Use appropriate car seat for the toddler. • Supervise the child closely to prevent injury. • Childproof the house to ensure that poisonous products, drugs, guns, and small objects are out of the toddler's reach. • Never leave the child alone and unsupervised outside. • Keep all hot items on the stove out of the child's reach.	Toddlers accomplish a wide variety of developmental tasks and progress to walking and talking. They become more independent and continue to explore their environment.
Preschooler Falls Cuts Burns Drowning Inhalation or ingestion Guns and weapons	• Teach the child to wear proper safety equipment when riding bicycles or scooters. • Ensure that playing areas are safe. • Begin to teach safety measures to the child. • Do not leave the child alone in the bathtub or near water. • Practice emergency evacuation measures. • Teach about fire safety.	Though more independent, preschoolers still have an immature understanding of dangerous behavior. They may strive to imitate adults and thus attempt dangerous behavior.

(continued)

Fundamentals Review 4-1 continued

PREVENTING ACCIDENTS AND PROMOTING SAFETY AT VARYING DEVELOPMENTAL STAGES

Developmental Stage/Safety Risks	Teaching Tip	Why Is This Important
School-aged child Burns Drowning Broken bones Concussions (TBI) Inhalation or ingestion Guns and weapons Substance abuse Bullying	• Teach accident prevention at school and home. • Teach the child to wear safety equipment when playing sports and when riding a bicycle. • Reinforce teaching about symptoms that require immediate attention. • Continue immunizations as scheduled. • Provide drug, alcohol, and sexuality education. • Reinforce the use of seatbelts and pedestrian safety. • Support social relationships and watch for changes in the child that may indicate bullying or being bullied.	School-aged children have developed more refined muscular coordination, but increasing involvement in sports and play activities increases their risk for injury. TBI can cause disruption in brain function and death. Cognitive maturity improves their ability to understand safety instructions.
Adolescent Motor vehicle accidents Drowning Guns and weapons Inhalation and ingestion Bullying	• Teach responsibilities of new freedoms that accompany being a teenager. • Enroll the teen in safety courses (driver education, water safety, emergency care measures). • Emphasize gun safety. • Get physical examination before participating in sports. • Make time to listen to and talk with your adolescent (helps with stress reduction). • Follow healthy lifestyle (nutrition, rest, etc.). • Teach about sexuality, intercourse sexually transmitted infections, and birth control. • Encourage the child to report any sexual harassment or abuse of any kind. • Engage in open dialogue about events relative to social media, personal relationships, and school activities.	Adolescence is a critical period in growth and development. The adolescent needs increasing freedom and responsibility to prepare for adulthood. During this time, the mind has a great ability to acquire and use knowledge. The teen's peer group is a greater influence than family during this stage.
Adult Stress Domestic violence Motor vehicle accidents Industrial accidents Drug and alcohol abuse	• Practice stress reduction techniques (e.g., meditation, exercise). • Enroll in a defensive driving course. • Evaluate the workplace for safety hazards and utilize safety equipment as prescribed. • Practice moderation when consuming alcohol. • Avoid the use of illegal drugs. • Provide options and referrals to those experiencing intimate partner violence (IPV).	As people progress through the adult years, visible signs of aging become apparent. Lifestyle behaviors and situational or family crises can also impact an adult's overall health and cause stress. Preventive health practices help adults improve the quality and duration of life.
Older Adult Falls Motor vehicle accidents Elder abuse Sensorimotor changes Fires	• Identify safety hazards in the environment. • Modify the environment as necessary. • Attend defensive driving courses on courses designed for older adult drivers. • Encourage regular vision and hearing tests. • Ensure that prescribed eyeglasses and hearing aids are available and functioning. • Wear appropriate footwear. • Have operational smoke detectors in place. • Objectively document and report any signs of neglect and abuse.	Accidental injuries occur more frequently in older adults because of decreased sensory abilities, slower reflexes and reaction times, changes in hearing and vision, and loss of strength and mobility. Collaboration between family/caregivers and health care providers can ensure a safe, comfortable environment and promote healthy aging.

Fundamentals Review 4-2

GENERAL GUIDELINES FOR RESTRAINT USE

- The patient has the right to be free from restraints that are not medically necessary. Restraints may be used only to protect the patient, staff, or others, and must be discontinued at the earliest possible time. Restraints *must not* be used for the convenience of staff or to punish a patient.
- The patient's family/caregivers must be involved in the plan of care. They must be consulted when the decision is made to use restraints. The family/caregivers must be instructed regarding the facility's restraint policy and alternatives to restraints that are available.
- Physical restraints should be considered only after assessment of the patient, environment, and the situation; interventions to relieve discomforting behaviors have been used, precipitating factors have been identified and eliminated, if possible; and consultation with other health care professionals has occurred.
- **Alternatives to restraints and less restrictive interventions must have been implemented and failed. All alternatives used must be documented.**
- Contradictions to physical restraints should be assessed.

- The benefit gained from using a restraint must outweigh the known risks for that patient.
- The restraints must be prescribed by a physician or other licensed practitioner who is responsible for the care of the patient. The order can never be for use on an "as-needed" basis.
- Once in place, the patient must be monitored and reassessed frequently, based on facility policy and patient status. The patient's vital signs must be assessed, and the patient must be visually observed every hour or according to facility policy.
- A physician or other licensed practitioner who is permitted to order restraint or seclusion in that health care facility and is responsible for the care of the patient must reevaluate and assess the patient every 24 hours (in the hospital setting) (CMS, 2006).
- Personal needs must be met. Provide fluids, nutrition, and toileting assistance every 2 hours.
- Skin integrity must be assessed, and range-of-motion exercises provided every 2 hours.
- Documentation regarding why, how, where, and for how long the restraints were placed, and patient monitoring is vital.

Source: Modified from Centers for Medicare & Medicaid Services (CMS). (2020a). Department of Health and Human Services. CMS manual system. Pub. 100–07. Appendix A. Survey protocol, regulations and interpretive guidelines for hospitals. §482.13. *Conditions of participation: Patients' rights.* https://www.cms.gov/Regulations-and-Guidance/Guidance/Manuals/downloads/som107ap_a_hospitals.pdf; Centers for Medicare & Medicaid Services (CMS). (2020b). Department of Health and Human Services. CMS manual system. Pub. 100–07. Appendix PP. Guidance to surveyors for long term care facilities. §482.10. *Resident rights.* https://www.cms.gov/Regulations-and-Guidance/Guidance/Manuals/downloads/som107ap_pp_guidelines_ltcf.pdf; and Centers for Medicare & Medicaid Services (CMS). (2006). Department of Health and Human Services. Federal Register. Part IV. 42 CFR Part 482. *Medicare and Medicaid programs; Hospital conditions of participation: Patients' rights; Final rule.* https://www.cms.gov/Regulations-and-Guidance/Legislation/CFCsAndCoPs/downloads/finalpatientrightsrule.pdf

Skill 4-1 ▶ Performing a Situational Assessment

Awareness of the patient's environment and of the patient's situation is an integral part of nursing care. Situational awareness in the patient care environment involves knowledge, attention, and responsiveness in relation to patient monitoring; knowing and understanding what's happening around you; and awareness of patient safety (Fore & Sculli, 2013; Fukuta & Iitsuka, 2018; Green et al., 2017; Large & Aldridge, 2018). Situational awareness in nursing includes routine use of a general survey (observation) of the patient, family/caregivers, and environment, using input from all senses (Cohen, 2013). These observations contribute to an understanding of the current situation and support anticipation of potential problems. Identifying and solving problems is essential to effective and safe nursing practice. Integration of situational awareness as part of routine nursing care allows nurses to anticipate patients' needs "by knowing what is going on, why it's happening and what's likely to happen next" (Cohen, 2013, p. 64). Situational awareness promotes a safer patient care environment, reduces risk for falls, and helps the nurse develop care priorities, acting correctly when things go as planned, and reacting appropriately when they don't (Cohen, 2013, p. 64; Fore & Sculli, 2013; Godlock et al., 2016; Large & Aldridge, 2018).

(continued on page 158)

Skill 4-1 ▶ Performing a Situational Assessment *(continued)*

DELEGATION CONSIDERATIONS	A situational assessment should not be delegated to assistive personnel (AP). However, the AP may notice some items while providing care. The nurse must then validate, analyze, document, communicate, and act on these findings, as appropriate. Depending on the state's nurse practice act and the organization's policies and procedures, the licensed practical/vocational nurses (LPN/LVNs) may perform some or all of the parts of a situational assessment. The decision to delegate must be based on careful analysis of the patient's needs and circumstances as well as the qualifications of the person to whom the task is being delegated. Refer to the Delegation Guidelines in Appendix A.
EQUIPMENT	• PPE, as indicated
ASSESSMENT	A situational assessment is completed during every encounter with the patient and periodically at planned intervals throughout the day. Observations should be modified based on the specific patient care setting (e.g., long-term care, school, home health, etc.) and circumstances.
ACTUAL OR POTENTIAL HEALTH PROBLEMS AND NEEDS	Many actual or potential health problems or needs may require the use of this skill as part of related interventions. An appropriate health problem or need may include: • Fall risk • Injury risk • Impaired Mobility
OUTCOME IDENTIFICATION AND PLANNING	The expected outcome to achieve is that a situational assessment is completed, the patient's needs are met, and the patient remains free from injury.

IMPLEMENTATION

ACTION	**RATIONALE**
1. Perform hand hygiene and put on PPE, if indicated.	Hand hygiene and PPE prevent the spread of microorganisms. PPE is required based on transmission precautions.
2. Identify the patient. Explain the purpose of the assessment to the patient.	Identifying the patient ensures the right patient receives the intervention and helps prevent errors. Explanation helps reduce anxiety and promotes engagement and understanding.
3. Assess for data that suggest a problem with the patient's airway, breathing, or circulation. If a problem is present, identify if it is urgent or nonurgent in nature. Refer to Chapter 3 for specific related assessments.	Problems with the patient's airway, breathing, or circulation may signal a situation requiring immediate action. It is important to determine the importance of information, focus on the most relevant and important data, act on that which is important and develop plans for interventions that can be justified in relation to their likelihood of success (Lasater, 2007).

ACTION

RATIONALE

4. Assess the patient's level of consciousness, orientation, and speech. Observe the patient's behavior and affect (Figure 1). If a problem is present, identify if it is urgent or nonurgent in nature. Refer to Chapter 3 for specific related assessments.

Problems with the patient's level of consciousness, orientation, speech, behavior, or affect may signal a situation requiring immediate action. It is important to determine the importance of information, focus on the most relevant and important data, act on that which is important and develop plans for interventions that can be justified in relation to their likelihood of success (Lasater, 2007).

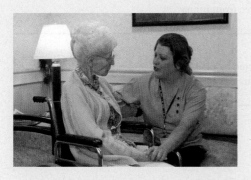

FIGURE 1. Observing the patient's behavior and affect. (Used with permission from Shutterstock. *Photo by Rick Brady.*)

5. Assess the patency of an oxygen delivery device, if in use. Refer to Chapter 14 for specific related assessments.

Properly functioning equipment is required to maintain delivery of oxygen.

6. Assess other relevant *priority* body systems as appropriate, based on individual patient circumstances.

Nurses must use clinical judgment to adapt this assessment for each patient, based on the individual circumstances of an individual patient (Henley Haugh, 2015).

7. Survey the patient's environment. Assess the bed position and call bell location. The bed should be in the lowest position, and the call bell (based on specific patient care setting) should be within the patient's reach.

Environmental survey identifies problems that may harm the patient (Cohen, 2013).

8. Assess for clutter and hazards. Remove excess equipment, supplies, furniture, and other objects from rooms and walkways. Pay particular attention to high traffic areas and the route to the bathroom.

All are possible hazards and could cause the patient to fall.

9. Note the presence and location of appropriate emergency equipment, based on individual patient situation.

Emergency equipment must be immediately available if needed.

10. Note the presence and location of appropriate assistive devices and mobility aids, based on individual patient situation. Ensure any devices are within the patient's reach.

Assistive devices should be available for patient use.

11. Assess for the presence of an intravenous (IV) access and/or infusion. Assess patency of the device and the insertion site. If an infusion is present, assess the solution and rate. Refer to Chapter 16 for specific related assessments.

Assessment allows for identification of problems and ensures administration of intravenous fluids as prescribed.

12. Assess for the presence of any tubes, such as gastric tubes, chest tubes, surgical drains, or urinary catheters. Assess patency of the device and insertion site. Refer to Chapter 8 and Chapters 11 through 14 for specific related assessments.

Assessment allows for identification of problems and ensures patency of devices.

13. Provide a bedside commode and/or urinal/bedpan, if appropriate. Ensure that it is near the bed at all times.

This prevents falls related to incontinence or trying to get to the bathroom.

14. Ensure that the bedside table, telephone, and other personal items are within the patient's reach at all times.

This prevents the patient from having to overreach for a device or items, and/or possibly attempt ambulation or transfer unassisted.

15. Consider what further assessments should be completed and additional interventions that may be indicated. Identify problems that need to be communicated and whom to contact.

Early detection of problems allows for corresponding interventions to prevent adverse occurrences, supporting improved patient outcomes (Large & Aldridge, 2018).

(continued on page 160)

Skill 4-1 ▶ Performing a Situational Assessment *(continued)*

ACTION

16. Remove PPE, if used. Perform hand hygiene.

RATIONALE

Proper removal of PPE reduces the risk for infection transmission and contamination of other items. Hand hygiene prevents transmission of microorganisms.

EVALUATION

The expected outcomes have been met when a situational assessment has been completed, the patient's needs are met, and the patient remains free from injury.

DOCUMENTATION

Guidelines

Document significant assessment findings as directed by facility policy and protocol. Include associated interventions and/or related communication.

DEVELOPING CLINICAL REASONING AND CLINICAL JUDGMENT

SPECIAL CONSIDERATIONS

Community-Based Care Considerations

• Examine the home for objects on the floor, the presence of wires or cords, objects on the steps, and loose or torn carpet. Encourage residents to keep walkways, floors, and stairs clear.
• Assess for adequate lighting, especially at the top and bottom of stairs and pathways from the bedroom to bathroom.
• Assess for the presence of working smoke detectors at a minimum on every floor of the home, ideally in every room. Provide education regarding safe use as appropriate.
• Assess for the presence of a carbon monoxide detector.
• Assess for the presence of firearms in the home. Provide education regarding safe storage as appropriate.
• Assess for the presence of space heaters. Provide education regarding safe use as appropriate.
• If there are children in the home, evaluate the method used to store medications, cleaning products, insecticides, and corrosives. Provide education regarding safe storage as appropriate and Poison Control Center contact information.

Skill 4-2 ▶ Fall Risk and Fall-Related Injury Risk Reduction

Falls are the second leading cause of unintentional injuries throughout life, with older adults and children being at highest risk (World Health Organization, 2018). In older adults, fall-related injuries are often serious and are associated with disability, loss of independence, social isolation, and death (National Council on Aging, n.d.). Falls are caused by and associated with multiple factors. Primary causes of falls include:

• Developmental stage/age group
• Balance problems or gait disturbance
• Lower body/muscle weakness
• Dizziness, syncope, and vertigo
• Cardiovascular changes, such as postural hypotension
• Change in vision or vision impairment
• Physical environment/environmental hazards
• Acute illness
• Neurologic disease, such as dementia or depression
• Language disorders that impair communication
• Polypharmacy

Many of these causes are within the realm of nursing responsibility. A team approach and engagement with patients, families and/or caregivers that utilizes an interdisciplinary, multifactorial approach to assessment, intervention, and evaluation leads to maximum prevention (Benning & Webb, 2019; Dykes et al., 2018; Jones et al., 2019; Stoeckle et al., 2019; Tucker et al., 2019; WHO, 2018). Identifying at-risk patients is crucial to planning appropriate interventions to prevent a fall. Fall risk assessment is discussed in the assessment section of this skill and includes an example of a fall-assessment tool. Table 4-1 identifies examples of fall risk reduction strategies for acute care based on fall risk assessment; interventions should be tailored based on patient-specific risk factors to develop a personalized plan (Dykes et al., 2018). The combination of an assessment tool with an individualized care/intervention plan sets the stage for best practice (Dykes et al., 2018; Grossman et al., 2018; Williams, 2018).

Providing patient education and a safer patient environment can reduce the incidence and severity of falls (The Joint Commission, 2015). Interventions to reduce fall-related injuries work in conjunction with strategies to decrease fall risk to reduce the physical and psychological injury and trauma experienced by patients and their families, caregivers, and significant others.

Table 4-1 Recommended Fall-Prevention Strategies by Fall Risk Level

LOW FALL RISK	MODERATE FALL RISK	HIGH FALL RISK
Fall Risk Score: 0–5 Points	*Fall Risk Score: 6–10 Points* *Color Code: Yellow*	*Fall Risk Score: >10 Points* *Color Code: Red*
Maintain safe unit environment, including: • Remove excess equipment/supplies/furniture from rooms and hallways. • Coil and secure excess electrical and telephone wires. • Clean all spills in patient room or in hallway immediately. Place signage to indicate wet floor danger. • Restrict window openings. The following are examples of basic safety interventions: • Orient patient to surroundings, including bathroom location, use of bed, and location of call bell. • Keep bed in lowest position during use unless impractical (as in ICU nursing or specialty beds). • Keep top two side rails up (excludes box beds). In ICU, keep all side rails up. • Secure locks on beds, stretchers, and wheelchairs. • Keep floors clutter/obstacle free (with attention to path between bed and bathroom/commode). • Place call bell and frequently needed objects within patient reach. Answer call bell promptly. • Encourage patients/families to call for assistance when needed. • Display special instructions for vision and hearing. • Ensure adequate lighting, especially at night. • Use properly fitting nonskid footwear.	• Institute flagging system: yellow card outside room and yellow sticker on health record. Hill ROM flag (if available), assignment board/electronic board. In addition to measures listed under low fall risk: • Monitor and assist patient in following daily schedules. • Supervise and/or assist bedside sitting, personal hygiene, and toileting, as appropriate. • Reorient confused patients, as necessary. • Establish elimination schedule, including use of bedside commode, if appropriate. • PT (physical therapy) consult if patient has a history of fall and/or mobility impairment. Evaluate need for: • OT (occupational therapy) consult • Slip-resistant chair mat (do *not* use in shower chair) • Use of seatbelt, when in wheelchair	• Institute flagging system: red card outside room and red sticker on health record, assignment board/electronic board: nurse call system flag, if available. In addition to measures listed under moderate and low fall risk: • Remain with patient while toileting. • Observe every 60 minutes unless patient is on activated bed/chair alarm. • If patient requires an air overlay, remove mattress (unless contraindicated by overlay type) or use side rail protectors. • When necessary, transport throughout hospital with assistance of staff or trained caregivers. Consider alternatives, for example, bedside procedure. Notify receiving area of high fall risk. Evaluate need for the following, starting with less restrictive to more restrictive measures in the listed order: • Moving patient to room with best visual access to nursing station • Bed/chair alarm • Specialty fall-prevention bed • 24-hour supervision/sitter • Physical restraint/enclosed bed (only if less restrictive alternatives have been considered and found to be ineffective)

Source: Recommended fall-prevention strategies by fall risk level. Reprinted with permission. © 2003, The Johns Hopkins Hospital.

(*continued on page 162*)

Skill 4-2 ▶ Fall Risk and Fall-Related Injury Risk Reduction *(continued)*

DELEGATION CONSIDERATIONS

After assessment of fall risk by the registered nurse (RN), activities related to reducing a patient's risk for falls may be delegated to assistive personnel (AP) as well as to licensed practical/vocational nurses (LPN/LVNs). The decision to delegate must be based on careful analysis of the patient's needs and circumstances as well as the qualifications of the person to whom the task is being delegated. Refer to the Delegation Guidelines in Appendix A.

EQUIPMENT

- Fall risk assessment tool, if available
- PPE, as indicated
- Additional intervention tools, as appropriate (refer to sample intervention equipment in this skill)

ASSESSMENT

At a minimum, fall risk assessment needs to occur on admission to a facility, during an initial home visit, following a change in the patient's condition, after a fall, when the patient is transferred between facilities, and during annual well-visits and health screenings. If it is determined that the patient is at risk for falling, regular assessment must continue. Assess the patient and the health record for factors that increase the patient's risk for falling. An objective, systematic fall risk assessment is made easier by the use of a fall risk assessment tool, combined with additional assessments to evaluate risks not captured by the tool (The Joint Commission, 2015). The Johns Hopkins Fall Risk Assessment Tool (Figure 1) is one example of a fall risk assessment tool. The Hendrich II Fall Risk Model (older adults) and the Humpty Dumpty Falls Scale (pediatric patients) are other tools to evaluate fall risk factors.

Assess for a history of a fall or falls. Once a person falls one time, the chance of falling again increases dramatically regardless of whether the patient is in a hospital, a long-term care facility, or the community (Grossman et al., 2018; Soh et al., 2020). If the patient has experienced a previous fall, assess the circumstances surrounding the fall and any associated symptoms (AGS, n.d.). Review the patient's medication history and medication record for medications that may increase the risk for falls. Assess for the following additional risk factors for falls (AGS, n.d.; Centers for Disease Control and Prevention [CDC], 2019d; CDC, 2017; WHO, 2018):

- Lower extremity muscle weakness
- Gait or balance deficit
- Mobility impairment
- Restraint use
- Use of an assistive device
- Presence of IV therapy
- Impaired activities of daily living (ADLs)
- Age older than 65 years/children
- Altered elimination
- History of falls
- Administration of high-risk drugs, such as narcotic analgesics, antiepileptics, benzodiazepines, and drugs with anticholinergic effects
- Use of four or more medications
- Alcohol or substance abuse
- Postural (orthostatic) hypotension
- Depression
- Visual deficit
- Arthritis
- Fear of falling
- History of cerebrovascular accident
- Cognitive impairment
- Secondary diagnosis/chronic disease
- Home/environmental hazards/dangers

Johns Hopkins
Fall Risk Assessment Tool

If patient has any of the following conditions, check the box and apply Fall Risk interventions as indicated.

High Fall Risk - Implement High Fall Risk interventions per protocol
- ☐ History of more than one fall within 6 months before admission
- ☐ Patient has experienced a fall during this hospitalization
- ☐ Patient is deemed high fall-risk per protocol (e.g., seizure precautions)

Low Fall Risk - Implement Low Fall Risk interventions per protocol
- ☐ Complete paralysis or completely immobilized

Do not continue with Fall Risk Score Calculation if any of the above conditions are checked.

FALL RISK SCORE CALCULATION – Select the appropriate option in each category. Add all points to calculate Fall Risk Score. (If no option is selected, score for category is 0)	Points
Age (single-select) ☐ 60 - 69 years (1 point) ☐ 70 -79 years (2 points) ☐ greater than or equal to 80 years (3 points)	
Fall History (single-select) ☐ One fall within 6 months before admission (5 points)	
Elimination, Bowel and Urine (single-select) ☐ Incontinence (2 points) ☐ Urgency or frequency (2 points) ☐ Urgency/frequency and incontinence (4 points)	
Medications: Includes PCA/opiates, anticonvulsants, anti-hypertensives, diuretics, hypnotics, laxatives, sedatives, and psychotropics (single-select) ☐ On 1 high fall risk drug (3 points) ☐ On 2 or more high fall risk drugs (5 points) ☐ Sedated procedure within past 24 hours (7 points)	
Patient Care Equipment: Any equipment that tethers patient (e.g., IV infusion, chest tube, indwelling catheter, SCDs, etc.) (single-select) ☐ One present (1 point) ☐ Two present (2 points) ☐ 3 or more present (3 points)	
Mobility (multi-select; choose all that apply and add points together) ☐ Requires assistance or supervision for mobility, transfer, or ambulation (2 points) ☐ Unsteady gait (2 points) ☐ Visual or auditory impairment affecting mobility (2 points)	
Cognition (multi-select; choose all that apply and add points together) ☐ Altered awareness of immediate physical environment (1 point) ☐ Impulsive (2 points) ☐ Lack of understanding of one's physical and cognitive limitations (4 points)	
Total Fall Risk Score (Sum of all points per category)	
SCORING: 6-13 Total Points = Moderate Fall Risk, >13 Total Points = High Fall Risk	

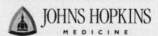

FIGURE 1. Johns Hopkins Fall Risk Assessment Tool. (Reprinted with permission. © 2003, The Johns Hopkins Hospital.)

(continued on page 164)

Skill 4-2 ▶ Fall Risk and Fall-Related Injury Risk Reduction *(continued)*

ACTUAL OR POTENTIAL HEALTH PROBLEMS AND NEEDS	Many actual or potential health problems or needs may require the use of this skill as part of related interventions. An appropriate health problem or need may include: • Fall risk • Injury risk • Impaired Walking
OUTCOME IDENTIFICATION AND PLANNING	The expected outcome to achieve is that the patient does not experience a fall and remains free of injury. Other outcomes that may be appropriate include the following: the patient's environment is free from hazards; patient, family, and/or caregiver demonstrates an understanding of appropriate interventions to prevent falls; the patient uses assistive devices correctly; the patient uses safe transfer procedures; and appropriate precautions are implemented related to the use of medications that increase the risk for falls.

IMPLEMENTATION

ACTION	RATIONALE
1. Perform hand hygiene and put on PPE, if indicated.	Hand hygiene and PPE prevent the spread of microorganisms. PPE is required based on transmission precautions.
2. Identify the patient. Assess fall risk as outlined above.	Identifying the patient ensures the right patient receives the intervention and helps prevent errors. Fall risk assessment aids in providing appropriate interventions for the individual patient.
3. Review the results of the fall risk assessment and fall risk factors with the patient, family, and/or caregivers (Figure 2).	Promotes person-centered, individualized care and engagement, continuity of care and understanding.
4. Explain the rationale for interventions to reduce the patient's risk for fall to the patient, family, and/or caregivers.	Explanation helps reduce anxiety and promotes engagement and understanding.
5. Include the patient, family, and/or caregivers in the plan of care.	Promotes person-centered, individualized care and engagement, continuity of care and understanding (CDC, 2017; CDC, 2019d; Hager et al., 2019; Stoeckle et al., 2019; Tucker et al., 2019; Williams, 2018).
6. Provide time for the patient, family, and/or caregivers to discuss concerns about falling, identify fall risk factors not identified by the risk assessment, confirm their understanding of risk factors and interventions, and to verbalize concerns or questions.	Promotes person-centered, individualized care and engagement, continuity of care and understanding. Active involvement on the part of patients, family, and/or caregivers is an important part of identification of fall risk and associated interventions (CDC, 2017; CDC, 2019d; Stoeckle et al., 2019; Tucker et al., 2019; Williams, 2018).
7. Provide adequate lighting. Use a night light during sleeping hours.	Good lighting reduces accidental tripping over and bumping into objects that may not be seen. Night light provides illumination in an unfamiliar environment.
8. Remove excess equipment, supplies, furniture, and other objects from rooms and walkways. Pay particular attention to high traffic areas and the route to the bathroom.	All are possible hazards.
9. Orient patient and significant others to new surroundings, including use of the telephone, call bell, patient bed, and room illumination. Indicate the location of the patient's bathroom.	Knowledge of proper use of equipment relieves anxiety and promotes engagement.

ACTION

10. Consider use of a low bed to replace regular hospital bed, as indicated (Figure 3). Low beds should be raised to the appropriate height for each patient to allow safe transition out of bed (Hester, 2015).

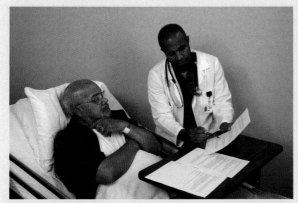

FIGURE 2. Reviewing the results of the fall risk assessment and fall risk factors with the patient. (From Eliopoulos, C. [2018]. *Gerontological nursing* [9th ed., p. 109]. Wolters Kluwer.)

11. Use floor mats if the patient is at risk for getting out of bed without calling for assistance and is at risk for injury (Quigley, 2015) (see Figure 3). Floor mats should only be on the floor by the bedside on the safest side of the bed for patient exit when the patient is resting in bed (Quigley, 2015).
12. Provide nonskid footwear and/or walking shoes (Figure 4).

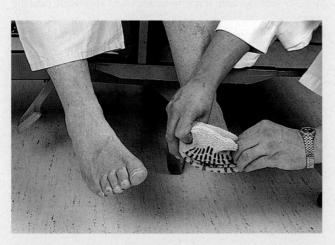

13. Institute a toileting regimen and/or continence program, if appropriate.
14. Provide a bedside commode and/or urinal/bedpan, if appropriate. Ensure that it is near the bed at all times, if appropriate for individual patient.

RATIONALE

The use of low beds is associated with decreased serious fall-related injuries (Hester, 2015).

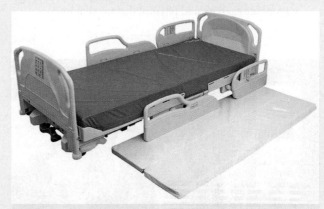

FIGURE 3. Low bed with floor mats. (Reprinted with permission from CHG Hospital Beds, London, ON.) *Note:* Mats should be in place on floor only when the patient is in the bed. Floor mats should be stored underneath the bed when the patient is not in the bed to reduce the risk of tripping. This image is for illustrative purposes only.

Floor mats cushion falls and may reduce trauma resulting from falls (Hester, 2015; Quigley 2015). Floor mats should be stored underneath the bed when the patient is not in the bed to reduce the risk of tripping (Quigley, 2015).

Nonskid footwear prevents slipping and walking shoes improve balance when ambulating or transferring.

FIGURE 4. Providing nonskid footwear.

Toileting on a regular basis decreases risk for falls.

This prevents falls related to incontinence or trying to get to the bathroom. It may be necessary to move the bedside commode out of sight to discourage attempts at independent transfer by patients with altered mobility, as appropriate.

(continued on page 166)

Skill 4-2 ▶ Fall Risk and Fall-Related Injury Risk Reduction *(continued)*

ACTION	RATIONALE
15. Ensure that the call bell, bedside table, telephone, and other personal items are within the patient's reach at all times.	This prevents the patient from having to overreach for a device or items, and/or possibly attempt ambulation or transfer unassisted.
16. Confer with the health care team regarding and encourage appropriate exercise and physical therapy (Figure 5).	Exercise programs, such as muscle strengthening, balance training, resistance training, and walking plans, promote improved balance and reduce the risk of falls and fall-related injuries (CDC, 2017; Thomas et al., 2019).

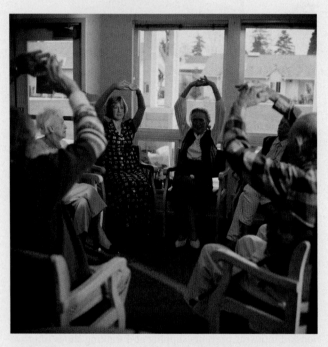

FIGURE 5. Encouraging appropriate exercise. (From Hinkle, J. L., & Cheever, K. H. [2018] *Brunner & Suddarth's textbook of medical-surgical nursing* [14th ed.]. Wolters Kluwer.)

ACTION	RATIONALE
17. Confer with the health care team regarding appropriate mobility aids, such as a cane or walker.	Mobility aids can help improve balance and steady the patient's gait.
18. Confer with the health care team regarding the use of bone-strengthening medications, such as calcium, vitamin D, and drugs to prevent/treat osteoporosis.	Bone strengthening has been suggested to reduce fracture with fall-related injuries (CDC, 2019a).
19. Encourage the patient to rise or change position slowly and sit for several minutes before standing.	Gradual position changes reduce the risk of falls related to orthostatic hypotension.
20. Evaluate the appropriateness of graduated compression stockings for lower extremities.	Graduated compression stockings minimize venous pooling and promote venous return.
21. Confer with the health care team to review medications for potential hazards.	Certain medications and combinations of medications have been associated with increased risk for falls.
22. Keep the bed in the lowest position. If elevated to provide care (to reduce caregiver strain) or when a patient is transferring out of bed, ensure that it is lowered when care is completed.	Keeping bed in lowest position reduces the risk of a fall and fall-related injury (AHRQ, 2013).

ACTION	RATIONALE
23. Make sure locks on the bed or wheelchair are secured at all times (Figure 6).	Locking prevents the bed or wheelchair from moving out from under the patient.
24. Use bed rails according to facility policy, when appropriate, based on individual patient assessment (Figure 7).	Inappropriate bed-rail use has been associated with patient injury and increased fall risk (FDA, 2018b). Side rails that are raised with the intent to prevent the patient from voluntarily attempting or actually getting out of bed are considered a restraint (The Joint Commission, 2017).

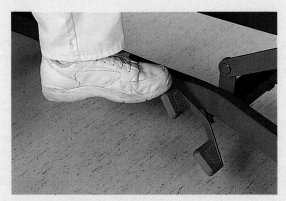

FIGURE 6. Engaging bed locks.

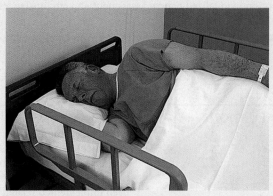

FIGURE 7. Raising side rails on bed at the patient's request.

25. Anticipate patient needs and provide assistance with activities instead of waiting for the patient to ask.	Patients whose needs are met sustain fewer falls.
26. Consider the use of an electronic personal alarm or pressure sensor alarm for the bed or chair (Figure 8).	The alarm helps alert staff to unassisted changes in position by the patient.

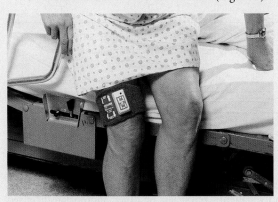

FIGURE 8. Patient wearing a personal alarm device.

27. Discuss the possibility of appropriate family member(s)/caregiver(s) staying with the patient.	The presence of a family member/caregiver provides familiarity and companionship.
28. Consider the use of a patient attendant or sitter.	An attendant or sitter can provide companionship and supervision; however, the effectiveness of this intervention on patient falls is unclear (Greeley et al., 2020).

(continued on page 168)

Skill 4-2 ▶ Fall Risk and Fall-Related Injury Risk Reduction *(continued)*

ACTION	**RATIONALE**
29. Increase the frequency of patient observation and surveillance. Utilize 1- or 2-hour patient care rounds/intentional rounding (hourly/nursing rounds), including pain assessment, toileting assistance, patient comfort, making sure personal items are in reach, and meeting patient needs.	Intentional rounding/patient care rounds anticipate and proactively address patient needs (Hicks, 2015; Ryan et al., 2019). Patient care rounds can reduce patient falls (Ryan et al., 2019; Spano-Szekely, 2018).
30. Assess for and make use of safe patient handling equipment (e.g., gait belt, lifts, transfer devices) as appropriate, based on individualized patient assessment and circumstances. Refer to Chapter 9.	Use of safe patient handling equipment facilitates safe patient transfers (lateral and vertical), repositioning, mobility, and transport (VHACEOSH, 2016).
31. Remove PPE, if used. Perform hand hygiene.	Proper removal of PPE reduces the risk for infection transmission and contamination of other items. Hand hygiene prevents transmission of microorganisms.

EVALUATION

The expected outcomes have been met when the patient has not experienced a fall and has remained uninjured; interventions to minimize risk factors that might precipitate a fall have been implemented; the patient's environment is free from hazards; the patient, family, and/or caregiver demonstrated an understanding of appropriate interventions to prevent falls; the patient uses assistive devices correctly; the patient uses safe transfer procedures; and appropriate precautions have been implemented related to the use of medications that increase the risk for falls.

DOCUMENTATION

Guidelines

Document patient fall risk assessment results. Include appropriate interventions to reduce fall risk in the plan of care. Document patient and family/caregiver teaching relative to fall risk reduction. Document interventions included in care.

Sample Documentation

> 11/1/25 1730 Patient admitted to room 650W; oriented to room. Fall assessment low risk. Basic safety interventions in place per facility Fall Prevention Guidelines. Will continue to monitor and reevaluate.
>
> —B. Clapp, RN

DEVELOPING CLINICAL REASONING AND CLINICAL JUDGMENT

UNEXPECTED SITUATIONS AND ASSOCIATED INTERVENTIONS

- *Patient experiences a fall:* Immediately assess the patient's condition. Provide care and interventions appropriate for status/injuries. Notify patient's physician or other appropriate licensed practitioner of the incident and your assessment of the patient. Ensure prompt follow-through for any orders for diagnostic tests, such as x-rays or CT scans, as prescribed. Evaluate circumstances of the fall and the patient's environment and institute appropriate measures to prevent further incidents. Document incident, assessments, and interventions in the patient's health record. Complete a **safety event report** per facility policy.

SPECIAL CONSIDERATIONS

General Considerations

- For each fall risk factor, identify specific interventions that relate directly to the risk. Interventions should be customized for each patient based on issues identified in the assessment (Grossman et al., 2018).

- If a low bed is used, patients who are weak may have trouble getting out of bed safely. Low beds should be raised to the appropriate height for each patient to allow safe transition out of bed (Hester, 2015).
- Empower patients to become active participants in fall risk reduction. Provide health care interventions that are patient centered to enable patients to be a partner in reduction of fall risk (Tucker et al., 2019).
- Implement and use injury-prevention strategies and devices to prevent or reduce injuries from falls.
  - Floor matting and compliant flooring provide a cushioned surface that reduces impact, decreasing the likelihood of injury if the patient falls (Hester, 2015; Quigley, 2015).
  - Hip protectors reduce impact from falls that could cause hip fracture (Hester, 2015; Korall et al., 2019).
- Enclosure bed can be used as part of a patient's plan of care to prevent falls and provide a safer environment (Harris, 2015). An enclosure bed is considered a restraint because it limits the patient's ability to get out of bed but is less restrictive than other types of restraints (Harris, 2015).

Infant and Child Considerations

- Pediatric patient falls include unique risk factors for consideration that include normal childhood behavior and development (Benning & Webb, 2019).
- Children fall for a variety of reasons that may not be captured adequately by any one assessment tool (Williams, 2018). All hospitalized children may be at risk for falling, reinforcing the need for increased emphasis on fall risk reduction, and minimization of fall-related injuries. Use of a validated assessment tool may help identify pediatric patients who may be at increased risk, but continuous assessment of the patient's health status, disease process, and effects of treatments, as well as reassessment over time, considering identified risks, is necessary to help keep pediatric patients safe from falls (Williams, 2018).
- Encourage parents and caregivers to use home safety devices, such as guards on windows that are above ground level, stair gates, and guard rails (CDC, 2019d).
- Encourage parents and caregivers to supervise young children at all times around fall hazards, such as stairs and playground equipment, whether at home or out in the community (CDC, 2019d).
- Parents and caregivers should never leave infants and young children on a bed or any other furniture unsupervised (Cronan, 2018).
- Provide education for parents and caregivers about home safety: never put an infant in a baby seat on top of a counter or other high surface; always strap young children into high chairs, changing tables, shopping carts, and strollers (Cronan, 2018).

Older Adult Considerations

- Encourage older adults to talk with their health care provider about a "falls checkup" on a regular basis (AGS, 2019).
- Encourage older adults to avoid wearing bifocal or multifocal glasses when walking; these types of lenses can make things seem closer or farther away than they really are. These patients should consider obtaining a pair of glasses with only the distance prescription for outdoor activities (CDC, 2017).
- Exercise improves balance and strengthens muscles in older adults (CDC, 2017).
- Exercise programs should be encouraged for older adults. Exercise has the potential to decrease falls in older adults (Hamed et al., 2018).
- Older adults may have a low self-perceived fall risk level; focused effort to disseminate information and increase patient engagement in fall prevention should be part of transition from health care facilities, such as the hospital, to home environments (Shuman et al., 2019).
- Older adults should assess their home environment to improve safety: remove times that are a tripping hazard (including throw rugs and small area rugs), add grab bars inside and outside the tub or shower and next to the toilet, install railings on both sides of any stairs, and use bright light bulbs (adding lights if needed) (CDC, 2017; National Institute on Aging, n.d.).

(continued on page 170)

Skill 4-2 ▶ Fall Risk and Fall-Related Injury Risk Reduction *(continued)*

Community-Based Care Considerations

- Patients are at risk for falls in their home. Assess for risk factors in the home and assess the home environment. Include patient teaching regarding falls as part of the plan of care. See Box 4-1 for possible interventions for the home setting.
- Exercise programs should be encouraged for community- dwelling adults 65 years or older who are at increased risk for falls (Grossman et al., 2018).
- Exercise should be included as part of home-based fall-prevention interventions to improve balance and performance of ADLs (Fahlström et al., 2018).
- Multifactorial interventions, based on assessment of modifiable risk factors for falls for an individual patient, should be offered for community-dwelling adults age 65 years or older who are at increased risk for falls (Grossman et al., 2018). Interventions could include behavioral therapy, nutrition therapy, education, medication management, urinary incontinence management, environmental modification, physical or occupational therapy, and referral to specialists (e.g., ophthalmologist, neurologist, cardiologist) (Grossman et al., 2018).
- Parents and caregivers should check that surfaces under playground equipment are safe, soft, and are of appropriate materials (such as wood chips or sand) (CDC, 2019d).

Box 4-1 ▍ Patient Education for Preventing Falls in the Home

- Talk with your health care provider about a plan for an exercise program. Regular exercise helps maintain strength and flexibility and can help slow bone loss.
- Have regular hearing and vision testing. Always wear glasses and hearing aids, if prescribed. Even small changes in sight and hearing can affect stability.
- Wear low-heeled, rubber-soled shoes. Avoid wearing only socks or shoes with smooth soles.
- Have handrails on both sides of stairs and make use of them when using the stairs. Try not to carry things when using the steps. When necessary, hold item in one hand and use the handrail with the other hand.
- Install safety gates at the bottom and top of staircases to keep children from tumbling down.
- Avoid using chairs and tables as ladders to reach items that are too high to reach.
- Keep electrical and telephone cords against the wall and out of walkways.
- Consider rails next to the toilet and in the shower or tub and raised toilet seats.

- Know the possible side effects of medications used. Some can affect coordination and balance.
- Use a cane, walking stick, or walker to help improve stability.
- Keep home temperature at a moderate level. Temperatures too hot or too cold can contribute to dizziness.
- Stand up slowly after eating, lying down, or resting. Standing too quickly can cause fainting or dizziness.
- Make sure there is good lighting, particularly at the stairs.
- Use a night light.
- Remove clutter from walkways inside and outside the house.
- Carpets should be fixed firmly to the floor to prevent slipping. Use no-slip strips on uncarpeted surfaces.
- Use nonskid mats, strips, or carpet on surfaces that get wet.
- Use rubber mats in the shower to prevent slips and falls from wet surfaces.
- Check all medications, including prescriptions, and over-the-counter drugs, herbs, and vitamins, with your health care provider and/or pharmacist to find out if any put you at risk for falling.

Source: Adapted from American Geriatrics Society (AGS) Health in Aging Foundation. (2019). *Tips for preventing serious falls.* AGS Geriatrics Healthcare Professionals. https://www.healthinaging.org/tools-and-tips/tips-preventing-serious-falls; American Geriatrics Society (AGS) Health in Aging Foundation. (n.d.). *Aging & health A-Z. Falls prevention.* AGS Geriatrics Healthcare Professionals. Retrieved June 15, 2020, from https://www.healthinaging.org/a-z-topic/falls-prevention; National Home Security Alliance. (2018). *Safety at home: 10 common safety hazards around the house.* https://staysafe.org/safety-at-home-10-common-safety-hazards-around-the-house/; and National Institute on Aging. (2017). *Health information. Prevent falls and fractures.* https://www.nia.nih.gov/health/prevent-falls-and-fractures; National Institute on Aging. (n.d.). *Fall-proofing your home.* https://www.nia.nih.gov/health/fall-proofing-your-home

EVIDENCE FOR PRACTICE ▶

ENGAGING PATIENTS IN FALL RISK ASSESSMENT
Providing patient education and a safer patient environment can reduce the incidence and severity of falls (Quigley, 2015; Stubbs et al., 2015; Tomita et al., 2014). Many prevention programs are not tailored for older patients transitioning home (Shuman et al., 2019). How can nurses engage older adults in fall prevention at home?

Related Research

Shuman, C. J., Montie, M., Hoffman, G. J., Powers, K. E., Doettl, S., Anderson, C. A., & Titler, M. G. (2019). Older adults' perceptions of their fall risk and prevention strategies after transitioning from hospital to home. *Journal of Gerontological Nursing, 45*(1), 23–30. https://doi. org/10.3928/00989134-20190102-04

This study explored patients' perceptions about falls and fall-related events after transitioning from hospital to home. Nine older adults designated as being at risk of falls during hospitalization and recently discharged (within 4 weeks) from a community medical center participated in this qualitative study. During face-to-face semi-structured interviews, participants were asked about their perceptions of fall risk and prevention. At the end of the interview, participants were shown three no-cost brochures from the Centers for Disease Control and Prevention's *Stopping Elderly Accidents, Deaths & Injuries* (STEADI) *Initiative* from the CDC (2017). These patient education tools provide a checklist for helping patients identify their risk for falls, identify four ways older adults can prevent falls, and help older adults identify and eliminate potential fall hazards in their homes. The interview audio recordings were transcribed verbatim and read twice and checked for accuracy against the recordings. Data were analyzed using constant comparative methods, and trustworthiness was established through credibility, dependability, and confirmability. Five major themes emerged from data analysis: sedentary behaviors and limited functioning, prioritization of social involvement, low perceived fall risk and attribution of risk to external factors, avoidance and caution as fall prevention, and limited fall-prevention information during transition from hospital to home. The researchers concluded that evidence-based patient and provider resources to prevent falls are not being routinely used to engage and educate older adults in fall prevention. The researchers suggested nurses must implement interventions to engage patients in fall prevention during the transition from hospital to home. Prevention programs adapted to the postdischarge period may engage patients in fall prevention and support well-being and independence.

Relevance to Nursing Practice

Limited awareness of and engagement in effective fall prevention may heighten recently discharged older adults' risks for falls. Nurses have a key role to play in engaging patients in their health care. Programs that provide patients with information related to fall risk and fall prevention should be implemented during care transitions to home and address gaps in the provision of fall-prevention information.

Skill 4-3 ▶ Implementing Alternatives to the Use of Restraints

Restraint-free care is the standard of practice and an indicator of quality care in all health care settings (American Nurses Association, 2012; Touhy & Jett, 2018, p. 210). Physical restraints do not prevent falls, and they increase the possibility of serious injury due to a fall (Taylor et al., 2023). Additional negative outcomes of restraint use include skin breakdown and contractures, incontinence, depression, delirium, anxiety, aspiration, and respiratory difficulties, and even death (Taylor et al., 2023). Federal guidelines reinforce that in all settings, the primary responsibility is to protect and promote patient's rights and that restraints may only be used to protect the patient, staff, or others (Taylor et al., 2023). Federal and state mandates as well as the Joint Commission recommend that acute care facilities use restraints only as a last resort (CMS, 2020a; Taylor et al., 2023). The current standard for long-term care facilities is to provide safe care without the use of physical or chemical restraints (Taylor et al., 2023).

(continued on page 172)

Skill 4-3 ▶ Implementing Alternatives to the Use of Restraints *(continued)*

Careful nursing assessment is the key to identifying appropriate alternatives to restraint use and finding an individualized solution (Taylor et al., 2023). The American Nurses Association (ANA, 2012) has approved a position statement defining the nurses' role in reducing restraint use in health care. Their recommendations are included in Box 4-2. Restraints should be used only after less restrictive methods have failed. The following skill outlines possible alternatives to restraint use.

Box 4-2 ANA Board of Directors Position Statement: Reduction of Patient Restraint and Seclusion in Health Care Settings

Recommendations: To ensure safe, quality care for all patients in the least restrictive environment, ANA supports nursing efforts to:

1. Educate nurses, nursing students, unlicensed personnel, other members of the interdisciplinary team, and family caregivers on the appropriate use of restraint and seclusion, and on the alternatives to these restrictive interventions;
2. Ensure sufficient nursing staff to monitor and individualize care with the goal of only using restraint when no other viable option is available;
3. Ensure policies and environment support services are in place to provide feasible alternatives to physical and chemical restraints;
4. Move progressively toward a restraint-free environment while providing a therapeutic sanctuary for all;
5. Enforce documentation requirements and education about what should be documented;
6. Explore the ethical implications of restraining patients with nursing students and discuss the need for institutional policy that clarifies when, where, and how patients are to be restrained and monitored while restrained;
7. Be aware of all implications of allowing the application of restraints in health care settings. The nurse administrator should make consultation available to nurses, including ethical consultation about decisions to restrain; and
8. Develop clear policies based on accepted national standards to guide decision making regarding restraints.

Source: American Nurses Association (ANA). (2012). ANA Position Statement: *Reduction of patient restraint and seclusion in health care settings.* https://www.nursingworld.org/practice-policy/nursing-excellence/official-position-statements/id/reduction-of-patient-restraint-and-seclusion-in-health-care-settings/. © 2012 by American Nurses Association. Reprinted with permission. All rights reserved.

DELEGATION CONSIDERATIONS

After assessment by the RN, activities related to the use of alternatives to restraints may be delegated to assistive personnel (AP) as well as to licensed practical/vocational nurses (LPN/LVNs). The decision to delegate must be based on careful analysis of the patient's needs and circumstances as well as the qualifications of the person to whom the task is being delegated. Refer to the Delegation Guidelines in Appendix A.

EQUIPMENT

- PPE, as indicated
- Additional intervention tools, as appropriate (refer to sample intervention equipment in this skill)

ASSESSMENT

Assess the patient's status. Determine whether the patient's pattern of behavior (wandering, fall risk, interfering with medical devices, resistive to care, danger to self or others) increases the potential need for restraint use. Assess to determine the meaning of the behavior and its cause. Assess for pain. Assess respiratory status, vital signs, blood glucose level, fluid and electrolyte issues, and medications. Assess the patient's functional, mental, and psychological status. Evaluate the patient's environment, including noise level, lighting, floor surfaces, design/suitability of equipment and furniture, visual cues, barriers to mobility, space for privacy, and clothing. Assess and evaluate the effectiveness of restraint alternatives.

ACTUAL OR POTENTIAL HEALTH PROBLEMS AND NEEDS

Many actual or potential health problems or needs may require the use of this skill as part of related interventions. An appropriate health problem or need may include:

- Acute confusion
- Injury risk

| OUTCOME IDENTIFICATION AND PLANNING | The expected outcome to achieve when implementing alternatives to restraints is that the use of restraints is avoided, and the patient and others remain free from injury. |

IMPLEMENTATION

ACTION	**RATIONALE**
1. Perform hand hygiene and put on PPE, if indicated.	Hand hygiene and PPE prevent the spread of microorganisms. PPE is required based on transmission precautions.
2. Identify the patient.	Identifying the patient ensures the right patient receives the intervention and helps prevent errors.
3. Explain the rationale for interventions to the patient and family/caregivers.	Explanation helps reduce anxiety and promotes engagement and understanding.
4. Include the patient's family and/or caregivers in the plan of care.	Promotes person-centered, individualized care and engagement, continuity of care and understanding.
5. Identify behavior(s) that place the patient at risk for restraint use. Assess the patient's status and environment, as outlined above.	Behaviors, such as interference with therapy or treatment, risk for falls, agitation/restlessness, resistance to care, wandering, and/or cognitive impairment, put the patient at risk for restraint use. Assessment and interpretation of patient behavior identifies unmet physiologic or psychosocial needs, acute changes in mental or physical status, provides for appropriate environments and individualized care, and respects patient's needs and rights.
6. Identify triggers or contributing factors to patient behaviors: a. Assess respiratory status, vital signs, blood glucose level, fluid, and electrolyte issues (Taylor et al., 2023). b. Evaluate medication usage for medications that can contribute to cognitive and movement dysfunction and to increased risk for falls (Taylor et al., 2023).	Changes in physiologic status and prescribed medications can be triggers and/or contributing factors. Removal of underlying issues triggering or contributing to patient behaviors can decrease or eliminate the need for restraint use.
7. Assess the patient's functional, mental, and psychological status and the environment, as outlined above.	Assessment provides a better understanding of the reason for the behavior, leading to individualized interventions that can eliminate restraint use and provide for patient safety.
8. Provide adequate lighting. Use a night light during sleeping hours.	Appropriate lighting can reduce disruptive behavior related to fear in an unfamiliar environment.
9. Consult with the health care team regarding the continued need for treatments/therapies and the use of the least invasive method to deliver care.	Exploring the possibility of administering treatment in a less intrusive manner or discontinuing treatment no longer needed can remove the stimulus for behavior that increases risk for the use of restraints.
10. Assess the patient for pain and discomfort. Provide appropriate pharmacologic and nonpharmacologic interventions. (Refer to Chapter 10.)	Unrelieved pain can contribute to behaviors that increase the risk for the use of restraints.
11. Ask a family member or caregiver to stay with the patient.	Having someone stay with the patient provides companionship and familiarity.
12. Reduce unnecessary environmental stimulation and noise.	Increased stimulation can contribute to behaviors that increase the risk for the use of restraints.
13. Provide simple, clear, and direct explanations for treatments and care. Repeat to reinforce, as needed.	Explanation helps reduce anxiety and promotes engagement and understanding.
14. Distract and redirect using a calm voice.	Distraction and redirection can reduce or remove behaviors that increase risk for the use of restraints.

(continued on page 174)

Skill 4-3 ▶ Implementing Alternatives to the Use of Restraints *(continued)*

ACTION	RATIONALE
15. Increase the frequency of patient observation and surveillance; utilize 1- or 2-hour patient care rounds/intentional rounding (hourly/nursing rounds), including pain assessment, toileting assistance, patient comfort, keeping personal items in reach, and meeting patient needs.	Patient care rounds/intentional rounding (hourly/nursing rounds) improve identification of unmet needs, which can decrease behaviors that increase risk for the use of restraints.
16. Implement fall-precaution interventions. Refer to Skill 4-2.	Behaviors that increase risk for the use of restraints also increase the risk for falls.
17. Camouflage tube and other treatment sites with clothing, elastic sleeves, or bandaging.	Camouflaging tubes and other treatment sites removes stimulus that can trigger behaviors that increase risk for the use of restraints. Assess sites regularly for complications (Taylor et al., 2023).
18. Investigate possibility of discontinuing bothersome treatment devices (e.g., IV line, catheter).	Remove invasive devices as early as possible (Lawson et al., 2020). Removes stimulus that can trigger behaviors that increase risk for the use of restraints.
19. Ensure the use of glasses and hearing aids, if necessary.	Glasses and hearing aids allow for correct interpretation of the environment and activities to reduce confusion.
20. Consider relocation to a room close to the nursing station.	Relocation close to the nursing station provides the opportunity for increased frequency of observation.
21. Encourage daily exercise/provide exercise and activities or relaxation techniques.	Activity provides an outlet for energy and stimulation, decreasing behaviors associated with increased risk for the use of restraints.
22. Make the environment as homelike as possible; provide familiar objects.	Familiarity provides reassurance and comfort, decreasing apprehension and reducing behaviors associated with increased risk for the use of restraints.
23. Allow restless patients to walk after ensuring that the environment is safe. Use a large plant or a piece of furniture as a barrier to limit wandering from the designated area.	Activity provides an outlet for energy and stimulation, decreasing behaviors associated with increased risk for the use of restraints.
24. Consider the use of a patient attendant or sitter.	An attendant or sitter provides companionship and supervision.
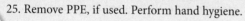 25. Remove PPE, if used. Perform hand hygiene.	Proper removal of PPE reduces the risk for infection transmission and contamination of other items. Hand hygiene prevents transmission of microorganisms.

EVALUATION The expected outcomes have been met when the use of restraints has been avoided, and the patient and others remained free from injury.

DOCUMENTATION

Guidelines Document patient assessment. Include appropriate interventions to reduce the need for restraints in the plan of care. Document patient and family/caregiver teaching relative to the use of interventions. Document interventions included in care.

Sample Documentation

1/1/25 2330 Patient pulling IV tubing and attempting to remove dressing at insertion site left antecubital. NPO status; IV necessary for hydration and medication. Explanation regarding IV access reinforced with patient and wife. IV site covered with gauze and tubing placed under top bed linen to minimize appearance. Wife provided CD of patient's favorite music and a puzzle. Rounding increased to every 30 minutes when family not present.

—B. Clapp, RN

DEVELOPING CLINICAL REASONING AND CLINICAL JUDGMENT

UNEXPECTED SITUATIONS AND ASSOCIATED INTERVENTIONS

- *Interventions to distract no longer effective. Patient continues to pull at IV site and tubing:* Reevaluate need for IV fluid infusion. Consult with health care team regarding possibility of converting to intermittent access. Reevaluate patient and environment; attempt additional/different interventions as outlined above.

SPECIAL CONSIDERATIONS

- An alternative approach for temporary restraint is therapeutic holding (hugging), which makes use of a secure, comfortable, temporary holding position that provides close physical contact with the parent or caregiver for 30 minutes or less (Kyle & Carman, 2021; Perry et al., 2018).
- Enclosure beds are a possible option for physical restraints (Kim et al., 2018). Enclosure bed can be used as part of a patient's plan of care to prevent falls and provide a safer environment (Harris, 2015). An enclosure bed is considered a restraint because it limits the patient's ability to get out of bed but is less restrictive than other types of restraints (Harris, 2015).
- Use of mechanical restraint in acute psychiatric/behavioral health environments can be reduced through increased frequency of direct registered nurse surveillance and assessment of restrained individuals (every 15 minutes to continue surveillance) (Allen et al., 2020).

EVIDENCE FOR PRACTICE ▶

MINIMIZING RESTRAINT USE

These resources summarize current best evidence on the topic of interventions to be used as alternatives to the use of restraints, as well as minimizing and eliminating the use of restraints.

- American Nurses Association (ANA). (2012). *Reduction of patient restraint and seclusion in health care settings.* https://www.nursingworld.org/practice-policy/nursing-excellence/official-position-statements/id/reduction-of-patient-restraint-and-seclusion-in-health-care-settings/
- American Psychiatric Nurses Association. (2018). *Positionstatement on the use of seclusion and restraint.* https://www.apna.org/resources/apna-seclusion-restraint-position-paper/
- Centers for Medicare & Medicaid Services (CMS). (2020a). Department of Health and Human Services. CMS manual system. Pub. 100–07. Appendix A. Survey protocol, regulations and interpretive guidelines for hospitals. §482.13. *Conditions of participation: Patients' rights.* https://www.cms.gov/Regulations-and-Guidance/Guidance/Manuals/downloads/som107ap_a_hospitals.pdf
- Centers for Medicare & Medicaid Services (CMS). (2020b). Department of Health and Human Services. CMS manual system. Pub. 100–07. Appendix PP. Guidance to surveyors for long term care facilities. §482.10. *Resident rights.* https://www.cms.gov/Regulations-and-Guidance/Guidance/Manuals/downloads/som107ap_pp_guidelines_ltcf.pdf
- Cotter, V. T., & Evans, L. K. (2021). *Consult Geri. Try this: Series. Avoiding restraints in patients with dementia. Issue #1 of dementia series.* The Hartford Institute for Geriatric Nursing. https://hign.org/consultgeri/try-this-series/avoiding-restraints-patients-dementia
- Grover Snook, A. (2017, March 31). *Physical restraint use.* CINAHL Information Systems. https://www.ebscohost.com/assets-sample-content/Physical_Restraint_Use.pdf
- Registered Nurses' Association of Ontario (RNAO). (2012). International affairs & best practice guidelines. *Promoting safety: Alternative approaches to the use of restraints.* https://rnao.ca/bpg/guidelines/promoting-safety-alternative-approaches-use-restraints

Skill 4-4 ▶ Applying an Extremity Restraint

Cloth extremity restraints immobilize one or more extremities. They may be indicated after other measures have failed to prevent a patient from removing therapeutic devices, such as intravenous (IV) access devices, endotracheal tubes, oxygen, or other treatment interventions. **Restraints should be used only after less restrictive methods have failed. Ensure compliance with ordering, assessment, and maintenance procedures. Restraints must be applied safely and appropriately to reduce risks of injury.** Federal guidelines reinforce that in all settings, the primary responsibility is to protect and promote patient's rights, and that restraints may only be used to protect the patient, staff, or others (Taylor et al., 2023). They must be discontinued at the earliest possible time (Taylor et al., 2023).

An extremity restraint may be applied to the hands, wrists, or ankles. Review the general guidelines for using restraints in the chapter introduction and in Fundamentals Review 4-2 and Box 4-2 in Skill 4-3. See also Evidence for Practice after Skill 4-3 for best evidence on the topic of interventions to be used as alternatives to the use of restraints, as well as minimizing and eliminating the use of restraints.

DELEGATION CONSIDERATIONS	After assessment of the patient by the RN, the application of an extremity restraint may be delegated to assistive personnel (AP) as well as to licensed practical/vocational nurses (LPN/LVNs). The decision to delegate must be based on careful analysis of the patient's needs and circumstances as well as the qualifications of the person to whom the task is being delegated. Refer to the Delegation Guidelines in Appendix A.
EQUIPMENT	• Appropriate cloth restraint for the extremity that is to be immobilized • Padding, if necessary, for bony prominences • PPE, as indicated
ASSESSMENT	Assess the patient's physical condition and the potential for injury to self or others. A confused patient who might remove devices needed to sustain life is considered at risk for injury to self and may require the use of restraints. Assess the patient's behavior, including the presence of confusion, agitation, and combativeness as well as the patient's ability to understand and follow directions. Evaluate the appropriateness of the least restrictive restraint device. For example, if the patient has had a stroke and cannot move the left arm, a restraint may be needed only on the right arm. Inspect the extremity where the restraint will be applied. Establish baseline skin condition for comparison at future assessments while the restraint is in place. Consider using another form of restraint if the restraint may cause further injury at the site. Before application, assess for adequate circulation in the extremity to which the restraint is to be applied, including capillary refill and proximal pulses.
ACTUAL OR POTENTIAL HEALTH PROBLEMS AND NEEDS	Many actual or potential health problems or needs may require the use of this skill as part of related interventions. An appropriate health problem or need may include: • Injury risk • Acute confusion
OUTCOME IDENTIFICATION AND PLANNING	The expected outcome to achieve is that the patient is constrained by the restraint and remains free from injury, and the restraint does not interfere with therapeutic devices. Other outcomes that may be appropriate include the following: the patient does not experience impaired skin integrity, the patient does not sustain injury due to the restraints, and the patient's family/caregivers will demonstrate an understanding about the use of the restraint and their role in the patient's care.

IMPLEMENTATION

ACTION

RATIONALE

1. Determine the need for restraints. Assess the patient's physical condition, behavior, and mental status. (Refer to Fundamentals Review 4-2 and Box 4-2 in Skill 4-3.)

Restraints should be used only as a last resort when alternative measures have failed, and the patient is at increased risk for harming self or others.

2. Confirm facility policy for the application of restraints. **Secure an order from the physician or other licensed practitioner who is permitted to order restraint or seclusion in that health care facility, or validate that the order has been obtained within the required time frame (CMS, 2020a).**

Policy protects the patient and the nurse and specifies guidelines for application as well as the type of restraint and duration. **Each order for restraint or seclusion used for the management of violent or self-destructive behavior that jeopardizes the immediate physical safety of the patient, a staff member, or others may only be renewed in accordance with the following limits for up to a total of 24 hours: (A) 4 hours for adults 18 years of age or older, (B) 2 hours for children and adolescents 9 to 17 years of age, or (C) 1 hour for children under 9 years of age. After 24 hours, before writing a new order for the use of restraint or seclusion for the management of violent or self-destructive behavior, a physician or other licensed practitioner who is permitted to order restraint or seclusion in that health care facility and responsible for the care of the patient must see and assess the patient (CMS, 2006).**

3. Perform hand hygiene and put on PPE, if indicated.

Hand hygiene and PPE prevent the spread of microorganisms. PPE is required based on transmission precautions.

4. Identify the patient.

Identifying the patient ensures the right patient receives the intervention and helps prevent errors.

5. Explain the reason for restraint use to patient and family/caregivers. Clarify how care will be given and how needs will be met. Explain that restraint is a temporary measure.

Explanation to the patient and family/caregivers may lessen confusion and anger and provide reassurance. A clearly stated facility policy on the application of restraints should be available for the patient and family/caregivers to read. In a long-term care facility, the family/caregivers must give consent before a restraint is applied.

6. Include the patient's family and/or caregivers in the plan of care.

Promotes person-centered, individualized care and engagement, continuity of care and understanding.

7. Inspect the restraint before use. Do not use a restraint that is soiled or damaged (TIDI Products, 2018a).

Always inspect the device before each use, checking for broken stitches or parts, torn, cut or frayed material; or locks, buckles or hook-and-loop fasteners that do not hold securely. Do not use soiled or damaged restraints to prevent injury or death (TIDI Products, 2018a).

8. Apply restraint according to the manufacturer's directions:

Proper application reduces the risk for injury.

   a. Choose the least restrictive type of device that allows the greatest possible degree of mobility.

This provides minimal restriction.

   b. Pad bony prominences.

Padding helps prevent skin injury.

(continued on page 178)

Skill 4-4 ▶ Applying an Extremity Restraint *(continued)*

ACTION	**RATIONALE**

ACTION

c. Wrap the restraint around the extremity with the soft part in contact with the skin (Figure 1). If a hand mitt is being used, pull over the hand with cushion to the palmar aspect of the hand (Figure 2).

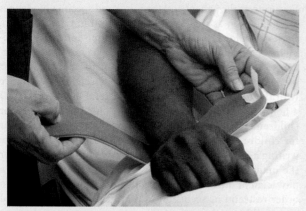

FIGURE 1. Wrapping the restraint around the extremity with the soft part in contact with the skin.

9. Secure in place with the hook-and-loop fastener straps or other mechanism, depending on specific restraint device (Figure 3). Depending on the characteristics of the specific restraint, close the quick-release buckle on the cuff.

10. **Ensure that one to two fingers can be inserted between the restraint and patient's extremity (Figure 4).**

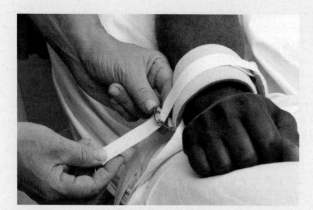

FIGURE 3. Securing restraint on extremity.

11. Maintain restrained extremity in normal anatomic position. **Use a quick-release knot to tie the restraint to the bed frame that moves with the patient, not side rail, bed rail, mattress, or head/footboard (Figure 5).** The restraint may also be attached to a chair frame. The site should not be readily accessible to the patient.

12. Remove PPE, if used. Perform hand hygiene.

RATIONALE

Prevents excess pressure on the extremity.

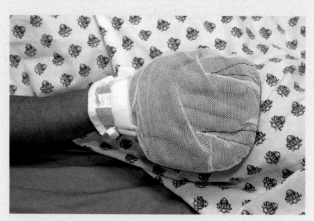

FIGURE 2. Using a hand mitt, with cushion to the palmar aspect of hand.

Proper application secures the restraint and ensures that there is no interference with the patient's circulation and potential alteration in neurovascular status.

The restraint must be snug, but not compromise circulation (TIDI Products, 2018b). Proper application ensures that nothing interferes with the patient's circulation and potential alteration in the neurovascular status.

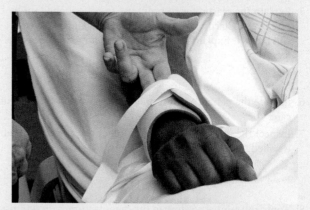

FIGURE 4. Ensuring that two fingers can be inserted between the restraint and the patient's extremity.

Maintaining a normal position lessens the possibility of an injury. A quick-release knot ensures that the restraint will not tighten when pulled and can be removed quickly in an emergency. Securing the restraint to a side rail may injure the patient when the side rail is lowered. Tying the restraint out of the patient's reach promotes security.

Proper removal of PPE reduces the risk for infection transmission and contamination of other items. Hand hygiene prevents transmission of microorganisms.

ACTION

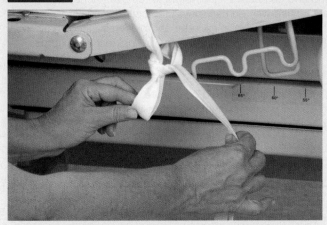

RATIONALE

FIGURE 5. Securing restraint to bed frame.

13. **Assess the patient according to facility policy, or more often, based on the individual patient circumstances and nursing judgment.** Assessment should include the placement of the restraint, neurovascular assessment of the affected extremity, and skin integrity. In addition, assess for signs of sensory deprivation, such as increased sleeping, daydreaming, anxiety, panic, and hallucinations. Monitor the patient's vital signs.

The condition of the restrained patient must be continually assessed, monitored, and reevaluated (CMS, 2006). The frequency of monitoring should be made on an individual basis, which includes a rationale that reflects consideration of the individual patient's medical needs and health status (CMS, 2006). Improperly applied restraints may cause skin tears, abrasions, or bruises. Decreased circulation may result in paleness, coolness, decreased sensation, tingling, numbness, or pain in extremity. The use of restraints may decrease environmental stimulation and result in sensory deprivation. Monitoring vital signs provides information about the status of the patient.

14. **Remove restraint at least every 2 hours or according to facility policy, individual patient circumstances, and nursing judgment. Remove the restraint at least every 2 hours for children 9 to 17 years of age and at least every 1 hour for children under 9 years of age, or according to facility policy, individual patient circumstances, and nursing judgment.** Perform range-of-motion (ROM) exercises. Provide for hydration, nutritional, and elimination needs.

Removal allows you to assess the patient and reevaluate the need for a restraint. It also allows interventions for toileting, provision of nutrition and liquids, exercise, and change of position. Exercise increases circulation in the restrained extremity.

15. **Evaluate the patient for continued need of restraint.** Reapply restraint only if continued need is evident and order is still valid.

Continued need must be documented for reapplication.

16. Reassure the patient at regular intervals. Provide continued explanation of rationale for interventions, reorientation if necessary, and plan of care. **Keep the call bell within the patient's easy reach.**

Reassurance demonstrates caring and provides an opportunity for sensory stimulation as well as ongoing assessment and evaluation. The patient can use the call bell to summon assistance quickly.

EVALUATION

The expected outcomes have been met when the patient has remained free from injury to self or others, circulation to extremity remained adequate, skin integrity was not impaired under the restraint, and the patient and family/caregivers were aware of rationale for restraints.

DOCUMENTATION

Guidelines

Document alternative measures attempted before application of the restraint and that less restrictive interventions have been determined to be ineffective. Document patient assessment before application. Record patient and family/caregiver education and understanding regarding restraint use. Document family/caregiver consent, if necessary, according to facility policy. Document reason for restraining patient, date and time of application, type of restraint, times when removed, and frequency and result of nursing assessments.

(continued on page 180)

Skill 4-4 ▶ Applying an Extremity Restraint *(continued)*

Sample Documentation

7/10/25 0830 Patient disoriented and combative. Attempting to remove tracheostomy and indwelling urinary catheter; verified with primary physician both devices are necessary at this time. Patient continued to tug at catheter and pull on tracheostomy while supervised at bedside. Family unwilling to sit with patient. Wrist restraints applied bilaterally as prescribed.

—K. Urhahn, RN

7/10/25 1030 Patient continues to be disoriented and combative. Wrist restraints removed for 30 minutes during patient's bath; skin intact, hands warm, even skin tone, +radial pulses, +movement; passive and active range of motion completed. Wrist restraints reapplied.

—K. Urhahn, RN

DEVELOPING CLINICAL REASONING AND CLINICAL JUDGMENT

UNEXPECTED SITUATIONS AND ASSOCIATED INTERVENTIONS

- *Patient has an IV catheter in the right wrist and is trying to remove a drain from a wound:* The left wrist may have a cloth restraint applied. Due to the IV in the right wrist, alternative forms of restraints could be tried, such as a cloth mitt or an elbow restraint.
- *Patient cannot move left arm:* Do not apply the restraint to an extremity that is immobile. If the patient cannot move the extremity, there is no need to apply a restraint. Restraint may be applied to right arm after obtaining an order from the physician or other licensed practitioner who is permitted to order restraint or seclusion in that health care facility and is responsible for the care of the patient.

SPECIAL CONSIDERATIONS
General Considerations

- Do not position patient with wrist restraints flat in a supine position due to an increased risk for aspiration (Springer, 2015). If supine position is necessary, be aware that constant monitoring may be required to reduce risk for complications for those at risk of vomiting while restrained (TIDI Products, 2018a).
- Check restraint for correct size before applying. Extremity restraints are available in different sizes. If restraint is too large, patient may free the extremity. If restraint is too small, circulation may be affected.
- Avoid use on an extremity restraint on a limb with a dislocation or fracture (TIDI Products, 2018b).
- Do not use on an extremity with an IV or wound site that could be compromised by the device (TIDI Products, 2018b).
- Always inspect the device before each use, checking for broken stitches or parts, torn, cut or frayed material; or locks, buckles or hook-and-loop fasteners that do not hold securely. Do not use soiled or damaged restraints (TIDI Products, 2018a).

Community-Based Care Considerations

- In long-term care facilities, patients have the right to be free from physical or chemical restraint not required to treat the resident's medical symptoms. When the use of restraints is indicated, the facility must use the least restrictive alternative for the least amount of time and document ongoing reevaluation of the need for restraints (CMS, 2020b).

EVIDENCE FOR PRACTICE ▶

MINIMIZING RESTRAINT USE
Several resources provide current best evidence on the topic of interventions to be used as alternatives to the use of restraints, as well as minimizing and eliminating the use of restraints. Refer to the Evidence for Practice in Skill 4-3.

Skill 4-5 ▶ Applying a Waist Restraint

Waist restraints are a form of restraint that is applied to the patient's torso. It is applied over the patient's clothes, gown, or pajamas. When using a waist restraint, patients can move their extremities, but cannot get out of the chair or bed. **Restraints should be used only after less restrictive methods have failed. Ensure compliance with ordering, assessment, and maintenance procedures. Historically, vest or jacket restraints were used to prevent similar patient movement, but their use has significantly decreased due to concerns for the potential risk for asphyxiation with these devices. However, research suggests that waist restraints pose the same potential risk for asphyxial death as vest restraints** (Berzlanovich et al., 2012; Capezuti et al., 2008). Federal guidelines reinforce that in all settings, the primary responsibility is to protect and promote patient's rights, and that restraints may only be used to protect the patient, staff, or others (Taylor et al., 2023). They must be discontinued at the earliest possible time (Taylor et al., 2023).

Health care providers need to be aware of the potential outcome of using this device and weigh it against possible benefit from its use. Review the general guidelines for using restraints in the chapter introduction and Fundamentals Review 4-2 and Box 4-2 in Skill 4-3. See also Evidence for Practice in Skill 4-3 for best evidence on the topic of interventions to be used as alternatives to the use of restraints, as well as minimizing and eliminating the use of restraints.

DELEGATION CONSIDERATIONS	After assessment of the patient by the RN, the application of a waist restraint may be delegated to assistive personnel (AP) as well as to licensed practical/vocational nurses (LPN/LVNs). The decision to delegate must be based on careful analysis of the patient's needs and circumstances as well as the qualifications of the person to whom the task is being delegated. Refer to the Delegation Guidelines in Appendix A.
EQUIPMENT	• Waist restraint • Additional padding as needed • PPE, as indicated
ASSESSMENT	Assess the patient's physical condition and for the potential for injury to self or others. A confused patient who is being treated with devices needed to sustain life, such as pulmonary intubation, might attempt to ambulate and is considered at risk for injury to self, and may require the use of restraints. Assess the patient's behavior, including the presence of confusion, agitation, combativeness, and ability to understand and follow directions. Evaluate the appropriateness of the least restrictive restraint device. Inspect the patient's torso for any wounds or therapeutic devices that may be affected by the waist restraint. Consider using another form of restraint if the restraint may cause further injury at the site. Assess the patient's respiratory effort. If applied incorrectly, the waist restraint can restrict the patient's ability to breathe.
ACTUAL OR POTENTIAL HEALTH PROBLEMS AND NEEDS	Many actual or potential health problems or needs may require the use of this skill as part of related interventions. An appropriate health problem or need may include: • Injury risk • Acute confusion
OUTCOME IDENTIFICATION AND PLANNING	The expected outcome to achieve is that the patient is constrained by the restraint, remains free from injury, and the restraint does not interfere with therapeutic devices. Other outcomes that may be appropriate include the following: the patient does not experience impaired skin integrity, the patient does not sustain injury due to the restraints, and the patient's family/caregivers demonstrate an understanding about the use of the restraint and their role in the patient's care.

(*continued on page 182*)

Skill 4-5 ▶ Applying a Waist Restraint *(continued)*

IMPLEMENTATION

ACTION	RATIONALE
1. Determine the need for restraints. Assess the patient's physical condition, behavior, and mental status. (Refer to Fundamentals Review 4-2 and Box 4-2 in Skill 4-3.)	Restraints should be used only as a last resort when alternative measures have failed, and the patient is at increased risk for harming self or others.
2. Confirm facility policy for application of restraints. **Secure an order from the physician or other licensed practitioner who is permitted to order restraint or seclusion in that health care facility, or validate that the order has been obtained within the required time frame (CMS, 2020a).**	Policy protects the patient and the nurse and specifies guidelines for application as well as type of restraint and duration. **Each order for restraint or seclusion used for the management of violent or self-destructive behavior that jeopardizes the immediate physical safety of the patient, a staff member, or others may only be renewed in accordance with the following limits for up to a total of 24 hours: (A) 4 hours for adults 18 years of age or older, (B) 2 hours for children and adolescents 9 to 17 years of age, or (C) 1 hour for children under 9 years of age. After 24 hours, before writing a new order for the use of restraint or seclusion for the management of violent or self-destructive behavior, a physician or other licensed practitioner who is permitted to order restraint or seclusion in that health care facility who is responsible for the care of the patient must see and assess the patient (CMS, 2006).**

ACTION	RATIONALE
3. Perform hand hygiene and put on PPE, if indicated.	Hand hygiene and PPE prevent the spread of microorganisms. PPE is required based on transmission precautions.

ACTION	RATIONALE
4. Identify the patient.	Identifying the patient ensures the right patient receives the intervention and helps prevent errors.
5. Explain reason for the use of restraint to patient and family/caregivers. Clarify how care will be given and how needs will be met. Explain that restraint is a temporary measure.	Explanation to patient and family/caregivers may lessen confusion and anger and provide reassurance. A clearly stated facility policy on the application of restraints should be available for patient and family/caregivers to read. In a long-term care facility, the family/caregivers must give consent before a restraint is applied.
6. Include the patient's family and/or caregivers in the plan of care.	Promotes person-centered, individualized care and engagement, continuity of care and understanding.
7. Inspect the restraint before use. Do not use a restraint that is soiled or damaged (TIDI Products, 2018a).	Always inspect the device before each use, checking for broken stitches or parts, torn, cut or frayed material; or locks, buckles or hook-and-loop fasteners that do not hold securely. Do not use soiled or damaged restraints to prevent injury or death (TIDI Products, 2018a).
8. Apply restraint according to the manufacturer's directions:	Proper application reduces the risk for injury. Proper application ensures that there is no interference with patient's respiration.
a. Choose the correct size of the least restrictive type of device that allows the greatest possible degree of mobility.	This provides minimal restriction.
b. Pad bony prominences that may be affected by the waist restraint.	Padding helps prevent injury.
c. Assist patient to a sitting position, if not contraindicated.	This will assist you in helping the patient into the waist restraint.
d. Place waist restraint on patient over gown. Bring ties through slots in restraint. Position slots at patient's back (Figure 1).	Placing the waist restraint over the gown protects the patient's skin. Positioning the slots with the ties at the back keeps them out of the patient's vision.
e. Pull the ties secure. **Ensure that the restraint is not too tight and has no wrinkles.**	Proper application secures the restraint and reduces risk for injury; securing too tightly could impede breathing. Wrinkles in the restraint may lead to skin impairment.

ACTION

f. Insert an open hand between restraint and patient to ensure that breathing is not constricted (TIDI Products, 2009). Assess respirations after restraint is applied.

9. Use a quick-release knot to tie the restraint to the bed frame that moves with the patient, not side rail, bed rail, mattress, or head/food board. (Refer to Figure 5 in Skill 4-4.) If patient is in a wheelchair, lock the wheels and place the ties under the arm rests and tie behind the chair (Figure 2). Site should not be readily accessible to the patient.

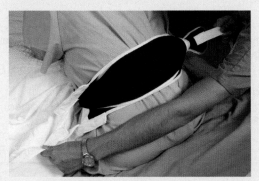

FIGURE 1. Positioning waist restraint.

 10. Remove PPE, if used. Perform hand hygiene.

11. Assess the patient according to facility policy, or more often, based on the individual patient circumstances and nursing judgment. Assessment should include the placement of the restraint, respirations, and skin integrity. Assess for signs of sensory deprivation, such as increased sleeping, daydreaming, anxiety, panic, and hallucinations. Monitor the patient's vital signs.

12. Remove restraint at least every 2 hours or according to facility policy, individual patient circumstances, and nursing judgment. Remove the restraint at least every 2 hours for children 9 to 17 years of age and at least every 1 hour for children under 9 years of age, or according to facility policy, individual patient circumstances, and nursing judgment. Provide for hydration, nutritional, and elimination needs. Provide exercise as appropriate for patient.

13. Evaluate patient for continued need of restraint. Reapply restraint only if continued need is evident and order is still valid.

14. Reassure patient at regular intervals. Provide continued explanation of rationale for interventions, reorientation if necessary, and plan of care. Keep the call bell within easy reach of the patient.

RATIONALE

The restraint must be snug, but not compromise the patient's breathing (TIDI Products, 2009).

A quick-release knot ensures that the restraint will not tighten when pulled and can be removed quickly in an emergency. Securing the restraint to a side rail may injure the patient when the side rail is lowered. Tying the restraint out of patient's reach promotes security.

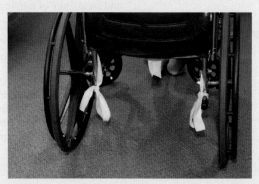

FIGURE 2. Restraint secured behind chair, out of the patient's reach.

Proper removal of PPE reduces the risk for infection transmission and contamination of other items. Hand hygiene prevents transmission of microorganisms.

The condition of the restrained patient must be continually assessed, monitored, and reevaluated (CMS, 2006). The frequency of monitoring should be made on an individual basis which includes a rationale that reflects consideration of the individual patient's medical needs and health status (CMS, 2006). Improperly applied restraints may cause difficulty breathing, skin tears, abrasions, or bruises. Decreased circulation can result in impaired skin integrity. The use of restraints may decrease environmental stimulation and result in sensory deprivation. Monitoring vital signs provides information about the status of the patient.

Removal allows you to assess patient and reevaluate need for restraint. It also allows interventions for toileting, provision of nutrition and liquids, exercise, and change of position. Exercise increases circulation and helps decrease risks associated with immobility.

Continued need must be documented for reapplication.

Reassurance demonstrates caring and provides an opportunity for sensory situation as well as ongoing assessment and evaluation. Patient can use call bell to summon assistance quickly.

(continued on page 184)

Skill 4-5 ▶ Applying a Waist Restraint *(continued)*

EVALUATION

The expected outcomes have been met when patient has remained free from injury to self or others, respirations have been easy and effortless, skin integrity has been maintained under the restraint, and the patient and family/caregivers demonstrated understanding of the rationale for using the restraints.

DOCUMENTATION

Guidelines

Document alternative measures attempted before applying restraint and that less restrictive interventions have been determined to be ineffective. Document patient assessment before application. Record patient and family/caregiver education and understanding regarding restraint use. Document family/caregiver consent, if necessary, according to facility policy. Document reason for restraining patient, date and time of application, type of restraint, times when removed, and result and frequency of nursing assessment.

Sample Documentation

9/30/25 2130 Patient continues to attempt to get out of bed without assistance. Waist restraint applied at night, as prescribed, when family leaves. Bed height low; side rails up ×2.
—B. Clapp, RN

9/30/25 2300 Waist restraint removed; skin intact; patient ambulated to restroom with assistance. Patient requested to ambulate to kitchen for snack; patient assisted to kitchen; graham crackers and milk obtained. Patient returned to bed and waist restraint reapplied after snack.
—B. Clapp, RN

DEVELOPING CLINICAL REASONING AND CLINICAL JUDGMENT

UNEXPECTED SITUATIONS AND ASSOCIATED INTERVENTIONS

- *Patient slides down and gets neck caught in the restraint:* Immediately release restraint. Determine alternate methods for restraining.
- *Patient slides down and out of the restraint:* Immediately release restraint. Ensure restraint is properly applied. Determine alternate methods for restraining.
- *Patient is exhibiting signs of respiratory distress:* Release restraint. Restraint may be applied too tightly and cause difficulty with chest expansion. Ensure restraint is properly applied. Determine alternate methods for restraining.

SPECIAL CONSIDERATIONS

- Do not use a waist restraint on patients with an ostomy, colostomy, or gastrostomy tube; hernias; pelvic fracture; severe chronic obstructive pulmonary disease (COPD); or who have postsurgery tubes, incisions, or monitoring lines. These could be disrupted by the restraint (TIDI Products, 2009).
- Do not position patient with wrist restraints flat in a supine position due to an increased risk for aspiration (Springer, 2015). If supine position is necessary, be aware that constant monitoring may be required to reduce risk for complications for those at risk of vomiting while restrained (TIDI Products, 2018a).
- Always inspect the device before each use, checking for broken stitches or parts, torn, cut or frayed material; or locks, buckles or hook-and-loop fasteners that do not hold securely. Do not use soiled or damaged restraints (TIDI Products, 2018a).

Community-Based Care Considerations

- In long-term care facilities, patients have the right to be free from physical or chemical restraint not required to treat the resident's medical symptoms. When the use of restraints is indicated, the facility must use the least restrictive alternative for the least amount of time and document ongoing reevaluation of the need for restraints (CMS, 2020b).

EVIDENCE FOR PRACTICE ▶

MINIMIZING RESTRAINT USE
Several resources provide current best evidence on the topic of interventions to be used as alternatives to the use of restraints, as well as minimizing and eliminating the use of restraints. Refer to the Evidence for Practice after Skill 4-3.

Skill 4-6 ▶ Applying an Elbow Restraint

Elbow restraints are generally used on infants and children but may be used with adults. They prevent the patient from bending the elbows and reaching incisions or therapeutic devices. The patient can move all joints and extremities except the elbow. **Restraints should be used only after less restrictive methods have failed. Ensure compliance with ordering, assessment, and maintenance procedures. Restraints must be applied safely and appropriately to reduce risks of injury.** Federal guidelines reinforce that in all settings, the primary responsibility is to protect and promote patient's rights, and that restraints may only be used to protect the patient, staff, or others (Taylor et al., 2023). They must be discontinued at the earliest possible time (Taylor et al., 2023).

Review the general guidelines for using restraints in the chapter introduction and Fundamentals Review 4-2 and Box 4-2 in Skill 4-3. See also Evidence for Practice in Skill 4-3 for best evidence on the topic of interventions to be used as alternatives to the use of restraints, as well as minimizing and eliminating the use of restraints.

DELEGATION CONSIDERATIONS	After assessment of the patient by the RN, the application of an elbow restraint may be delegated to assistive personnel (AP) as well as to licensed practical/vocational nurses (LPN/LVNs). The decision to delegate must be based on careful analysis of the patient's needs and circumstances as well as the qualifications of the person to whom the task is being delegated. Refer to the Delegation Guidelines in Appendix A.
EQUIPMENT	• Elbow restraint • Padding, as necessary • PPE, as indicated
ASSESSMENT	Assess the patient's physical condition and for the potential for injury to self or others. A confused patient who might remove devices needed to sustain life is considered at risk for injury to self and may require the use of restraints. Assess the patient's behavior, including the presence of confusion, agitation, combativeness, and ability to understand and follow directions. Evaluate the appropriateness of the least restrictive restraint device. Inspect the arm where the restraint will be applied. Baseline skin condition should be established for comparison at future assessments while the restraint is in place. Consider using another form of restraint if the restraint may cause further injury at the site. Assess capillary refill and proximal pulses in the arm to which the restraint is to be applied. This helps to determine the circulation in the extremity before applying the restraint. The restraint should not interfere with circulation. Measure the distance from the patient's shoulder to wrist and limb circumference to determine the appropriate size of elbow restraint to apply.
ACTUAL OR POTENTIAL HEALTH PROBLEMS AND NEEDS	Many actual or potential health problems or needs may require the use of this skill as part of related interventions. An appropriate health problem or need may include: • Injury risk • Acute confusion
OUTCOME IDENTIFICATION AND PLANNING	The expected outcome to achieve when applying an elbow restraint is that the patient is constrained by the restraint and remains free from injury, and the restraint does not interfere with therapeutic devices. Other outcomes that may be appropriate include the following: the patient does not experience impaired skin integrity, and the patient's family/caregivers demonstrate an understanding about the use of the restraint and its role in the patient's care.

IMPLEMENTATION

ACTION	RATIONALE
1. Determine the need for restraints. Assess the patient's physical condition, behavior, and mental status. (Refer to Fundamentals Review 4-2 and Box 4-2 in Skill 4-3.)	Restraints should be used only as a last resort when alternative measures have failed, and the patient is at increased risk for harming self or others.

(continued on page 186)

Skill 4-6 ▶ Applying an Elbow Restraint *(continued)*

ACTION

2. Confirm facility policy for application of restraints. **Secure an order from the physician or other licensed practitioner who is permitted to order restraint or seclusion in that health care facility, or validate that the order has been obtained within the required time frame (CMS, 2020a).**

3. Perform hand hygiene and put on PPE, if indicated.

4. Identify the patient.

5. Explain the reason for use to the patient and family/caregivers. Clarify how care will be given and how needs will be met. Explain that restraint is a temporary measure.

6. Include the patient's family and/or caregivers in the plan of care.

7. Inspect the restraint before use. Do not use a restraint that is soiled or damaged (TIDI Products, 2018a).

8. Apply the restraint according to the manufacturer's directions:

   a. Choose the correct size of the least restrictive type of device that allows the greatest possible degree of mobility.

   b. Pad bony prominences that may be affected by the restraint.

   c. Spread elbow restraint out flat. Place the middle of the elbow restraint behind the patient's elbow. **The restraint should not extend below the wrist or place pressure on the axilla.**

   d. **Wrap the restraint snugly around the patient's arm.** Secure hook-and-loop straps around the restraint (Figure 1). **Ensure that two fingers can be inserted between the restraint and the patient's arm.**

RATIONALE

Policy protects the patient and the nurse and specifies guidelines for application as well as the type of restraint and duration of use. **Each order for restraint or seclusion used for the management of violent or self-destructive behavior that jeopardizes the immediate physical safety of the patient, a staff member, or others may only be renewed in accordance with the following limits for up to a total of 24 hours: (A) 4 hours for adults 18 years of age or older, (B) 2 hours for children and adolescents 9 to 17 years of age, or (C) 1 hour for children under 9 years of age. After 24 hours, before writing a new order for the use of restraint or seclusion for the management of violent or self-destructive behavior, a physician or other licensed practitioner who is permitted to order restraint or seclusion in that health care facility who is responsible for the care of the patient must see and assess the patient (CMS, 2006).**

Hand hygiene and PPE prevent the spread of microorganisms. PPE is required based on transmission precautions.

Identifying the patient ensures the right patient receives the intervention and helps prevent errors.

Explanation to patient and family/caregivers may lessen confusion and anger and provide reassurance. A clearly stated facility policy on application of restraints should be available for the patient and family/caregivers to read. In a long-term care facility, the family/caregivers must give consent before a restraint is applied.

Promotes person-centered, individualized care and engagement, continuity of care and understanding.

Always inspect the device before each use, checking for broken stitches or parts, torn, cut or frayed material; or locks, buckles or hook-and-loop fasteners that do not hold securely. Do not use soiled or damaged restraints to prevent injury or death (TIDI Products, 2018a).

Proper application reduces the risk for injury. Proper application ensures that there is no interference with patient's circulation.

This provides minimal restriction.

Padding helps prevent injury.

Elbow restraint should be placed in the middle of the arm to ensure that the patient cannot bend the elbow. The patient should be able to move the wrist. Pressure on the axilla may lead to skin impairment.

Wrapping snugly ensures that the patient will not be able to remove the device. Hook-and-loop straps will hold the restraint in place and prevent removal of the restraint. Being able to insert two fingers helps to prevent impaired circulation and potential alterations in neurovascular status.

ACTION

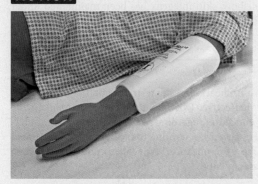

FIGURE 1. Child with elbow restraint secured in place.

e. **Ensure that one to two fingers can be inserted between the restraint and patient's extremity.**

f. Apply a restraint to the opposite arm if the patient can move the arm.

9. **Assess circulation to fingers and hand.** Refer to Chapter 3.

10. Remove PPE, if used. Perform hand hygiene.

11. **Assess the patient according to facility policy, or more often, based on the individual patient circumstances and nursing judgment.** Assessment should include the placement of the restraint, neurovascular assessment of the affected extremity, and skin integrity. Assess for signs of sensory deprivation, such as increased sleeping, daydreaming, anxiety, panic, and hallucinations. Monitor the patient's vital signs.

12. **Remove restraint at least every 2 hours or according to facility policy, individual patient circumstances, and nursing judgment. Remove the restraint at least every 2 hours for children 9 to 17 years of age and at least every 1 hour for children under 9 years of age, or according to facility policy, individual patient circumstances, and nursing judgment.** Perform range-of-motion (ROM) exercises. Provide for hydration, nutritional, and elimination needs.

13. **Evaluate the patient for continued need of restraint.** Reapply the restraint only if continued need is evident and order is still valid.

14. Reassure the patient at regular intervals. Provide continued explanation of rationale for interventions, reorientation if necessary, and plan of care. **Keep the call bell within easy reach of the patient.**

RATIONALE

The restraint must be snug, but not compromise circulation (TIDI Products, 2019). Proper application ensures that nothing interferes with the patient's circulation and potential alteration in the neurovascular status.

Bilateral elbow restraints are needed if the patient can move both arms.

Circulation should not be impaired by the elbow restraint.

Proper removal of PPE reduces the risk for infection transmission and contamination of other items. Hand hygiene prevents transmission of microorganisms.

The condition of the restrained patient must be continually assessed, monitored, and reevaluated (CMS, 2006). The frequency of monitoring should be made on an individual basis which includes a rationale that reflects consideration of the individual patient's medical needs and health status (CMS, 2006). Improperly applied restraints may cause skin tears, abrasions, or bruises. Decreased circulation may result in paleness, coolness, decreased sensation, tingling, numbness, or pain in extremity. The use of restraints may decrease environmental stimulation and result in sensory deprivation. Monitoring vital signs provides information about the status of the patient.

Removal allows you to assess patient and reevaluate the need for a restraint. Allows interventions for toileting; provision of nutrition and liquids, and exercise; and change of position. Exercise increases circulation in the restrained extremity.

Continued need must be documented for reapplication.

Reassurance demonstrates caring and provides opportunity for sensory situation as well as ongoing assessment and evaluation. The patient or family/caregiver can use a call bell can use it to summon assistance quickly.

(continued on page 188)

Skill 4-6 ▶ Applying an Elbow Restraint *(continued)*

EVALUATION

The expected outcome has been met when the restraint prevented injury to the patient or others. In addition, the patient was unable to bend the elbow, skin integrity has been maintained under the restraint, and the family/caregivers demonstrated an understanding of the rationale for the elbow restraint.

DOCUMENTATION

Guidelines

Document alternative measures attempted before application of the restraint and that less restrictive interventions have been determined to be ineffective. Document patient assessment before application. Record patient and family/caregiver education regarding restraint use and their understanding. Document family/caregiver consent, if necessary, according to facility policy. Document the reason for restraining patient, date and time of application, type of restraint, times when removed, and result and frequency of nursing assessment.

Sample Documentation

> 9/1/25 0800 Elbow restraints removed while am personal care performed (45 minutes). Skin warm, dry, even tone; + radial and brachial pulses, equal bilaterally, capillary refill <3 seconds. Patient moving arms appropriately. Continues to pick at colostomy bag. Distraction techniques used to no avail.
>
> —B. Clapp, RN
>
> 9/1/25 0855 Skin intact and warm. Elbow restraints reapplied. Will remove when family arrives at bedside or every 2 hours as per policy.
>
> —B. Clapp, RN

DEVELOPING CLINICAL REASONING AND CLINICAL JUDGMENT

UNEXPECTED SITUATIONS AND ASSOCIATED INTERVENTIONS

- *Skin breakdown is noted on elbows:* Ensure that restraints are being removed routinely for at least 30 minutes and a skin inspection is done. If restraints are still needed, a padded dressing should be applied under the elbow restraint. Ensure restraint is properly applied. Determine possible alternate methods for restraining.
- *Patient reports discomfort and pain or cries when elbow is moved:* Restraints need to be removed more frequently, with active and/or passive ROM. If elbow is not moved, it will become stiff and painful. Ensure restraint is properly applied. Determine possible alternate methods for restraining.
- *Application of elbow restraint does not control the patient's body movement to allow for needed examination or treatment:* Reassess situation and consider continued need for restraint and possible use of a more restrictive type of restraint.

Community-Based Care Considerations

- In long-term care facilities, patients have the right to be free from physical or chemical restraint not required to treat the resident's medical symptoms. When the use of restraints is indicated, the facility must use the least restrictive alternative for the least amount of time and document ongoing re-evaluation of the need for restraints (CMS, 2020b).

EVIDENCE FOR PRACTICE ▶

MINIMIZING RESTRAINT USE

Several resources provide current best evidence on the topic of interventions to be used as alternatives to the use of restraints, as well as minimizing and eliminating the use of restraints. Refer to the Evidence for Practice after Skill 4-3.

Skill 4-7 ▶ Applying a Mummy Restraint

A mummy restraint is appropriate for short-term restraint and temporary immobilization of an infant or small child to control the child's movements during examination or to provide care for the head and neck or care to one extremity. **Restraints should be used only after less restrictive methods have failed. Ensure compliance with ordering, assessment, and maintenance procedures. Restraints must be applied safely and appropriately to reduce risks of injury.** Federal guidelines reinforce that in all settings, the primary responsibility is to protect and promote patient's rights, and that restraints may only be used to protect the patient, staff, or others (Taylor et al., 2023). They must be discontinued at the earliest possible time (Taylor et al., 2023).

Review the general guidelines for using restraints in the chapter introduction and Fundamentals Review 4-2 and Box 4-2 in Skill 4-3. See also Evidence for Practice after Skill 4-3 for best evidence on the topic of interventions to be used as alternatives to the use of restraints, as well as minimizing and eliminating the use of restraints.

DELEGATION CONSIDERATIONS

After assessment of the patient by the RN, the application of a mummy restraint may be delegated to assistive personnel (AP) as well as to licensed practical/vocational nurses (LPN/LVNs). The decision to delegate must be based on careful analysis of the patient's needs and circumstances as well as the qualifications of the person to whom the task is being delegated. Refer to the Delegation Guidelines in Appendix A.

EQUIPMENT

- Small blanket or sheet
- PPE, as indicated

ASSESSMENT

Assess the patient's behavior and need for a restraint. Assess for wounds or therapeutic devices that may be affected by the restraint. Evaluate the appropriateness of the least restrictive restraint device. Another form of restraint may be more appropriate to prevent injury.

ACTUAL OR POTENTIAL HEALTH PROBLEMS AND NEEDS

Many actual or potential health problems or needs may require the use of this skill as part of related interventions. An appropriate health problem or need may include:
- Injury risk
- Acute anxiety

OUTCOME IDENTIFICATION AND PLANNING

The expected outcome to achieve is that the patient is constrained by the restraint and remains free from injury, and that the restraint does not interfere with therapeutic devices. Other outcomes that may be appropriate include the following: examination and/or treatment is provided without incident, and the patient's family/caregivers demonstrate an understanding about the use of the restraint and its role in the patient's care.

IMPLEMENTATION

ACTION

1. Determine the need for restraints. Assess the patient's physical condition, behavior, and mental status. (Refer to Fundamentals Review 4-2 and Box 4-2 in Skill 4-3.)

RATIONALE

Restraints should be used only as a last resort when alternative measures have failed, and the patient is at increased risk for harming self or others.

(continued on page 190)

Skill 4-7 ▶ Applying a Mummy Restraint *(continued)*

ACTION	**RATIONALE**
2. Confirm facility policy for application of restraints. **Secure an order from the physician or other licensed practitioner who is permitted to order restraint or seclusion in that health care facility, or validate that the order has been obtained within the required time frame (CMS, 2020a).**	This policy protects the patient and the nurse and specifies guidelines for application as well as the type of restraint and duration. **Each order for restraint or seclusion used for the management of violent or self-destructive behavior that jeopardizes the immediate physical safety of the patient, a staff member, or others may only be renewed in accordance with the following limits for up to a total of 24 hours: (A) 4 hours for adults 18 years of age or older, (B) 2 hours for children and adolescents 9 to 17 years of age, or (C) 1 hour for children under 9 years of age. After 24 hours, before writing a new order for the use of restraint or seclusion for the management of violent or self-destructive behavior, a physician or other licensed practitioner who is permitted to order restraint or seclusion in that health care facility who is responsible for the care of the patient must see and assess the patient (CMS, 2006).**
3. Perform hand hygiene and put on PPE, if indicated.	Hand hygiene and PPE prevent the spread of microorganisms. PPE is required based on transmission precautions.
4. Identify the patient.	Identifying the patient ensures the right patient receives the intervention and helps prevent errors.
5. Explain the reason for use to the patient and family/caregivers. Clarify how care will be given and how needs will be met. Explain that restraint is a temporary measure.	Explanation to the patient and family/caregivers may lessen confusion and anger and provide reassurance. A clearly stated facility policy on application of restraints should be available for patient and family/caregivers to read. In a long-term care facility, the family/caregivers must give consent before a restraint is applied.
6. Include the patient's family and/or caregivers in the plan of care.	Promotes person-centered, individualized care and engagement, continuity of care and understanding.
7. Open the blanket or sheet. Place the child on the blanket, with the edge of the blanket at or above neck level.	This positions the child correctly on the blanket.
8. Position the child's right arm alongside the child's body. Left arm should not be constrained at this time. Pull the right side of the blanket tightly over the child's right shoulder and chest. Secure under the left side of the child's body (Figure 1).	Wrapping snugly ensures that the child will not be able to wriggle out.
9. Position the left arm alongside the child's body. Pull the left side of the blanket tightly over the child's left shoulder and chest. Secure under the right side of the child's body (Figure 2).	Wrapping snugly ensures that the child will not be able to wriggle out.
10. Fold the lower part of the blanket up and pull over the child's body. Secure under the child's body on each side or with safety pins (Figure 3).	This ensures that the child will not be able to wriggle out.

ACTION	RATIONALE

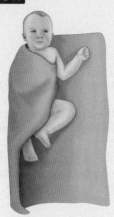

FIGURE 1. Pulling blanket over right shoulder and chest and securing under patient's left side.

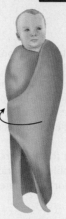

FIGURE 2. Securing blanket under right side of body.

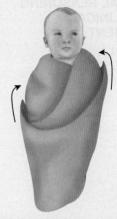

FIGURE 3. Securing lower corner of blanket under each side of patient's body.

11. Stay with the child while the mummy wrap is in place. Reassure the child and parents at regular intervals. Once examination or treatment is completed, unwrap the child.

Remaining with the child prevents injury. Reassurance demonstrates caring and provides opportunity for ongoing assessment and evaluation.

12. Remove PPE, if used. Perform hand hygiene.

Proper removal of PPE reduces the risk for infection transmission and contamination of other items. Hand hygiene prevents transmission of microorganisms.

EVALUATION

The expected outcome has been met when the restraint has prevented injury to the patient and others. In addition, the examination or treatment has been provided without incident, and the family/caregiver demonstrated an understanding of the rationale for the mummy restraint.

DOCUMENTATION

Guidelines

Document alternative measures attempted before applying a restraint and that less restrictive interventions have been determined to be ineffective. Document patient assessment before application. Record patient and family/caregiver education and understanding regarding restraint use. Document family/caregiver consent, if necessary, according to facility policy. Document the reason for restraining patient, date and time of application, type of restraint, times when removed, and result and frequency of nursing assessment.

Sample Documentation

6/9/25 0230 Patient requires suturing of forehead. Parent attempted to hold child for procedure without success. Need to restrain child explained to parents. Mummy restraint applied with parents' consent. Restraint removed after 20 minutes; sutures intact. Wound care instructions (verbal and written) provided to parents; parents verbalize understanding.

—D. Dunn, RN

(continued on page 192)

Skill 4-7 ▶ Applying a Mummy Restraint *(continued)*

DEVELOPING CLINICAL REASONING AND CLINICAL JUDGMENT

SPECIAL CONSIDERATIONS

- Mummy restraints should be used only for the duration of the procedure because it is a total body restraint (Sibert-Flagg, 2018)
- For the infant who needs continuous observation for respiratory status, fold the mummy restraint so the chest is exposed (Sibert-Flagg, 2018)
- Mummy restraint secures the child's entire body or every extremity except for one; one extremity may be left unsecured if exposure is necessary to provide care involving the one extremity (Kyle & Carman, 2021).
- An alternative approach for temporary restraint is therapeutic holding (hugging), which makes use of a secure, comfortable, temporary holding position that provides close physical contact with the parent or caregiver for 30 minutes or less (Kyle & Carman, 2021; Perry et al., 2018).

EVIDENCE FOR PRACTICE ▶

MINIMIZING RESTRAINT USE

Several resources provide current best evidence on the topic of interventions to be used as alternatives to the use of restraints, as well as minimizing and eliminating the use of restraints. Refer to the Evidence for Practice after Skill 4-3.

Enhance Your Understanding

Focusing on Patient Care: Developing Clinical Reasoning and Clinical Judgment

Consider the case scenarios at the beginning of the chapter as you answer the following questions to enhance your understanding and apply what you have learned.

QUESTIONS

1. Megan Lewis, an 18-month-old with an IV access in her left forearm, is continually picking at the IV and dressing. What interventions would be appropriate as alternatives to restraints? If unsuccessful, what restraint(s) would be appropriate for Megan?

2. Kevin Mallory, a 35-year-old body builder with a closed head injury, is extremely strong. The fear is that he will rip the cloth restraints and extubate himself. What other type of restraints could be tried?

3. John Frawley, a 72-year-old patient with Alzheimer disease, continually tries to get out of bed without assistance. He has an unsteady gait and has one broken hip due to a fall. What are the appropriate interventions to try with Mr. Frawley?

You can find suggested answers after the Bibliography at the end of this chapter.

Integrated Case Study Connection

The case studies in the back of the book focus on integrating concepts. Refer to the following case studies to enhance your understanding of the concepts and skills in this chapter.

- Basic Case Studies: Abigail Cantonelli, page 1193; Claudia Tran, page 1201.
- Intermediate Case Studies: Olivia Greenbaum, page 1209; Kent Clark, page 1217.

Bibliography

Agency for Healthcare Research and Quality (AHRQ). (2013). *Preventing falls in hospitals.* https://www.ahrq.gov/professionals/systems/hospital/fallpxtoolkit/fallpxtk3.html

Agency for Healthcare Research and Quality (AHRQ). (2018a). *Preventing falls in hospitals.* https://www.ahrq.gov/professionals/systems/hospital/fallpxtoolkit/index.html

Agency for Healthcare Research and Quality (AHRQ). (2018b). *AHRQ's safety program for nursing homes: On-time falls prevention.* https://www.ahrq.gov/patient-safety/settings/long-term-care/resource/ontime/fallspx/index.html

Allen, D. E., Fetzer, S. J., & Cummings, K. S. (2020). Decreasing duration of mechanical restraint episodes by increasing registered nurse assessment and surveillance in an acute psychiatric hospital. *Journal of the American Psychiatric Nurses Association, 26*(3), 245–249. https://doi.org/10.1177/1078390319878776

American Geriatrics Society (AGS) Health in Aging Foundation. (n.d.). *Aging & health A-Z. Falls prevention.* AGS Geriatrics Healthcare Professionals. Retrieved June 15, 2020, from https://www.healthinaging.org/a-z-topic/falls-prevention

American Geriatrics Society (AGS) Health in Aging Foundation. (2019). *Tips for preventing serious falls.* AGS Geriatrics Healthcare Professionals. https://www.healthinaging.org/tools-and-tips/tips-preventing-serious-falls

American Nurses Association (ANA). (2012). *Reduction of patient restraint and seclusion in health care settings.* https://www.nursingworld.org/practice-policy/nursing-excellence/official-position-statements/id/reduction-of-patient-restraint-and-seclusion-in-health-care-settings/#:~:text=The%20American%20Nurses%20Association%20(ANA,seclusion%20in%20health%20care%20settings.&text=Nurses%20struggle%20to%20balance%20their,harm%20to%20patients%20and%20staff

American Psychiatric Nurses Association (APNA). (2018). *APNA position statement on the use of seclusion and restraint.* https://www.apna.org/resources/apna-seclusion-restraint-position-paper/

Bak, J., Zoffmann, V., Sestoft, D. M., Almivk, R., Philos, D., & Brandt-Christensen, M. (2014). Mechanical restraint in psychiatry: Preventive factors in theory and practice. A Danish-Norwegian Association study. *Perspectives in Psychiatric Care, 50*(3), 155–166. https://doi.org/10.1111/ppc.12036

Benning, S., & Webb, T. (2019). Taking the fall for kids: A journey to reducing pediatric falls. *Journal of Pediatric Nursing, 46,* 100–108. https://doi.org/10.1016/j.pedn.2019.03.008

Bergen, G., Stevens, M. R., Kakara, R., & Burns, E. R. (2019). Understanding modifiable and unmodifiable older adult fall risk factors to create effective prevention strategies. *Journal of American Lifestyle Medicine.* https://doi.org/10.1177%2F1559827619880529

Berzlanovich, A. M., Schöpfer, J., & Keil, W. (2012). Deaths due to physical restraint. *Deutsches Arzteblatt International, 109*(3), 27–32. https://doi.org/10.3238/arztebl.2012.0027

Cangany, M., Peters, L., Gregg, K., Welsh, T., & Jimison, B. (2018). Preventing falls: Is no toileting alone the answer? *Medsurg Nursing, 27*(6), 379–382.

Capezuti, E., Brush, B. L., Won, R. M, Wagner, L. M., & Lawson, W. T. (2008). Least restrictive or least understood? Waist restraints, provider practices, and risk of harm. *Journal of Aging & Social Policy, 20*(3), 305–322. https://doi.org/10.1080/08959420802050967

Centers for Disease Control and Prevention (CDC). (2017). *Home and recreational safety. Important facts about falls.* https://www.cdc.gov/homeandrecreationalsafety/falls/adultfalls.html

Centers for Disease Control and Prevention (CDC). (2019a). *STEADI. Stopping elderly accidents, deaths & injuries.* https://www.cdc.gov/steadi/index.html

Centers for Disease Control and Prevention (CDC). (2019b). *STEADI. Algorithm for fall risk screening, assessment, and intervention among community-dwelling adults 65 years and older.* https://www.cdc.gov/steadi/pdf/STEADI-Algorithm-508.pdf

Centers for Disease Control and Prevention (CDC). (2019c). *Injury prevention & control. Injuries among children and teens. National action plan for child injury prevention.* https://www.cdc.gov/injury/features/child-injury/

Centers for Disease Control and Prevention (CDC). (2019d). *Child safety publications. National action plan.* https://www.cdc.gov/safechild/publications.htmll

Centers for Disease Control and Prevention (CDC). (2020a). *Emergency preparedness and response. Health Alert Network (HAN).* https://emergency.cdc.gov/han/

Centers for Disease Control and Prevention (CDC). (2020b). *Injury prevention & control. Injury and violence prevention and control.* https://www.cdc.gov/injury/

Centers for Medicare & Medicaid Services (CMS). (n.d.). *Rights & protections for everyone with Medicare.* Department of Health and Human Services. https://www.medicare.gov/claims-appeals/your-medicare-rights/rights-protections-for-everyone-with-medicare

Centers for Medicare & Medicaid Services (CMS). (2006). Department of Health and Human Services. Federal Register. Part IV. 42 CFR Part 482. *Medicare and Medicaid programs; Hospital conditions of participation: Patients' rights; Final rule.* https://www.cms.gov/Regulations-and-Guidance/Legislation/CFCsAndCoPs/downloads/finalpatientrightsrule.pdf

Centers for Medicare & Medicaid Services (CMS). (2020a). Department of Health and Human Services. CMS manual system. Pub. 100–07. Appendix A. Survey protocol, regulations and interpretive guidelines for hospitals. §482.13. *Conditions of participation: Patients' rights.* https://www.cms.gov/Regulations-and-Guidance/Guidance/Manuals/downloads/som107ap_a_hospitals.pdf

Centers for Medicare & Medicaid Services (CMS). (2020b). Department of Health and Human Services. CMS manual system. Pub. 100–07. Appendix PP. Guidance to surveyors for long term care facilities. §482.10. *Resident rights.* https://www.cms.gov/Regulations-and-Guidance/Guidance/Manuals/downloads/som107ap_pp_guidelines_ltcf.pdf

Cohen, N. L. (2013). Using the ABCs of situational awareness for patient safety. *Nursing, 43*(4), 64–65.

Cotter, V. T., & Evans, L. K. (2021). *Consult Geri. Try this: Series. Avoiding restraints in patients with dementia. Issue #1 of dementia series.* The Hartford Institute for Geriatric Nursing. https://hign.org/consultgeri/try-this-series/avoiding-restraints-patients-dementia

Cronan, K. M. (2018). *KidsHealth/for parents. First aid: Falls.* The Nemours Foundation. https://kidshealth.org/en/parents/falls-sheet.html

Delgado, S. A. (2020). Physical restraints: Protecting patients or devices? *American Journal of Critical Care, 29*(2), 103. https://doi.org/10.4037/ajcc2020742

Dykes, P. C., Adelman, J., Adkison, L., Bogaisky, M., Carroll, D. L., Carter, E., Duckworth, M., Herlihy, L., Hurley, A. C., Khasnabish, S., Kurian, S., Lindros, M. E., Marsh, K. F., McNinney, T., Ryan, V., Scanlan, M., Spivack, L., Shelley A., & Yu, S. P. (2018). Preventing falls in hospitalized patients. Engage patients and families in a three-step prevention process to reduce the risk of falls. *American Nurse Today, 13*(9), 8–13.

Eliopoulos, C. (2018). *Gerontological nursing* (9th ed.). Wolters Kluwer.

Fahlström, G., Kamwendo, K., Forsberg, J., & Bodin, L. (2018). Fall prevention by nursing assistants among community-living elderly people. A randomised controlled trial. *Scandinavian Journal of Caring Sciences, 32*(2), 575–585. https://doi.org/10.1111/scs.12481

Fore, A. M., & Sculli, G. L. (2013). A concept analysis of situational awareness in nursing. *Journal of Advanced Nursing, 69*(12), 2613–2621.

Fukuta, D., & Iitsuka, M. (2018). Nontechnical skills training and patient safety in undergraduate nursing education: A systematic review. *Teaching and Learning in Nursing, 13*(4), 233–239. https://doi.org/10.1016/j.teln.2018.06.004

Godlock, G., Christiansen, M., & Feider, L. (2016). Implementation of an evidence-based patient safety team to prevent falls in inpatient medical units. *Medsurg Nursing, 25*(1), 17–23.

Greeley, A. M., Tanner, P., Mak, S., Begashaw, M. M., Miake-Lye I. M., & Shekelle, P. G. (2020). Sitters as a patient safety strategy to reduce hospital falls. A systematic review. *Annals of Internal Medicine, 172*(5), 317–324. https://doi.org/10.7326/M19-2628

Green, B., Parry, D., Oeppen, R. S., Plint, S., Dale, T., & Brennan, P. A. (2017). Situational awareness—what it means for clinicians, its recognition and importance in patient safety. *Oral Diseases, 23,* 721–725. doi:10.1111/odi.12547

Grossman, D. C., Curry, S. J., Owens, D. K., Barry, M. J., Caughey, A. B., Davidson, K. W., Doubeni, C. A., Epling, J. W. Jr, Kemper, A. R., Krist, A. H., Kubik, M., Landefeld, S., Mangione, C. M., Pignone, M., Silverstein, M., Simon, M. A., & Tseng, C. W. (2018). Interventions to prevent falls in community-dwelling older adults: U. S. Preventive Services Task Force Recommendation Statement. *JAMA, 319*(16), 1696–1704. https://doi.org/10.1001/jama.2018.3097

Hamed, A., Bohm, S., Mersmann, F., & Arampatzis, A. (2018). Follow-up efficacy of physical exercise interventions on fall incidence and fall risk in healthy older adults: A systematic review and meta-analysis. *Sports Medicine Open, 4*(1), 56. https://doi.org/10.1186/s40798-018-0170-z

Harris, J. L. (2015). Enclosure bed: A protective and calming restraint. *American Nurse Today, 10*(1), 30–31.

Hendrich, A. (2007). Predicting patient falls. *American Journal of Nursing, 107*(11), 50–58.

Henley Haugh, K. (2015). Head-to-toe: Organizing your baseline patient physical assessment. *Nursing, 45*(12), 58–61.

Hester, A. L. (2015). Preventing injuries from patient falls. *American Nurse Today, 10*(7), 36–37.

Hicks, D. (2015). Can rounding reduce patient falls in acute care? An integrative literature review. *Medsurg Nursing, 24*(1), 51–55.

Hinkle, J. L., & Cheever, K. H. (2018). *Brunner & Suddarth's textbook of medical-surgical nursing* (14th ed.). Wolters Kluwer.

The Joint Commission (TJC). (2020). National patient safety goals. 2020 Home care National Patient Safety Goals. https://www.jointcommission.org/-/media/tjc/documents/standards/national-patient-safety-goals/2020/npsg_chapter_ome_jul2020.pdf

The Joint Commission. (2015) *Fact sheets. Preventing falls and fall-related injuries in health care facilities. Sentinel Event Alert,* (55). https://www.jointcommission.org/-/media/tjc/documents/resources/patient-safety-topics/sentinel-event/sea_55_falls_4_26_16.pdf

The Joint Commission. (2017). *Restraint and seclusion—Enclosure beds, side rails and mitts.* https://www.jointcommission.org/en/standards/standard-faqs/critical-access-hospital/provision-of-care-treatment-and-services-pc/000001668/

Jones, K. J., Crowe, J., Allen, J. A., Skinner, A. M., High, R., Kennel, V., & Reiter-Palmon, R. (2019). The impact of post-gall huddles on repeat fall rates and perceptions of safety culture: A quasi-experimental evaluation of a patient safety demonstration project. *BMC Health Services Research, 19*(1), 650. https://doi.org/10.1186/s12913-019-4453-y

Kersey-Matusiak, G. (2019). *Delivering culturally competent nursing care. Working with diverse and vulnerable populations* (2nd ed.). Springer Publishing Company.

Kim, C., Hughes, M., & Fields, W. (2018). Nurses' reactions to enclosure beds. *Medsurg Nursing, 27*(2), 87–92.

Korall, A. M. B., Feldman, F., Yang, Y., Cameron, I. D., Leung, P. M., Sims-Gould, J., & Robinovitch, S. N. (2019). Effectiveness of hip protectors to reduce risk for hip fracture from falls in long-term care. *The Journal of Post-Acute and Long-Term Care Medicine, 20*(11), 1397–1403. https://doi.org/10.1016/j.jamda.2019.07.010

Kyle, T., & Carman, S. (2021). *Essentials of pediatric nursing* (4th ed.). Wolters Kluwer.

Lach, H. W. (2019). *ConsultGeri. Try this: Series. Home safety inventory for older adults with dementia. Issue #12 of dementia series.* The Hartford Institute for Geriatric Nursing. https://hign.org/consultgeri/try-this-series/home-safety-inventory-older-adults-dementia

Large, C., & Aldridge, M. (2018). Non-technical skills required to recognise and escalate patient deterioration in acute hospital settings. *Nursing Management (Harrow), 25*(2), 24–30.

Lasater, K. (2007). Clinical judgment development: Using simulation to create an assessment rubric. *Journal of Nursing Education, 46*(11), 496–503.

Lawson, T. N., Tan, A., Thrane, S. E., Happ, M. B., Mion, L. C., Tate, J., & Balas, M. C. (2020). Predictors of new-onset physical restraint use in critically ill adults. *American Journal of Critical Care, 29*(2), 92–102. https://doi.org/10.4037/ajcc2020361

MedlinePlus. (2020). *Use of restraints.* U.S. National Library of Medicine. https://medlineplus.gov/ency/patientinstructions/000450.htm

Minnier, W., Leggett, M., Persaud, I., & Breda, K. (2019). Patient safety. Four smart steps: Fall Prevention for community-dwelling older adults. *Creative Nursing, 25*(2), 169–175. https://doi.org/10.1891/1078-4535.25.2.169

Mittaz Hager, A. G., Mathieu, N., Lenoble-Hoskovec, C., Swaenburg J., de Bie, R., & Hilfiker, R. (2019). Effects of three home-based exercise programmes regarding falls, quality of life and exercise-adherence in older adults at risk of falling: Protocol for a randomized controlled trial. *BMC Geriatrics, 19*(1), 13. https://doi.org/10.1186/s12877-018-1021-y

Morse, J. M., Tylko, S. J., & Dixon, H. A. (1987). Characteristics of the fall-prone patient. *Gerontologist, 27*(4), 516–522. https://doi.org/10.1093/geront/27.4.516

Morton, P. G., & Fontaine, D. K. (2018). *Critical care nursing. A holistic approach* (11th ed.). Wolters Kluwer.

National Council on Aging (NCOA). (2021, July 14). *Get the facts on falls prevention.* https://www.ncoa.org/article/get-the-facts-on-falls-prevention

National Home Security Alliance. (2018). *Safety at home: 10 common safety hazards around the house.* https://staysafe.org/safety-at-home-10-common-safety-hazards-around-the-house/

National Institute on Aging. (n.d.). *Fall-proofing your home.* https://www.nia.nih.gov/health/fall-proofing-your-home

National Institute on Aging. (2017). *Health information. Prevent falls and fractures.* https://www.nia.nih.gov/health/prevent-falls-and-fractures

National Safety Council. (n.d.). Safety at home. Top causes of preventable injuries, death off the job. Retrieved June 16, 2020, from https://www.nsc.org/home-safety

Patient Safety Network (PSNet). (2019a). *Patient safety primer. Culture of safety.* Agency for Healthcare Research and Quality. https://psnet.ahrq.gov/primer/culture-safety

Patient Safety Network (PSNet). (2019b). *Patient safety primer. Never events.* https://psnet.ahrq.gov/primer/never-events

Perry, S. E., Hockenberry, M. J., Lowdermilk, D. L., Wilson, D., Cashion, K., Rodgers, C. C., & Rhodes Alden, K. (2018). *Maternal child nursing care* (6th ed.). Elsevier.

Poh, F. J. X., & Shorey, S. (2020). A literature review of factors influencing injurious falls. *Clinical Nursing Research, 29*(3), 141–148. https://doi.org/10.1177/1054773818802187

Public Health Facility of Canada. (2015). The safe living guide–A guide to home safety for seniors. https://www.canada.ca/en/public-health/services/health-promotion/aging-seniors/publications/publications-general-public/safe-living-guide-a-guide-home-safety-seniors.html

Quigley, P. A. (2015). Evidence levels: Applied to select fall and fall injury prevention practices. *Rehabilitation Nursing, 41*(1), 5–15. https://doi.org/10.1002/rnj.253

Registered Nurses' Association of Ontario (RNAO). (2012). *Best practice guidelines. Promoting safety: Alternative approaches to the use of restraints.* https://rnao.ca/bpg/guidelines/promoting-safety-alternative-approaches-use-restraints

Rochon, R., & Salazar, L. (2019). Partnering with the patient to reduce falls in a medical-surgical unit. *International Journal of Safe Patient Handling & Mobility, 9*(4), 135–142.

Ryan, L., Jackson, D., Woods, C., & Usher, K. (2019). Intentional rounding–An integrative literature review. *Journal of Advance Nursing, 75*(6), 1151–1161. https://doi.org/10.1111/jan.13897

Shuman, C. J., Montie, M., Hoffman, G. J., Powers, K. E., Doettl, S., Anderson, C. A., & Titler, M. G. (2019). Older adults' perceptions of their fall risk and prevention strategies after transitioning from hospital to home. *Journal of Gerontological Nursing, 45*(1), 23–30. https://doi.org/10.3928/00989134-20190102-04

Silbert-Flagg, J., & Pillitteri, A. (2018). *Maternal & child health nursing* (8th ed.). Wolters Kluwer.

Soh, S., Barker, A. L., Morello, R. T., & Ackerman, I. N. (2020). Applying the International Classification of Functioning, Disability and Health framework to determine the predictors of falls and fractures in people with osteoarthritis or at high risk of developing osteoarthritis: Data from the Osteoarthritis Initiative. *BMC Musculoskeletal Disorders, 21*(1), 138. https://doi.org/10.1186/s12891-020-3160-5

Spano-Szekely, L., Winkler, A., Waters, C., Dealmeida, S., Brandt, K., Williamson, M., Blum, C., Gasper, L., & Wright, F. (2018). Individualized fall prevention program in an acute care setting. *Journal of Nursing Care Quality, 34*(2), 127–132. https://doi.org/10.1097/NCQ.0000000000000344

Springer, G. (2015). When and how to use restraints. *American Nurse Today, 10*(1), 26–27. https://www.myamericannurse.com/wp-content/uploads/2015/01/ant1-Restraints-1218.pdf

Stoeckle, A., Iseler, J. I., Havey, R., & Aebersold, C. (2019). Catching quality before it falls. Preventing falls and injuries in the adult emergency department. *Journal of Emergency Nursing, 45*(3), 257–264. https://doi.org/10.1016/j.jen.2018.08.001

Struth, D. (2009). *The 60 second situational assessment.* Quality and Safety Education for Nurses (QSEN) Institute. https://qsen.org/the-60-second-situational-assessment/

Stubbs, B., Brefka, S., & Denkinger, M. D. (2015). What works to prevent falls in community-dwelling older adults? Umbrella review of meta-analyses of randomized controlled trials. *Physical Therapy, 95*(8), 1095–1110.

Taylor, C., Lynn, P., & Bartlett, J. (2023). *Fundamentals of nursing: The art and science of person-centered care* (10th ed.). Wolters Kluwer.

Thomas, E., Battaglia, G., Patti, A., Brusa, J., Leonardi, V., Palma, A., & Bellafiore, M. (2019). Physical activity programs for balanced and fall prevention in elderly. A systematic review. *Medicine, 98*(27), e16218. https://doi.org/10.1097/MD.0000000000016218

TIDI Products. (2009, April 6). *Posey® soft belt. Application instructions.* https://f.hubspotusercontent40.net/hubfs/8218994/IFU/Restraints%20and%20Restraint%20Alternatives/Posey-Soft-Belt.pdf

TIDI Products. (2018a, December 4). *Posey®. Safety information for the use of Posey® restraining products.* https://f.hubspotusercontent40.net/hubfs/8218994/IFU/Restraints%20and%20Restraint%20Alternatives/Posey-Soft-Limb-Holder-2530-2540-25281.pdf

TIDI Products. (2018b, November 29). *Posey® limb holders. Application instructions for wrist and ankle.* https://f.hubspotusercontent40.net/hubfs/8218994/IFU/Restraints%20and%20Restraint%20Alternatives/Posey-Soft-Limb-Holder-2530-2540-25281.pdf

TIDI Products. (2019, September 20). *Posey® SecureSleeve® Protector. Application instructions.* https://f.hubspotusercontent40.net/hubfs/8218994/IFU/Restraints%20and%20Restraint%20Alternatives/Posey-Secure-Sleeve.pdf

Tomita, M. R., Saharan, S., Rajendran, S., Mochajski, S. M., & Schweitzer, J. A. (2014). Psychometrics of the Home Safety Self-Assessment Tool (HSSAT) to prevent falls in community-swelling older adults. *The American Journal of Occupational Therapy, 68*(6), 711–718. DOI: 10.5014/ajot.2014.010801

Toughy, T. A., & Jett, K. (2018). *Ebersol and Hess' Gerontological nursing & healthy aging* (5th ed.). Elsevier.

Tucker, S., Sheikholeslami, D., Farrington, M., Picone, D., Johnson, J., Matthews, G., Evans, R., Gould, R., Bohlken, D., Comried, L., Petrulevich, K., Perkhounkove, E., & Cullen, L. (2019). Patient, nurse and organizational factors that influence evidence-based fall preention for hospitalized oncology patients: An exploratory study. *Worldviews on Evidence-Based Nursing, 16*(2), 111–120. https://doi.org/10.1111/wvn.12353

U.S. Food and Drug Administration (FDA). (2017). *A guide to bed safety bed rails in hospitals, nursing homes, and home health care: The facts.* https://www.fda.gov/medical-devices/hospital-beds/guide-bed-safety-bed-rails-hospitals-nursing-homes-and-home-health-care-facts

U.S. Food and Drug Administration (FDA). (2018a). *Bed rail safety.* https://www.fda.gov/medical-devices/consumer-products/bed-rail-safety?source=govdelivery&utm_medium=email&utm_source=govdelivery

U.S. Food and Drug Administration (FDA). (2018b). *Hospital beds.* https://www.fda.gov/medical-devices/general-hospital-devices-and-supplies/hospital-beds

VHA Center for Engineering & Occupational Safety and Health (CEOSH) (VHACEOSH). (2016). *Safe patient handling and mobility guidebook.* http://www.tnpatientsafety.com/pubfiles/Initiatives/workplace-violence/sphm-pdf.pdf

Williams, L. (2018). Identifying risk for falls in pediatric patients. *AACN Advanced Critical Care, 29*(3), 343–347. https://doi.org/10.4037/aacnacc2018936

World Health Organization (WHO). (2018, January 16). *Fact sheets. Falls.* https://www.who.int/news-room/fact-sheets/detail/falls#:~:text=Falls%20are%20the%20second%20leading,greatest%20number%20of%20fatal%20falls

SUGGESTED ANSWERS FOR FOCUSING ON PATIENT CARE: DEVELOPING CLINICAL REASONING AND CLINICAL JUDGMENT

1. Nursing interventions for Megan should include the use of distraction, such as play, toys, music, games, and so forth. (Refer to Skill 4-3.) Megan's parent should be encouraged to stay with her to provide supervision and distraction, also. Cover the IV access site with a dressing and gauze, or other covering. If all other alternatives to restraints are attempted, and it is necessary to maintain the IV infusion, an elbow restraint (Skill 4-6) or hand mitt (Skill 4-4) would be the least restrictive restraints to prevent dislodgement of Megan's IV access.

2. You must implement as many alternatives to restraints as possible for Mr. Mallory. Refer to Skill 4-3. In addition, consult

with the health care team to discuss a possible time frame for extubation. Increase frequency of monitoring, repeat explanations, and provide distraction as part of the plan of care for this patient. Elbow restraints (Skill 4-6) would be a possible solution if it is determined that restraints are required.

3. Fall prevention is best achieved through the implementation of multiple strategies. Begin by assessing the patient's motivation for attempting activity unassisted. Provide reassurance and explanations related to care. If possible, Mr. Frawley could be moved to a room closer to the nursing station to allow increased monitoring. Additional nursing interventions to try could include asking family members to stay with Mr. Frawley, providing distraction based on information from the family regarding favorite activities, more frequent rounding to ensure that his toileting needs are met, as well as need for hydration. Provide a low bed for the patient, as well as floor mats, to reduce the risk for serious injury if Mr. Frawley should fall. Refer to Skill 4-2 for additional intervention suggestions.

5

Medications

Focusing on Patient Care

This chapter will help you develop the skills needed to administer medications safely to the following patients:

Cooper Jackson, age 2, does not want to take his ordered oral antibiotic.

Erika Jenkins, age 20, is extremely afraid of needles and is at the clinic for her birth-control injection.

Jonah Dinerman, age 63, was recently diagnosed with diabetes and needs to be taught how to give himself insulin injections.

Refer to Focusing on Patient Care: Developing Clinical Reasoning and Clinical Judgment at the end of the chapter to apply what you learn.

Learning Outcomes

After completing the chapter, you will be able to accomplish the following:

1. Prepare medications for administration in a safe manner.
2. Administer oral medications.
3. Administer medications via a gastric tube.
4. Remove medication from an ampule.
5. Remove medication from a vial.
6. Mix medications from two vials in one syringe.
7. Identify appropriate needle size and angle of insertion for intradermal, subcutaneous, and intramuscular injections.
8. Locate appropriate sites for intradermal injection.
9. Administer an intradermal injection.
10. Locate appropriate sites for a subcutaneous injection.
11. Administer a subcutaneous injection.
12. Locate appropriate sites for an intramuscular injection.
13. Administer an intramuscular injection.
14. Administer a continuous subcutaneous infusion: Applying an insulin pump.
15. Administer medications by intravenous bolus or push through a continuous intravenous infusion.
16. Administer medications by intravenous bolus or push through a medication or drug-infusion lock.
17. Administer a piggyback, intermittent, intravenous infusion of medication.
18. Administer an intermittent intravenous infusion of medication via a mini-infusion pump.

19. Apply a transdermal patch.
20. Administer eye drops.
21. Administer eye irrigation.
22. Administer ear drops.
23. Administer ear irrigation.
24. Administer a nasal spray.
25. Administer a vaginal cream.
26. Administer a rectal suppository.
27. Administer medication via a metered-dose inhaler.
28. Administer medication via a dry-powder inhaler.
29. Administer medication via a small-volume nebulizer.

Nursing Concepts

- Assessment
- Clinical decision making/clinical judgment
- Safety
- Teaching and learning/patient education

Medication administration is a core nursing function that involves skillful technique and consideration of safety principles that consider the patient's developmental state, individual characteristics, and health status. The nurse administering medications needs to have knowledge of drugs, including drug names, preparations, classifications, adverse effects, and physiologic factors that affect drug action (Fundamentals Review 5-1).

Use of the three checks and the rights of medication administration when administering medications can assist with safe administration of medications. The use of technology, such as bar-code medication administration (BCMA) and medication dispensing systems, does not relieve the nurse of responsibility for ensuring safe medication administration. Check the label on the medication package or container three times during medication preparation and administration (Fundamentals Review 5-2).

The rights of medication administration (Fundamentals Review 5-3) can help to ensure accuracy when administering medications. However, the Institute for Safe Medication Practices (2007) reiterated a position taken in 1999 that the rights of medication administration "are merely broadly stated goals or desired outcomes of safe medication practices" (para. 1). The rights themselves do not ensure medication safety. The nurse assumes individual accountability for safe drug administration by collaborating with the patient and interprofessional team and engaging in behavior that follows standards of best practice and behaviors prescribed by the institution to achieve the goals of the rights (Frandsen & Pennington, 2021; Hanson & Haddad, 2020; Rohde & Domm, 2017). Suggested rights of administration vary slightly between references, spanning from the classic 5 rights (Rights 1 through 5 in Fundamentals Review 5-3) to up to 10 or 11 rights of medication administration identified in the evidence for practice (Frandsen & Pennington, 2021; Hanson & Haddad, 2020; McCuistion et al., 2021; Smeulers et al., 2015). The first five rights (Fundamentals Review 5-3) are included in most references to the rights of medication administration and are the ones verified at each of the three checks (Taylor et al., 2023). Nurses should integrate reliance on embedded, sometime rote, processes with intentional decision making grounded in clinical judgment (Taylor et al., 2023).

In addition, it is important to acknowledge that medication administration is a process with many interconnected players, including clinical nurses, physicians, advanced practice professionals, pharmacists, and patients. All involved in the process share the responsibility for a safe medication system (Hanson & Haddad, 2020). Education and training should focus on interprofessional roles and responsibilities, communication techniques, and other initiatives that foster the teamwork required to promote patient safety in medication administration processes (Bartlett & Kinsey, 2020).

When administering medication, consider factors that may affect drug action, such as age-related considerations. For example, physiologic changes associated with the aging process, including decreased gastric motility, muscle mass, acid production, and blood flow affect drug action (Rochon, 2020). Older adults may also be more susceptible to certain **adverse drug reactions**. Drug interactions in older adults are a very real and dangerous problem because older adults are more likely to take multiple drugs simultaneously and because of age-related declines in hepatic and renal function (Cahir et al., 2019).

Nursing responsibilities for drug administration are summarized in Fundamentals Review 5-4. This chapter covers skills that the nurse needs to administer medications safely via multiple routes. Proper use of equipment and proper technique are imperative. Fundamentals Review 5-5 and Figure 5-1 review important guidelines related to administering parenteral medications. Nurses should be aware of the higher risk of making an error when their workflow is disrupted from either a distraction or interruption; effective reduction and management of distractions and interruptions is critical to safe medication administration and increased patient safety (Bravo et al., 2016; Hanson & Haddad, 2020; Williams et al., 2014). Medication errors predominately occur during the phases of preparing and administering medications (Hanson & Haddad, 2020).

Fundamentals Review 5-1

KNOW YOUR MEDICATIONS

Before administering any medication, know the following:

- Mode of action and purpose of medication (making sure that this medication is appropriate for the patient with consideration to the patient's developmental state, individual characteristics, and health status)

- Adverse effects of and contraindications for the medication
- Antagonist of medication (as appropriate)
- Safe dosage range for medication
- Potential interactions with other medications
- Precautions to take before administration
- Proper administration technique

Fundamentals Review 5-2

THE THREE CHECKS

"Three Checks" denotes that the label on the medication package or container should be checked three times during medication preparation and administration.

1. Read the Electronic Medication Administration Record (eMAR) or Medication Administration Record (MAR); **read the label** when reaching for the unit dose package or container and selecting the proper medication from the patient's medication drawer or medication supply system. This is the *first check* of the medication label.
2. After retrieving the medication from the drawer, **read the label** and compare the medication label with the eMAR/MAR. Note: Compare with the

eMAR/MAR immediately before pouring from a multidose container. This is the *second check* of the medication label.

3. The *third check* can be performed in one of two ways, depending on facility policy:
   - Most commonly, at the bedside, **read the label** and recheck the label with the eMAR/MAR after identifying the patient and before administration.
   - When all medications for one patient have been prepared, **read the label** and recheck the labels with the eMAR/MAR before replacing the multidose container in the drawer or shelf before taking the medication to the patient.

Fundamentals Review 5-3

RIGHTS OF MEDICATION ADMINISTRATION

The "Rights of Medication Administration" can help to ensure accuracy when administering medications. To prevent medication errors, always ensure that the:

1. **Right medication** is given to the
2. **Right patient** in the
3. **Right dosage** (in the right form) through the
4. **Right route** at the
5. **Right time** for the
6. **Right reason** based on the

7. **Right (appropriate) assessment** data using the
8. **Right documentation** and monitoring for the
9. **Right response** by the patient.

Additional rights have been suggested to include (10) the **right to education**, ensuring patients receive accurate and thorough information about the medication, and (11) the **right to refuse**, acknowledging that patients can and do refuse to take a medication.

Fundamentals Review 5-4

NURSING RESPONSIBILITIES FOR ADMINISTERING DRUGS

- Assessing the patient and understanding the clinical purpose (indication); understanding the desire outcome for administration of a particular medication
- Preparing the medication to be administered (checking labels, preparing injections, observing proper asepsis techniques with needles and syringes)
- Calculating accurate dosages
- Validating medication calculations with another nurse
- Administering the medication (e.g., proper injection techniques, aids to help swallowing, topical methods, and so on)

- Documenting the medications given
- Monitoring the patient's reaction and evaluating the patient's response
- Collaborating with other members of the health care team involved in the patient's care.
- Educating the patient regarding their medications and medication regimen

Fundamentals Review 5-5

NEEDLE/SYRINGE SELECTION

- The route of administration directs the choice of needle length. Refer to the discussion related to each particular route for specific guidelines regarding needle length.
- Body size is also taken into consideration in relation to needle length. An obese person requires a longer needle to reach muscle tissue than does a thin person. A thin person or an older adult with decreased muscle mass or subcutaneous tissue requires a shorter needle.
- When looking at a needle package, the first number is the needle gauge or diameter of the needle (e.g., 18, 20) and the second number is the length in inches (e.g., 1, 1.5).
- As the gauge number becomes larger, the size of the needle becomes smaller; for instance, a 24-gauge needle is smaller than an 18-gauge needle.
- When giving an injection, the viscosity of the medication directs the choice of gauge (diameter). A

thicker medication is given through a needle with a larger gauge, and a thinner-consistency medication is given through a needle with a smaller gauge, such as a 24-gauge.
- The amount of medication to be administered directs the choice of the size of the syringe. Smaller syringes should be used as needed for precise dosing because they provide smaller increments of measurement—never estimate a dose. For example, a 1-mL syringe provides increments of 0.01 mL, but a 5-mL syringe allows for precise measures only down to 0.2 mL.
- The type of medication also influences the choice of syringe. There are special syringes for certain uses. An example is the insulin syringe used only to inject insulin.

Fundamentals Review 5-5 continued

NEEDLE/SYRINGE SELECTION

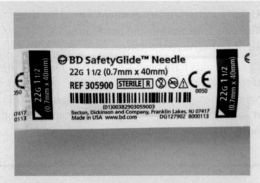

Needle package showing first number (gauge or diameter of the needle) and second number (length of the needle in inches).

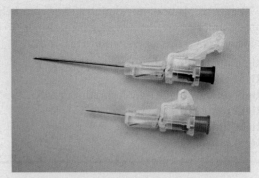

Different needle sizes. An 18-gauge needle (*top*) and a 24-gauge needle (*bottom*).

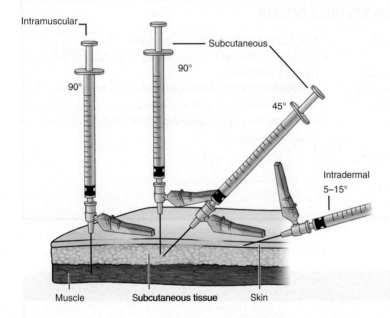

FIGURE 5-1. Comparison of insertion angles for intramuscular, subcutaneous, and intradermal injections.

Skill 5-1 ▶ Administering Oral Medications

Drugs given orally are intended for absorption in the stomach and small intestine. The oral route is the most common route of administration and is usually the most convenient and comfortable route for the patient. Drugs administered orally have a slower onset and a more prolonged, but less potent, effect compared to drugs given via other routes of administration.

DELEGATION CONSIDERATIONS

The administration of oral medications is not delegated to assistive personnel (AP). The administration of specified oral medications to stable patients in some long-term care settings may be delegated to AP who have received appropriate training. Depending on the state's nurse practice act and the organization's policies and procedures, the administration of oral medications may be delegated to licensed practical/vocational nurses (LPN/LVNs). The decision to delegate must be based on careful analysis of the patient's needs and circumstances as well as the qualifications of the person to whom the task is being delegated. Refer to the Delegation Guidelines in Appendix A.

EQUIPMENT	
	• Medication in disposable cup or oral syringe
	• Liquid (e.g., water, juice) with straw, if not contraindicated
	• Electronic Medication Administration Record (eMAR) or Medication Administration Record (MAR)
	• PPE, as indicated

ASSESSMENT

Assess the appropriateness of the drug for the patient. Review the medical history and allergy, assessment, and laboratory data that may influence drug administration. Check the expiration date. Assess the patient's ability to swallow medications; check the gag reflex, if indicated. If the patient cannot swallow, is unconscious or NPO, does not have gag reflex, or is experiencing nausea or vomiting, withhold the medication, notify the health care team, and complete proper documentation. Assess the patient's knowledge of the medication. If the patient has a knowledge deficit about the medication, this may be the appropriate time to begin education about the medication. If the medication may affect the patient's vital signs, assess them before administration. If the medication is for pain relief, assess the patient's pain level before and after administration. Verify the patient's name as well as the dose, route, and time of administration.

ACTUAL OR POTENTIAL HEALTH PROBLEMS AND NEEDS

Many actual or potential health problems or issues may require the use of this skill as part of related interventions. An appropriate health problem or issue may include:
• Knowledge deficiency
• Polypharmacy
• Aspiration risk

OUTCOME IDENTIFICATION AND PLANNING

The expected outcomes to achieve when administering an oral medication include that the medication is successfully administered via the oral route, the patient experiences the desired effect from the medication, the patient does not aspirate, the patient does not experience adverse effects, and the patient understands and complies with the medication regimen.

IMPLEMENTATION

ACTION	**RATIONALE**
1. Gather equipment. Check each medication prescribed against the original in the health record, depending on facility policy and the medication order system in place. Clarify any inconsistencies. Check the patient's health record for allergies.	The prescription is the legal record of prescribed medication interventions. This comparison helps to identify errors that may have occurred when orders were transcribed. Computer provider order-entry (CPOE) systems allow prescribers to send electronic medication prescriptions directly to the pharmacy located in a health care facility and to outpatient pharmacies.
2. Know the actions, special nursing considerations, safe dose ranges, purpose of administration, and potential adverse effects of the medications to be administered. Consider the appropriateness of the medication for this patient.	This knowledge aids the nurse in evaluating the therapeutic effect of the medication in relation to the patient's health status and can also be used to educate the patient about the medication.
3. Perform hand hygiene.	Hand hygiene prevents the spread of microorganisms.
4. Move the medication supply system to the outside of the patient's room or prepare for administration at the medication supply system in the medication area. Alternatively, access the medication administration supply system at or inside the patient's room.	Organization facilitates error-free administration and saves time.

(*continued on page 202*)

Skill 5-1 ▶ Administering Oral Medications *(continued)*

ACTION

5. Unlock the medication supply system or drawer. Enter the passcode into the computer and scan employee identification, if required.

6. **Prepare medications for one patient at a time.**

7. Read the eMAR/MAR and read the label when selecting the proper medication from the medication supply system or patient's medication drawer.

8. Read the label and compare the medication label with the eMAR/MAR (Figure 1). Check expiration dates and perform calculations, if necessary. Scan the bar code on the package, if required.

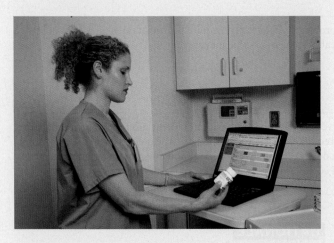

9. Prepare the required medications:

   a. *Unit dose packages:* **Do not open the wrapper until at the bedside.** Keep opioids and medications that require special nursing assessments separate from other medication packages.

   b. *Multidose containers:* When removing tablets or capsules from a multidose bottle, pour the necessary number into the bottle cap and then place the tablets or capsules in a medication cup. Break only scored tablets, if necessary, to obtain the proper dosage. Do not touch tablets or capsules with your hands.

   c. *Liquid medication in multidose bottle:* When pouring liquid medications out of a multidose bottle, hold the bottle so the label is against the palm. Use the appropriate measuring device when pouring liquids and read the amount of medication at the bottom of the meniscus at eye level (Figure 2). Wipe the lip of the bottle with a paper towel.

RATIONALE

Locking the medication supply system or drawer safeguards each patient's medication supply. Facility accrediting organizations require medication supply systems to be locked when not in use. Entering the passcode and scanning ID allows only authorized users into the computer system and identifies the user for documentation by the computer.

This prevents errors in medication administration.

This is the *first* check of the medication label.

This is the *second* check of the label. Verify calculations with another nurse to ensure safety, if necessary.

FIGURE 1. Comparing medication label with eMAR.

Wrapper is kept intact because the label is needed for an additional safety check. Special assessments may be required before giving certain medications. These may include assessing vital signs and checking laboratory test results.

Pouring medication into the cap allows for easy return of excess medication to the bottle. Pouring tablets or capsules into your hand is unsanitary.

Liquid that may drip onto the label makes the label difficult to read. Accuracy is possible when the appropriate measuring device is used and then read accurately.

ACTION

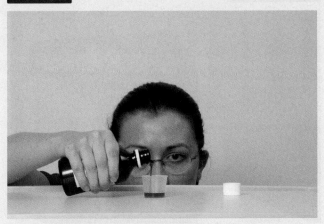

FIGURE 2. Measuring at eye level. (*Source:* Used with permission from Shutterstock. *Photo by B. Proud.*)

10. **Depending on facility policy, the third check of the label may occur at this point. If so, when all medications for one patient have been prepared, read the label and recheck the labels with the eMAR/MAR before taking the medications to the patient. However, many facilities require the third check to occur at the bedside, after identifying the patient.**

11. Replace any multidose containers in the patient's drawer or medication supply system. **Log out of and/or lock the medication supply system before leaving it.**

12. Transport medications to the patient's bedside carefully and keep the medications in sight at all times.

13. **Ensure that the patient receives the medications at the correct time.**

 14. Perform hand hygiene and put on PPE, if indicated.

 15. **Identify the patient. Compare the information with the eMAR/MAR. The patient should be identified using at least two of the following methods** (The Joint Commission, 2021):

a. Check the name on the patient's identification band (Figure 3).

b. Check the identification number on the patient's identification band.

c. Check the birth date on the patient's identification band.

d. Ask the patient to state their name and birth date, based on facility policy.

16. **Complete necessary assessments before administering medications. Check the patient's allergy bracelet, if present, or ask the patient about allergies. Explain the purpose and action of each medication to the patient.**

17. Scan the patient's bar code on the identification band, if required (Figure 4) (The Joint Commission, 2021).

RATIONALE

This *third* check ensures accuracy and helps to prevent errors. *Note:* Many facilities require the third check to occur at the bedside, after identifying the patient and before administration.

Locking the medication supply system or drawer safeguards the patient's medication supply. Facility accrediting organizations require medication supply systems to be locked when not in use.

Careful handling and close observation prevent accidental or deliberate disarrangement of medications.

Check facility policy, which may allow for administration within a period of 30 minutes before or 30 minutes after the designated time.

Hand hygiene and PPE prevent the spread of microorganisms. PPE is required based on transmission precautions.

Identifying the patient ensures the right patient receives the medications and helps prevent errors. The patient's room number or physical location is not used as an identifier (The Joint Commission, 2021). Replace the identification band if it is missing or inaccurate in any way.

This requires a response from the patient, but illness and strange surroundings often cause patients to be confused.

Assessment is a prerequisite to administration of medications.

The bar code provides an additional check to ensure that the medication is given to the right patient.

(*continued on page 204*)

Skill 5-1 ▶ Administering Oral Medications *(continued)*

ACTION	RATIONALE

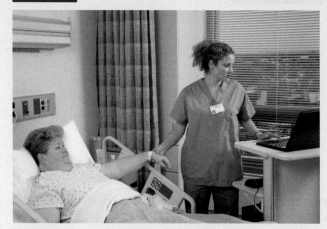

FIGURE 3. Comparing patient's name and identification number with eMAR.

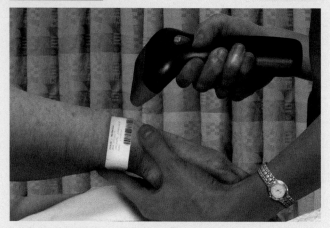

FIGURE 4. Scanning bar code on patient's identification bracelet. (*Photo by B. Proud.*)

18. **Based on facility policy, the third check of the medication label may occur at this point. If so, read the label and recheck the label with the eMAR/MAR before administering the medications to the patient.**

Many facilities require the *third* check to occur at the bedside, after identifying the patient and before administration. If facility policy directs the *third* check at this time, this *third* check ensures accuracy and helps prevent errors.

19. Assist the patient to an upright or lateral (side-lying) position.

Swallowing is facilitated by proper positioning. An upright or side-lying position protects the patient from aspiration.

20. Administer medications:

a. Offer water or other permitted fluids with pills, capsules, tablets, and some liquid medications.

Liquids facilitate swallowing of solid drugs. Some liquid drugs are intended to adhere to the pharyngeal area, in which case liquid is not offered with the medication.

b. Ask whether the patient prefers to take the medications by hand or in a cup.

This encourages the patient's participation in taking the medications.

21. **Remain with the patient until each medication is swallowed. Never leave medication at the patient's bedside (Figure 5).**

Unless you have seen the patient swallow the drug, the drug cannot be recorded as administered. The patient's health record is a legal record. Medications can be left at the bedside only with a prescriber's order.

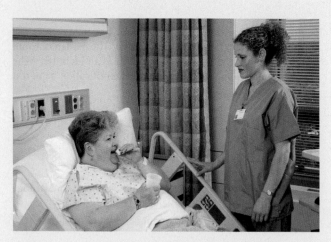

FIGURE 5. Remaining with patient until each medication is swallowed.

22. Assist the patient to a comfortable position. Remove PPE, if used. Perform hand hygiene.

Promotes patient comfort. Proper removal of PPE prevents transmission of microorganisms. Hand hygiene deters the spread of microorganisms.

ACTION

23. Document the administration of the medication immediately after administration. See Documentation section below.

24. Evaluate the patient's response to the medication within the appropriate time frame.

RATIONALE

Timely documentation helps to ensure patient safety.

The patient needs to be evaluated for therapeutic and adverse effects from the medication.

EVALUATION

The expected outcomes have been met when the patient has swallowed the medication, did not aspirate, verbalized an understanding of the medication, experienced the desired effect from the medication, and did not experience adverse effects.

DOCUMENTATION

Guidelines

Record each medication immediately after it is administered on the eMAR/MAR or health record using the required format. Include the date and time of administration (Figure 6). If using a bar-code system, medication administration is automatically recorded when the bar code is scanned. PRN medications require documentation of the reason for administration. Prompt recording avoids the possibility of accidentally repeating the administration of the drug. If the drug was refused or omitted, record this in the appropriate area on the medication record and notify the health care team as appropriate. This verifies the reason medication was omitted and ensures that health care personnel providing care for the patient are aware of the occurrence. Recording administration of an opioid may require additional documentation on a controlled-substance record, stating drug count and other specific information. A record of fluid intake and output measurement is required.

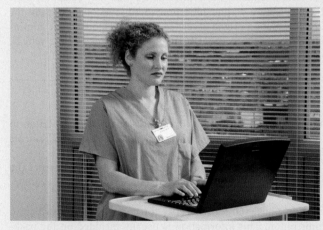

FIGURE 6. Recording each medication administered on eMAR.

Sample Documentation

Lippincott
DocuCare

Practice documenting medication administration in *Lippincott DocuCare*.

8/6/25 0835 Patient states he is having constant stabbing leg pains. Rates pain as an 8/10. Percocet 2 tabs administered.

—*K. Sanders, RN*

8/6/25 0905 Patient resting comfortably. Rates leg pain as a 1/10.

—*K. Sanders, RN*

8/6/25 1300 Patient states he does not want pain medication, despite return of leg pain. States, "It made me feel woozy last time." Feelings discussed with patient. Patient agrees to take Percocet 1 tab at this time.

—*K. Sanders, RN*

8/6/25 1320 Percocet, 1 tablet given PO.

—*K. Sanders, RN*

(continued on page 206)

Skill 5-1 ▶ Administering Oral Medications   *(continued)*

**DEVELOPING
CLINICAL REASONING
AND CLINICAL
JUDGMENT**
**UNEXPECTED
SITUATIONS AND
ASSOCIATED
INTERVENTIONS**

- *Patient states that it feels like medication is lodged in throat:* Offer the patient more fluids to drink. If allowed, offer the patient bread or crackers to help move the medication to the stomach.
- *It is unclear whether the patient swallowed the medication:* Check in the patient's mouth, under their tongue, and between their cheek and gum. Patients with altered cognition may not be aware that the medication was not swallowed. Also, patients may "cheek" medications to avoid taking the medication or to save it for later use.
- *Patient vomits immediately or shortly after receiving oral medication:* Assess vomit, looking for pills or fragments. Do not readminister the medication without notifying the health care team. If a whole pill is seen and can be identified, the prescriber may ask that the medication be administered again. If a pill is not seen or medications cannot be identified, do not readminister the medication in order to prevent the patient from receiving too large a dose.
- *Child refuses to take oral medications:* Some medications may be mixed in a small amount of food, such as pudding or ice cream. Do not add the medication to liquids because the medication may alter the taste of liquids; if the child then refuses to drink the rest of the liquid, you will not know how much of the medication was ingested. Use creativity when devising ways to administer medications to a child. See the section below, Infant and Child Considerations, for suggestions.
- *Capsule or tablet falls to the floor during administration:* Discard and obtain a new dose for administration. This prevents contamination and transmission of microorganisms.
- *Patient refuses medication:* Explore the reason for the patient's refusal. Review the rationale for use of the drug, explain the risk of refusal, and any other information that may be appropriate. If you are unable to administer the medication despite education and discussion, document the omission and any education and/or explanation provided related to attempts to facilitate administration according to facility policy. The health care team should be informed of the refusal, especially when the omission poses a specific threat to the patient (McCuistion et al., 2021).

**SPECIAL
CONSIDERATIONS**
General Considerations

- Some liquid medication preparations, such as suspensions and emulsions, require agitation to ensure even distribution of medication in the solution. Be familiar with the specific requirements for medications you are administering.
- Place medications intended for sublingual absorption under the patient's tongue. Instruct the patient to allow the medication to dissolve completely. Reinforce the importance of not swallowing the medication tablet.
- Some oral medications are provided in powdered forms. Verify the correct liquid in which to dissolve the medication for administration. This information is usually included on the package. Verify any unclear instructions with a pharmacist or medication reference. If there is more than one possible liquid in which to dissolve the medication, include the patient in the decision process; patients may find one choice more palatable than another.
- Ongoing assessment is an important part of nursing care for both evaluation of patient response to administered medications and early detection of adverse drug reactions. If an adverse effect is suspected, withhold further medication doses and notify the health care team. Additional intervention is based on type of reaction and patient assessment.
- If the patient questions a medication order or states the medication is different from the usual dose, always recheck and clarify with the original prescription and/or prescriber.
- If the patient's level of consciousness is altered or their swallowing is impaired, check with the health care team to clarify the route of administration or alternative forms of medication. This may also be a solution for a pediatric or a confused patient who is refusing to take a medication.
- Patients with poor vision can request large-type labels on medication containers. A magnifying lens also may be helpful.

- Provide written medication information to reinforce discussion and education in the appropriate language, if the patient is literate. If the patient is unable to read, provide written information to family or caregiver, if appropriate. Written information should be at a 4th- to 6th-grade level, using short sentences and simple words, and incorporate pictures to increase ease of understanding (Patient Safety Network, 2019).
- If the patient has difficulty swallowing tablets, it may be appropriate to crush the medication to facilitate administration. Not all medications can be crushed or altered; long-acting and slow-release drugs are examples of medications that cannot be crushed. Check manufacturer's recommendations and/or with a pharmacist to verify (Anderson, 2019; Boullata, 2021; White & Bradnam, 2015).
- If the medication can be crushed, use a pill-crusher or mortar and pestle to grind the tablet into a powder. Crush each pill one at a time. Dissolve the powder with water or other recommended liquid in a liquid medication cup, keeping each medication separate from the others. Keep the package label with the medication cup for future comparison of information. Combine the crushed medication with a small amount of soft food, such as applesauce or pudding, to facilitate administration.
- Liquid medication not dispensed as unit dose should be administered in an oral syringe when available (ISMP, 2020) (Figure 7).

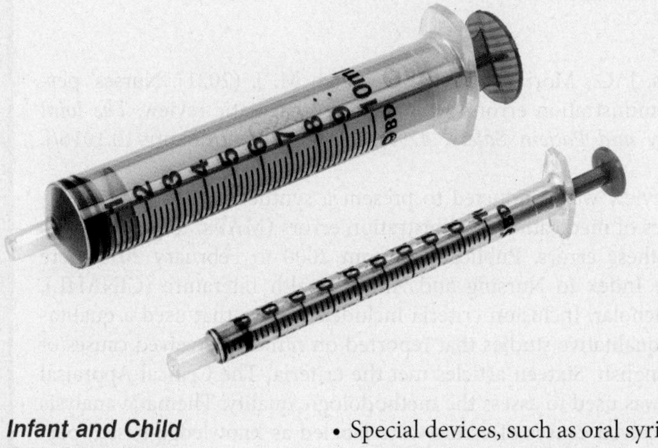

FIGURE 7. Monoject™ oral syringe. Note that specific syringes are designed for "ORAL USE ONLY." (Courtesy and © Becton, Dickinson and Company. Reprinted with permission.)

Infant and Child Considerations

- Special devices, such as oral syringes and calibrated nipples, are available in a pharmacy to ensure accurate dose calculations for young children and infants.
- Some creative ways to administer medications to children include the following: have a "tea party" with medicine cups; place a designated oral tip syringe or dropper in the space between the cheek and gum and slowly administer the medication (Kyle & Carman, 2021); save a special treat for after the medication administration (e.g., movie, playroom time, or a special food, if allowed).
- If a medication has an objectionable taste, warn the child if they are old enough to understand. Failing to warn the child is likely to decrease the child's trust in the nurse. Do not lie to a child about medication administration.
- Caution caregivers to remove and dispose of plastic syringe caps present on the end of syringes before drug administration to reduce the risk of choking. Companies manufacture syringes labeled "oral use" without the caps on them and should be considered for use (ISMP, 2020).

Older Adult Considerations

- Older adults with arthritis may have difficulty opening childproof caps. On request, the pharmacist can substitute a cap that is easier to open. A rubber band twisted around the cap may provide a more secure grip for older adults.
- Consider large-print written medication information, when appropriate.
- Physiologic changes associated with the aging process, including decreased gastric motility, muscle mass, acid production, and blood flow, can affect the patient's response to the medication, including drug absorption and increased risk of adverse effects. Older adults are more likely to take multiple drugs. As a result, drug interactions in the older adult are a significant consideration that may affect mental status (Frandsen & Pennington, 2021).

(continued on page 208)

Skill 5-1 ▶ Administering Oral Medications (continued)

Community-Based Care Considerations

- Encourage the patient to discard expired prescription medications based on label instructions or community guidelines.
- Discuss safe storage of medications when there are children and pets in the home environment.
- Discuss with parents the difference in over-the-counter medications made for infants and medications made for children. Many times, parents do not realize that there are different strengths to the actual medications, leading to under- or overdosing.
- Encourage patients to carry a card listing all medications they take, including dosage and frequency, in case of an emergency.
- Discuss the importance of using an appropriate measuring device for liquid medications. Caution patients not to use eating utensils for measuring medications; use a liquid medication cup, oral syringe, or measuring spoon to provide accurate dosing.

EVIDENCE FOR PRACTICE ▶

MEDICATION ADMINISTRATION ERRORS

Medication errors occur frequently and are a serious problem in health care. Medication errors may have serious consequences. Health care providers, including nurses, have a responsibility to prevent medication errors. What insights can nurses provide to guide interventions to help improve the medication administration process?

Related Research

Schroers, G., Niehoff, M., Ross, J. G., Moriarty, H., & Crescenz, M. J. (2021). Nurses' perceived causes of medication administration errors: A qualitative systematic review. *The Joint Commission Journal on Quality and Patient Safety, 47*(1), 38–53. https://doi.org/10.1016/j.jcjq.2020.09.010

This qualitative systematic review was conducted to present a synthesis of qualitative evidence of nurses' perceived causes of medication administration errors (MAEs) to guide efforts to mitigate the occurrence of these errors. Publications from 2000 to February 2019 were searched using the Cumulative Index to Nursing and Allied Health Literature (CINAHL), PubMed, Scopus, and Google Scholar. Inclusion criteria included studies that used a qualitative or mixed methods design, qualitative studies that reported on nurses' perceived causes of MAEs and were published in English. Sixteen articles met the criteria. The Critical Appraisal Skills Programme (CASP) tool was used to assess the methodologic quality. Thematic analysis of the data was performed. Perceived causes of errors were labeled as knowledge-based, personal, and contextual factors. Results indicated the primary knowledge-based factor was lack of medication knowledge. Personal factors included fatigue and complacency. Contextual factors identified included heavy workloads and interruptions. Contextual factors were reported in all reviewed studies and were often interconnected with personal and knowledge-based factors. The authors concluded nurses perceive the causes of MAEs as being multifactorial and interconnected and often stem from systemic issues. The authors suggest system changes are necessary to address and mitigate medication administration errors and must include multifactorial interventions directed at the factors contributing to medication administration errors.

Relevance to Nursing Practice

Medication administration is an important nursing responsibility. Nurses and health care systems need to be aware of the factors that contribute to medication errors and work to identify and reduce these factors in their practice.

Skill 5-2 ▶ Administering Medications via a Gastric Tube

Patients with a gastrointestinal (GI) tube (nasogastric, nasointestinal, percutaneous endoscopic gastrostomy [PEG], or jejunostomy [J] tube) often receive medication through the tube. Care of the patient with an enteral feeding tube is described in Chapter 11.

Flush the tube with at least 15 mL (purified) water (at least 5 mL for children) before giving each medication and immediately after giving each medication (Boullata, 2021; Boullata et al., 2017; Zoeller et al., 2020). Flushing helps to maintain tube patency.

A patient access connector called ENFit® has been made available on enteral administration sets, enteral syringes, and enteral access devices (Boullata et al., 2017). These connectors are not interconnectable with other therapy connections, such as those on intravenous, respiratory, neuraxial or limb-cuff pressure devices, decreasing the risk of inadvertent connection between an enteral feeding system and a nonenteral system (such as an intravascular catheter, peritoneal dialysis catheter, or tracheostomy) (Boullata et al., 2017). Guidelines for safe practices from the American Society for Parenteral and Enteral Nutrition (ASPEN) recommend use of a clean enteral syringe (≥20 mL) to administer medication through an enteral access device (Boullata et al., 2017). Figure 1 shows a selection of various sizes of the enteral syringes with the ENFit® connection.

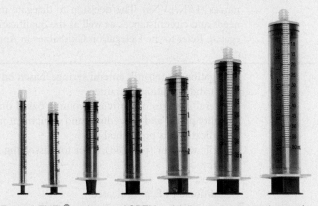

FIGURE 1. Enteral ENFit® syringes. ASPEN guidelines recommend use of a clean enteral ≥20-mL syringe to administer medication through an enteral access device. (Courtesy of Medline Industries, LP.)

Use liquid medications, when possible and if they are appropriate for enteral administration, because they are readily absorbed and less likely to cause tube occlusions. Liquid medications not specifically formulated for enteral administration may contain sugars, preservatives, and agents that thicken the solution and may cause GI disturbances and impact on medication absorption (Bandy et al., 2019; Boullata et al., 2017; Zoeller et al., 2020). Dilute thick suspensions as needed with an equal amount of (purified) water taking into consideration the overall fluid volume permitted for the patient (Boullata, 2021; Boullata et al., 2017; White & Bradnam, 2015). Pediatric patients require less volume and should have medications diluted to a 50/50 concentration with a minimum volume of 5 mL (Zoeller et al., 2020).

Certain solid immediate-release dosage medications can be crushed and combined with liquid to make a slurry. Crush each pill, one at a time, grinding to a fine powder and mix with at least 30 mL of (purified) water immediately before administration through the tube, keeping each medication separate from the others and flushing with water between each medication (Bandy et al., 2019; Boullata, 2021; Zoeller et al., 2020). The medications may not be physically or chemically compatible; mixing them can lead to tube obstruction from precipitate formation or altered therapeutic actions (Boullata, 2021; White & Bradnam, 2015). Sterile water or purified water is recommended for use as a diluent to eliminate the presence of pathogenic contaminants (Boullata, 2021; White & Bradnam, 2015; Zoeller et al., 2020). In addition, sterile water should be used for tube flushes in immunocompromised or critically ill patients (Allen, 2015; Boullata et al., 2017).

Certain capsules may be opened, emptied into (purified) water, and administered through the enteral tube; however, dose accuracy should be a consideration (Boullata, 2021; Boullata et al., 2017; White & Bradnam, 2015). **Not all medications can be crushed or altered; long-acting and slow-release drugs are examples of medications that cannot be crushed.** Check the

(continued on page 210)

Skill 5-2 ▶ Administering Medications via a Gastric Tube   *(continued)*

manufacturer's recommendations and/or with a pharmacist to verify (Anderson, 2019; Boullata, 2021; White & Bradnam, 2015).

If the patient is receiving tube feedings, review information about the drugs to be administered. Absorption of some drugs (e.g., phenytoin) and/or effect (e.g., carbidopa/levodopa) is affected by tube-feeding formulas (Boullata, 2021; Frandsen & Pennington, 2021). Discontinue a continuous tube feeding and leave the tube clamped for the required period of time before and after the medication has been given, according to the reference and facility protocol.

Health care providers must know policies and procedures regarding administration of medications via the enteral route to prevent administration errors and maximize therapeutic effectiveness (Boullata, 2021). Once prepared, keep the package label with the medication dispensing instrument for future comparison of information.

DELEGATION CONSIDERATIONS	The administration of medications via a gastric tube is not delegated to assistive personnel (AP). Depending on the state's nurse practice act and the organization's policies and procedures, the administration of medications via a gastric tube may be delegated to licensed practical/vocational nurses (LPN/LVNs). The decision to delegate must be based on careful analysis of the patient's needs and circumstances as well as the qualifications of the person to whom the task is being delegated. Refer to the Delegation Guidelines in Appendix A.
EQUIPMENT	• Irrigation set (60-mL enteral syringe, based on facility policy and procedures and equipment in use) and irrigation container) • Enteral syringes of sufficient volume based on medications to be administered, depending on facility policy and procedures and equipment in use • Medications as prescribed • Sterile water or (purified) water for dissolving medications and irrigation depending on facility policy • Gloves • Additional PPE, as indicated
ASSESSMENT	Assess the appropriateness of the drug for the patient. Review the medical history and allergy, assessment, and laboratory data that may influence drug administration. Research each medication to be given, especially for mode of action, side effects, nursing implications, ability to be crushed, and whether the medication should be given with or without food. Verify patient name, dose, route, and time of administration. Assess the patient's knowledge of the medication and the reason for its administration. If the patient has a knowledge deficit about the medication, this may be the appropriate time to begin educating the patient about the medication. Auscultate the abdomen for evidence of bowel sounds. Palpate the abdomen for tenderness and distention. Ascertain the time of the patient's last bowel movement and measure abdominal girth, if appropriate. If the medication may affect the patient's vital signs, assess them before administration. If the medication is for pain relief, assess the patient's pain level before and after administration.
ACTUAL OR POTENTIAL HEALTH PROBLEMS AND NEEDS	Many actual or potential health problems or issues may require the use of this skill as part of related interventions. An appropriate health problem or issue may include: • Knowledge deficiency • Injury risk • Aspiration risk
OUTCOME IDENTIFICATION AND PLANNING	The expected outcomes to achieve are that the patient receives the medication via the tube and experiences the intended effect of the medication. In addition, the patient verbalizes knowledge of the medications given, the patient remains free from adverse effects and injury, and the gastric tube remains patent.

IMPLEMENTATION

ACTION

1. Gather equipment. Check each medication prescribed against the original in the health record, depending on facility policy and the medication order system in place. Clarify any inconsistencies. Check the patient's health record for allergies.

2. Know the actions, special nursing considerations, safe dose ranges, purpose of administration, and adverse effects of the medications to be administered. Consider the appropriateness of the medication for this patient.

 3. Perform hand hygiene.

4. Move the medication supply system to the outside of the patient's room or prepare for administration at the medication supply system in the medication area. Alternatively, access the medication administration supply system at or inside the patient's room.

5. Unlock the medication supply system or drawer. Enter the passcode into the computer and scan employee identification, if required.

6. **Prepare medications for one patient at a time.**

7. Read the eMAR/MAR and read the label when selecting the proper medication from the medication supply system or patient's medication drawer.

8. Read the label and compare the label with the eMAR/MAR. Check expiration dates and perform calculations, if necessary. Scan the bar code on the package, if required.

9. Check to see if medications to be administered come in a liquid form. **If the medication was supplied as a pill or capsule, check with the pharmacy or drug reference to verify the ability to crush tablets or open capsules.**

10. Prepare the medication.
    Pills: Using a pill crusher, crush each pill one at a time. Dissolve the powder with at least 30 mL of (purified) water in a liquid medication cup, keeping each medication separate from the others. Keep the package label with the medication, for future comparison of information. Draw the mixture into an enteral syringe, based on facility policy and procedure and type of equipment in use (Boullata et al., 2017).

RATIONALE

The prescription is the legal record of prescribed medication interventions. This comparison helps to identify errors that may have occurred when orders were transcribed. Computer provider order-entry (CPOE) systems allow prescribers to send electronic medication prescriptions directly to the pharmacy located in a health care facility and to outpatient pharmacies.

This knowledge aids the nurse in evaluating the therapeutic effect of the medication in relation to the patient's health status and can also be used to educate the patient about the medication.

Hand hygiene prevents the spread of microorganisms.

Organization facilitates error-free administration and saves time.

Locking the medication supply system or drawer safeguards each patient's medication supply. Facility accrediting organizations require medication supply systems to be locked when not in use. Entering the passcode and scanning ID allows only authorized users into the computer system and identifies the user for documentation by the computer.

This prevents errors in medication administration.

This is the *first* check of the label.

This is the *second* check of the label. Verify calculations with another nurse to ensure safety, if necessary.

To prevent the tube from becoming clogged, all medications should be given in liquid form whenever possible. Not all medications can be crushed or altered; long-acting and slow-release drugs are examples of medications that cannot be crushed. Check manufacturer's recommendations and/or with a pharmacist to verify (Anderson, 2019; Boullata, 2021; White & Bradnam, 2015).

The medications may not be physically or chemically compatible; mixing them can lead to tube obstruction or altered therapeutic actions (Anderson, 2019; Boullata, 2021). The label is needed for an additional safety check. Some medications require pre-administration assessments. Guidelines for safe practices from the American Society for Parenteral and Enteral Nutrition (ASPEN) recommend use of a clean enteral syringe (≥20 mL) to administer medication through an enteral access device (Boullata et al., 2017).

(continued on page 212)

Skill 5-2 ▶ Administering Medications via a Gastric Tube *(continued)*

ACTION	RATIONALE
Liquid: When pouring liquid medications from a multidose bottle, hold the bottle with the label against the palm. Use the appropriate measuring device when pouring liquids and read the amount of medication at the bottom of the meniscus at eye level (refer to Skill 5-1). Wipe the lip of the bottle with a paper towel. Draw the mixture into an enteral syringe, based on facility policy and procedure and type of equipment in use (Boullata et al., 2017).	Liquid that may drip onto the label makes the label difficult to read. Accuracy is possible when the appropriate measuring device is used and then read accurately. Guidelines for safe practices from the American Society for Parenteral and Enteral Nutrition (ASPEN) recommend use of a clean enteral syringe (≥20 mL) to administer medication through an enteral access device (Boullata et al., 2017).

11. **Depending on facility policy, the third check of the label may occur at this point. If so, when all medications for one patient have been prepared, read the label and recheck the labels with the eMAR/MAR before taking the medications to the patient. However, many facilities require the third check to occur at the bedside, after identifying the patient.**

This *third* check ensures accuracy and helps to prevent errors. *Note:* Many facilities require the *third* check to occur at the bedside, after identifying the patient and before administration.

12. Label the enteric syringe or medication cup with the medication's name, dose, and amount (The Joint Commission, 2021).

Unlabeled medications are unidentifiable and may lead to a medication administration error (The Joint Commission, 2021).

13. Replace any multidose containers in the patient's drawer or medication supply system.

Proper storage safeguards medications.

14. **Log out of and/or lock the medication supply system before leaving it.**

Locking the medication supply system or drawer safeguards the patient's medication supply. Facility accrediting organizations require medication supply systems to be locked when not in use.

15. Transport medications to the patient's bedside carefully and keep the medications in sight at all times.

Careful handling and close observation prevent accidental or deliberate disarrangement of medications.

16. **Ensure that the patient receives the medications at the correct time.**

Check facility policy, which may allow for administration within a period of 30 minutes before or 30 minutes after the designated time.

 17. Perform hand hygiene and put on PPE, if indicated.

Hand hygiene and PPE prevent the spread of microorganisms. PPE is required based on transmission precautions.

18. **Identify the patient. Compare the information with the eMAR/MAR. The patient should be identified using at least two of the following methods** (The Joint Commission, 2021):

Identifying the patient ensures the right patient receives the medications and helps prevent errors. The patient's room number or physical location is not used as an identifier (The Joint Commission, 2021). Replace the identification band if it is missing or inaccurate in any way.

a. Check the name on the patient's identification band.

This requires a response from the patient, but illness and strange surroundings often cause patients to be confused.

b. Check the identification number on the patient's identification band.

c. Check the birth date on the patient's identification band.

d. Ask the patient to state their name and birth date, based on facility policy.

19. **Complete necessary assessments before administering medications. Check the patient's allergy bracelet, if present, or ask the patient about allergies. Explain what you are going to do, and the reason for doing it, to the patient.**

Assessment is a prerequisite to administration of medications. Explanation relieves anxiety and facilitates patient engagement.

20. Scan the patient's bar code on the identification band, if required (Figure 2) (The Joint Commission, 2021).

This provides an additional check to ensure that the medication is given to the right patient.

ACTION

21. **Based on facility policy, the third check of the label may occur at this point. If so, read the label and recheck the labels with the eMAR/MAR before administering the medications to the patient.**

22. Assist the patient to the high-Fowler's position, unless contraindicated.

23. Put on gloves.

24. If patient is receiving continuous tube feedings, pause the tube-feeding pump (Figure 3).

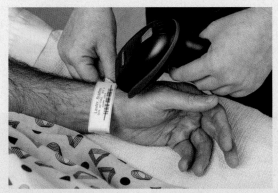

FIGURE 2. Scanning bar code on the patient's identification bracelet. (*Source:* Used with permission from Shutterstock. *Photo by B. Proud.*)

25. Pour the water into the irrigation container. Measure 30 mL of water. Apply clamp on feeding tube, if present. Alternatively, pinch gastric tube below port with fingers, or position stopcock to correct direction. Open ENFit® connector (Boullata et al., 2017) or medication port on gastric tube delegated to medication administration (Figure 4) or disconnect tubing for feeding from gastric tube and place cap on end of feeding tubing.

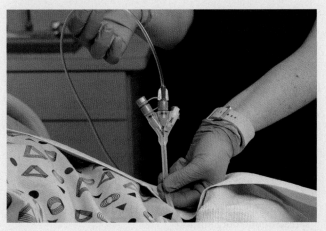

RATIONALE

Many facilities require the *third* check to occur at the bedside, after identifying the patient and before administration. If facility policy directs the *third* check at this time, this *third* check ensures accuracy and helps to prevent errors.

This reduces the risk of aspiration.

Gloves prevent contact with mucous membranes and body fluids.

If the pump is not stopped, tube feeding will flow out of the tube and onto the patient.

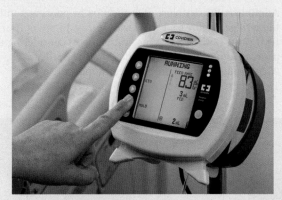

FIGURE 3. Pausing feeding pump.

Fluid is ready for flushing of the tube. Applying clamp, folding the tube over, and clamping, or the correct positioning of the stopcock prevents any backflow of gastric drainage. Covering end of feeding tubing prevents contamination. Use of ENFit® connectors decreases the risk of inadvertent connection between an enteral feeding system and a nonenteral system (Boullata et al., 2017).

FIGURE 4. Pinching (or clamping) gastric tubing to prevent backflow of gastric drainage and opening medication administration port.

(continued on page 214)

Skill 5-2 ▶ Administering Medications via a Gastric Tube *(continued)*

ACTION	RATIONALE
26. **Check tube placement, depending on type of tube and facility policy.** Refer to Skill 11-2, Chapter 11.	Tube placement must be confirmed before administering anything through the tube to avoid inadvertent instillation in the respiratory tract.
27. Apply clamp on feeding tube, if present. Alternatively, pinch the gastric tube below port with fingers, or position stop-cock to correct direction. Remove irrigation syringe from the gastric tube. Remove the plunger of the syringe. Reinsert the syringe in the gastric tube without the plunger. Pour at least 15 mL of purified water into the syringe (Figure 5). **Unclamp the tube and allow the water to enter the stomach via gravity infusion.**	Clamping prevents backflow of gastric drainage. Flushing the tube ensures that all the residual is cleared from the tube.
28. Administer the first dose of medication by pouring it into the syringe (Figure 6). Follow with at least 15 mL of (purified) water flush between medication doses considering the patient's intake restrictions or fluid status (Zoeller et al., 2020). Follow the last dose of medication with at least 15 mL of (purified) water flush (Boullata et al., 2017; Zoeller et al., 2020).	Flushing between medications prevents any possible interactions between the medications. Flushing at the end maintains tube patency, prevents blockage by medication particles, and ensures all doses enter the stomach (Boullata, 2021).

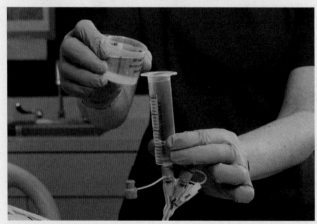

FIGURE 5. Pouring water into syringe inserted in gastric tube.

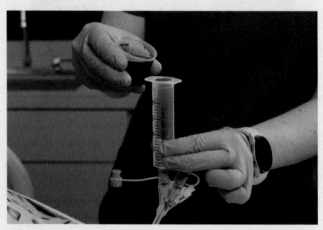

FIGURE 6. Pouring medication into syringe inserted in gastric tube.

ACTION	RATIONALE
29. Clamp the tube, remove the syringe, and replace the feeding tubing. If a stopcock is used, position it to correct direction. If a ENFit® connector or tube medication port was used, cap the port. Unclamp the gastric tube and restart tube feeding, if appropriate for medications administered.	Some medications require the holding of the tube feeding for a certain period of time after administration. Consult a drug reference or a pharmacist.
30. Remove gloves. Perform hand hygiene. Assist the patient to a comfortable position. If receiving a tube feeding, position the patient as upright as possible with the head of the bed elevated at least 30 to 45 degrees or as near normal position for eating as possible (Boullata et al., 2017; Roveron et al., 2018).	Removing gloves and performing hand hygiene reduces the risk of the spread of microorganisms and contamination of other items. Assisting the patient to a comfortable position ensures patient comfort. Keeping the head of the bed elevated helps prevent aspiration.
31. Remove additional PPE, if used. Perform hand hygiene.	Proper removal of PPE reduces the risk of infection transmission and contamination of other items. Hand hygiene prevents the spread of microorganisms.

ACTION

32. Document the administration of the medication immediately after administration. See Documentation section below.

33. Evaluate the patient's response to the medication within the appropriate time frame.

RATIONALE

Timely documentation helps to ensure patient safety.

The patient needs to be evaluated for therapeutic and adverse effects from the medication.

EVALUATION

The expected outcomes have been met when the patient has received the prescribed medications and experienced the intended effects of the medications administered. In addition, the patient has demonstrated a patent and functioning gastric tube, verbalized knowledge of the medications given, and remained free from adverse effects and injury.

DOCUMENTATION
Guidelines

Document the administration of the medication immediately after administration, including date, time, dose, and route of administration on the eMAR/MAR or record using the required format. If using a bar-code system, medication administration is automatically recorded when the bar code is scanned. PRN medications require documentation of the reason for administration. Prompt recording avoids the possibility of accidentally repeating the administration of the drug. Record the amount of gastric residual, if appropriate. Record the amount of liquid given on the intake and output record. If the drug was refused or omitted, record this in the appropriate area on the medication record and notify the health care team as appropriate. This verifies the reason medication was omitted and ensures that health care personnel providing care for the patient are aware of the occurrence.

DEVELOPING CLINICAL REASONING AND CLINICAL JUDGMENT

UNEXPECTED SITUATIONS AND ASSOCIATED INTERVENTIONS

- *Medication enters tube and then tube becomes clogged:* Attach a 60-mL syringe onto the end of the tube. Pull back and then lightly apply pressure to the plunger in a repetitive motion. This may dislodge the medication. Try using warm water and gentle pressure to remove the clog. Carbonated sodas, such as colas, and meat tenderizers have not been shown effective in removing clogs in feeding tubes. Zoeller et al. (2020) suggest a pancreatic enzyme solution of uncoated pancreatic enzyme and sodium bicarbonate in 5 mL of purified water to unclog enteral tubes. Never use a stylet to unclog tubes. If the medication does not move through the tube, notify the health care team. The tube may have to be replaced.

SPECIAL CONSIDERATIONS
General Considerations

- If medications are being administered via a nasogastric tube that is attached to suction, the tube should remain clamped, off suction, for a period of time after medication administration. This allows for medication absorption before returning to suction. Check facility policy and drug reference for specific drug requirements.
- If the patient is receiving a tube feeding after medication administration, once the appropriate amount of time has lapsed after administration of the medication, position the patient as upright as possible with the head of the bed elevated at least 30 to 45 degrees or as near normal position for eating as possible (Boullata et al., 2017; Roveron et al., 2018). Refer to Skill 11-3 in Chapter 11 for additional details related to administration of enteral tube feedings.
- Document the water intake and liquid medication by tube on the intake and output record. Adjust the amount of water used if the patient's fluid intake is restricted (Taylor et al., 2023; Zoeller et al., 2020).
- If necessary to use a plunger in the irrigation syringe to administer medications, instill gently and slowly. Gravity administration is considered best to avoid excess pressure.

(continued on page 216)

Skill 5-2 ▶ Administering Medications via a Gastric Tube *(continued)*

- If the patient is receiving tube feedings, review information about the drugs to be administered. Discontinue a continuous tube feeding and leave the tube clamped for the required period of time before and after the medication has been given, according to the reference and facility protocol.
- Ongoing assessment is an important part of nursing care for both evaluation of patient response to administered medications and early detection of adverse drug reactions. If an adverse effect is suspected, withhold further medication doses and notify the health care team. Additional intervention is based on type of reaction and patient assessment.

Infant and Child Considerations

- Pediatric patients require less volume; flush the tube with at least 5 mL of (purified) water for children before and immediately after giving each medication (Boullata et al., 2017; Zoeller et al., 2020). The last dose of medication should be followed by 15 mL of (purified) water (Zoeller et al., 2020).

EVIDENCE FOR PRACTICE ▶

ASPEN SAFE PRACTICES FOR ENTERAL NUTRITION THERAPY
Boullata, J. I., Carrera, A. L., Harvey, L., Escuro, A. A., Hudson, L., Mays, A., Wessel, J. J., Bajpai, S., Beebe, M. L., Kinn, T. J., Klang, M. G., Lord, L., Martin, K., Pompeii-Wolfe, C., Sullivan, J., Wood, A., Malone, A., & Guenter, P., & ASPEN Safe Practices for Enteral Nutrition Therapy, American Society for Parenteral and Enteral Nutrition. (2017). ASPEN safe practices for enteral nutrition therapy. *Journal of Parenteral and Enteral Nutrition, 41*(1), 15–103. https://doi.org/10.1177/0148607116673053

The American Society for Parenteral and Enteral Nutrition (ASPEN) *Safe Practices for Enteral Nutrition Therapy* guideline provides recommendations based on the available evidence and expert consensus for safe practices for patients receiving enteral nutrition, including medication administration and enteral access devices.

Skill 5-3 ▶ Removing Medication From an Ampule

An **ampule** is a glass flask that contains a single dose of medication for parenteral administration. Because there is no way to prevent contamination of any unused portion of medication after the ampule is opened, discard any remaining medication if not all the medication is used for the prescribed dose. You must break the thin neck of the ampule to remove the medication.

DELEGATION CONSIDERATIONS

The preparation of medication from an ampule is not delegated to assistive personnel (AP). Depending on the state's nurse practice act and the organization's policies and procedures, the preparation of medication from an ampule may be delegated to a licensed practical/vocational nurse (LPN/LVN). The decision to delegate must be based on careful analysis of the patient's needs and circumstances as well as the qualifications of the person to whom the task is being delegated. Refer to the Delegation Guidelines in Appendix A.

EQUIPMENT

- Sterile syringe and filter needle
- New needle for replacing filter needle, if indicated
- Ampule of medication
- Antimicrobial swab
- Small, sterile gauze pad
- Gloves
- Electronic Medication Administration Record (eMAR) or Medication Administration Record (MAR)

ASSESSMENT

Assess the appropriateness of the drug for the patient. Review the medical history and allergy, assessment, and laboratory data that may influence drug administration. Assess the medication in the ampule for any particles or discoloration. Assess the ampule for any cracks or chips. Check the expiration date before administering the medication. Assess the patient's knowledge of the medication. If the patient has a knowledge deficit about the medication, this may be the appropriate time to begin education about the medication. If the medication may affect the patient's vital signs, assess them before administration. If the medication is for pain relief, assess the patient's pain level before and after administration. Verify patient name, dose, route, and time of administration.

ACTUAL OR POTENTIAL HEALTH PROBLEMS AND NEEDS	Many actual or potential health problems or issues may require the use of this skill as part of related interventions. An appropriate health problem or issue may include: • Infection risk • Knowledge deficiency • Injury risk
OUTCOME IDENTIFICATION AND PLANNING	The expected outcomes to achieve when removing medication from an ampule are that the medication is removed in a sterile manner, the medication is free from glass shards and contamination, and the proper dose is prepared.

IMPLEMENTATION

ACTION

1. Gather equipment. Check each medication prescribed against the original in the health record, depending on facility policy and the medication order system in place. Clarify any inconsistencies. Check the patient's health record for allergies.

2. Know the actions, special nursing considerations, safe dose ranges, purpose of administration, and adverse effects of the medications to be administered. Consider the appropriateness of the medication for this patient.

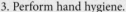
3. Perform hand hygiene.

4. Move the medication supply system to the outside of the patient's room or prepare for administration at the medication supply system in the medication area. Alternatively, access the medication administration supply system at or inside the patient's room.

5. Unlock the medication supply system or drawer. Enter the passcode and scan employee identification, if required.

6. **Prepare medications for one patient at a time.**

7. Read the eMAR/MAR and read the label when selecting the proper medication from the medication supply system or the patient's medication drawer.

8. Read the label and compare the label with the eMAR/MAR. Check expiration dates and perform calculations, if necessary. Scan the bar code on the package, if required.

RATIONALE

The prescription is the legal record of prescribed medication interventions. This comparison helps to identify errors that may have occurred when orders were transcribed. Computer provider order-entry (CPOE) systems allow prescribers to send electronic medication prescriptions directly to the pharmacy located in a health care facility and to outpatient pharmacies.

This knowledge aids the nurse in evaluating the therapeutic effect of the medication in relation to the patient's health status and can also be used to educate the patient about the medication.

Hand hygiene prevents the spread of microorganisms.

Organization facilitates error-free administration and saves time.

Locking the medication supply system or drawer safeguards each patient's medication supply. Facility accrediting organizations require medication supply systems to be locked when not in use. Entering the passcode and scanning ID allows only authorized users into the computer system and identifies the user for documentation by the computer.

This prevents errors in medication administration.

This is the *first* check of the label.

This is the *second* check of the label. Verify calculations with another nurse to ensure safety, if necessary.

(*continued on page 218*)

Skill 5-3 ▶ Removing Medication From an Ampule *(continued)*

ACTION	**RATIONALE**
9. Tap the stem of the ampule (Figure 1) or twist your wrist quickly (Figure 2) while holding the ampule vertically.	This facilitates movement of medication in the stem to the body of the ampule.

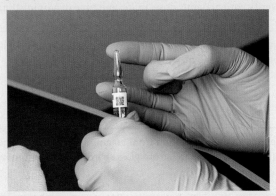

FIGURE 1. Tapping stem of the ampule.

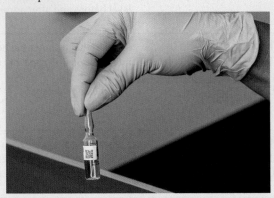

FIGURE 2. Twisting wrist quickly while holding ampule vertically.

10. Put on gloves. Using the antimicrobial swab, scrub the neck of the ampule. Wrap a small sterile gauze pad around the neck of the ampule.

Gloves reduce risk of injury to hands from glass (Innovation Compounding, 2020). Scrubbing the neck is necessary to reduce the risk of contamination (Dolan et al., 2016; Innovation Compounding, 2020). Wrapping the neck of the ampule with gauze protects your fingers from the glass as the ampule is broken.

11. Breaking away from your body, use a snapping motion to break off the top of the ampule along the scored line at its neck (Figure 3). **Always break away from your body.**

This protects your face and fingers from any shattered glass fragments.

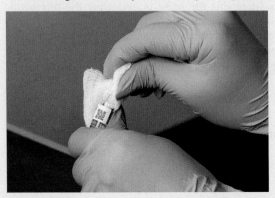

FIGURE 3. Using a snapping motion to break top of ampule.

12. Attach the filter needle to the syringe. Remove the cap from the filter needle by pulling it straight off.

Use of a filter needle prevents the accidental withdrawing of small glass particles with the medication (Innovation Compounding, 2020). Pulling the cap off in a straight manner prevents accidental needlestick.

13. Withdraw the medication in the amount ordered plus a small amount more (approximately 30% more). **Do not inject air into the solution. While inserting the filter needle into the ampule, be careful not to touch the rim.** Use either of the following methods to withdraw the medication:

a. Insert the tip of the needle into the ampule, which is upright on a flat surface, and withdraw fluid into the syringe (Figure 4). **Touch the plunger only at the knob.**

b. Insert the tip of the needle into the ampule and invert the ampule. Keep the needle centered and not touching the sides of the ampule. Withdraw fluid into the syringe (Figure 5). **Touch the plunger only at the knob.**

By withdrawing an additional small amount of medication, any air bubbles in the syringe can be displaced once the syringe is removed while allowing ample medication to remain in the syringe. The contents of the ampule are not under pressure; therefore, air is unnecessary and will cause the contents to overflow. The rim of the ampule is considered contaminated.

Handling the plunger only at the knob will keep the shaft of the plunger sterile.

Surface tension holds the fluids in the ampule when inverted. If the needle touches the sides or is removed and then reinserted into the ampule, surface tension is broken, and fluid runs out. Handling the plunger only at the knob will keep the shaft of the plunger sterile.

ACTION

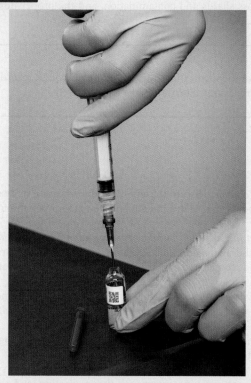

FIGURE 4. Withdrawing medication from upright ampule.

RATIONALE

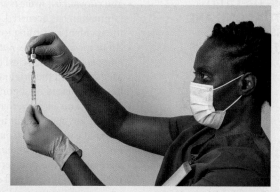

FIGURE 5. Withdrawing medication from inverted ampule.

14. Wait until the needle has been withdrawn to tap the syringe and expel the air carefully by pushing on the plunger. **Check the amount of medication in the syringe with the medication dose and discard any surplus, according to facility policy.**

15. **Depending on facility policy, the third check of the label may occur at this point. If so, when all medications for one patient have been prepared, read the label and recheck the labels with the eMAR/MAR before taking the medications to the patient. However, many facilities require the third check to occur at the bedside, after identifying the patient.**

16. Label the syringe with the medication name, dose, and amount (The Joint Commission, 2021).

17. **Engage the safety guard on the filter needle and remove the needle. Discard the filter needle in a suitable container. Attach the appropriate administration device to the syringe.**

18. Discard the ampule in a suitable container. Remove gloves and perform hand hygiene.

19. **Log out of and/or lock the medication supply system before leaving it.**

20. Perform hand hygiene.

21. Proceed with administration, based on prescribed route.

Ejecting air into the solution increases pressure in the ampule and can force the medication to spill out over the ampule. Ampules may have overfill. Careful measurement ensures that the correct dose is withdrawn.

This *third* check ensures accuracy and helps to prevent errors. *Note:* Many facilities require the *third* check to occur at the bedside, after identifying the patient and before administration.

Unlabeled syringes are unidentifiable and may lead to a medication administration error (The Joint Commission, 2021).

The filter needle used to draw up medication should not be used to administer the medication. This will prevent any glass shards from entering the patient during administration.

Any medication that has not been removed from the ampule must be discarded because sterility of contents cannot be maintained in an opened ampule. Removing gloves and performing hand hygiene deters the spread of microorganisms

Locking the medication supply system safeguards the patient's medication supply. Facility accrediting organizations require medication supply systems to be locked when not in use.

Hand hygiene deters the spread of microorganisms.

See appropriate skill for prescribed route.

(continued on page 220)

Skill 5-3 ▶ Removing Medication From an Ampule   *(continued)*

EVALUATION

The expected outcomes have been met when the medication was removed from the ampule in a sterile manner, it remained free from glass shards and contamination, and the proper dose was prepared.

DOCUMENTATION

Guidelines

It is not necessary to record the removal of the medication from the ampule. Prompt recording of administration of the medication is required immediately after it is administered.

DEVELOPING CLINICAL REASONING AND CLINICAL JUDGMENT

UNEXPECTED SITUATIONS AND ASSOCIATED INTERVENTIONS

- *You cut yourself while trying to open the ampule:* Discard the ampule and medication in case contamination has occurred. Clean and bandage the wound and obtain a new ampule. Communicate the incident according to facility policy.
- *All of medication was not removed from the stem and insufficient medication remains in body of ampule:* Discard the ampule and drawn medication. Obtain a new ampule and start over. Medication in the original ampule stem is considered contaminated once the neck of the ampule has been placed on a nonsterile surface.
- *You inject air into inverted ampule, spraying medication:* Wash your hands to remove any medication. If any medication has gotten into your eyes, perform eye irrigation. Obtain a new ampule for medication dose. Communicate the incident according to facility policy.
- *Plunger becomes contaminated before inserted into ampule:* Discard the needle and syringe and start over. If the plunger is contaminated after medication is drawn into the syringe, it is not necessary to discard and start over. The contaminated plunger will enter the barrel of the syringe when pushing the medication out, will not come in contact with the medication, and will not contaminate the medication.

SPECIAL CONSIDERATIONS

- When mixing medications in one syringe, preparation of medications in one syringe depends on how the medication is supplied. When preparing medications from an ampule and a vial, prepare the medication in the vial first. Draw up the medication in the ampule *after* the medication in the vial (see Skill 5-4).

Skill 5-4 ▶ Removing Medication From a Vial

Skill Variation: *Reconstituting Powdered Medication in a Vial*

A **vial** is a glass bottle with a self-sealing stopper through which medication is removed. For safety in transporting and storing, the vial top is usually covered with a metal or plastic cap that can be removed easily. The self-sealing stopper that is then exposed is the means of entrance into the vial. Single-dose vials are used once, and then discarded, regardless of the amount of the drug that is used from the vial. Multidose vials contain several doses of medication and can be used multiple times. The Centers for Disease Control and Prevention (CDC) recommends that medications packaged as multiuse vials be assigned to a single patient whenever possible (CDC, 2019). If the medication enters the patient treatment area, the vial should be designated as a single patient use vial (CDC, 2019). In addition, it is recommended that the top of the vial be cleaned before each entry, and that a new sterile needle and syringe are used for each entry (CDC, 2019).

The medication contained in a vial can be in liquid or powder form. Powdered forms must be dissolved in an appropriate diluent before administration. The following skill reviews removing liquid medication from a vial. Refer to the accompanying Skill Variation for steps to reconstitute powdered medication.

DELEGATION CONSIDERATIONS	The preparation of medication from a vial is not delegated to assistive personnel (AP). Depending on the state's nurse practice act and the organization's policies and procedures, the preparation of medication from a vial may be delegated to licensed practical/vocational nurses (LPN/LVNs). The decision to delegate must be based on careful analysis of the patient's needs and circumstances as well as the qualifications of the person to whom the task is being delegated. Refer to the Delegation Guidelines in Appendix A.
EQUIPMENT	• Sterile syringe and needle or blunt cannula (size depends on medication being administered) • Needleless access device (if available) • Vial of medication • Antimicrobial swab • Second needle (optional) • Filter needle (optional) • Electronic Medication Administration Record (eMAR) or Medication Administration Record (MAR)
ASSESSMENT	Assess the appropriateness of the drug for the patient. Review the medical history and allergy, assessment, and laboratory data that may influence drug administration. Assess the medication in the vial for any discoloration or particles. Check the expiration date before administering medication. Assess the patient's knowledge of the medication. If the patient has a knowledge deficit about the medication, this may be the appropriate time to begin education about the medication. If the medication may affect the patient's vital signs, assess them before administration. If the medication is for pain relief, assess the patient's pain level before and after administration. Verify patient name, dose, route, and time of administration.
ACTUAL OR POTENTIAL HEALTH PROBLEMS AND NEEDS	Many actual or potential health problems or issues may require the use of this skill as part of related interventions. An appropriate health problem or issue may include: • Infection risk • Knowledge deficiency • Injury risk
OUTCOME IDENTIFICATION AND PLANNING	The expected outcomes to achieve when removing medication from a vial are withdrawal of the medication into a syringe in a sterile manner, the medication is free from contamination, and the proper dose is prepared.

IMPLEMENTATION

ACTION	**RATIONALE**
1. Gather equipment. Check each medication prescribed against the original in the health record, depending on facility policy and the medication order system in place. Clarify any inconsistencies. Check the patient's health record for allergies.	The prescription is the legal record of prescribed medication interventions. This comparison helps to identify errors that may have occurred when orders were transcribed. Computer provider order-entry (CPOE) systems allow prescribers to send electronic medication prescriptions directly to the pharmacy located in a health care facility and to outpatient pharmacies.
2. Know the actions, special nursing considerations, safe dose ranges, purpose of administration, and adverse effects of the medications to be administered. Consider the appropriateness of the medication for this patient.	This knowledge aids the nurse in evaluating the therapeutic effect of the medication in relation to the patient's health status and can also be used to educate the patient about the medication.
3. Perform hand hygiene.	Hand hygiene deters the spread of microorganisms.
4. Move the medication supply system to the outside of the patient's room or prepare for administration at the medication supply system in the medication area. Alternatively, access the medication administration supply system at or inside the patient's room.	Organization facilitates error-free administration and saves time.

(continued on page 222)

Skill 5-4 ▶ Removing Medication From a Vial *(continued)*

ACTION	RATIONALE
5. Unlock the medication supply system or drawer. Enter the passcode and scan employee identification, if required.	Locking the medication supply system or drawer safeguards each patient's medication supply. Facility accrediting organizations require medication supply systems to be locked when not in use. Entering the passcode and scanning ID allows only authorized users into the system and identifies the user for documentation by the computer.
6. **Prepare medications for one patient at a time.**	This prevents errors in medication administration.
7. Read the eMAR/MAR and read the label when selecting the proper medication from the medication supply system or the patient's medication drawer.	This is the *first* check of the label.
8. Read the label and compare the label with the eMAR/MAR. Check expiration dates and perform calculations, if necessary. Scan the bar code on the package, if required.	This is the *second* check of the label. Verify calculations with another nurse to ensure safety, if necessary.
9. Remove the metal or plastic cap on the vial that protects the self-sealing stopper.	The cap needs to be removed to access the medication in the vial.
10. **Scrub the self-sealing stopper top with the antimicrobial swab and allow to dry.**	The antimicrobial swab removes surface microbial contamination. Allowing the antimicrobial solution to dry completely (5 to 20 seconds) ensures complete antimicrobial effectiveness (Gorski et al., 2021; Slater et al., 2018). Drying also prevents antimicrobial solution from entering the vial on the needle.
11. Remove the cap from the needle or blunt cannula by pulling it straight off. **If the vial in use is a multidose vial**, touch the plunger only at the knob and draw back an amount of air into the syringe that is equal to the specific dose of medication to be withdrawn. If the vial in use is a single-use vial, there is no need to draw air into the syringe.	Pulling the cap off in a straight manner prevents accidental needlestick injury. Handling the plunger only at the knob will keep the shaft of the plunger sterile. Because a vial is a sealed container, injection of an equal amount of air (before fluid is removed) is required to prevent the formation of a partial vacuum. If not enough air is injected, the negative pressure makes it difficult to withdraw the medication after repeated use.
12. Hold the vial on a flat surface. Pierce the self-sealing stopper in the center with the needle tip (Figure 1) or blunt cannula; alternatively, insert a needleless access device (Figure 2) into the stopper on the vial and connect the syringe. Inject the measured air into the space above the solution **Do not inject air into the solution.** If the vial in use is a single-use vial, there is no need to inject air into the vial.	Air bubbled through the solution could result in withdrawal of an inaccurate amount of medication. Needleless access devices may be used to prevent needlestick injuries based on facility policy (Frandsen & Pennington, 2021).

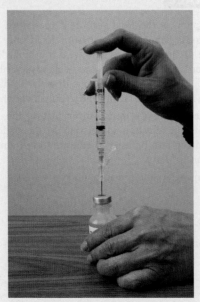

FIGURE 1. Injecting air with vial upright.

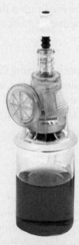

FIGURE 2. Example of a needleless system to access a medication vial.

ACTION

13. Invert the vial. **Keep the tip of the needle or blunt cannula below the fluid level if in use (Figure 3).**

14. Hold the vial in one hand and use the other to withdraw the medication. **Touch the plunger only at the knob. Draw up the prescribed amount of medication while holding the syringe vertically and at eye level (Figure 4).**

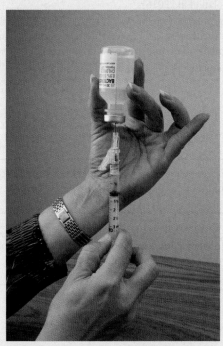

FIGURE 3. Positioning needle tip in solution.

15. If any air bubbles accumulate in the syringe, tap the barrel of the syringe sharply and move the needle past the fluid into the air space to re-inject the air bubble into the vial. Return the needle tip to the solution and continue withdrawal of the medication.

16. After the correct dose is withdrawn, remove the needle or needleless access device from the vial; carefully replace the sterile cap over the needle if used. Alternatively, carefully attach a needle or syringe cap. Some facilities require changing the needle, if one was used to withdraw the medication, before administering the medication.

17. **Check the amount of medication in the syringe with the medication dose and discard any surplus.**

18. **Depending on facility policy, the third check of the label may occur at this point. If so, when all medications for one patient have been prepared, read the label and recheck the labels with the eMAR/MAR before taking the medications to the patient. However, many facilities require the third check to occur at the bedside, after identifying the patient.**

19. **Label the syringe with the medication's name, dose, and amount (The Joint Commission, 2021).**

RATIONALE

This prevents air from being aspirated into the syringe.

Handling the plunger only at the knob will keep the shaft of the plunger sterile. Holding the syringe at eye level facilitates accurate reading, and the vertical position makes removal of air bubbles from the syringe easy.

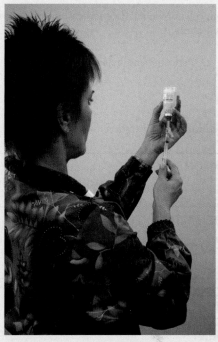

FIGURE 4. Withdrawing medication at eye level.

Removal of air bubbles is necessary to ensure an accurate dose of medication.

Capping prevents contamination and protects against accidental needlesticks. A one-handed recap method may be used as long as care is taken not to contaminate the needle during the process. Changing the needle may be necessary because passing the needle through the stopper on the vial may dull the needle. In addition, it ensures the tip of the needle is free from medication residue, significantly reducing pain intensity associated with the injection (Ağaç & Günes, 2010).

Careful measurement ensures that the correct dose is withdrawn.

This *third* check ensures accuracy and helps to prevent errors. *Note:* Many facilities require the *third* check to occur at the bedside, after identifying the patient and before administration.

Unlabeled syringes are unidentifiable and may lead to a medication administration error (The Joint Commission, 2021).

(continued on page 224)

Skill 5-4 ▶ Removing Medication From a Vial *(continued)*

ACTION	**RATIONALE**
20. If a multidose vial is being used, label the vial with the date and time opened and the beyond-use date (see Special Considerations), and store the vial containing the remaining medication according to facility policy. Limit the use of multiple-dose vials and dedicate them to a single patient whenever possible (CDC, 2019).	Because the vial is sealed, the medication inside remains sterile and can be used for future injections. Labeling the opened vials with a date, time, and beyond-use date limits its use after a specific time period. Limiting use of multiple-dose vials and dedicating their use to a single patient when possible limits risk of contamination and transfer of microorganisms (CDC, 2019; Dolan et al., 2016).
21. Log out of and/or lock the medication supply system before leaving it.	Locking the medication supply system or drawer safeguards the patient's medication supply. Facility accrediting organizations require medication supply systems to be locked when not in use.
22. Perform hand hygiene.	Hand hygiene deters the spread of microorganisms.
23. Proceed with administration, based on prescribed route.	See appropriate skill for prescribed route.

EVALUATION

The expected outcomes have been met when the medication was withdrawn into the syringe in a sterile manner, it remained free from contamination, and the proper dose was prepared.

DOCUMENTATION

Guidelines

It is not necessary to record the removal of the medication from a vial. Prompt recording of administration of the medication is required immediately after it is administered.

DEVELOPING CLINICAL REASONING AND CLINICAL JUDGMENT

UNEXPECTED SITUATIONS AND ASSOCIATED INTERVENTIONS

- *A piece of self-sealing stopper is noticed floating in the medication in the syringe:* Discard the syringe, needle, and vial. Obtain a new vial, syringe, and needle and prepare the dose as ordered.
- *As the needle attached to the syringe filled with air is inserted into vial, the plunger is immediately pulled down:* If possible to withdraw medication, continue steps as explained above. If such a vacuum has formed that this is impossible, remove the syringe and inject more air into the vial.
- *Plunger is contaminated before injecting air into vial:* Discard the needle and syringe and start over.
- *Plunger is contaminated after medication is drawn into syringe:* It is not necessary to discard the needle and syringe and start over. The contaminated plunger will enter the barrel of the syringe when pushing the medication out, will not come in contact with the medication, and will not contaminate the medication.

SPECIAL CONSIDERATIONS

- When mixing medications in one syringe, preparation of medications in one syringe depends on how the medication is supplied. When using a single-dose vial and a multidose vial, inject air into the multidose vial and draw the medication from the multidose vial into the syringe first. This prevents the contents of the multidose vial from being contaminated with the medication in the single-dose vial. The steps to follow when preparing medications from two multidose vials in one syringe are outlined in Skill 5-5.
- Vials used to draw two or more medications into a single syringe must be discarded after use (Dolan et al., 2016).
- Do not administer medication from a single-dose vial to multiple patients (CDC, 2019).
- Limit the use of multiple-dose vials and dedicate them to a single patient whenever possible (CDC, 2019).
- Multiple-dose vials must be labeled with a beyond-use date when first opened, as indicated by facility policy (CDC, 2019).

Skill Variation ▶ Reconstituting Powdered Medication in a Vial

Drugs that are unstable in liquid form are often provided in a dry powder form. The powder must be mixed with the correct amount of appropriate solution (diluent) to prepare the medication for administration (*reconstitution*). Verify the correct amount and correct solution type for the specific medication prescribed. This information is found on the vial label, package insert, in a drug reference, an on-line pharmacy source, medication database, or from the pharmacist. To reconstitute powdered medication:

1. Gather equipment. Check each medication prescribed against the original in the health record, depending on facility policy and the medication order system in place. Clarify any inconsistencies. Check the patient's health record for allergies.
2. Know the actions, special nursing considerations, safe dose ranges, purpose of administration, and adverse effects of the medications to be administered. Consider the appropriateness of the medication for this patient.

3. Perform hand hygiene.

4. Move the medication supply system to the outside of the patient's room or prepare for administration at the medication supply system in the medication area. Alternatively, access the medication administration supply system at or inside the patient's room.
5. Unlock the medication supply system or drawer. Enter the passcode and scan employee identification, if required.
6. **Prepare medications for one patient at a time.**
7. Read the eMAR/MAR and read the label when selecting the proper medication and diluent from medication supply system or from the patient's medication drawer. This is the *first* check of the medication label.
8. Read the label and compare the labels with the eMAR/MAR. This is the *second* check of the medication label. Check expiration dates and perform calculations, check medication calculation with another nurse. Scan the bar code on the package, if required.
9. Remove the metal or plastic cap on the medication vial and diluent vial that protects the self-sealing stoppers.
10. Scrub the self-sealing tops on both the diluent and powdered medication vials with the antimicrobial swab and allow to dry.
11. **Draw up the appropriate amount of diluent into the syringe.**
12. Insert the needle, needleless access device or blunt cannula through the center of the self-sealing stopper on the powdered medication vial.
13. Inject the diluent into the powdered medication vial.
14. Remove the needle, needleless access device or blunt cannula from the vial and replace sterile cap.

15. Gently agitate the vial to mix the powdered medication and the diluent completely. Do not shake the vial.
16. Draw up the prescribed amount of medication, as described in Steps 10–15 in Skill 5-4, while holding the syringe vertically and at eye level.
17. After the correct dose is withdrawn, remove the needle or needleless access device from the vial; carefully replace the sterile cap over the needle if used. Alternatively, carefully attach a needle or syringe cap. Some facilities require changing the needle, if one was used to withdraw the medication, before administering the medication.
18. **Check the amount of medication in the syringe with the medication dose and discard any surplus.**
19. **Depending on facility policy, the *third* check of the label may occur at this point. If so, read the label and recheck the labels with the eMAR/MAR before taking the medications to the patient. However, many facilities require the third check to occur at the bedside, after identifying the patient.**
20. Label the syringe with the medication's name, dose, and amount (The Joint Commission, 2021).
21. **Log out of and/or lock the medication supply system before leaving it.**

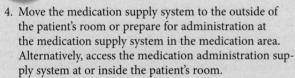

22. Perform hand hygiene.

23. Proceed with administration, based on prescribed route.

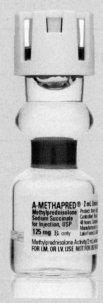

FIGURE A. Example of a specially designed vial that has the diluent and powder separated by a rubber stopper within the vial.

Note: Powdered medications may be supplied in specially designed vials that have the diluent and powder in the same vial, separated by a rubber stopper within the vial (Figure A). When the nurse is ready to administer the medication, the rubber stopper is deployed, and the vial is agitated gently to mix the diluent and powder.

Skill 5-5 ▶ Mixing Medications From Two Vials in One Syringe

Preparation of two medications in one syringe depends on how the medication is supplied. When using two multidose vials, air is injected into both vials before withdrawing the first medication, to prevent the accidental injection of medication into the second vial. When using a single-dose vial and a multidose vial, air is injected into the multidose vial and the medication in the multidose vial is drawn into the syringe first. This prevents the contents of the multidose vial from being contaminated with the medication in the single-dose vial. The CDC recommends that medications packaged as multiuse vials be assigned to a single patient whenever possible (CDC, 2019). In addition, it is recommended that the top of the vial be cleaned before each entry, and that a new sterile needle and syringe are used before each entry (CDC, 2019).

When considering mixing two medications in one syringe, you must ensure that the two drugs are compatible. Be aware of drug incompatibilities when preparing medications in one syringe. Certain medications are incompatible with other drugs in the same syringe. Other drugs have limited compatibility and should be administered within 15 minutes of preparation. Mixing more than two drugs in one syringe is not recommended (Taylor et al., 2023). If it must be done, contact the pharmacist to determine the compatibility of the three drugs, as well as the compatibility of their pH values and the preservatives that may be present in each drug. A drug-compatibility table should be available to nurses who are preparing medications.

Insulin, with many types available for use, is an example of a medication that may be combined together in one syringe for injection. Insulins vary in their onset and duration of action and are classified as rapid acting, short acting, intermediate acting, and long acting (Frandsen & Pennington, 2021). Before administering any insulin, be aware of the onset time, peak, and duration of effects, and ensure that proper food is available. Be aware that some insulins, such as glargine and detemir, cannot be mixed with other insulins. Refer to a drug reference for a listing of the different types of insulin and action specific to each type.

Insulin is used as the sample medication in the steps outlined below for mixing two medications in one syringe. Insulin is typically available in multidose vials, and dosages are calculated in units. The scale commonly used is U100, which is based on 100 units of insulin contained in 1 mL of solution. An insulin syringe is also calibrated in units. Insulin is also available in injection pens, which eliminate the need to prepare two medications in one syringe. Insulin injection pens are prefilled devices that combine the insulin container and syringe. Patients attach a needle for each administration, dial a dose of insulin, and depress a plunger to administer the dose. Use of an insulin injection pen is outlined in the Skill Variation in Skill 5-7 on page 244.

DELEGATION CONSIDERATIONS	The preparation of medication from two vials is not delegated to assistive personnel (AP). Depending on the state's nurse practice act and the organization's policies and procedures, the preparation of medication from two vials may be delegated to licensed practical/vocational nurses (LPN/LVNs). The decision to delegate must be based on careful analysis of the patient's needs and circumstances as well as the qualifications of the person to whom the task is being delegated. Refer to the Delegation Guidelines in Appendix A.
EQUIPMENT	The preparation of two types of insulin in one syringe is used as the example in the following procedure. • Two vials of medication (insulin in this example) • Sterile syringe (insulin syringe in this example) • Sterile needle (if not already packaged with syringe) • Antimicrobial swabs • Electronic Medication Administration Record (eMAR) or Medication Administration Record (MAR)
ASSESSMENT	Assess the appropriateness of the drug for the patient. Review the medical history and allergy, assessment, and laboratory data that may influence drug administration. Determine the compatibility of the two medications. Not all insulins can be mixed together. Assess the contents of each vial of insulin. It is very important to be familiar with the particular drug's properties to be able to assess the quality of the medication in the vial before withdrawal. Unmodified preparations of insulin typically appear as clear substances, so they should be without particles or foreign

matter. Modified preparations of insulin are typically suspensions, so they do not appear as clear substances. Check the expiration date before administering the medication. Assess the patient's knowledge of the medication. If the patient has a knowledge deficit about the medication, this may be the appropriate time to begin education about the medication. Check the patient's blood glucose level, if appropriate, before administering the insulin. Verify patient name, dose, route, and time of administration.

ACTUAL OR POTENTIAL HEALTH PROBLEMS AND NEEDS	Many actual or potential health problems or issues may require the use of this skill as part of related interventions. An appropriate health problem or issue may include: • Infection risk • Knowledge deficiency • Hyperglycemia
OUTCOME IDENTIFICATION AND PLANNING	The expected outcomes to achieve when mixing two different types of medication in one syringe are the accurate withdrawal of each medication into a syringe in a sterile manner, the medication is free from contamination, and the proper dose is prepared.

IMPLEMENTATION

ACTION	RATIONALE
1. Gather equipment. Check each medication prescribed against the original in the health record, depending on facility policy and the medication order system in place. Clarify any inconsistencies. Check the patient's health record for allergies.	The prescription is the legal record of prescribed medication interventions. This comparison helps to identify errors that may have occurred when orders were transcribed. Computer provider order-entry (CPOE) systems allow prescribers to send electronic medication prescriptions directly to the pharmacy located in a health care facility and to outpatient pharmacies.
2. Know the actions, special nursing considerations, safe dose ranges, purpose of administration, and adverse effects of the medications to be administered. Confirm the compatibility of the medications in one syringe. Consider the appropriateness of the medication for this patient.	This knowledge aids the nurse in evaluating the therapeutic effect of the medication in relation to the patient's health status and can also be used to educate the patient about the medication.
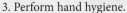3. Perform hand hygiene.	Hand hygiene prevents the spread of microorganisms.
4. Move the medication supply system to the outside of the patient's room or prepare for administration at the medication supply system in the medication area. Alternatively, access the medication administration supply system at or inside the patient's room.	Organization facilitates error-free administration and saves time.
5. Unlock the medication supply system or drawer. Enter the passcode and scan employee identification, if required.	Locking the supply system or drawer safeguards each patient's medication supply. Facility accrediting organizations require medication supply systems to be locked when not in use. Entering the passcode and scanning ID allows only authorized users into the system and identifies the user for documentation by the computer.
6. **Prepare medications for one patient at a time.**	This prevents errors in medication administration.
7. Read the eMAR/MAR and read the label when selecting the proper medications from the medication supply system or the patient's medication drawer.	This is the *first* check of the label.
8. Read the label and compare the labels with the eMAR/MAR. Check expiration dates and perform dosage calculations, if necessary. Scan the bar code on the package, if required.	This is the *second* check of the labels. Verify calculations with another nurse to ensure safety, if necessary.

(continued on page 228)

Skill 5-5 ▶ Mixing Medications From Two Vials in One Syringe (continued)

ACTION	RATIONALE
9. If necessary, remove the cap that protects the self-sealing stopper on each vial.	The cap protects the self-sealing top.
10. **If the medication is a suspension (e.g., a modified insulin, such as NPH insulin), roll and agitate the vial to mix it well.**	There is controversy regarding how to mix insulin in suspension. Some sources advise rolling the vial; others advise shaking the vial. Consult facility policy or pharmacist. Regardless of the method used, it is essential that the suspension be mixed well to avoid administering an inconsistent dose.
11. **Scrub the self-sealing stopper top with the antimicrobial swab and allow it to dry.**	The antimicrobial swab removes surface microbial contamination. Allowing the antimicrobial solution to dry completely (5 to 20 seconds) ensures complete antimicrobial effectiveness (Gorski et al., 2021; Slater et al., 2018). Drying also prevents antimicrobial solution from entering the vial on the needle.
12. Remove the cap from the needle by pulling it straight off. Touch the plunger only at the knob. Draw back an amount of air into the syringe that is equal to the dose of modified insulin to be withdrawn.	Pulling the cap off in a straight manner prevents accidental needlestick. Handling the plunger only by the knob ensures sterility of the shaft of the plunger. Before fluid is removed, injection of an equal amount of air is required to prevent the formation of a partial vacuum, because a vial is a sealed container. If not enough air is injected, the negative pressure makes it difficult to withdraw the medication with repeated use.
13. Hold the modified vial on a flat surface. Pierce the self-sealing stopper in the center with the needle tip and inject the measured air into the space above the solution (Figure 1). Do not inject air into the solution. Withdraw the needle.	Unmodified insulin should never be contaminated with modified insulin. Placing air in the modified insulin first without allowing the needle to contact the insulin ensures that the second vial-entered (unmodified) insulin is not contaminated by the medication in the other vial. Air bubbled through the solution could result in withdrawal of an inaccurate amount of medication.
14. Draw back an amount of air into the syringe that is equal to the dose of unmodified insulin to be withdrawn.	A vial is a sealed container. Therefore, injection of an equal amount of air (before fluid is removed) is required to prevent the formation of a partial vacuum. If not enough air is injected, the negative pressure makes it difficult to withdraw the medication.
15. Hold the unmodified vial on a flat surface. Pierce the self-sealing stopper in the center with the needle tip and inject the measured air into the space above the solution (Figure 2). Do not inject air into the solution. Keep the needle in the vial.	Air bubbled through the solution could result in withdrawal of an inaccurate amount of medication.

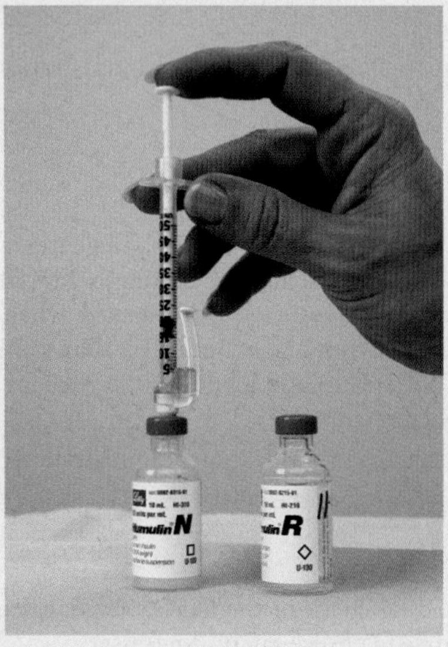

FIGURE 1. Injecting air into modified insulin preparation.

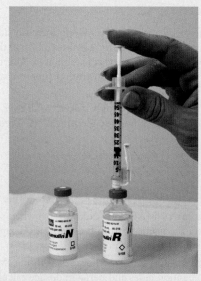

FIGURE 2. Injecting air into unmodified insulin vial.

ACTION

16. Invert the vial of unmodified insulin. Hold the vial in one hand and use the other to withdraw the medication. **Touch the plunger only at the knob. Draw up the prescribed amount of medication while holding the syringe at eye level and vertically (Figure 3).** Turn the vial over and then remove the needle from the vial.

17. Check that there are no air bubbles in the syringe.

18. **Check the amount of medication in the syringe with the medication dose and discard any surplus.**

19. **Recheck the vial label with the eMAR/MAR.**

20. Calculate the endpoint on the syringe for the combined insulin amount by adding the number of units for each dose together.

21. Insert the needle into the modified vial and invert it, **taking care not to push the plunger and inject medication from the syringe into the vial.** Invert the vial of modified insulin. Hold the vial in one hand and use the other to withdraw the medication. **Touch the plunger only at the knob. Draw up the prescribed amount of medication while holding the syringe at eye level and vertically (Figure 4). Take care to withdraw only the prescribed amount.** Turn the vial over and then remove the needle from the vial. Carefully recap the needle. Carefully replace the cap over the needle.

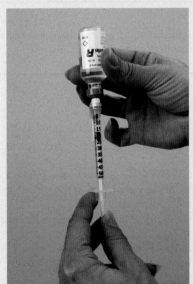

FIGURE 3. Withdrawing prescribed amount of unmodified insulin.

22. **Check the amount of medication in the syringe with the medication dose.**

RATIONALE

Holding the syringe at eye level facilitates accurate reading, and the vertical position allows easy removal of air bubbles from the syringe. First dose is prepared and is not contaminated by insulin that contains modifiers.

The presence of air in the syringe would result in an inaccurate dose of medication.

Careful measurement ensures that the correct dose is withdrawn.

This is the *third* check to ensure accuracy and to prevent errors. It must be checked now for the first medication in the syringe, as it is not possible to ensure accuracy once a second drug is in the syringe.

This allows for accurate withdrawal of the second dose.

The previous addition of air eliminates the need to create positive pressure. Holding the syringe at eye level facilitates accurate reading. Capping the needle prevents contamination and protects the nurse against accidental needlesticks. A one-handed recap method may be used as long as care is taken to ensure that the needle remains sterile.

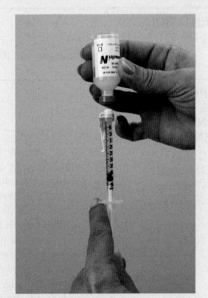

FIGURE 4. Withdrawing modified insulin.

Careful measurement ensures that correct dose is withdrawn.

(*continued on page 230*)

Skill 5-5 ▶ Mixing Medications From Two Vials in One Syringe *(continued)*

ACTION	RATIONALE
23. Depending on facility policy, the third check of the label may occur at this point. If so, read the label and recheck the labels with the MAR before taking the medications to the patient. However, many facilities require the third check to occur at the bedside, after identifying the patient.	This *third* check ensures accuracy and helps to prevent errors. *Note:* Many facilities require the *third* check to occur at the bedside, after identifying the patient and before administration.
24. Label the vials with the date and time opened and beyond-use date, and store the vials containing the remaining medication, according to facility policy.	Because the vial is sealed, the medication inside remains sterile and can be used for future injections. Labeling the opened vials with a date and time limits its use after a specific time period. The CDC recommends that medications packaged as multiuse vials be assigned to a single patient whenever possible (CDC, 2019; Dolan et al., 2016).
25. Label the syringe with the medication's name, dose, and amount date (The Joint Commission, 2021).	Unlabeled syringes are unidentifiable and may lead to a medication administration error (The Joint Commission, 2021).
26. **Log out of and/or lock the medication supply system before leaving it.**	Locking the medication supply system or drawer safeguards the patient's medication supply. Facility accrediting organizations require medication supply systems to be locked when not in use.
27. Perform hand hygiene.	Hand hygiene deters the spread of microorganisms.
28. Proceed with administration, based on prescribed route.	See appropriate skill for prescribed route.

EVALUATION

The expected outcomes have been met when the medication was withdrawn into the syringe in a sterile manner, it was free from contamination, and the proper dose was prepared.

DOCUMENTATION

Guidelines

It is not necessary to record the removal of the medication from the vials. Prompt recording of administration of the medication is required immediately after it is administered.

DEVELOPING CLINICAL REASONING AND CLINICAL JUDGMENT

UNEXPECTED SITUATIONS AND ASSOCIATED INTERVENTIONS

- *You contaminate the plunger before injecting air into the insulin vial:* Discard the needle and syringe and start over.
- *The plunger is contaminated after medication is drawn into the syringe:* It is not necessary to discard and start over. The contaminated plunger will enter the barrel of the syringe when pushing the medication out and will not contaminate the medication.
- *You allow modified insulin to come in contact with the needle before entering the unmodified insulin vial:* Discard the needle and syringe and start over.
- *You notice that the combined amount is not the ordered amount (i.e., you have less or more units in combined syringe than ordered):* Discard the syringe and start over. There is no way to know for sure which dosage is wrong or which medication should be expelled.
- *You inject medication from the first vial (in syringe) into the second vial:* Discard the vial and syringe and start over.

SPECIAL CONSIDERATIONS

General Considerations

- A patient with diabetes who is visually impaired may find it helpful to use a magnifying apparatus that fits around the syringe.
- Before attempting to explain or demonstrate devices that help low-vision diabetic patients to prepare their medication, attempt to use the device yourself under similar circumstances. To detect any difficulties the patient may experience, practice using the aid with your eyes closed or in a poorly lit room.

Infant and Child Considerations

- School-age children are generally able to prepare and administer their own injections, such as insulin, with supervision (American Academy of Pediatrics, 2020). Parents/caregivers and the child should be involved in teaching.

Skill 5-6 ▶ Administering an Intradermal Injection

Intradermal injections are administered into the dermis, just below the epidermis. The intradermal route has the longest absorption time of all parenteral routes. For this reason, intradermal injections are used for sensitivity tests, such as tuberculin and allergy tests, and local anesthesia. The advantage of the intradermal route for these tests is that the body's reaction to substances is easily visible, and degrees of reaction are discernible by comparative study.

Sites commonly used are the inner surface of the forearm, the upper chest, and the upper back, under the scapula. Equipment used for an intradermal injection includes a tuberculin syringe calibrated in tenths and hundredths of a milliliter and a ⅜- to ½-inch, 26- or 27-gauge needle (Taylor et al., 2023). The dosage given intradermally is small, usually less than 0.5 mL (Taylor et al., 2023). The angle of administration for an intradermal injection is 5 to 15 degrees (see Figure 5-1 in the chapter opener on page 200).

DELEGATION CONSIDERATIONS

The administration of an intradermal injection is not delegated to assistive personnel (AP). Depending on the state's nurse practice act and the organization's policies and procedures, the administration of an intradermal injection may be delegated to licensed practical/vocational nurses (LPN/LVNs). The decision to delegate must be based on careful analysis of the patient's needs and circumstances as well as the qualifications of the person to whom the task is being delegated. Refer to the Delegation Guidelines in Appendix A.

EQUIPMENT

- Prescribed medication
- Sterile syringe, usually a tuberculin syringe calibrated in tenths and hundredths, and a ⅜″ to ½″, 26- or 27-gauge needle
- Antimicrobial swab
- Disposable gloves
- Small gauze square
- Electronic Medication Administration Record (eMAR) or Medication Administration Record (MAR)
- PPE, as indicated
- Marking pen for indicating area for future assessment, if indicated

ASSESSMENT

Assess the appropriateness of the drug for the patient. Review the medical history and allergy, assessment, and laboratory data that may influence drug administration. Check the expiration date before administering medication. Assess the site on the patient where the injection is to be given. Avoid areas of broken or open skin. Avoid areas that are highly pigmented, and those that have lesions, bruises, or scars and are hairy. Assess the patient's knowledge of the medication. If the patient has a knowledge deficit about the medication, this may be the appropriate time to begin education about the medication Verify the patient's name, dose, route, and time of administration.

(continued on page 232)

Skill 5-6 ▶ Administering an Intradermal Injection *(continued)*

ACTUAL OR POTENTIAL HEALTH PROBLEMS AND NEEDS	Many actual or potential health problems or issues may require the use of this skill as part of related interventions. An appropriate health problem or issue may include: • Knowledge deficiency • Infection risk • Injury risk

OUTCOME IDENTIFICATION AND PLANNING	The expected outcomes to achieve when administering an intradermal injection are that the medication is injected, and a wheal appears at the injection site. Other outcomes that may be appropriate include the following: the patient refrains from rubbing the site, the patient does not experience adverse effects, and the patient understands and engages with the medication regimen.

IMPLEMENTATION

ACTION

1. Gather equipment. Check each medication prescribed against the original in the health record, depending on facility policy and the medication order system in place. Clarify any inconsistencies. Check the patient's health record for allergies.

2. Know the actions, special nursing considerations, safe dose ranges, purpose of administration, and adverse effects of the medications to be administered. Consider the appropriateness of the medication for this patient.

3. Perform hand hygiene.

4. Move the medication supply system to the outside of the patient's room or prepare for administration at the medication supply system in the medication area. Alternatively, access the medication administration supply system at or inside the patient's room.

5. Unlock the medication supply system or drawer. Enter the passcode and scan employee identification, if required.

6. **Prepare medications for one patient at a time.**

7. Read the eMAR/MAR and read the label when selecting the proper medication from the medication supply system or the patient's medication drawer.

8. Read the label and compare the label with the eMAR/MAR. Check expiration dates and perform calculations, if necessary. Scan the bar code on the package, if required.

9. If necessary, withdraw the medication from an ampule or vial as described in Skills 5-3 and 5-4.

10. **Depending on facility policy, the third check of the label may occur at this point. If so, when all medications for one patient have been prepared, read the label and recheck the labels with the eMAR/MAR before taking the medications to the patient. However, many facilities require the third check to occur at the bedside, after identifying the patient.**

RATIONALE

The prescription is the legal record of prescribed medication interventions. This comparison helps to identify errors that may have occurred when orders were transcribed. Computer provider order-entry (CPOE) systems allow prescribers to send electronic medication prescriptions directly to the pharmacy located in a health care facility and to outpatient pharmacies.

This knowledge aids the nurse in evaluating the therapeutic effect of the medication in relation to the patient's health status and can also be used to educate the patient about the medication.

Hand hygiene deters the spread of microorganisms.

Organization facilitates error-free administration and saves time.

Locking the medication supply system or drawer safeguards each patient's medication supply. Facility accrediting organizations require medication supply systems to be locked when not in use. Entering the passcode and scanning ID allows only authorized users into the system and identifies the user for documentation by the computer.

This prevents errors in medication administration.

This is the *first* check of the label.

This is the *second* check of the label. Verify calculations with another nurse to ensure safety.

This *third* check ensures accuracy and helps to prevent errors. *Note:* Many facilities require the *third* check to occur at the bedside, after identifying the patient and before administration.

ACTION

11. Label the syringe with the medication's name, dose, and amount (The Joint Commission, 2021).

12. **Log out of and/or lock the medication supply system before leaving it.**

13. Transport medications to the patient's bedside carefully and keep the medications in sight at all times.

14. **Ensure that the patient receives the medications at the correct time.**

15. Perform hand hygiene and put on PPE, if indicated.

16. **Identify the patient. Compare the information with the eMAR/MAR. The patient should be identified using at least two of the following methods** (The Joint Commission, 2021):

   a. Check the name on the patient's identification band.

   b. Check the identification number on the patient's identification band.

   c. Check the birth date on the patient's identification band.

   d. Ask the patient to state their name and birth date, based on facility policy.

17. Close the door to the room or pull the bedside curtain.

18. **Complete necessary assessments before administering medications. Check the patient's allergy bracelet, if present, or ask the patient about allergies. Explain the purpose and action of the medication to the patient.**

19. Scan the patient's bar code on the identification band, if required (The Joint Commission, 2021).

20. **Based on facility policy, the third check of the label may occur at this point. If so, read the label and recheck the labels with the eMAR/MAR before administering the medications to the patient.**

21. Put on gloves.

22. Select an appropriate administration site. Assist the patient to the appropriate position for the site chosen. Drape, as needed, to expose only site area to be used.

23. Cleanse the site with an antimicrobial swab while wiping with a firm, circular motion and moving outward from the injection site. Allow the skin to dry.

24. Remove the needle cap with the nondominant hand by pulling it straight off.

25. Use the nondominant hand to spread the skin taut over the injection site (Figure 1).

RATIONALE

Unlabeled syringes are unidentifiable and may lead to a medication administration error (The Joint Commission, 2021).

Locking the medication supply system or drawer safeguards the patient's medication supply. Facility accrediting organizations require medication supply systems to be locked when not in use.

Careful handling and close observation prevent accidental or deliberate disarrangement of medications.

Check facility policy, which may allow for administration within a period of 30 minutes before or 30 minutes after the designated time.

Hand hygiene and PPE prevent the spread of microorganisms. PPE is required based on transmission precautions.

Identifying the patient ensures the right patient receives the medications and helps prevent errors. The patient's room number or physical location is not used as an identifier (The Joint Commission, 2021). Replace the identification band if it is missing or inaccurate in any way.

This requires a response from the patient, but illness and strange surroundings often cause patients to be confused.

This provides patient privacy.

Assessment is a prerequisite to administration of medications. Explanation provides rationale, increases knowledge, promotes patient engagement, and reduces anxiety.

This provides an additional check to ensure that the medication is given to the right patient.

Many facilities require the *third* check to occur at the bedside, after identifying the patient and before administration. If facility policy directs the *third* check at this time, this *third* check ensures accuracy and helps to prevent errors.

Gloves help prevent exposure to contaminants.

Using the appropriate site prevents injury and allows for accurate reading of the test site at the appropriate time. Draping provides privacy and warmth.

Pathogens on the skin can be forced into the tissues by the needle. Moving from the center outward prevents contamination of the site. Allowing the antimicrobial solution to dry completely (5 to 20 seconds) ensures complete antimicrobial effectiveness (Gorski et al., 2021; Slater et al., 2018), and prevents introducing alcohol into the tissue, which can be irritating and uncomfortable.

This technique lessens the risk of an accidental needlestick.

Taut skin provides an easy entrance into intradermal tissue.

(continued on page 234)

Skill 5-6 ▶ Administering an Intradermal Injection *(continued)*

ACTION	**RATIONALE**

26. Hold the syringe in the dominant hand, between the thumb and forefinger with the bevel of the needle up.

Using the dominant hand allows for easy, appropriate handling of the syringe. Having the bevel up allows for smooth piercing of the skin and introduction of medication into the dermis.

27. Hold the syringe at a 5- to 15-degree angle from the site. Place the needle almost flat against the patient's skin (Figure 2), bevel side up, and insert the needle into the skin. Insert the needle only about ⅛ inch with entire bevel under the skin.

The dermis is entered when the needle is held as nearly parallel to the skin as possible and is inserted about ⅛ inch.

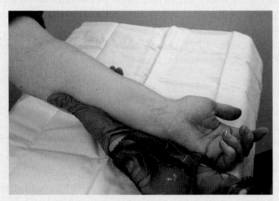

FIGURE 1. Spreading skin taut over injection site.

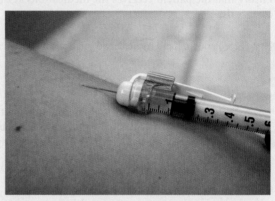

FIGURE 2. Inserting needle almost flat against the skin.

28. Once the needle is in place, steady the lower end of the syringe. Slide your dominant hand to the end of the plunger.

This prevents injury and inadvertent advancement or withdrawal of needle.

29. Slowly inject the agent while watching for a small wheal to appear (Figure 3).

The appearance of a wheal indicates the medication is in the dermis.

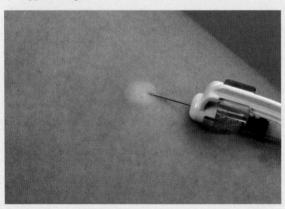

FIGURE 3. Observing for wheal while injecting medication.

30. Withdraw the needle quickly at the same angle that it was inserted. Do not recap the used needle. Engage the safety shield or needle guard.

Withdrawing the needle quickly and at the angle at which it entered the skin minimizes tissue damage and discomfort for the patient. Safety shield or needle guard prevents accidental needlestick injury.

31. **Do not massage the area after removing needle. Tell the patient not to rub or scratch the site. If necessary, gently blot the site with a dry gauze square. Do not apply pressure or rub the site.** Use the marking pen to mark the area for further assessment, if indicated.

Massaging or rubbing the area where an intradermal injection is given may spread the medication to underlying subcutaneous tissue.

32. Remove gloves and perform hand hygiene. Assist the patient to a position of comfort.

Removing gloves and performing hand hygiene reduces risk for contamination of other items and the spread of microorganisms. Assisting the patient to a position of comfort promotes patient comfort.

ACTION	**RATIONALE**
33. Discard the needle and syringe in an appropriate container, such as a sharps receptacle.	Proper disposal of the needle prevents injury.
34. Remove additional PPE, if used. Perform hand hygiene.	Proper removal of PPE reduces the risk of infection transmission and contamination of other items. Hand hygiene prevents the spread of microorganisms.
35. Document the administration of the medication immediately after administration. See Documentation section below.	Timely documentation helps to ensure patient safety.
36. Evaluate the patient's response to the medication within the appropriate time frame.	The patient needs to be evaluated for therapeutic and adverse effects from the medication.
37. Observe the area for signs of a reaction at determined intervals after administration. Inform the patient of the need for inspection.	With many intradermal injections, you need to look for a localized reaction in the area of the injection at the appropriate interval(s) determined by the type of medication and purpose. Explanation provides rationale, increases knowledge, promotes patient engagement, and reduces anxiety.
38. If medication is intended for allergy skin testing, observe the patient for sensitivity to the injected allergen (Hoy & Ng, 2021).	Sensitivity to an allergen places the patient at risk for the development of anaphylaxis and may require the administration of epinephrine subcutaneously (Hoy & Ng, 2021). (Refer to Skill 5-7.)

EVALUATION

The expected outcomes have been met when the medication has been injected and a wheal has formed at the injection site, the patient has refrained from rubbing the site, the patient did not experience adverse effects, and the patient has verbalized an understanding of the medication regimen.

DOCUMENTATION

Guidelines

Record each medication administered on the eMAR/MAR or health record using the required format, including date, time, and the site of administration, immediately after administration. Some facilities recommend circling the injection site with ink. Circling the injection site easily identifies the intradermal injection site and allows for future careful observation of the exact area. If using a bar-code system, medication administration is automatically recorded when the bar code is scanned. PRN medications require documentation of the reason for administration. Prompt recording avoids the possibility of accidentally repeating the administration of the drug. If the drug was refused or omitted, record this in the appropriate area on the medication record and notify the health care team as appropriate. This verifies the reason medication was omitted and ensures that health care personnel providing care for the patient are aware of the occurrence.

DEVELOPING CLINICAL REASONING AND CLINICAL JUDGMENT

UNEXPECTED SITUATIONS AND ASSOCIATED INTERVENTIONS

- *You do not note a wheal or blister at the injection site:* The medication has been inadvertently injected subcutaneously. Document according to facility policy and notify the health care team as appropriate. You may need to obtain an order to repeat the procedure.
- *Medication leaks out of the injection site before the needle is withdrawn:* The needle was inserted less than ⅛ inch. Document according to facility policy and notify the health care team as appropriate. You may need to obtain an order to repeat the procedure.
- *You stick yourself with the needle before injection:* Discard the needle and syringe appropriately. Follow facility policy regarding needlestick injury. Prepare a new syringe with medication and administer to the patient. Communicate and document the incident according to facility policy.
- *You stick yourself with the needle after injection:* Discard the needle and syringe appropriately. Follow facility policy regarding needlestick injury. Communicate and document the incident according to facility policy.

(continued on page 236)

Skill 5-6 ▶ Administering an Intradermal Injection   *(continued)*

SPECIAL
CONSIDERATIONS

- Fluzone® Intradermal is the only vaccine in the United States administered by the intradermal route and is available for patients ages 18 to 64 years (CDC, 2015b; Prescriber's Digital Reference [PDR], 2021; Sanofi Pasteur, 2017). The site of administration for this vaccine is the deltoid region of the upper arm, and the needle is inserted perpendicular to the skin (PDR, 2021). **This vaccine should not be administered into the forearm or other site used to administer other intradermal medications.** The single-dose prefilled microinjection syringe administers a 0.1-mL dose (Sanofi Pasteur, 2017). **No other influenza vaccine formulations should be administered by the intradermal route.** Follow the manufacturer's directions for appropriate administration.
- Ongoing assessment is an important part of nursing care for both evaluation of patient response to administered medications and early detection of adverse reactions. If an adverse effect is suspected, withhold further medication doses and notify the health care team. Additional intervention is based on type of reaction and patient assessment.

Skill 5-7 ▶ Administering a Subcutaneous Injection

Skill Variation: *Using an Insulin Injection Pen to Administer Insulin via the Subcutaneous Route*

Subcutaneous injections are administered into the adipose tissue layer just below the epidermis and dermis. This tissue has few blood vessels, so drugs administered here have a slow, sustained rate of absorption into the capillaries. Various sites may be used for subcutaneous injections, including the outer aspect of the upper arm, the abdomen (from below the costal margin to the iliac crests), the anterior aspects of the thigh, the upper back, and the upper ventral- or dorsogluteal area. Figure 1 displays the sites on the body where subcutaneous injections can be given. Absorption rates differ among the various sites. Injections in the abdomen are absorbed most rapidly; ones in the arms are absorbed somewhat more slowly; those in the thighs, even more slowly; and those in the ventral or dorsogluteal areas have the slowest absorption (American Diabetes Association [ADA], 2020).

It is important to choose the right equipment to ensure depositing the medication into the intended subcutaneous tissue and not the underlying muscle. Equipment used for a subcutaneous injection includes a syringe of appropriate volume for the amount of drug being administered. A 25- to 30-gauge, ⅜- to 1-inch needle can be used; the 25-gauge, ⅝-inch needles are most commonly used for subcutaneous injections for adults (Taylor et al., 2023). Needle length ranges exist because patients present with different amounts of subcutaneous tissue that varies based on age, body mass index, and general build—choose the needle length based on the amount of subcutaneous tissue present (Shepherd, 2018b) and that ensures the needle terminates in the subcutaneous tissue (Taylor et al., 2023). Some medications are packaged in prefilled cartridges with a needle attached. One example is an insulin injection pen, which may be used for subcutaneous injection of insulin (see the accompanying Skill Variation for technique). Confirm that the provided needle is appropriate for the patient before use. If not, the medication will have to be transferred to another syringe and the appropriate needle attached.

Subcutaneous injections are administered at a 45- or 90-degree angle, with the 45-degree angle used only for patients with a limited amount of subcutaneous tissue. Choose the angle of needle insertion based on the amount of subcutaneous tissue present and the length of the needle. In general, insert the shorter, ⅜-inch needle, at a 90-degree angle (common on prefilled and insulin syringes). The longer, ⅝-inch needle, may be inserted at a 45-degree angle. Figure 5-1 in the chapter opener on page 200 shows the angles of insertion for subcutaneous injections.

Usually, no more than 1 mL of solution is given subcutaneously. Giving larger amounts adds to the patient's discomfort and may predispose to poor absorption. It is necessary to rotate sites or areas for injection if the patient is to receive frequent injections. This helps to prevent buildup of fibrous/adipose tissue and permits complete absorption of the medication. Further information regarding insulin administration and rotation of injection sites can be found in the General Considerations at the end of this skill.

Box 5-1 discusses techniques for reducing discomfort when injecting medications subcutaneously or intramuscularly.

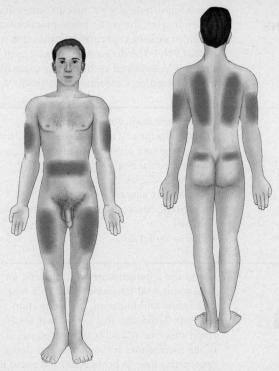

FIGURE 1. Body sites where subcutaneous injections can be given.

Box 5-1 Reducing Discomfort in Subcutaneous and Intramuscular Administrations

The following are recommended techniques for reducing discomfort when injecting medications subcutaneously or intramuscularly:

- Select a needle of the smallest gauge that is appropriate for the site and solution to be injected and select the correct needle length.
- Be sure the needle is free of medication that may irritate superficial tissues as the needle is inserted. The recommended procedure is to use two needles—one to remove the medication from the vial or ampule and a second one to inject the medication. If medication is in a prefilled syringe with a nonremovable needle and has dripped back on the needle during preparation, gently tap the barrel to remove the excess solution.
- Consider application of manual pressure at the insertion site by pressing the insertion site firmly for 10 seconds before needle insertion. It has been suggested that this action stimulates the surrounding nerve endings, leading to a reduction in the sensory input from the injection and resulting decreased pain intensity (Chung et al., 2002; Öztürk et al., 2017).
- Use the Z-track technique for intramuscular injections to prevent leakage of medication into the needle track, thus minimizing discomfort.
- Inject the medication into relaxed muscles. More pressure and discomfort occur when the medication is injected into a contracted muscle.
- Do not inject areas that feel hard on palpation or tender to the patient.

- Insert the needle with a dartlike motion without hesitation and remove it quickly at the same angle at which it was inserted. These techniques reduce discomfort and tissue irritation.
- Do not administer more solution in one injection than is recommended for the site. Injecting more solution creates excess pressure in the area and increases discomfort.
- Inject the solution slowly so that it may be dispersed more easily into the surrounding tissue (10 seconds per 1 mL).
- Apply gentle pressure after injection, unless this technique is contraindicated.
- Allow the patient who is fearful of injections to talk about their fears. Answer the patient's questions truthfully and explain the nature and purpose of the injection. Taking the time to offer support often allays fears and decreases discomfort.
- Rotate sites when the patient is to receive repeated injections. Injections in the same site may cause undue discomfort, irritation, or abscesses in tissues.
- Consider age-appropriate nonpharmacologic methods for infants and children (American Academy of Pediatrics, 2019; CDC, 2020, 2021), such as breastfeeding, the administration of sweet solutions, front-to-front upright holding, rapid injection without aspiration, administration of the most painful vaccine last, tactile stimulation, and other distractions. Consider use of pain-relieving ointments or sprays at the injection site (American Academy of Pediatrics, 2019; CDC, 2020). Involve the child's parent/family/caregiver for support when possible (CDC, 2020).

(continued on page 238)

Skill 5-7 ▶ Administering a Subcutaneous Injection *(continued)*

DELEGATION CONSIDERATIONS	The administration of a subcutaneous injection is not delegated to assistive personnel (AP). Depending on the state's nurse practice act and the organization's policies and procedures, the administration of a subcutaneous injection may be delegated to licensed practical/vocational nurses (LPN/LVNs). The decision to delegate must be based on careful analysis of the patient's needs and circumstances as well as the qualifications of the person to whom the task is being delegated. Refer to the Delegation Guidelines in Appendix A.
EQUIPMENT	• Prescribed medication • Sterile syringe and needle. Needle size depends on the medication to be administered and patient body type (see previous discussion). • Antimicrobial swab • Nonlatex, disposable gloves • Small gauze square • Electronic Medication Administration Record (eMAR) or Medication Administration Record (MAR) • PPE, as indicated
ASSESSMENT	Assess the appropriateness of the drug for the patient. Review the medical history and allergy, assessment, and laboratory data that may influence drug administration. Check the expiration date before administering the medication. Assess the site on the patient where the injection is to be given. Avoid sites that are bruised, tender, hard, swollen, inflamed, or scarred. These conditions could affect the reliability of absorption (ADA, 2020; Gelder, 2014). Assess the patient's knowledge of the medication. If the patient has deficient knowledge about the medication, this may be the appropriate time to begin education about it. If the medication may affect the patient's vital signs, assess them before administration. If the medication is for pain relief, assess the patient's pain before and after administration. Verify patient name, dose, route, and time of administration.
ACTUAL OR POTENTIAL HEALTH PROBLEMS AND NEEDS	Many actual or potential health problems or issues may require the use of this skill as part of related interventions. An appropriate health problem or issue may include: • Knowledge deficiency • Infection risk • Injury risk
OUTCOME IDENTIFICATION AND PLANNING	The expected outcomes to achieve are that the patient receives the medication via the subcutaneous route and experiences the intended effect of the medication. Other outcomes that may be appropriate include the following: the patient does not experience adverse effects, and the patient understands and engages with the medication regimen.

IMPLEMENTATION

ACTION	RATIONALE
1. Gather equipment. Check each medication prescribed against the original in the health record, depending on facility policy and the medication order system in place. Clarify any inconsistencies. Check the patient's health record for allergies.	The prescription is the legal record of prescribed medication interventions. This comparison helps to identify errors that may have occurred when orders were transcribed. Computer provider order-entry (CPOE) systems allow prescribers to send electronic medication prescriptions directly to the pharmacy located in a health care facility and to outpatient pharmacies.
2. Know the actions, special nursing considerations, safe dose ranges, purpose of administration, and adverse effects of the medications to be administered. Consider the appropriateness of the medication for this patient.	This knowledge aids the nurse in evaluating the therapeutic effect of the medication in relation to the patient's health status and can also be used to educate the patient about the medication.
3. Perform hand hygiene.	Hand hygiene prevents the spread of microorganisms.

ACTION	**RATIONALE**
4. Move the medication supply system to the outside of the patient's room or prepare for administration at the medication supply system in the medication area. Alternatively, access the medication administration supply system at or inside the patient's room.	Organization facilitates error-free administration and saves time.
5. Unlock the medication supply system or drawer. Enter the passcode and scan employee identification, if required.	Locking the medication supply system or drawer safeguards each patient's medication supply. Facility accrediting organizations require medication supply systems to be locked when not in use. Entering the passcode and scanning ID allows only authorized users into the computer system and identifies the user for documentation by the computer.
6. **Prepare medications for one patient at a time.**	This prevents errors in medication administration.
7. Read the eMAR/MAR and read the label when selecting the proper medication from the medication supply system or the patient's medication drawer.	This is the *first* check of the label.
8. Read the label and compare the medication label with the eMAR/MAR. Check expiration dates and perform calculations, if necessary. Scan the bar code on the package, if required.	This is the *second* check of the label. Verify calculations with another nurse to ensure safety, if necessary.
9. If necessary, withdraw the medication from an ampule or vial as described in Skills 5-3 and 5-4.	
10. **Depending on facility policy, the third check of the label may occur at this point. If so, when all medications for one patient have been prepared, read the label and recheck the labels with the eMAR/MAR before taking the medications to the patient. However, many facilities require the third check to occur at the bedside, after identifying the patient.**	This *third* check ensures accuracy and helps to prevent errors. *Note:* Many facilities require the *third* check to occur at the bedside, after identifying the patient and before administration.
11. Label the syringe with the medication's name, dose, and amount (The Joint Commission, 2021).	Unlabeled syringes are unidentifiable and may lead to a medication administration error (The Joint Commission, 2021).
12. **Log out of and/or lock the medication supply system before leaving it.**	Locking the medication supply system or drawer safeguards the patient's medication supply. Facility accrediting organizations require medication supply systems to be locked when not in use.
13. Transport medications to the patient's bedside carefully and keep the medications in sight at all times.	Careful handling and close observation prevent accidental or deliberate disarrangement of medications.
14. **Ensure that the patient receives the medications at the correct time.**	Check facility policy, which may allow for administration within a period of 30 minutes before or 30 minutes after the designated time.
15. Perform hand hygiene and put on PPE, if indicated.	Hand hygiene and PPE prevent the spread of microorganisms. PPE is required based on transmission precautions.
16. **Identify the patient. Compare the information with the eMAR/MAR. The patient should be identified using at least two of the following methods** (The Joint Commission, 2021):	Identifying the patient ensures the right patient receives the medications and helps prevent errors. The patient's room number or physical location is not used as an identifier (The Joint Commission, 2021). Replace the identification band if it is missing or inaccurate in any way.
a. Check the name on the patient's identification band.	
b. Check the identification number on the patient's identification band.	
c. Check the birth date on the patient's identification band.	
d. Ask the patient to state their name and birth date, based on facility policy.	This requires a response from the patient, but illness and strange surroundings often cause patients to be confused.

(continued on page 240)

Skill 5-7 ▸ Administering a Subcutaneous Injection *(continued)*

ACTION	**RATIONALE**

17. Close the door to the room or pull the bedside curtain.

This provides patient privacy.

18. Complete necessary assessments before administering medications. Check the patient's allergy bracelet, if present, or ask the patient about allergies. Explain the purpose and action of the medication to the patient.

Assessment is a prerequisite to administration of medications. Explanation provides rationale, increases knowledge, promotes patient engagement, and reduces anxiety.

19. Scan the patient's bar code on the identification band, if required (The Joint Commission, 2021) (Figure 2).

Scanning provides an additional check to ensure that the medication is given to the right patient.

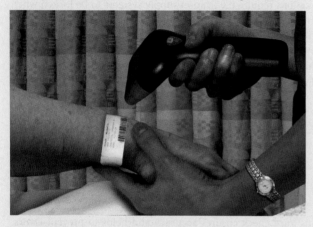

FIGURE 2. Scanning bar code on the patient's identification bracelet. (*Source:* Used with permission from Shutterstock. *Photo by B. Proud.*)

20. Based on facility policy, the third check of the label may occur at this point. If so, read the label and recheck the labels with the eMAR/MAR before administering the medications to the patient.

Many facilities require the *third* check to occur at the bedside, after identifying the patient and before administration. If facility policy directs the *third* check at this time, this *third* check ensures accuracy and helps to prevent errors.

21. Put on gloves.

Gloves help prevent exposure to contaminants.

22. Select an appropriate administration site. Assist the patient to the appropriate position for the site chosen. Drape, as needed, to expose only site area to be used.

Using an appropriate site and positioning prevent injury. Draping helps maintain the patient's privacy.

23. Identify the appropriate landmarks for the site chosen.

Good visualization is necessary to establish the correct site location and to avoid complications (Taylor et al., 2023).

24. Cleanse the area around the injection site with an antimicrobial swab. Use a firm, circular motion while moving outward from the injection site (Figure 3). Allow the area to dry.

Pathogens on the skin can be forced into the tissues by the needle. Moving from the center outward prevents contamination of the site. Allowing the antimicrobial solution to dry completely (5 to 20 seconds) ensures complete antimicrobial effectiveness (Gorski et al., 2021; Slater et al., 2018), and prevents introducing alcohol into the tissue, which can be irritating and uncomfortable.

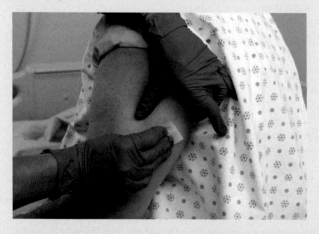

FIGURE 3. Cleaning injection site.

25. Remove the needle cap with the nondominant hand, pulling it straight off.

The cap protects the needle from contact with microorganisms. This technique lessens the risk of an accidental needlestick.

ACTION

26. Hold the syringe in the dominant hand between the thumb and forefinger. Use the thumb, index finger and middle finger on the nondominant hand to pinch up the skin and underlying fatty tissue (Figure 4). Inject the needle quickly at a 45- or 90-degree angle, depending on the amount of underlying subcutaneous tissue. (Figure 5).

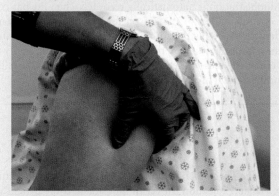

FIGURE 4. Pinching up the skin and underlying fatty tissue.

27. Move your nondominant hand to the lower end of the syringe and slide your dominant hand to the end of the plunger, taking care to avoid moving the syringe. Alternatively, move your middle finger into place on the syringe, holding the syringe with your thumb and middle finger, and move your index finger to the end of the plunger; taking care to avoid moving the syringe.

28. Inject the medication. Withdraw the needle quickly at the same angle at which it was inserted, while supporting the surrounding tissue with your nondominant hand.

29. Do not recap the used needle. Engage the safety shield or needle guard.

30. If blood or clear fluid appears at the site after withdrawing the needle, use a gauze square to apply gentle pressure to the site. **Do not massage the site.**

 31. Remove gloves and perform hand hygiene. Assist the patient to a position of comfort.

32. Discard the needle and syringe in an appropriate container, such as a sharps receptacle.

 33. Remove additional PPE, if used. Perform hand hygiene.

34. Document the administration of the medication immediately after administration.

35. Evaluate the patient's response to the medication within the appropriate time frame for the particular medication.

RATIONALE

Pinching up the skin and underlying fatty tissue lifts the adipose tissue away from underlying muscle and tissue (Shepherd, 2018b; Wolicki & Miller, 2020). Inserting the needle quickly causes less pain to the patient. For a person with a limited amount of subcutaneous tissue, insert the needle at a 45-degree angle (Shepherd, 2018b).

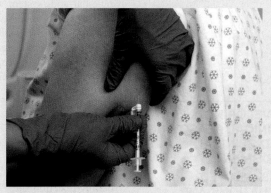

FIGURE 5. Inserting needle.

This allows for stabilization of the syringe and avoids movement. Moving the syringe could cause damage to the tissues and inadvertent administration into an incorrect area.

Slow withdrawal of the needle pulls the tissues and causes discomfort. Applying counter traction around the injection site helps to prevent pulling on the tissue as the needle is withdrawn. Removing the needle at the same angle at which it was inserted minimizes tissue damage and discomfort for the patient.

Safety shield or needle guard prevents accidental needlestick.

Massaging the site can damage underlying tissue and increase the absorption of the medication (Taylor et al., 2023). Massaging after heparin administration can contribute to hematoma formation.

Removing gloves and performing hand hygiene reduces the risk of contamination of other items and the spread of microorganisms. Assisting the patient to a position of comfort promotes patient comfort.

Proper disposal of the needle prevents injury.

Proper removal of PPE reduces the risk of infection transmission and contamination of other items. Hand hygiene prevents the spread of microorganisms.

Timely documentation helps to ensure patient safety.

The patient needs to be evaluated for therapeutic and adverse effects from the medication.

(continued on page 242)

Skill 5-7 ▶ Administering a Subcutaneous Injection *(continued)*

EVALUATION

The expected outcomes have been met when the patient has received the medication via the subcutaneous route and has experienced the intended effect of the medication, the patient did not experience adverse effects, and the patient has verbalized an understanding of the medication regimen.

DOCUMENTATION

Guidelines

Record each medication given on the eMAR/MAR or health record using the required format immediately after administration, including date, dose, time, and the site of administration. If using a bar-code system, medication administration is automatically recorded when the bar code is scanned. PRN medications require documentation of the reason for administration. Prompt recording avoids the possibility of accidentally repeating the administration of the drug. If the drug was refused or omitted, record this in the appropriate area on the medication record and notify the health care team as appropriate. This verifies the reason medication was omitted and ensures that health care personnel providing care for the patient are aware of the occurrence.

DEVELOPING CLINICAL REASONING AND CLINICAL JUDGMENT

UNEXPECTED SITUATIONS AND ASSOCIATED INTERVENTIONS

- *Patient refuses to let you administer medication in a different location:* Explain the rationale behind rotating injection sites. Discuss other available injection sites with the patient. If the patient will still not allow injection in another area, administer medication to patient, document the patient's refusal of rotation of the injection site and discussion, and notify the health care team.
- *You stick yourself with the needle before injection:* Discard the needle and syringe appropriately. Follow facility policy regarding needlestick injury. Prepare a new syringe with medication and administer to the patient. Communicate and document the incident according to facility policy.
- *You stick yourself with the needle after injection:* Discard the needle and syringe appropriately. Communicate and document the incident according to facility policy.
- *During injection, patient pulls away from the needle before the medication is delivered fully:* Remove and appropriately discard the needle. Attach a new needle to the syringe and administer the remaining medication at a different site. Document events and interventions according to facility policy.

SPECIAL CONSIDERATIONS

General Considerations

- Ongoing assessment is an important part of nursing care for both evaluation of patient response to administered medications and early detection of adverse drug reactions. If an adverse effect is suspected, withhold further medication doses and notify the health care team. Additional intervention is based on type of reaction and patient assessment.
- Injection speed does not seem to influence pain sensation associated with subcutaneous injection (Heise et al., 2014; Mohammady et al., 2017; Pich, 2020; Zijlstra et al., 2018).
- Because absorption rates vary from site to site, it is recommended that patients administering their own insulin use the same area of the body at the same time every day to ensure more consistent absorption and prevent tissue changes from repeated use of the same site (ADA, 2020; Frandsen & Pennington, 2021; Karch, 2020). For instance, every morning the patient may use the abdomen for insulin injection, and every evening before dinner, the patient may inject the insulin into the arms or thighs. Keep in mind that the best absorption occurs in the abdomen. In each case, the injections should be given an inch away from the previous injection site. A small spot bandage or piece of tape can be used to mark the first injection site, with subsequent injections rotated in a circle around that site. After this area has been used, an adjacent site, an inch away, can be selected, using the same rotation format. A marked diagram incorporated into the patient's plan of care is also helpful for noting alternative sites. Patients should be encouraged to not rely on memory. The patient cannot always recall the site of the previous injection, therefore, the site of administration should be recorded. When the patient is receiving care from a health care provider, the site of administration must be recorded in the patient's health record.
- Heparin is administered subcutaneously. The abdomen is the most commonly used administration site. Avoid the area 2 inches around the umbilicus and the belt line.

- Certain medications have specific manufacturer-recommended administration requirements. For example, enoxaparin (low–molecular-weight heparin) should be administered alternating between the left and right anterolateral and left and right posterolateral abdominal wall (Sanofi-Aventis, 2020) (Figure 6). To administer the medication, pinch the tissue gently to form a skin fold and insert the needle at a 90-degree angle (Sanofi-Aventis, 2020). Enoxaparin is packaged in a prefilled syringe with an air bubble. **Do not expel the air bubble before administration** (Sanofi-Aventis, 2020).

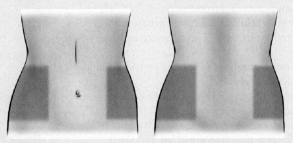

Anterior view   Posterior view

FIGURE 6. Sites for administration of enoxaparin.

Infant and Child Considerations	- Do not tell a child that an injection will not hurt. Describe the feel of the injection as a pinch or a sting. A child who believes you have been dishonest is less likely to cooperate with future procedures.
Older Adult Considerations	- Many older adults have less adipose tissue. Adjust the needle length and insertion angle accordingly. (Refer to discussion earlier in Skill.) You do not want to inadvertently give a subcutaneous medication intramuscularly.
Community-Based Care Considerations	- Reuse of syringes in the home setting is not recommended. - The use of antimicrobial swabs to clean the injection site in home environments may be unnecessary; patients may use soap and water to clean the site if the area is visibly soiled (Sexson et al., 2016). - Because absorption rates vary from site to site, it is recommended that patients administering their own insulin use the same area of the body at the same time every day to ensure more consistent absorption and prevent tissue changes from repeated use of the same site (ADA, 2020; Frandsen & Pennington, 2021). Refer to the information discussed in the "General Considerations" section of this Skill. - Encourage patients to consult the policies of their local government regarding contaminated and sharps waste disposal. - The U.S. Food & Drug Administration (FDA, 2021) recommends a two-step process for properly disposing of used needles and other sharps by patients, family members, and caregivers: (1) Needles and other sharps should be placed in a sharps disposal container immediately after they have been used to reduce the risk of needle sticks, cuts, and punctures from loose sharps. (2) Used sharps disposal containers should be disposed of according to community guidelines; guidelines and disposal programs vary depending on location. Patients should consult local trash removal services and the local health department to identify available disposal methods. Never use glass containers. - Sharps disposal methods (depending on community location) include drop boxes or supervised collection sites, household hazardous waste collection sites, mail-back programs, and residential special waste pick-up services (FDA, 2021). - If a patient, family member, or caregiver does not want to purchase a sharps container, an empty laundry detergent or bleach bottle may be used. It must be a strong plastic container with a screw-on lid, *not* an empty plastic water or soda bottle or other type of thin plastic container (SafeNeedleDisposal.org, 2021). Label the container as sharps and not for recycling. The screw-on top should be used to close the container for disposal, and containers should be sealed with strong tape (e.g., duct tape) (SafeNeedleDisposal.org, 2021). - Sharps disposal containers should be kept out of reach of children and pets (FDA, 2021). - The Safe Needle Disposal resource page provides information on needle disposal takeback programs and an interactive tool to locate state waste links (FDA, 2021; SafeNeedleDisposal.org, 2022).

(continued on page 244)

Skill 5-7 ▶ Administering a Subcutaneous Injection *(continued)*

Skill Variation ▶ Using an Insulin Injection Pen to Administer Insulin via the Subcutaneous Route

Prepare medication as outlined in Steps 1–23 above (Skill 5-7).

1. Remove the pen cap.
2. Insert an insulin cartridge into the pen, if necessary, following the manufacturer's directions.
3. If administering an insulin suspension, gently roll the pen 10 times and invert the pen 10 times to mix the insulin.
4. Scrub the self-sealing seal end of the pen cartridge holder with an antimicrobial swab.
5. Remove the protective paper tab from the needle.
6. Screw the needle onto the reservoir.
7. Remove the outer and inner needle caps. (Patients at home should reserve the outer shield for later use.)
8. Dial the dose selector to 2 units to prime the pen (perform an *air shot*) to get rid of air and make certain the pen is working properly.
9. Hold the pen upright and tap to force any air bubbles to the top.
10. Hold the pen upright and press the injection button or plunger firmly. Watch for a drop of insulin at the needle tip.
11. Check the drug reservoir to make sure sufficient insulin is available for the dose.
12. Check that the dose selector is at 0, then dial the units of insulin for the dose.
13. Put on gloves.
14. Clean the injection site. If the pen needle is longer than 5 mm, gently pinch the skin at the injection site to form a skin fold (Becton, Dickinson and Company, 2021a).
15. Hold the pen in the palm of the hand, perpendicular to the forearm, with the thumb at the injection button end of the pen. Use the thumb for injection (Figure A).
16. Administer the subcutaneous injection. Press the injection button on the pen all the way in. Keep the button depressed and count to 10 before removing from the skin.
17. The safety shield automatically covers the needle when needle is removed from the skin. Remove the needle from the pen; a second safety shield automatically covers

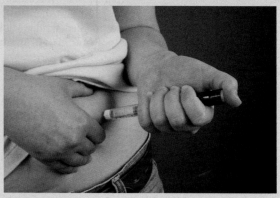

FIGURE A. Patient using insulin pen. (*Source:* Used with permission from Shutterstock. *Photo by B. Proud.*)

the back end of the needle when removed from the pen. Dispose of the needle in a sharps container.

18. Alternatively, patients at home should replace the reserved outer shield on the needle before removing the needle from the pen. Other needle removal devices and procedures exist; patients should follow the instructions provided by their health care provider related to their specific insulin pen.
19. Remove gloves and additional PPE, if used.
 20. Perform hand hygiene.

21. Document administration on the eMAR/MAR, including the injection site.

Source: Adapted from Becton, Dickinson and Company. (2021a). Injecting insulin with a pen. https://www.bd.com/en-uk/products/diabetes/diabetes-learning-centre/injection-technique/injecting-insulin-with-a-pen; Becton, Dickinson and Company. (2021b). BD AutoShield Duo™ pen needle. https://www.bd.com/en-us/offerings/capabilities/diabetes-care/pen-needles/bd-autoshield-duo-pen-needle-x857469.

Skill 5-8 ▶ Administering an Intramuscular Injection

Intramuscular injections deliver medication through the skin and subcutaneous tissues into certain muscles. Muscles have a larger and a greater number of blood vessels than subcutaneous tissue, allowing faster onset of action than with subcutaneous injections. An intramuscular injection is chosen when a reasonably rapid systemic uptake of the drug is needed by the body and when a relatively prolonged action is required. Some medications administered intramuscularly are formulated to have a longer duration of effect. The deposit of medication creates a depot at the injection site, designed to deliver slow, sustained release over hours, days, or weeks.

It is important to choose the right needle length for a particular intramuscular injection. Needle length should be based on the individual patient. (See Table 5-1 for intramuscular needle length recommendations.) Patients who are obese may require a longer needle (Wolicki & Miller, 2020), and emaciated patients may require a shorter needle. Appropriate gauge is determined by the medication being administered. In general, biologic agents and medications in aqueous solutions should be administered with a 20- to 25-gauge needle. Medications in oil-based solutions should be administered with an 18- to 25-gauge needle. Many medications come in prefilled syringe units. If a needle is provided on the prefilled unit, ensure that the needle on the unit is the appropriate length for the patient and situation.

To avoid complications, the nurse must be able to identify anatomic landmarks and site boundaries. See Figure 1 for a depiction of anatomic landmarks and site boundaries for potential intramuscular injection sites. Consider the age of the patient, medication type, and medication volume when selecting an intramuscular injection site. (See Table 5-2 for information related to intramuscular site selection.) Rotate the sites used to administer intramuscular medications when therapy requires repeated injections. Depending on the site selected, it may be necessary to reposition the patient (refer to Table 5-3).

Administer the intramuscular injection so that the needle is perpendicular to the patient's body. This ensures it is given using a 90-degree angle of injection (CDC, 2021). Figure 5-1 in the chapter opener on page 200 shows the angle of insertion for intramuscular injections.

Table 5-1   Intramuscular Injection Needle Length

SITE/AGE	NEEDLE LENGTH
Vastus lateralis (Anterolateral thigh)	5/8″ to 1.5″
Deltoid (children)	5/8″ to 1″
Deltoid (adults)	1″ to 1.5″
Ventrogluteal (adults)	1″ to 1½″

Note: Biologic sex and weight are directly related to needle length choice; the size of the muscle, the adipose tissue thickness at the injection site, the volume of medication to be administered, and the injection technique also need to be considered (Wolicki, J., & Miller, E. [2020]. Chapter 6. Vaccine administration. In J. Hamborsky, A. Kroger, & C. Wolf [Eds.], Epidemiology and prevention of vaccine-preventable diseases. *The pink book* [13th ed.]. Centers for Disease Control and Prevention. Public Health Foundation. https://www.cdc.gov/vaccines/pubs/pinkbook/vac-admin.html).

Source: Adapted from Centers for Disease Control and Prevention (CDC). (2021, May 4). *Vaccine recommendations and guidelines of the ACIP. General best practice guidelines for immunization: Best practices guidance of the Advisory Committee on Immunization Practices (ACIP).* https://www.cdc.gov/vaccines/hcp/acip-recs/general-recs/administration. html; Wolicki, J., & Miller, E. (2020). Chapter 6. Vaccine administration. In J. Hamborsky, A. Kroger, & C. Wolf (Eds.), Epidemiology and prevention of vaccine-preventable diseases. *The pink book* (13th ed.). Centers for Disease Control and Prevention. Public Health Foundation. https://www.cdc.gov/vaccines/pubs/pinkbook/vac-admin.html

Table 5-2   Intramuscular Site Selection

AGE OF PATIENT	RECOMMENDED SITE
Infants	Vastus lateralis (Anterolateral thigh)
Toddlers (1–2 years)	Vastus lateralis (Anterolateral thigh) (preferred) or deltoid if muscle size is large enough
Child/Adolescent (3–18 years)	Deltoid (preferred) or vastus lateralis (anterolateral thigh)
Adults	Deltoid (vaccines); ventrogluteal or vastus lateralis (anterolateral thigh) (general IM injections)

Source: Adapted from Arslan, G. G., & Özden, D. (2018). Creating a change in the use of ventrogluteal site for intramuscular injection. *Patient Preference and Adherence, 12,* 1749–1756. https://doi.org/10.2147/PPA.S168885; Centers for Disease Control and Prevention (CDC). (2021, May 4). *Vaccine recommendations and guidelines of the ACIP. General best practice guidelines for immunization: Best practices guidance of the Advisory Committee on Immunization Practices (ACIP).* https://www.cdc.gov/vaccines/hcp/acip-recs/general-recs/administration.html; Şanlialp Zeyrek, A., Takmak, Ş., Kurban, N. K., & Arslan, S. (2019). Systematic review and meta-analysis: Physical-procedural interventions used to reduce pain during intramuscular injections in adults. *Journal of Advanced Nursing, 75*(12), 3346–3361. https://doi.org/10.1111/jan.14183; Wolicki, J., & Miller, E. (2020). Chapter 6. Vaccine administration. In J. Hamborsky, A. Kroger, & C. Wolf (Eds.), Epidemiology and prevention of vaccine-preventable diseases. *The pink book* (13th ed.). Centers for Disease Control and Prevention. Public Health Foundation. https://www.cdc.gov/vaccines/pubs/pinkbook/vac-admin.html.

(*continued on page 246*)

Skill 5-8 ▶ Administering an Intramuscular Injection *(continued)*

Table 5-3 Patient Positioning

INJECTION SITE	PATIENT POSITION
Deltoid	Patient may sit or stand. A child may be held in an adult's lap.
Ventrogluteal	Patient may lie on the back, abdomen, or side.
Vastus lateralis (Anterolateral thigh)	Patient may sit or lie supine. Infants and young children may lie cuddled on an adult's lap, lying on the back; or be held in an upright in an adult's lap.

Source: Adapted from Taylor, C., Lynn, P., & Bartlett, J. (2023). *Fundamentals of nursing: The art and science of person-centered care* (10th ed.). Wolters Kluwer.

Wolicki, J., & Miller, E. (2020). Chapter 6. Vaccine administration. In J. Hamborsky, A. Kroger, & C. Wolf (Eds.), Epidemiology and prevention of vaccine-preventable diseases. *The pink book* (13th ed.). Centers for Disease Control and Prevention. Public Health Foundation. https://www.cdc.gov/vaccines/pubs/pinkbook/vac-admin.html.

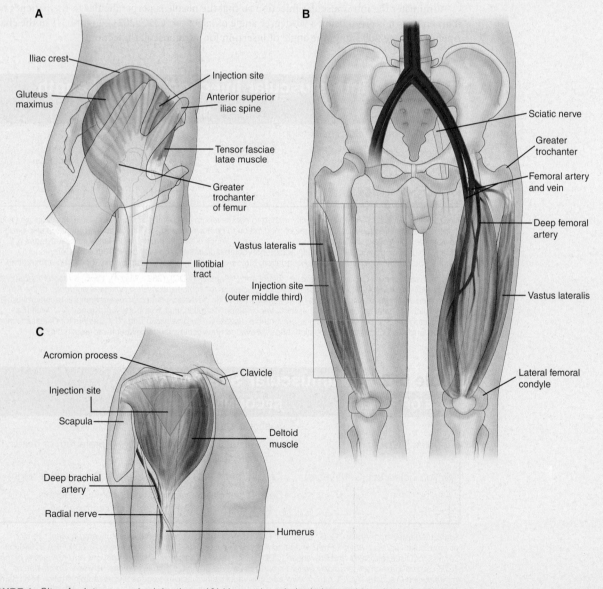

FIGURE 1. Sites for intramuscular injections. (**A**) Ventrogluteal site is located by placing palm on greater trochanter and index finger on the anterosuperior iliac spine and extend the middle finger dorsally, palpating the iliac crest; administer in the center of the triangle formed with the fingers. (**B**) Vastus lateralis site is identified by dividing the thigh into thirds, horizontally and vertically; and administer in the outer middle third. (**C**) Deltoid muscle site is located by palpating lower edge of acromion process and forming a triangle at the midpoint in line with the axilla on the lateral aspect of the upper arm, with the base of the triangle at the acromion process; administer in the center of the triangle.

The medication volume that can be administered intramuscularly varies based on the intended site. In general, 1 to 5 mL is the accepted volume range, with a limitation of 1 mL of solution at the deltoid site. However, up to 2 mL may be administered at the deltoid site, depending on the size of the individual patient's muscle (Gutierrez & Munakomi, 2021). The less-developed muscles of children and older people limit the intramuscular injection to 1 to 2 mL.

Many of the drugs given intramuscularly can cause irritation to subcutaneous tissues when backflow into the tissues occurs along the injection track. Therefore, the Z-track technique is recommended for all intramuscular injections (particularly nonvaccine injections) to ensure that medication does not leak back along the needle track and into the subcutaneous tissue (Hopkins & Arias, 2013; Karch, 2020; Yilmaz et al., 2016). This technique reduces pain and discomfort (Şanlialp Zeyrek et al., 2019), particularly for patients receiving injections over an extended period. The Z-track method is also suggested for older adults who have decreased muscle mass. Some medications, such as iron, are best given via the Z-track method due to the irritation and discoloration associated with the medication (Karch, 2020). An alternative method for intramuscular injection is to stretch the skin flat between two fingers and hold it taut for needle insertion. The decision regarding use of the Z-track method or stretching the skin at the site is based on the individual patient and nursing judgment (Taylor et al., 2023). Knowledge of landmarks and risks, along with an assessment of muscle size and consideration of the medication itself are of paramount importance for the nurse.

Aspiration, or pulling back on the plunger to check if a blood vessel has been entered, is not necessary and has not proved to be a reliable indicator of needle placement. The use of correct technique and recommended anatomic injection sites results in a very small likelihood of injecting into a blood vessel and there is no scientific evidence to support aspiration (CDC, 2021; Davidson & Rourke, 2013; Sisson, 2015). The World Health Organization (WHO, 2020) and CDC (2015a) do not include aspiration in the steps for intramuscular injection of vaccines. The wide-spread use of auto-disable (AD) syringes encouraged by the WHO (2020) further reinforces no aspiration with intramuscular vaccine administration, since most AD syringes are not designed to aspirate (Sepah et al., 2017). Some medication manufacturers indicate that aspiration may be recommended when administering certain medications, at certain dosages and certain rates, but more research needs to be done on this topic (Mraz et al., 2018; Sepah et al., 2017; Thomas et al., 2016). Consult facility policy and manufacturer recommendations to ensure safe administration.

Refer to Box 5-1 in Skill 5-7 on page 237 for techniques for reducing discomfort when injecting medications subcutaneously or intramuscularly.

The following skill outlines administration of an intramuscular injection using the Z-track technique. If, based on assessment of the particular circumstances for an individual patient, the nurse decides not to use the Z-track technique, the skin should be stretched flat between two fingers and held taut for needle insertion.

DELEGATION CONSIDERATIONS

The administration of an intramuscular injection is not delegated to assistive personnel (AP). Depending on the state's nurse practice act and the organization's policies and procedures, the administration of an intramuscular injection may be delegated to licensed practical/vocational nurses (LPN/LVNs). The decision to delegate must be based on careful analysis of the patient's needs and circumstances as well as the qualifications of the person to whom the task is being delegated. Refer to the Delegation Guidelines in Appendix A.

EQUIPMENT

- Gloves
- Additional PPE, as indicated
- Prescribed medication
- Sterile syringe and needle of appropriate size and gauge
- Antimicrobial swab
- Small gauze square
- Electronic Medication Administration Record (eMAR) or Medication Administration Record (MAR)

ASSESSMENT

Assess the appropriateness of the drug for the patient. Review the medical history and allergy, assessment, and laboratory data that may influence drug administration. Check the expiration date. Assess the site on the patient where the injection is to be given. Avoid any site that is bruised, tender, hard, swollen, inflamed, or scarred. Assess the patient's knowledge of the medication. If the patient has deficient knowledge about the medication, this may be the appropriate time to begin

(continued on page 248)

Skill 5-8 ▶ Administering an Intramuscular Injection *(continued)*

education about it. If the medication may affect the patient's vital signs, assess them before administration. If the medication is intended for pain relief, assess the patient's pain before and after administration. Verify patient name, dose, route, and time of administration.

ACTUAL OR POTENTIAL HEALTH PROBLEMS AND NEEDS	Many actual or potential health problems or issues may require the use of this skill as part of related interventions. An appropriate health problem or issue may include: • Knowledge deficiency • Injury risk • Infection risk
OUTCOME IDENTIFICATION AND PLANNING	The expected outcomes to achieve when administering an intramuscular injection are that the patient receives the medication via the intramuscular route and experiences the intended effect of the medication, the patient does not experience adverse effects, and the patient verbalizes an understanding of the medication regimen.

IMPLEMENTATION

ACTION	RATIONALE
1. Gather equipment. Check each medication prescribed against the original in the health record, depending on facility policy and the medication order system in place. Clarify any inconsistencies. Check the patient's health record for allergies.	The prescription is the legal record of prescribed medication interventions. This comparison helps to identify errors that may have occurred when orders were transcribed. Computer provider order-entry (CPOE) systems allow prescribers to send electronic medication prescriptions directly to the pharmacy located in a health care facility and to outpatient pharmacies.
2. Know the actions, special nursing considerations, safe dose ranges, purpose of administration, and adverse effects of the medications to be administered. Consider the appropriateness of the medication for this patient.	This knowledge aids the nurse in evaluating the therapeutic effect of the medication in relation to the patient's health status and can also be used to educate the patient about the medication.
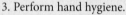3. Perform hand hygiene.	Hand hygiene prevents the spread of microorganisms.
4. Move the medication supply system to the outside of the patient's room or prepare for administration at the medication supply system in the medication area. Alternatively, access the medication administration supply system at or inside the patient's room.	Organization facilitates error-free administration and saves time.
5. Unlock the medication supply system or drawer. Enter the passcode and scan employee identification, if required.	Locking the medication supply system or drawer safeguards each patient's medication supply. Facility accrediting organizations require medication supply systems to be locked when not in use. Entering the passcode and scanning ID allows only authorized users into the system and identifies the user for documentation by the computer.
6. **Prepare medications for one patient at a time.**	This prevents errors in medication administration.
7. Read the eMAR/MAR and read the label when selecting the proper medication from the medication supply system or the patient's medication drawer.	This is the *first* check of the label.
8. Read the label and compare the label with the eMAR/MAR. Check expiration dates and perform calculations, if necessary. Scan the bar code on the package, if required.	This is the *second* check of the label. Verify calculations with another nurse to ensure safety, if necessary.
9. If necessary, withdraw the medication from an ampule or vial as described in Skills 5-3 and 5-4.	

ACTION

10. **Depending on facility policy, the third check of the label may occur at this point. If so, when all medications for one patient have been prepared, read the label and recheck the labels with the eMAR/MAR before taking the medications to the patient. However, many facilities require the third check to occur at the bedside, after identifying the patient.**

11. Label the syringe with the medication's name, dose, and amount (The Joint Commission, 2021).

12. **Log out of and/or lock the medication supply system before leaving it.**

13. Transport medications to the patient's bedside carefully and keep the medications in sight at all times.

14. **Ensure that the patient receives the medications at the correct time.**

 15. Perform hand hygiene and put on PPE, if indicated.

 16. **Identify the patient. Compare the information with the eMAR/MAR. The patient should be identified using at least two of the following methods** (The Joint Commission, 2021):

a. Check the name on the patient's identification band.

b. Check the identification number on the patient's identification band.

c. Check the birth date on the patient's identification band.

d. Ask the patient to state their name and birth date, based on facility policy.

17. Close the door to the room or pull the bedside curtain.

18. **Complete necessary assessments before administering medications. Check the patient's allergy bracelet, if present, or ask the patient about allergies. Explain the purpose and action of the medication to the patient.**

19. Scan the bar code on the patient's identification band, if required (Figure 2) (The Joint Commission, 2021).

RATIONALE

This *third* check ensures accuracy and helps to prevent errors. *Note:* Many facilities require the *third* check to occur at the bedside, after identifying the patient and before administration.

Unlabeled syringes are unidentifiable and may lead to a medication administration error (The Joint Commission, 2021).

Locking the medication supply system or drawer safeguards the patient's medication supply. Facility accrediting organizations require medication supply systems to be locked when not in use.

Careful handling and close observation prevent accidental or deliberate disarrangement of medications.

Check facility policy, which may allow for administration within a period of 30 minutes before or 30 minutes after the designated time.

Hand hygiene and PPE prevent the spread of microorganisms. PPE is required based on transmission precautions.

Identifying the patient ensures the right patient receives the medications and helps prevent errors. The patient's room number or physical location is not used as an identifier (The Joint Commission, 2021). Replace the identification band if it is missing or inaccurate in any way.

This requires a response from the patient, but illness and strange surroundings often cause patients to be confused.

This provides patient privacy.

Assessment is a prerequisite to administration of medications. Explanation provides rationale, increases knowledge, promotes patient engagement, and reduces anxiety.

This provides an additional check to ensure that the medication is given to the right patient.

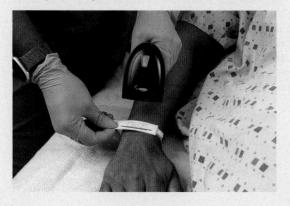

FIGURE 2. Scanning bar code on the patient's identification bracelet.

(continued on page 250)

Skill 5-8 ▶ Administering an Intramuscular Injection *(continued)*

ACTION	RATIONALE
20. **Based on facility policy, the third check of the label may occur at this point. If so, read the label and recheck the labels with the eMAR/MAR before administering the medications to the patient.**	Many facilities require the *third* check to occur at the bedside, after identifying the patient and before administration. If facility policy directs the *third* check at this time, this *third* check ensures accuracy and helps to prevent errors.
21. Put on gloves.	Gloves help prevent exposure to contaminants.
22. Select an appropriate administration site. Assist the patient to the appropriate position for the site chosen. Refer to Table 5-3. Drape, as needed, to expose only the site area being used.	Selecting the appropriate site and appropriate positioning prevent injury. Draping provides privacy and warmth.
23. **Identify the appropriate landmarks and site boundaries for the site chosen (Figure 3).**	Good visualization is necessary to establish the correct site location and to avoid complications (Taylor et al., 2023).

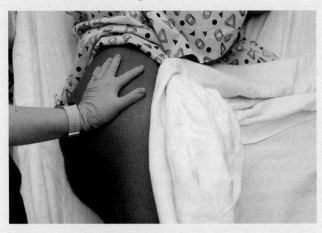

FIGURE 3. Identifying the appropriate landmarks.

ACTION	RATIONALE
24. Cleanse the site with an antimicrobial swab while wiping with a firm, circular motion and moving outward from the injection site. Consider leaving the alcohol pad on the skin with the tip of the pad pointing toward the center of the area you just prepared. Allow the skin to dry.	Pathogens on the skin can be forced into the tissues by the needle. Moving from the center outward prevents contamination of the site. Allowing the antimicrobial solution to dry completely (5 to 20 seconds) ensures complete antimicrobial effectiveness (Gorski et al., 2021; Slater et al., 2018), and prevents introducing alcohol into the tissue, which can be irritating and uncomfortable.
25. Remove the needle cap by pulling it straight off. Hold the syringe in your dominant hand between the thumb and forefinger.	This technique lessens the risk of an accidental needlestick and also prevents inadvertently unscrewing the needle from the barrel of the syringe.
26. Displace the skin in a Z-track manner. Pull or shift the skin and underlying tissue down or to one side 1 to 2 cm (Karch, 2020; Yilmaz et al., 2016) with your nondominant hand and hold the skin and tissue in this position (Figure 4). Alternatively, based on assessment of the particular circumstances for an individual patient, if the nurse decides not to use the Z-track technique, the skin should be stretched flat between two fingers and held taut for needle insertion.	Z-track technique is recommended for all intramuscular injections to ensure medication does not leak back along the needle track and into the subcutaneous tissue (Hopkins & Arias, 2013; Yilmaz et al., 2016). This technique reduces pain and discomfort, particularly for patients receiving injections over an extended period. The Z-track method is also suggested for older adults who have decreased muscle mass. Some agents, such as iron, are best given via the Z-track method due to the irritation and discoloration associated with this agent.

ACTION	RATIONALE

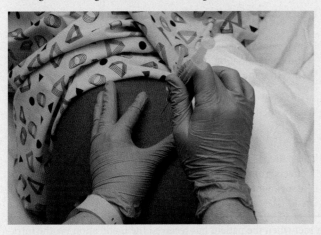

FIGURE 4. Z-track or zigzag technique is recommended for intramuscular injections. (**A**) Normal skin and tissues. (**B**) Pulling or shifting the skin and underlying tissue down or to one side. (**C**) Needle is inserted at a 90-degree angle. (**D**) Once needle is withdrawn, displaced tissue is allowed to return to its normal position, preventing solution from escaping from muscle tissue. Hand and finger positioning is adjusted for the specific administration site for accurate identification of landmarks and use of safe injection technique.

27. Quickly dart the needle into the tissue so that the needle is perpendicular to the patient's body, administering at an angle of 90 degrees (CDC, 2021) (Figure 5).	A quick injection is less painful. Inserting the needle at a 90-degree angle facilitates entry into muscle tissue.

FIGURE 5. Darting needle into tissue.

28. As soon as the needle is in place, use the thumb and forefinger of your nondominant hand to hold the lower end of the syringe, taking care to maintain the displacement of the skin and tissue. Slide your dominant hand to the end of the plunger. Inject the solution slowly.	Moving the syringe could cause damage to the tissues and inadvertent administration into an incorrect area. Rapid injection of the solution creates pressure in the tissues, resulting in discomfort.
29. Once the medication has been instilled, wait 10 seconds before withdrawing the needle.	This allows medication to begin to diffuse into the surrounding muscle tissue (Gutierrez & Munakomi, 2021).
30. Withdraw the needle smoothly and steadily at the same angle at which it was inserted, supporting tissue around the injection site with your nondominant hand. **Remove the hand holding the displaced skin and tissue only after removal of the needle, allowing the displaced skin and tissue to return to its normal position.**	Slow withdrawal of the needle pulls the tissues and causes discomfort. Applying counter traction around the injection site helps to prevent pulling on the tissue as the needle is withdrawn. Removing the needle at the same angle at which it was inserted minimizes tissue damage and discomfort for the patient. Allowing displaced skin and tissue to move back into place while needle is still inserted causes damage to the tissues.
31. Do not recap the used needle. Engage the safety shield or needle guard.	A safety shield or needle guard prevents accidental needlestick.

(continued on page 252)

Skill 5-8 ▶ Administering an Intramuscular Injection *(continued)*

ACTION	RATIONALE
32. Apply gentle pressure at the site with a dry gauze (Figure 6). **Do not massage the site.**	Light pressure causes less trauma and irritation to the tissues. Massaging can force medication into subcutaneous tissues and increase discomfort.

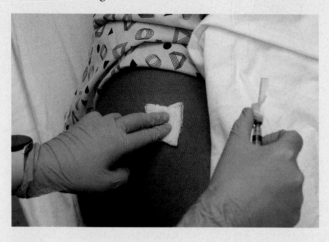

FIGURE 6. Applying gentle pressure at injection site.

ACTION	RATIONALE
33. Remove gloves and perform hand hygiene. Assist the patient to a position of comfort.	Removing gloves and performing hand hygiene reduces the risk of contamination of other items and the spread of microorganisms. Assisting the patient to a position of comfort promotes patient comfort.
34. Discard the needle and syringe in the appropriate container, such as a sharps receptacle.	Proper disposal of the needle prevents injury.
35. Remove gloves and additional PPE, if used. Perform hand hygiene.	Proper removal of PPE reduces the risk of infection transmission and contamination of other items. Hand hygiene prevents the spread of microorganisms.
36. Document the administration of the medication immediately after administration. See Documentation section below.	Timely documentation helps to ensure patient safety.
37. Evaluate the patient's response to the medication within the appropriate time frame. Assess site, if possible, within 2 to 4 hours after administration.	The patient needs to be evaluated for therapeutic and adverse effects from the medication. Visualization of the site allows for assessment of any untoward effects.

EVALUATION

The expected outcomes have been met when the patient has received the medication via the intramuscular route and experienced the intended effect of the medication, the patient did not experience adverse effects, and the patient has verbalized an understanding of the medication regimen.

DOCUMENTATION

Guidelines

Record each medication given on the eMAR/MAR or record using the required format, including date, time, and the site of administration, immediately after administration. If using a bar-code system, medication administration is automatically recorded when the bar code is scanned. PRN medications require documentation of the reason for administration. Prompt recording avoids the possibility of accidentally repeating the administration of the drug. If the drug was refused or omitted, record this in the appropriate area on the medication record and notify the health care team as appropriate. This verifies the reason medication was omitted and ensures that health care personnel providing care for the patient are aware of the occurrence.

DEVELOPING CLINICAL REASONING AND CLINICAL JUDGMENT

UNEXPECTED SITUATIONS AND ASSOCIATED INTERVENTIONS

- *You stick yourself with the needle before injection:* Discard the needle and syringe appropriately. Follow facility policy regarding needlestick injury. Prepare a new syringe with the medication and administer to the patient. Communicate and document the incident according to facility policy.
- *You stick yourself with the needle after injection:* Discard the needle and syringe appropriately. Follow facility policy regarding needlestick injury. Communicate and document the incident according to facility policy.
- *During injection, the patient pulls away from the needle before the medication is delivered fully:* Remove and appropriately discard the needle. Attach a new needle to the syringe and administer the remaining medication at a different site. Document events and interventions, according to facility policy.
- *While injecting the needle into the patient, you hit patient's bone:* Withdraw and discard the needle. Apply a new needle to the syringe and administer in an alternate site. Document the incident in the patient's health record. Notify the health care team. Communicate and document the incident according to facility policy.

SPECIAL CONSIDERATIONS

General Considerations

- Ongoing assessment is an important part of nursing care for both evaluation of patient response to administered medications and early detection of adverse drug reactions. If an adverse effect is suspected, withhold further medication doses and notify the health care team. Additional intervention is based on the type of reaction and patient assessment.
- The deltoid is the recommended site for vaccines for adults and may be used for children ages 3 to 18 years for vaccine administration (CDC, 2021).

Infant and Child Considerations

- The vastus lateralis is the preferred site for intramuscular injections in infants (age 12 months and younger) and young children (ages 1 to 2 years) (CDC, 2021). The deltoid can be used in children ages 1 to 2 years if the deltoid muscle mass is adequate (CDC, 2021).
- The deltoid is the preferred site for children ages 3 to 18 years (CDC, 2021).

Older Adult Considerations

- Muscle mass atrophies as a person ages. Take care to evaluate the patient's muscle mass and body composition. Use an appropriate needle length and gauge for patient's body composition. Choose an appropriate site based on the patient's body composition.

Community-Based Care Considerations

- The use of antimicrobial swabs to clean the injection site in home environments may be unnecessary; patients may use soap and water to clean the site if the area is visibly soiled (Sexson et al., 2016).
- Encourage patients to consult the policies of their local government regarding contaminated and sharps waste disposal.
- The U.S Food & Drug Administration (FDA, 2021) recommends a two-step process for properly disposing of used needles and other sharps by patients, family members, and caregivers. (1) Needles and other sharps should be placed in a sharps disposal container immediately after they have been used to reduce the risk of needle sticks, cuts, and punctures from loose sharps. (2) Used sharps disposal containers should be disposed of according to community guidelines; guidelines and disposal programs vary depending on location. Patients should consult local trash removal services and the local health department to identify available disposal methods. Never use glass containers.
- Sharps disposal methods (depending on community location) include drop boxes or supervised collection sites, household hazardous waste collection sites; mail-back programs, and residential special waste pick-up services (FDA, 2021).

(continued on page 254)

Skill 5-8 ▶ Administering an Intramuscular Injection *(continued)*

- If a patient, family member, or caregiver does not want to purchase a sharps container, an empty laundry detergent or bleach bottle may be used; it must be a strong plastic container with a screw-on lid, *not* an empty plastic water or soda bottle or other type of thin plastic container (SafeNeedleDisposal.org, 2021). Label the container as sharps and not for recycling. The screw-on top should be used to close the container for disposal, and containers should be sealed with strong tape (e.g., duct tape) (SafeNeedleDisposal.org, 2021).
- Sharps disposal containers should be kept out of reach of children and pets (FDA, 2021).
- The Safe Needle Disposal resource page provides information on needle disposal takeback programs and an interactive tool to locate state waste links (FDA, 2021; SafeNeedleDisposal.org, 2021).

Skill 5-9 ▶ Administering a Continuous Subcutaneous Infusion: Applying an Insulin Pump

Some medications, such as insulin and morphine, may be administered continuously via the subcutaneous route. Continuous subcutaneous insulin infusion (CSII, or insulin pump) allows for multiple preset rates of insulin delivery. These delivery systems consist of a small pump with a reservoir that delivers insulin through infusion tubing to a small plastic cannula or needle (Figure 1) or a wireless patch-pump system, which uses wireless communication to control insulin delivery into the subcutaneous tissue (Nimri et al., 2020) (Figure 2). Pumps can be programmed to deliver a continuous dose of insulin (basal) and on-demand (bolus) administration as needed for meals or an elevation in blood glucose. The settings may be adjusted as needed for things such as exercise and illness. This type of insulin administration more closely mirrors the body's normal function and promotes better blood glucose control, increases quality of life, and reduces potential microvascular and macrovascular complications of diabetes (ADCES, 2021; Nimri et al., 2020). Many insulin pumps are waterproof and interface with a smartphone. It is recommended that the site is changed every 2 to 3 days according to the manufacturer's recommendations to prevent tissue damage or absorption problems (ADCES, 2021).

Another example of a medication given via continuous subcutaneous infusion is morphine. Subcutaneous morphine infusion can be used for palliative dyspnea and pain management. Advantages of continuous subcutaneous medication infusion include the sustained rate of absorption via the subcutaneous route and convenience for the patient.

The following skill outlines steps in applying an insulin pump utilizing infusion tubing and a small needle-insertion device. There are many different manufacturers of insulin pumps. **Nurses need to be familiar with the particular pump in use by their patient and to refer to the specific manufacturer's recommendations for use.**

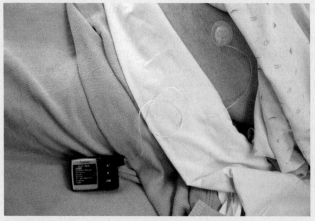

FIGURE 1. Insulin pump utilizing infusion tubing and a small needle-insertion device.

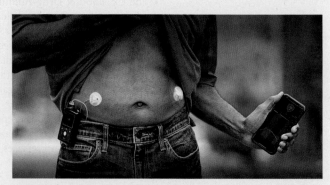

FIGURE 2. Insulin pump utilizing a wireless patch-pump system.

DELEGATION CONSIDERATIONS

The administration of a continuous subcutaneous infusion using an insulin pump is not delegated to assistive personnel (AP). Depending on the state's nurse practice act and the organization's policies and procedures, the management of an insulin pump in some settings may be delegated to licensed practical/vocational nurses (LPN/LVNs) who have received appropriate training. The decision to delegate must be based on careful analysis of the patient's needs and circumstances as well as the qualifications of the person to whom the task is being delegated. Refer to the Delegation Guidelines in Appendix A.

EQUIPMENT

- Insulin pump
- Pump syringe and vial of insulin or prefilled cartridge, as ordered
- Sterile infusion set
- Insertion (triggering) device
- Needle (24- or 22-gauge, or blunt-ended needle)
- Antimicrobial swabs
- Sterile nonocclusive dressing
- Electronic Medication Administration Record (eMAR) or Medication Administration Record (MAR)
- Disposable gloves
- Additional PPE, as indicated

ASSESSMENT

Assess the appropriateness of the drug for the patient. Review the medical history and allergy, assessment, and laboratory data that may influence drug administration. Check the expiration date. Assess the infusion site. Typical infusion sites include those areas used for subcutaneous insulin injection. Assess the area where the pump is to be applied. Do not place the pump on skin that is irritated or not intact. Assess the patient's knowledge of the medication. If the patient has a knowledge deficit about the medication, this may be the appropriate time to begin education about it. Assess the patient's blood glucose level as appropriate or as ordered. Verify patient name, dose, route, and time of administration.

ACTUAL OR POTENTIAL HEALTH PROBLEMS AND NEEDS

Many actual or potential health problems or issues may require the use of this skill as part of related interventions. An appropriate health problem or issue may include:
- Knowledge deficiency
- Risk for medication side effect
- Hyperglycemia

OUTCOME IDENTIFICATION AND PLANNING

The expected outcomes to achieve are that the device is applied successfully using aseptic technique, the medication is administered correctly, and the patient experiences the intended effect of the medication. Other outcomes that may be appropriate include the following: the patient verbalizes an understanding of the rationale for the pump use and mechanism of action, the patient's skin remains intact, and the patient does not experience unstable blood glucose levels or adverse effect.

IMPLEMENTATION

ACTION

1. Gather equipment. Check each medication prescribed against the original in the health record, depending on facility policy and the medication order system in place. Clarify any inconsistencies. Check the patient's health record for allergies.

2. Know the actions, special nursing considerations, safe dose ranges, purpose of administration, and adverse effects of the medications to be administered. Consider the appropriateness of the medication for this patient.

RATIONALE

The prescription is the legal record of prescribed medication interventions. This comparison helps to identify errors that may have occurred when orders were transcribed. Computer provider order-entry (CPOE) systems allow prescribers to send electronic medication prescriptions directly to the pharmacy located in a health care facility and to outpatient pharmacies.

This knowledge aids the nurse in evaluating the therapeutic effect of the medication in relation to the patient's health status and can also be used to educate the patient about the medication.

(continued on page 256)

Skill 5-9 ▶ Administering a Continuous Subcutaneous Infusion: Applying an Insulin Pump *(continued)*

ACTION	RATIONALE
3. Perform hand hygiene.	Hand hygiene prevents the spread of microorganisms.
4. Move the medication supply system to the outside of the patient's room or prepare for administration at the medication supply system in the medication area. Alternatively, access the medication administration supply system at or inside the patient's room.	Organization facilitates error-free administration and saves time.
5. Unlock the medication supply system or drawer. Enter the passcode and scan employee identification, if required.	Locking the medication supply system or drawer safeguards each patient's medication supply. Facility accrediting organizations require medication supply systems to be locked when not in use. Entering the passcode and scanning ID allows only authorized users into the system and identifies the user for documentation by the computer.
6. **Prepare medications for one patient at a time.**	This prevents errors in medication administration.
7. Read the eMAR/MAR and read the label when selecting the proper medication from the medication supply system or the patient's medication drawer.	This is the *first* check of the label.
8. Read the label and compare the label with the eMAR/MAR. Check expiration dates and perform calculations, if necessary. Scan the bar code on the package, if required.	This is the *second* check of the label. Verify calculations with another nurse to ensure safety, if necessary.
9. If using a prepackaged insulin syringe or cartridge, remove from packaging. Follow Skill 5-4 to prepare insulin from a vial, if necessary. Prepare enough insulin to last the patient 2 to 3 days, plus 30 units for priming tubing.	Patient will wear pump for up to 3 days without changing syringe or tubing.
10. **Depending on facility policy, the third check of the label may occur at this point. If so, when all medications for one patient have been prepared, read the label and recheck the labels with the eMAR/MAR before taking the medications to the patient. However, many facilities require the third check to occur at the bedside, after identifying the patient.**	This *third* check ensures accuracy and helps to prevent errors. *Note:* Many facilities require the *third* check to occur at the bedside, after identifying the patient and before administration.
11. Label the syringe/cartridge with the medication's name, dose, and amount (The Joint Commission, 2021).	Unlabeled syringes are unidentifiable and may lead to a medication administration error (The Joint Commission, 2021).
12. **Log out of and/or lock the medication supply system before leaving it.**	Locking the medication supply system or drawer safeguards the patient's medication supply. Facility accrediting organizations require medication supply systems to be locked when not in use.
13. Transport medications to the patient's bedside carefully and keep the medications in sight at all times.	Careful handling and close observation prevent accidental or deliberate disarrangement of medications.
14. Ensure that the patient receives the medications at the correct time.	Check facility policy, which may allow for administration within a period of 30 minutes before or 30 minutes after the designated time.
15. Perform hand hygiene and put on PPE, if indicated.	Hand hygiene and PPE prevent the spread of microorganisms. PPE is required based on transmission precautions.

ACTION	RATIONALE

16. Identify the patient. Compare the information with the eMAR/MAR. The patient should be identified using at least two of the following methods (The Joint Commission, 2021):

a. Check the name on the patient's identification band.

b. Check the identification number on the patient's identification band.

c. Check the birth date on the patient's identification band.

d. Ask the patient to state their name and birth date, based on facility policy.

17. Close the door to the room or pull the bedside curtain.

18. Complete necessary assessments before administering medications. Check the patient's allergy bracelet, if present, or ask the patient about allergies. Explain the purpose and action of the medication to the patient.

19. Scan the patient's bar code on the patient's identification band, if required (The Joint Commission, 2021) (Figure 3).

Identifying the patient ensures the right patient receives the medications and helps prevent errors. The patient's room number or physical location is not used as an identifier (The Joint Commission, 2021). Replace the identification band if it is missing or inaccurate in any way.

This requires a response from the patient, but illness and strange surroundings often cause patients to be confused.

This provides patient privacy.

Assessment is a prerequisite to administration of medications. Explanation provides rationale, increases knowledge, and reduces anxiety.

This provides an additional check to ensure that the medication is given to the right patient.

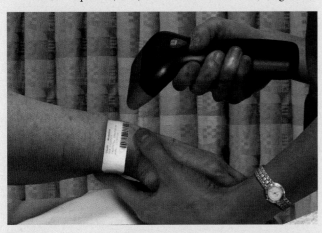

FIGURE 3. Scanning bar code on patient's identification bracelet. (*Source:* Used with permission from Shutterstock. *Photo by B. Proud.*)

20. Based on facility policy, the third check of the label may occur at this point. If so, read the label and recheck the labels with the eMAR/MAR before administering the medications to the patient.

21. Put on gloves.

22. Remove the cap from the syringe or insulin cartridge (Figure 4). Attach sterile tubing to the syringe or insulin cartridge. Open the pump and place the syringe or cartridge in compartment according to the manufacturer's directions (Figure 5). Close the pump.

Many facilities require the *third* check to occur at the bedside, after identifying the patient and before administration. If facility policy directs the *third* check at this time, this *third* check ensures accuracy and helps to prevent errors.

Gloves prevent contact with blood and body fluids.

Tubing must be attached correctly, and the syringe must be placed in pump correctly for insulin delivery.

(continued on page 258)

Skill 5-9 ▶ Administering a Continuous Subcutaneous Infusion: Applying an Insulin Pump *(continued)*

ACTION	RATIONALE

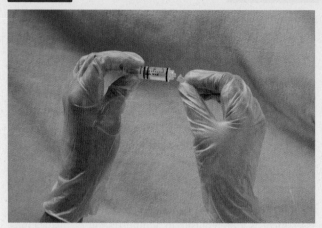

FIGURE 4. Removing cap from syringe or insulin cartridge.

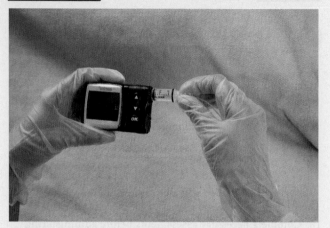

FIGURE 5. Placing syringe or cartridge in compartment according to the manufacturer's directions.

23. Initiate priming of the tubing, according to the manufacturer's directions. Program the pump according to the manufacturer's recommendations following prescribed insulin regimen (Figure 6). **Check for any bubbles in the tubing.**

Removing all the air from the tubing and correct programming of pump ensures the patient receives the correct dose of insulin.

24. Activate the delivery device. Place the needle between prongs of the insertion device with the sharp edge facing out. Push the insertion set down until a click is heard.

To ensure correct placement of insulin pump needle, an insertion device must be used.

25. Select an appropriate administration site. Assist the patient to the appropriate position for the site chosen. Drape, as needed, to expose only the site area to be used.

Using the appropriate site and appropriate positioning prevents injury. Draping maintains privacy and warmth.

26. **Identify the appropriate landmarks for the site chosen.**

Good visualization is necessary to establish the correct site location and to avoid complications (Taylor et al., 2023).

27. Cleanse the site with an antimicrobial swab while wiping with a firm, circular motion and moving outward from the injection site (Figure 7). Allow the skin to dry.

Pathogens on the skin can be forced into the tissues by the needle. Moving from the center outward prevents contamination of the site. Allowing the antimicrobial solution to dry completely ensures complete antimicrobial effectiveness (Gorski et al., 2021; Slater et al., 2018), and prevents introducing alcohol into the tissue, which can be irritating and uncomfortable.

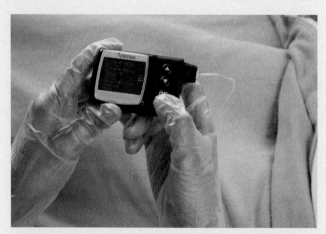

FIGURE 6. Programming pump according to prescribed insulin dosing following manufacturer's guidelines for the device.

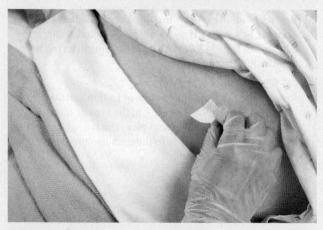

FIGURE 7. Cleansing area around injection site with antimicrobial swab.

ACTION

28. Remove paper from adhesive backing. Remove the needle guard. Pinch skin at the insertion site, press the insertion device on the site, and press the release button to insert the needle. Remove the triggering device. Alternatively, if a needle was used to introduce a subcutaneous catheter and then withdrawn, engage the safety shield or needle guard.

29. Apply a sterile occlusive dressing over the insertion site, if not part of the insertion device (Figure 8). Attach the pump to patient's clothing, as desired.

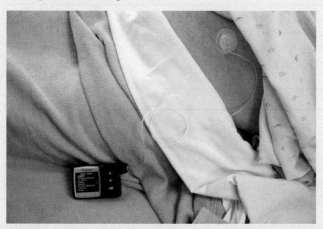

30. Remove gloves and perform hand hygiene. Assist the patient to a position of comfort.

31. If a needle was used to introduce a subcutaneous catheter and then withdrawn, discard the needle and syringe in the appropriate receptacle, such as a sharps receptacle.

32. Remove additional PPE, if used. Perform hand hygiene.

33. Document the administration of the medication immediately after administration. See Documentation section below.

34. Evaluate the patient's response to the medication within the appropriate time frame. Monitor the patient's blood glucose levels, as appropriate, or as ordered.

RATIONALE

To ensure delivery of insulin into subcutaneous tissue, a skin fold is made with a pinch *before* insertion of the medication. Safety shield or needle guard prevents accidental needlestick.

Dressing prevents contamination of site. The pump can be dislodged easily if not attached securely to patient.

FIGURE 8. Insulin pump in place.

Removing gloves and performing hand hygiene reduces the risk of contamination of other items and the spread of microorganisms. Assisting the patient to a position of comfort promotes patient comfort.

Proper disposal of the needle prevents injury.

Proper removal of PPE reduces the risk of infection transmission and contamination of other items. Hand hygiene prevents the spread of microorganisms.

Timely documentation helps to ensure patient safety.

The patient needs to be evaluated to ensure that the pump is delivering the drug appropriately. The patient needs to be evaluated for therapeutic and adverse effects from the medication.

EVALUATION

The expected outcomes have been met when the device was applied successfully, the medication was administered correctly, the patient has experienced the intended effect of the medication, the patient has verbalized an understanding of the rationale for the pump use and mechanism of action, the patient's skin remained intact, and the patient did not experience unstable blood glucose levels or adverse effect.

(continued on page 260)

Skill 5-9 ▶ Administering a Continuous Subcutaneous Infusion: Applying an Insulin Pump *(continued)*

DOCUMENTATION

Guidelines

Document the application of the pump, the type of insulin used, pump settings, insertion site, and any teaching done with the patient on the eMAR/MAR or record using the required format, including date, time, and the site of administration, immediately after administration. If using a bar-code system, medication administration is automatically recorded when the bar code is scanned. PRN medications require documentation of the reason for administration. Prompt recording avoids the possibility of accidentally repeating the administration of the drug. If the drug was refused or omitted, record this in the appropriate area on the medication record and notify the health care team. This verifies the reason medication was omitted and ensures that health care personnel providing care for the patient are aware of the occurrence.

Sample Documentation

9/22/25 1000 Insulin pump inserted by patient on left upper quadrant of abdomen with minimal assistance. Pump filled with 300 units (3 mL) of lispro insulin. Rate set at 1 unit per hour. Patient verbalized desire to apply pump without assistance when site next changed.

—B. Clapp, RN

DEVELOPING CLINICAL REASONING AND CLINICAL JUDGMENT

UNEXPECTED SITUATIONS AND ASSOCIATED INTERVENTIONS

- *After the pump is attached to the patient, a large amount of air is noted in tubing:* Remove the pump from the patient. Obtain a new sterile tubing with insertion needle. Prime the tubing and reinsert.
- *Patient must rotate site more frequently than every 2 to 3 days due to insulin usage:* Check the manufacturer's recommendations. Most pumps are initially set in a smaller mode but can be changed for a larger amount of insulin delivery.
- *Patient expresses unwillingness to rotate site at least every 3 days:* Inform the patient that absorption of medication decreases after 3 days, which may increase their need for insulin. Rotating sites prevents this decrease in absorption from developing. In addition, site rotation reduces risk of infection at the site.
- *You note that the insertion site is now erythematous:* Remove the stylet, obtain a new pump setup, and insert at a different site at least 1 inch from the old site.
- *Occlusive dressing will not stick due to perspiration:* Apply a skin barrier around the insertion site but not over the insertion site.

SPECIAL CONSIDERATIONS

General Considerations

- The U.S. FDA has approved an insulin pump that responds to sensor data to adjust basal rates, suspend on low or impending low rates, and give automatic correction bolus doses when glucose is approaching predetermined targets (ADCES, 2021).
- Assess infusion site areas routinely for inflammation, allergic reactions, infection, and lipodystrophy (ADCES, 2021).
- Good hygiene and frequent catheter site changes reduce the risk of site complications. Change the catheter site every 2 to 3 days (ADCES, 2021).
- Adverse cutaneous reactions, such as contact dermatitis and allergic contact dermatitis, are sometimes an issue with insulin pumps (Herman et al., 2020). Routine assessment of insertion and pump sites is important for early detection and intervention (Ahrensbøll-Friis et al., 2021; Herman et al., 2020).
- In an in-patient setting, insulin self-administered by the patient through the insulin pump should be communicated to the nurse at the time of administration. This allows for accurate documentation of insulin requirements.

- Patient and family/caregiver education should include information about the technical components of the insulin pump, including how to insert/change the battery, filling and inserting the insulin cartridge/reservoir, how to insert/change the infusion set and tubing (if applicable), how to input information for the pump to calculate appropriate insulin dosages, noting program basal rate changes, how to review the pump history, and how to troubleshoot to solve potential problems with the pump (ADCES, 2021).
- Ongoing assessment is an important part of nursing care for both evaluation of patient response to administered medications and early detection of adverse reactions. If an adverse effect is suspected, withhold further medication doses and notify the health care team. Additional intervention is based on type of reaction and patient assessment.

Community-Based Care Considerations

- Encourage patients to consult the policies of their local government regarding contaminated and sharps waste disposal.
- The U.S Food & Drug Administration (FDA, 2021) recommends a two-step process for properly disposing of used needles and other sharps by patients, family members and caregivers. (1) Needles and other sharps should be placed in a sharps disposal container immediately after they have been used to reduce the risk of needle sticks, cuts, and punctures from loose sharps. (2) Used sharps disposal containers should be disposed of according to community guidelines; guidelines and disposal programs vary depending on location. Patients should consult local trash removal services and the local health department to identify available disposal methods. Never use glass containers.
- Sharps disposal methods (depending on community location) include drop boxes or supervised collection sites, household hazardous waste collection sites, mail-back programs, and residential special waste pick-up services (FDA, 2021).
- If a patient, family member, or caregiver does not want to purchase a sharps container, an empty laundry detergent or bleach bottle may be used; it must be a strong plastic container with a screw-on lid, *not* an empty plastic water or soda bottle or other type of thin plastic container (SafeNeedleDisposal.org, 2021). Label the container as sharps and not for recycling. The screw-on top should be used to close the container for disposal, and containers should be sealed with strong tape (e.g., duct tape) (SafeNeedleDisposal.org, 2021).
- Sharps disposal containers should be kept out of reach of children and pets (FDA, 2021).
- The Safe Needle Disposal resource page provides information on needle disposal takeback programs and an interactive tool to locate state waste links (FDA, 2021; SafeNeedleDisposal.org, 2021).

EVIDENCE FOR PRACTICE ▶

CONTINUOUS SUBCUTANEOUS INSULIN INFUSION (CSII)

Association of Diabetes Care & Education Specialists (ADCES). (2021, March). ADCES practice paper. Continuous subcutaneous insulin infusion (CSII) without and with sensor integration. https://www.diabeteseducator.org/docs/default-source/default-document-library/continuous-subcutaneous-insulin-infusion-2018-v2.pdf?sfvrsn=4

This practice paper provides information to support maintaining a high level of expertise in patient care and education for health care professionals who include insulin pump and sensor training in their professional practice. The paper also outlines topics that should be covered by diabetes care and education specialists when teaching people with diabetes and their family/caregivers. These guidelines are directed to diabetes nurse educators but provide best-practice guidelines for all nurses caring for patients with diabetes considering or using continuous subcutaneous insulin infusion (CSII).

Skill 5-10

Administering Medications by Intravenous Bolus or Push Through an Intravenous Infusion

A medication can be administered via the **intravenous (IV) route** as an IV bolus or push through a venous access device being used for continuous infusion of fluid. This involves a single injection of a concentrated solution directly into an IV access. Drugs given by IV push are used for intermittent dosing or to treat emergencies. The drug is administered at the rate recommended by the manufacturer, supported by evidence for practice, or in accordance with approved institutional guidelines (Institute for Safe Medication Practices, 2015, p. 13). **Confirm exact administration times by consulting a drug reference, package insert, or a pharmacist. Appropriately label all clinician-prepared syringes of IV push medications or solutions, unless the medication or solution is prepared at the patient's bedside and is immediately administered to the patient** (ISMP, 2015, p. 12).

DELEGATION CONSIDERATIONS

The administration of medications by intravenous bolus is not delegated to assistive personnel (AP). Depending on the state's nurse practice act and the organization's policies and procedures, the administration of specified intravenous medications in some settings may be delegated to licensed practical/vocational nurses (LPN/LVNs) who have received appropriate training. The decision to delegate must be based on careful analysis of the patient's needs and circumstances as well as the qualifications of the person to whom the task is being delegated. Refer to the Delegation Guidelines in Appendix A.

EQUIPMENT

- Antimicrobial swab
- Watch or clock with second hand
- Gloves
- Additional PPE, as indicated
- Prescribed medication
- Two normal saline flushes prepared in a syringe (3 to 10 mL) according to facility policy
- Passive disinfection caps (based on facility policy)
- Syringe with a needleless device or 23- to 25-gauge, 1-inch needle (follow facility policy)
- Electronic Medication Administration Record (eMAR) or Medication Administration Record (MAR)

ASSESSMENT

Assess the appropriateness of the drug for the patient. Review the medical history and allergy, assessment, and laboratory data that may influence drug administration. Check the expiration date. Assess the compatibility of the ordered medication and the IV fluid. Assess the patient's IV site for signs of any complications. (Refer to Fundamentals Review 16-3 and Box 16-2 in Chapter 16 on pages 1005 and 1021.) Assess the patient's knowledge of the medication. If the patient has a knowledge deficit about the medication, this may be the appropriate time to begin education about the medication. If the medication may affect the patient's vital signs, assess them before administration. If the medication is for pain relief, assess the patient's pain before and after administration. Verify the patient's name, dose, route, and time of administration.

ACTUAL OR POTENTIAL HEALTH PROBLEMS AND NEEDS

Many actual or potential health problems or issues may require the use of this skill as part of related interventions. An appropriate health problem or issue may include:
- Injury risk
- Risk for adverse medication interaction
- Knowledge deficiency

OUTCOME IDENTIFICATION AND PLANNING

The expected outcomes to achieve are that the medication is given safely via the IV route, and the patient experiences the intended effect of the medication. Other outcomes that may be appropriate include the following: the patient experiences no adverse effects, and the patient verbalizes an understanding of and engages with the medication regimen.

IMPLEMENTATION

ACTION	RATIONALE

1. Gather equipment. Check each medication prescribed against the original in the health record, depending on facility policy and the medication order system in place. Clarify any inconsistencies. Check the patient's health record for allergies. Check a drug resource to clarify whether the medication needs to be diluted before administration. Check the administration rate.

The prescription is the legal record of prescribed medication interventions. This comparison helps to identify errors that may have occurred when orders were transcribed. Computer provider order-entry (CPOE) systems allow prescribers to send electronic medication prescriptions directly to the pharmacy located in a health care facility and to outpatient pharmacies. Compatibility of medication and solution prevents complications. Delivers the correct dose of medication as prescribed.

2. Know the actions, special nursing considerations, safe dose ranges, purpose of administration, and adverse effects of the medications to be administered. Consider the appropriateness of the medication for this patient.

This knowledge aids the nurse in evaluating the therapeutic effect of the medication in relation to the patient's health status and can also be used to educate the patient about the medication.

3. Perform hand hygiene.

Hand hygiene prevents the spread of microorganisms.

4. Move the medication supply system to the outside of the patient's room or prepare for administration at the medication supply system in the medication area. Alternatively, access the medication administration supply system at or inside the patient's room.

Organization facilitates error-free administration and saves time.

5. Unlock the medication supply system or drawer. Enter the passcode and scan employee identification, if required.

Locking the medication supply system or drawer safeguards each patient's medication supply. Facility accrediting organizations require medication supply systems to be locked when not in use. Entering the passcode and scanning ID allows only authorized users into the system and identifies the user for documentation by the computer.

6. **Prepare medications for one patient at a time.**

This prevents errors in medication administration.

7. Read the eMAR/MAR and select the proper medication from the medication supply system or the patient's medication drawer.

This is the *first* check of the label.

8. Compare the label with the eMAR/MAR. Check expiration dates and perform calculations, if necessary. Scan the bar code on the package, if required.

This is the *second* check of the label. Verify calculations with another nurse to ensure safety, if necessary.

9. If necessary, withdraw the medication from an ampule or vial as described in Skills 5-3 and 5-4.

10. **Depending on facility policy, the third check of the label may occur at this point. If so, when all medications for one patient have been prepared, recheck the labels with the eMAR/MAR before taking the medications to the patient. However, many facilities require the third check to occur at the bedside, after identifying the patient.**

This *third* check ensures accuracy and helps to prevent errors. *Note:* Many facilities require the *third* check to occur at the bedside, after identifying the patient and before administration.

11. Label the syringe with the medication's name, dose, and amount (The Joint Commission, 2021).

Unlabeled syringes are unidentifiable and may lead to a medication administration error (The Joint Commission, 2021). Appropriately label all clinician-prepared syringes of IV push medications or solutions, unless the medication or solution is prepared at the patient's bedside and is immediately administered to the patient (ISMP, 2015, p. 12).

12. **Log out of and/or lock the medication supply system before leaving it.**

Locking the medication supply system or drawer safeguards the patient's medication supply. Facility accrediting organizations require medication supply systems to be locked when not in use.

(*continued on page 264*)

Skill 5-10 ▶ Administering Medications by Intravenous Bolus or Push Through an Intravenous Infusion *(continued)*

ACTION	RATIONALE
13. Transport medications and equipment to the patient's bedside carefully and keep the medications in sight at all times.	Careful handling and close observation prevent accidental or deliberate disarrangement of medications. Having equipment available saves time and facilitates performance of the task.
14. **Ensure that the patient receives the medications at the correct time.**	Check facility policy, which may allow for administration within a period of 30 minutes before or 30 minutes after the designated time.
15. Perform hand hygiene and put on PPE, if indicated.	Hand hygiene and PPE prevent the spread of microorganisms. PPE is required based on transmission precautions.
16. **Identify the patient. Compare the information with the eMAR/MAR. The patient should be identified using at least two of the following methods** (The Joint Commission, 2021):	Identifying the patient ensures the right patient receives the medications and helps prevent errors. The patient's room number or physical location is not used as an identifier (The Joint Commission, 2021). Replace the identification band if it is missing or inaccurate in any way.
a. Check the name on the patient's identification band.	This requires a response from the patient, but illness and strange surroundings often cause patients to be confused.
b. Check the identification number on the patient's identification band.	
c. Check the birth date on the patient's identification band.	
d. Ask the patient to state their name and birth date, based on facility policy.	
17. Close the door to the room or pull the bedside curtain.	This provides patient privacy.
18. **Complete necessary assessments before administering medications. Check the patient's allergy bracelet, if present, or ask the patient about allergies. Explain the purpose and action of the medication to the patient.**	Assessment is a prerequisite to administration of medications. Explanation provides rationale, increases knowledge, and reduces anxiety.
19. Scan the patient's bar code on the identification band, if required (The Joint Commission, 2021).	This provides an additional check to ensure that the medication is given to the right patient.
20. **Based on facility policy, the third check of the label may occur at this point. If so, recheck the label with the eMAR/MAR before administering the medications to the patient.**	Many facilities require the *third* check to occur at the bedside, after identifying the patient and before administration. If facility policy directs the *third* check at this time, this *third* check ensures accuracy and helps to prevent errors.
21. Assess the IV site for the presence of inflammation or infiltration or other signs of complications.	IV medication must be given directly into a vein for safe administration.
22. If the IV infusion is being administered via an infusion pump, pause the pump.	Pausing prevents infusion of fluid during bolus administration and activation of pump occlusion alarms.
23. Put on gloves.	Gloves prevent contact with blood and body fluids.
24. Select the injection port on the administration set that is closest to the patient. Close the clamp on the administration set immediately above the injection port (Figure 1). Do not disconnect the administration set from the venous access device hub (Gorski et al., 2021).	Using the port closest to the needle insertion site minimizes dilution of the medication. Closing the clamp immediately above the access port ensures the medication is administered to the patient and prevents the medication from backing up the tubing.

ACTION

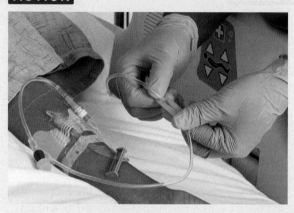

FIGURE 1. Closing the clamp on the administration set.

25. Remove the passive disinfection cap from the needleless connector or end cap on the infusion set injection port (Figure 2). Alternatively, if a passive disinfection cap is not in place, use an antimicrobial swab to vigorously disinfect the connection surface and sides of the needleless connector or end cap on the injection port and allow it to dry.

26. Uncap the saline flush syringe. Insert the saline flush syringe into the needleless connector or end cap on the injection port on the administration tubing (Figure 3).

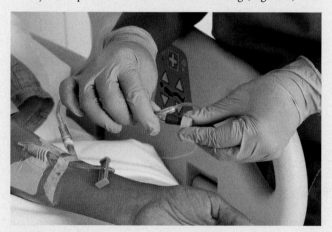

FIGURE 2. Removing the passive disinfection cap.

27. Pull back on the syringe plunger to aspirate the catheter for positive blood return (Figure 4). If positive, instill the solution over 1 minute or according to facility policy. Remove the syringe.

RATIONALE

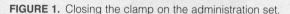

The passive disinfection caps contain an antiseptic-impregnated sponge that dispenses the antiseptic over the connector's top and threads, and provides continuous disinfection of the needleless connection versus intermittent disinfection when using antimicrobial wipes (Barton, 2019; Casey et al., 2018). Venous access device entry points, end caps, and needleless connectors must be vigorously scrubbed and disinfected prior to each access to reduce the risk for introduction of microorganisms and prevent venous access device–related infection (Flynn et al., 2019; Gorski et al., 2021). Friction is needed to physically remove microorganisms from the top, sides, and threads of the needleless connector or end cap. Allow the antiseptic to dry completely to ensure complete effectiveness (Gorski et al., 2021; Slater et al., 2018).

Assessing patency of the venous access device is necessary to ensure IV administration of the medication.

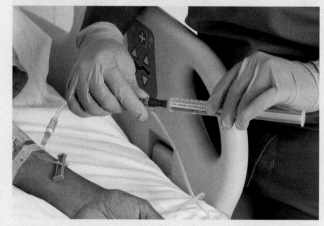

FIGURE 3. Inserting the saline flush syringe into the injection port.

Positive blood return confirms patency before administration of medications and solutions (Gorski et al., 2021). Flushing without incident ensures patency of the IV line and administration of the medication into the bloodstream.

(continued on page 266)

Skill 5-10 ▶ Administering Medications by Intravenous Bolus or Push Through an Intravenous Infusion *(continued)*

ACTION	RATIONALE

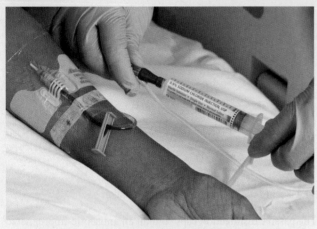

FIGURE 4. Pulling back on the plunger to aspirate for a blood return.

28. Use an antimicrobial swab to vigorously disinfect the connection surface and sides of the needleless connector or end cap on the injection port and allow it to dry.

Venous access device entry points, end caps, and needleless connectors must be vigorously scrubbed and disinfected prior to each access to reduce the risk for introduction of microorganisms and prevent venous access device–related infection (Flynn et al., 2019; Gorski et al., 2021). Friction is needed to physically remove microorganisms from the top, sides, and threads of the needleless connector or end cap. Allow the antiseptic to dry completely to ensure complete effectiveness (Gorski et al., 2021; Slater et al., 2018).

29. Uncap the medication syringe. Insert the medication syringe into the needleless connector or end cap on the injection port. Using a watch or clock with a second-hand to time the rate, **inject the medication at the recommended rate (Figure 5).**

This delivers the correct amount of medication at the proper interval.

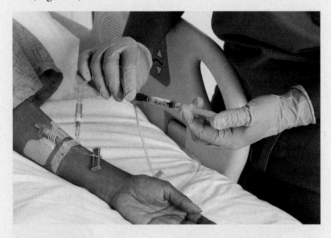

FIGURE 5. Injecting medication at the recommended rate.

30. While administering the medication, observe the infusion site and assess the patient for any adverse reaction. If signs of adverse reaction occur, stop the infusion immediately and notify the health care team.

Signs of adverse reaction, such as peripheral IV infiltration, rash or itching, or pain at the infusion site, necessitate stopping administration of the drug (Gorski et al., 2021).

ACTION

31. Detach the medication syringe. Use a new antimicrobial swab to vigorously disinfect the connection surface and sides of the needleless connector or end cap on the injection port and allow it to dry. Uncap the second saline flush syringe. Insert the saline flush syringe into the needleless connector or end cap on the injection port. Instill the flush solution at the same rate as the administered medication (Gorski et al., 2021).

32. Remove the flush syringe. Unclamp the administration set above the injection port.

33. Using an antimicrobial swab, vigorously disinfect the connection surface and sides of the needleless connector or end cap on the injection port and allow it to dry. Attach a passive disinfection cap to the needleless connector or end cap on the extension tubing or the injection port on the administration set (Figure 6).

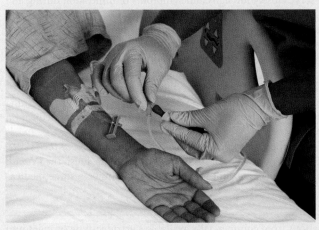

34. Remove gloves and perform hand hygiene. Restart the infusion pump and check IV fluid infusion rate.

35. Discard the syringe in the appropriate receptacle.

36. Remove additional PPE, if used. Perform hand hygiene.

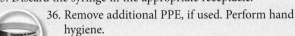

37. Document the administration of the medication immediately after administration. See Documentation section below.

38. Evaluate the patient's response to the medication within the appropriate time frame.

RATIONALE

Venous access device entry points, end caps, and needleless connectors must be vigorously scrubbed and disinfected prior to each access to reduce the risk for introduction of microorganisms and prevent venous access device–related infection (Flynn et al., 2019; Gorski et al., 2021). Friction is needed to physically remove microorganisms from the top, sides, and threads of the needleless connector or end cap. Allow the antiseptic to dry completely to ensure complete effectiveness (Gorski et al., 2021; Slater et al., 2018). Flushing after medication administration ensures the entire drug dose has been cleared from the extension tubing on the venous access device or from the infusion system and prevents precipitation due to solution/medication incompatibility (Gorski et al., 2021).

Clamping prevents air from entering the extension set on a capped venous access device. Unclamping the administration set allows for resumption of the continuous IV infusion.

Venous access device entry points, end caps, and needleless connectors must be vigorously scrubbed and disinfected prior to each access to reduce the risk for introduction of microorganisms and prevent venous access device–related infection (Flynn et al., 2019; Gorski et al., 2021). Friction is needed to physically remove microorganisms from the top, sides, and threads of the needleless connector or end cap. Allow the antiseptic to dry completely to ensure complete effectiveness (Gorski et al., 2021; Slater et al., 2018). Passive disinfection caps contain an antiseptic-impregnated sponge that dispenses the antiseptic over the connector's top and threads and protect the hub from contamination by touch or airborne sources (Barton, 2019; Casey et al., 2018).

FIGURE 6. Attaching a passive disinfection cap.

Removing gloves and performing hand hygiene prevents the spread of microorganisms. Restarting the infusion pump resumes the prescribed continuous infusion of fluid. Checking the IV fluid infusion rate assures accuracy in administration.

Proper disposal prevents injury and spread of microorganisms.

Proper removal of PPE reduces the risk of infection transmission and contamination of other items. Hand hygiene prevents the spread of microorganisms.

Timely documentation helps to ensure patient safety.

The patient needs to be evaluated for therapeutic and adverse effects from the medication.

(continued on page 268)

Skill 5-10 ▶ Administering Medications by Intravenous Bolus or Push Through an Intravenous Infusion   *(continued)*

EVALUATION

The expected outcomes have been met when the medication was administered safely via the IV route, the patient has experienced the intended effect of the medication, the patient experienced no adverse effects, and the patient has verbalized an understanding of and engages with the medication regimen.

DOCUMENTATION

Guidelines

Document the administration of the medication immediately after administration, including date, time, dose, route of administration, site of administration, and rate of administration on the eMAR/MAR or record using the required format. If using a bar-code system, medication administration is automatically recorded when the bar code is scanned. PRN medications require documentation of the reason for administration. Prompt recording avoids the possibility of accidentally repeating the administration of the drug. If the drug was refused or omitted, record this in the appropriate area on the medication record and notify the health care team as appropriate. This verifies the reason medication was omitted and ensures that health care personnel providing care for the patient are aware of the occurrence.

DEVELOPING CLINICAL REASONING AND CLINICAL JUDGMENT

UNEXPECTED SITUATIONS AND ASSOCIATED INTERVENTIONS

- *Upon assessing the IV site before administering medication, no blood return is visible upon aspiration:* If the IV appears patent, without signs of infiltration, and IV fluid infuses without difficulty, proceed with administration. Observe closely for signs and symptoms of infiltration during and after administration.
- *Upon assessing the patient's IV site before administering medication, you note that IV has infiltrated:* Stop the IV fluid and remove the IV from the patient's extremity. Restart the IV in a different location. Continue to monitor the new IV site as medication is administered.
- *While administering medication, you note a cloudy, white substance forming in the IV tubing:* Stop administering the medication. Clamp the IV at the site nearest to the patient. Change the administration tubing and restart the infusion. Check a drug resource or consult a pharmacist regarding compatibility of the medication and IV fluid before continuing with administration. Medication infusion may require a second IV site.
- *While you are administering the medication, the patient begins to complain of pain at the IV site:* Stop the medication. Assess the IV site for any signs of infiltration or phlebitis. Flush the IV with normal saline to check for patency. If the IV site appears within normal limits, resume medication administration at a slower rate.

SPECIAL CONSIDERATIONS

- Do not withdraw IV push medications from commercially available, cartridge-type syringes into another syringe for administration. Using the cartridge as a vial can lead to contamination and/or dosing errors, drug mix-ups, and other medication errors (ISMP, 2015, p. 11).
- Do not dilute or reconstitute IV push medications by drawing up the contents into a commercially available, prefilled flush syringe of 0.9% sodium chloride. These devices have been approved for flushing of vascular access devices, but have not been approved for the reconstitution, dilution, and/or subsequent administration of IV push medications (ISMP, 2015, p. 11).
- Appropriately label all clinician-prepared syringes of IV push medications or solutions, unless the medication or solution is prepared at the patient's bedside and is immediately administered to the patient (ISMP, 2015, p. 12).
- If the IV is a small gauge (22 to 24 gauge) placed in a small vein, a blood return may not occur even if the IV is intact. Also, the patient may report stinging and pain at the site while medication is being administered due to irritation of the vein. Slowing the rate of administration may relieve discomfort.
- Ongoing assessment is an important part of nursing care for both evaluation of patient response to administered medications and early detection of adverse drug reactions. If an adverse effect is suspected, withhold further medication doses and notify the health care team. Additional intervention is based on type of reaction and patient assessment.

**EVIDENCE
FOR PRACTICE ▶**

INFUSION NURSING STANDARDS OF PRACTICE
Infusion Nurses Society (INS). (2021). Infusion therapy. Standards of practice. *Journal of Infusion Nursing, 44*(Suppl 1), S1–S224. https://doi.org/10.1097/NAN.0000000000000396
The Infusion Nurses Society is recognized as the global authority in infusion therapy. The *Infusion Nursing Standards of Practice* is an evidence-based document, providing guidelines for nurses related to infusion therapy for use in all patient settings and addressing all patient populations.

Skill 5-11 ▶ Administering Medications by Intravenous Bolus or Push Through a Medication or Drug-Infusion Lock

A medication or drug-infusion lock, also known as an intermittent peripheral venous access device or saline lock, is used for patients who require intermittent IV medication, but not a continuous IV infusion. This device consists of a catheter connected to a short length of tubing capped with a sealed injection port. After the catheter is in place in the patient's vein, the catheter and tubing are anchored to the patient's arm so that the catheter remains in place until the patient no longer requires the repeated medication intravenously. Medication administration involves a single injection of a concentrated solution directly into an IV access. Drugs given by IV push are used for intermittent dosing or to treat emergencies. The drug is administered at the rate recommended by the manufacturer, supported by evidence for practice, or in accordance with approved institutional guidelines (Institute for Safe Medication Practices, 2015, p. 13). **Confirm exact administration times by consulting a drug reference, package insert, or a pharmacist. Appropriately label all clinician-prepared syringes of IV push medications or solutions, unless the medication or solution is prepared at the patient's bedside and is immediately administered to the patient** (ISMP, 2015, p. 12).

The medication or drug-infusion lock is kept patent (working) by flushing with small amounts of saline pushed through the device on a routine basis. The nurse must confirm IV placement before administration of medication. It is important to flush the drug-infusion lock before and after the medication is administered to clear the vein of any medication and to prevent clot formation in the device. If infiltration or phlebitis occurs, the lock is removed and replaced in a new site. Refer to Chapter 16 for a more detailed discussion of intravenous access devices and associated nursing skills.

DELEGATION CONSIDERATIONS

The administration of medications through an intermittent peripheral venous access device is not delegated to assistive personnel (AP). Depending on the state's nurse practice act and the organization's policies and procedures, the administration of specified IV medications in some settings may be delegated to licensed practical/vocational nurses (LPN/LVNs) who have received appropriate training. The decision to delegate must be based on careful analysis of the patient's needs and circumstances as well as the qualifications of the person to whom the task is being delegated. Refer to the Delegation Guidelines in Appendix A.

EQUIPMENT

- Prescribed medication
- Two normal saline flushes prepared in a syringe (3 to 10 mL) according to facility policy
- Antimicrobial swabs
- Passive disinfection caps (based on facility policy)
- Syringe with a needleless device or 23- to 25-gauge, 1-inch needle (follow facility policy)
- Watch or clock with a second hand
- Disposable gloves
- Electronic Medication Administration Record (eMAR) or Medication Administration Record (MAR)
- Additional PPE, as indicated

(*continued on page 270*)

Skill 5-11 ▶ Administering Medications by Intravenous Bolus or Push Through a Medication or Drug-Infusion Lock *(continued)*

ASSESSMENT

Assess the appropriateness of the drug for the patient. Review the medical history and allergy, assessment, and laboratory data that may influence drug administration. Check the expiration date. Assess the patient's IV site for signs of any complications. (Refer to Fundamentals Review 16-3 and Box 16-2 in Chapter 16 on pages 1005 and 1021.) Assess the patient's knowledge of the medication. If the patient has a knowledge deficit about the medication, this may be the appropriate time to begin education about the medication. If the medication may affect the patient's vital signs, assess them before administration. If the medication is for pain relief, assess the patient's pain before and after administration. Verify the patient's name, dose, route, and time of administration.

ACTUAL OR POTENTIAL HEALTH PROBLEMS AND NEEDS

Many actual or potential health problems or issues may require the use of this skill as part of related interventions. An appropriate health problem or issue may include:

- Risk for medication side effect
- Knowledge deficiency
- Injury risk

OUTCOME IDENTIFICATION AND PLANNING

The expected outcomes to achieve when administering medication via a medication or drug-infusion lock are that the medication is delivered via the IV route, and the patient experiences the intended effect of the medication. Other outcomes that may be appropriate include the following: the patient experiences no adverse effects, and the patient verbalizes an understanding of and engages with the medication regimen.

IMPLEMENTATION

ACTION	**RATIONALE**
1. Gather equipment. Check each medication prescribed against the original in the health record, depending on facility policy and the medication order system in place. Clarify any inconsistencies. Check the patient's health record for allergies. Check a drug resource to clarify whether medication needs to be diluted before bolus administration. Verify the recommended administration rate.	The prescription is the legal record of prescribed medication interventions. This comparison helps to identify errors that may have occurred when orders were transcribed. Computer provider order-entry (CPOE) systems allow prescribers to send electronic medication prescriptions directly to the pharmacy located in a health care facility and to outpatient pharmacies. Recommended administration rate delivers the correct dose of medication as prescribed.
2. Know the actions, special nursing considerations, safe dose ranges, purpose of administration, and adverse effects of the medications to be administered. Consider the appropriateness of the medication for this patient.	This knowledge aids the nurse in evaluating the therapeutic effect of the medication in relation to the patient's health status and can also be used to educate the patient about the medication.
3. Perform hand hygiene.	Hand hygiene prevents the spread of microorganisms.
4. Move the medication supply system to the outside of the patient's room or prepare for administration at the medication supply system in the medication area. Alternatively, access the medication administration supply system at or inside the patient's room.	Organization facilitates error-free administration and saves time.
5. Unlock the medication supply system or drawer. Enter the passcode and scan employee identification, if required.	Locking the medication supply system or drawer safeguards each patient's medication supply. Facility accrediting organizations require medication supply systems to be locked when not in use. Entering the passcode and scanning ID allows only authorized users into the system and identifies the user for documentation by the computer.
6. **Prepare medications for one patient at a time.**	This prevents errors in medication administration.

ACTION

7. Read the eMAR/MAR and select the proper medication from the medication supply system or the patient's medication drawer.

8. Compare the label with the eMAR/MAR. Check expiration dates and perform calculations, if necessary. Scan the bar code on the package, if required.

9. If necessary, withdraw the medication from an ampule or vial as described in Skills 5-3 and 5-4.

10. **Depending on facility policy, the third check of the label may occur at this point. If so, when all medications for one patient have been prepared, recheck the labels with the eMAR/MAR before taking the medications to the patient. However, many facilities require the third check to occur at the bedside, after identifying the patient.**

11. Label the syringe with the medication's name, dose, and amount (The Joint Commission, 2021).

12. **Log out of and/or lock the medication supply system before leaving it.**

13. Transport medications and equipment to the patient's bedside carefully and keep the medications in sight at all times.

14. **Ensure that the patient receives the medications at the correct time.**

15. Perform hand hygiene and put on PPE, if indicated.

16. **Identify the patient. Compare the information with the eMAR/MAR. The patient should be identified using at least two of the following methods** (The Joint Commission, 2021):

a. Check the name on the patient's identification band.

b. Check the identification number on the patient's identification band.

c. Check the birth date on the patient's identification band.

d. Ask the patient to state their name and birth date, based on facility policy.

17. Close the door to the room or pull the bedside curtain.

18. **Complete necessary assessments before administering medications. Check the patient's allergy bracelet, if present, or ask the patient about allergies. Explain the purpose and action of the medication to the patient.**

19. Scan the bar code on the patient's identification band, if required (The Joint Commission, 2021) (Figure 1).

20. **Based on facility policy, the third check of the label may occur at this point. If so, recheck the labels with the eMAR/MAR before administering the medications to the patient.**

RATIONALE

This is the *first* check of the label.

This is the *second* check of the label. Verify calculations with another nurse to ensure safety, if necessary.

Allows administration of medication.

This *third* check ensures accuracy and helps to prevent errors. *Note:* Many facilities require the *third* check to occur at the bedside, after identifying the patient and before administration.

Unlabeled syringes are unidentifiable and may lead to a medication administration error (The Joint Commission, 2021).

Locking the medication supply system or drawer safeguards the patient's medication supply. Facility accrediting organizations require medication supply systems to be locked when not in use.

Careful handling and close observation prevent accidental or deliberate disarrangement of medications. Having equipment available saves time and facilitates performance of the task.

Check facility policy, which may allow for administration within a period of 30 minutes before or 30 minutes after the designated time.

Hand hygiene and PPE prevent the spread of microorganisms. PPE is required based on transmission precautions.

Identifying the patient ensures the right patient receives the medications and helps prevent errors. The patient's room number or physical location is not used as an identifier (The Joint Commission, 2021). Replace the identification band if it is missing or inaccurate in any way.

This requires a response from the patient, but illness and strange surroundings often cause patients to be confused.

This provides patient privacy.

Assessment is a prerequisite to administration of medications. Explanation provides rationale, increases knowledge, and reduces anxiety.

Scanning provides an additional check to ensure that the medication is given to the right patient.

Many facilities require the *third* check to occur at the bedside, after identifying the patient and before administration. If facility policy directs the *third* check at this time, this *third* check ensures accuracy and helps to prevent errors.

(continued on page 272)

Skill 5-11 ▶ Administering Medications by Intravenous Bolus or Push Through a Medication or Drug-Infusion Lock *(continued)*

ACTION

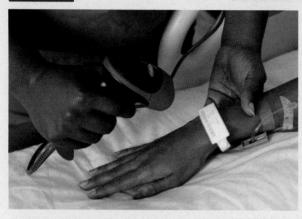

FIGURE 1. Scanning bar code on patient's identification bracelet.

RATIONALE

21. Assess the IV site for the presence of inflammation or infiltration.

22. Put on gloves.

23. Remove the passive disinfection cap from the needleless connector or access port of the medication lock (Figure 2). Alternatively, if a passive disinfection cap is not in place, use an antimicrobial swab to vigorously disinfect the connection surface and sides of the needleless connector or end cap on the injection port and allow it to dry.

24. Uncap the saline flush syringe. Stabilize the port with your nondominant hand and insert the saline flush syringe into the needleless connector or end cap on the access port of the medication lock (Figure 3).

IV medication must be given directly into a vein for safe administration.

Gloves protect the nurse's hands from contact with the patient's blood.

Passive disinfection caps contain an antiseptic-impregnated sponge that dispenses the antiseptic over the connector's top and threads and protects the hub from contamination by touch or airborne sources (Barton, 2019; Casey et al., 2018). Venous access device entry points, end caps, and needleless connectors must be vigorously scrubbed and disinfected prior to each access to reduce the risk for introduction of microorganisms and prevent venous access device–related infection (Flynn et al., 2019; Gorski et al., 2021). Friction is needed to physically remove microorganisms from the top, sides, and threads of the needleless connector or end cap. Allow the antiseptic to dry completely to ensure complete effectiveness (Gorski et al., 2021; Slater et al., 2018).

Assessing patency of the venous access device is necessary to ensure IV administration of the medication.

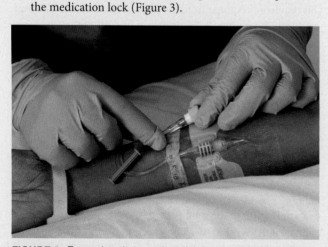

FIGURE 2. Removing the passive disinfection cap from the access port.

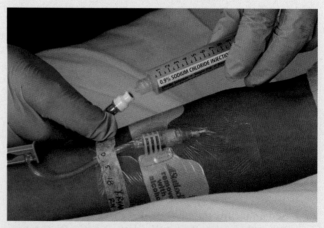

FIGURE 3. Inserting the saline flush syringe into the access port.

ACTION

25. Release the clamp on the extension tubing of the medication lock (Figure 4). Pull back on the syringe plunger to aspirate the catheter for positive blood return (Figure 5). If positive, instill the solution over 1 minute or according to facility policy. Observe the insertion site while inserting the saline. Remove the syringe.

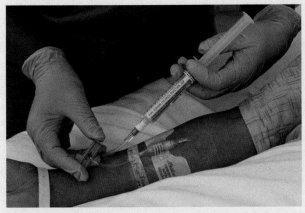

FIGURE 4. Releasing the clamp on the extension tubing.

26. Use an antimicrobial swab to vigorously disinfect the connection surface and sides of the needleless connector or end cap on the injection port and allow it to dry.

27. Uncap the medication syringe. Insert the medication syringe into the needleless connector or end cap on the access port of the medication lock. Using a watch or clock with a second-hand to time the rate, **inject the medication at the recommended rate (Figure 6). Do not force the injection if resistance is felt.**

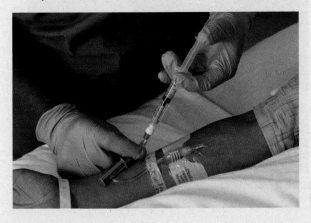

RATIONALE

Positive blood return confirms patency before administration of medications and solutions (Gorski et al., 2021). Flushing without incident ensures patency of the IV line and administration of the medication into the bloodstream. Puffiness, pain, or swelling as the site is flushed could indicate infiltration of the catheter.

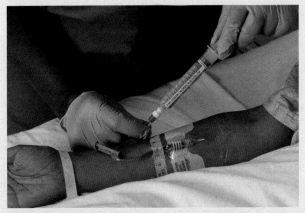

FIGURE 5. Pulling back on the plunger to aspirate for a blood return.

Venous access device entry points, end caps, and needleless connectors must be vigorously scrubbed and disinfected prior to each access to reduce the risk for introduction of microorganisms and prevent venous access device–related infection (Flynn et al., 2019; Gorski et al., 2021). Friction is needed to physically remove microorganisms from the top, sides, and threads of the needleless connector or end cap. Allow the antiseptic to dry completely to ensure complete effectiveness (Gorski et al., 2021; Slater et al., 2018).

This delivers the correct amount of medication at the proper interval. Easy installation of medication usually indicates that the lock is still patent and in the vein. If force is used against resistance, a clot may break away and cause a blockage elsewhere in the body.

FIGURE 6. Injecting the medication at the recommended rate.

(continued on page 274)

Skill 5-11 ▶ Administering Medications by Intravenous Bolus or Push Through a Medication or Drug-Infusion Lock *(continued)*

ACTION	RATIONALE
28. While administering the medication, observe the infusion site and assess the patient for any adverse reaction. If signs of adverse reaction occur, stop the infusion immediately and notify the health care team.	Signs of adverse reaction, such as peripheral IV infiltration, rash or itching, or pain at the infusion site, necessitate stopping administration of the drug (Gorski et al., 2021).
29. Remove the medication syringe from the access port. Use a new antimicrobial swab to vigorously disinfect the connection surface and sides of the needleless connector or end cap on the injection port and allow it to dry. Stabilize the port with your nondominant hand. Uncap the second saline flush syringe. Insert the saline flush syringe into the needleless connector or end cap on the access port. Instill the flush solution at the same rate as the administered medication (Gorski et al., 2021).	Venous access device entry points, end caps, and needleless connectors must be vigorously scrubbed and disinfected prior to each access to reduce the risk for introduction of microorganisms and prevent venous access device–related infection (Flynn et al., 2019; Gorski et al., 2021). Friction is needed to physically remove microorganisms from the top, sides, and threads of the needleless connector or end cap. Allow the antiseptic to dry completely to ensure complete effectiveness (Gorski et al., 2021; Slater et al., 2018). Flushing after medication administration ensures the entire drug dose has been cleared from the extension tubing on the venous access device or from the infusion system and prevents precipitation due to solution/medication incompatibility (Gorski et al., 2021).
30. If the medication lock is capped with a positive pressure valve/device, remove the syringe, and then clamp the extension tubing (Figure 7). Alternatively, to gain positive pressure if positive pressure valve/device is not present, clamp the extension tubing as you are still flushing the last of the saline into the medication lock. Remove the syringe.	Positive pressure prevents blood from backing into the catheter and causing the medication lock to clot off.
31. Using an antimicrobial swab, vigorously disinfect the connection surface and sides of the needleless connector or end cap on the injection port and allow it to dry. Attach a passive disinfection cap to the needleless connector or end cap on the access port of the medication lock (Figure 8).	Venous access device entry points, end caps, and needleless connectors must be vigorously scrubbed and disinfected prior to each access to reduce the risk for introduction of microorganisms and prevent venous access device–related infection (Flynn et al., 2019; Gorski et al., 2021). Friction is needed to physically remove microorganisms from the top, sides, and threads of the needleless connector or end cap. Allow the antiseptic to dry completely to ensure complete effectiveness (Gorski et al., 2021; Slater et al., 2018). Passive disinfection caps contain an antiseptic-impregnated sponge that dispenses the antiseptic over the connector's top and threads and protect the hub from contamination by touch or airborne sources (Barton, 2019; Casey et al., 2018).

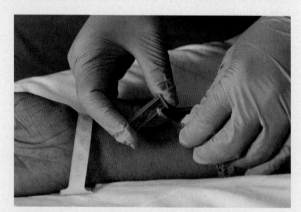

FIGURE 7. Clamping the extension tubing.

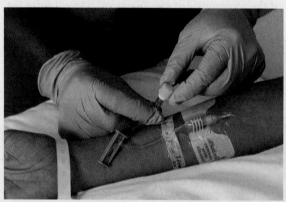

FIGURE 8. Attaching a passive disinfection cap to the access port.

ACTION

32. Discard the syringe in the appropriate receptacle.

33. Remove gloves and additional PPE, if used. Perform hand hygiene.

34. Document the administration of the medication immediately after administration. See Documentation section below.

35. Evaluate the patient's response to the medication within an appropriate time frame.

RATIONALE

Proper disposal prevents injury and the spread of microorganisms.

Proper removal of PPE reduces the risk of infection transmission and contamination of other items. Hand hygiene prevents the spread of microorganisms.

Timely documentation helps to ensure patient safety.

The patient needs to be evaluated for therapeutic and adverse effects from the medication.

EVALUATION

The expected outcomes have been met when the medication was delivered via the IV route, the patient has experienced the intended effect of the medication, the patient has experienced no adverse effects, and the patient has verbalized an understanding of and engages with the medication regimen.

DOCUMENTATION

Guidelines

Document the administration of the medication and saline flush, including date, time, dose, route of administration, site of administration, and rate of administration on the eMAR/MAR or record using the required format, immediately after administration. If using a bar-code system, medication administration is automatically recorded when the bar code is scanned. PRN medications require documentation of the reason for administration. Prompt recording avoids the possibility of accidentally repeating the administration of the drug. If the drug was refused or omitted, record this in the appropriate area on the medication record and notify the health care team as appropriate. This verifies the reason medication was omitted and ensures that the health care personnel providing care for the patient are aware of the occurrence.

DEVELOPING CLINICAL REASONING AND CLINICAL JUDGMENT

UNEXPECTED SITUATIONS AND ASSOCIATED INTERVENTIONS

- *Upon assessing the medication lock site before administering the medication, you note that the medication lock has infiltrated:* Remove the medication lock from the extremity. Restart the peripheral venous access in a different location. Continue to monitor the new site as the medication is administered.
- *While you are administering medication, the patient begins to complain of pain at the site:* Stop the medication. Assess the medication lock site for signs of infiltration and phlebitis. Flush the medication lock with normal saline again to recheck patency. If the IV site appears within normal limits, resume medication administration at a slower rate. If pain persists, stop, remove the medication lock, and restart in a different location.
- *As you are attempting to access the lock, the syringe tip touches the patient's arm:* Discard the syringe. Prepare a new dose for administration.
- *No blood return is noted upon aspiration:* If the medication lock appears patent, without signs of infiltration, and normal saline fluid infuses without difficulty, proceed with administration. Observe closely for signs and symptoms of infiltration during and after administration.

(continued on page 276)

Skill 5-11 ▶ Administering Medications by Intravenous Bolus or Push Through a Medication or Drug-Infusion Lock (continued)

SPECIAL CONSIDERATIONS

General Considerations

- Vascular access devices should also be "locked" after completion of the flush solution at each use to decrease the risk of occlusion and catheter-related bloodstream infection (Gorski et al., 2021). According to the guidelines from the INS, vascular access devices are locked with normal saline solution (Gorski et al., 2021). If the device is not in use, periodic flushing according to facility policy is required to keep the catheter patent.
- Previously, recommendations suggested routine rotation of insertions sites at various intervals, usually 72 to 96 hours. Current research and guidelines support maintaining peripheral IV access devices until no longer clinically indicated or until a complication develops (Gorski et al., 2021; Weston, 2019). Nurses should use clinical assessment and judgment in deciding when to replace or discontinue a peripheral venous access device.
- The clinical need for the IV catheter should be assessed on a daily basis (Gorski et al., 2021). The device insertion site and dressing should be assessed every 4 hours at a minimum (Gorski et al., 2021; Weston, 2019).
- A peripheral venous access device that is no longer necessary should not be kept in place just in case it may be needed in a few days (Weston, 2019).
- Ongoing assessment is an important part of nursing care to evaluate patient response to administered medications and early detection of adverse reactions. If an adverse effect is suspected, withhold further medication doses and notify the health care team. Additional intervention is based on type of reaction and patient assessment.

Infant and Child Considerations

- The primary method for IV medication administration for infants and children is a mini-infusion (syringe) pump (Kyle & Carman, 2021). Refer to Skill 5-13.
- Administration of IV bolus or push medication is usually reserved for emergency situations and when therapeutic blood levels must be reached quickly to achieve the desired effect (Kyle & Carman, 2021).

EVIDENCE FOR PRACTICE ▶

INFUSION NURSING STANDARDS OF PRACTICE

Infusion Nurses Society (INS). (2021). Infusion therapy. Standards of practice. *Journal of Infusion Nursing, 44*(Suppl 1), S1–S224. https://doi.org/10.1097/NAN.0000000000000396
Refer to details in Skill 5-10, Evidence for Practice.

Skill 5-12 ▶ Administering a Piggyback Intermittent Intravenous Infusion of Medication

Medications can be administered by intermittent IV infusion. The drug is mixed with a small amount of an IV solution, such as 50 to 100 mL, and administered over a short period at the prescribed interval (e.g., every 8 hours). The administration is most often performed using an electronic infusion device (IV or infusion pump), which requires the nurse to program the infusion rate (mL/hr) into the pump. *Smart (computerized) pumps* are increasingly being used by many facilities for IV infusions, including intermittent infusions. Smart pumps also require programming of infusion rates by the nurse, but also are able to identify dosing limits and practice guidelines to aid in safe administration (ISMP, 2020). These smart IV pumps use computerized dose error-reduction software with IV drug therapy libraries that calculates infusion rates and provides an alert to the user when infusion rate limits are exceeded (Giuliano et al., 2018). Smart pumps are used in the majority (88.1%) of hospital settings in the United States (Schneider et al., 2018). Administration of an intermittent infusion may also be achieved by gravity infusion, which requires the nurse to calculate the infusion rate in drops per minute. The best practice, however, is to use a program-mable electronic infusion device utilizing dose-error reduction computer software (ISMP, 2020). Additional information about intravenous infusions and Smart pumps is provided in Chapter 16.

Although newer infusion pumps allow for more flexibly (including concurrent programming of primary and secondary/piggyback lines), some IV piggyback delivery systems still require the container with the intermittent or additive solution to be placed higher than the primary solution container. An extension hook provided by the manufacturer provides for easy lowering of the main IV container. The port on the primary IV line has a back-check valve that automatically stops the flow of the primary solution, allowing the secondary or piggyback solution to flow when con-nected. Because **manufacturers' designs vary, it is important to check the directions carefully for the systems used in the facility.**

DELEGATION CONSIDERATIONS

The administration of medications by intermittent IV infusion is not delegated to assistive person-nel (AP). Depending on the state's nurse practice act and the organization's policies and procedures, the administration of specified IV medications in some settings may be delegated to licensed practical/vocational nurses (LPN/LVNs) who have received appropriate training. The decision to delegate must be based on careful analysis of the patient's needs and circumstances as well as the qualifications of the person to whom the task is being delegated. Refer to the Delegation Guidelines in Appendix A.

EQUIPMENT

- Medication prepared in labeled small-volume IV bag
- Short secondary infusion tubing
- Infusion pump
- Antimicrobial swab
- Needleless connector, if required, based on facility procedure
- Metal or plastic hook
- IV pole
- Watch or clock with a second hand (gravity infusion)
- Date label for tubing
- Electronic Medication Administration Record (eMAR) or Medication Administration Record (MAR)
- PPE, as indicated

ASSESSMENT

Assess the appropriateness of the drug for the patient. Review the medical history and allergy, assessment, and laboratory data that may influence drug administration. Check the expiration date. **Assess the compatibility of the ordered medication, diluent, and the infusing IV fluid.** Assess the patient's IV site for signs of any complications. (Refer to Fundamentals Review 16-3 and Box 16-2 in Chapter 16 on pages 1005 and 1021.) Assess the patient's knowledge of the medication. If the patient has a knowledge deficit about the medication, this may be the appropriate time to begin education about the medication. If the medication may affect the patient's vital signs, assess them before administration. Verify patient name, dose, route, and time of administration.

ACTUAL OR POTENTIAL HEALTH PROBLEMS AND NEEDS

Many actual or potential health problems or issues may require the use of this skill as part of related interventions. An appropriate health problem or issue may include:
- Risk for medication side effect
- Risk for adverse medication interaction
- Knowledge deficiency

OUTCOME IDENTIFICATION AND PLANNING

The expected outcomes to achieve are that the medication is delivered via the IV route, and the patient experiences the intended effect of the medication. Other outcomes that may be appropri-ate include the following: the patient experiences no adverse effects, and the patient verbalized an understanding of and engages with the medication regimen.

(continued on page 278)

Skill 5-12 ▶ Administering a Piggyback Intermittent Intravenous Infusion of Medication *(continued)*

IMPLEMENTATION

ACTION	RATIONALE
1. Gather equipment. Check each medication prescribed against the original in the health record, depending on facility policy and the medication order system in place. Clarify any inconsistencies. Check the patient's health record for allergies. Check the administration rate.	The prescription is the legal record of prescribed medication interventions. This comparison helps to identify errors that may have occurred when orders were transcribed. Computer provider order-entry (CPOE) systems allow prescribers to send electronic medication prescriptions directly to the pharmacy located in a health care facility and to outpatient pharmacies.
2. Know the actions, special nursing considerations, safe dose ranges, purpose of administration, and adverse effects of the medications to be administered. Consider the appropriateness of the medication for this patient. **Assess the compatibility of the ordered medication, diluent, and the infusing IV fluid.**	This knowledge aids the nurse in evaluating the therapeutic effect of the medication in relation to the patient's health status and can also be used to educate the patient about the medication. Compatibility of medication and solutions prevents complications.
3. Perform hand hygiene.	Hand hygiene prevents the spread of microorganisms.
4. Move the medication supply system to the outside of the patient's room or prepare for administration at the medication supply system in the medication area. Alternatively, access the medication administration supply system at or inside the patient's room.	Organization facilitates error-free administration and saves time.
5. Unlock the medication supply system or drawer. Enter the passcode and scan employee identification, if required.	Locking the medication supply system or drawer safeguards each patient's medication supply. Facility accrediting organizations require medication supply systems to be locked when not in use. Entering the passcode and scanning ID allows only authorized users into the system and identifies the user for documentation by the computer.
6. **Prepare medications for one patient at a time.**	This prevents errors in medication administration.
7. Read the eMAR/MAR and read the label when selecting the proper medication from the medication supply system or the patient's medication drawer.	This is the *first* check of the label.
8. Read the label and compare the label with the eMAR/MAR. Check expiration dates. Confirm the prescribed or appropriate infusion rate. Calculate the drip rate if using a gravity system. Scan the bar code on the package, if required.	This is the *second* check of the label. Verify calculations with another nurse to ensure safety, if necessary. Infusing medication at an appropriate rate prevents injury.
9. **Depending on facility policy, the third check of the label may occur at this point. If so, when all medications for one patient have been prepared, read the label and recheck the labels with the eMAR/MAR before taking the medications to the patient. However, many facilities require the third check to occur at the bedside, after identifying the patient.**	This *third* check ensures accuracy and helps to prevent errors. *Note:* Many facilities require the *third* check to occur at the bedside, after identifying the patient and before administration.
10. **Log out of and/or lock the medication supply system before leaving it.**	Locking the medication supply system or drawer safeguards the patient's medication supply. Facility accrediting organizations require medication supply systems to be locked when not in use.
11. Transport medications to the patient's bedside carefully and keep the medications in sight at all times.	Careful handling and close observation prevent accidental or deliberate disarrangement of medications.
12. **Ensure that the patient receives the medications at the correct time.**	Check facility policy, which may allow for administration within a period of 30 minutes before or 30 minutes after the designated time.
13. Perform hand hygiene and put on PPE, if indicated.	Hand hygiene and PPE prevent the spread of microorganisms. PPE is required based on transmission precautions.

ACTION	RATIONALE

14. **Identify the patient. Compare the information with the eMAR/MAR. The patient should be identified using at least two of the following methods** (The Joint Commission, 2021):

Identifying the patient ensures the right patient receives the medications and helps prevent errors. The patient's room number or physical location is not used as an identifier (The Joint Commission, 2021). Replace the identification band if it is missing or inaccurate in any way.

a. Check the name on the patient's identification band.

This requires a response from the patient, but illness and strange surroundings often cause patients to be confused.

b. Check the identification number on the patient's identification band.

c. Check the birth date on the patient's identification band.

d. Ask the patient to state their name and birth date, based on facility policy.

15. Close the door to the room or pull the bedside curtain.

This provides patient privacy.

16. **Complete necessary assessments before administering medications. Check the patient's allergy bracelet, if present, or ask the patient about allergies. Explain the purpose and action of the medication to the patient.**

Assessment is a prerequisite to administration of medications. Explanation provides rationale, increases knowledge, and reduces anxiety.

17. Scan the patient's bar code on the identification band, if required (The Joint Commission, 2021).

Scanning provides an additional check to ensure that the medication is given to the right patient.

18. **Based on facility policy, the third check of the label may occur at this point. If so, read the label and recheck the labels with the eMAR/MAR before administering the medications to the patient.**

Many facilities require the *third* check to occur at the bedside, after identifying the patient and before administration. If facility policy directs the *third* check at this time, this *third* check ensures accuracy and helps to prevent errors.

19. Assess the IV site for the presence of inflammation or infiltration or other signs of complications.

IV medication must be given directly into a vein for safe administration.

20. Close the clamp on the short secondary infusion tubing. Using aseptic technique, remove the cap on the tubing spike and the cap on the port of the medication container, taking care to avoid contaminating either end.

Closing the clamp prevents fluid from entering the system until the nurse is ready. Maintaining sterility of the tubing and the medication port prevents contamination.

21. Attach the infusion tubing to the medication container by inserting the tubing spike into the port with a firm push and twisting motion, taking care to avoid contaminating either end.

Maintaining sterility of the tubing and medication port prevents contamination.

22. Hang the piggyback container on the IV pole, positioning it higher than the primary IV if necessary, based on the type of IV infusion device in use and according to the manufacturer's recommendations. If necessary for the particular infusion pump in use, use the metal or plastic hook to lower the primary IV fluid container (Figure 1). If using gravity infusion, the primary IV fluid container must be lowered.

The position of the containers influences the flow of IV fluid into the primary setup.

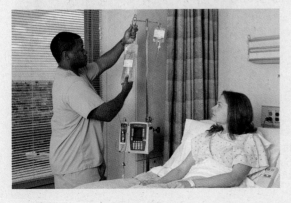

FIGURE 1. Lowering the primary IV fluid container to position the piggyback container higher than primary IV fluid container. (*Source:* Used with permission from Shutterstock. *Photo by B. Proud.*)

(continued on page 280)

Skill 5-12 ▶ Administering a Piggyback Intermittent Intravenous Infusion of Medication *(continued)*

ACTION	RATIONALE
23. If the secondary infusion tubing is being used for the first time, place a label on the administration tubing with the current date.	Most facilities allow the reuse of tubing, reducing the risk for contamination. The frequency of administration set tubing changes varies. Refer to Box 16-3 in Skill 16-3 for recommended administration set change guidelines. The label identifies the date of the first use of the tubing. Intermittent administration sets disconnected after use should be replaced every 24 hours; repeated disconnection and reconnection increase the risk of contamination at the spike end, catheter hub, needleless connector, and the end of the administration set, potentially increasing the risk for catheter-related bloodstream infection (Gorski et al., 2021).
24. Squeeze the drip chamber on the administration tubing and release. Fill the chamber to the line or about half full. Open the clamp on the administration tubing and prime the tubing. Close the clamp. Place the needleless connector on the end of the tubing, using sterile technique, if required.	This removes air from tubing and preserves the sterility of the setup.
25. Remove the passive disinfection cap from the needleless connector or end cap on the infusion set injection port. Alternatively, if a passive disinfection cap is not in place, use an antimicrobial swab to vigorously disinfect the connection surfaces and sides of the access port or stopcock on the administration set above where the tubing enters the infusion pump or above the roller clamp on the primary IV infusion tubing (gravity infusion) (Figure 2).	Passive disinfection caps contain an antiseptic-impregnated sponge that dispenses the antiseptic over the connector's top and threads and protects the hub from contamination by touch or airborne sources (Barton, 2019; Casey et al., 2018). Venous access device entry points, end caps, and needleless connectors must be vigorously scrubbed and disinfected prior to each access to reduce the risk for introduction of microorganisms and prevent venous access device–related infection (Flynn et al., 2019; Gorski et al., 2021). Friction is needed to physically remove microorganisms from the top, sides, and threads of the needleless connector or end cap. Allow the antiseptic to dry completely to ensure complete effectiveness (Gorski et al., 2021; Slater et al., 2018). The backflow valve in the primary line secondary port stops flow of the primary infusion while the piggyback solution is infusing. Once completed, the backflow valve opens, and flow of the primary solution resumes.
26. Connect the piggyback setup to the access port (Figure 3) or stopcock. If using, turn the stopcock to the open position.	Needleless systems and a stopcock setup eliminate the need for a needle and are recommended by the CDC.

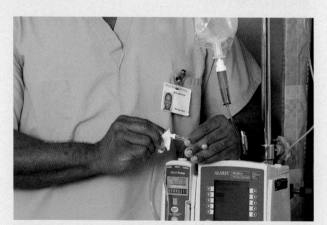

FIGURE 2. Vigorously scrubbing the access port. (*Source:* Used with permission from Shutterstock. *Photo by B. Proud.*)

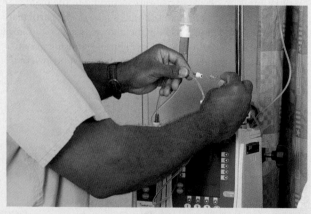

FIGURE 3. Connecting piggyback administration set to access port. (*Source:* Used with permission from Shutterstock. *Photo by B. Proud.*)

ACTION	RATIONALE
27. Alternatively, if the administration set is in place from a previous infusion, there is no need to disconnect the secondary tubing to connect the current dose of medication. The secondary tubing will be primed via "backfill" or "back prime" of the secondary tubing.	Most facilities allow the reuse of tubing, reducing the risk for contamination. "Back prime" is recommended as the method to use to prime a secondary administration set when there is compatibility with the primary fluid (Gorski et al., 2021). The frequency of administration set tubing changes varies. Refer to Box 16-3 in Skill 16-3 for recommended administration set change guidelines.
28. Clamp the secondary infusion tubing and remove the previous, empty medication bag. Attach the current medication dose bag to the secondary infusion tubing, as outlined in Steps 20–22. Lower the medication bag below the main IV solution container and open the clamp on the secondary infusion tubing. This allows the primary IV solution to flow up the secondary tubing to the drip chamber, "back priming" or "backfilling" the tubing. Allow the solution to enter the drip chamber until the drip chamber is half full. Close the clamp on the secondary tubing and hang the medication container on the IV pole.	This "backfill" method keeps the infusion system intact, preventing both introduction of microorganisms and loss of medication when the tubing is primed. "Back prime" is recommended as the method to use to prime a secondary administration set when there is compatibility with the primary fluid (Gorski et al., 2021). Check facility policy regarding the use of "back prime."
29. Open the clamp on the secondary infusion tubing. Set the rate for the secondary infusion on the infusion pump and begin the infusion (Figure 4). If using gravity infusion, use the roller clamp on the primary infusion tubing to regulate the flow at the prescribed delivery rate (Figure 5). Monitor medication infusion at periodic intervals.	The backflow valve in the primary line secondary port stops the flow of the primary infusion while the piggyback solution is infusing. Once completed, the backflow valve opens, and flow of the primary solution resumes. It is important to verify the safe administration rate for each drug to prevent adverse effects.

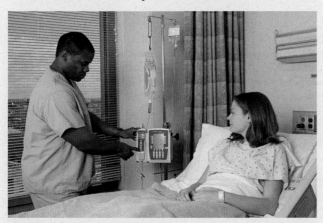

FIGURE 4. Setting rate for secondary infusion on infusion pump. (*Source:* Used with permission from Shutterstock. *Photo by B. Proud.*)

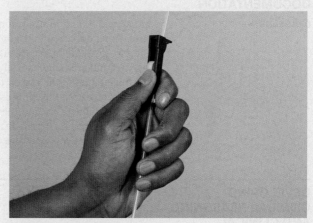

FIGURE 5. Using roller clamp on primary infusion tubing to regulate gravity flow. (*Source:* Used with permission from Shutterstock. *Photo by B. Proud.*)

ACTION	RATIONALE
30. Clamp the tubing on the piggyback set when the solution is infused and leave the setup in place.	Most facilities allow the reuse of tubing, reducing the risk for contamination. Leaving the secondary tubing and medication bag in place until the next dose keeps the infusion system intact, preventing both introduction of microorganisms and loss of medication when the tubing is primed. "Back prime" is recommended as the method to use to prime a secondary administration set when there is compatibility with the primary fluid (Gorski et al., 2021). Check facility policy regarding the use of "back prime." The frequency of administration set tubing changes varies. Refer to Box 16-3 in Skill 16-3 for recommended administration set change guidelines.

(*continued on page 282*)

Skill 5-12 ▶ Administering a Piggyback Intermittent Intravenous Infusion of Medication *(continued)*

ACTION	RATIONALE
31. Raise the primary IV fluid container to the original height, if lowered for the infusion. **Check the primary infusion rate on the infusion pump. If using gravity infusion, readjust the flow rate of the primary IV.**	Most infusion pumps automatically restart the primary infusion at the previous rate after the secondary infusion is completed. If using gravity infusion, piggyback medication administration may interrupt the normal flow rate of the primary IV. Rate readjustment may be necessary.
32. Remove PPE, if used. Perform hand hygiene.	Proper removal of PPE reduces the risk of infection transmission and contamination of other items. Hand hygiene prevents the spread of microorganisms.
33. Document the administration of the medication immediately after administration. See Documentation section below. Document the volume of fluid administered on the intake and output record, if necessary.	Timely documentation helps to ensure patient safety.
34. Evaluate the patient's response to the medication within an appropriate time frame.	The patient needs to be evaluated for therapeutic and adverse effects from the medication.

EVALUATION

The expected outcomes have been met when the medication was delivered via the IV route, the patient has experienced the intended effect of the medication, the patient experienced no adverse effects, and the patient has verbalized an understanding of and engages with the medication regimen.

DOCUMENTATION

Guidelines

Document the administration of the medication immediately after administration, including date, time, dose, route of administration, site of administration, and rate of administration on the eMAR/MAR or record using the required format. If using a bar-code system, medication administration is automatically recorded when the bar code is scanned. PRN medications require documentation of the reason for administration. Prompt recording avoids the possibility of accidentally repeating the administration of the drug. If the drug was refused or omitted, record this in the appropriate area on the medication record and notify the health care team as appropriate. This verifies the reason medication was omitted and ensures that health care personnel providing care for the patient are aware of the occurrence. Document the volume of fluid administered on the intake and output record.

DEVELOPING CLINICAL REASONING AND CLINICAL JUDGMENT

UNEXPECTED SITUATIONS AND ASSOCIATED INTERVENTIONS

- *Upon assessing the IV site before administering medication, you note that the IV has infiltrated:* Stop the IV fluid and remove the IV from the extremity. Restart the IV in a different location. Continue to monitor the new IV site as the medication is administered.
- *While administering medication, you note a cloudy, white substance forming in the IV tubing:* Stop the IV from flowing and stop administering the medication to prevent precipitate from entering the patient's circulation. Clamp the IV at the site nearest to the patient. Replace tubing on primary and secondary infusions. Check a drug resource or consult a pharmacist regarding compatibility of the medication and IV fluid before continuing with administration. Medication infusion may require a second IV site or administration through an access port closer to the IV site and flushing of the tubing before and after administration.
- *While you are administering medication, the patient begins to complain of pain at the IV site:* Stop the medication. Assess the IV site for any signs of complications. Flush the IV with normal saline to check for patency. If the IV site appears within normal limits, resume medication administration at a slower rate.

SPECIAL CONSIDERATIONS

General Considerations

- Intermittent administration sets disconnected after use should be replaced every 24 hours; repeated disconnection and reconnection increases risk of contamination at the spike end, catheter hub, needleless connector, and the end of the administration set, potentially increasing the risk for catheter-related bloodstream infection (Gorski et al., 2021).
- Ongoing assessment is an important part of nursing care for both evaluation of patient response to administered medications and early detection of adverse reactions. If an adverse effect is suspected, withhold further medication doses and notify the patient's health care team. Additional intervention is based on type of reaction and patient assessment.

Infant and Child Considerations

- The primary method for IV medication administration for infants and children is a mini-infusion (syringe) pump (Kyle & Carman, 2021). Refer to Skill 5-13.
- Infants and small children with fluid restrictions may not tolerate the added IV fluid needed for administration with piggyback systems. For these children, consider using the mini-infusion pump (see Skill 5-13).

EVIDENCE FOR PRACTICE ▶

INFUSION NURSING STANDARDS OF PRACTICE

Infusion Nurses Society (INS). (2021). Infusion therapy. Standards of practice. *Journal of Infusion Nursing, 44*(Suppl 1), S1–S224. https://doi.org/10.1097/NAN.0000000000000396
Refer to details in Skill 5-10, Evidence for Practice.

Skill 5-13 ▶ Administering an Intermittent Intravenous Infusion of Medication via a Mini-Infusion Pump

Medications can be administered by intermittent IV infusion. The mini-infusion pump (syringe pump) for intermittent infusion is battery- or electrical-operated; medication mixed in a syringe is connected to the primary line and delivered by mechanical pressure applied to the syringe plunger and provides a highly precise rate of infusion (Kyle & Carman, 2021). Mini-infusion pumps may use a smart pump design; *smart (computerized) pumps* are increasingly being used by many facilities for IV infusions, including intermittent infusions. Smart pumps require programming of infusion rates by the nurse, but also are able to identify dosing limits and practice guidelines to aid in safe administration (ISMP, 2020). These smart IV pumps use computerized dose error-reduction software with IV drug therapy libraries that calculates infusion rates and provides an alert to the user when infusion rate limits are exceeded (Giuliano et al., 2018). Because **manufacturers' designs vary, it is important to check the directions carefully for the systems used in the facility.**

DELEGATION CONSIDERATIONS

The administration of medications by intermittent IV infusion is not delegated to assistive personnel (AP). Depending on the state's nurse practice act and the organization's policies and procedures, the administration of specified IV medications in some settings may be delegated to licensed practical/vocational nurses (LPN/LVNs) who have received appropriate training. The decision to delegate must be based on careful analysis of the patient's needs and circumstances as well as the qualifications of the person to whom the task is being delegated. Refer to the Delegation Guidelines in Appendix A.

EQUIPMENT

- Medication prepared in labeled syringe
- Mini-infusion pump and tubing
- Needleless connector, if required, based on facility system
- Antimicrobial swab
- Date label for tubing
- Electronic Medication Administration Record (eMAR) or Medication Administration Record (MAR)
- PPE, as indicated

(*continued on page 284*)

Skill 5-13 ▶ Administering an Intermittent Intravenous Infusion of Medication via a Mini-Infusion Pump *(continued)*

ASSESSMENT	Assess the appropriateness of the drug for the patient. Review the medical history and allergy, assessment, and laboratory data that may influence drug administration. Check the expiration date. **Assess the compatibility of the ordered medication, diluent, and the infusing IV fluid.** Assess the patient's IV site for signs of any complications. (Refer to Fundamentals Review 16-3 and Box 16-2 in Chapter 16 on pages 1005 and 1021.) Assess the patient's/family's/caregiver's knowledge of the medication. If the patient/family/caregiver has a knowledge deficit about the medication, this may be the appropriate time to begin education about the medication. If the medication may affect the patient's vital signs, assess them before administration. Verify patient name, dose, route, and time of administration. Assess the patient's knowledge of the medication.
ACTUAL OR POTENTIAL HEALTH PROBLEMS AND NEEDS	Many actual or potential health problems or issues may require the use of this skill as part of related interventions. An appropriate health problem or issue may include: • Risk for medication side effect • Risk for adverse medication interaction • Knowledge deficiency
OUTCOME IDENTIFICATION AND PLANNING	The expected outcomes to achieve are that the medication is delivered via the IV route, and the patient experiences the intended effect of the medication. Other outcomes that may be appropriate include the following: the patient experiences no adverse effects, and the patient verbalizes an understanding of and engages with the medication regimen.

IMPLEMENTATION

ACTION	**RATIONALE**
1. Gather equipment. Check each medication prescribed against the original in the health record, depending on facility policy and the medication order system in place. Clarify any inconsistencies. Check the patient's health record for allergies.	The prescription is the legal record of prescribed medication interventions. This comparison helps to identify errors that may have occurred when orders were transcribed. Computer provider order-entry (CPOE) systems allow prescribers to send electronic medication prescriptions directly to the pharmacy located in a health care facility and to outpatient pharmacies. Compatibility of medication and solution prevents complications.
2. Know the actions, special nursing considerations, safe dose ranges, purpose of administration, and adverse effects of the medications to be administered. Consider the appropriateness of the medication for this patient. **Assess the compatibility of the ordered medication, diluent, and the infusing IV fluid.**	This knowledge aids the nurse in evaluating the therapeutic effect of the medication in relation to the patient's health status and can also be used to educate the patient about the medication. Compatibility of medication and solutions prevents complications.
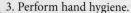 3. Perform hand hygiene.	Hand hygiene prevents the spread of microorganisms.
4. Move the medication supply system to the outside of the patient's room or prepare for administration at the medication supply system in the medication area. Alternatively, access the medication administration supply system at or inside the patient's room.	Organization facilitates error-free administration and saves time.
5. Unlock the medication supply system or drawer. Enter the passcode and scan employee identification, if required.	Locking the medication supply system or drawer safeguards each patient's medication supply. Facility accrediting organizations require medication supply systems to be locked when not in use. Entering the passcode and scanning ID allows only authorized users into the system and identifies the user for documentation by the computer.
6. **Prepare medications for one patient at a time.**	This prevents errors in medication administration.

ACTION	**RATIONALE**

7. Read the eMAR/MAR and read the label when selecting the proper medication from the medication supply system or the patient's medication drawer.

This is the *first* check of the label.

8. Read the label and compare the label with the eMAR/MAR. Check expiration dates. Confirm the prescribed or appropriate infusion rate. Scan the bar code on the package, if required.

This is the *second* check of the label. Verify calculations with another nurse to ensure safety, if necessary. Infusing medication at appropriate rate prevents injury.

9. **Depending on facility policy, the third check of the label may occur at this point. If so, when all medications for one patient have been prepared, read the label and recheck the labels with the eMAR/MAR before taking the medications to the patient. However, many facilities require the third check to occur at the bedside, after identifying the patient.**

This *third* check ensures accuracy and helps to prevent errors. *Note:* Many facilities require the *third* check to occur at the bedside, after identifying the patient and before administration.

10. **Log out of and/or lock the medication supply system before leaving it.**

Locking the medication supply system or drawer safeguards the patient's medication supply. Facility accrediting organizations require medication supply systems to be locked when not in use.

11. Transport medications to the patient's bedside carefully and keep the medications in sight at all times.

Careful handling and close observation prevent accidental or deliberate disarrangement of medications.

12. **Ensure that the patient receives the medications at the correct time.**

Check facility policy, which may allow for administration within a period of 30 minutes before or 30 minutes after the designated time.

 13. Perform hand hygiene and put on PPE, if indicated.

Hand hygiene and PPE prevent the spread of microorganisms. PPE is required based on transmission precautions.

 14. **Identify the patient. Compare the information with the eMAR/MAR. The patient should be identified using at least two of the following methods** (The Joint Commission, 2021):

Identifying the patient ensures the right patient receives the medications and helps prevent errors. The patient's room number or physical location is not used as an identifier (The Joint Commission, 2021). Replace the identification band if it is missing or inaccurate in any way.

a. Check the name on the patient's identification band.

This requires a response from the patient, but illness and strange surroundings often cause patients to be confused.

b. Check the identification number on the patient's identification band.

c. Check the birth date on the patient's identification band.

d. Ask the patient to state their name and birth date, based on facility policy.

15. Close the door to the room or pull the bedside curtain.

This provides patient privacy.

16. **Complete necessary assessments before administering medications. Check the patient's allergy bracelet, if present, or ask the patient about allergies. Explain the purpose and action of the medication to the patient/family/caregiver.**

Assessment is a prerequisite to administration of medications. Explanation provides rationale, increases knowledge, and reduces anxiety.

17. Scan the bar code on the patient's identification band, if required (The Joint Commission, 2021).

This provides an additional check to ensure that the medication is given to the right patient.

18. **Based on facility policy, the third check of the label may occur at this point. If so, read the label and recheck the labels with the eMAR/MAR before administering the medications to the patient.**

Many facilities require the *third* check to occur at the bedside, after identifying the patient and before administration. If facility policy directs the *third* check at this time, this *third* check ensures accuracy and helps to prevent errors.

19. Assess the IV site for the presence of inflammation or infiltration or other signs of complications.

IV medication must be given directly into a vein for safe administration.

(continued on page 286)

Skill 5-13 ▶ Administering an Intermittent Intravenous Infusion of Medication via a Mini-Infusion Pump   *(continued)*

ACTION	RATIONALE
20. Using aseptic technique, remove the cap on the administration tubing and the cap on the medication syringe, taking care not to contaminate either end.	Maintaining sterility of the tubing and medication port prevents contamination.
21. Attach the administration tubing to the syringe, taking care not to contaminate either end.	Maintaining sterility of the tubing and medication port prevents contamination.
22. Place a label on the tubing with the current date.	The label identifies the date of the first use of the tubing. Most facilities allow the reuse of tubing, reducing the risk for contamination. The frequency of administration set tubing changes varies. Refer to Box 16-3 in Skill 16-3 for recommended administration set change guidelines. Intermittent administration sets disconnected after use should be replaced every 24 hours; repeated disconnection and reconnection increases risk of contamination at the spike end, catheter hub, needleless connector, and the end of the administration set, potentially increasing the risk for catheter-related bloodstream infection (Gorski et al., 2021).
23. Fill the administration tubing (priming) with medication and purge the air from the tubing by applying gentle pressure to the syringe plunger (Kyle & Carman, 2021). Place the needleless connector on the end of the tubing, if required, using sterile technique.	This removes air from the tubing and maintains sterility.
24. Insert the syringe into the mini-infusion pump according to the manufacturer's directions (Figure 1).	The syringe must fit securely in the pump apparatus for proper operation.
25. Remove the passive disinfection cap from the needleless connector or end cap on the access port on the primary IV infusion tubing, closest to the IV insertion site (Figure 2). Alternatively, if a passive disinfection cap is not in place, use an antimicrobial swab to vigorously disinfect the connection surface and sides of the access port or stopcock above the roller clamp on the primary IV infusion tubing, usually the port closest to the IV insertion site.	The passive disinfection caps contain an antiseptic-impregnated sponge that dispenses the antiseptic over the connector's top and threads and protects the hub from contamination by touch or airborne sources (Barton, 2019; Casey et al., 2018). Venous access device entry points, end caps, and needleless connectors must be vigorously scrubbed and disinfected prior to each access to reduce the risk for introduction of microorganisms and prevent venous access device–related infection (Flynn et al., 2019; Gorski et al., 2021). Friction is needed to physically remove microorganisms from the top, sides, and threads of the needleless connector or end cap. Allow the antiseptic to dry completely to ensure complete effectiveness (Gorski et al., 2021; Slater et al., 2018).

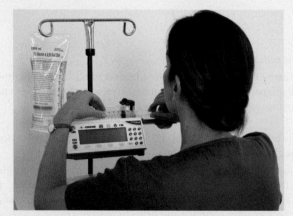

FIGURE 1. Inserting syringe into mini-infusion pump.

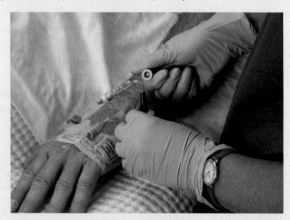

FIGURE 2. Removing the passive disinfection cap from the access port closest to IV insertion site.

ACTION	RATIONALE
26. Connect the secondary infusion to the primary infusion at the access port (Figure 3).	This allows for delivery of the medication.
27. Program the mini-infusion pump to the appropriate rate and begin infusion (Figure 4). Set the alarm if recommended by the manufacturer.	The pump delivers medication at a controlled rate. The alarm is recommended for use with medication or a drug-infusion lock.

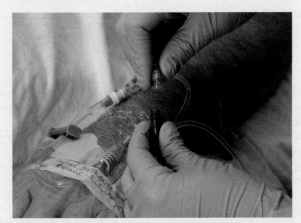

FIGURE 3. Connecting secondary infusion tubing the access port.

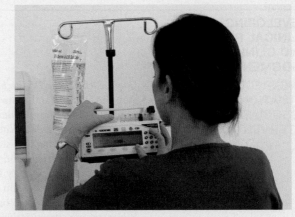

FIGURE 4. Programming mini-infusion pump.

ACTION	RATIONALE
28. When the infusion is completed, flush the syringe pump tubing, according to facility policy and procedure (Kyle & Carman, 2021).	Flushing the syringe pump tubing delivers any medication remaining in the tubing (Kyle & Carman, 2021).
29. Clamp the tubing on the syringe pump tubing.	Most facilities allow the reuse of tubing, reducing the risk for contamination. The frequency of administration set tubing changes varies. Refer to Box 16-3 in Skill 16-3 for recommended administration set change guidelines.
30. Check the rate of the primary infusion.	Administration of a secondary infusion may interfere with the primary infusion rate.
31. Remove PPE, if used. Perform hand hygiene.	Proper removal of PPE reduces the risk of infection transmission and contamination of other items. Hand hygiene prevents the spread of microorganisms.
32. Document the administration of the medication immediately after administration. See Documentation section below. Document the volume of fluid administered on the intake and output record, if necessary.	Timely documentation helps to ensure patient safety.
33. Evaluate the patient's response to the medication within the appropriate time frame. Monitor the IV site at periodic intervals.	The patient needs to be evaluated for therapeutic and adverse effects from the medication.

EVALUATION

The expected outcomes have been met when the medication was delivered via the IV route, the patient has experienced the intended effect of the medication, the patient experienced no adverse effects, and the patient has verbalized an understanding of and engaged with the medication regimen.

DOCUMENTATION

Guidelines

Document the administration of the medication immediately after administration, including date, time, dose, route of administration, site of administration, and rate of administration on the eMAR/MAR or record using the required format. If using a bar-code system, medication administration is

(*continued on page 288*)

Skill 5-13 ▶ Administering an Intermittent Intravenous Infusion of Medication via a Mini-Infusion Pump *(continued)*

automatically recorded when the bar code is scanned. PRN medications require documentation of the reason for administration. Prompt recording avoids the possibility of accidentally repeating the administration of the drug. If the drug was refused or omitted, record this in the appropriate area on the medication record and notify the health care team as appropriate. This verifies the reason medication was omitted and ensures that health care personnel providing care for the patient are aware of the occurrence. Document the volume of fluid administered on the intake and output record, if necessary.

DEVELOPING CLINICAL REASONING AND CLINICAL JUDGMENT

UNEXPECTED SITUATIONS AND ASSOCIATED INTERVENTIONS

- *Upon assessing the IV site before administering medication, you note that the IV has infiltrated:* Stop the IV fluid and remove the IV from the extremity. Restart the IV in a different location. Continue to monitor the new IV site as medication is administered.
- *While administering medication, you note a cloudy, white substance forming in the IV tubing:* Stop the IV from flowing and stop administering the medication to prevent precipitate from entering the patient's circulation. Clamp the IV at the site nearest to the patient. Replace the tubing on primary and secondary infusions. Check a drug resource or consult a pharmacist regarding compatibility of medication and IV fluid before continuing with administration. The medication infusion may require a second IV site or flushing of tubing before and after administration.
- *While you are administering medication, the patient begins to complain of pain at the IV site:* Stop the medication. Assess the IV site for any signs of complications. Flush the IV with normal saline to check for patency. If the IV site appears within normal limits, resume medication administration at a slower rate and continue to monitor.

SPECIAL CONSIDERATIONS

General Considerations

- If the medication is delivered via intermittently through a medication or drug-infusion lock, flush the peripheral IV access device before and after medication administration as outlined in Skill 5-11. Once the post-infusion flush is completed, attach a passive disinfection cap to the needleless connector or end cap on the access port of the medication lock, based on facility policy.
- Intermittent administration sets disconnected after use should be replaced every 24 hours; repeated disconnection and reconnection increases the risk of contamination at the spike end, catheter hub, needleless connector, and the end of the administration set, potentially increasing the risk for catheter-related bloodstream infection (Gorski et al., 2021)
- Ongoing assessment is an important part of nursing care for both evaluation of patient response to administered medications and early detection of adverse drug reactions. If an adverse effect is suspected, withhold further medication doses and notify the health care team. Additional intervention is based on type of reaction and patient assessment.

Infant and Child Considerations

- The primary method for IV medication administration for infants and children is a mini-infusion (syringe) pump (Kyle & Carman, 2021).

EVIDENCE FOR PRACTICE ▶

INFUSION NURSING STANDARDS OF PRACTICE

Infusion Nurses Society (INS). (2021). Infusion therapy. Standards of practice. *Journal of Infusion Nursing, 44*(Suppl 1), S1–S224. https://doi.org/10.1097/NAN.0000000000000396
Refer to details in Skill 5-10, Evidence for Practice.

Skill 5-14 ▶ Applying a Transdermal Patch

The transdermal route is being used more frequently to deliver medication. A disk or patch that contains medication intended for daily use or longer is applied to the patient's skin. Medications delivered via a transdermal patch have a slow onset of action and maintain consistent serum drug levels. Transdermal patches are commonly used to deliver hormones, opioid analgesics, cardiac medications, and nicotine. Medication errors have occurred when patients apply multiple patches at once or fail to remove the overlay on the patch that exposes the skin to the medication. Opioid analgesic patches are associated with the most adverse drug effects and require careful monitoring for advancing sedation and respiratory depression (Jungquist et al., 2020). Clear patches have a cosmetic advantage, but they can be difficult to find on the patient's skin when they need to be removed or replaced.

DELEGATION CONSIDERATIONS

The administration of medication via a transdermal patch is not delegated to assistive personnel (AP). Depending on the state's nurse practice act and the organization's policies and procedures, the administration of a transdermal patch may be delegated to licensed practical/vocational nurses (LPN/LVNs). The decision to delegate must be based on careful analysis of the patient's needs and circumstances as well as the qualifications of the person to whom the task is being delegated. Refer to the Delegation Guidelines in Appendix A.

EQUIPMENT

- Medication patch
- Gloves
- Scissors (optional)
- Disposable washcloth or washcloth, soap, and water
- Electronic Medication Administration Record (eMAR) or Medication Administration Record (MAR)
- Additional PPE, as indicated

ASSESSMENT

Assess the appropriateness of the drug for the patient. Review the medical history and allergy, assessment, and laboratory data that may influence drug administration. Check the expiration date before administering the medication. Assess the skin at the location where the patch will be applied. Many patches have different and specific instructions for where the patch is to be placed. For example, transdermal patches that contain estrogen cannot be placed on breast tissue. Check the manufacturer's instructions for the appropriate location for the patch. The site should be clean, dry, and free of hair. Do not place transdermal patches on irritated or broken skin (Cohrs & Kerns, 2020). Assess the patient for any old patches. Do not place a new transdermal patch until old patches have been removed. Verify the application frequency for the specific medication. Assess the patient's knowledge of the medication. If the patient has a knowledge deficit about the medication, this may be the appropriate time to begin education about the medication. If the medication may affect the patient's vital signs, assess them before administration. If the medication is for pain relief, assess the patient's pain before and after administration. Verify patient name, dose, route, and time of administration.

ACTUAL OR POTENTIAL HEALTH PROBLEMS AND NEEDS

Many actual or potential health problems or issues may require the use of this skill as part of related interventions. An appropriate health problem or issue may include:
- Risk for medication side effect
- Risk for adverse medication interaction
- Knowledge deficiency

OUTCOME IDENTIFICATION AND PLANNING

The expected outcomes to achieve are that the medication is delivered via the transdermal route and the patient experiences the intended effect of the medication. Other outcomes that may be appropriate include the following: the patient experiences no adverse effect, the patient's skin remains free from alterations in integrity, and the patient verbalizes an understanding of and engages with the medication regimen.

(continued on page 290)

Skill 5-14 ▶ Applying a Transdermal Patch *(continued)*

IMPLEMENTATION

ACTION	RATIONALE
1. Gather equipment. Check each medication prescribed against the original in the health record, depending on facility policy and the medication order system in place. Clarify any inconsistencies. Check the patient's health record for allergies.	The prescription is the legal record of prescribed medication interventions. This comparison helps to identify errors that may have occurred when orders were transcribed. Computer provider order-entry (CPOE) systems allow prescribers to send electronic medication prescriptions directly to the pharmacy located in a health care facility and to outpatient pharmacies.
2. Know the actions, special nursing considerations, safe dose ranges, purpose of administration, and adverse effects of the medications to be administered. Consider the appropriateness of the medication for this patient.	This knowledge aids the nurse in evaluating the therapeutic effect of the medication in relation to the patient's health status and can also be used to educate the patient about the medication.
3. Perform hand hygiene.	Hand hygiene prevents the spread of microorganisms.
4. Move the medication supply system to the outside of the patient's room or prepare for administration at the medication supply system in the medication area. Alternatively, access the medication administration supply system at or inside the patient's room.	Organization facilitates error-free administration and saves time.
5. Unlock the medication supply system or drawer. Enter the passcode and scan employee identification, if required.	Locking the medication supply system or drawer safeguards each patient's medication supply. Facility accrediting organizations require medication supply systems to be locked when not in use. Entering the passcode and scanning ID allows only authorized users into the system and identifies the user for documentation by the computer.
6. **Prepare medications for one patient at a time.**	This prevents errors in medication administration.
7. Read the eMAR/MAR and read the label when selecting the proper medication from the medication supply system or the patient's medication drawer.	This is the *first* check of the label.
8. Read the label and compare the label with the eMAR/MAR. Check expiration dates and perform calculations, if necessary. Scan the bar code on the package, if required.	This is the *second* check of the label. Verify calculations with another nurse to ensure safety, if necessary.
9. **Depending on facility policy, the third check of the label may occur at this point. If so, when all medications for one patient have been prepared, read the label and recheck the labels with the eMAR/MAR before taking the medications to the patient. However, many facilities require the third check to occur at the bedside, after identifying the patient.**	This *third* check ensures accuracy and helps to prevent errors. *Note:* Many facilities require the *third* check to occur at the bedside, after identifying the patient and before administration.
10. **Log out of and/or lock the medication supply system before leaving it.**	Locking the medication supply system or drawer safeguards the patient's medication supply. Facility accrediting organizations require medication supply systems to be locked when not in use.
11. Transport medications to the patient's bedside carefully and keep the medications in sight at all times.	Careful handling and close observation prevent accidental or deliberate disarrangement of medications.
12. **Ensure that the patient receives the medications at the correct time.**	Check facility policy, which may allow for administration within a period of 30 minutes before or 30 minutes after the designated time.
13. Perform hand hygiene and put on PPE, if indicated.	Hand hygiene and PPE prevent the spread of microorganisms. PPE is required based on transmission precautions.

ACTION	RATIONALE

14. **Identify the patient. Compare the information with the eMAR/MAR. The patient should be identified using at least two of the following methods** (The Joint Commission, 2021):

Identifying the patient ensures the right patient receives the medications and helps prevent errors. The patient's room number or physical location is not used as an identifier (The Joint Commission, 2021). Replace the identification band if it is missing or inaccurate in any way.

a. Check the name on the patient's identification band.

This requires a response from the patient, but illness and strange surroundings often cause patients to be confused.

b. Check the identification number on the patient's identification band.

c. Check the birth date on the patient's identification band.

d. Ask the patient to state their name and birth date, based on facility policy.

15. **Complete necessary assessments before administering medications. Check the patient's allergy bracelet, if present, or ask the patient about allergies. Explain the purpose and action of each medication to the patient.**

Assessment is a prerequisite to administration of medications.

16. Scan the bar code on the patient's identification band, if required (The Joint Commission, 2021) (Figure 1).

This provides an additional check to ensure that the medication is given to the right patient.

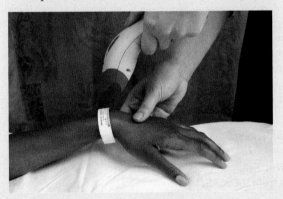

FIGURE 1. Scanning bar code on patient's identification bracelet.

17. **Based on facility policy, the third check of the label may occur at this point. If so, read the label and recheck the labels with the eMAR/MAR before administering the medications to the patient.**

Many facilities require the *third* check to occur at the bedside, after identifying the patient and before administration. If facility policy directs the *third* check at this time, this *third* check ensures accuracy and helps to prevent errors.

18. Put on gloves.

Gloves protect the nurse when handling the medication on the transdermal patch.

19. Assess the patient's skin where patch is to be placed, looking for any signs of irritation or breakdown. Site should be clean, dry, and free of hair. Rotate application sites.

Transdermal patches should not be placed on skin that is irritated or broken down. Hair can prevent the patch from sticking to the skin. Rotating sites reduces risk for skin irritation.

20. **Remove any old transdermal patches of the same kind from the patient's skin.** Fold the old patch in half with the adhesive sides sticking together and discard according to facility policy. Gently wash the area where the old patch was with a disposable washcloth or soap and water.

Leaving old patches on a patient while applying new ones may lead to delivery of a toxic level of the drug. Folding sides together prevents accidental contact with remaining medication. Washing the area with soap and water removes all traces of medication in that area.

21. Remove the patch from its protective covering. Remove the covering on the patch without touching the medication surface (Figure 2). Apply the patch to the patient's skin (Figure 3). Use the palm of your hand to press firmly for a minimum of 30 seconds. Do not massage. Use your fingers to go around the edges of the patch to press edges firmly to the skin (MedlinePlus, 2019).

Touching the adhesive side may alter the amount of medication left on the patch. Pressing firmly for a minimum of 30 seconds ensures that the patch stays on the patient's skin (Lindauer et al., 2017; MedlinePlus, 2019; MFMER, 2021a). Massaging the site may increase absorption of the medication.

(continued on page 292)

Skill 5-14 ▶ Applying a Transdermal Patch *(continued)*

ACTION

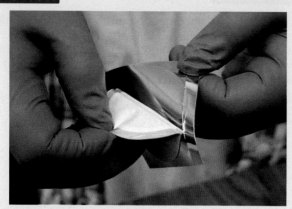

FIGURE 2. Removing protective covering on patch.

22. Remove gloves. Perform hand hygiene.

23. Depending on facility policy, initial and write the date and time of administration on a piece of medical tape. Apply the tape to the patient's skin in close proximity to the patch. **Do not write directly on the medication patch.**

24. Remove additional PPE, if used. Perform hand hygiene.

25. Document the administration of the medication immediately after administration. See Documentation section below.

26. Evaluate the patient's response to the medication within the appropriate time frame.

RATIONALE

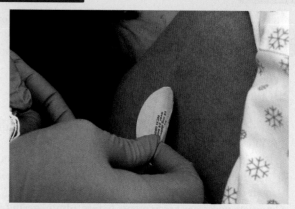

FIGURE 3. Applying patch to patient's skin.

Removing gloves and performing hand hygiene prevents the spread of microorganisms.

Most manufacturers recommend against writing on patches due to insufficient data on the practice. Writing on the patch could damage or tear it. Moreover, if ink is used, it may leach through and come into contact with the medication, and it is not known whether ink might interact with a given medication or impede its delivery (Durand et al., 2012).

Proper removal of PPE reduces the risk of infection transmission and contamination of other items. Hand hygiene prevents the spread of microorganisms.

Timely documentation helps to ensure patient safety.

The patient needs to be evaluated for therapeutic and adverse effects from the medication.

EVALUATION

The expected outcomes have been met when the medication was delivered via the transdermal route, the patient has experienced the intended effect of the medication, the patient experienced no adverse effect, the patient's skin has remained free from alterations in integrity, and the patient has verbalized an understanding of and engaged with the medication regimen.

DOCUMENTATION

Guidelines

Document the administration of the medication immediately after administration, including date, time, dose, route of administration, and site of administration on the eMAR/MAR or record using the required format. If using a bar-code system, medication administration is automatically recorded when the bar code is scanned. PRN medications require documentation of the reason for administration. Prompt recording avoids the possibility of accidentally repeating the administration of the drug. If the drug was refused or omitted, record this in the appropriate area on the medication record and notify the health care team as appropriate. This verifies the reason the medication was omitted and ensures that health care personnel providing care for the patient are aware of the occurrence.

DEVELOPING CLINICAL REASONING AND CLINICAL JUDGMENT

UNEXPECTED SITUATIONS AND ASSOCIATED INTERVENTIONS

- *You did not wear gloves while applying the transdermal patch:* Immediately perform good hand hygiene using soap and water to remove any medication that may be on the skin. You may feel the effects of the medication if any came into contact with your skin.
- *You find more than one old transdermal patch while applying a new transdermal patch:* Remove all old patches of the same kind; remember that more than one medication may be delivered via a transdermal patch. Check orders in the health record to ensure that the patient is still receiving the medication. Failure to remove old transdermal patches is considered a medication error and special event. Notify the health care team of potential medication overdose. Follow facility policy regarding documentation for special events.
- *When removing an old transdermal patch, you note the skin underneath is erythematosus and swollen:* Wash the skin with soap and water and assess the patient for any latex or adhesive allergies. Discuss with the patient whether the patch site has been rotated. Notify the health care team before applying a new patch.

SPECIAL CONSIDERATIONS

General Considerations

- Transdermal drug products have specific application sites, application intervals, and considerations. It is important to be knowledgeable about the specific drug administered. For example, fentanyl may be applied to the chest, back, flank, and upper arm; it is reapplied every 3 days; and patients may experience increased absorption with increased body temperature (Janssen Pharmaceuticals, Inc., 2018). Nitroglycerin transdermal may be placed on any hairless surface, except on extremities below the knees or elbows, with the chest being the preferred site; it is reapplied every 12 to 14 hours; patients should have a nitrate-free interval each day of 10 to 12 hours to ensure nitrate tolerance does not develop (Aroesty & Kannam, 2020; Holden, 2013; MFMER, 2021b).
- Apply the patch at the same time of day, according to the prescribed instructions and medication specifications.
- Check for dislodgement of the patch if the patient is active. Refer to manufacturer information about the patch or consult with the pharmacist to determine reapplication schedule and procedure.
- Aluminum backing on a patch necessitates precautions if defibrillation is required. Avoid placing AED pads in contact with or on top of a medication patch. The patch may block the delivery of energy to the heart and cause small burns to the skin. If it will not delay shock delivery, wear gloves or other barrier (to avoid transfer of medication from the patch to you) to quickly remove the patch and wipe the area before attaching the AED pad (AHA, 2020).Burns and smoke may result. In addition, these patches should be removed before magnetic resonance imaging is performed to avoid burning of the skin.
- Assess for any skin irritation at the application site. If necessary, remove the patch, wash the area carefully with soap and water, and allow the skin to air dry. Apply a new patch at a different site. Assess the potential for adverse reaction.
- Ongoing assessment is an important part of nursing care to evaluate patient response to administered medications and early detection of adverse drug reactions. If an adverse effect is suspected, withhold further medication doses and notify the patient's health care team. Additional intervention is based on type of reaction and patient assessment.

Community-Based Care Considerations

- Some manufacturers recommend that patients wearing patches avoid external heat sources (e.g., heating pads, electric blankets, heat lamps, saunas, hot tubs, sunlight), as heat may promote drug absorption through the skin (Cohrs & Kerns, 2020). Consult specific information from the manufacturer related to a particular medication.
- Caregivers and patients should be instructed to be certain to remove an old transdermal medication before applying a new one, as many patches have residual drug content even after the recommended application time.
- Instruct patients and caregivers to rotate application sites to decrease the risk of skin irritation.
- Instruct patients and caregivers to wash their hands thoroughly after the application of a transdermal medication to avoid inadvertent eye contact.
- Instruct patients and caregivers to discard used transdermal medications folded in half according to the manufacturer's instructions in household trash and out of reach of children, to avoid inadvertent exposure by children and pets (Cohrs & Kerns, 2020; Lampert et al., 2018).

Skill 5-15 ▶ Administering Eye Drops

Skill Variation: *Administering Eye Ointment*

Eye drops are instilled for their local effects, such as for pupil dilation or constriction when examining the eye, for infection treatment, or for controlling intraocular pressure (e.g., for patients with glaucoma). The type and amount of solution administered depends on the purpose of the instillation. If a patient is using more than one type of eye drop, scheduled at the same time, wait 3 to 5 minutes between the different kinds of medication (Gudgel, 2021; NIH, 2020). Consult a drug reference, package insert, or pharmacist for details for specific medications.

The eye is a delicate organ, highly susceptible to infection and injury. Although the eye is never free of microorganisms, the secretions of the conjunctiva protect against many pathogens. For maximal safety for the patient, the equipment, solutions, and ointments introduced into the conjunctival sac should be sterile. If this is not possible, follow careful guidelines for medical asepsis.

Refer to the accompanying Skill Variation for the steps to administer eye ointment.

DELEGATION CONSIDERATIONS

The administration of medication via drops in the eye is not delegated to assistive personnel (AP). Depending on the state's nurse practice act and the organization's policies and procedures, the administration of eye drops may be delegated to licensed practical/vocational nurses (LPN/LVNs). The decision to delegate must be based on careful analysis of the patient's needs and circumstances as well as the qualifications of the person to whom the task is being delegated. Refer to the Delegation Guidelines in Appendix A.

EQUIPMENT

- Gloves
- Additional PPE, as indicated
- Eye drop medication
- Tissues
- Normal saline solution
- Disposable washcloth, washcloth, cotton balls, or gauze squares
- Electronic Medication Administration Record (eMAR) or Medication Administration Record (MAR)

ASSESSMENT

Assess the appropriateness of the drug for the patient. Review the medical history and allergy, assessment, and laboratory data that may influence drug administration. Check the expiration date before administering the medication. Assess the affected eye for any drainage, erythema, or swelling. Assess the patient's knowledge of the medication. If the patient has a knowledge deficit about the medication, this may be the appropriate time to begin education about the medication. Verify patient name, dose, route, and time of administration.

ACTUAL OR POTENTIAL HEALTH PROBLEMS AND NEEDS

Many actual or potential health problems or issues may require the use of this skill as part of related interventions. An appropriate health problem or issue may include:
- Risk for medication side effect
- Knowledge deficiency
- Injury risk

OUTCOME IDENTIFICATION AND PLANNING

The expected outcomes to achieve when administering eye drops are that the medication is delivered successfully into the eye, and the patient experiences the intended effect of the medication. Other outcomes that may be appropriate include the following: the patient experiences no allergic response, the patient does not exhibit systemic effects of the medication, the patient's eye remains free from injury, and patient verbalizes an understanding of and engages with the medication regimen.

IMPLEMENTATION

ACTION	RATIONALE
1. Gather equipment. Check each medication prescribed against the original in the health record, depending on facility policy and the medication order system in place. Clarify any inconsistencies. Check the patient's health record for allergies.	The prescription is the legal record of prescribed medication interventions. This comparison helps to identify errors that may have occurred when orders were transcribed. Computer provider order-entry (CPOE) systems allow prescribers to send electronic medication prescriptions directly to the pharmacy located in a health care facility and to outpatient pharmacies.

ACTION	**RATIONALE**
2. Know the actions, special nursing considerations, safe dose ranges, purpose of administration, and adverse effects of the medications to be administered. Consider the appropriateness of the medication for this patient.	This knowledge aids the nurse in evaluating the therapeutic effect of the medication in relation to the patient's health status and can also be used to educate the patient about the medication.
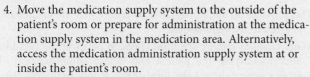 3. Perform hand hygiene.	Hand hygiene prevents the spread of microorganisms.
4. Move the medication supply system to the outside of the patient's room or prepare for administration at the medication supply system in the medication area. Alternatively, access the medication administration supply system at or inside the patient's room.	Organization facilitates error-free administration and saves time.
5. Unlock the medication supply system or drawer. Enter the passcode and scan employee identification, if required.	Locking the medication supply system or drawer safeguards each patient's medication supply. Facility accrediting organizations require medication supply systems to be locked when not in use. Entering the passcode and scanning ID allows only authorized users into the system and identifies the user for documentation by the computer.
6. **Prepare medications for one patient at a time.**	This prevents errors in medication administration.
7. Read the eMAR/MAR and read the label when selecting the proper medication from the patient's medication drawer or medication supply system.	This is the *first* check of the label.
8. Read the label and compare the label with the eMAR/MAR. Check expiration dates and perform calculations, if necessary. Scan the bar code on the package, if required.	This is the *second* check of the label. Verify calculations with another nurse to ensure safety, if necessary.
9. **Depending on facility policy, the third check of the label may occur at this point. If so, when all medications for one patient have been prepared, read the label and recheck the labels with the eMAR/MAR before taking the medications to the patient. However, many facilities require the third check to occur at the bedside, after identifying the patient.**	This *third* check ensures accuracy and helps to prevent errors. *Note:* Many facilities require the *third* check to occur at the bedside, after identifying the patient and before administration.
10. **Log out of and/or lock the medication supply system before leaving it.**	Locking the medication supply system or drawer safeguards the patient's medication supply. Facility accrediting organizations require medication supply systems to be locked when not in use.
11. Transport medications to the patient's bedside carefully and keep the medications in sight at all times.	Careful handling and close observation prevent accidental or deliberate disarrangement of medications.
12. **Ensure that the patient receives the medications at the correct time.**	Check facility policy, which may allow for administration within a period of 30 minutes before or 30 minutes after the designated time.
13. Perform hand hygiene and put on PPE, if indicated.	Hand hygiene and PPE prevent the spread of microorganisms. PPE is required based on transmission precautions.
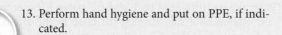 14. **Identify the patient. Compare the information with the eMAR/MAR. The patient should be identified using at least two of the following methods** (The Joint Commission, 2011):	Identifying the patient ensures the right patient receives the medications and helps prevent errors. The patient's room number or physical location is not used as an identifier (The Joint Commission, 2021). Replace the identification band if it is missing or inaccurate in any way.
a. Check the name on the patient's identification band.	This requires a response from the patient, but illness and strange surroundings often cause patients to be confused.

(continued on page 296)

Skill 5-15 ▶ Administering Eye Drops *(continued)*

ACTION	**RATIONALE**

    b. Check the identification number on the patient's identification band.

    c. Check the birth date on the patient's identification band.

    d. Ask the patient to state their name and birth date, based on facility policy.

15. Close the door to the room or pull the bedside curtain.

    This provides patient privacy.

16. **Complete necessary assessments before administering medications. Check the patient's allergy bracelet, if present, or ask the patient about allergies. Explain the purpose and action of each medication to the patient.**

    Assessment is a prerequisite to administration of medications.

17. Scan the bar code on the patient's identification band, if required (The Joint Commission, 2021) (Figure 1).

    This provides an additional check to ensure that the medication is given to the right patient.

18. **Based on facility policy, the third check of the label may occur at this point. If so, read the label and recheck the labels with the eMAR/MAR before administering the medications to the patient.**

    Many facilities require the third *check to occur at the bedside, after identifying the patient and before administration. If facility policy directs the* third *check at this time, this* third *check ensures accuracy and helps to prevent errors.*

19. Put on gloves.

    Gloves protect the nurse from potential contact with mucous membranes and body fluids.

20. Offer a tissue to the patient. Patients wearing contact lenses should remove them, unless prescribed medication instructions indicate the lenses should be left in during administration (Gudgel, 2021).

    Solution and tears may spill from the eye during the procedure.

21. If indicated, cleanse the eyelids and eyelashes of any drainage with a washcloth, cotton balls, or gauze squares moistened with water or normal saline solution, as indicated by the patient's condition. Use each area of the cleaning surface once, moving from the inner toward the outer canthus (Figure 2).

    Debris can be carried into the eye when the conjunctival sac is exposed. Using each area of the gauze once and moving from the inner canthus to the outer canthus prevents carrying debris to the lacrimal ducts.

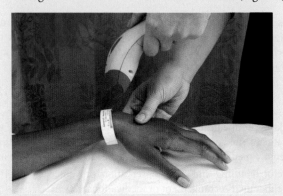

FIGURE 1. Scanning bar code on patient's identification bracelet.

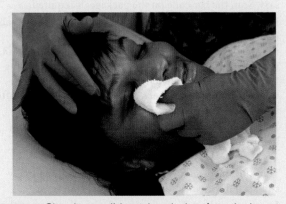

FIGURE 2. Cleaning eyelids and eyelashes from the inner toward the outer canthus.

22. Tilt the patient's head back slightly if they are sitting, or place the patient's head over a pillow if they are lying down. **Tilting the patient's head should be avoided if the patient has a cervical spine injury or other condition resulting in limited range of notion.** The head may be turned slightly to the affected side to prevent the solution or tears from flowing toward the opposite eye (Figure 3).

    Tilting the patient's head back slightly makes it easier to reach the conjunctival sac. Turning the head to the affected side helps to prevent the solution or tears from flowing toward the opposite eye.

23. Remove the cap from the medication bottle, being careful not to touch the inside of the cap or the tip of the container. (See the accompanying Skill Variation for administering eye ointment.)

    Touching the inside of the cap or tip of container may contaminate the bottle of medication.

ACTION

RATIONALE

24. Have the patient look up and focus on something on the ceiling. Place your thumb or two fingers near the margin of the lower eyelid immediately below eyelashes and apply pressure downward over the bony cheek prominence. The lower conjunctival sac is exposed as the lower lid is pulled down (Figure 4).

By having the patient look up and focus on something else, the procedure is less traumatic and keeps the eye still. The eye drop should be placed in the conjunctival sac, not directly on the eyeball.

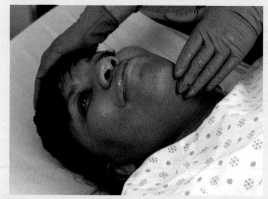

FIGURE 3. Turning head slightly to affected side.

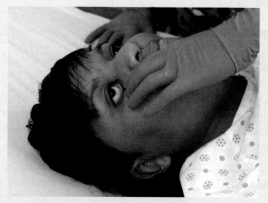

FIGURE 4. Applying pressure downward over bony cheek prominence to expose lower conjunctival sac.

25. Rest the lateral side of your hand on the patient's forehead, just above the eyebrow. Invert the monodrip plastic container that is commonly used to instill eye drops.

Stabilizing your hand on the patient's forehead prevents accidental contamination of the bottle tip and injury to the eye.

26. **Hold the dropper close to the eye but avoid touching eyelids or lashes.** Squeeze the container according to the manufacturer's recommendations and allow the prescribed number of drops to fall into the lower conjunctival sac (Figure 5). Alternatively, use the technique indicated in the product insert to release the drop of medication.

Touching the eye, eyelids, or lashes can contaminate the medication in the bottle; startle the patient, causing blinking; or injure the eye. Do not allow the medication to fall onto the cornea. This may injure the cornea or cause the patient to have an unpleasant sensation. Some ophthalmic solutions have unique dispensing bottles that require tapping or pressing the base of the bottle to release the drop of medication as opposed to squeezing the sides; compressing the sides will result in too much medication being expelled (Cohen, 2017; NPS Medicinewise, 2020).

27. Release the lower lid after the eye drops are instilled. Ask the patient to close their eyes gently.

This allows the medication to be distributed over the entire eye.

28. Apply or ask the patient to apply as appropriate, gentle pressure over the inner canthus (where the eyelid meets the nose) to prevent eye drops from flowing into the tear duct (Gudgel, 2021) (Figure 6).

This maximizes absorption by the eye (Gudgel, 2021) and minimizes the risk of systemic effects from the medication.

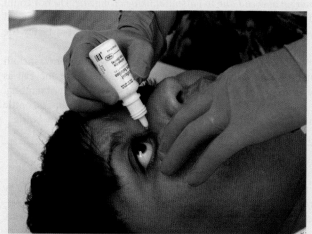

FIGURE 5. Squeezing container to administering drops into conjunctival sac.

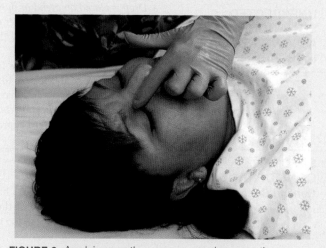

FIGURE 6. Applying gentle pressure over inner canthus.

(*continued on page 298*)

Skill 5-15 ▶ Administering Eye Drops *(continued)*

ACTION	**RATIONALE**
29. Instruct the patient not to rub the affected eye. Replace the cover on the medication bottle.	This prevents injury and irritation to the eye. The cover prevents contamination.
30. Remove gloves. Perform hand hygiene. Assist the patient to a comfortable position.	Removing gloves and performing hand hygiene prevents the spread of microorganisms. Assisting the patient to a position of comfort promotes patient comfort.
31. Remove additional PPE, if used. Perform hand hygiene.	Proper removal of PPE reduces the risk of infection transmission and contamination of other items. Hand hygiene prevents the spread of microorganisms.
32. Document the administration of the medication immediately after administration. See Documentation section below.	Timely documentation helps to ensure patient safety.
33. Evaluate the patient's response to the medication within an appropriate time frame.	The patient needs to be evaluated for therapeutic and adverse effects from the medication.

EVALUATION

The expected outcomes have been met when the medication was delivered successfully into the eye, the patient has experienced the intended effect of the medication, the patient experienced no allergic response, the patient did not exhibit systemic effects of the medication, the patient's eye has remained free from injury, and the patient has verbalized an understanding of and engaged with the medication regimen.

DOCUMENTATION

Guidelines

Document the administration of the medication immediately after administration, including date, time, dose, route of administration, and site of administration, specifically right, left, or both eyes, on the eMAR/MAR or health record using the required format. If using a bar-code system, medication administration is automatically recorded when the bar code is scanned. PRN medications require documentation of the reason for administration. Prompt recording avoids the possibility of accidentally repeating the administration of the drug. If the drug was refused or omitted, record this in the appropriate area on the medication record and notify the health care team. This verifies the reason medication was omitted and ensures that that health care personnel providing care for the patient are aware of the occurrence.

DEVELOPING CLINICAL REASONING AND CLINICAL JUDGMENT

UNEXPECTED SITUATIONS AND ASSOCIATED INTERVENTIONS

- *Drop is placed on eyelid or outer margin of eyelid due to patient blinking or moving:* Do not count this drop in the total number of drops administered. Allow the patient to regain composure and proceed with application of the medication. Consider approaching the patient from below the line of sight.
- *You cannot open eyelids due to dried crust and matting of eyelids:* Place a warm, wet washcloth over the eye and allow it to remain there for approximately 3 minutes. Cleanse the eye as described previously. You may need to repeat this procedure if there is a large amount of matting.
- *Bottle or tube of medication comes in contact with the eyeball when applying medication:* The bottle is contaminated; discard appropriately. Notify the pharmacy to obtain or retrieve a new bottle.

SPECIAL CONSIDERATIONS

General Considerations

- Some ophthalmic solutions have unique dispensing bottles that require tapping or pressing the base of the bottle to release the drop of medication as opposed to squeezing the sides; compressing the sides will result in too much medication being expelled (Cohen, 2017; NPS Medicinewise, 2020).

- Ongoing assessment is an important part of nursing care to evaluate patient response to administered medications and early detection of adverse drug reactions. If an adverse effect is suspected, withhold further medication doses and notify the patient's health care team. Additional intervention is based on type of reaction and patient assessment.

Infant and Child Considerations

- To apply eye drops in a small child, two or more people may be needed to restrain the child. Make sure the child does not reach up to the eye, causing the nurse to jab the medication bottle into the eye.

Community-Based Care Considerations

- Elderly patients may have difficulty with self-administration of eye drops. Poor vision and functional status may lead to poor administration technique, resulting in ineffective treatment (Choy et al., 2019).
- Patients who wear contact lenses should be instructed to remove the lenses before administration of eye drops, unless instructed by the ophthalmologist to leave the lenses in (Gudgel, 2021).

Skill Variation ▶ Administering Eye Ointment

Prepare medication as outlined in Steps 1–21 above (Skill 5-15).

1. Have the patient look up and focus on something on the ceiling.
2. Place thumb or two fingers near the margin of the lower eyelid immediately below eyelashes and exert pressure downward over the bony cheek prominence. The lower conjunctival sac is exposed as the lower lid is pulled down.
3. Hold the ointment tube close to eye but avoid touching eyelids or lashes. Squeeze the container and apply about 0.5 inch of ointment from the tube along the exposed sac. Apply the medication, moving from the inner canthus to the outer canthus. Twist the tube to break off a ribbon of ointment. **Do not touch the tip to the eye.**
4. Release the lower lid after ointment is instilled. Ask the patient to close their eyes gently.
5. The patient's body warmth helps to liquefy the ointment. Instruct the patient to keep the eye closed and move the

eye in the socket to help spread the ointment under the lids and over the surface of the eyeball. The patient may then open the eye.

6. Remove gloves and perform hand hygiene. Assist the patient to a comfortable position. Explain that the ointment may temporarily blur vision; encourage the patient not to rub the eye.

7. Remove additional PPE, if used. Perform hand hygiene.

8. Document administration of the medication on the eMAR/MAR or health record immediately after administering the medication.
9. Evaluate the patient's response to the medication within an appropriate time frame.

Skill 5-16 ▶ Administering an Eye Irrigation

Eye irrigation is performed to remove secretions or foreign bodies or to cleanse and soothe the eye. In an emergency, eye irrigation can be used to remove chemicals or other substances that may burn or injure the eye. When irrigating one eye, take care that the overflowing irrigation fluid does not contaminate the other eye. Eye flush stations may be available in emergency departments to aid in irrigation of the eye; many work environments, such as a lab where chemicals are used, in which there is risk for accidental exposure also have eye flush stations as well.

DELEGATION CONSIDERATIONS

The administration of an eye irrigation is not delegated to nursing assistive personnel (AP). Depending on the state's nurse practice act and the organization's policies and procedures, the administration of an eye irrigation may be delegated to licensed practical/vocational nurses (LPN/LVNs). The decision to delegate must be based on careful analysis of the patient's needs and circumstances as well as the qualifications of the person to whom the task is being delegated. Refer to the Delegation Guidelines in Appendix A.

(continued on page 300)

Skill 5-16 ▸ Administering an Eye Irrigation *(continued)*

EQUIPMENT

- Sterile irrigation solution as prescribed at room temperature (sterile water, normal saline solution, Ringer's lactate, clean water) (Gwenhure, 2020; Stevens, 2016)
- Local anesthetic eye drops
- Sterile irrigation set (sterile container and irrigating or bulb syringe) or intravenous infusion administration tubing, depending on circumstances and prescribed irrigant

- Emesis basin or irrigation basin
- Washcloth
- Waterproof pad
- Towel
- Gloves
- Face shield and splash guard
- Additional PPE, as indicated

ASSESSMENT

Assess the appropriateness of the irrigation solution for the patient. Review the medical history and allergy, assessment, and laboratory data that may influence drug administration. Check the expiration date of the irrigant. Assess the patient's eyes for redness, erythema, edema, drainage, or tenderness. Assess the patient's knowledge of the procedure. If the patient has a knowledge deficit about the procedure, this may be an appropriate time to begin patient education. Assess the patient's ability to participate in the procedure. Verify patient name, dose, route, and time of administration.

ACTUAL OR POTENTIAL HEALTH PROBLEMS AND NEEDS

Many actual or potential health problems or issues may require the use of this skill as part of related interventions. An appropriate health problem or issue may include:
- Knowledge deficiency
- Infection risk
- Acute pain

OUTCOME IDENTIFICATION AND PLANNING

The expected outcome to achieve is that the eye is cleansed successfully. Other outcomes that may be appropriate include the following: the patient verbalizes an understanding of the procedure and is able to participate, the patient's pain and discomfort are reduced/relieved, and the patient's eye remains free from additional injury.

IMPLEMENTATION

ACTION	RATIONALE
1. Gather equipment. Check each irrigation intervention prescribed against the original in the health record, depending on facility policy and the medication order system in place. Clarify any inconsistencies. Check the patient's health record for allergies.	The prescription is the legal record of prescribed medication interventions. This comparison helps to identify errors that may have occurred when orders were transcribed. Computer provider order-entry (CPOE) systems allow prescribers to send electronic medication prescriptions directly to the pharmacy located in a health care facility and to outpatient pharmacies.
2. Know the actions, special nursing considerations, purpose of administration, and potential adverse effects of the medications to be administered. Consider the appropriateness of the medication for this patient.	This knowledge aids the nurse in evaluating the therapeutic effect of the medication in relation to the patient's health status and can also be used to educate the patient about the medication.
3. Perform hand hygiene and put on PPE, if indicated.	Hand hygiene and PPE prevent the spread of microorganisms. PPE is required based on transmission precautions.
4. Move the medication supply system to the outside of the patient's room or prepare for administration at the medication supply system in the medication area. Alternatively, access the medication administration supply system at or inside the patient's room.	Organization facilitates error-free administration and saves time.

44

44

ACTION

5. Unlock the medication supply system or drawer. Enter the passcode into the computer and scan employee identification, if required.

6. **Prepare medications for one patient at a time.**
7. Read the eMAR/MAR and read the label when selecting the proper irrigation solution from the medication supply system or patient's medication drawer.

8. Read the label and compare the medication label with the eMAR/MAR. Check expiration dates and perform calculations, if necessary. Scan the bar code on the package, if required.

9. **Depending on facility policy, the third check of the label may occur at this point. If so, when all medications for one patient have been prepared, read the label and recheck the labels with the eMAR/MAR before taking the medications to the patient. However, many facilities require the third check to occur at the bedside, after identifying the patient.**

10. **Log out of and/or lock the medication supply system before leaving it.**

11. Transport medications to the patient's bedside carefully and keep the medications in sight at all times.
12. **Ensure that the patient receives the medications at the correct time.**

 13. Perform hand hygiene and put on PPE, if indicated.

 14. **Identify the patient. Compare the information with the eMAR/MAR. The patient should be identified using at least two of the following methods** (The Joint Commission, 2021):

a. Check the name on the patient's identification band.

b. Check the identification number on the patient's identification band.

c. Check the birth date on the patient's identification band.

d. Ask the patient to state their name and birth date, based on facility policy.

15. Close the door to the room or pull the bedside curtain.
16. **Complete necessary assessments before administering medications. Check the patient's allergy bracelet, if present, or ask the patient about allergies. Explain the purpose and action of each medication to the patient.**

17. Scan the patient's bar code on the identification band, if required (The Joint Commission, 2021).
18. Assemble equipment at the patient's bedside.

RATIONALE

Locking the medication supply system or drawer safeguards each patient's medication supply. Facility accrediting organizations require medication supply systems to be locked when not in use. Entering the passcode and scanning ID allows only authorized users into the computer system and identifies the user for documentation by the computer.

This prevents errors in administration.

This is the *first* check of the medication label.

This is the *second* check of the label. Verify calculations with another nurse to ensure safety, if necessary.

This *third* check ensures accuracy and helps to prevent errors. *Note:* Many facilities require the third check to occur at the bedside, after identifying the patient and before administration.

Locking the medication supply system or drawer safeguards the patient's medication supply. Facility accrediting organizations require medication supply systems to be locked when not in use.

Careful handling and close observation prevent accidental or deliberate disarrangement of medications.

Check facility policy, which may allow for administration within a period of 30 minutes before or 30 minutes after the designated time.

Hand hygiene and PPE prevent the spread of microorganisms. PPE is required based on transmission precautions.

Identifying the patient ensures the right patient receives the medications and helps prevent errors. The patient's room number or physical location is not used as an identifier (The Joint Commission, 2021). Replace the identification band if it is missing or inaccurate in any way.

This requires a response from the patient, but illness and strange surroundings often cause patients to be confused.

This provides patient privacy.

Assessment is a prerequisite to administration of medications. Explanation provides rationale, increases knowledge, promotes patient engagement, and reduces anxiety.

This provides an additional check to ensure that the medication is given to the right patient.

This provides for an organized approach to the task.

(*continued on page 302*)

Skill 5-16 ▶ Administering an Eye Irrigation *(continued)*

ACTION	RATIONALE

ACTION

19. **Based on facility policy, the third check of the medication label may occur at this point. If so, read the label and recheck the label with the eMAR/MAR before administering the medications to the patient.**

20. Administer the local anesthetic eye drops to the affected eye(s) (Stevens, 2016).

21. Have the patient sit or lie with their head tilted toward the side of the affected eye (Figure 1). Protect the patient and bed with a waterproof pad.

22. Put on gloves. Clean lids and lashes with a washcloth moistened with water or normal saline or the solution ordered for the irrigation, as indicated by the patient's condition. Wipe from the inner canthus toward outer canthus (Figure 2). Use a different corner of the washcloth with each wipe.

RATIONALE

Many facilities require the *third* check to occur at the bedside, after identifying the patient and before administration. If facility policy directs the *third* check at this time, this *third* check ensures accuracy and helps prevent errors.

Anesthetic eye drops can make the procedure less painful and uncomfortable (Gwenhure, 2020).

Gravity aids the flow of the solution away from the unaffected eye and from the inner canthus of the affected eye toward the outer canthus.

Gloves protect the nurse from contact with mucous membranes, body fluids, and contaminants. Materials lodged on lids or in lashes may be washed into the eye. Wiping from the inner to outer canthus protects the nasolacrimal duct and the other eye. Use of a different part of the washcloth prevents transmission of bacteria.

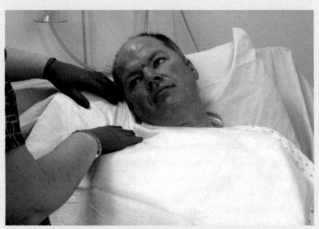

FIGURE 1. Tilting head toward affected eye.

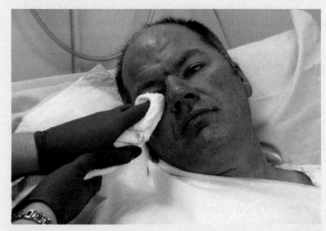

FIGURE 2. Cleaning eyelids and eyelashes from inner canthus to outer canthus.

23. Put on a face shield/splash guard. Place the curved basin at the patient's cheek on the side of the affected eye to receive the irrigating solution (Figure 3). If the patient is able, ask them to support the basin.

The face shield/splash guard protects the nurse from contact with splashed body fluids and contaminants. Gravity aids the flow of the solution.

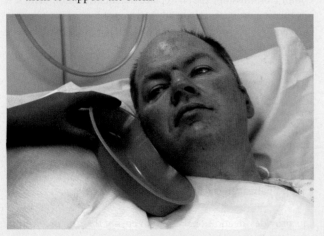

FIGURE 3. Placing basin to catch irrigating fluid.

ACTION

24. Fill the irrigation syringe with the prescribed fluid. Place your thumb near the margin of the lower eyelid immediately below eyelashes and two fingers above the eye. Apply pressure downward over the bony cheek prominence to expose the lower conjunctival sac as the lower lid is pulled down. Hold the upper lid open with your fingers (Figure 4).

25. **Hold the irrigation syringe (Figure 5) or tip of the IV tubing 3 to 4 cm but no more than 5 cm from the eye** (Stevens, 2016). **Tell the patient the irrigation is going to start. Direct the flow of the solution from the inner to outer canthus along the conjunctival sac.**

RATIONALE

The solution is directed only into the lower conjunctival sac because the cornea is sensitive and easily injured. This also prevents reflex blinking.

This minimizes the risk for injury to the cornea. Directing the solution toward the outer canthus helps prevent the spread of contamination from the eye to the lacrimal sac, the lacrimal duct, and the nose.

A distance of 3 to 4 cm and no more than 5 cm prevents damage to the eye from the force of fluid (Gwenhure, 2020; Stevens, 2016).

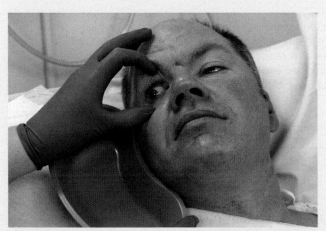

FIGURE 4. Exposing lower conjunctival sac and holding upper lid open.

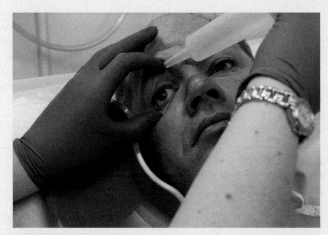

FIGURE 5. Holding irrigation syringe 3 to 4 cm but no more than 5 cm from eye.

26. Ask the patient to move the eye in all directions, if possible, while the irrigation is maintained (Stevens, 2016). Irrigate until the solution is clear or all the solution has been used. **Use only enough force to remove secretions gently from the conjunctiva. Avoid touching any part of the eye with the irrigating tip.**

27. Pause the irrigation and have the patient close their eye periodically during the procedure.

28. Dry the periorbital area after irrigation with a gauze sponge. Offer a towel to the patient if their face and/or neck is wet.

 29. Remove gloves. Perform hand hygiene. Assist the patient to a comfortable position.

30. Remove the face shield and splash guard and additional PPE, if used. Perform hand hygiene.

31. Evaluate the patient's response to the medication within an appropriate time frame.

Directing solutions with force may cause injury to the tissues of the eye as well as to the conjunctiva. Touching the eye is uncomfortable for the patient and may cause damage to the cornea.

Movement of the eye when the lids are closed helps to move secretions from the upper to the lower conjunctival sac.

Leaving the skin moist after irrigation is uncomfortable for the patient.

Removing gloves and performing hand hygiene prevents the spread of microorganisms. Assisting the patient to a position of comfort promotes patient comfort.

Proper removal of PPE reduces the risk of infection transmission and contamination of other items. Hand hygiene prevents the spread of microorganisms.

The patient needs to be evaluated for therapeutic and adverse effects from the medication.

(continued on page 304)

Skill 5-16 ▶ Administering an Eye Irrigation *(continued)*

EVALUATION

The expected outcomes have been met when the eye was irrigated successfully, the patient has verbalized an understanding of the procedure and was able to participate, the patient's pain and discomfort were reduced/relieved, and the patient's eye has remained free from additional injury.

DOCUMENTATION

Guidelines

Document the procedure, site, the type of solution and volume used, length of time irrigation performed, pre- and post-procedure assessments, characteristics of any drainage, and the patient's response to the treatment on the eMAR/MAR or record using the required format. If using a bar-code system, medication administration is automatically recorded when the bar code is scanned. PRN medications require documentation of the reason for administration. Prompt recording avoids the possibility of accidentally repeating the administration of the drug. If the drug was refused or omitted, record this in the appropriate area on the medication record and notify the health care team. This verifies the reason medication was omitted and ensures that that health care personnel providing care for the patient are aware of the occurrence.

Sample Documentation

8/26/25 1820 Sclera of left eye reddened, with periorbital edema and erythema. Thick, yellow liquid draining from left eye. Irrigation of left eye performed using 500 mL of sterile saline. Patient's sclera remains reddened, with slight periorbital edema and erythema. No drainage noted from left eye after irrigation. Patient tolerated procedure with minimal discomfort. Denies need for pain medication at this time. Patient rates pain at present as 1/10.

—B. Clapp, RN

DEVELOPING CLINICAL REASONING AND CLINICAL JUDGMENT

UNEXPECTED SITUATIONS AND ASSOCIATED INTERVENTIONS

- *Patient reports significant pain during the procedure:* Stop the procedure and notify the health care team. Consult with the health care team regarding the need for an ophthalmology consult to check for any foreign objects, such as glass, before proceeding with irrigation.
- *Patient cannot keep the eye open during the procedure:* You may need assistance to help the patient keep the eye open.

SPECIAL CONSIDERATIONS

- For foreign body removal, a minute or so of irrigation should be sufficient to remove any foreign bodies (Stevens, 2016).
- For severe acid or alkali burns, emergency irrigation should continue for at least 15 minutes, and 30 minutes is better (Stevens, 2016).
- Ongoing assessment is an important part of nursing care to evaluate patient response to administered treatments and early detection of adverse drug reactions. If an adverse effect is suspected, notify the health care team. Provide additional intervention based on type of reaction and patient assessment.
- In some instances where chemical contamination is suspected, the pH of the eye may need to be checked to facilitate treatment. When only one eye is contaminated, both eyes should be checked to use the noncontaminated eye as a control (Gwenhure, 2020).

Skill 5-17 ▶ Administering Ear Drops

Drugs are instilled into the auditory canal for their local effect and are used to soften wax, relieve pain, apply local anesthesia, and treat infections. If the tympanic membrane is ruptured or has been opened by surgical intervention, the middle ear and the inner ear have a direct passage to the external ear. When this occurs, perform instillations with the greatest of care to prevent forcing materials from the outer ear into the middle ear and the inner ear. In this circumstance, use sterile technique to prevent infection.

DELEGATION CONSIDERATIONS	The administration of medication via drops in the ear is not delegated to assistive personnel (AP). Depending on the state's nurse practice act and the organization's policies and procedures, the administration of ear drop may be delegated to licensed practical/vocational nurses (LPN/LVNs). The decision to delegate must be based on careful analysis of the patient's needs and circumstances as well as the qualifications of the person to whom the task is being delegated. Refer to the Delegation Guidelines in Appendix A.

EQUIPMENT

- Ear drop medication
- Tissue
- Cotton balls (optional)
- Gloves
- Additional PPE, as indicated

- Disposable washcloth or washcloth (optional)
- Normal saline solution or warm water
- Electronic Medication Administration Record (eMAR) or Medication Administration Record (MAR)

ASSESSMENT

Assess the appropriateness of the drug for the patient. Review the medical history and allergy, assessment, and laboratory data that may influence drug administration. Assess the affected ear for redness, erythema, edema, drainage, or tenderness. Assess the patient's knowledge of the medication and procedure. If the patient has a knowledge deficit about the medication, this may be an appropriate time to begin education about the medication. Assess the patient's ability to participate with the procedure. Verify patient name, dose, route, and time of administration.

ACTUAL OR POTENTIAL HEALTH PROBLEMS AND NEEDS

Many actual or potential health problems or issues may require the use of this skill as part of related interventions. An appropriate health problem or issue may include:
- Knowledge deficiency
- Injury risk
- Acute pain

OUTCOME IDENTIFICATION AND PLANNING

The expected outcomes to achieve are that drops are administered successfully, and the patient experiences the intended effect of the medication. Other outcomes that may be appropriate include the following: the patient verbalizes an understanding of the rationale for the ear drop instillation, and the patient does not experience injury.

IMPLEMENTATION

ACTION	**RATIONALE**
1. Gather equipment. Check each medication prescribed against the original in the health record, depending on facility policy and the medication order system in place. Clarify any inconsistencies. Check the patient's health record for allergies.	The prescription is the legal record of prescribed medication interventions. This comparison helps to identify errors that may have occurred when orders were transcribed. Computer provider order-entry (CPOE) systems allow prescribers to send electronic medication prescriptions directly to the pharmacy located in a health care facility and to outpatient pharmacies.
2. Know the actions, special nursing considerations, safe dose ranges, purpose of administration, and adverse effects of the medication to be administered. Consider the appropriateness of the medication for this patient.	This knowledge aids the nurse in evaluating the therapeutic effect of the medication in relation to the patient's health status and can also be used to educate the patient about the medication.
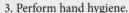 3. Perform hand hygiene.	Hand hygiene prevents the spread of microorganisms.
4. Move the medication supply system to the outside of the patient's room or prepare for administration at the medication supply system in the medication area. Alternatively, access the medication administration supply system at or inside the patient's room.	Organization facilitates error-free administration and saves time.

(continued on page 306)

Skill 5-17 ▶ Administering Ear Drops *(continued)*

ACTION	**RATIONALE**
5. Unlock the medication supply system or drawer. Enter the passcode and scan employee identification, if required.	Locking the medication supply system or drawer safeguards each patient's medication supply. Facility accrediting organizations require medication supply systems to be locked when not in use. Entering the passcode and scanning ID allows only authorized users into the system and identifies the user for documentation by the computer.
6. **Prepare medications for one patient at a time.**	This prevents errors in medication administration.
7. Read the eMAR/MAR and read the label when selecting the proper medication from the patient's medication drawer or medication supply system.	This is the *first* check of the label.
8. Read the label and compare the label with the eMAR/MAR. Check expiration dates and perform calculations, if necessary. Scan the bar code on the package, if required.	This is the *second* check of the label. Verify calculations with another nurse to ensure safety, if necessary.
9. **Depending on facility policy, the third check of the label may occur at this point. If so, when all medications for one patient have been prepared, read the label and recheck the labels with the eMAR/MAR before taking the medications to the patient. However, many facilities require the third check to occur at the bedside, after identifying the patient.**	This *third* check ensures accuracy and helps to prevent errors. *Note:* Many facilities require the *third* check to occur at the bedside, after identifying the patient and before administration.
10. **Log out of and/or lock the medication supply system before leaving it.**	Locking the medication supply system or drawer safeguards the patient's medication supply. Facility accrediting organizations require medication supply systems to be locked when not in use.
11. Transport medications to the patient's bedside carefully and keep the medications in sight at all times.	Careful handling and close observation prevent accidental or deliberate disarrangement of medications.
12. **Ensure that the patient receives the medications at the correct time.**	Check facility policy, which may allow for administration within a period of 30 minutes before or 30 minutes after the designated time.
13. Perform hand hygiene and put on PPE, if indicated.	Hand hygiene and PPE prevent the spread of microorganisms. PPE is required based on transmission precautions.
14. **Identify the patient. Compare the information with the eMAR/MAR. The patient should be identified using at least two of the following methods** (The Joint Commission, 2021):	Identifying the patient ensures the right patient receives the medications and helps prevent errors. The patient's room number or physical location is not used as an identifier (The Joint Commission, 2021). Replace the identification band if it is missing or inaccurate in any way.
a. Check the name on the patient's identification band.	This requires a response from the patient, but illness and strange surroundings often cause patients to be confused.
b. Check the identification number on the patient's identification band.	
c. Check the birth date on the patient's identification band.	
d. Ask the patient to state their name and birth date, based on facility policy.	
15. Close the door to the room or pull the bedside curtain.	This provides patient privacy.
16. **Complete necessary assessments before administering medications. Check the patient's allergy bracelet, if present, or ask the patient about allergies. Explain the purpose and action of each medication to the patient.**	Assessment is a prerequisite to administration of medications.
17. Scan the bar code on the patient's identification band, if required (The Joint Commission, 2021).	This provides an additional check to ensure that the medication is given to the right patient.

ACTION

18. **Based on facility policy, the third check of the label may occur at this point. If so, read the label and recheck the labels with the eMAR/MAR before administering the medications to the patient.**

19. Warm the bottle of medication by rubbing between the palms of your hands, holding the bottle in your hands for 1 to 2 minutes, or by placing it in warm water (American Academy of Pediatrics, 2013; MFMER, 2021c). Put on gloves.

20. Cleanse the external ear of any drainage with a cotton ball or washcloth moistened with normal saline or water (Figure 1).

21. Place the patient on their unaffected side in bed, or, if ambulatory, have them sit with their head well tilted to the side so that the affected ear is facing upward (Figure 2).

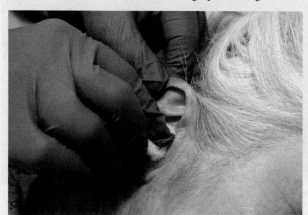

FIGURE 1. Cleaning external ear.

22. Remove the cap from the medication bottle, being careful not to touch the inside of the cap or the tip of the container (Figure 3).

23. Straighten the auditory canal by pulling the cartilaginous portion of the pinna up and back for an adult. (See Infant and Child Considerations for correct positioning for this age group.)

24. Invert and hold the medication bottle in the ear with its tip above the auditory canal (Figure 4). Do not touch the dropper to the ear.

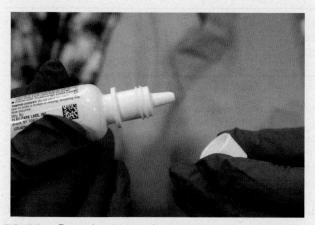

FIGURE 3. Removing the cap from the medication bottle.

RATIONALE

Many facilities require the *third* check to occur at the bedside, after identifying the patient and before administration. If facility policy directs the *third* check at this time, this *third* check ensures accuracy and helps to prevent errors.

Administration of cold solution in the ear is uncomfortable and could cause the patient to become dizzy (MFMER, 2021c). Gloves protect the nurse from potential contact with mucous membranes and body fluids.

Debris and drainage may prevent some of the medication from entering the ear canal.

This positioning prevents the drops from escaping from the ear.

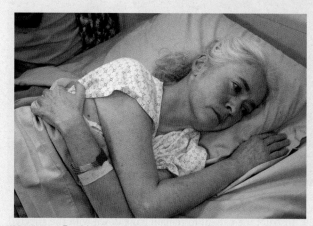

FIGURE 2. Positioning patient on unaffected side.

Touching the inside of the cap or tip of container may contaminate the bottle of medication.

Pulling on the pinna as described helps to straighten the canal properly for ear drop instillation.

By holding the medication bottle in the ear, the medication will enter the ear canal. Touching the bottle to the ear contaminates the bottle and medication. The hard tip of the medication bottle can damage the tympanic membrane if it is jabbed into the ear.

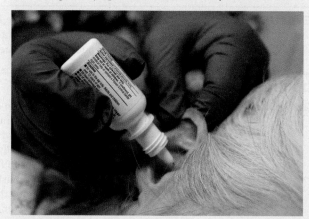

FIGURE 4. Pulling the pinna up and back and placing dropper tip above auditory canal.

(*continued on page 308*)

Skill 5-17 ▶ Administering Ear Drops *(continued)*

ACTION	**RATIONALE**
25. **Squeeze the container and allow drops to fall on the side of the canal. Avoid instilling in the middle of the canal, to avoid instilling directly onto the tympanic membrane.**	It is uncomfortable for the patient if the drops fall directly onto the tympanic membrane.
26. Release the pinna after instilling the drops, and have the patient maintain their head position to prevent escape of medication.	The medication should remain in the ear canal for at least 5 minutes.
27. Gently press on the tragus a few times (Figure 5).	Pressing on the tragus causes the medication to move from the canal toward the tympanic membrane.
28. If prescribed, loosely insert a cotton ball into the ear canal (Figure 6).	A cotton ball can help prevent the medication from leaking out of the ear canal.

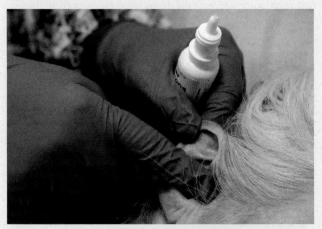

FIGURE 5. Applying pressure to tragus.

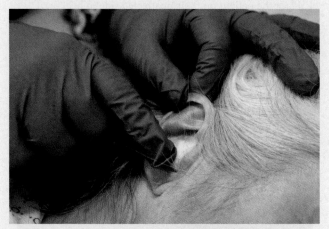

FIGURE 6. Inserting cotton ball into ear canal.

ACTION	**RATIONALE**
29. Instruct the patient to remain lying down with the affected ear upward for 5 to 20 minutes, based on specifics for prescribed medication and/or facility policy.	This ensures the medication remains in the ear canal and maximizes medication absorption (Frandsen & Pennington, 2021; MFMER, 2021c).
30. Replace the cap on the medication bottle. Remove gloves and additional PPE, if used. Perform hand hygiene.	Replacing the cap prevents contamination of the tip of the bottle. Proper removal of PPE reduces the risk of infection transmission and contamination of other items. Hand hygiene prevents the spread of microorganisms.
31. Document the administration of the medication immediately after administration. See Documentation section below.	Timely documentation helps to ensure patient safety.
32. Evaluate the patient's response to the medication within an appropriate time frame.	The patient needs to be evaluated for therapeutic and adverse effects from the medication.

EVALUATION
The expected outcomes have been met when the ear drops were administered successfully, the patient has experienced the intended effect of the medication, the patient has verbalized an understanding of and engaged in the medication regimen, and the patient did not experience injury.

DOCUMENTATION

Guidelines
Document the administration of the medication immediately after administration, including date, time, dose, route of administration, and site of administration, specifically right, left, or both ears, on the eMAR/MAR or record using the required format. If using a bar-code system, medication administration is automatically recorded when the bar code is scanned. PRN medications require documentation of the reason for administration. Prompt recording avoids the possibility of accidentally repeating the administration of the drug. Document pre- and post-administration assessments, characteristics of any drainage, and the patient's response to the treatment, if appropriate. If the drug was refused or omitted, record this in the appropriate area on the medication record and notify the health care team as appropriate. This verifies the reason medication was omitted and ensures that health care personnel providing care for the patient are aware of the occurrence.

DEVELOPING CLINICAL REASONING AND CLINICAL JUDGMENT

UNEXPECTED SITUATIONS AND ASSOCIATED INTERVENTIONS

- *Medication runs from ear into eye:* Notify the health care team and check with the pharmacy. Eye irrigation may need to be performed.
- *Patient reports extreme pain when you press on the tragus:* Allow the patient to press on the tragus. If pressure causes too much pain, this part may be deferred.

SPECIAL CONSIDERATIONS

General Considerations

- If both ears are to be treated, wait 5 to 20 minutes before having the patient turn over to instill drops into the second ear (Frandsen & Pennington, 2021; MFMER, 2021c).
- Ongoing assessment is an important part of nursing care to evaluate the patient response to administered treatments and early detection of adverse drug reactions. If an adverse effect is suspected, notify the health care team. Additional intervention is based on type of reaction and patient assessment.

Infant and Child Considerations

- Pull the pinna up and back for a child older than age 3 years (Figure 7) and down and back for an infant or a child younger than age 3 years (Figure 8) to straighten the ear canal (American Academy of Pediatrics, 2013; Kyle & Carman, 2021).
- Soothe, comfort, and distract the child after administration to keep the child still after administration (Kyle & Carman, 2021).

Community-Based Care Considerations

- Teach the patient/family member/caregiver to warm the ear drops before administration by holding the container in the hand or placing it in a pocket for 5 minutes (Bauldoff et al., 2020).
- Teach the patient/family member/caregiver to use the nondominant hand to straighten the ear canal and the dominant hand to administer the drops (Bauldoff et al., 2020).
- Caution the patient/family member/caregiver to avoid touching the applicator/tip of the bottle to any surface, including the ear, to avoid contamination (MFMER, 2021c).

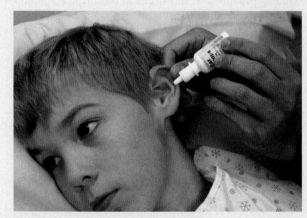

FIGURE 7. Pulling pinna up and back for a child older than age 3 years.

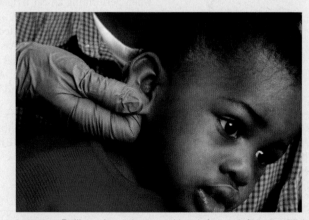

FIGURE 8. Pulling pinna down and back for an infant or child younger than age 3 years.

Skill 5-18 ▶ Administering an Ear Irrigation

Irrigations of the external auditory canal are ordinarily performed for cleaning purposes or for applying heat to the area. Typically, a normal saline solution is used, although an antiseptic solution may be indicated for local action. To prevent pain and/or dizziness, make sure the irrigation solution is warmed to body temperature (Schumann et al., 2021). An irrigation syringe is used most commonly; however, an irrigation container with tubing and an ear tip (Taylor et al., 2023) or pulsating water devices may also be used (Schumann et al., 2021). The following skill outlines use of an irrigation syringe.

DELEGATION CONSIDERATIONS

The administration of an irrigation of the ear is not delegated to assistive personnel (AP). Depending on the state's nurse practice act and the organization's policies and procedures, the irrigation of the ear may be delegated to licensed practical/vocational nurses (LPN/LVNs). The decision to delegate must be based on careful analysis of the patient's needs and circumstances as well as the qualifications of the person to whom the task is being delegated. Refer to the Delegation Guidelines in Appendix A.

EQUIPMENT

- Prescribed irrigating solution (warmed to 98.6°F [37°C]) (Schumann et al., 2021)
- Irrigation set (container and irrigation syringe, tubing and ear tip, or pulsating water device)
- Waterproof pad
- Emesis basin
- Gloves
- Additional PPE, as indicated
- Cotton balls, disposable washcloth, or washcloth
- Normal saline or water
- Electronic Medication Administration Record (eMAR) or Medication Administration Record (MAR)

ASSESSMENT

Assess the appropriateness of the irrigation solution/medication and procedure for the patient. Review the medical history and allergy, assessment, and laboratory data that may influence drug administration. Check expiration dates. Assess for the presence of conditions that indicate irrigation is contraindicated, such as complications from a previous ear irrigation; ear surgery; suspected or actual tympanic puncture or perforation; cleft palate (Harkin, 2015; Hayter, 2016; Schumann et al., 2021). Assess for the presence of conditions that indicate the need for increased caution when performing an ear irrigation, including patients with anticoagulant use, diabetes, immunocompromised, dizziness and tinnitus or patients who had radiation therapy to the ear (Schwartz et al., 2017). Assess the affected ear for redness, erythema, edema, drainage, or tenderness. Assess the patient's ability to hear. Assess the patient's knowledge of the medication and procedure. If the patient has a knowledge deficit about the medication, this may be an appropriate time to begin education about the medication. Assess the patient's ability to participate with the procedure. Verify patient name, dose, route, and time of administration.

ACTUAL OR POTENTIAL HEALTH PROBLEMS AND NEEDS

Many actual or potential health problems or issues may require the use of this skill as part of related interventions. An appropriate health problem or issue may include:
- Acute pain
- Injury risk
- Knowledge deficiency

OUTCOME IDENTIFICATION AND PLANNING

The expected outcomes to achieve are that the irrigation is administered successfully, and the patient experiences the intended effect of the procedure. Other outcomes that may be appropriate include the following: the patient remains free from injury, and the patient verbalizes an understanding of and engages with the therapeutic regimen.

IMPLEMENTATION

ACTION

1. Gather equipment. Check each medication prescribed against the original in the health record, depending on facility policy and the medication order system in place. Clarify any inconsistencies. Check the patient's health record for allergies.

2. Know the actions, special nursing considerations, safe dose ranges, purpose of administration, and adverse effects of the medication to be administered. Consider the appropriateness of the medication for this patient.

3. Perform hand hygiene.

4. Move the medication supply system to the outside of the patient's room or prepare for administration at the medication supply system in the medication area. Alternatively, access the medication administration supply system at or inside the patient's room.

5. Unlock the medication supply system or drawer. Enter the passcode and scan employee identification, if required.

6. **Prepare medications for one patient at a time.**

7. Read the eMAR/MAR and read the label when selecting the proper medication from the medication supply system or the patient's medication drawer.

8. Read the label and compare the label with the eMAR/MAR. Check expiration dates and perform calculations, if necessary. Scan the bar code on the package, if required.

9. **Depending on facility policy, the third check of the label may occur at this point. If so, when all medications for one patient have been prepared, read the label and recheck the labels with the eMAR/MAR before taking the medications to the patient. However, many facilities require the third check to occur at the bedside, after identifying the patient.**

10. **Log out of and/or lock the medication supply system before leaving it.**

11. Transport medications to the patient's bedside carefully and keep the medications in sight at all times.

12. **Ensure that the patient receives the medications at the correct time.**

13. Perform hand hygiene and put on PPE, if indicated.

RATIONALE

The prescription is the legal record of prescribed medication interventions. This comparison helps to identify errors that may have occurred when orders were transcribed. Computer provider order-entry (CPOE) systems allow prescribers to send electronic medication prescriptions directly to the pharmacy located in a health care facility and to outpatient pharmacies.

This knowledge aids the nurse in evaluating the therapeutic effect of the medication in relation to the patient's health status and can also be used to educate the patient about the medication.

Hand hygiene prevents the spread of microorganisms.

Organization facilitates error-free administration and saves time.

Locking the medication supply system or drawer safeguards each patient's medication supply. Facility accrediting organizations require medication supply systems to be locked when not in use. Entering the passcode and scanning ID allows only authorized users into the computer system and identifies the user for documentation by the computer.

This prevents errors in medication administration.

This is the *first* check of the label.

This is the *second* check of the label. Verify calculations with another nurse to ensure safety, if necessary.

This *third* check ensures accuracy and helps to prevent errors. *Note:* Many facilities require the *third* check to occur at the bedside, after identifying the patient and before administration.

Locking the medication supply system or drawer safeguards the patient's medication supply. Facility accrediting organizations require medication supply systems to be locked when not in use.

Careful handling and close observation prevent accidental or deliberate disarrangement of medications.

Check facility policy, which may allow for administration within a period of 30 minutes before or 30 minutes after the designated time.

Hand hygiene and PPE prevent the spread of microorganisms. PPE is required based on transmission precautions.

(*continued on page 312*)

Skill 5-18 ▶ Administering an Ear Irrigation *(continued)*

ACTION	**RATIONALE**
14. **Identify the patient. Compare the information with the eMAR/MAR. The patient should be identified using at least two of the following methods** (The Joint Commission, 2021):	Identifying the patient ensures the right patient receives the medications and helps prevent errors. The patient's room number or physical location is not used as an identifier (The Joint Commission, 2021). Replace the identification band if it is missing or inaccurate in any way.
a. Check the name on the patient's identification band.	This requires a response from the patient, but illness and strange surroundings often cause patients to be confused.
b. Check the identification number on the patient's identification band.	
c. Check the birth date on the patient's identification band.	
d. Ask the patient to state their name and birth date, based on facility policy.	
15. Close the door to the room or pull the bedside curtain.	This provides patient privacy.
16. **Complete necessary assessments before administering medications. Check the patient's allergy bracelet, if present, or ask the patient about allergies. Explain the purpose and action of the medication to the patient.**	Assessment is a prerequisite to administration of medications. Explanation provides rationale, increases knowledge, promotes patient engagement, and reduces anxiety.
17. Scan the bar code on the patient's identification band, if required (The Joint Commission, 2021).	This provides an additional check to ensure that the medication is given to the right patient.
18. **Based on facility policy, the third check of the label may occur at this point. If so, read the label and recheck the labels with the eMAR/MAR before administering the medications to the patient.**	Many facilities require the *third* check to occur at the bedside, after identifying the patient and before administration. If facility policy directs the *third* check at this time, this *third* check ensures accuracy and helps to prevent errors.
19. Assemble equipment at the patient's bedside.	This provides for an organized approach to the task.
20. Put on gloves.	Gloves protect the nurse from potential contact with contaminants and body fluids.
21. Assist the patient to sit up or lie with their head tilted slightly toward the side of the affected ear. Protect the patient and the bed with a waterproof pad. If the patient is able, have them support the basin under the ear to receive the irrigating solution.	Gravity causes the irrigating solution to flow from the ear to the basin.
22. Cleanse the external ear of any drainage with a cotton ball or washcloth moistened with normal saline or water.	Debris and drainage on the external ear may be washed into the ear and/or may prevent some of the medication from entering the ear canal.
23. Pretreat the ear with 2 to 4 drops of warm water or irrigating solution (refer to Skill 5-17) and wait 15 minutes.	Pretreating softens any cerumen that may be present and enhances the effectiveness of the ear irrigation (Schumann et al., 2021; Schwartz et al., 2017).
24. Fill the irrigating or bulb syringe with the warmed solution. If an irrigating container is used, prime the tubing.	Priming the tubing allows air to escape from the tubing. Air forced into the ear canal is noisy and therefore unpleasant for the patient.
25. Straighten the auditory canal by pulling the cartilaginous portion of pinna up and back for an adult (Figure 1). (See Infant and Child Considerations for correct positioning for this age group.)	Straightening the ear canal allows the solution to reach all areas of the canal easily.
26. Point the syringe tip superiorly and posteriorly toward the upper back to the ear canal wall. Use a gentle squirting motion to **direct a steady, slow stream of solution against the roof of the auditory canal, using only enough force to remove secretions (Figure 2). Do not occlude the auditory canal with the irrigating nozzle.** Allow the solution to flow out unimpeded.	Use of a gentle squirting motion and directing the solution at the roof of the canal help separate cerumen from the ear canal and prevent tympanic membrane injury or perforation (Schumann et al., 2021). Continuous in-and-out flow of the irrigating solution helps to prevent pressure in the canal.

ACTION

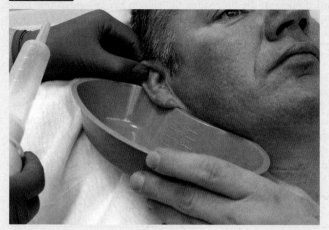

FIGURE 1. Pulling pinna up and back to straighten the ear canal.

27. When irrigation is complete, place a cotton ball loosely in the auditory meatus (Figure 3) and have the patient lie on the side of the affected ear on a towel or absorbent pad.

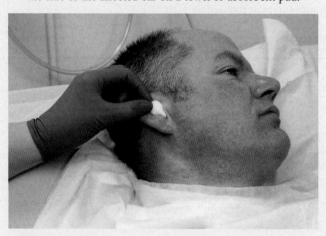

28. Remove gloves and any additional PPE, if used. Perform hand hygiene.

29. Document the administration of the medication immediately after administration. See Documentation section below.

30. Evaluate the patient's response to the procedure. Return in 10 to 15 minutes. Put on gloves, remove the cotton ball, and assess drainage.

31. Remove gloves and perform hand hygiene. Assist the patient to a position of comfort.

32. Evaluate the patient's response to the medication within an appropriate time frame.

RATIONALE

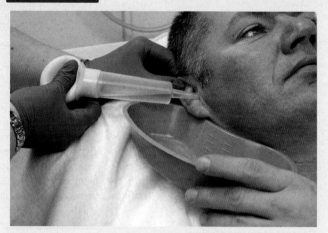

FIGURE 2. Instilling irrigation fluid.

The cotton ball absorbs excess fluid, and gravity allows the remaining solution in the canal to escape from the ear.

FIGURE 3. Placing cotton ball in ear.

Proper removal of PPE reduces the risk of infection transmission and contamination of other items. Hand hygiene prevents the spread of microorganisms.

Timely documentation helps to ensure patient safety.

The patient needs to be evaluated for any adverse effects from the procedure. Drainage or pain may indicate injury to the tympanic membrane.

Removing gloves and performing hand hygiene reduces the risk of contamination of other items and the spread of microorganisms. Assisting the patient to a position of comfort promotes patient comfort.

The patient needs to be evaluated for therapeutic and adverse effects from the medication.

(continued on page 314)

Skill 5-18 ▶ Administering an Ear Irrigation *(continued)*

EVALUATION

The expected outcomes have been met when the irrigation has been administered successfully, the patient has experienced the intended effect of the procedure, the patient has remained free from injury, and the patient has verbalized an understanding of the rationale for the procedure.

DOCUMENTATION

Guidelines

Document pre- and post-administration assessments, the procedure, site, the type of solution and volume used, length of time irrigation performed, characteristics of any drainage, and the patient's response to the treatment on the eMAR/MAR or record using the required format. If using a bar-code system, medication administration is automatically recorded when the bar code is scanned. PRN medications require documentation of the reason for administration. Prompt recording avoids the possibility of accidentally repeating the administration of the drug. If the procedure was refused or omitted, record this in the appropriate area on the medication record and notify the health care team as appropriate. This verifies the reason medication was omitted and ensures that health care personnel providing care for the patient are aware of the occurrence.

Sample Documentation

> 7/6/25 1830 Right ear noted to be without external edema and redness. No drainage noted. Patient reports slightly decreased hearing in right ear. Slight tenderness noted on palpation. Irrigation of right ear performed using 100 mL of warmed normal saline. Clear return with particles of cerumen noted. Patient tolerated procedure with minimal discomfort. Patient reports no change in hearing in right ear. Denies need for pain medication at this time. Patient rates pain at present as 1/10.
>
> —B. Clapp, RN

DEVELOPING CLINICAL REASONING AND CLINICAL JUDGMENT

UNEXPECTED SITUATIONS AND ASSOCIATED INTERVENTIONS

- *Patient reports significant pain during irrigation:* Stop the irrigation. Check the temperature of the solution. If the solution has cooled, rewarm it and try again. If the patient still reports pain, stop the irrigation and notify the health care team.

SPECIAL CONSIDERATIONS

General Considerations

- Ongoing assessment is an important part of nursing care to evaluate patient response to administered medications and early detection of adverse drug reactions. If an adverse effect is suspected, withhold further medication doses and notify the health care team. Additional intervention is based on type of reaction and patient assessment.

Infant and Child Considerations

- Pull the pinna up and back for a child older than age 3 years (Figure 4) and down and back for an infant or a child younger than age 3 years (Figure 5) to straighten the ear canal (American Academy of Pediatrics, 2013; Kyle & Carman, 2021).

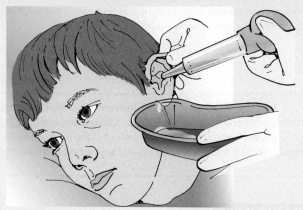

FIGURE 4. Pulling pinna up and back for child older than age 3 years.

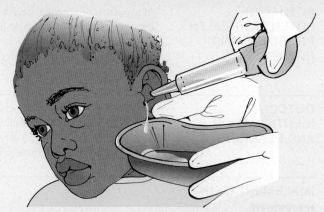

FIGURE 5. Pulling pinna down and back for an infant or child younger than age 3 years.

Skill 5-19 ▶ Administering a Nasal Spray

Skill Variation: *Administering Medication via Nasal Drops*

Nasal instillations are used to treat allergies, sinus infections, and nasal congestion. Medications with a systemic effect, such as vasopressin or naloxone, may also be prepared as a nasal instillation. The nose is normally not a sterile cavity, but because of its connection with the sinuses, it is important to observe medical asepsis carefully when using nasal instillations.

The following skill describes the steps to administer a nasal spray. Medications may also be applied to the nasal mucous membrane via nasal drops. Refer to the accompanying Skill Variation for guidelines to administer medication via nasal drops.

DELEGATION CONSIDERATIONS

The administration of medication using a nasal spray is not delegated to assistive personnel (AP). Depending on the state's nurse practice act and the organization's policies and procedures, administration of a nasal spray may be delegated to licensed practical/vocational nurses (LPN/LVNs). The decision to delegate must be based on careful analysis of the patient's needs and circumstances as well as the qualifications of the person to whom the task is being delegated. Refer to the Delegation Guidelines in Appendix A.

EQUIPMENT

- Prescribed medication in nasal spray bottle
- Gloves
- Additional PPE, as indicated
- Tissue
- Electronic Medication Administration Record (eMAR) or Medication Administration Record (MAR)

ASSESSMENT

Assess the appropriateness of the drug for the patient. Review the medical history and allergy, assessment, and laboratory data that may influence drug administration. Assess the nares for redness, erythema, edema, drainage, or tenderness. Assess the patient's knowledge of the medication and the procedure. If the patient has a knowledge deficit about the medication, this may be an appropriate time to begin education about the procedure. Assess the patient's ability to participate with the procedure. Verify patient name, dose, route, and time of administration.

(continued on page 316)

Skill 5-19 ▶ Administering a Nasal Spray *(continued)*

ACTUAL OR POTENTIAL HEALTH PROBLEMS AND NEEDS	Many actual or potential health problems or issues may require the use of this skill as part of related interventions. An appropriate health problem or issue may include: • Knowledge deficiency • Risk for medication side effect • Impaired comfort

OUTCOME IDENTIFICATION AND PLANNING	The expected outcomes to achieve are that the medication is administered successfully into the nose, and the patient experiences the intended effect of the medication. Other outcomes that may be appropriate include the following: the patient verbalizes an understanding of the medication regimen, the patient experiences no allergic response, and the patient experiences minimal discomfort.

IMPLEMENTATION

ACTION	RATIONALE
1. Gather equipment. Check each medication prescribed against the original in the health record, depending on facility policy and the medication order system in place. Clarify any inconsistencies. Check the patient's health record for allergies.	The prescription is the legal record of prescribed medication interventions. This comparison helps to identify errors that may have occurred when orders were transcribed. Computer provider order-entry (CPOE) systems allow prescribers to send electronic medication prescriptions directly to the pharmacy located in a health care facility and to outpatient pharmacies.
2. Know the actions, special nursing considerations, safe dose ranges, purpose of administration, and adverse effects of the medication to be administered. Consider the appropriateness of the medication for this patient.	This knowledge aids the nurse in evaluating the therapeutic effect of the medication in relation to the patient's health status and can also be used to educate the patient about the medication.
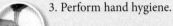 3. Perform hand hygiene.	Hand hygiene prevents the spread of microorganisms.
4. Move the medication supply system to the outside of the patient's room or prepare for administration at the medication supply system in the medication area. Alternatively, access the medication administration supply system at or inside the patient's room.	Organization facilitates error-free administration and saves time.
5. Unlock the medication supply system or drawer. Enter the passcode and scan employee identification, if required.	Locking the medication supply system or drawer safeguards each patient's medication supply. Facility accrediting organizations require medication supply systems to be locked when not in use. Entering the passcode and scanning ID allows only authorized users into the system and identifies the user for documentation by the computer.
6. **Prepare medications for one patient at a time.**	This prevents errors in medication administration.
7. Read the eMAR/MAR and read the label when selecting the proper medication from the patient's medication drawer or medication supply system.	This is the *first* check of the label.
8. Read the label and compare the label with the eMAR/MAR. Check expiration dates and perform calculations, if necessary. Scan the bar code on the package, if required.	This is the *second* check of the label. Verify calculations with another nurse to ensure safety, if necessary.
9. **Depending on facility policy, the third check of the label may occur at this point. If so, when all medications for one patient have been prepared, read the label and recheck the labels with the eMAR/MAR before taking the medications to the patient. However, many facilities require the third check to occur at the bedside, after identifying the patient.**	This *third* check ensures accuracy and helps to prevent errors. *Note:* Many facilities require the *third* check to occur at the bedside, after identifying the patient and before administration.

ACTION

10. **Log out of and/or lock the medication supply system before leaving it.**

11. Transport medications to the patient's bedside carefully and keep the medications in sight at all times.

12. **Ensure that the patient receives the medications at the correct time.**

13. Perform hand hygiene and put on PPE, if indicated.

14. **Identify the patient. Compare the information with the eMAR/MAR. The patient should be identified using at least two of the following methods** (The Joint Commission, 2021):

a. Check the name on the patient's identification band.

b. Check the identification number on the patient's identification band.

c. Check the birth date on the patient's identification band.

d. Ask the patient to state their name and birth date, based on facility policy.

15. Close the door to the room or pull the bedside curtain.

16. **Complete necessary assessments before administering medications. Check the patient's allergy bracelet, if present, or ask the patient about allergies. Explain the purpose and action of each medication to the patient.**

17. Scan the bar code on the patient's identification band, if required (The Joint Commission, 2021) (Figure 1).

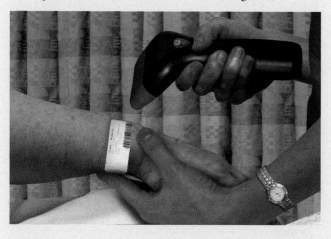

FIGURE 1. Scanning bar code on the patient's identification bracelet.

18. **Based on facility policy, the third check of the label may occur at this point. If so, read the label and recheck the labels with the eMAR/MAR before administering the medications to the patient.**

19. Put on gloves.

RATIONALE

Locking the medication supply system or drawer safeguards the patient's medication supply. Facility accrediting organizations require medication supply systems to be locked when not in use.

Careful handling and close observation prevent accidental or deliberate disarrangement of medications.

Check facility policy, which may allow for administration within a period of 30 minutes before or 30 minutes after the designated time.

Hand hygiene and PPE prevent the spread of microorganisms. PPE is required based on transmission precautions.

Identifying the patient ensures the right patient receives the medications and helps prevent errors. The patient's room number or physical location is not used as an identifier (The Joint Commission, 2021). Replace the identification band if it is missing or inaccurate in any way.

This requires a response from the patient, but illness and strange surroundings often cause patients to be confused.

This provides patient privacy.

Assessment is a prerequisite to administration of medications.

This provides an additional check to ensure that the medication is given to the right patient.

Many facilities require the *third* check to occur at the bedside, after identifying the patient and before administration. If facility policy directs the *third* check at this time, this *third* check ensures accuracy and helps to prevent errors.

Gloves protect the nurse from potential contact with contaminants and body fluids.

(continued on page 318)

Skill 5-19 ▶ Administering a Nasal Spray *(continued)*

ACTION

20. Provide the patient with paper tissues and ask them to blow their nose.

21. Assist the patient to the appropriate position for the specific medication; some nasal sprays are administered with the patient's head tilted back, while others are administered with the patient's head tilted forward. Refer to the package insert or a drug resource for the specific medication, or consult a pharmacist. **Tilting the patient's head should be avoided if the patient has a cervical spine injury or other condition resulting in limited range of notion.**

22. Instruct the patient that it is necessary to inhale gently through the nose as the spray is being administered or not to inhale gently as the spray is being administered. Your instruction to the patient will depend on the medication being administered. Consult the manufacturer's instructions for each medication.

23. Agitate the bottle gently, if required for the specific medication. Insert the tip of the nosepiece of the bottle into one nostril (Figure 2). Close the opposite nostril with a finger. Instruct the patient to breathe in gently through the nostril, if required. Compress or activate the bottle to release one spray at the same time the patient breathes in.

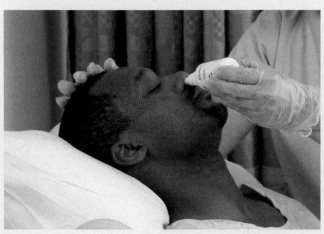

24. Keep the medication container compressed and remove it from the nostril. Release the container from the compressed state. Do not allow the container to return to its original position until it is removed from the patient's nose.

25. Have the patient hold their breath for a few seconds, and then breathe out slowly through their mouth. Repeat in the other nostril, as prescribed or indicated.

26. Wipe the outside of the bottle nose piece with a clean, dry tissue or cloth and replace the cap. Instruct the patient to avoid blowing their nose for 5 to 10 minutes, depending on the medication.

27. Remove gloves. Perform hand hygiene. Assist the patient to a comfortable position.

RATIONALE

Blowing the nose clears the nasal mucosa prior to medication administration.

This positioning allows the spray to flow into the nares and maximize absorption. Patients requiring administration of intranasal corticosteroids are asked to tilt their head forward while the nurse sprays the medication laterally away from the septum (Sedaghat, 2017). Tilting the head is contraindicated with cervical spine injury.

Inhalation helps to distribute the spray in the nares. Inhalation during administration is not recommended for some medications.

This mixes the medication thoroughly to ensure a consistent dose of medication.

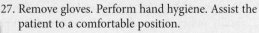
FIGURE 2. Inserting tip of bottle into one nostril.

This prevents contamination of the contents of the container.

This allows the medication to remain in contact with nasal mucous membranes.

This keeps the end of the bottle clean. Avoiding nose blowing keeps the medication in contact with nasal mucous membranes.

Removing gloves and performing hand hygiene reduces the risk of contamination of other items and the spread of microorganisms. Assisting the patient to a comfortable position promotes patient comfort.

ACTION

28. Remove additional PPE, if used. Perform hand hygiene.

29. Document the administration of the medication immediately after administration. See Documentation section below.

30. Evaluate the patient's response to the procedure and medication within an appropriate time frame.

RATIONALE

Proper removal of PPE reduces the risk of infection transmission and contamination of other items. Hand hygiene prevents the spread of microorganisms.

Timely documentation helps to ensure patient safety.

The patient needs to be evaluated for therapeutic and adverse effects from the medication.

EVALUATION

The expected outcomes have been met when the medication was administered successfully into the nose, the patient has experienced the intended effect of the medication, the patient has verbalized an understanding of the medication regimen, the patient experienced no allergic response, and the patient experienced minimal discomfort.

DOCUMENTATION

Guidelines

Document the administration of the medication, including date, time, dose, route of administration, and site of administration, specifically right, left, or both nares, on the eMAR/MAR or record using the required format. If using a bar-code system, medication administration is automatically recorded when the bar code is scanned. PRN medications require documentation of the reason for administration. Prompt recording avoids the possibility of accidentally repeating the administration of the drug. Document pre- and post-administration assessments, characteristics of any drainage, and the patient's response to the treatment, if appropriate. If the drug was refused or omitted, record this in the appropriate area on the medication record and notify the health care team as appropriate. This verifies the reason medication was omitted and ensures that health care personnel providing care for the patient are aware of the occurrence.

DEVELOPING CLINICAL REASONING AND CLINICAL JUDGMENT

UNEXPECTED SITUATIONS AND ASSOCIATED INTERVENTIONS

- *Patient sneezes immediately after receiving nose spray:* Do not repeat the dosage, because you cannot determine how much medication was actually absorbed.

SPECIAL CONSIDERATIONS

- Ongoing assessment is an important part of nursing care to evaluate patient response to administered medications and early detection of adverse drug reactions. If an adverse effect is suspected, withhold further medication doses and notify the patient's health care team. Additional intervention is based on type of reaction and patient assessment.
- Naloxone is a medication used to rapidly reverse opioid overdose (SAMHSA, 2020). Naloxone is given immediately when a suspected or known opioid overdose has occurred (MFMER, 2021d). **Do not prime or test the nasal spray; it contains a single dose of naloxone and cannot be reused.** The medication is inserted into each naris until the side of the nozzle is against the naris (MFMER, 2021d). The plunger is compressed to administer the dose and may be repeated every 2 to 3 minutes until the patient is responsive or additional emergency medical personnel arrive (MFMER, 2021d). Naloxone is also available for intramuscular, subcutaneous, and IV administration (SAMHSA, 2020).

(continued on page 320)

Skill 5-19 ▶ Administering a Nasal Spray *(continued)*

Skill Variation ▶ Administering Medication via Nasal Drops

Prepare medication as outlined in Steps 1–18 above (Skill 5-19).

1. Put on gloves. Assist the patient to an upright position with their head tilted back.
2. Draw sufficient solution into the dropper for both nares. Do not return excess solution to the bottle to avoid contamination.
3. Have the patient breathe through their mouth. Hold the tip of the nose up and place the dropper just above the naris, about 1/3 inch. Instill the prescribed number of drops in one naris and then into the other. Avoid touching the naris with the dropper.

4. Have the patient remain in position with their head tilted back for 5 minutes to prevent the escape of the medication.

5. Remove gloves and any additional PPE, if used. Perform hand hygiene.

6. Document administration of the medication on the eMAR/MAR immediately after administering the medication. Document the site, if only one nostril is used.
7. Evaluate the patient's response to the medication within an appropriate time frame.

Skill 5-20 ▶ Administering a Vaginal Cream

Skill Variation: *Administering a Vaginal Suppository*

Creams, foams, and tablets can be applied intravaginally using a narrow, tubular applicator with an attached plunger. Suppositories that melt when exposed to body heat are also administered by vaginal insertion (see the accompanying Skill Variation on page 325). Refrigerate suppositories for storage. Time the administration of vaginal medications to allow the patient to lie down afterward to retain the medication.

DELEGATION CONSIDERATIONS

The administration of medication as a vaginal cream is not delegated to assistive personnel (AP). Depending on the state's nurse practice act and the organization's policies and procedures, administration of a vaginal cream may be delegated to licensed practical/vocational nurses (LPN/LVNs). The decision to delegate must be based on careful analysis of the patient's needs and circumstances as well as the qualifications of the person to whom the task is being delegated. Refer to the Delegation Guidelines in Appendix A.

EQUIPMENT

• Prescribed medication with applicator, if appropriate
• Water-soluble lubricant
• Perineal pad
• Disposable washcloth or washcloth, skin cleanser, and warm water
• Waterproof disposable pad
• Gloves
• Additional PPE, as indicated
• Electronic Medication Administration Record (eMAR) or Medication Administration Record (MAR)

ASSESSMENT

Assess the appropriateness of the drug for the patient. Review the medical history and allergy, assessment, and laboratory data that may influence drug administration. Check the expiration date. Assess the external genitalia and vaginal canal for redness, erythema, edema, drainage, or tenderness. Assess the patient's knowledge of the medication and procedure. If the patient has a knowledge deficit about the medication, this may be an appropriate time to begin education about the medication. Assess the patient's ability to participate with the procedure. Verify patient name, dose, route, and time of administration.

ACTUAL OR POTENTIAL HEALTH PROBLEMS AND NEEDS	Many actual or potential health problems or issues may require the use of this skill as part of related interventions. An appropriate health problem or issue may include: • Knowledge deficiency • Risk for medication side effect • Risk for injury
OUTCOME IDENTIFICATION AND PLANNING	The expected outcomes to achieve are that the medication is administered successfully into the vagina, and the patient experiences the intended effect of the medication. Other outcomes that may be appropriate include the following: the patient verbalizes an understanding of the medication regimen, the patient experiences no allergic response, and the patient experiences minimal discomfort.

IMPLEMENTATION

ACTION	**RATIONALE**
1. Gather equipment. Check each medication prescribed against the original in the health record, depending on facility policy and the medication order system in place. Clarify any inconsistencies. Check the patient's health record for allergies.	The prescription is the legal record of prescribed medication interventions. This comparison helps to identify errors that may have occurred when orders were transcribed. Computer provider order-entry (CPOE) systems allow prescribers to send electronic medication prescriptions directly to the pharmacy located in a health care facility and to outpatient pharmacies.
2. Know the actions, special nursing considerations, safe dose ranges, purpose of administration, and adverse effects of the medication to be administered. Consider the appropriateness of the medication for this patient.	This knowledge aids the nurse in evaluating the therapeutic effect of the medication in relation to the patient's health status and can also be used to educate the patient about the medication.
3. Perform hand hygiene.	Hand hygiene prevents the spread of microorganisms.
4. Move the medication supply system to the outside of the patient's room or prepare for administration at the medication supply system in the medication area. Alternatively, access the medication administration supply system at or inside the patient's room.	Organization facilitates error-free administration and saves time.
5. Unlock the medication supply system or drawer. Enter the passcode and scan employee identification, if required.	Locking of the medication supply system or drawer safeguards each patient's medication supply. Facility accrediting organizations require medication supply systems to be locked when not in use. Entering the passcode and scanning ID allows only authorized users into the system and identifies the user for documentation by the computer.
6. **Prepare medications for one patient at a time.**	This prevents errors in medication administration.
7. Read the eMAR/MAR and read the label when selecting the proper medication from the medication supply system or the patient's medication drawer.	This is the *first* check of the label.
8. Read the label and compare the label with the eMAR/MAR. Check expiration dates and perform calculations, if necessary. Scan the bar code on the package, if required.	This is the *second* check of the label. Verify calculations with another nurse to ensure safety, if necessary.
9. **Depending on facility policy, the third check of the label may occur at this point. If so, when all medications for one patient have been prepared, read the label and recheck the labels with the eMAR/MAR before taking the medications to the patient. However, many facilities require the third check to occur at the bedside, after identifying the patient.**	This *third* check ensures accuracy and helps to prevent errors. *Note:* Many facilities require the *third* check to occur at the bedside, after identifying the patient and before administration.

(continued on page 322)

Skill 5-20 ▶ Administering a Vaginal Cream *(continued)*

ACTION	RATIONALE
10. **Log out of and/or lock the medication supply system before leaving it.**	Locking the medication supply system or drawer safeguards the patient's medication supply. Facility accrediting organizations require medication supply systems to be locked when not in use.
11. Transport medications to the patient's bedside carefully and keep the medications in sight at all times.	Careful handling and close observation prevent accidental or deliberate disarrangement of medications.
12. **Ensure that the patient receives the medications at the correct time.**	Check facility policy, which may allow for administration within a period of 30 minutes before or 30 minutes after the designated time.

 13. Perform hand hygiene and put on PPE, if indicated.

Hand hygiene and PPE prevent the spread of microorganisms. PPE is required based on transmission precautions.

 14. **Identify the patient. Compare the information with the eMAR/MAR. The patient should be identified using at least two of the following methods** (The Joint Commission, 2021):

Identifying the patient ensures the right patient receives the medications and helps prevent errors. The patient's room number or physical location is not used as an identifier (The Joint Commission, 2021). Replace the identification band if it is missing or inaccurate in any way.

a. Check the name on the patient's identification band.

This requires a response from the patient, but illness and strange surroundings often cause patients to be confused.

b. Check the identification number on the patient's identification band.

c. Check the birth date on the patient's identification band.

d. Ask the patient to state their name and birth date, based on facility policy.

15. Close the door to the room or pull the bedside curtain.	This provides patient privacy.
16. **Complete necessary assessments before administering medications. Check the patient's allergy bracelet, if present, or ask the patient about allergies. Explain the purpose and action of each medication to the patient.**	Assessment is a prerequisite to administration of medications. Explanation provides rationale, increases knowledge, promotes patient engagement, and reduces anxiety.
17. Scan the bar code on the patient's identification band, if required (The Joint Commission, 2021) (Figure 1).	This provides an additional check to ensure that the medication is given to the right patient.

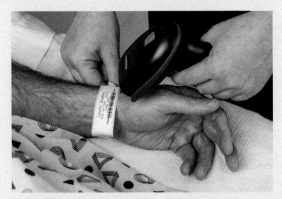

FIGURE 1. Scanning bar code on patient's identification bracelet. (*Source:* Used with permission from Shutterstock. Photo by B. Proud.)

| 18. **Based on facility policy, the third check of the label may occur at this point. If so, read the label and recheck the labels with the eMAR/MAR before administering the medications to the patient.** | Many facilities require the *third* check to occur at the bedside, after identifying the patient and before administration. If facility policy directs the *third* check at this time, this *third* check ensures accuracy and helps to prevent errors. |
| 19. Ask the patient to void before inserting the medication. | Voiding empties the bladder and helps to minimize pressure and discomfort during administration. |

ACTION

20. Put on gloves.

21. Position the patient so they are lying on their back with their knees flexed. Maintain privacy with draping. Place a waterproof disposable pad under their hips. Provide adequate light to visualize the vaginal opening.

22. Perform perineal care. Spread the labia with your fingers, and cleanse the area at the vaginal orifice with a disposable washcloth or washcloth and warm water, using a different corner of the washcloth with each stroke. Wipe from above the vaginal orifice downward toward the sacrum (front to back) (Figure 2).

23. Remove gloves and put on new gloves.

24. Fill the vaginal applicator with the prescribed amount of cream (Figure 3). (See the accompanying Skill Variation for administering a vaginal **suppository**.)

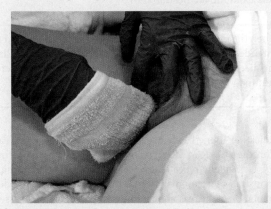

FIGURE 2. Performing perineal care.

25. Lubricate the applicator with the lubricant, as necessary.

26. Spread the labia with your nondominant hand and gently introduce the applicator with your dominant hand, in a rolling manner, while directing it downward and backward.

27. After the applicator is properly positioned (Figure 4), the labia may be allowed to fall in place if necessary to free the hand for manipulating the plunger. Push the plunger to its full length and then gently remove the applicator with the plunger depressed.

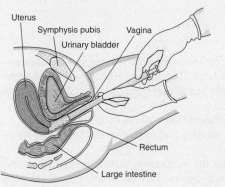

FIGURE 4. Positioning applicator in vagina for administration of medication.

RATIONALE

Gloves protect the nurse from potential contact with contaminants and body fluids.

This position provides access to vaginal canal and helps to retain medication in the canal. The waterproof pad prevents soiling or dampening of bed linen. Draping limits exposure of the patient and promotes warmth and privacy. Adequate light facilitates ease of administration.

These techniques prevent contamination of the vaginal orifice with debris surrounding the anus.

Changing gloves prevents spread of microorganisms.

This ensures the correct dosage of medication will be administered.

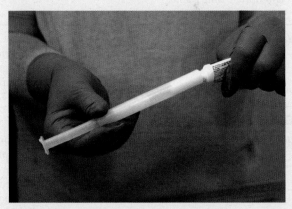

FIGURE 3. Filling vaginal applicator with cream.

Ordinarily, lubrication is unnecessary, but it may be used to reduce friction while inserting the applicator.

This follows the normal contour of the vagina for its full length.

Pushing the plunger will gently deploy the cream into the vaginal orifice.

(*continued on page 324*)

Skill 5-20 ▶ Administering a Vaginal Cream (continued)

ACTION	**RATIONALE**
28. **Ask the patient to remain in the supine position for a minimum of 10 to 15 minutes after insertion (Karch, 2020). Some medications are administered prior to lying down to go to bed.** Offer the patient a perineal pad to collect drainage; the patient should not use a tampon (MFMER, 2021e).	This gives the medication time to be absorbed in the vaginal cavity. As the medication heats up, some may leak from the vaginal orifice.
29. Dispose of the applicator in an appropriate receptacle or clean the nondisposable applicator according to the manufacturer's directions.	Disposal prevents transmission of microorganisms. Cleaning prepares the applicator for future use by the same patient for continuing treatment.
30. Remove gloves and additional PPE, if used. Perform hand hygiene.	Proper removal of PPE reduces the risk of infection transmission and contamination of other items. Hand hygiene prevents the spread of microorganisms.
31. Document the administration of the medication immediately after administration. See Documentation section below.	Timely documentation helps to ensure patient safety.
32. Evaluate the patient's response to the medication within an appropriate time frame.	The patient needs to be evaluated for therapeutic and adverse effects from the medication.

EVALUATION

The expected outcomes have been met when the medication was administered successfully into the vagina, the patient has experienced the intended effect of the medication, the patient has verbalized an understanding of and engages with the medication regimen, the patient experienced no allergic response, and the patient experienced minimal discomfort.

DOCUMENTATION

Guidelines

Document the administration of the medication immediately after administration, including date, time, dose, and route of administration on the eMAR/MAR or record using the required format. Prompt recording avoids the possibility of accidentally repeating the administration of the drug. If using a bar-code system, medication administration is automatically recorded when the bar code is scanned. PRN medications require documentation of the reason for administration. Document assessment, characteristics of any drainage, and the patient's response to the treatment, if appropriate. If the drug was refused or omitted, record this in the appropriate area on the medication record and notify the health care team as appropriate. This verifies the reason medication was omitted and ensures that health care personnel providing care for the patient are aware of the occurrence.

Sample Documentation

> 7/23/25 2300 Monistat vaginal cream administered as ordered. Small amount of curdlike, white discharge noted from vagina. Perineal skin remains erythematous. Patient states, "It doesn't itch as much as it has been."
>
> —K. Sanders, RN

DEVELOPING CLINICAL REASONING AND CLINICAL JUDGMENT

SPECIAL CONSIDERATIONS

- Ongoing assessment is an important part of nursing care to evaluate patient response to administered medications and early detection of adverse reactions. If an adverse effect is suspected, withhold further medication doses and notify the patient's health care team. Additional intervention is based on type of reaction and patient assessment.
- Instruct patients to avoid using tampons during treatment time (MFMER, 2021e).
- Explain to the patient that they may want to use a sanitary pad to protect clothing from stains from the medication.
- Instruct the patient that they should not stop using the medication if their menstrual period begins during the treatment time; the patient should use sanitary pads rather than tampons (MFMER, 2021e).

Skill Variation ▶ Administering a Vaginal Suppository

Prepare medication and patient as outlined in Steps 1–23 above (Skill 5-20).

1. Remove the suppository from its wrapper and lubricate the round end with the water-soluble lubricant (Figure A). Lubricate your gloved index finger on your dominant hand.

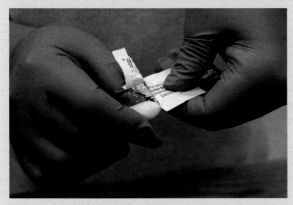

FIGURE A. Lubricating suppository.

2. Spread the labia with your nondominant hand.
3. Insert the rounded end of the suppository along the posterior wall of the canal (Figure B). Insert to the length of your finger.

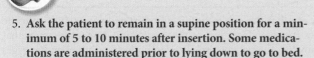

4. Remove gloves. Perform hand hygiene.

5. **Ask the patient to remain in a supine position for a minimum of 5 to 10 minutes after insertion. Some medications are administered prior to lying down to go to bed.**
6. Offer the patient a perineal pad to collect drainage.

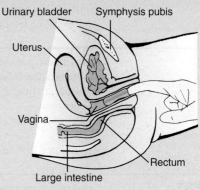

FIGURE B. Inserting suppository into vagina.

7. Remove additional PPE, if used. Perform hand hygiene.

8. Document administration of the medication on the eMAR/MAR immediately after administering the medication.
9. Evaluate the patient's response to the medication within an appropriate time frame.
10. Assist the patient to a comfortable position after the **required 10 to 15 minutes in the supine position** (Karch, 2020).

Unexpected Situations and Associated Interventions

- *Upon assessing the patient after administering a vaginal suppository, you note the suppository is not in the vagina but instead is between the labia:* Put on gloves and reinsert the suppository, ensuring that it is inserted fully.

Skill 5-21 ▶ Administering a Rectal Suppository

Rectal suppositories are used primarily for their local action, such as laxatives and fecal softeners. Systemic effects are also achieved with rectal suppositories, such as antiemetic or antipyretic effect. Suppositories may be used when it is difficult or not possible for a patient to take medications orally. It is important to ensure the suppository is placed past the internal anal sphincter and against the rectal mucosa.

Rectal suppositories should not be administered to patients who have had recent rectal or prostate surgery, patients who have thrombocytopenia or who are neutropenic, patients with a paralytic ileus, and patients at risk for cardiac arrhythmias due to the risk of a vasovagal response (Taylor et al., 2023). Rectal suppositories are contraindicated, unless prescribed by the surgeon, physician, or advance practice practitioner, following gastrointestinal or gynecological surgery (Dougherty & Lister, 2015, as cited in Mitchell, 2019, p. 288).

(continued on page 326)

Skill 5-21 ▶ Administering a Rectal Suppository   *(continued)*

DELEGATION CONSIDERATIONS	The administration of medication as a rectal suppository is not delegated to assistive personnel (AP). Depending on the state's nurse practice act and the organization's policies and procedures, administration of a vaginal cream may be delegated to licensed practical/vocational nurses (LPN/LVNs). The decision to delegate must be based on careful analysis of the patient's needs and circumstances as well as the qualifications of the person to whom the task is being delegated. Refer to the Delegation Guidelines in Appendix A.
EQUIPMENT	• Prescribed medication suppository (rectal) • Water-soluble lubricant • Nonlatex, disposable gloves • Toilet tissue • Electronic Medication Administration Record (eMAR) or Medication Administration Record (MAR) • Additional PPE, as indicated
ASSESSMENT	Assess the appropriateness of the drug for the patient. Review the medical history and allergy, assessment, and laboratory data that may influence drug administration, particularly the patient's white blood cell and platelet counts. Check the expiration date. Assess for the presence of conditions that would indicate the suppository may be contraindicated; refer to the details in the introduction to this Skill. Assess relevant body systems for the particular medication being administered. Assess the rectal area for any alterations in integrity. Assess the patient's knowledge of the medication and procedure. If the patient has a knowledge deficit about the medication, this may be an appropriate time to begin education about the medication. Assess the patient's ability to participate with the procedure. Verify patient name, dose, route, and time of administration.
ACTUAL OR POTENTIAL HEALTH PROBLEMS AND NEEDS	Many actual or potential health problems or issues may require the use of this skill as part of related interventions. An appropriate health problem or issue may include: • Knowledge deficiency • Infection risk • Constipation
OUTCOME IDENTIFICATION AND PLANNING	The expected outcomes to achieve are that the medication is administered successfully into the rectum, and the patient experiences the intended effect of the medication. Other outcomes that may be appropriate include the following: the patient verbalizes an understanding of and engages with the medication regimen, and the patient experienced minimal discomfort.

IMPLEMENTATION

ACTION	**RATIONALE**
1. Gather equipment. Check each medication prescribed against the original in the health record, depending on facility policy and the medication order system in place. Clarify any inconsistencies. Check the patient's health record for allergies.	The prescription is the legal record of prescribed medication interventions. This comparison helps to identify errors that may have occurred when orders were transcribed. Computer provider order-entry (CPOE) systems allow prescribers to send electronic medication prescriptions directly to the pharmacy located in a health care facility and to outpatient pharmacies.
2. Know the actions, special nursing considerations, safe dose ranges, purpose of administration, and adverse effects of the medication to be administered. Consider the appropriateness of the medication for this patient.	This knowledge aids the nurse in evaluating the therapeutic effect of the medication in relation to the patient's mucosa and health status and can also be used to educate the patient about the medication.
3. Perform hand hygiene.	Hand hygiene prevents the spread of microorganisms.

ACTION

4. Move the medication supply system to the outside of the patient's room or prepare for administration at the medication supply system in the medication area. Alternatively, access the medication administration supply system at or inside the patient's room.

5. Unlock the medication supply system or drawer. Enter the passcode and scan employee identification, if required.

6. **Prepare medications for one patient at a time.**

7. Read the eMAR/MAR and read the label when selecting the proper medication from the medication supply system or the patient's medication drawer.

8. Read the label and compare the label with the eMAR/MAR. Check expiration dates and perform calculations, if necessary. Scan the bar code on the package, if required.

9. **Depending on facility policy, the third check of the label may occur at this point. If so, when all medications for one patient have been prepared, read the label and recheck the labels with the eMAR/MAR before taking the medications to the patient. However, many facilities require the third check to occur at the bedside, after identifying the patient.**

10. **Log out of and/or lock the medication supply system before leaving it.**

11. Transport medications to the patient's bedside carefully and keep the medications in sight at all times.

12. **Ensure that the patient receives the medications at the correct time.**

13. Perform hand hygiene and put on PPE, if indicated.

14. **Identify the patient. Compare the information with the eMAR/MAR. The patient should be identified using at least two of the following methods** (The Joint Commission, 2021):

a. Check the name on the patient's identification band.

b. Check the identification number on the patient's identification band.

c. Check the birth date on the patient's identification band.

d. Ask the patient to state their name and birth date, based on facility policy.

15. Close the door to the room or pull the bedside curtain.

16. **Complete necessary assessments before administering medications. Check the patient's allergy bracelet, if present, or ask the patient about allergies. Explain the purpose and action of each medication to the patient.**

RATIONALE

Organization facilitates error-free administration and saves time.

Locking the medication supply system or drawer safeguards each patient's medication supply. Facility accrediting organizations require medication supply systems to be locked when not in use. Entering the passcode and scanning ID allows only authorized users into the system and identifies the user for documentation by the computer.

This prevents errors in medication administration.

This is the *first* check of the label.

This is the *second* check of the label. Verify calculations with another nurse to ensure safety, if necessary.

This *third* check ensures accuracy and helps to prevent errors. *Note:* Many facilities require the *third* check to occur at the bedside, after identifying the patient and before administration.

Locking the medication supply system or drawer safeguards the patient's medication supply. Facility accrediting organizations require medication supply systems to be locked when not in use.

Careful handling and close observation prevent accidental or deliberate disarrangement of medications.

Check facility policy, which may allow for administration within a period of 30 minutes before or 30 minutes after the designated time.

Hand hygiene and PPE prevent the spread of microorganisms. PPE is required based on transmission precautions.

Identifying the patient ensures the right patient receives the medications and helps prevent errors. The patient's room number or physical location is not used as an identifier (The Joint Commission, 2021). Replace the identification band if it is missing or inaccurate in any way.

This requires a response from the patient, but illness and strange surroundings often cause patients to be confused.

This provides patient privacy.

Assessment is a prerequisite to administration of medications.

(continued on page 328)

Skill 5-21 ▶ Administering a Rectal Suppository *(continued)*

ACTION	RATIONALE
17. Scan the patient's bar code on the identification band, if required (The Joint Commission, 2021) (Figure 1).	This provides an additional check to ensure that the medication is given to the right patient.
18. **Based on facility policy, the third check of the label may occur at this point. If so, read the label and recheck the labels with the eMAR/MAR before administering the medications to the patient.**	Many facilities require the *third* check to occur at the bedside, after identifying the patient and before administration. If facility policy directs the *third* check at this time, this *third* check ensures accuracy and helps to prevent errors.
19. Put on gloves.	Gloves protect the nurse from potential contact with contaminants and body fluids.
20. Assist the patient to their left side in a Sims' position. Drape accordingly to expose only the buttocks.	Sims' positioning allows for easy access to the anal area. Lying on their left side decreases the chance of expulsion of the suppository. Proper draping maintains privacy.
21. Remove the suppository from its wrapper. Apply lubricant to the rounded end (Figure 2). Lubricate the index finger of your dominant hand.	The lubricant reduces friction on administration and increases patient comfort.

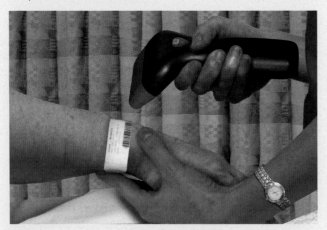

FIGURE 1. Scanning bar code on patient's identification bracelet. (*Source:* Used with permission from Shutterstock. Photo by B. Proud.)

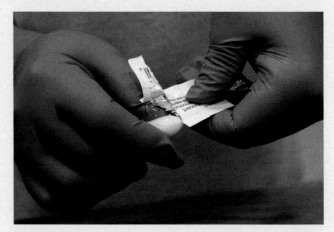

FIGURE 2. Applying lubricant to rounded end of suppository.

22. Separate the buttocks with your nondominant hand and instruct the patient to breathe slowly and deeply through their mouth while the suppository is being inserted.	Slow, deep breaths help to relax the anal sphincter and reduce discomfort.
23. Using your index finger, insert the suppository, round end first, **along the rectal wall.** Insert about 3 to 4 inches (Figure 3).	The suppository must make contact with the rectal mucosa for absorption to occur. If inserted into stool, it will be ineffective (Peate, 2015).

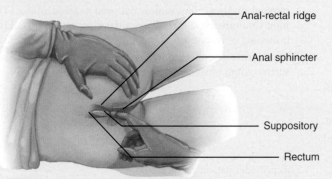

Anal-rectal ridge

Anal sphincter

Suppository

Rectum

FIGURE 3. Inserting suppository round end first along rectal wall.

ACTION	**RATIONALE**
24. Use toilet tissue to clean any stool or lubricant from around the anus. Release the buttocks. Encourage the patient to remain on their side for at least 5 minutes (Taylor et al., 2023) and retain the suppository for the appropriate amount of time for the specific medication.	Cleaning prevents skin irritation. Side-lying for at least 5 minutes prevents accidental expulsion of the suppository and ensures absorption of the medication.
25. Remove gloves and any additional PPE, if used. Perform hand hygiene.	Proper removal of PPE reduces the risk of infection transmission and contamination of other items. Hand hygiene prevents the spread of microorganisms.
26. Document the administration of the medication immediately after administration. See Documentation section below.	Timely documentation helps to ensure patient safety.
27. Evaluate the patient's response to the medication within an appropriate time frame.	The patient needs to be evaluated for therapeutic and adverse effects from the medication.

EVALUATION

The expected outcomes have been met when the medication was administered into the rectum, the patient has experienced the intended effect of the medication, the patient has verbalized an understanding of and engaged with the medication regimen, and the patient experienced minimal discomfort.

DOCUMENTATION

Guidelines

Document the administration of the medication immediately after administration, including date, time, dose, and route of administration on the eMAR/MAR or record using the required format. If using a bar-code system, medication administration is automatically recorded when the bar code is scanned. PRN medications require documentation of the reason for administration. Prompt recording avoids the possibility of accidentally repeating the administration of the drug. Document your assessments, and the patient's response to the treatment, if appropriate. If the drug was refused or omitted, record this in the appropriate area on the medication record and notify the health care team as appropriate. This verifies the reason medication was omitted and ensures that health care personnel providing care for the patient are aware of the occurrence.

DEVELOPING CLINICAL REASONING AND CLINICAL JUDGMENT

UNEXPECTED SITUATIONS AND ASSOCIATED INTERVENTIONS

- *Patient expels the suppository before it is absorbed:* Put on gloves and apply additional lubricant to the suppository. Reinsert past the internal sphincter. If the suppository has warmed and become too soft, discard it and notify the health care team. An additional dose may be ordered.

SPECIAL CONSIDERATIONS

General Considerations

- If the suppository is for laxative purposes, it must remain in position for 35 to 45 minutes, or until the patient feels the urge to defecate (Taylor et al., 2023).
- Ongoing assessment is an important part of nursing care to evaluate patient response to administered medications and early detection of adverse reactions. If an adverse effect is suspected, withhold further medication doses and notify the patient's health care team. Additional intervention is based on type of reaction and patient assessment.

Infant and Child Considerations

- For an infant or child younger than age 3 years, use the fifth finger for insertion. For an older child, use the index finger (Kyle & Carman, 2021).
- It may be necessary to hold the buttocks together for a few minutes to relieve pressure on the anal sphincter and expulsion of the suppository.

Older Adult Considerations

- Older adults may have difficulty retaining rectal suppositories because of decreased muscle tone and loss of sphincter control.

Skill 5-22 ▶ Administering Medication via a Metered-Dose Inhaler (MDI)

Skill Variation: *Administering Medication via a Metered-Dose Inhaler Without a Spacer*

Drugs for **inhalation** may be administered via a **metered-dose inhaler (MDI)**. An MDI is a hand-held inhaler that uses an aerosol spray or mist to deliver a controlled dose of medication with each compression of the canister that is then breathed in by the patient. The medication is then absorbed rapidly through the lung tissue, resulting in local and systemic effects. There are two methods for using an MDI; the preferred method is with a device called a valved holding chamber or spacer and is outlined in the steps in this skill (Center for Disease Control, 2018; Quaranta, 2018). An MDI can also be used without a chamber. Refer to the accompanying Skill Variation at the end of this skill. Patients should discuss which method is most appropriate for use with their health care provider. There are a number of different medication inhaler devices, which increases the risk of administration error (Quaranta, 2018). As a result, using the proper technique for the prescribed inhaler is imperative, or therapy will not be effective (Price et al., 2017; Quaranta, 2018).

DELEGATION CONSIDERATIONS	The administration of medication via a metered-dose inhaler is not delegated to assistive personnel (AP). Depending on the state's nurse practice act and the organization's policies and procedures, administration of a metered-dose inhaler may be delegated to licensed practical/vocational nurses (LPN/LVNs). The decision to delegate must be based on careful analysis of the patient's needs and circumstances as well as the qualifications of the person to whom the task is being delegated. Refer to the Delegation Guidelines in Appendix A.
EQUIPMENT	• Stethoscope • Prescribed medication in an MDI • Spacer or holding chamber • Electronic Medication Administration Record (eMAR) or Medication Administration Record (MAR) • PPE, as indicated
ASSESSMENT	Assess the appropriateness of the drug for the patient. Review the medical history and allergy, assessment, and laboratory data that may influence drug administration. Assess respiratory rate, rhythm, effort, and depth to establish a baseline. Assess lung sounds before and after use to establish a baseline and determine the effectiveness of the medication. Assess the peak flow before and after administration to establish a baseline and determine the effectiveness of the medication. If appropriate and/or prescribed, assess oxygen saturation level before and after medication administration. The oxygenation level usually increases after the medication is administered. Assess the patient's ability to manage an MDI; young and older adults may have dexterity problems. Assess the patient's knowledge and understanding of the medication's purpose and action. If the patient has a knowledge deficit about the medication, this may be the appropriate time to begin education about the medication Verify patient name, dose, route, and time of administration.
ACTUAL OR POTENTIAL HEALTH PROBLEMS AND NEEDS	Many actual or potential health problems or issues may require the use of this skill as part of related interventions. An appropriate health problem or issue may include: • Activity intolerance • Impaired gas exchange • Knowledge deficiency
OUTCOME IDENTIFICATION AND PLANNING	The expected outcomes to achieve when using an MDI are that the medication is administered and breathed in by the patient, and the patient experiences the intended effect of the medication. Other outcomes that may be appropriate include the following: the patient verbalizes an understanding of and engages in the medication regimen, and the patient demonstrates correct use of the MDI.

IMPLEMENTATION

ACTION

1. Gather equipment. Check each medication prescribed against the original in the health record, depending on facility policy and the medication order system in place. Clarify any inconsistencies. Check the patient's health record for allergies.

2. Know the actions, special nursing considerations, safe dose ranges, purpose of administration, and adverse effects of the medications to be administered. Consider the appropriateness of the medication for this patient.

 3. Perform hand hygiene.

4. Move the medication supply system to the outside of the patient's room or prepare for administration at the medication supply system in the medication area. Alternatively, access the medication administration supply system at or inside the patient's room.

5. Unlock the medication supply system or drawer. Enter the passcode and scan employee identification, if required.

6. **Prepare medications for one patient at a time.**

7. Read the eMAR/MAR and read the label when selecting the proper medication from the patient's medication drawer or medication supply system.

8. Read the label and compare the label with the eMAR/MAR. Check expiration dates and perform calculations, if necessary. Scan the bar code on the package, if required.

9. **Depending on facility policy, the third check of the label may occur at this point. If so, when all medications for one patient have been prepared, read the label and recheck the labels with the eMAR/MAR before taking the medications to the patient. However, many facilities require the third check to occur at the bedside, after identifying the patient.**

10. **Log out of and/or lock the medication supply system before leaving it.**

11. Transport medications to the patient's bedside carefully and keep the medications in sight at all times.

12. **Ensure that the patient receives the medications at the correct time.**

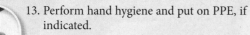 13. Perform hand hygiene and put on PPE, if indicated.

RATIONALE

The prescription is the legal record of prescribed medication interventions. This comparison helps to identify errors that may have occurred when orders were transcribed. Computer provider order-entry (CPOE) systems allow prescribers to send electronic medication prescriptions directly to the pharmacy located in a health care facility and to outpatient pharmacies.

This knowledge aids the nurse in evaluating the therapeutic effect of the medication in relation to the patient's health status and can also be used to educate the patient about the medication.

Hand hygiene prevents the spread of microorganisms.

Organization facilitates error-free administration and saves time.

Locking the medication supply system or drawer safeguards each patient's medication supply. Facility accrediting organizations require medication supply systems to be locked when not in use. Entering the passcode and scanning ID allows only authorized users into the computer system and identifies the user for documentation by the computer.

This prevents errors in medication administration.

This is the *first* check of the label.

This is the *second* check of the label. Verify calculations with another nurse to ensure safety, if necessary.

This *third* check ensures accuracy and helps to prevent errors. *Note:* Many facilities require the *third* check to occur at the bedside, after identifying the patient and before administration.

Locking the medication supply system or drawer safeguards the patient's medication supply. Facility accrediting organizations require medication supply systems to be locked when not in use.

Careful handling and close observation prevent accidental or deliberate disarrangement of medications.

Check facility policy, which may allow for administration within a period of 30 minutes before or 30 minutes after the designated time.

Hand hygiene and PPE prevent the spread of microorganisms. PPE is required based on transmission precautions.

(continued on page 332)

Skill 5-22 ▶ Administering Medication via a Metered-Dose Inhaler (MDI) *(continued)*

ACTION

14. **Identify the patient. Compare the information with the eMAR/MAR. The patient should be identified using at least two of the following methods** (The Joint Commission, 2021):

    a. Check the name on the patient's identification band.

    b. Check the identification number on the patient's identification band.

    c. Check the birth date on the patient's identification band.

    d. Ask the patient to state their name and birth date, based on facility policy.

15. Close the door to the room or pull the bedside curtain.

16. **Complete necessary assessments before administering medications. Check the patient's allergy bracelet, if present, or ask the patient about allergies. Explain what you are going to do and the reason for doing it to the patient.**

17. Scan the bar code on the patient's identification band, if required (The Joint Commission, 2021) (Figure 1).

18. **Based on facility policy, the third check of the label may occur at this point. If so, read the label and recheck the labels with the eMAR/MAR before administering the medications to the patient.**

19. Remove the MDI mouthpiece cover. Shake the inhaler, if necessary; refer to the details for the individual drug and inhaler in use (Allergy & Asthma Network, 2020a).

20. If the MDI is new or has not been used recently (several days or weeks), the device should be primed (Asthma Initiative of Michigan, n.d.; Hess et al., 2021); priming refers to actuating the device several times before use. Refer to specific details for the individual drug in use.

21. Remove the cover from each end of the spacer. Attach the MDI to the spacer by inserting in the open end of the spacer, opposite the mouthpiece. (Refer to the accompanying Skill Variation for using an MDI without a spacer.)

22. The patient should take a deep breath in, then breathe out completely, and place the spacer's mouthpiece into their mouth, grasping it securely with their teeth and above the tongue, and sealing the lips tightly around the mouthpiece (Figure 2).

RATIONALE

Identifying the patient ensures the right patient receives the medications and helps prevent errors. The patient's room number or physical location is not used as an identifier (The Joint Commission, 2021). Replace the identification band if it is missing or inaccurate in any way.

This requires a response from the patient, but illness and strange surroundings often cause patients to be confused.

This provides patient privacy.

Assessment is a prerequisite to administration of medications. Explanation provides rationale, increases knowledge, promotes patient engagement, and reduces anxiety.

This provides an additional check to ensure that the medication is given to the right patient.

Many facilities require the *third* check to occur at the bedside, after identifying the patient and before administration. If facility policy directs the *third* check at this time, this *third* check ensures accuracy and helps to prevent errors.

Shaking requirements and amount of shaking differ based on type of medication and inhaler (Allergy & Asthma Network, 2020a). The medication and propellant may separate when the canister is not in use. Shaking well ensures that the patient is receiving the correct dosage of medication.

Priming the metering chamber is required to ensure accurate delivery of the medication (Hess et al., 2021).

The use of a spacer or valved holding chamber is preferred because it traps the medication and aids in delivery of the correct dose.

The tongue should be kept under the mouthpiece so it does not block the opening of the mouthpiece (Gerald & Dhand, 2020). Medication should not leak out around the mouthpiece.

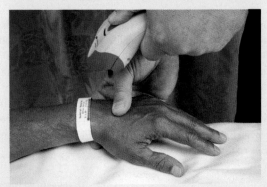

FIGURE 1. Scanning bar code on patient's identification bracelet.

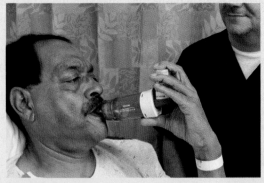

FIGURE 2. Placing spacer with MDI into mouth.

ACTION

RATIONALE

23. The patient should then depress the canister once, releasing one puff into the spacer, then inhale slowly and deeply through the mouth, until their lungs are full (Allergy & Asthma Network, 2020a).

The spacer will hold the medication in suspension for a short period so that the patient can receive more of the prescribed medication than if it had been projected into the air. Breathing slowly and deeply distributes the medication deep into the airways.

24. **Instruct the patient to hold their breath for 5 to 10 seconds, or as long as possible; the patient should remove the spacer from their mouth and then exhale slowly through pursed lips** (Allergy & Asthma Network, 2020a; American Lung Association, 2021).

This allows better distribution of the medication to the airways and longer absorption time for the medication.

25. Wait 1 to 5 minutes, as prescribed, before administering the next puff, if prescribed.

This ensures that both puffs are absorbed as much as possible. Bronchodilation after the first puff allows for deeper penetration by subsequent puffs.

26. After the prescribed number of puffs has been administered, have the patient remove the MDI from the spacer and replace the caps on both MDI and spacer.

By replacing the caps, the patient is preventing any dust or dirt from entering and being propelled into the bronchioles with later doses.

27. Have the patient gargle and rinse with tap water after using an MDI, as necessary. Clean the MDI according to the manufacturer's directions.

Rinsing removes medication residue from the mouth. Rinsing is necessary when using inhaled steroids because oral fungal infections can occur. The buildup of medication in the device can attract bacteria and affect how the medication is delivered.

28. Remove PPE, if used. Perform hand hygiene.

Proper removal of PPE reduces the risk of infection transmission and contamination of other items. Hand hygiene prevents the spread of microorganisms.

29. Document the administration of the medication immediately after administration. See Documentation section below.

Timely documentation helps to ensure patient safety.

30. Evaluate the patient's response to the medication within an appropriate time frame. Reassess lung sounds, oxygen saturation level, peak flow, and respirations, as indicated.

The patient needs to be evaluated for therapeutic and adverse effects from the medication.

EVALUATION

The expected outcomes have been met when the medication was administered and breathed in by the patient, the patient has experienced the intended effect of the medication, the patient has verbalized an understanding of and engaged with the medication regimen, and the patient has demonstrated correct use of the MDI.

DOCUMENTATION

Guidelines

Document the administration of the medication immediately after administration, including date, time, dose, route of administration and any teaching done with the patient on the eMAR/MAR or record using the required format. If using a bar-code system, medication administration is recorded automatically when the bar code is scanned. PRN medications require documentation of the reason for administration. Prompt recording avoids the possibility of accidentally repeating the administration of the drug. Document respiratory rate, oxygen saturation, if applicable, peak flow measurements and lung assessment, and the patient's response to the treatment, if appropriate. If the drug was refused or omitted, record this in the appropriate area on the medication record and notify the health care team. This verifies the reason medication was omitted and ensures that health care personnel providing care for the patient are aware of the occurrence.

(continued on page 334)

Skill 5-22 ▶ Administering Medication via a Metered-Dose Inhaler (MDI) *(continued)*

Sample Documentation

9/29/25 0820 Wheezes noted bilaterally, during expiration in all lung fields, O$_2$ saturation 92%, respiratory rate 24 breaths per minute, patient reports shortness of breath and cough. After albuterol MDI administration, lung sounds are clear to auscultation bilaterally in all lung fields, O$_2$ saturation 97%, respiratory rate 18 breaths per minute with no cough or report of shortness of breath. Patient able to demonstrate accurately the use of an MDI and spacer and verbalizes understanding of medication purpose and action.

—C. Bausler, RN

DEVELOPING CLINICAL REASONING AND CLINICAL JUDGMENT

UNEXPECTED SITUATIONS AND ASSOCIATED INTERVENTIONS

- *Patient uses MDI, but symptoms are not relieved:* Check to make sure that the inhaler still contains medication. The patient may have received only propellant, without medication. If necessary, obtain a new medication inhaler and administer dose as prescribed. If the inhaler is not empty and symptoms persist, contact the health care team to discuss appropriate interventions.
- *Patient is unable to use MDI:* Many companies have adaptive devices that assist patients to use MDIs.
- *Patient reports that relief of symptoms has decreased, even with increased number of puffs:* Have the patient demonstrate the technique they are using. Because it is common for patients to have knowledge gaps regarding the correct use of an MDI, it is imperative to review the technique with each patient (Frandsen & Pennington, 2021; Quaranta, 2018). Poor administration technique can lead to a decrease in effectiveness and a need for an increased dosage of medication.

SPECIAL CONSIDERATIONS

General Considerations

- Effective use of the MDI depends on proper technique (Hess et al., 2021). Education on correct use of inhaler is critical to reduce errors in use and improve efficacy of medication and patient outcomes (Hess et al., 2021; Price et al., 2017). Education should include brief, repeated MDI practice for motor learning to promote mastery (Gao et al., 2020; Schmitz et al., 2019).
- The plastic holder and cap provided with the inhaler should be cleaned at least weekly. Remove the medication canister and clean with warm running water. Shake the holder and allow it to air dry.
- Some medication canisters cannot be removed from the plastic holder. Wipe the mouthpiece with a cloth or dry cotton swab and/or refer to the manufacturer's directions for cleaning (Cleveland Clinic, 2014).
- Store the MDI in a location that is not exposed to heat (Frandsen & Pennington, 2021).
- Clean the spacer (valved holding chamber) once a week by soaking in warm water with a mild detergent for 15 minutes. Rinse well and shake off excess water. Allow it to air dry (Allergy & Asthma Network, 2020c; Cleveland Clinic, 2014).
- Do not store the spacer (valved holding chamber) in a plastic bag to prevent moisture retention and possible resulting microorganism growth.
- If the medication being administered is a steroid, the patient should rinse their mouth with water after administration to prevent throat irritation and secondary infection to the oral mucosa (MFMER, 2021f).
- Ongoing assessment is an important part of nursing care to evaluate patient response to administered medications and early detection of adverse reactions. If an adverse effect is suspected, withhold further medication doses and notify the patient's health care team. Additional intervention is based on type of reaction and patient assessment.

Infant and Child Considerations

- Young children usually require a spacer to use an MDI. A spacer is recommended for any child who has difficulty squeezing the canister and inhaling at the right time, particularly children younger than ages 5 to 6 years (Moore, 2020). Spacers with masks are available for young children. The mask must fit securely over both the nose and the mouth to ensure a good seal and prevent medication from escaping.
- Children must be able to seal their lips around the mouthpiece in order to use a spacer without a mask.
- Many medications can also be administered as a nebulizer (see Skill 5-24).

Community-Based Care Considerations

- It is important for patients to know how to tell when MDI medication levels are getting low. The most reliable method is to look on the canister and see how many puffs the canister contains. Divide this number by the number of puffs used daily to ascertain how many days the MDI will last. For instance, if the MDI contains 200 puffs and the patient takes 6 puffs per day, the MDI should last for 33 days. Keep a diary or record of inhaler use and discard the inhaler on reaching the labeled number of doses. This method may be cumbersome and impractical for some patients, but it is a reliable way to determine how much medication remains in an MDI. Another accurate way to know when the canister is depleted is to use a dose counter, which counts down each time the canister is activated (Gerald & Dhand, 2020). **Floating the canister in water is not reliable and is no longer recommended** (Gerald & Dhand, 2020; MedlinePlus, 2020).

Skill Variation ▶ Administering Medication via a Metered-Dose Inhaler Without a Spacer

There is inconsistency in the evidence for practice related to use of an MDI without a spacer. Some sources identify that the mouthpiece should be held in the mouth, with lips sealed around the inhaler, and other sources identify that the mouthpiece should be held two finger breadths from the mouth for use (CDC, 2018; Cleveland Clinic, 2014; Hess et al., 2021; MedlinePlus, 2020). Patients should refer to the specific instructions provided with the MDI or from their health care provider.

Prepare medication as outlined in Steps 1–20 above (Skill 5-22).

1. Remove the cap from the MDI.
2. Have the patient take a deep breath and exhale.
3. Have the patient hold the inhaler 1 to 2 inches away from the mouth (about the width of two fingers [Quaranta, 2018]) (Figure A). Alternatively, have the patient place the inhaler mouthpiece in their mouth, grasping it securely with teeth and above the tongue, and sealing the lips tightly around the mouthpiece.
4. Have the patient begin to inhale slowly and deeply, depress the medication canister, and continue to inhale until their lungs are full.
5. **Instruct the patient to hold their breath for 5 to 10 seconds, or as long as possible, and then remove the spacer from their mouth and exhale slowly through pursed lips.**
6. **Wait 1 to 5 minutes, as prescribed, before administering the next puff.**

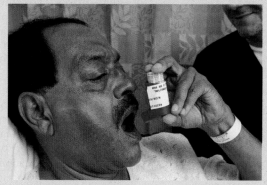

FIGURE A. Holding the MDI 1 to 2 inches from the mouth.

7. After the prescribed number of puffs has been administered, have the patient replace the cap on the MDI.

 8. Remove PPE, if used. Perform hand hygiene.

9. Document administration of the medication on the eMAR/MAR immediately after administering the medication.
10. Evaluate the patient's response to the medication within an appropriate time frame. Reassess lung sounds, oxygen saturation level, peak flow, and respirations, as indicated.

(continued on page 336)

Skill 5-22 ▶ Administering Medication via a Metered-Dose Inhaler (MDI) *(continued)*

EVIDENCE FOR PRACTICE ▶

PATIENT EDUCATION AND INHALED MEDICATIONS

Correct use of an inhaler is critical to ensure accurate dosing of medication. Nurses play a key role in educating patients and their family/caregivers and validating mastery of knowledge to improve patient outcomes.

Related Research

Gao, G., Liao, Y., Mo, L., Gong, Y., Shao, X., & Li, J. (2020). A randomized controlled trial of a nurse-led education pathway for asthmatic children from outpatient to home. *International Journal of Nursing Practice, 26*(3), e12823. https://doi.org/10.1111/ijn.12823

The purpose of this randomized controlled trial was to evaluate the efficacy of a nurse-led pathway, a standard education program, on children with asthma. A convenience sample of children with asthma was recruited from an outpatient department of a hospital in China. Participants experienced asthma symptoms during the day or night, experienced limitation in daily activities or sports because of asthma, had a need for rescue medication or unscheduled visits to their health care provider, and had a need emergency department visits because of exacerbations in the 3 months prior to initiation of study. The 125 participants were randomly assigned to either the control group or the intervention group. The intervention group ($n = 73$) received predetermined step-by-step education sessions based on a self-designed education pathway, including four visits by a clinical nurse with expertise in pediatric asthma management (two outpatient sessions, one home visit, and one telephone visit). Each visit had specific education items and addressed tailored interventions for problems identified by the patient during the visit. Visits focused on education about asthma management, trigger avoidance, peak flow measurement and asthma diary use, inhaler training, medication adherence, and management of asthma attacks. The control group ($n = 52$) received usual care, consisting of one routine education session. Asthma control, health-related quality of life, and health care utilization measures were taken at baseline and at follow-up visits (3 months and 6 months). Results indicated significantly higher scores in the intervention group for health-related quality of life ($P = .026$) and inhaler technique ($P = .002$) at the 3-month visit and asthma control test ($P = .002$) at the 6-month visit. The numbers of unscheduled physician visits and school absences were lower in the intervention group than in the control group within 6 months. There were no significant differences observed in emergency department visits and hospitalizations. The researchers concluded a nurse-led education pathway was more effective than usual care to provide information and support in asthma self-management from the outpatient clinic to home to improve asthma control, health-related quality of life, inhaler technique, and health care utilization. The authors suggest a nurse-led education pathway is an effective intervention for children with asthma.

Relevance to Nursing Practice

Nurses play a large role in patient education and in designing interventions to positively impact patient outcomes. Accurate dosing of inhaled medications, and therefore control of symptoms and disease treatment, depends on correct use of the delivery device. Providing patient education related to self-administration of medications and other aspects of disease management provides a comprehensive education model for improving patient outcomes.

EVIDENCE FOR PRACTICE ▶

INHALED MEDICATIONS

Correct use of a metered-dose inhaler is critical to ensure accurate dosing of medication. Patients who are prescribed medications delivered with an MDI must have accurate knowledge and demonstrate appropriate technique regarding use to ensure accurate medication delivery. Nurses play a key role in patient education and must have adequate knowledge to provide appropriate educational intervention.

Related Research

De Tratto, K., Gomez, C., Ryan, C. J., Bracken, N., Steffen, A., & Corbridge, S. J. (2014). Nurses' knowledge of inhaler technique in the inpatient hospital setting. *Clinical Nurse Specialist: The Journal for Advanced Nursing Practice, 28*(3), 156–160. https://doi.org/10.1097/NUR.0000000000000047

The purpose of this study was to examine inpatient staff nurses' self-perceptions of their inhaler technique knowledge, frequency of providing patient education, and responsibility for providing education. The study also assessed the nurses demonstrated inhaler technique using both a metered-dose inhaler (MDI) and diskus (a dry powder inhaler). A total of 100 nurses at a large urban academic medical center working on inpatient medical units agreed to participate. Participants completed a Likert-scale written survey to measure self-perceptions of inhaler technique and frequency and responsibility of patient education regarding MDI and diskus inhaler discharge teaching. Participating nurses then demonstrated inhaler-use technique to a data collector who utilized a detailed, validated checklist outlining the steps for use of both types of inhalers to evaluate the nurses' performance. Misuse of both MDI and diskus technique was defined for the study as having less than 75% of the steps correct (<9 of 12 steps for MDI and <8 steps for diskus). Overall misuse rates for both MDI (82%) and diskus (92%) devices were high, with poor correlation between perceived ability and investigator-measured level of performance of inhaler technique. Key steps missed in use of the devices included breathing out fully prior to inhaling with both devices. Ninety percent of participants missed keeping the device horizontal, and 78% did not breathe in quickly during use of the diskus. Frequency of teaching for the diskus device by nurses was correlated with higher scores on the validated checklist, but this was not the case with the MDI. The researchers concluded that although nurses are a key component of patient education, nursing staff lack adequate knowledge of inhaler technique.

Relevance to Nursing Practice

Nurses play a large role in patient education and in designing interventions to positively impact patient outcomes. Accurate dosing of inhaled medications, and therefore control of symptoms and disease treatment, depends on correct use of the delivery device. Providing patient education related to self-administration of medications, leading to accurate medication dosing, is a very important nursing intervention. Nurses must take responsibility for acquiring and maintaining accurate knowledge with regard to use of these devices in order to provide accurate patient teaching. Nurses may advocate for education regarding inhaler technique as part of facility-wide professional development interventions.

Skill 5-23 ▶ Administering Medication via a Dry Powder Inhaler

Drugs for inhalation may be administered via a dry powder inhaler (DPI). A DPI is a handheld inhaler (diskus) that uses a dry powder form of medication, either in a small capsule or disk inserted into the DPI, or in a compartment inside the DPI. DPIs are breath activated and create aerosols by drawing air through a dose of powdered medication (Hess et al., 2021). A quick breath by the patient activates the flow of medication, eliminating the need to coordinate activating the inhaler (spraying the medicine) while inhaling the medicine. However, the drug output and size distribution of the aerosol from a DPI is at least partly dependent on the flow rate through the device, so the patient must be able to take a powerful, deep inspiration (Alismail et al., 2016; Price et al., 2017; Quaranta, 2018). The medication is then absorbed rapidly through the lung tissue, resulting in local and systemic effects.

(continued on page 338)

Skill 5-23 ▶ Administering Medication via a Dry Powder Inhaler *(continued)*

Many types of DPIs are available, with distinctive operating instructions. Some have to be loaded with a dose of medication each time they are used, and some hold a number of preloaded doses. **It is important to understand the particular instructions both for the medication and for the particular delivery device being used.**

DELEGATION CONSIDERATIONS	The administration of medication via a dry powder inhaler is not delegated to assistive personnel (AP). Depending on the state's nurse practice act and the organization's policies and procedures, administration of medication using a dry powder inhaler may be delegated to licensed practical/vocational nurses (LPN/LVNs). The decision to delegate must be based on careful analysis of the patient's needs and circumstances as well as the qualifications of the person to whom the task is being delegated. Refer to the Delegation Guidelines in Appendix A.
EQUIPMENT	• Stethoscope • DPI and prescribed medication • Electronic Medication Administration Record (eMAR) or Medication Administration Record (MAR) • PPE, as indicated
ASSESSMENT	Assess the appropriateness of the drug for the patient. Review the medical history and allergy, assessment, and laboratory data that may influence drug administration. Assess respiratory rate, rhythm, effort, and depth to establish a baseline. Assess lung sounds before and after use to establish a baseline and determine the effectiveness of the medication. Assess the peak flow before and after administration to establish a baseline and determine the effectiveness of the medication. If appropriate and/or prescribed, assess oxygen saturation level before and after medication administration. The oxygenation level usually increases after the medication is administered. Assess the patient's ability to manage a DPI. Assess the patient's knowledge and understanding of the medication's purpose and action. If the patient has a knowledge deficit about the medication, this may be the appropriate time to begin education about the medication Verify patient name, dose, route, and time of administration.
ACTUAL OR POTENTIAL HEALTH PROBLEMS AND NEEDS	Many actual or potential health problems or issues may require the use of this skill as part of related interventions. An appropriate health problem or issue may include: • Activity intolerance • Impaired gas exchange • Knowledge deficiency
OUTCOME IDENTIFICATION AND PLANNING	The expected outcomes to achieve are that the medication is administered and breathed in by the patient, and the patient experiences the intended effect of the medication. Other outcomes that may be appropriate include the following: the patient verbalizes an understanding of and engages with the medication regimen, and the patient demonstrates correct use of the DPI.

IMPLEMENTATION

ACTION	**RATIONALE**
1. Gather equipment. Check each medication prescribed against the original in the health record, depending on facility policy and the medication order system in place. Clarify any inconsistencies. Check the patient's health record for allergies.	The prescription is the legal record of prescribed medication interventions. This comparison helps to identify errors that may have occurred when orders were transcribed. Computer provider order-entry (CPOE) systems allow prescribers to send electronic medication prescriptions directly to the pharmacy located in a health care facility and to outpatient pharmacies.
2. Know the actions, special nursing considerations, safe dose ranges, purpose of administration, and adverse effects of the medications to be administered. Consider the appropriateness of the medication for this patient.	This knowledge aids the nurse in evaluating the therapeutic effect of the medication in relation to the patient's health status and can also be used to educate the patient about the medication.

ACTION	**RATIONALE**

 3. Perform hand hygiene.

Hand hygiene prevents the spread of microorganisms.

4. Move the medication supply system to the outside of the patient's room or prepare for administration at the medication supply system in the medication area. Alternatively, access the medication administration supply system at or inside the patient's room.

Organization facilitates error-free administration and saves time.

5. Unlock the medication supply system or drawer. Enter the passcode and scan employee identification, if required.

Locking the medication supply system or drawer safeguards each patient's medication supply. Facility accrediting organizations require medication supply systems to be locked when not in use. Entering the passcode and scanning ID allows only authorized users into the system and identifies the user for documentation by the computer.

6. **Prepare medications for one patient at a time.**

This prevents errors in medication administration.

7. Read the eMAR/MAR and read the label when selecting the proper medication from the patient's medication drawer or medication supply system.

This is the *first* check of the label.

8. Read the label and compare the label with the eMAR/MAR. Check expiration dates and perform calculations, if necessary. Scan the bar code on the package, if required.

This is the *second* check of the label. Verify calculations with another nurse to ensure safety, if necessary.

9. **Depending on facility policy, the third check of the label may occur at this point. If so, when all medications for one patient have been prepared, read the label and recheck the labels with the eMAR/MAR before taking the medications to the patient. However, many facilities require the third check to occur at the bedside, after identifying the patient.**

This *third* check ensures accuracy and helps to prevent errors. *Note:* Many facilities require the *third* check to occur at the bedside, after identifying the patient and before administration.

10. **Log out of and/or lock the medication supply system before leaving it.**

Locking the medication supply system or drawer safeguards the patient's medication supply. Facility accrediting organizations require medication supply systems to be locked when not in use.

11. Transport medications to the patient's bedside carefully and keep the medications in sight at all times.

Careful handling and close observation prevent accidental or deliberate disarrangement of medications.

12. **Ensure that the patient receives the medications at the correct time.**

Check facility policy, which may allow for administration within a period of 30 minutes before or 30 minutes after the designated time.

 13. Perform hand hygiene and put on PPE, if indicated.

Hand hygiene and PPE prevent the spread of microorganisms. PPE is required based on transmission precautions.

 14. **Identify the patient. Compare the information with the eMAR/MAR. The patient should be identified using at least two of the following methods** (The Joint Commission, 2021):

Identifying the patient ensures the right patient receives the medications and helps prevent errors. The patient's room number or physical location is not used as an identifier (The Joint Commission, 2021). Replace the identification band if it is missing or inaccurate in any way.

a. Check the name on the patient's identification band.

b. Check the identification number on the patient's identification band.

c. Check the birth date on the patient's identification band.

d. Ask the patient to state their name and birth date, based on facility policy.

This requires a response from the patient, but illness and strange surroundings often cause patients to be confused.

(continued on page 340)

Skill 5-23 ▶ Administering Medication via a Dry Powder Inhaler *(continued)*

ACTION	RATIONALE
15. Close the door to the room or pull the bedside curtain.	This provides patient privacy.
16. **Complete necessary assessments before administering medications. Check the patient's allergy bracelet, if present, or ask the patient about allergies. Explain what you are going to do, and the reason for doing it, to the patient.**	Assessment is a prerequisite to administration of medications. Explanation provides rationale, increases knowledge, and reduces anxiety.
17. Scan the patient's bar code on the identification band, if required (The Joint Commission, 2021) (Figure 1).	This provides an additional check to ensure that the medication is given to the right patient.
18. **Based on facility policy, the third check of the label may occur at this point. If so, read the label and recheck the labels with the eMAR/MAR before administering the medications to the patient.**	Many facilities require the *third* check to occur at the bedside, after identifying the patient and before administration. If facility policy directs the *third* check at this time, this *third* check ensures accuracy and helps to prevent errors.
19. Remove the mouthpiece cover or remove the device from the storage container. Load a dose into the device as directed by the manufacturer, if necessary. Alternatively, activate the inhaler, if necessary, according to the manufacturer's directions. Once prepared for inhalation, do not point the DPI downward because the dose may fall out (Hess et al., 2021).	This is necessary to deliver the medication.
20. Have the patient breathe out slowly and completely, without breathing into the DPI.	This allows for deeper inhalation with the medication dose. Moisture from the patient's breath can clog the inhaler.
21. Instruct the patient to place their teeth over, and seal lips around, the mouthpiece (Figure 2). **It is important to not block the opening with the tongue or teeth.**	This prevents medication from escaping and allows for a tight seal, ensuring maximal dosing of medication. Blocking the opening interferes with medication delivery.

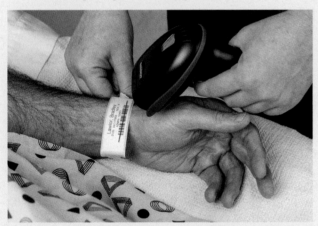

FIGURE 1. Scanning bar code on patient's identification bracelet.

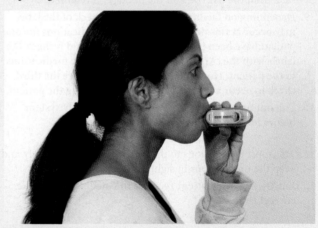

FIGURE 2. Patient with teeth over and lips sealed around DPI mouthpiece.

ACTION	RATIONALE
22. **Instruct the patient to breathe in forcefully, steadily, and deeply through the mouth, until their lungs are full** (Hess et al., 2021).	This activates the flow of medication. Deep inhalation allows for maximal distribution of medication to lung tissue.
23. Instruct the patient to remove the inhaler from mouth. Instruct the patient to hold their breath for 5 to 10 seconds, or as long as possible, and then to exhale normally (Hess et al., 2021).	This allows better distribution and longer absorption time for the medication.
24. Have the patient take a few normal breaths, then breathe in through the device a second time, based on the DPI in use. If a second dose is prescribed, reload and repeat (Allergy & Asthma Network, 2020b; Cleveland Clinic, 2020).	This ensures that both puffs are absorbed as much as possible. Some types of DPIs require a second inhalation for an individual dose (Hess et al., 2021).
25. After the prescribed number of puffs has been administered, have the patient replace the cap or storage container.	By replacing the cap, the patient is preventing any dust or dirt from entering the inhaler and being propelled into their bronchioles with later doses and from clogging the inhaler.

ACTION

26. Have the patient gargle and rinse with tap water after using the DPI. Clean the DPI according to the manufacturer's directions.

 27. Remove gloves and additional PPE, if used. Perform hand hygiene.

28. Document the administration of the medication immediately after administration. See Documentation section below.

29. Evaluate the patient's response to the medication within an appropriate time frame. Reassess lung sounds, oxygen saturation level, and respirations, as indicated.

RATIONALE

Rinsing is necessary when using inhaled steroids because oral fungal infections can occur. Rinsing removes medication residue from the mouth. Medication buildup in the device can affect how the medication is delivered as well as attract bacteria.

Proper removal of PPE reduces the risk of infection transmission and contamination of other items. Hand hygiene prevents the spread of microorganisms.

Timely documentation helps to ensure patient safety.

The patient needs to be evaluated for therapeutic and adverse effects from the medication. Lung sounds and oxygen saturation level may improve after DPI use. Respirations may decrease after DPI use.

EVALUATION

The expected outcomes have been met when the medication was administered and breathed in by the patient, the patient has experienced the intended effect of the medication, the patient has verbalized an understanding of and engaged in the medication regimen, and the patient has demonstrated correct use of the DPI.

DOCUMENTATION

Guidelines

Document the administration of the medication immediately after administration, including date, time, dose, and route of administration on the eMAR/MAR or record using the required format. If using a bar-code system, medication administration is automatically recorded when the bar code is scanned. PRN medications require documentation of the reason for administration. Prompt recording avoids the possibility of accidentally repeating the administration of the drug. Document respiratory rate, oxygen saturation and peak flow measurements, if applicable, lung assessment, and the patient's response to the treatment, if appropriate. If the drug was refused or omitted, record this in the appropriate area on the medication record and notify the health care team, as appropriate. This verifies the reason medication was omitted and ensures that health care personnel providing care for the patient are aware of the occurrence.

Sample Documentation

12/22/25 1715 Breath sounds slightly decreased in bases of lung pretreatment, respirations 18 breaths per minute and regular. After DPI, lung sounds remain diminished bilaterally in bases, O_2 saturation 97%, respiratory rate 16 breaths per minute. Patient able to demonstrate accurately the use of a DPI and verbalizes understanding of medication purpose and action.

—C. Bausler, RN

DEVELOPING CLINICAL REASONING AND CLINICAL JUDGMENT

UNEXPECTED SITUATIONS AND ASSOCIATED INTERVENTIONS

• *Patient reports that relief of symptoms has decreased:* Have the patient demonstrate the technique they are using. Because it is common for patients to have knowledge gaps regarding the correct use of a dry powered inhaler, it is imperative to review the technique with each patient at each encounter (Alsomali et al., 2017; Quaranta, 2018). Poor administration technique can lead to a decrease in effectiveness of the medication.

(continued on page 342)

Skill 5-23 ▶ Administering Medication via a Dry Powder Inhaler (continued)

SPECIAL CONSIDERATIONS

General Considerations

- Instruct the patient never to exhale into the mouthpiece or shake the inhaler (Allergy & Asthma Network, 2020b; Cleveland Clinic, 2020).
- If mist can be seen from the mouth or nose, the DPI is being used incorrectly.
- Follow the manufacturer's directions to clean the DPI.
- Store inhaler, capsules, and disks away from moisture at room temperature.
- Explain to the patient that there may not be any taste, smell, or feel associated with inhalation of the medication, which may be different from what they have experienced with another inhaler. As long as the directions for use of the DPI are followed, the patient will receive the full dose of medication (Cleveland Clinic, 2020).
- Ongoing assessment is an important part of nursing care to evaluate patient response to administered medications and early detection of adverse drug reactions. If an adverse effect is suspected, withhold further medication doses and notify the patient's health care team. Additional intervention is based on type of reaction and patient assessment.

Older Adult Considerations

- Older adults may experience poor DPI technique related to issues with dexterity, cognition and inspiratory ability. Poor technique errors may lead to poor clinical outcomes. Assessment of inhaler technique performance is important, and placebo device training should be considered (Maricoto et al., 2020).

Community-Based Care Considerations

- Many DPIs have dosage counters to keep track of remaining doses or indicators to alert when the device is almost empty (Allergy & Asthma Network, 2020b).
- If a particular DPI does not have a dose counter, teach patients how to tell when medication levels are getting low. The most reliable method is to look on the package and see how many doses the DPI contains. Divide this number by the number of doses used daily to ascertain how many days the DPI will last. Keep a diary or record of DPI use and discard the DPI on reaching the labeled number of doses.

EVIDENCE FOR PRACTICE ▶

PATIENT EDUCATION AND INHALED MEDICATIONS

Correct use of an inhaler is critical to ensure accurate dosing of medication. Nurses play a key role in educating patients and their family/caregivers and validating mastery of knowledge to improve patient outcomes.

Related Research

Gao, G., Liao, Y., Mo, L., Gong, Y., Shao, X., & Li, J. (2020). A randomized controlled trial of a nurse-led education pathway for asthmatic children from outpatient to home. *International Journal of Nursing Practice*, 26(3), e12823. https://doi.org/10.1111/ijn.12823
   Refer to details in Skill 5-22, Evidence for Practice.

EVIDENCE FOR PRACTICE ▶

INHALED MEDICATIONS

Correct use of a dry powder inhaler (DPI; diskus) is critical to ensure accurate dosing of medication. Patients who are prescribed medications delivered with a DPI must have accurate knowledge and demonstrate appropriate technique regarding use to ensure accurate medication delivery. Nurses play a key role in patient education and must have adequate knowledge to provide appropriate educational intervention.

Related Research

De Tratto, K., Gomez, C., Ryan, C. J., Bracken, N., Steffen, A., & Corbridge, S. J. (2014). Nurses' knowledge of inhaler technique in the inpatient hospital setting. *Clinical Nurse Specialist: The Journal for Advanced Nursing Practice*, 28(3), 156–160. https://doi.org/10.1097/NUR.0000000000000047
   Refer to details in Skill 5-22, Evidence for Practice.

Skill 5-24 ▶ Administering Medication via a Small-Volume Nebulizer

Drugs for inhalation may be administered via a small-volume **nebulizer**. Nebulizers utilize the force of high-flow oxygen or compressed air through a fluid medication to disperse fine particles of liquid medication into the deeper passages of the respiratory tract, where absorption occurs. The nebulizer medication treatment continues until all the medication in the nebulizer cup has been inhaled.

DELEGATION CONSIDERATIONS	The administration of medication via a nebulizer is not delegated to assistive personnel (AP). Depending on the state's nurse practice act and the organization's policies and procedures, administration of medication using a nebulizer may be delegated to licensed practical/vocational nurses (LPN/LVNs). The decision to delegate must be based on careful analysis of the patient's needs and circumstances as well as the qualifications of the person to whom the task is being delegated. Refer to the Delegation Guidelines in Appendix A.

EQUIPMENT

- Stethoscope
- Prescribed medication
- Nebulizer tubing and chamber
- Air compressor or oxygen hookup
- Sterile saline (if medication is not premeasured)
- Electronic Medication Administration Record (eMAR) or Medication Administration Record (MAR)
- PPE, as indicated

ASSESSMENT	Assess the appropriateness of the drug for the patient. Review the medical history and allergy, assessment, and laboratory data that may influence drug administration. Assess respiratory rate, rhythm, effort, and depth to establish a baseline. Assess lung sounds before and after use to establish a baseline and determine the effectiveness of the medication. Assess the peak flow before and after administration to establish a baseline and determine the effectiveness of the medication. If appropriate and/or prescribed, assess oxygen saturation level before and after medication administration. The oxygenation level usually increases after the medication is administered. Assess the patient's ability to manage a nebulizer. Assess the patient's knowledge and understanding of the medication's purpose and action. If the patient has a knowledge deficit about the medication, this may be the appropriate time to begin education about the medication Verify patient name, dose, route, and time of administration.
ACTUAL OR POTENTIAL HEALTH PROBLEMS AND NEEDS	Many actual or potential health problems or issues may require the use of this skill as part of related interventions. An appropriate health problem or issue may include: - Altered breathing pattern - Impaired gas exchange - Knowledge deficiency
OUTCOME IDENTIFICATION AND PLANNING	The expected outcomes to achieve are that the medication is administered and breathed in by the patient, and the patient experiences the intended effect of the medication. Other outcomes that may be appropriate include the following: the patient verbalizes an understanding of and engages with the medication regimen, and the patient demonstrates correct use of the nebulizer.

IMPLEMENTATION

ACTION	RATIONALE
1. Gather equipment. Check each medication prescribed against the original in the health record, depending on facility policy and the medication order system in place. Clarify any inconsistencies. Check the patient's health record for allergies.	The prescription is the legal record of prescribed medication interventions. This comparison helps to identify errors that may have occurred when orders were transcribed. Computer provider order-entry (CPOE) systems allow prescribers to send electronic medication prescriptions directly to the pharmacy located in a health care facility and to outpatient pharmacies.

(continued on page 344)

Skill 5-24 ▶ Administering Medication via a Small-Volume Nebulizer *(continued)*

ACTION	**RATIONALE**
2. Know the actions, special nursing considerations, safe dose ranges, purpose of administration, and adverse effects of the medications to be administered. Consider the appropriateness of the medication for this patient.	This knowledge aids the nurse in evaluating the therapeutic effect of the medication in relation to the patient's health status and can also be used to educate the patient about the medication.
3. Perform hand hygiene.	Hand hygiene prevents the spread of microorganisms.
4. Move the medication supply system to the outside of the patient's room or prepare for administration at the medication supply system in the medication area. Alternatively, access the medication administration supply system at or inside the patient's room.	Organization facilitates error-free administration and saves time.
5. Unlock the medication supply system or drawer. Enter the passcode and scan employee identification, if required.	Locking the medication supply system or drawer safeguards each patient's medication supply. Facility accrediting organizations require medication supply systems to be locked when not in use. Entering the passcode and scanning ID allows only authorized users into the system and identifies the user for documentation by the computer.
6. **Prepare medications for one patient at a time.**	This prevents errors in medication administration.
7. Read the eMAR/MAR and read the label when selecting the proper medication from the medication supply system or the patient's medication drawer.	This is the *first* check of the label.
8. Read the label and compare the label with the eMAR/MAR. Check expiration dates and perform calculations, if necessary. Scan the bar code on the package, if required.	This is the *second* check of the label. Verify calculations with another nurse to ensure safety, if necessary.
9. **Depending on facility policy, the third check of the label may occur at this point. If so, when all medications for one patient have been prepared, read the label and recheck the labels with the eMAR/MAR before taking the medications to the patient. However, many facilities require the third check to occur at the bedside, after identifying the patient.**	This *third* check ensures accuracy and helps to prevent errors. *Note:* Many facilities require the *third* check to occur at the bedside, after identifying the patient and before administration.
10. **Log out of and/or lock the medication supply system before leaving it.**	Locking the medication supply system or drawer safeguards the patient's medication supply. Facility accrediting organizations require medication supply systems to be locked when not in use.
11. Transport medications to the patient's bedside carefully and keep the medications in sight at all times.	Careful handling and close observation prevent accidental or deliberate disarrangement of medications.
12. **Ensure that the patient receives the medications at the correct time.**	Check facility policy, which may allow for administration within a period of 30 minutes before or 30 minutes after the designated time.
13. Perform hand hygiene and put on PPE, if indicated.	Hand hygiene and PPE prevent the spread of microorganisms. PPE is required based on transmission precautions.
14. **Identify the patient. Compare the information with the eMAR/MAR. The patient should be identified using at least two of the following methods (The Joint Commission, 2021):**	Identifying the patient ensures the right patient receives the medications and helps prevent errors. The patient's room number or physical location is not used as an identifier (The Joint Commission, 2021). Replace the identification band if it is missing or inaccurate in any way.
a. Check the name on the patient's identification band.	This requires a response from the patient, but illness and strange surroundings often cause patients to be confused.
b. Check the identification number on the patient's identification band.	

ACTION

   c. Check the birth date on the patient's identification band.

   d. Ask the patient to state their name and birth date, based on facility policy.

15. Close the door to the room or pull the bedside curtain.

16. **Complete necessary assessments before administering medications. Check the patient's allergy bracelet, if present, or ask the patient about allergies. Explain what you are going to do, and the reason for doing it, to the patient.**

17. Scan the patient's bar code on the identification band, if required (The Joint Commission, 2021).

18. **Based on facility policy, the third check of the label may occur at this point. If so, read the label and recheck the labels with the eMAR/MAR before administering the medications to the patient.**

19. Remove the nebulizer cup from the device and open it. Place a premeasured unit-dose medication in the bottom section of the cup or use a dropper to place a concentrated dose of medication in the cup (Figure 1). Add prescribed diluent (usually saline), if required.

20. Screw the top portion of the nebulizer cup back in place and attach the cup to the nebulizer. Attach one end of tubing to the stem on the bottom of the nebulizer cuff and the other end to the air compressor or oxygen source.

21. Turn on the air compressor or oxygen (flow of 6 to 8 L/min [Hess et al., 2021]). Check that a fine medication mist is produced by opening the valve. Have the patient place the mouthpiece into the mouth and grasp securely with their teeth and lips.

22. **Instruct the patient to breathe normally through the mouth with occasional deep breaths (Figure 2). A nose clip may be necessary if the patient is also breathing through the nose.**

RATIONALE

This provides patient privacy.

Assessment is a prerequisite to administration of medications. Explanation provides rationale, increases knowledge, promotes patient engagement, and reduces anxiety.

Scanning provides an additional check to ensure that the medication is given to the right patient.

Many facilities require the *third* check to occur at the bedside, after identifying the patient and before administration. If facility policy directs the *third* check at this time, this *third* check ensures accuracy and helps to prevent errors.

To get enough volume to make a fine mist, normal saline may need to be added to the concentrated medication.

Air or oxygen must be forced through the nebulizer to form a fine mist.

If there is no fine mist, make sure that medication has been added to the cup and that the tubing is connected to the air compressor or oxygen outlet. Adjust flow meter if necessary.

While the patient inhales, the medication comes in contact with the respiratory tissue and is absorbed.

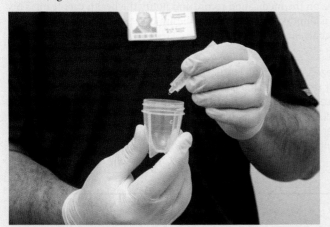

FIGURE 1. Putting medication into nebulizer.

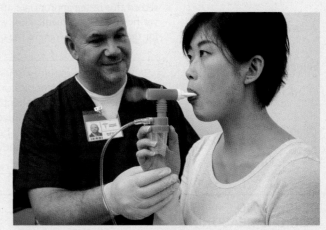

FIGURE 2. Inhaling slowly and deeply through the mouth.

23. Continue this inhalation technique until all medication in the nebulizer cup has been aerosolized (usually about 15 minutes). Once the fine mist decreases in amount, gently flick the sides of the nebulizer cup.

Once the fine mist stops, the medication is no longer being aerosolized. By gently flicking the cup sides, any medication that is stuck to the sides is knocked into the bottom of the cup, where it can become aerosolized.

(continued on page 346)

Skill 5-24 ▶ Administering Medication via a Small-Volume Nebulizer *(continued)*

ACTION	RATIONALE
24. When the medication in the nebulizer cup has been completely aerosolized, the cup will be empty and no more aerosol will be produced. Have the patient remove the nebulizer from their mouth and gargle and rinse with tap water, as indicated. Clean and store the nebulizer and equipment according to the manufacturer's directions and facility policy.	Rinsing is necessary when using inhaled steroids because oral fungal infections can occur. Rinsing removes medication residue from the mouth. The buildup of medication in the device can affect how the medication is delivered as well as attract bacteria.
25. Remove gloves and additional PPE, if used. Perform hand hygiene.	Proper removal of PPE reduces the risk of infection transmission and contamination of other items. Hand hygiene prevents the spread of microorganisms.
26. Document the administration of the medication immediately after administration. See Documentation section below.	Timely documentation helps to ensure patient safety.
27. Evaluate the patient's response to the medication within an appropriate time frame. Reassess lung sounds, oxygen saturation level, peak flow, and respirations, as indicated.	The patient needs to be evaluated for therapeutic and adverse effects from the medication. Lung sounds and oxygen saturation level may improve after nebulizer use. Respirations may decrease after nebulizer use.

EVALUATION

The expected outcomes have been met when the medication was administered and breathed in by the patient, the patient has experienced the intended effect of the medication, the patient has verbalized an understanding of and engaged with the medication regimen, and the patient has demonstrated correct use of the nebulizer.

DOCUMENTATION

Guidelines

Document the administration of the medication immediately after administration, including date, time, dose, and route of administration on the eMAR/MAR or record using the required format. If using a bar-code system, medication administration is automatically recorded when the bar code is scanned. PRN medications require documentation of the reason for administration. Prompt recording avoids the possibility of accidentally repeating the administration of the drug. Document respiratory rate, oxygen saturation and peak flow measurements, if applicable, lung assessment, and the patient's response to the treatment, if appropriate. If the drug was refused or omitted, record this in the appropriate area on the medication record and notify the health care team. This verifies the reason medication was omitted and ensures that health care personnel providing care for the patient are aware of the occurrence.

Sample Documentation

> 9/29/25 2300 Expiratory wheezes noted in all lungs fields before albuterol nebulizer, O_2 saturation 92%, respiratory rate 24 breaths per minute, patient reports "feeling like I can't get my breath." Patient reassessed 20 minutes after albuterol nebulizer treatment; lung sounds are clear to auscultation and equal in all lung fields, O_2 saturation 97%, respiratory rate 18 breaths per minute unlabored. Patient verbalized relief of shortness of breath and an understanding of medication purpose and action.
>
> —*C. Bausler, RN*

DEVELOPING CLINICAL REASONING AND CLINICAL JUDGMENT

UNEXPECTED SITUATIONS AND ASSOCIATED INTERVENTIONS

• *Patient is unable to hold nebulizer in mouth and/or is unable to keep lips closed around device:* A plain oxygen mask can be attached to the nebulizer device and used to deliver the nebulized medication, eliminating the need to hold the device in the mouth.

SPECIAL
CONSIDERATIONS

General Considerations

- Ongoing assessment is an important part of nursing care to evaluate patient response to administered medications and early detection of adverse drug reactions. If an adverse effect is suspected, withhold further medication doses and notify the patient's health care team. Additional intervention is based on type of reaction and patient assessment.

Infant and Child Considerations

- A small child may use a mask instead of a mouthpiece. The mask must fit securely over both the nose and the mouth to ensure a good seal and prevent medication escaping.
- Children must be able to seal their lips around the mouthpiece to use a nebulizer without a mask.

Community-Based Care Considerations

- After each dose, the medicine cup and mouthpiece should be washed with water and air dried, while the medicine cup, mouthpiece, or mask should be washed with a mild detergent daily (Cleveland Clinic, 2019). Weekly disinfection is recommended.

Enhance Your Understanding

Focusing on Patient Care: Developing Clinical Reasoning and Clinical Judgment

Consider the case scenarios at the beginning of the chapter as you answer the following questions to enhance your understanding and apply what you have learned.

QUESTIONS

1. When entering Cooper Jackson's room with the antibiotic, Cooper becomes visibly upset and runs to his mother. What is the best technique to administer liquid medication to an uncooperative 2-year-old? Thirty minutes after receiving an oral medication, Cooper vomits. Should the nurse re-administer the medication?

2. What are some ways that the nurse can make Erika Jenkins feel more relaxed about receiving her injection?

3. What are some priority points that the nurse needs to discuss with Jonah Dinerman, the patient with type 1 diabetes, if the education needs to be completed in a short time?

You can find suggested answers after the Bibliography at the end of this chapter.

Integrated Case Study Connection

The case studies in the back of the book focus on integrating concepts. Refer to the following case studies to enhance your understanding of the concepts and skills in this chapter.

Bibliography

Ağaç, E., & Günes, Ü. Y. (2010). Effect on pain of changing the needle prior to administering medicine intramuscularly: A randomized controlled trial. *Journal of Advanced Nursing, 67*(3), 563–568. https://doi.org/10.1111/j.1365-2648.2010.05513

Ahrensbøll-Friis, U., Simonsen, A. B., Zachariae, C., Thyssen, J. P., & Johansen, J. D. (2021). Contact dermatitis caused by glucose sensors, insulin pumps, and tapes: Results from a 5-year period. *Contact Dermatitis, 84*(2), 75–81. https://doi.org/10.1111/cod.13664

Alismail, A., Song, C. A., Terry, M. H., Daher, N., Almutairi, W. A., & Lo, T. (2016). Diverse inhaler devices: A big challenge for health-care professionals. *Respiratory Care, 61*(5), 593–599.

Allen, S. M. (2015). As a flushing agent for enteral nutrition, does sterile water compared to tap water affect the associated risk of infection in critically ill patients? *The Alabama Nurse, 42*(1), 5–6.

Allergy & Asthma Network. (2020a). *How to use a metered-dose inhaler (MDI).* https://allergyasthmanetwork.org/what-is-asthma/how-is-asthma-treated/how-to-use-a-metered-dose-inhaler/

Allergy & Asthma Network. (2020b). *How to use a dry powder inhaler (DPI).* https://allergyasthmanetwork.org/what-is-asthma/how-is-asthma-treated/how-to-use-a-dry-powder-inhaler/

Allergy & Asthma Network. (2020c). *How to clean your asthma spacer.* https://allergyasthmanetwork.org/news/why-and-how-wash-your-valved-holding-chamber/

Alsomali, H. J., Vines, D. L., Stein, B. D., & Becker, E. A. (2017). Evaluating the effectiveness of written dry powder inhaler instructions and health literacy in subjects diagnosed with COPD. *Respiratory Care, 62*(2), 172–178. https://doi.org/10.4187/respcare.04686

American Academy of Pediatrics. (2013, February 13). *How to give ear drops.* Healthychildren.org. https://www.healthychildren.org/English/safety-prevention/at-home/medication-safety/Pages/How-to-Give-Ear-Drops.aspx

American Academy of Pediatrics. (2019, November 12). *Tear-free vaccination tips.* https://www.healthychildren.org/English/safety-prevention/immunizations/Pages/Tear-Free-Vaccination-Tips.aspx

American Academy of Pediatrics. (2020, December 7). *Diabetes in children.* https://www.healthychildren.org/English/health-issues/conditions/chronic/Pages/Diabetes.aspx

American Diabetes Association (ADA). (2022). *Insulin routines.* Retrieved April 29, 2022, from https://www.diabetes.org/healthy-living/medication-treatments/insulin-other-injectables/insulin-routines

American Heart Association (AHA). (2020). *2020 CPR & ECC guidelines. BLS provider manual.* AHA product number: 20–1102.

American Lung Association. (2021, January 27). *How to use a metered-dose inhaler with a spacer or valved holding chamber.* [Video]. https://www.lung.org/lung-health-diseases/lung-disease-lookup/asthma/patient-resources-and-videos/videos/how-to-use-a-metered-dose-inhaler

Anderson, L. (2019). Enteral feeding tubes: an overview of nursing care. *British Journal of Nursing, 28*(12):748–754. https://doi.10.12968/bjon.2019.28.12.748

Andrews, M., Boyle, J. S., & Collins, J. (2020). *Transcultural concepts in nursing care* (8th ed.). Wolters Kluwer.

Aroesty, J. M., & Kannam, J. P. (2020, August 27). *Patient education: Medication for angina (Beyond the basics).* UpToDate. https://www.uptodate.com/contents/medications-for-angina-beyond-the-basics

Arslan, G. G., & Özden, D. (2018). Creating a change in the use of ventrogluteal site for intramuscular injection. *Patient Preference and Adherence, 12*, 1749–1756. https://doi.org/10.2147/PPA.S168885

Association of Diabetes Care & Education Specialists (ADCES). (2021, March). *ADCES practice paper. Continuous subcutaneous insulin infusion (CSII) without and with sensor integration.* https://www.diabeteseducator.org/docs/default-source/default-document-library/continuous-subcutaneous-insulin-infusion-2018-v2.pdf?sfvrsn=4

Asthma Initiative of Michigan (AIM). (n.d.). *How to use a metered-dose inhaler the right way.* https://getasthmahelp.org/inhalers-how-to.aspx#

Bandy, K. S., Albrecht, S., Parag, B., & McClave, S. A. (2019). Practices involved in the enteral delivery of drugs. *Current Nutrition Reports, 8*(4), 356–362. https://doi.org/10.1007/s13668-019-00290-4

Bartlett, J. L., & Kinsey, J. D. (2020). Large-group, asynchronous, interprofessional simulation: Identifying roles and improving communication with student pharmacists and student nurses. *Currents in Pharmacy Teaching and Learning, 12*(6), 763–770. https://doi.org/10.1016/j.cptl.2020.01.023

Barton, A. (2019). The case for using a disinfecting cap for needle free connectors. *British Journal of Nursing, 24*(14), S22–S27. https://doi.org/10.12968/bjon.2019.28.14.S22

Bauldoff, G., Gubrud, P., & Carno, M. A. (2020). *LeMone and Burke's medical-surgical nursing: Clinical reasoning in patient care* (7th ed.). Pearson.

Becton, Dickinson and Company. (2021a). *Injecting insulin with a pen.* https://www.bd.com/en-uk/products/diabetes/diabetes-learning-centre/injection-technique/injecting-insulin-with-a-pen

Becton, Dickinson and Company. (2021b). *BD AutoShield Duo™ pen needle.* https://www.bd.com/en-us/offerings/capabilities/diabetes-care/pen-needles/bd-autoshield-duo-pen-needle-x857469

Boullata, J. (2021). Enteral medication for the tube-fed patient: making this route safe and effective. *Nutrition in Clinical Practice, 36*(1), 111–132. https://doi.org/10.1002/ncp.10615

Boullata, J. I., Carrera, A. L., Harvey, L., Escuro, A. A., Hudson, L., Mays, A., Wessel, J. J., Bajpai, S., Beebe, M. L., Kinn, T. J., Klang, M. G., Lord, L., Martin, K., Pompeii-Wolfe, C., Sullivan, J., Wood, A., Malone, A., Guenter, P., & ASPEN Safe Practices for Enteral Nutrition Therapy, American Society for Parenteral and Enteral Nutrition. (2017). ASPEN safe practices for enteral nutrition therapy. *Journal of Parenteral and Enteral Nutrition, 41*(1), 15–103. https://doi.org/10.1177/0148607116673053

Bravo, K., Cochran, G., & Barrett, R. (2016). Nursing strategies to increase medication safety in inpatient settings. *Journal of Nursing Care Quality, 31*(4), 335–341. https://doi.org/10.1097/NCQ.0000000000000181

Cahir, C., Wallace, E., Cummins, A., Telijeur, C., Byrne, C., Bennett, K., & Fahey, T. (2019). Identifying adverse drug events in older community-swelling patients. *Annals of Family Medicine, 17*(2), 133–140. https://doi.org/10.1370/afm.2359

Casey, A. L., Karpanen, T. J., Nightingale, P., & Elliot, T. S. (2018). An in vitro comparison of standard cleaning to a continuous passive disinfection cap for the decontamination of needle-free connectors. *Antimicrobial Resistance & Infection Control, 7,* Article number: 50. https://doi.org/10.1186/s13756-018-0342-0

Centers for Disease Control and Prevention (CDC), Hamborsky, J., Kroger, A., & Wolfe, C. (Eds.). (2015a). Epidemiology and prevention of vaccine-preventable diseases. *The pink book* (13th ed.). Public Health Foundation. https://www.cdc.gov/vaccines/pubs/pinkbook/index.html

Centers for Disease Control and Prevention (CDC), Hamborsky, J., Kroger, A., & Wolfe, C. (Eds.). (2015b). Appendix A. Schedules and recommendation. In *Epidemiology and prevention of vaccine-preventable diseases. The pink book* (13th ed.). Public Health Foundation. https://www.cdc.gov/vaccines/pubs/pinkbook/appendix/appdx-a.html

Centers for Disease Control and Prevention (CDC). (2018, March 7). *Know how to use your asthma inhaler.* https://www.cdc.gov/asthma/inhaler_video/default.htm

Centers for Disease Control and Prevention (CDC). (2019, June 2017). *Medication preparation questions.* https://www.cdc.gov/injectionsafety/providers/provider_faqs_med-prep.html

Centers for Disease Control and Prevention (CDC). (2020, July 27). *Make shots less stressful.* https://www.cdc.gov/vaccines/parents/visit/less-stressful.html

Centers for Disease Control and Prevention (CDC). (2021, May 4). *Vaccine recommendations and guidelines of the ACIP. General best practice guidelines for immunization: Best practices guidance of the Advisory Committee on Immunization Practices (ACIP).* https://www.cdc.gov/vaccines/hcp/acip-recs/general-recs/administration.html

Choy, B. N. K., Zhu, M. M., Pang, J. C. S., Chan, J. C. H., Ng, A. L. K., Fan, M. C. Y., Iu, L. P. L., Kwan, J. S. K., Lai, J. S. M., & Chiu, P. K. C. (2019). Factors associated with poor eye drop administration technique and the role of patient education among Hong Kong elderly population. *Journal of Ophthalmology*, Article ID 5962065. https://doi.org/10.1155/2019/5962065

Chung, J. W., Ng, W. M., & Wong, T. K. (2002). An experimental study on the use of manual pressure to reduce pain in intramuscular injections. *Journal of Clinical Nursing, 11*(4), 457–461. https://doi.org/10.1046/j.1365-2702.2002.00645

Cleveland Clinic. (2014, May 21). *Inhalers.* https://my.clevelandclinic.org/health/drugs/8694-inhalers

Cleveland Clinic. (2019, November 20). *Home nebulizer.* https://my.clevelandclinic.org/health/drugs/4254-home-nebulizer

Cleveland Clinic. (2020, December 21). *Dry powder inhaler (DPI): Diskus®.* https://my.clevelandclinic.org/health/drugs/6439-dry-powder-inhaler-dpi-diskus

Cohen, M. R. (2017). Medication errors. *Nursing, 47*(12), 72. https://doi.org/10.1097/01.NURSE.0000526894.07627.3c

Cohrs, J., & Kerns, R. (2020). Using transdermal patches to treat neuropathic pain. *Nursing, 50*(4), 15–16. https://doi.org/10.1097/01.NURSE.0000657076.10174.66

Davidson, K. M., & Rourke, L. (2013). Teaching best-evidence: Deltoid intramuscular injection technique. *Journal of Nursing Education and Practice, 3*(7), 120–128. https://doi.org/10.5430/jnep.v3n7p120

De Tratto, K., Gomez, C., Ryan, C. J., Bracken, N., Steffen, A., & Corbridge, S. J. (2014). Nurses' knowledge of inhaler technique in the inpatient hospital setting. *Clinical Nurse Specialist: The Journal for Advanced Nursing Practice, 28*(3), 156–160. https://doi.org/10.1097/NUR.0000000000000047.

Dolan, S. A., Arias, K. M., Felizardo, G., Barnes, S., Kraska, S., Patrick, M., Bumsted, A. (2016). APIC position paper: Safe injection, infusion, and medication vial practices in health care. *American Journal of Infection Control, 44*(7), 750–757. https://doi.org/10.1016/j.ajic.2016.02.033

Dudek, S. (2018). *Nutrition essentials for nursing practice* (8th ed.). Wolters Kluwer.

Durand, C., Alhammad, A., & Willett, K. C. (2012). Practical considerations for optimal transdermal drug delivery. *American Journal of Health-System Pharmacy, 69*(2), 116–124. https://doi.org/10.2146/ajhp110158

Eliopoulos, C. (2018). *Gerontological nursing* (9th ed.). Wolters Kluwer.

Fischbach, F. T., & Fischbach, M. A. (2018). *A manual of laboratory and diagnostic tests* (10th ed.). Wolters Kluwer.

Flynn, J. M., Larsen, E. N., Keogh, S., Ullman, A. J., & Rickard, C. M. (2019). Methods for microbial needleless connector decontamination: A systematic review and meta-analysis. *American Journal of Infection Control, 47*(8), 956–965. https://doi.org/10.1016/j.ajic.2019.01.002

Frandsen, G., & Pennington, S. S. (2021). *Abrams' clinical drug therapy: Rationales for nursing practice* (12th ed.). Wolters Kluwer.

Gao, G., Liao, Y., Mo, L., Gong, Y., Shao, X., & Li, J. (2020). A randomized controlled trial of a nurse-led education pathway for asthmatic children from outpatient to home. *International Journal of Nursing Practice, 26*(3), e12823. https://doi.org/10.1111/ijn.12823

Gelder, C. (2014). Best practice injection technique for children and young people with diabetes. *Nursing Children and Young People, 26*(7), 32–36. https://doi.org/10.7748/ncyp.26.7.32.e458

Gerald, L. B., & Dhand, R. (2020, September 29). *Patient education: Inhaler techniques in adults (Beyond the basics).* UpToDate. https://www.uptodate.com/contents/inhaler-techniques-in-adults-beyond-the-basics?topicRef=1173&source=see_link

Giuliano, K. K., Su, W., Degnan, D. D., Fitzgerald, K., Zink, R. J., & DeLaurentis, P. (2018). Intravenous smart pump drug library compliance: A descriptive study of 44 hospitals. *Journal of Patient Safety, 14*(4), e76–e82. https://doi.org/10.1097/PTS.0000000000000383

Gorski, L. A., Hadaway, L., Hagle, M. E., Broadhurst, D., Clare, S., Kleidon, T., Meyer, B. M., Nickel, B.,

Rowley, S., Sharpe, E., & Alexander, M. Infusion Nurses Society. (2021). Infusion therapy. Standards of practice. *Journal of Infusion Nursing, 44*(Suppl 1), S1–S224. https://doi.org/10.1097/NAN.0000000000000396

Gudgel, D. T. (2021, March 10). How to put in eye drops. *American Academy of Ophthalmology*. https://www.aao.org/eye-health/treatments/how-to-put-in-eye-drops

Gutierrez, J. J. P., & Munakomi, S. (2021). *Intramuscular injection*. StatPearls. https://www.ncbi.nlm.nih.gov/books/NBK556121/

Gwenhure, T. (2020). Procedure for eye irrigation to treat ocular chemical injury. *Nursing, 116*(2), 46–48. https://www.nursingtimes.net/clinical-archive/accident-and-emergency/procedure-for-eye-irrigation-to-treat-ocular-chemical-injury-03-02-2020/

Hanson, A., & Haddad, L. M. (2020, November). Nursing rights of medication administration. In *StatPearls*. StatPearls Publishing. https://www.ncbi.nlm.nih.gov/books/NBK560654/

Harkin, H. (2015). Ear care and irrigation with water: An update. *Practice Nurse, 45*(7), 24–26.

Hayter, K. L. (2016). Listen up for safe ear irrigation. *Nursing, 46*(6), 62–65. https://doi.org/10.1097/01.NURSE.0000481437.02178.3b

Heise, T., Nosek, L., Dellweg, S., Zijlstra, E., Praestmark, K. A., Kildegaard, J., Nielsen, G., & Sparre, T. (2014). Impact of injection speed and volume on perceived pain during subcutaneous injections into the abdomen and thigh: A single-centre, randomized controlled trial. *Diabetes Obesity and Metabolism, 16*(10), 971–976. https://doi.org/10.1111/dom.12304

Herman, A., de Montjoye, L., & Baeck, M. (2020). Adverse cutaneous reaction to diabetic glucose sensors and insulin pumps: Irritant contact dermatitis or allergic contact dermatitis? *Contact Dermatitis, 83*(1), 25–30. https://doi.org/10.1111/cod.13529

Hess, D. R., MacIntyre, N. R., Galvin, W. F., & Mishoe, S. C. (2021). *Respiratory care. Principles and practice* (4th ed.). Jones & Bartlett Learning.

Hinkle, J. L., & Cheever, K. H. (2018). *Brunner & Suddarth's textbook of medical-surgical nursing* (14th ed.). Wolters Kluwer.

Holden, D. N. (2013, October 11). *Are nitrate-free intervals really needed?* Medscape Nurses. https://www.medscape.com/viewarticle/812374_1

Hopkins, U., & Arias, C. (2013). Large-volume IM injections: A review of best practices. *Oncology Nurse Advisor*, 32–37.

Hoy, H., & Ng, Y. C. (2021). Immune responses and transplantation. In M. Harding (Ed.), *Lewis's medical and surgical nursing: assessment and management of clinical problems* (11th ed.). Elsevier.

Innovation Compounding. (2020). *Instructional guide. Ampules. Aseptic technique.* [Video]. https://innovationcompounding.com/patient-tutorials/

Institute for Safe Medication Practices (ISMP). (2015). *ISMP safe practice guidelines for adult IV push medications.* https://www.ismp.org/sites/default/files/attachments/2017-11/ISMP97-Guidelines-071415-3.%20FINAL.pdf

Institute for Safe Medication Practices (ISMP). (2020, February 21). *2020–2021 ISMP targeted medication safety best practices for hospitals.* https://www.ismp.org/sites/default/files/attachments/2020-02/2020-2021%20TMSBP-%20FINAL_1.pdf

International Council of Nurses (ICN). (2019). *Nursing diagnosis and outcome statements.* https://www.icn.ch/sites/default/files/inline-files/ICNP2019-DC.pdf

Janssen Pharmaceuticals, Inc. (2018, July). *Instructions for use. Duragesic®. Fentanyl transdermal system.* https://www.janssenlabels.com/package-insert/product-instructions-for-use/DURAGESIC-ifu.pdf

Jarvis, C., & Echkardt, A. (2020). *Physical examination & health assessment* (8th ed.). Elsevier.

Jensen, S. (2019). *Nursing health assessment. A best practice approach* (3rd ed.). Wolters Kluwer.

The Joint Commission. (2021). *Hospital: 2021 National Patient Safety Goals.* https://www.jointcommission.org/standards/national-patient-safety-goals/hospital-national-patient-safety-goals/

Jungquist, C. R., Quinlan-Colwell, A., Vallerand, A., Carlisle, H. L., Cooney, M., Dempsey, S. J., Dunwoody, D., Maly, A., Meloche, K., Meyers, A., Sawyer, J., Singh, N., Sullivan, D., Watson, C., & Polomano, R. C. (2020). American Society for Pain Management nursing guidelines on monitoring for opioid-induced advancing sedation and respiratory depression: Revisions. *Pain Management Nursing, 21*(1), 7–25. https://doi.org/10.1016/j.pmn.2019.06.007

Kaiser Permanente. (2020, October 26). *Using a metered-dose inhaler: Care instructions.* https://healthy.kaiserpermanente.org/health-wellness/health-encyclopedia/he.using-a-metered-dose-inhaler-care-instructions.ud1565

Karch, A. M. (2020). *Focus on nursing pharmacology* (8th ed.). Wolters Kluwer.

Kyle, T., & Carman, S. (2021). *Essentials of pediatric nursing* (4th ed.). Wolters Kluwer.

Lampert, A., Kessler, J., Washington-Dorando, P., Bardenheuer, H. J., Bocek Eknes, E.M., Krisam, J., Haefeli, W. E., & Seidling, H. M. (2018). Patient experiences with handling of analgesic transdermal patches and challenges in correct drug administration: A pilot study on patient education. *Journal of Patient Safety, 14*(4), e97–e101. https://doi.org/10.1097/PTS.0000000000000538

Lindauer, A., Sexson, K., & Harvath, T. (2017). Teaching caregivers to administer eye drops, transdermal patches, and suppositories. *American Journal of Nursing. 117*(1), 54–59. https://doi.org/10.1097/01.NAJ.0000511568.58187.36

Maricoto, T., Santos, D., Carvalho, C., Teles, I., Correia-de-Sousa, J., & Taborda-Barata, L. (2020). Assessment of poor inhaler technique in older patients with asthma or COPD: A predictive tool for clinical risk and inhaler performance. *Drugs & Aging, 37*(8), 605–616. https://doi.org/10.1007/s40266-020-00779-6

Mayo Foundation for Medical Education and Research (MFMER). (2021a, April 1). *Fentanyl (Transdermal route).* https://www.mayoclinic.org/drugs-supplements/fentanyl-transdermal-route/proper-use/drg-20068152

Mayo Foundation for Medical Education and Research (MFMER). (2021b, February 1). *Nitroglycerin (Transdermal route).* https://www.mayoclinic.org/drugs-supplements/nitroglycerin-transdermal-route/side-effects/drg-20072959?p=1

Mayo Foundation for Medical Education and Research (MFMER). (2021c, May 1). *Ofloxacin (Otic route).* https://www.mayoclinic.org/drugs-supplements/ofloxacin-otic-route/proper-use/drg-20065162

Mayo Foundation for Medical Education and Research (MFMER). (2021d). *Naloxone (Intranasal).* https://www.mayoclinic.org/drugs-supplements/naloxone-nasal-route/proper-use/drg-20165181#:~:text=Gently%20insert%20the%20tip%20of,nostril%20after%20giving%20the%20dose

Mayo Foundation for Medical Education and Research (MFMER). (2021e). *Terconazole (Vaginal route).* https://www.mayoclinic.org/drugs-supplements/terconazole-vaginal-route/proper-use/drg-20061411

Mayo Foundation for Medical Education and Research (MFMER). (2021f). *Corticosteroid (Inhalation route).* https://www.mayoclinic.org/drugs-supplements/corticosteroid-inhalation-route/proper-use/drg-20070533?p=1

McCuistion, L. E., DiMaggio, K. V., Winton, M. B., & Yeager, J. J. (2021). *Pharmacology: A patient-centered nursing process approach* (10th ed.). Elsevier.

MedlinePlus. (2019, April 15). *Methylphenidate transdermal patch.* U.S. National Library of Medicine. https://medlineplus.gov/druginfo/meds/a606014.html

MedlinePlus. (2020, January 13). *How to use an inhaler-no spacer.* U.S. National Library of Medicine. https://medlineplus.gov/ency/patientinstructions/000041.htm

Mitchell, A. (2019). Administering a suppository: Types, considerations and procedure. *British Journal of Nursing, 28*(5), 288–289. https://doi.org/10.12968/bjon.2019.28.5.288

Mohammady, M., Janani, L., & Akbari Sari, A. (2017). Slow versus fast subcutaneous heparin injections for prevention of bruising and site pain intensity. *Cochrane Database of Systematic Reviews. 11*(11), CD008077. https://doi.org/10.1002/14651858.CD008077.pub4

Moore, R. H. (2020, January 10). Patient education: Asthma inhaler techniques in children (Beyond the basics). UpToDate. https://www.uptodate.com/contents/asthma-inhaler-techniques-in-children-beyond-the-basics

Mraz, M., Thomas, C., & Rajcan, L. (2018). Intramuscular injection CLIMAT pathway: A clinical practice guideline. *British Journal of Nursing, 27*(13), 752–756. https://doi.org/10.12968/bjon.2018.27.13.752

National Institutes of Health. National Library of Medicine. DailyMed. (2020, October 22). *Label: Ilevro. Nepafenac suspension.* https://dailymed.nlm.nih.gov/dailymed/lookup.cfm?setid=6c212466-ff8d-ecfc-ede2-ef8bdcaaf114

Nimri, R., Nir, J., & Phillip, M. (2020). Insulin pump therapy. *American Journal of Therapeutics, 27*(1), e30–e41. https://doi.org/10.1097/MJT.0000000000001097

Norris, T. L. (2020). *Porth's essentials of pathophysiology* (5th ed.). Wolters Kluwer.

NPS Medicinewise. (2020, October). *Consumer medicine information.* Ilevro. Nepafenac. https://www.nps.org.au/medicine-finder/ilevro-eye-drops

Öztürk, D., Baykara, Z. G., Karadag, A., & Eyikara, E. (2017). The effect of the application of manual pressure before the administration of intramuscular injections on students' perceptions of postinjection pain: A semi-experimental study. *Journal of Clinical Nursing, 26*(11–12), 1632–1638. https://doi.org/10.1111/jocn.13530

Patient Safety Network (PSNet). (2019, September). *Health literacy.* Agency for Healthcare Research and Quality (AHRQ). https://psnet.ahrq.gov/primer/health-literacy

Peate, I. (2015). How to administer suppositories. *Nursing Standard, 30*(1), 34–36. https://doi.org/10.7748/ns.30.1.34.e9483

Pich, J. (2020). Slow versus fast subcutaneous heparin injections for prevention of bruising and site pain intensity: A Cochrane review summary. *International Journal of Nursing Studies, 103*, 103–238. https://doi.org/10.1016/j.ijnurstu.2018.12.001

Prescriber's Digital Reference (PDR). (2021). *Influenza vaccine-drug summary.* https://www.pdr.net/drug-summary/Fluzone-Intradermal-influenza-vaccine-3091

Price, D. B., Román-Rodríguez, M., McQueen, R. B., Bosnic-Anticevich, S., Carter, V., Gruffydd-Jones, K., Haughney, J., Henrichsen, S., Hutton, C., Infantino, A., Lavorini, F., Law, L. M., Lisspers, K., Papi, A., Ryan, D., Ställberg, B., van der Molen, T., & Chrystyn, H. (2017). Inhaler errors in the CRITIKAL Study: Type, frequency, and association with asthma outcomes. *The Journal of Allergy and Clinical Immunology. In Practice, 5*(4), 1071–1081.e9. https://doi.org/10.1016/j.jaip.2017.01.004

Problem-based care plans. (2020). In *Lippincott advisor*. Wolters Kluwer. https://advisor.lww.com/lna/home.do

Pyl, J., Dendooven, E., Van Eekelen, I., den Brinker, M., Dotremont, H., France, A., Foubert, K., Pieters, L., Lambert, J., De Block, C., & Aerts, O. (2020). Prevalence and prevention of contact dermatitis caused by FreeStyle Libre: A monocentric experience. *Diabetes Care, 43*(4), 918–920.

Quaranta, J. (2018). *Asthma management in children and adults* (2nd ed.). S.C. Publishing.

Rochon, P. A. (2020, April 26). *Drug prescribing for older adults.* UpToDate. https://www.uptodate.com/contents/drug-prescribing-for-older-adults/print

Rohde, E., & Domm, E. (2017). Nurses' clinical reasoning practices that support safe medication administration: an integrative review of the literature. *Journal of Clinical Nursing, 27*, e402–e411. https://doi.org/10.1111/jocn.14077

Roveron, G., Antonini, M., Barbierato, M., Calandrino, V., Canese, G., Chiurazzi, L. F., Coniglio, G., Gentini, G., Marchetti, M., Minucci, A., Nembrini, L., Neri, V., Trovato, P., & Ferrara, F. (2018). Clinical practice guidelines for the nursing management of percutaneous endoscopic gastrostomy and jejunostomy (PEG/PEJ) in adult patients. *Journal of Wound, Ostomy, and Continence Nursing, 45*(4), 326–334. https://doi.org/10.1097/WON.0000000000000442

SafeNeedleDisposal.org. (2021). Download educational materials. https://safeneedledisposal.org/resource-center/online-brochures/

SafeNeedleDisposal.org. (2022, January 21). How to dispose of used sharps. https://safeneedledisposal.org/

Şanlialp Zeyrek, A., Takmak, Ş., Kurban, N. K., & Arslan, S. (2019). Systematic review and meta-analysis: Physical-procedural interventions used to reduce pain during intramuscular injections in adults. *Journal of*

Advanced Nursing, 75(12), 3346–3361. https://doi.org/ 10.1111/jan.14183

Sanofi-Aventis. (2020, May 20). *Lovenox: Highlights of prescribing information.* http://products.sanofi.us/ Lovenox/Lovenox.pdf

Sanofi Pasteur. (2017). *476 Fluzone® intradermal quadrivalent (Influenza vaccine).* https://www.fda.gov/ media/106170/download

Schmitz, D. C., Ivancie, R. A., Rhee, K. E., Pierce, H. C., Cantu, A. O., & Fisher, E. S. (2019). Imperative instruction for pressurized metered-dose inhalers: Provide perspectives. *Respiratory Care, 64*(3), 292–298.

Schneider, P. J., Pedersen, C. A., & Scheckelhoff, D. J. (2018). ASHP national survey of pharmacy practice in hospital settings: Dispensing and administration–2017. *American Journal of Health-System Pharmacy, 75*(16), 1203–1226. https://doi.org/10.2146/ajhp180151

Schroers, G., Niehoff, M., Ross, J. G., Moriarty, H., & Crescenz, M. J.(2021). Nurses' perceived causes of medication administration errors: A qualitative systematic review. *The Joint Commission Journal on Quality and Patient Safety, 47*(1), 38–53. https://doi.org/10.1016/j. jcjq.2020.09.010

Schumann, J. A., Toscano, M. L., & Pfleghaar, N. (2021, January 12). *Ear irrigation.* StatPearls. https://www.ncbi.nlm.nih.gov/books/NBK459335/

Schwartz, S. R., Magit, A. E., Rosenfeld, R. M., Ballachanda, B. B., Hackell, J. M., Krouse, H. J., Lawlor, C. M., Lin, K., Parham, K., Stutz, D. R., Walsh, S., Woodson, E. A., Yanagisawa, K., & Cunningham, E. R. (2017). Clinical practice guideline (Update): Earwax (Cerumen impaction). *Otolaryngology Head Neck Surgery, 156*(1S), S1–S29. https://doi. org/10.1177/0194599816671491

Sedaghat A. R. (2017). Chronic Rhinosinusitis. *American Family Physician, 96*(8), 500–506.

Sepah, Y., Samad, L., Altaf, A., Halim, M. S., Rajagopalan, N., & Javed Khan, A. (2017). Aspiration in injections: Should we continue or abandon the practice? *F1000Research, 3,* 157. https://doi.org/10.12688/f1000-research.1113.3

Sexson, K., Lindauer, A., & Harvath, T. A. (2016). Administration of subcutaneous injections. *American Journal of Nursing, 116*(12), 49–52. https://doi. org/10.1097/01.NAJ.0000508671.49210.ba

Shepherd, E. (2018a). Injection technique 1: Administering drugs via the intramuscular route. *Nursing Times, 114*(8), 23–25. https://www. nursingtimes.net/clinical-archive/assessment-skills/ injection-technique-1-administering-drugs-via-the-intramuscular-route-23-07-2018/

Shepherd, E. (2018b). Injection technique 2: Administering drugs via the subcutaneous route. *Nursing Times, 114*(9), 55–57. https://cdn.ps.emap.com/wp-content/ uploads/sites/3/2018/08/182808-injection-technique-2-administering-drugs-via-the-subcutaneous-route.pdf

Silbert-Flagg, J., & Pillitteri, A. (2018). *Maternal and child health nursing* (8th ed.). Wolters Kluwer.

Sisson, H. (2015). Aspirating during the intramuscular injection procedure: A systematic literature review. *Journal of Clinical Nursing, 24*(17–18), 2368–2375. https://doi.org/10.1111/jocn.12824

Slater, K., Fullerton, F., Cooke, M., Snell, S., & Rickard, C. M. (2018). Needleless connector drying time-how long does it take? *American Journal of Infection Control, 46,* 1080–1081. https://doi. org/10.1016/j.ajic.2018.05.007

Smeulers, M., Verweij, L., Maaskant, M. M., de Boer, M., Kerdiet, T. T. P., van Dijkum, E. J. M. N., & Vermeulen, H. (2015). Quality indicators for safe medication preparation and administration: A systematic review. *PLoS ONE, 10*(4), 1–14. https://doi.org/10.1371/journal.pone.0122695

Stevens, S. (2016). Clinical skills for ophthalmology. How to irrigate the eye. *Community Eye Health Journal, 29*(95), 56. https://www.ncbi.nlm.nih.gov/pmc/articles/ PMC5340106/pdf/jceh_29_95_056.pdf

Substance Abuse and Mental Health Services Administration (SAMHSA). (2020, August 19). Naloxone. https://www.samhsa.gov/medication-assisted-treatment/ medications-counseling-related-

Taylor, C., Lynn, P., & Bartlett, J. (2023). *Fundamentals of nursing: The art and science of person-centered care* (10th ed.). Wolters Kluwer.

Thomas, C. M., Mraz, M., & Rajcan, L. (2016). Blood aspiration during IM injection. *Clinical Nursing Research, 25*(5), 549–559. https://doi. org/10.1177/1054773815575074

Toughy, T. A., & Jett, K. (2018). *Ebersol and Hess' gerontological nursing & healthy aging* (5th ed.). Elsevier.

U.S. Food and Drug Administration (FDA). (2021, April 28). *Best way to get rid of used needles and other sharps.* https://www.fda.gov/medical-devices/safely-using-sharps-needles-and-syringes-home-work-and-travel/best-way-get-rid-used-needles-and-other-sharps

VHA Center for Engineering & Occupational Safety and Health (CEOSH). (2016). *Safe patient handling and mobility guidebook.* http://www.tampavaref.org/safe-patient-handling.htm

Weber, J. R., & Kelley, J. H. (2018). *Health assessment in nursing* (6th ed.). Wolters Kluwer.

Weston, V. (2019). Assessment for catheter function, dressing adherence and device necessity. In N. L. Moureau (Ed.), *Vessel health and preservation: The right approach for vascular access.* Springer. https://link. springer.com/book/10.1007/978-3-030-03149-7

White, R., & Bradnam, V. (2015). *Handbook of drug administration via enteral feeding tubes* (3rd ed.). Pharmaceutical Press. https://rudiapt.files.wordpress. com/2017/11/handbook-of-drug-administration-via-enteral-feeding-tubes-2015.pdf

Williams, T., King, M. W., Thompson, J. A., & Champagne, M. T. (2014). Implementing evidence-based medication safety interventions on a progressive care unit. *American Journal of Nursing, 114*(11), 53–62. https://doi.org/10.1097/01. NAJ.0000456433.07343.7f

Wolicki, J., & Miller, E. (2020). Chapter 6. Vaccine administration. In J. Hamborsky, A. Kroger, and C. Wolf (Eds.), *Epidemiology and prevention of vaccine-preventable diseases. The pink book* (13th ed.). Centers for Disease Control and Prevention. Public Health Foundation. https://www.cdc.gov/vaccines/pubs/ pinkbook/vac-admin.html

World Health Organization (WHO). (2020). *Immunization in practice: A practical guide for health staff–Module 5: Managing and immunization session.* http://www.who.int/immunization/documents/ training/en

Yilmaz, D., Khorshid, L., & Dedeoğlu, Y. (2016). The effect of the Z-track technique on pain and drug leakage in intramuscular injections. *Clinical Nurse Specialist, 30*(6), E7–E12. https://doi.org/10.1097/ NUR.0000000000000245

Zijlstra, E., Jahnke, J., Fischer, A., Kapitza, C., & Forst, T. (2018). Impact of injection speed, volume and site on pain sensation. *Journal of diabetes science and technology, 12*(1), 163–168. https://doi. org/10.1177/1932296817735121

Zimmerman, P. G. (2010). Revisiting IM injections. *American Journal of Nursing, 110*(2), 60–61.

Zoeller, S., Bechtold, M. L., Burns, B., Cattell, T., Grenda, B., Haffke, L., Larimer, C., Powers, J., Reuning, F., Tweel, L., Guenter, P., & ASPEN Enteral Nutrition Task Force. (2020). Dispelling myths and unfounded practices about enteral nutrition. *Nutrition in Clinical Practice, 35*(2), 196–204. https://doi.org/10.1002/ ncp.10456

SUGGESTED ANSWERS FOR FOCUSING ON PATIENT CARE: DEVELOPING CLINICAL REASONING AND CLINICAL JUDGMENT

1. Discuss routines and rituals typically used at home with Cooper's mother. Incorporating these routines and rituals if they are safe and positive can provide a positive way to administer medication. Offer simple choices to Cooper, such as allowing him the choice of having the nurse or his mother administer the medication. A toddler may enjoy using an oral syringe to squirt the medicine into his own mouth. The nurse could also allow Cooper to act out medication administration with a favorite toy, pretending to administer liquid medication to the toy.

2. Explore Erika's feelings related to injections and assess her knowledge of the procedure. Allow patients who are fearful of injections to talk about their fears. Answer the patient's questions truthfully and explain the nature and purpose of the injection. Taking the time to offer support often allays fears and decreases discomfort. Explain to Erika how the injection will be given. Discuss possible injection sites and allow Erika to have a say in the location used for the injection, if possible. It is very important that the nurse selects the appropriate needle length and gauge for the medication and patient criteria, including site location, patient's body size, and age. The nurse must use the correct technique to administer the injection and minimize pain. The nurse should consider use of the Z-track technique to reduce pain and discomfort related to the injection.

3. Diabetes is a chronic illness that requires life-long self-management behaviors. However, it is important that, initially, Jonah learns the "survival skills." "Survival skills" are basic information that patients must know to survive. Jonah should have a basic understanding of the definition of diabetes, normal blood glucose ranges and target levels; the effect of insulin and exercise; the effect of food and stress; basic treatment approaches; administration of prescribed medications, including subcutaneous insulin and oral antidiabetes medications; and meal planning. Jonah must also have an understanding of how to recognize, treat, and prevent hypoglycemia and hyperglycemia before discharge. The nurse should include information related to the importance of continued diabetes education, once the basic skills are mastered and information understood. Patient knowledge and engagement with treatment are crucial to preventing complications related to diabetes.

6

Perioperative Nursing

Focusing on Patient Care

This chapter will help you develop the skills related to safe perioperative nursing care for the following patients:

Josie McKeown, a 2-day-old girl who needs surgery to correct a heart defect.

Tatum Kelly, a 28-year-old woman having outpatient surgery for breast reduction.

Dorothy Gibbs, an 81-year-old woman having surgery to remove a bowel obstruction.

Refer to Focusing on Patient Care: Developing Clinical Reasoning and Clinical Judgment at the end of the chapter to apply what you learn.

Learning Outcomes

After completing the chapter, you will be able to accomplish the following:

1. Provide patient teaching regarding deep-breathing exercises, coughing, and splinting of an incision.
2. Provide patient teaching regarding leg exercises.
3. Provide safe and effective care for the preoperative patient.
4. Provide safe and effective care for the postoperative patient.
5. Apply a forced-air warming device.

Nursing Concepts

- Assessment
- Clinical Decision Making/Clinical Judgment
- Comfort
- Safety

Awide range of illnesses and injuries may require treatment that includes some type of operative or invasive procedure that is performed in the operating room or surgical suite and are referred to as *surgery* (AORN, 2020). Surgical procedures may be inpatient, performed in a hospital; or ambulatory or outpatient, performed in a hospital-based surgical center, a freestanding surgical center, or a surgeon's office. In an ambulatory or outpatient center, the patient goes to the surgical area the day of surgery and returns home on the same day.

Nursing care provided for the patient before, during, and after surgery is called **perioperative nursing**. Perioperative nursing involves providing care for the patient during the **perioperative phase**; before (*preoperative*), during (*intraoperative*), and after surgery (*postoperative*). The nursing process is used during each phase to meet physical and psychosocial needs and to facilitate the patient's return to health.

Whether the surgery is performed in the inpatient or outpatient setting, one of the most significant roles of the perioperative nurse is that of collaborator—the nurse working directly and indirectly with other nurses, surgeons, support personnel, anesthesia professionals, perioperative services executives, quality improvement personnel, and risk management experts (Taylor et al., 2020). Evidence-based practice that considers patient and family/caregiver preferences, clinical expertise of the health care provider, and the best evidence available informs decision making at all stages of the perioperative process. The ultimate, shared goal is to provide safe, quality care for the vulnerable perioperative patient (AORN, 2020).

The nurse follows specific criteria and guidelines while conducting the preadmission assessment, preparation, and patient education. This preoperative care can be provided through a telephone call or a face-to-face interview with the patient. A preoperative teaching plan should include preoperative instructions and patient preparation. This teaching should include both the patient and the patient's family members/caregivers or guardian/significant others. For certain types of **elective surgery**, such as joint replacements, patients may participate in a group patient teaching session before their admission to the hospital. Refer to Fundamentals Review 6-1, 6-2, and 6-3.

The postoperative care of the patient begins immediately after the surgical procedure is completed. This involves a short stay in the **postanesthesia care unit (PACU)** or other recovery area for about 1 to 2 hours, depending on the type of surgery and the patient's condition. After this time period and when the patient's condition is stabilized, the patient may be transferred either to the intensive care unit (ICU), to the surgical unit in the hospital, or, if the surgery was ambulatory, the patient will be discharged to home. Nursing care throughout the postoperative period includes ongoing assessments, monitoring for complications, implementing specific nursing interventions, and patient and family/caregiver teaching, as needed (Hinkle et al., 2022; Robertson & Ford, 2020). Before discharge from either the hospital or the ambulatory care unit, all patients will receive both oral and written discharge instructions and information about follow-up care (Hinkle et al., 2022). In addition, to ensure early identification of complications and address any patient concerns, the patient may receive a follow-up telephone call the next day after discharge.

With an increasing trend toward short-stay or same-day surgical treatment, the nursing interventions in each phase of perioperative nursing care may vary somewhat, but they remain basically the same. While caring for the surgical patient, the nurse should keep in mind that a surgical procedure of any extent is a stressor that requires physical and psychosocial adaptations for both the patient and the family/caregivers (Fundamentals Review 6-4).

This chapter will cover the skills the nurse needs to provide safe perioperative nursing care in the pre- and postoperative phases.

Fundamentals Review 6-1

NURSING ASSESSMENT AND INTERVENTION BEFORE SURGERY

The nurse assesses for the following during preadmission or upon admission:

- Baseline physical status
- Baseline mental status
- Allergies and sensitivities
- Signs of abuse or neglect
- Cultural, emotional, and socioeconomic factors
- Pain (comprehensive assessment)
- Medication history, including non-prescription medications and supplements
- Previous surgeries, complications, and implants
- Anesthetic history
- Results of radiologic examinations and other preoperative testing

- Referrals
- Physical alterations that require additional equipment or supplies

The nurse also:

- Provides preoperative patient teaching
- Determines informed consent and/or knowledge of planned procedure
- Asks about advance directives
- Develops a plan of care
- Documents and communicates all information per facility policy

Source: From Taylor, C., Lynn, P., & Bartlett, J. (2020). *Fundamentals of nursing: The art and science of person-centered care* (10th ed.). Wolters Kluwer; Association of periOperative Registered Nurses (AORN). (2020). Guidelines for perioperative practice. https://www. aorn.org/guidelines.

Fundamentals Review 6-2

PREOPERATIVE INFORMATION FOR OUTPATIENT/SAME DAY SURGERY

Provide verbal and written instructions, in simple language the patient can understand, for patients having ambulatory surgery.

Ask the patient to:

- List all medications routinely taken and ask the health care provider which medicines should be taken or omitted the morning of surgery.
- Notify the surgeon's office if a cold or infection develops before surgery.
- List all allergies and be sure the operating staff is aware of these.

- Follow all instructions from your health care provider regarding bathing or showering with a special soap solution.
- Remove nail polish and do not wear makeup on the day of the procedure.
- Leave all jewelry and valuables at home.
- Have someone available for transportation home after recovery from anesthesia.

Inform patient of:

- Limitations on eating or drinking before surgery, with a specific time to begin the limitations.
- When and where to arrive for the procedure, as well as the estimated time when the procedure will be performed.

Fundamentals Review 6-3

SAMPLE PREOPERATIVE TEACHING: ACTIVITIES AND EVENTS FOR IN-PATIENT SURGERY PREOPERATIVE PHASE

- Exercises and physical activities:
  - Deep-breathing exercises
  - Coughing
  - Incentive spirometry
  - Turning
  - Leg exercises
  - Early mobility
  - Pneumatic/graduated compression stockings
- Pain management:
  - Meaning of PRN orders for medications
  - Patient-controlled analgesia (PCA), as appropriate

- Timing for best effect of medications
- Splinting incision
- Nonpharmacologic pain management options
- Visit by anesthesiologist
- Physical preparation:
  - Nothing by mouth (NPO)
  - Medications the night before and day of surgery
  - Preoperative checklist (review items)
- Visitors and waiting room
- Transport to operating room by stretcher

(continued)

Fundamentals Review 6-3   continued

SAMPLE PREOPERATIVE TEACHING: ACTIVITIES AND EVENTS FOR IN-PATIENT SURGERY PREOPERATIVE PHASE

INTRAOPERATIVE PHASE

- Holding area:
  - Skin preparation
  - Intravenous lines and fluids
  - Medications
- Operating room:
  - Operating room bed
  - Lights and common equipment (e.g., cardiac monitor, pulse oximeter, warming device)
  - Safety belt
  - Sensations
  - Staff

POSTOPERATIVE PHASE

- Postanesthesia care unit:
  - Frequent vital signs, assessments (e.g., orientation, movement of extremities, strength of grasp)

- Dressings, drains, tubes, catheters
- Intravenous lines
- Pain medications, comfort measures
- Family/caregiver notification
- Sensations
- Airway, oxygen therapy, pulse oximetry
- Staff
- Transfer to unit (on stretcher):
  - Frequent vital signs
  - Sensations
  - Pain medications, nonpharmacologic strategies
  - NPO, diet progression
  - Exercises
  - Early ambulation
  - Family/caregiver visits

Fundamentals Review 6-4

NURSING INTERVENTIONS TO MEET PSYCHOSOCIAL NEEDS OF PATIENTS HAVING SURGERY

- Establish and maintain a therapeutic relationship, allowing the patient to verbalize fears and concerns.
- Use active listening skills to identify and validate verbal and nonverbal messages revealing anxiety and fear.
- Use touch, as appropriate, to demonstrate genuine empathy and caring.
- Be prepared to respond to common patient questions about surgery:
  - Will I lose control of my body functions while I'm having surgery?

- How long will I be in the operating room and PACU?
- Where will my family be?
- Will I have pain when I wake up?
- Will the anesthetic make me sick?
- Will I need a blood transfusion?
- How long will it be before I can eat?
- What kind of scar will I have?
- When will I be able to be sexually active?
- When can I go back to work?

Skill 6-1 ▶ Teaching Deep-Breathing Exercises, Coughing, and Splinting

During surgery, the cough reflex is suppressed, mucus accumulates in the tracheobronchial passages, and the lungs do not ventilate fully. After surgery, respirations are often less effective as a result of anesthesia, pain medication, and decreased respiratory effort because of incisional, particularly thoracic and high abdominal incisions, or other pain. Alveoli do not inflate or may collapse. Along with retained secretions, this increases the risk for **atelectasis** and respiratory infection.

Deep-breathing exercises hyperventilate the alveoli and prevent them from collapsing again, improve lung expansion and volume, help to expel **anesthetic** gases and mucus, and facilitate tissue oxygenation (Hess et al., 2021; Hinkle et al., 2022). Coughing, which helps to remove mucus from the respiratory tract, usually is taught in conjunction with deep breathing. Because coughing is often painful for the patient with a thoracic or abdominal incision, it is important to teach the patient how to splint the incision when coughing. This technique provides support to the incision and helps reduce pain during coughing, deep breathing, and movement (Milotte et al., 2018). Some

Box 6-1 The I COUGH Multidisciplinary Program

The focus of this program is to reduce postoperative respiratory complications.

I COUGH stands for

I. *Incentive Spirometry*: Deep-breathing exercises will help keep your lungs healthy and prevent lung problems. This breathing exercise needs to be done 10 times each hour.

C. *Cough and Deep Breathe*: After surgery taking deep breaths and coughing helps to clear your lungs. This helps the lungs do the vital job of delivering oxygen to the tissues in your body.

O. *Oral Care*: Brushing your teeth and using mouthwash twice a day keeps your mouth clean from germs.

U. *Understanding Patient Education*: Is important for you and your family to take an active part in your recovery. We want your pain to be controlled so you can take deep breaths, cough, get out of bed for a walk and be sitting up at mealtime.

G. *Get Out of Bed*: Walking will help clear secretions from your lungs, help your circulation and help to regain your strength.

H. *Head of Bed Elevated*: It is important to keep the head of the bed elevated between 30 and 45 degrees. Being in an upright position after your operation will help with your breathing.

Source: Used with permission. From Boston Medical Center and Boston University School of Medicine. (n.d.). I COUGH. http://www.bumc.bu.edu/surgery/quality-safety/i-cough

facilities have implemented the I COUGH program to reduce postoperative pulmonary complications (Boston Medical Center and Boston University School of Medicine, n.d.; Cassidy et al., 2013, 2020; Lumb, 2019). This multidisciplinary pulmonary care program is outlined in Box 6-1.

DELEGATION CONSIDERATIONS

Preoperative assessment and teaching are not delegated to assistive personnel (AP). Depending on the state's nurse practice act and the organization's policies and procedures, preoperative teaching may be delegated to licensed practical/vocational nurses (LPN/LVNs) after an assessment of education needs by the registered nurse. The decision to delegate must be based on careful analysis of the patient's needs and circumstances as well as the qualifications of the person to whom the task is being delegated. Refer to the Delegation Guidelines in Appendix A.

EQUIPMENT

- Small pillow or folded bath blanket
- PPE, as indicated

ASSESSMENT

Identify patients who are considered at greater risk for respiratory complications after surgery, such as the very young and very old; obese or malnourished patients; patients with fluid and electrolyte imbalances; patients with chronic disease; patients who have underlying lung or cardiac disease; patients who have decreased mobility; and patients who are at risk for decreased engagement with postoperative activities, such as those with alterations in cognitive function (Hinkle et al., 2022). Depending on the particular at-risk patient, specific assessments and interventions may be warranted. Assess the patient's current level of knowledge regarding deep breathing, coughing, and splinting.

ACTUAL OR POTENTIAL HEALTH PROBLEMS AND NEEDS

Many actual or potential health problems or issues may require the use of this skill as part of related interventions. An appropriate health problem or issue may include:
- Knowledge deficiency
- Altered breathing pattern
- Impaired mobility

OUTCOME IDENTIFICATION AND PLANNING

The expected outcomes to achieve when teaching deep breathing, coughing, and splinting of an incision are that the patient verbalizes an understanding of the instructions and is able to accurately demonstrate the activities.

(continued on page 356)

Skill 6-1 ▶ Teaching Deep-Breathing Exercises, Coughing, and Splinting *(continued)*

IMPLEMENTATION

ACTION

1. Check the patient's health record for the type of surgery and review the prescribed interventions. Gather the necessary supplies.

2. Perform hand hygiene and put on PPE, if indicated.

3. Identify the patient.

4. Close the curtains around the bed and close the door to the room, if possible. Explain what you are going to do and why you are going to do it to the patient. Place necessary supplies on the bedside stand, overbed table, or other surface within easy reach.

5. Identify the patient's learning needs and the patient's level of knowledge regarding deep-breathing exercises, coughing, and splinting of the incision. If the patient has had surgery before, ask about this experience.

6. Explain the rationale for performing deep-breathing exercises, coughing, and splinting of the incision.

7. Teach the patient how to perform deep-breathing exercises and explain their importance.

   a. Assist or ask the patient to sit up (semi- or high-Fowler's position) (Figure 1), with the neck and shoulders supported. Ask the patient to place the palms of both hands along the lower anterior rib cage.

   b. Ask the patient to exhale gently and completely.

   c. Instruct the patient to breathe in through the nose as deeply as possible and hold breath for 3 to 5 seconds.

   d. Instruct the patient to exhale through the mouth, pursing the lips like when whistling.

RATIONALE

This check ensures that the care will be provided for the right patient and any specific teaching based on the type of surgery will be addressed. Preparation promotes efficient time management and an organized approach to the task.

Hand hygiene and PPE prevent the spread of microorganisms. PPE is required based on transmission precautions.

Identifying the patient ensures the right patient receives the intervention and helps prevent errors.

Closing the curtains and door ensures the patient's privacy. Explanation relieves anxiety and facilitates engagement. Bringing everything to the bedside conserves time and energy. Arranging items nearby is convenient, saves time, and avoids unnecessary stretching and twisting of muscles on the part of the nurse.

Identification of baseline knowledge contributes to individualized teaching. Previous surgical experience may impact pre-operative/postoperative care positively or negatively, depending on this experience.

Explanation facilitates patient engagement. An understanding of the rationale may contribute to increased engagement.

Deep-breathing exercises improve lung expansion and volume, help expel anesthetic gases and mucus from the airway, and facilitate the oxygenation of body tissues.

The upright position promotes chest expansion and lessens exertion of the abdominal muscles. Positioning the hands on the rib cage allows the patient to feel the chest rise and the lungs expand as the diaphragm descends.

Deep inhalation promotes lung expansion.

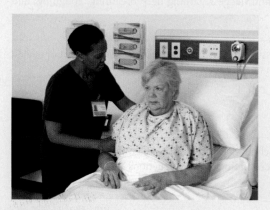

FIGURE 1. Assisting patient to semi- or high-Fowler's position.

ACTION

e. Have the patient practice the breathing exercise three times. Instruct the patient that this exercise should be performed every 1 to 2 hours for the first 24 hours after surgery, and every 2 hours thereafter (Cassidy et al., 2020), depending on risk factors and pulmonary status.

8. Provide teaching regarding coughing and splinting.

a. Ask the patient to sit up (semi-Fowler's position), leaning forward. Apply a folded bath blanket or small pillow against the part of the body where the incision will be (e.g., abdomen or chest) (Figure 2).

b. Ask the patient to inhale deeply and slowly through the nose and exhale through the mouth three times.

c. Ask the patient to take a deep breath and hold it for 3 seconds (Figure 3) and then cough out three short times (Figure 4).

d. Ask the patient to take a deep breath through the mouth and strongly and deeply cough again one or two times.

e. Ask the patient to take another deep breath, then relax and breathe normally.

f. Instruct the patient that they should perform these actions every 2 hours when awake after surgery (Cassidy et al., 2020; Hinkle et al., 2022).

RATIONALE

Return demonstration ensures that the patient is able to perform the exercises properly. Practice promotes effectiveness and engagement.

Coughing helps remove retained mucus from the respiratory tract. Splinting minimizes pain while coughing or moving.

These interventions aim to decrease discomfort while coughing.

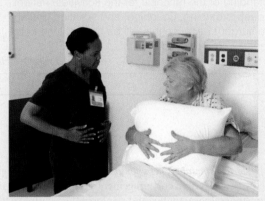

FIGURE 2. Having patient splint chest or abdominal incision by holding a folded bath blanket or small pillow against the incision.

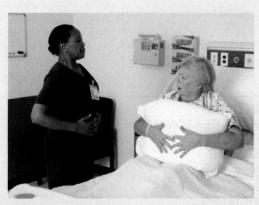

FIGURE 3. Telling patient to take a deep breath and hold for 3 seconds.

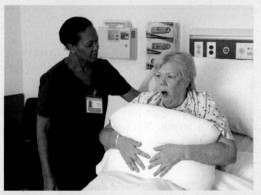

FIGURE 4. Encouraging patient to cough out three short times after holding breath.

(*continued on page 358*)

Skill 6-1 ▶ Teaching Deep-Breathing Exercises, Coughing, and Splinting *(continued)*

ACTION	RATIONALE
9. Validate the patient's understanding of the information. Ask the patient to give a return demonstration. Ask the patient if they have any questions. Encourage the patient to practice the activities and ask questions, if necessary.	Validation facilitates patient's understanding of information and performance of activities.
10. Remove PPE, if used. Perform hand hygiene.	Proper removal of PPE reduces the risk for infection transmission and contamination of other items. Hand hygiene prevents the spread of microorganisms.

EVALUATION

The expected outcomes have been met when the patient has verbalized an understanding of the instructions related to deep breathing, coughing, and splinting and has accurately demonstrated the activities.

DOCUMENTATION

Guidelines

Document the components of teaching related to deep-breathing exercises, coughing, and splinting that were reviewed with the patient and family/caregivers, if present. Record the patient's ability to demonstrate deep-breathing exercises, coughing, and splinting and their response to the teaching; note if any follow-up instruction needs to be performed.

Sample Documentation

> 4/2/25 1030 Perioperative teaching points related to deep breathing, coughing, and splinting reviewed with patient and his wife, including the rationale for each of these points. Patient verbalized an understanding of the rationale for the activities. Patient demonstrated proper technique for deep breathing, coughing, and splinting. Patient stated that he was anxious about the surgery because this will be his first time to the OR. Emotional support and reassurance were provided.
>
> —J. Lance, RN

DEVELOPING CLINICAL REASONING AND CLINICAL JUDGMENT

UNEXPECTED SITUATIONS AND ASSOCIATED INTERVENTIONS

- *Patient verbalizes concern about being able to remember steps for deep breathing and coughing:* Discuss with the patient why they feel this way. Offer encouragement and support. Reinforce that nurses will assist the patient with postoperative activities and reinforce the required actions. Provide written instructions as necessary to reinforce material.

SPECIAL CONSIDERATIONS

General Considerations

- Respiratory disorders, such as pneumonia, bronchitis, asthma, and chronic obstructive pulmonary diseases increase the risk for respiratory depression from anesthesia as well as postoperative pneumonia and atelectasis (Hinkle et al., 2022).

Infant and Child Considerations

- Deep breathing and coughing can be accomplished through play such as blowing bubbles or a whistle to enhance a child's participation (Kyle & Carman, 2017).

EVIDENCE FOR PRACTICE ▶

REDUCING POSTOPERATIVE PULMONARY COMPLICATIONS

A wide variety of factors increase the risk of postoperative complications. Potential respiratory complications include pulmonary embolus, atelectasis, and pneumonia. It is important to implement ongoing postoperative interventions to decrease the risk for postoperative complications.

Related Evidence

Cassidy, M. R., Rosenkranz, P., Macht, R. D., Talutis, S., & McAneny, D. (2020). The I COUGH Multidisciplinary Perioperative Pulmonary Care Program: One decade of experience. *The Joint Commission Journal on Quality and patient Safety, 46*(5), 241–249. https://doi.org/10.1016/j.jcjq.2020.01.005

This study aimed to identify a long-term perspective of the implementation of a standardized postoperative program to improve care, including special challenges and factors involved in sustaining success. A multidisciplinary team developed and implemented a strategy based on comprehensive patient and family/caregiver education and a set of standardized electronic prescribed interventions to specify early postoperative mobilization and pulmonary care to reduce postoperative pulmonary complications. The I COUGH program emphasizes **I**ncentive spirometry, **C**oughing and deep breathing, **O**ral care (brushing teeth and using mouthwash twice a day), **U**nderstanding (patient and family/caregiver education), **G**etting out of bed (at least three times a day), and **H**ead-of-bed elevation. The I COUGH program was implemented for all patients undergoing general or vascular surgery. This before-after study audited clinical practices and compared them to actual and risk-adjusted pulmonary outcomes. Results revealed improvements in compliance with the I COUGH elements were initially promising, but baseline behaviors eventually returned. Adverse outcomes were inversely correlated with adherence to the program in "sawtooth" patterns. Coordinated efforts and interventions to rededicate to the use of the I COUGH program were effective and resulted in improved patient outcomes. Compliance with getting patients out of bed was initially 20%, improved to 69% after implementation, returned to baseline 2 years after implementation (29%) and increased to 60% after rededication. Availability of incentive spirometry initially increased from 53% to 77% after I COUGH, dropped to 41% two years later, but improved to 94% with redirection to the program. Immediately after introduction of I COUGH, the incidence of postoperative pneumonia decreased from 3% (preimplementation) to 1.8% but climbed to 2.2% before improving and dropping to 0.4% with rejuvenated program implementation. The incidence of unplanned intubations was 2.3% before initial implementation of I COUGH and declined to 1.4% after its introduction, rebounded to 1.8% two years later, and improved to 0% after renewed efforts to implement the program.

The researchers concluded the I COUGH program reduces postoperative pulmonary complications within institutional culture is optimized around adherence to its principles. The success and sustainability of the I COUGH program depends on the commitment and interaction of dedicated stakeholders, financial support, human resources, and a supportive organizational environment. Momentum can be sustained by establishing a commitment to quality as an essential part of an institution's culture.

Relevance for Nursing Practice

Implementation of recommended postoperative interventions to prevent pulmonary complications is an important part of patient care. Basic postoperative patient care can favorably affect patient outcomes (Cassidy et al., 2013). Nurses must include preventative nursing interventions and patient education as part of the plan of care for patients undergoing surgical procedures.

Skill 6-2 ▶ Teaching Leg Exercises

During surgery, venous blood return from the legs slows (Hinkle et al., 2022). In addition, some patient positions used during surgery decrease venous return (AORN, 2018). **Thrombophlebitis, deep vein thrombosis (DVT)**, and the risk for emboli are potential complications from circulatory stasis in the legs (AORN, 2018). Leg exercises increase venous return through flexion and contraction of the quadriceps and gastrocnemius muscles and should be initiated early in the postoperative period to stimulate circulation (Hinkle et al., 2022). It is important to individualize leg exercises to patient needs, physical condition, health care provider preference, and facility protocol.

DELEGATION CONSIDERATIONS	Preoperative assessment and teaching are not delegated to assistive personnel (AP). Depending on the state's nurse practice act and the organization's policies and procedures, preoperative teaching may be delegated to licensed practical/vocational nurses (LPN/LVNs) after an assessment of education needs by the registered nurse. The decision to delegate must be based on careful analysis of the patient's needs and circumstances as well as the qualifications of the person to whom the task is being delegated. Refer to the Delegation Guidelines in Appendix A.
EQUIPMENT	• PPE, as indicated
ASSESSMENT	It is important to identify patients who are considered at greater risk, such as those with chronic disease; patients who are obese or who have underlying cardiovascular disease; patients who have decreased mobility; older adults; and patients who are at risk for decreased engagement with postoperative activities, such as those with alterations in cognitive function (Hinkle et al., 2022). Depending on the particular at-risk patient, specific assessments and interventions may be warranted. Assess the patient's current level of knowledge regarding leg exercises.
OUTCOME IDENTIFICATION AND PLANNING	The expected outcomes to achieve when teaching leg exercises are that the patient verbalizes an understanding of the instructions and is able to demonstrate the activity.
ACTUAL OR POTENTIAL HEALTH PROBLEMS AND NEEDS	Many actual or potential health problems or issues may require the use of this skill as part of related interventions. An appropriate health problem or issue may include: • Knowledge deficiency • Anxiety • Impaired mobility

IMPLEMENTATION

ACTION	**RATIONALE**
1. Check the patient's health record for the type of surgery and review the prescribed interventions. Gather the necessary supplies.	This check ensures that the care will be provided for the right patient and any specific teaching based on the type of surgery will be addressed. Preparation promotes efficient time management and an organized approach to the task.
2. Perform hand hygiene and put on PPE, if indicated.	Hand hygiene and PPE prevent the spread of microorganisms. PPE is required based on transmission precautions.
3. Identify the patient.	Identifying the patient ensures the right patient receives the intervention and helps prevent errors.

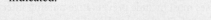

ACTION

4. Close the curtains around the bed and close the door to the room, if possible. Explain what you are going to do and why you are going to do it to the patient. Place necessary supplies on the bedside stand, overbed table, or other surface within easy reach.

5. Identify the patient's learning needs. Identify the patient's level of knowledge regarding leg exercises. If the patient has had surgery before, ask about this experience.

6. Explain the rationale for performing leg exercises.

7. Teach leg exercises and explain their purpose.

   a. Assist or ask the patient to sit up (semi-Fowler's position) (Figure 1) and explain to the patient that you will first demonstrate, and then coach them to exercise one leg at a time.
   b. Bend the patient's knee, raise the foot, and keep it elevated for a few seconds. Then, extend the lower leg, and hold this position for a few seconds (Figure 2). Lower the entire leg (Figure 3). Practice this exercise with the other leg.

RATIONALE

Closing the curtains and door ensures the patient's privacy. Explanation relieves anxiety and facilitates engagement. Bringing everything to the bedside conserves time and energy. Arranging items nearby is convenient, saves time, and avoids unnecessary stretching and twisting of muscles on the part of the nurse.

Identification of baseline knowledge contributes to individualized teaching. Previous surgical experience may impact preoperative/postoperative care positively or negatively, depending on this experience.

Explanation facilitates patient engagement. An understanding of rationale may contribute to increased engagement.

Leg exercises assist in preventing muscle weakness, promote venous return, and decrease complications related to venous stasis (Hinkle et al., 2022).

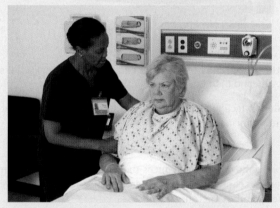

FIGURE 1. Assisting patient to semi-Fowler's position.

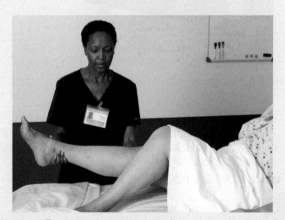

FIGURE 2. Extending lower portion of the leg and holding for a few seconds.

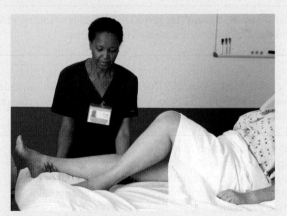

FIGURE 3. Lowering entire leg to bed.

(continued on page 362)

Skill 6-2 ▶ Teaching Leg Exercises *(continued)*

ACTION

RATIONALE

c. Assist or ask the patient to point the toes of both legs toward the foot of the bed, then relax them (Figure 4). Next, flex or pull the toes toward the chin (Figure 5).

d. Assist or ask the patient to keep legs extended and to make circles with both ankles, first circling to the left and then to the right (Figure 6). Instruct the patient to repeat these exercises three to five times with each leg. Instruct the patient to perform leg exercises every 2 to 4 hours when awake after surgery.

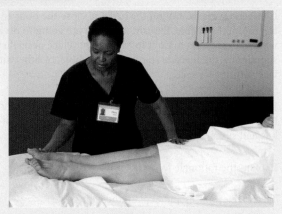

FIGURE 4. Pointing toes of both feet toward foot of bed.

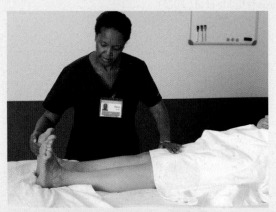

FIGURE 5. Pulling toes toward chin.

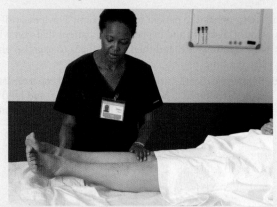

FIGURE 6. Having patient make circles with both ankles, first one way and then the other.

8. Validate the patient's understanding of the information. Ask the patient for a return demonstration. Ask the patient if they have any questions. Encourage the patient to practice the activities and ask questions, if necessary.

Validation facilitates the patient's understanding of information and performance of activities.

9. Remove PPE, if used. Perform hand hygiene.

Proper removal of PPE reduces the risk for infection transmission and contamination of other items. Hand hygiene prevents the spread of microorganisms.

EVALUATION

The expected outcomes have been met when the patient has verbalized an understanding of the instructions related to leg exercises and has accurately demonstrated the activities.

DOCUMENTATION

Guidelines

Document the components of teaching related to leg exercises that were reviewed with the patient and family/caregivers, if present. Record the patient's ability to demonstrate the leg exercises and response to the teaching; note if any follow-up instruction needs to be performed.

Sample Documentation

11/2/25 2230 Perioperative teaching points related to leg exercises reviewed with patient and her husband, including the rationale for each of these points. Patient verbalized an understanding of the rationale for the activities. Patient demonstrated proper technique for leg exercises and asked appropriate questions. Patient stated that she was anxious about the surgery because this will be her first surgical experience. Emotional support and reassurance were provided.

—J. Lynn, RN

DEVELOPING CLINICAL REASONING AND CLINICAL JUDGMENT

UNEXPECTED SITUATIONS AND ASSOCIATED INTERVENTIONS

• *Patient is unable to complete full range of motion of lower extremities due to pain from arthritis or other health issue:* Modify exercises based on patient's abilities. Encourage patient to perform to the best of their abilities. Document patient's range of motion and limitations related to exercises.

SPECIAL CONSIDERATIONS

• All postoperative patients are at some risk for thromboembolism and pulmonary embolism, but some risk factors, including a history of thrombosis, malignancy, trauma, obesity, indwelling venous catheters, and hormone use (e.g., estrogen) increase the risk (Hinkle et al., 2022).
• Certain types of surgeries are associated with a higher risk of deep vein thrombosis and pulmonary embolism, including orthopedic, bariatric, cardiothoracic, vascular, abdominal, pelvic, major plastic surgery, and genitourinary surgery involving the abdomen or pelvis (AORN, 2018).

EVIDENCE FOR PRACTICE ▶

PREVENTION OF DEEP VEIN THROMBOSIS
American Association of Critical Care Nurses. (2016). AACN practice alert: Preventing venous thromboembolism in adults. *Critical Care Nurse, 36*(5), e20–e23.

Association of periOperative Registered Nurses (AORN). (2018). Guideline summary: Prevention of venous thromboembolism. *AORN Journal, 107*(6), 750–754. http://doi.org/10.1002/aorn.12147

These guidelines outline expected nursing practice related to the prevention of venous thromboembolism (VTE) in adults. Depending on the individual patient's level of risk for VTE, appropriate interventions include anticoagulant therapy and mechanical prophylaxis including graduated compression stockings and intermittent pneumatic compression devices as well as daily interprofessional rounds to review each patient's VTE risk factors, current status, and response to treatment.

Skill 6-3 ▶ Providing Preoperative Patient Care

The preoperative phase consists of the time from when it is decided that surgery is needed until the patient is transferred to the operating room (OR) (Hinkle et al., 2022). Preoperative nursing care is focused on addressing key aspects of care involving (Hinkle et al., 2022; Turunen et al., 2017):
• Holistic preoperative screening—complete medical, physical, psychosocial, and personal assessments
• Coordination—collaborate with the entire interprofessional team
• Communication—promote open, clear communication
• Patient and family/caregiver education—provide specific pre- and postoperative instructions
• Individual patient- and family/caregiver-centered care—promote empowerment and emotional support/comfort
• Preoperative contact—engage with the patient prior to surgery for screening and patient preparation, providing last-minute instruction as needed
• Scheduling—prioritize and communicate surgical scheduling plans

Preoperative nursing care is affected by the length of the preoperative phase. Refer to Fundamentals Review 6-1, 6-2, and 6-3. There may not be enough time for comprehensive assessments and teaching for patients who enter the hospital through the emergency department needing immediate surgery and those who have outpatient/same-day surgery. In such cases, the nurse individualizes the plan of care for the particular patient and family/caregivers, utilizing nursing interventions that are designed to meet the priority needs of individual patients and situations (Hinkle et al., 2022).

(continued on page 364)

Skill 6-3 ▶ Providing Preoperative Patient Care *(continued)*

DELEGATION CONSIDERATIONS	Preoperative assessment and teaching are not delegated to assistive personnel (AP). Depending on the state's nurse practice act and the organization's policies and procedures, preoperative teaching may be delegated to licensed practical/vocational nurses (LPN/LVNs) after an assessment of education needs by the registered nurse. The decision to delegate must be based on careful analysis of the patient's needs and circumstances as well as the qualifications of the person to whom the task is being delegated. Refer to the Delegation Guidelines in Appendix A.

EQUIPMENT (Varies, Depending on the Type of Surgery and Surgical Setting)

- Blood pressure cuff
- Electronic blood pressure monitor/ sphygmomanometer
- Pulse oximeter
- IV infusion device
- Graduated compression stockings
- Pneumatic compression device
- Tubes, drains, vascular access tubing
- Incentive spirometer
- Small pillow
- PPE, as indicated

ASSESSMENT

The preoperative nursing assessment, which includes a complete baseline health assessment, is completed upon admission to the surgical facility. This assessment may begin in various settings, such as the surgeon's office, in the patient's home or by phone, or an inpatient unit, and is often conducted several days before surgery as part of preoperative laboratory screening and teaching. Interview the patient to determine the health history; identify risk factors for surgical adverse events and allergies; and determine any emotional, socioeconomic, cultural, and spiritual factors that may influence the patient's care. Ask about and review all medications the patient is taking, including non-prescription drugs, herbs, and supplements, as well as illicit drugs. Determine the teaching and psychosocial needs of the patient and family/caregivers. If the patient has a preferred speaking language other than English, it is essential to note this in the patient's record.

Perform assessments of skin, respiratory, cardiovascular, abdominal, neurologic, and musculoskeletal function. Take the patient's vital signs. Communicate any assessment abnormalities or areas of concern to the health care team. It is important for the nurse to identify patients who are considered at greater risk, such as the very young and very old; obese or malnourished patients; patients with fluid and electrolyte imbalances; patients with chronic health problems (such as cardiovascular disease, hepatic disease, pulmonary and renal disease); and patients taking certain medications (e.g., anticoagulants or analgesics) (Hinkle et al., 2022). Depending on the particular at-risk patient, additional specific assessments and interventions may be warranted.

ACTUAL OR POTENTIAL HEALTH PROBLEMS AND NEEDS

Many actual or potential health problems or issues may require the use of this skill as part of related interventions. An appropriate health problem or issue may include:

- Anxiety
- Venous thromboembolism risk
- Knowledge deficiency

OUTCOME IDENTIFICATION AND PLANNING

The expected outcome to achieve when providing preoperative patient care is that the patient will safely proceed to surgery. Other outcomes that may be appropriate include the following: the patient verbalizes physical- and emotional-readiness for surgery, and the patient verbalizes an understanding of measures to minimize the postoperative risks associated with surgery.

IMPLEMENTATION

ACTION	**RATIONALE**
1. Check the patient's health record for the type of surgery and review the prescribed interventions. Review the nursing database, history, and physical examination. Check that the baseline data are recorded; communicate any assessment abnormalities or areas of concern to the health care team.	These checks ensure that the care will be provided for the right patient and any specific teaching based on the type of surgery will be addressed. Also, this review helps to identify patients who are at increased surgical risk.
2. **Check that all diagnostic testing has been completed and results are available; identify and communicate abnormal results to the health care team.** Gather the necessary supplies.	This check may influence the type of surgery performed and anesthetic used, as well as the timing of surgery or the need for additional consultation. Preparation promotes efficient time management and an organized approach to the task.

ACTION

3. Perform hand hygiene and put on PPE, if indicated.

4. Identify the patient.

5. Close the curtains around the bed and close the door to the room, if possible. Explain what you are going to do and why you are going to do it to the patient and significant other. Place necessary supplies on the bedside stand, overbed table, or other surface within easy reach.

6. Explore the psychological needs of the patient and family/caregivers related to the surgery.

   a. Establish a therapeutic relationship, encouraging the patient to verbalize concerns or fears.

   b. Use active listening skills, answering questions, and clarifying any misinformation.

   c. Use touch, as appropriate, to convey genuine empathy.

   d. Offer to contact spiritual counselor (e.g., priest, minister, rabbi) to meet spiritual needs.

7. **Identify learning needs of patient and family/caregivers.** Ensure that the informed consent of the patient for the surgery has been signed, timed, dated, and witnessed. Inquire if the patient has any questions regarding the surgical procedure (Figure 1). Check the patient's record to determine if an advance directive has been completed. If an advance directive has not been completed, discuss with the patient the possibility of completing it, as appropriate. If patient has had surgery before, ask about this experience.

RATIONALE

Hand hygiene and PPE prevent the spread of microorganisms. PPE is required based on transmission precautions.

Identifying the patient ensures the right patient receives the intervention and helps prevent errors.

Closing the curtains and door ensures the patient's privacy. Explanation relieves anxiety and facilitates engagement. Bringing everything to the bedside conserves time and energy. Arranging items nearby is convenient, saves time, and avoids unnecessary stretching and twisting of muscles on the part of the nurse.

Meeting the psychological needs of the patient and family/caregivers before surgery can have a beneficial effect on the postoperative course.

Use of therapeutic communication skills decreases anxiety (Croke, 2020a), promotes healing, enhances safety, and improves clinical outcomes.

Spiritual beliefs for some patients and family/caregivers can provide a source of support over the perioperative course.

Patient education enhances surgical recovery and allays anxiety by preparing the patient for postoperative convalescence, discharge plans, and self-care (Croke, 2020b). The surgeon is responsible for explaining the details of the surgical procedure and potential risks and complications. The nurse is responsible for clarifying what the surgeon has explained to the patient and contacting the surgeon if the patient does not understand or has further questions. An advance directive provides written communication of the patient's wishes to the health care team related to the patient's desire for extraordinary life-sustaining treatments if the patient's condition is deemed unsalvageable. Previous surgical experience may impact preoperative care positively or negatively, depending on the patient's experience.

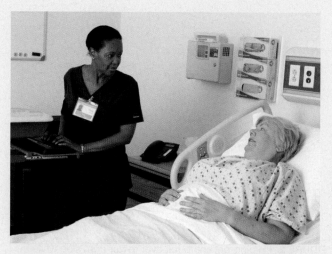

FIGURE 1. Identifying needs of patient and answering questions.

(*continued on page 366*)

Skill 6-3 ▶ Providing Preoperative Patient Care *(continued)*

ACTION	RATIONALE
8. Teach deep-breathing exercises. Refer to Skill 6-1.	Deep-breathing exercises improve lung expansion and volume, help expel anesthetic gases and mucus from the airway, and facilitate the oxygenation of body tissues.
9. Teach coughing and splinting. Refer to Skill 6-1.	Coughing helps remove retained mucus from the respiratory tract. Splinting minimizes pain while coughing or moving.
10. Teach use of incentive spirometer, as prescribed or indicated. (Refer to Skill 14-3 in Chapter 14.)	Incentive spirometry improves lung expansion, helps expel anesthetic gases and mucus from the airway, and facilitates oxygenation of body tissues. Use of incentive spirometry may be based on patient risk factors and/or health care provider preference; evidence of effectiveness in prevention of postoperative pulmonary complications is controversial (Branson, 2013; Cassidy et al., 2020; Lumb, 2019; Strickland et al., 2013).
11. Teach leg exercises, as appropriate. Refer to Skill 6-2.	Physical activity reduces the risk of postoperative complications. Leg exercises assist in preventing muscle weakness, promote venous return, and decrease complications related to venous stasis. Leg exercises may be contraindicated for patients with certain conditions, such as lower extremity fractures.
12. Teach about early ambulation, as appropriate.	Physical activity reduces the risk of postoperative complications. Early ambulation has positive effects on the respiratory, cardiovascular, integumentary, musculoskeletal, gastrointestinal, and renal systems (Hinkle et al., 2022). Discussing the benefits during the preoperative period help patients fully engage in this activity (as appropriate) despite expected pain and discomfort postoperatively.
13. Assist the patient in putting on graduated compression stockings. Refer to Skill 9-10 in Chapter 9 for specific information. Demonstrate how the pneumatic compression device operates. Refer to Skill 9-11 in Chapter 9 for specific information.	Graduated compression stockings and pneumatic compression devices are used postoperatively for patients who are at risk for a deep vein thrombosis (DVT) and pulmonary embolism (AORN, 2018; Fan et al., 2020; Hinkle et al., 2022; Tubog, 2019).
14. Teach about turning in the bed.	Turning and repositioning of the patient is important to prevent postoperative complications and to minimize pain.

a. Instruct the patient to use a pillow or bath blanket to splint where the incision will be. Ask the patient to raise their left knee and reach across to grasp the right side rail of the bed. If the patient is turning to the left side, they will bend the right knee and grasp the left side rail.

b. When turning the patient onto the right side, ask the patient to push with bent left leg and pull on the right side rail (Figure 2). Explain to the patient that you will place a pillow behind their back to provide support, and that the call bell will be placed within easy reach.

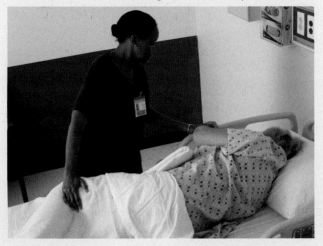

FIGURE 2. Helping patient to roll over to her right side while she pushes with left bent leg and pulls on the side rail.

ACTION

c. Explain to the patient that position change is recommended every 2 hours.

15. Provide individualized, developmentally appropriate teaching about pain management options, plans, and goals.

a. Discuss past experiences with pain and interventions that the patient has used to reduce pain.

b. Discuss the availability of analgesic medication postoperatively.

c. Discuss the use of PCA, as appropriate. Refer to Skill 10-4 in Chapter 10.

d. Explore the use of other alternative and nonpharmacologic methods to reduce pain, such as position change, massage, relaxation/diversion, guided imagery, and meditation. Refer to Skills 10-1 and 10-2 in Chapter 10.

16. Review equipment that may be used after surgery.

a. Show the patient various equipment, such as IV infusion devices, electronic blood pressure cuff, tubes, urinary catheters, and surgical drains.

17. Provide skin preparation.

a. **Ask the patient to bathe or shower with the antibacterial soap or solution. Remind the patient to clean the surgical site.** An antiseptic shower, bath, or cleansing with antimicrobial-impregnated wipes may be prescribed the evening before surgery and repeated the morning of surgery to begin the process of preparing the skin before surgery and to prevent infection (Mok et al., 2019; Parry, 2018). The skin is cleaned at the operative site with an antibacterial soap or solution to remove microorganisms. The patient can do this while taking a bath or shower. The specific choice of soap or antiseptic product depends on the patient, the procedure, and the manufacturer recommendations (AORN, 2020). This skin antiseptic eliminates skin microorganisms and leaves an antimicrobial film on their skin.

18. Provide teaching about and follow dietary/fluid restrictions. **Explain to the patient that both food and fluid will be restricted before surgery to ensure that the stomach contains a minimal amount of gastric secretions. This restriction is important to reduce the risk of aspiration. Emphasize to the patient the importance of avoiding food and fluids during the prescribed time period, because failure to adhere may necessitate cancellation of the surgery.**

RATIONALE

Individualized use of pharmacologic and nonpharmacologic methods of pain management is an important part of pain management guidelines related to surgery (Chou et al., 2016). Adequate pain control is important; continuing or unresolved pain can increase the patient's length of recovery and delay discharge.

Past experiences with pain can impact the patient's ability to manage surgical pain. Pain is a subjective experience and the interventions effective in reducing pain vary from patient to patient.

Depending on the prescribed interventions, the patient may need to request analgesic medication, as needed, or a patient-controlled analgesia (PCA) or epidural analgesia may be prescribed, for which the patient will need specific instruction on how to use. (see Chapter 10 for more information.)

Patient understanding of the use of PCA is crucial for effective, safe administration.

These measures may reduce anxiety and may decrease the amount of pain medication that is needed. Analgesic therapy should involve a multimodal approach influenced by age, weight, and comorbidity.

Knowledge can reduce anxiety about equipment and upcoming experiences. The patient may need an indwelling urinary catheter during and after surgery to keep the bladder empty and to monitor urinary output. Drains are frequently used to remove excess fluid around the surgical incision.

Evidence-based practice advises against hair removal at the surgical site due to increased potential for infection. If hair removal is necessary, it should be accomplished using hair clippers and be performed immediately before the surgery, in a patient care room outside the operating room, using disposable supplies and aseptic technique (AORN, 2020, as cited in Spruce, 2020a, p. 82). Follow facility policy regarding skin preparation of the surgical patient. In addition, immediately before the surgical procedure, the skin of the patient's operative site will be cleansed with a product that is compatible with the antiseptic used for showering.

Ensure that fluid and dietary restrictions (NPO), as prescribed or as per facility protocol, have been followed. These restrictions assist in preventing aspiration (Hinkle et al., 2022).

(continued on page 368)

Skill 6-3 ▶ Providing Preoperative Patient Care *(continued)*

ACTION	RATIONALE
19. Provide intestinal preparation, as appropriate. In certain situations, such as surgery of the lower gastrointestinal tract or pelvic surgery, the bowel will need to be prepared by administering enemas or laxatives.	A prescribed bowel prep and cleansing enema may be prescribed if the patient is scheduled for surgery of the lower gastrointestinal tract to evacuate the bowel and to reduce the intestinal bacteria to help prevent contamination of the surgical area during surgery. Peristalsis may not return for 24 to 48 hours after the bowel is handled, so preoperative cleansing also helps to decrease postoperative constipation.
a. As needed, explain the purpose of enemas or laxatives before surgery. If the patient will be administered an enema, clarify the steps as needed. Refer to Skills 13-1 and 13-2 in Chapter 13.	Enemas can be stressful, especially when repeated enemas are required to obtain a clear fluid return. Repeated enemas may cause fluid and electrolyte imbalance, orthostatic hypotension, and weakness.
20. **Check and verify administration of regularly scheduled medications.** Review with the patient routine medications, over-the-counter medications, and herbal supplements that are taken regularly. Check the prescribed interventions and review with the patient which medications they should take and those they should not take the day of surgery.	Many patients take medications for a variety of chronic medical conditions. Adjustments in taking these medications may be needed before surgery. Certain medications, such as aspirin, are stopped days before surgery due to their anticoagulant effect. Certain cardiac and respiratory drugs may be taken the day of surgery per prescribed intervention. If the patient has diabetes, oral hypoglycemic agent and/or insulin dosages may be reduced.
21. Provide information to the patient and family/caregivers regarding timing of surgical events and potential sensations that may be experienced. Explain to patients and their families how long the surgery and postanesthesia care will last, as well as what will be done before, during, and after surgery (e.g., procedures, medications, equipment). Explain to patients that they may not drive themselves home or take public transportation alone if they have had any anesthesia or sedation.	Patients and their families require this information to plan activities accordingly. Explanation and knowledge relieve anxiety and facilitates engagement.
22. Remove PPE, if used. Perform hand hygiene.	Proper removal of PPE reduces the risk for infection transmission and contamination of other items. Hand hygiene prevents the spread of microorganisms.

EVALUATION

The expected outcomes have been met when the patient has proceeded safely to surgery, the patient and/or family/caregivers have verbalized physical- and emotional-readiness for surgery, and the patient and/or family/caregivers have verbalized an understanding of measures to minimize the postoperative risks associated with surgery.

DOCUMENTATION

Guidelines

Document that the patient's health records were reviewed, including the history, physical assessment, and any laboratory values and diagnostic studies. Record that the health care team was notified of any abnormal values. Document the components of perioperative teaching that were reviewed with the patient and family/caregivers, if present, such as use of the incentive spirometer, deep-breathing exercises, splinting, leg exercises, graduated compression stockings, and pneumatic compression devices. Record the patient's ability to demonstrate the skills and response to the teaching, and note if any follow-up instruction needs to be performed. Document other preoperative teaching, including pain management, intestinal preparation, medications, and preoperative skin preparation. Record any patient concerns about the surgery and whether the surgeon/health care team was contacted to provide any further explanations. Document the emotional support that was offered to the patient and if a spiritual counselor was notified per request of patient.

Sample Documentation

> 4/2/25 1030 Patient's health records were reviewed, and no abnormal results were identified. Perioperative teaching points reviewed with patient and his wife, including the rationale for each of these points. Patient demonstrated proper deep breathing, splinting while coughing, and leg exercises. Reviewed pain management, intestinal preparation, medications, and preoperative skin preparation. Patient stated that he was anxious about the surgery because this will be his first time to the OR. Emotional support and reassurance were provided.
>
> —*J. Grabes, RN*

DEVELOPING CLINICAL REASONING AND CLINICAL JUDGMENT

UNEXPECTED SITUATIONS AND ASSOCIATED INTERVENTIONS

- *Patient's laboratory results are noted to be abnormal:* Notify health care team. Some abnormalities, such as an elevated international normalized ratio (INR) or abnormalities in the complete blood count (CBC), may postpone the surgery.
- *Patient says to you, "I'm not sure I really want this surgery":* Ask the patient to elaborate on their concerns. Discuss with the patient why they feel this way. Notify the health care team. Patients should not undergo surgery until any questions or doubts are resolved and they are sure that surgery is what they want.

SPECIAL CONSIDERATIONS

General Considerations

- Patients who are obese are at increased risk for respiratory and cardiovascular compromise as well as an increased incidence of gastroesophageal reflex disease, hiatal hernia, and abdominal pressure that puts them at increased risk for aspiration of stomach contents (AORN, 2020). In taking the history of these patients, be alert for other medical conditions, such as diabetes, cardiovascular disease, respiratory disease, kidney disease, and liver disease, which also increase the risk of surgical complications (Taylor et al., 2020).
- Current recommendations caution against routine opioid prescription postoperatively, focusing on oral opioid administration with acetaminophen and/or nonsteroidal anti-inflammatory drugs (NSAIDs) as needed, or the use of patient-controlled analgesia (PCA) when the parenteral route is necessary (Chou et al., 2016).

Infant and Child Considerations

- Children have special needs related to their overall health, age, and size. Easing preoperative anxiety of the child is crucial and includes using simple and concrete terms when providing information (Aranha & Dsouza, 2019; Kyle & Carman, 2021).
- The nurse needs to be sensitive to the anxiety level of the parent and provide support, explanations, and patient teaching, as needed (Aranha & Dsouza, 2019; Kyle & Carman, 2021).
- Accurate weights are essential for correct medication dosages (Kyle & Carman, 2021).
- Developmentally appropriate pain assessment and management needs to be initiated to ensure adequate pain management (Kyle & Carman, 2021).

Older Adult Considerations

- Age-related changes and preexisting chronic conditions can affect the postoperative course of the older adult patient (Eliopoulos, 2018).
- It is important to present preoperative teaching information slowly with reinforcement, because processing of information can be slower (Bastable, 2017).
- Management of postoperative pain in older adults may be complicated by a number of factors, including a higher risk of age- and disease-related changes in physiology and disease–drug and drug–drug interactions (Karch, 2020).

(continued on page 370)

Skill 6-3 ▶ Providing Preoperative Patient Care (continued)

EVIDENCE FOR PRACTICE ▶

REDUCING POSTOPERATIVE PULMONARY COMPLICATIONS

Cassidy, M. R., Rosenkranz, P., Macht, R. D., Talutis, S., & McAneny, D. (2020). The I COUGH Multidisciplinary Perioperative Pulmonary Care Program: One decade of experience. *The Joint Commission Journal on Quality and patient Safety, 46*, 241–249. https://doi.org/10.1016/j.jcjq.2020.01.005

Refer to details in Skill 6-1, Evidence for Practice.

EVIDENCE FOR PRACTICE ▶

PREVENTION OF DEEP VEIN THROMBOSIS

American Association of Critical Care Nurses. (2016). AACN practice alert: Preventing venous thromboembolism in adults. *Critical Care Nurse, 36*(5), e20–e23.

Association of periOperative Registered Nurses (AORN). (2018). Guideline summary: Prevention of venous thromboembolism. *AORN Journal, 107*(6), 750–754. http://doi.org/10.1002/aorn.12147

Refer to details in Skill 6-2, Evidence for Practice.

Skill 6-4 ▶ Providing Preoperative Patient Care: Day of Surgery

Due to the variety of outpatient and inpatient settings where elective surgery is performed, the day before surgery may be spent at home or in the hospital. If the patient will be arriving the morning of surgery to the surgical setting, they will receive a phone call the day before from a health care professional reminding the patient of the scheduled surgery, and key points, such as showering with an antiseptic cleansing agent, NPO restrictions, and any other pertinent information related to the particular procedure. In addition, the nurse will clarify any questions that the patient may have. If the patient is a hospitalized patient, the nurse will review the same information, clarify any concerns, and reinforce any perioperative instructions, as needed. A preoperative checklist is often used to outline the nurse's responsibilities on the day of surgery; some of the activities outlined in Skill 6-3 are part of this checklist and are completed and documented before the patient is transported to surgery. Refer as well to Fundamentals Review 6-1, 6-2, and 6-3.

DELEGATION CONSIDERATIONS

Preoperative measurement of vital signs may be delegated to assistive personnel (AP) as well as to licensed practical/vocational nurses (LPN/LVNs). Preoperative assessment and teaching are not delegated to AP. Depending on the state's nurse practice act and the organization's policies and procedures, preoperative teaching may be delegated to LPN/LVNs after an assessment of education needs by the registered nurse. The decision to delegate must be based on careful analysis of the patient's needs and circumstances as well as the qualifications of the person to whom the task is being delegated. Refer to the Delegation Guidelines in Appendix A.

EQUIPMENT

- Blood pressure cuff
- Electronic blood pressure monitor/sphygmomanometer
- Thermometer
- Pulse oximeter
- IV infusion device, IV solution, vascular access tubing

- Graduated compression stockings (as prescribed/indicated)
- Pneumatic compression device (as prescribed/indicated)
- Incentive spirometer (as prescribed/indicated)
- PPE, as indicated

ASSESSMENT

Immediately prior to the surgery, assess the patient's vital signs and communicate any abnormalities in vital signs as well as any abnormalities in laboratory and diagnostic results to the surgeon/health care team. Also, review and complete the preoperative checklist (see below) and inquire if the patient or family members/caregivers have any questions. Provide clarification as needed.

ACTUAL OR POTENTIAL HEALTH PROBLEMS AND NEEDS	Many actual or potential health problems or issues may require the use of this skill as part of related interventions. An appropriate health problem or issue may include: • Anxiety • Knowledge deficiency • Aspiration risk
OUTCOME IDENTIFICATION AND PLANNING	The expected outcome to achieve when providing preoperative patient care on the day of surgery is that the patient will safely proceed to surgery. Other outcomes that may be appropriate include: the patient and/or family/caregivers verbalize physical- and emotional-readiness for surgery, and the patient and/or family/caregivers verbalize an understanding of measures to minimize the postoperative risks associated with surgery and of what to expect over the remainder of the pre- and postoperative course.

IMPLEMENTATION

ACTION

1. Check the patient's health record for the type of surgery and review the prescribed interventions. Review the nursing database, history, and physical examination. Check that the baseline data are recorded; communicate those that are abnormal. Gather the necessary supplies.

 2. Perform hand hygiene and put on PPE, if indicated.

 3. Identify the patient.

4. Close the curtains around the bed and close the door to the room, if possible. Explain what you are going to do and why you are going to do it to the patient and significant other. Place necessary supplies on the bedside stand or overbed table, within easy reach.

5. Check that preoperative consent forms are signed, witnessed, and correct; verify that advance directives are in the health record (as applicable); and that the patient's health record is in order.

6. Measure vital signs (Figure 1). Notify the health care team and surgeon of any pertinent changes (e.g., rise or drop in blood pressure, elevated temperature, cough, symptoms of infection).

RATIONALE

A review of the health record ensures that the care will be provided for the right patient and any specific teaching based on the type of surgery will be addressed. Also, review identifies patients who are at surgical risks. Preparation promotes efficient time management and an organized approach to the task.

Hand hygiene and PPE prevent the spread of microorganisms. PPE is required based on transmission precautions.

Identifying the patient ensures the right patient receives the intervention and helps prevent errors.

Closing the curtains and door ensures the patient's privacy. Explanation relieves anxiety and facilitates engagement. Bringing everything to the bedside conserves time and energy. Arranging items nearby is convenient, saves time, and avoids unnecessary stretching and twisting of muscles on the part of the nurse.

These steps fulfill legal requirements related to informed consent and educate the patient regarding advance directives.

Vital signs taken now provide baseline data for comparison. Significant findings may require interventions and/or result in postponement of surgery.

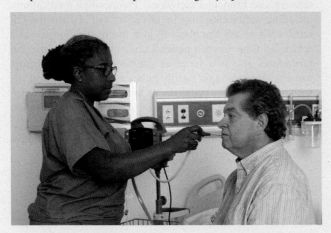

FIGURE 1. Obtaining preoperative vital signs.

(continued on page 372)

Skill 6-4 ▶ Providing Preoperative Patient Care: Day of Surgery *(continued)*

ACTION	RATIONALE
7. Provide hygiene and oral care. Assess for loose teeth and caps. **Verify adherence to food and fluid restrictions before surgery.**	These steps promote comfort and prevent intraoperative complications during anesthesia induction.
8. Facilitate/verify bathing was completed the morning of or night before surgery. **Complete any skin antiseptic preparation per surgical protocol or bundle or as prescribed.**	Skin antiseptic preparation the night before or the day of surgery eliminates skin microorganisms and leaves an antimicrobial film on the skin to minimize skin contamination and decrease the risk for postoperative surgical site infection (Taylor et al., 2020). Many facilities have specific surgical bundles or protocols that include preoperative showers or baths using soap, followed by an antiseptic wash using some combination of U.S. Food and Drug Administration (FDA)-approved iodine-, alcohol-, and/or chlorhexidine gluconate (CHG)-based products (AORN, 2020).
9. Instruct the patient to remove all personal clothing, including underwear, and to put on a hospital gown.	Having the patient wear only a gown permits access to the operative area and ease of assessment during the operative period.
10. Ask the patient to remove cosmetics, jewelry including body-piercing, nail polish, and prostheses (e.g., contact lenses, false eyelashes, dentures, and so forth). Some facilities allow a wedding band to be left in place depending on the type of surgery, provided it is secured to the finger with tape.	These items interfere with assessment during surgery. Some hospital policies advise having the patient wear eyeglasses and leave hearing aids in place, if needed. Document use of eyeglasses and hearing aids and that these items were sent with the patient.
11. If possible, give valuables to a family member/caregiver or place them in an appropriate area, such as the hospital safe, if this is not possible.	This ensures safety of valuables and personal possessions. Document where valuables have been secured.
12. Have the patient empty the bladder and bowels before surgery.	An empty bladder and bowels minimize risk for injury or complications during and after surgery.
13. Attend to any special preoperative orders, such as starting an IV line.	This prepares the patient for the operative procedure.
14. Complete preoperative checklist and record of patient's preoperative preparation.	This step ensures accurate documentation and communication with the perioperative nurse caring for patient.
15. Question the patient regarding the location of the operative site. Document the location in the health record according to facility policy. The actual site will be marked on the patient before the procedure is performed and, if possible, with the patient involved, by a licensed independent practitioner who is ultimately accountable for the procedure and will be present when the procedure is performed (The Joint Commission, n.d.).	The Universal Protocol for Preventing Wrong Site, Wrong Procedure, Wrong Person Surgery (part of the National Patient Safety Goals) requires marking and documentation to validate the intended site for the procedure (The Joint Commission, n.d., 2020).
16. Administer preoperative medication as prescribed.	Medication reduces anxiety, provides sedation, and diminishes salivary and bronchial secretions. Preoperative medications, including antibiotics, may be given "on call" (when the OR nurse calls to tell the nurse to give the medication) or at a scheduled time. Certain patients undergoing specific surgical procedures also may be given antibiotic prophylaxis before surgery; depending on facility policy and procedure and the specific medication, prophylactic antibiotics may be administered sent to the OR with the patient for administration immediately prior to the surgery.
17. Raise the bed side rails, based on facility policy; place the bed in lowest position. Instruct the patient to remain in bed or on the stretcher. If necessary, use a safety belt.	These actions ensure the patient's safety once the preoperative medication has been given.

ACTION

18. Help move the patient from the bed to the transport stretcher, if necessary. Reconfirm patient identification and ensure that all preoperative events and measures are documented.

19. Tell the patient's family/caregivers where the patient will be taken after surgery and the location of the waiting area where the surgeon will come to explain the outcome of the surgery. If possible, take the family/caregivers to the waiting area.

20. After the patient leaves for the OR, prepare the room for patients returning to a room on a hospital patient care unit and make a postoperative bed for the patient (Figure 2). Anticipate any necessary equipment based on the type of surgery and the patient's history and place at the bedside.

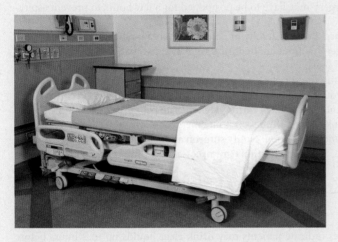

FIGURE 2. Postoperative bed, ready for patient's return.

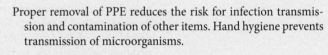

21. Remove PPE, if used. Perform hand hygiene.

RATIONALE

Helping the patient move prevents injury. Reconfirming the patient identity helps to ensure that the correct patient is being transported to surgery.

Informing the family members/caregivers of what to expect helps allay anxiety and avoid confusion.

Preparing for the patient's return helps to promote efficient care in the postoperative period.

Proper removal of PPE reduces the risk for infection transmission and contamination of other items. Hand hygiene prevents transmission of microorganisms.

EVALUATION   The expected outcomes have been met when the patient has safely proceeded to surgery, the patient and/or family/caregivers have verbalized physical- and emotional-readiness for surgery, and the patient and/or family/caregivers have verbalized an understanding of measures to minimize the postoperative risks associated with surgery and of what to expect over the remainder of the pre- and postoperative course.

DOCUMENTATION

Guidelines   Document that the preoperative checklist was completed, time of patient's last void, preoperative medications administered, intended procedure site, and any special interventions that were prescribed before sending the patient to the OR. Record if there were any abnormal results that were communicated to the surgeon/surgical team or the OR nurse. Note if the patient's valuables were given to a family member/caregiver or safe storage. Document that the patient was safely transferred onto the stretcher and escorted to the OR without incident. Record that the patient's family members/caregivers were instructed as to where to wait to meet the surgeon after the surgery is performed.

(continued on page 374)

Skill 6-4 ▶ Providing Preoperative Patient Care: Day of Surgery *(continued)*

Sample Documentation

> 4/3/25 1045 Preoperative checklist completed with no abnormalities noted, patient voided, and operative permit signed. Patient states surgical site is left knee. Maintained NPO status throughout night. IV started into right forearm, #18-gauge needle inserted without difficulty. IV solution of 1,000 mL of D5.45 sodium chloride at 80/mL/hr initiated. No preoperative medications prescribed. Patient verbalized that he will be glad when the surgery is over. Patient assisted onto stretcher for transfer to OR without difficulty. Family accompanied and instructed to wait in surgical waiting lounge.
> —A. Lynn, RN

DEVELOPING CLINICAL REASONING AND CLINICAL JUDGMENT

UNEXPECTED SITUATIONS AND ASSOCIATED INTERVENTIONS

- *Patient admits he ate "just a little bit" this morning upon waking from sleep:* Notify the surgeon/ surgical team. The patient's surgery may have to be postponed for a few hours to prevent aspiration during surgery.
- *Identification band is not in place:* Ensure identity of patient and obtain new identification band. Patient cannot proceed to surgery without an identification band. Two patient identifiers are required to meet patient safety goals.
- *Consent form is not signed:* Notify the surgeon/surgical team. It is the responsibility of the provider performing the procedure to obtain consent for surgery and anesthesia. Preoperative medications cannot be given until the consent form is signed. The patient should not proceed to surgery without a signed consent form (unless it is an emergency).
- *Patient refuses to take preoperative medication:* Notify surgeon and anesthesiologist/surgical team before patient goes to the OR. Many medications are necessary to protect the patient pre- or postoperatively.

SPECIAL CONSIDERATIONS

General Considerations

- Preoperative practice guidelines indicate patients may drink clear liquids up to 2 hours before procedures requiring general anesthesia, regional anesthesia, or procedural sedation and analgesia, as prescribed (American Society of Anesthesiologists, 2017). If clear liquids are allowed, they should be carefully defined for the patient, and include water, fruit juices without pulp, carbonated beverages, clear tea, and black coffee. These liquids do not include any alcohol. Light meals such as clear liquid and toast may be consumed up to 6 hours before elective procedures requiring general anesthesia, regional anesthesia, or procedural sedation and analgesia; regular meals should be finished 8 hours before elective procedures requiring general anesthesia, regional anesthesia, or procedural sedation, and analgesia (American Society of Anesthesiologists, 2017).
- Bariatric equipment, such as blood pressure cuffs, wide stretchers, and lift devices, need to be available for patients who are obese.

Infant and Child Considerations

- In many institutions, the parents are allowed to enter the preoperative area with the child. This has been shown to decrease the child's and the parents' anxiety.
- Infants may receive breastmilk 4 hours and/or infant formula 6 hours before elective procedures requiring general anesthesia, regional anesthesia, or procedural sedation and analgesia (American Society of Anesthesiologists, 2017).

Older Adult Considerations

- Due to the prevalence of hearing and vision loss in this age group, the necessity of wearing eyeglasses and hearing aids is essential for processing preoperative teaching and throughout the postoperative course. The patient who requires glasses and hearing aids to understand and/or read instructions should be sent to the preoperative area with the glasses and/or hearing aid in place and then remove them before entering the OR.

Skill 6-5 ▶ Providing Postoperative Care

Postoperative care facilitates recovery from surgery and supports the patient in coping with physical changes or alterations. Nursing assessments and interventions are consistent with those in the preoperative and intraoperative phases and are carried out to maintain function, promote recovery, and facilitate coping with alterations in structure or function.

After surgery, patients spend time on the postanesthesia care unit (PACU). After this time period and when the patient's condition is stabilized, the patient may be transferred either to the intensive care unit (ICU) if more in-depth monitoring and nursing care is required, or to the surgical unit in the hospital. If the surgery was ambulatory, the patient will be discharged to home.

Nursing care throughout the postoperative period includes ongoing assessments, monitoring for complications, implementing specific nursing interventions, and patient and family/caregiver teaching, as needed. Before discharge from either the hospital or the ambulatory care unit, all patients will receive both oral and written discharge instructions and information regarding appropriate follow-up appointments, usually with the surgeon at a minimum. Discharge teaching focuses on patient teaching to support and encourage continuation of interventions to prevent postoperative complications. In addition, the patient may receive a follow-up telephone call the next day after discharge to ensure early identification of complications and address any patient concerns.

Ongoing assessments are crucial for early identification of postoperative complications.

DELEGATION CONSIDERATIONS

Postoperative measurement of vital signs may be delegated to assistive personnel (AP) as well as to licensed practical/vocational nurses (LPN/LVNs). Postoperative assessment and teaching are not delegated to AP. Depending on the state's nurse practice act and the organization's policies and procedures, postoperative teaching may be delegated to LPN/LVNs after an assessment of education needs by the registered nurse. The decision to delegate must be based on careful analysis of the patient's needs and circumstances as well as the qualifications of the person to whom the task is being delegated. Refer to the Delegation Guidelines in Appendix A.

EQUIPMENT (Varies, Depending on the Surgery)

- Electronic blood pressure monitor/sphygmomanometer
- Blood pressure cuff
- Electronic thermometer
- Pulse oximeter
- Stethoscope
- IV infusion device, IV solutions
- Graduated compression stockings (as prescribed/indicated)

- Pneumatic compression devices (as prescribed/indicated)
- Tubes, drains, vascular access tubing
- Incentive spirometer (as prescribed/indicated)
- PPE, as indicated
- Blankets and/or forced-air warming device, as needed

ASSESSMENT

Assess the patient's mental status, positioning, and vital signs. Assess the patient's oxygen saturation level, skin color, respiratory status, and cardiovascular status. Assess the patient's neurovascular status, depending on the type of surgery. Assess the operative site, drains/tubes, and IV site(s). Perform a pain assessment. A wide variety of factors increase the risk for postoperative complications. Ongoing postoperative assessments and interventions are used to decrease the risk for postoperative complications. Assessment of the patient's and family's/caregiver's learning needs is also important.

ACTUAL OR POTENTIAL HEALTH PROBLEMS AND NEEDS

Many actual or potential health problems or issues may require the use of this skill as part of related interventions. An appropriate health problem or issue may include:
- Acute pain
- Impaired gas exchange
- Fluid imbalance

OUTCOME IDENTIFICATION AND PLANNING

The expected outcome to achieve when providing postoperative care to a patient is that the patient will recover from the surgery. Other outcomes that may be appropriate include the following: the patient's temperature remains between 97.7°F and 99.5°F (36.5°C and 37.5°C), the patient's vital signs remain stable, the patient remains free from infection, the patient does not experience any skin breakdown, the patient regains mobility, the patient's pain is managed appropriately, and the patient is comfortable with their body image. Specific expected outcomes are individualized based on risk factors, the surgical procedure, and the patient's unique needs.

(continued on page 376)

Skill 6-5 ▶ Providing Postoperative Care *(continued)*

IMPLEMENTATION

| ACTION | RATIONALE |

Immediate Care

1. When the patient returns from the PACU, participate in hand-off report from the PACU nurse and review the OR and PACU data. Gather the necessary supplies.

Obtaining a hand-off report ensures accurate communication and promotes continuity of care. Preparation promotes efficient time management and an organized approach to the task.

2. Perform hand hygiene and put on PPE, if indicated.

Hand hygiene and PPE prevent the spread of microorganisms. PPE is required based on transmission precautions.

3. Identify the patient.

Identifying the patient ensures the right patient receives the intervention and helps prevent errors.

4. Close the curtains around the bed and close the door to the room, if possible. Explain what you are going to do and why you are going to do it to the patient or significant other. Place necessary supplies on the bedside stand, over-bed table, or other surface within easy reach.

Closing the curtains and door ensures the patient's privacy. Explanation relieves anxiety and facilitates engagement. Bringing everything to the bedside conserves time and energy. Arranging items nearby is convenient, saves time, and avoids unnecessary stretching and twisting of muscles on the part of the nurse.

5. **Place the patient in safe position (semi- or high-Fowler's or side-lying). Note level of consciousness.**

A head of bed (HOB)-elevated position facilitates deep breathing; the side-lying position with neck slightly extended prevents aspiration and airway obstruction. Alternate positions may be appropriate based on the type of surgery.

6. **Obtain vital signs. Monitor and record vital signs frequently.** Prescribed assessment frequency may vary, but usual frequency includes taking vital signs every 15 minutes the first hour, every 30 minutes the next 2 hours, every hour for 4 hours, and finally every 4 hours. Refer to facility policy and adjust based on patient circumstances and nursing clinical judgment (AORN, 2019). Temperature measurement should be obtained using the same site and method of measurement (AORN, 2019). If continuous vital sign monitoring is used, apply monitor per manufacturer's directions.

Comparison with baseline preoperative vital signs may indicate impending shock, respiratory compromise, or hemorrhage. Although protocols are used as guidelines in the immediate postoperative period, the nurse is responsible for adjusting the frequency and priorities of assessment to the specific needs of each patient. Temperature measurement can vary significantly when temperatures are measured at different sites or by different methods; the same site and method of temperature measurement should be used throughout the perioperative phases when clinically feasible (AORN, 2019). Wireless continuous vital sign monitoring maybe used to aid in early detection of changes in the patient's condition (Downey et al., 2018; Verillo et al, 2019).

7. Assess the patient's respiratory status. (Refer to Skill 3-5 in Chapter 3.) Measure the patient's oxygen saturation level (Figure 1). If oxygen is prescribed or warranted, ensure accurate delivery device and flow rate. Measure and monitor the patient's end-tidal carbon dioxide levels as prescribed or based on facility policy.

Comparison with baseline preoperative respiratory assessment may indicate impending respiratory complications. Pulse oximetry provides information about the patient's oxygenation status. Measurement of end-tidal carbon dioxide levels (capnography) provides information about the patient's ventilation status and may be used to monitor patients with known or suspected obstructive sleep apnea and those who receive sedation and opioids or other CNS depressants (Borczynski & Worobel-Luk, 2019; Burns & Delgado, 2019; Hess et al., 2021).

8. Assess the patient's cardiovascular status. (Refer to Skills 3-6 and 3-10 in Chapter 3.)

Comparison with baseline preoperative cardiovascular assessment may indicate impending cardiovascular complications.

9. Assess the patient's neurovascular status, based on the type of surgery performed. (Refer to Skill 3-10 in Chapter 3.)

Comparison with baseline preoperative neurovascular assessment may indicate impending neurovascular complications.

10. Provide for warmth, using heated or extra blankets, or forced-air warming device as necessary. Refer to Skill 6-6. Assess skin color and condition.

The OR is a cold environment. All perioperative patients are at risk for hypothermia (AORN, 2019). **Hypothermia** is uncomfortable; is associated with prolonged postoperative recovery, cardiac arrhythmias, impaired renal function, and impaired wound healing (Hinkle et al., 2022; Link, 2020; Nieh & Su, 2018; Xu et al., 2019).

ACTION

11. Put on gloves. Assess the surgical site. Check dressings for color, odor, presence of drains, and amount of drainage (Figure 2). Mark the drainage on the dressing by circling the amount and include the time. Assess dependent areas, such as turning the patient to assess visually under the patient, for bleeding from the surgical site.

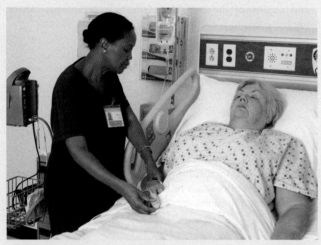

FIGURE 1. Obtaining postoperative oxygen saturation level.

12. Verify that all tubes and drains are patent and the equipment is working; note the amount of drainage in collection device. If an indwelling urinary catheter is in place, note urinary output.

13. Verify and maintain IV infusion at prescribed rate.

14. Assess for pain (refer to Chapter 10). Check health record to verify if analgesic medication was administered in the PACU. Administer analgesics as indicated, prescribed, and appropriate. If the patient has been instructed in the use of PCA for pain management, review its use. Institute nonpharmacologic pain management interventions as appropriate and indicated (Refer to Skill 10-1).

15. Assess for nausea and vomiting. Administer antiemetic medication as indicated, prescribed, and appropriate. Institute nonpharmacologic management interventions as appropriate and indicated.

16. Provide for a safe environment. Keep the bed in low position with the side rails up, based on facility policy. Have the call bell within patient's reach.

17. Remove PPE, if used. Perform hand hygiene.

 RATIONALE

Hemorrhage and shock are life-threatening complications of surgery and early recognition is essential.

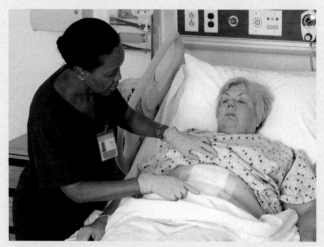

FIGURE 2. Checking dressings for color, odor, and amount of drainage.

This ensures function of drainage devices.

This replaces fluid loss and prevents dehydration and electrolyte imbalances.

Use a facility-approved pain scale (Chou et al., 2016). Observe for nonverbal behavior that may indicate pain, such as grimacing, crying, and restlessness. Analgesics and other nonpharmacologic pain strategies are used for relief of postoperative pain.

General anesthesia can cause postoperative nausea and vomiting. Vomiting can lead to serious complications, including pulmonary aspiration, dehydration, and dysrhythmias secondary to electrolyte imbalances (Koyuncu et al., 2020). Aromatherapy has been suggested as a complementary intervention to decrease postoperative nausea and vomiting (Abril et al., 2019; Karaman et al., 2019; Spruce, 2020b).

This adjustment to the bed prevents accidental injury. Easy access to the call bell permits the patient to call for nurse when necessary.

Proper removal of PPE reduces the risk for infection transmission and contamination of other items. Hand hygiene prevents transmission of microorganisms.

(continued on page 378)

Skill 6-5 ▶ Providing Postoperative Care *(continued)*

ACTION	**RATIONALE**

Ongoing Care

18. Promote optimal respiratory function.

The patient is at risk for respiratory complications postoperatively. Interventions can be implemented to prevent respiratory complications.

a. Assess respiratory rate, depth, quality, color, and capillary refill. Ask if the patient is experiencing any difficulty breathing.

The patient is at risk for pulmonary complications postoperatively. Postoperative analgesic medication can reduce the rate and quality of the respiratory effort. Interventions can be implemented to prevent cardiovascular complications.

b. Assist with coughing and deep-breathing exercises. (Refer to Skill 6-1.)

c. Assist with incentive spirometry, as indicated/prescribed. (Refer to Skill 14-3 in Chapter 14.)

d. Assist with early ambulation.

e. Provide frequent position changes.

f. Administer oxygen, as prescribed.

g. Monitor pulse oximetry. (Refer to Skill 14-1 in Chapter 14.)

19. Promote optimal cardiovascular function:

Patient is at risk for cardiovascular complications postoperatively. Interventions can be implemented to prevent cardiovascular complications.

a. Assess apical rate, rhythm, and quality and compare with peripheral pulses, color, and blood pressure. Ask if the patient has any chest pains or shortness of breath.

b. Provide frequent position changes.

c. Assist with early ambulation.

d. Apply graduated compression stockings or pneumatic compression devices, if prescribed and not in place. If in place, assess for integrity. (Refer to Skills 9-10 and 9-11 in Chapter 9.)

e. Provide leg and range-of-motion exercises if not contraindicated. (Refer to Skill 6-2.)

20. Promote optimal neurologic function:

Anesthetic and pain management agents can alter neurologic function. Sedation scales are used to assess sedation levels and provide nurses with a useful tool to make decisions about the timing of medication interventions and when to intervene based on patients' sedation levels (Hall & Stanley, 2019).

a. Assess level of consciousness, movement, and sensation. Assess and monitor the patient's level of sedation using a sedation scale, particularly if opioids are used to treat postoperative pain (Hall & Stanley, 2019).

b. Determine the level of orientation to person, place, and time.

c. Test motor ability by asking the patient to move each extremity.

Anesthesia alters motor and sensory function.

d. Evaluate sensation by asking the patient if they can feel your touch on an extremity.

21. Promote optimal renal and urinary function and fluid and electrolyte status. Assess intake and output, evaluate for urinary retention and monitor serum electrolyte levels.

Anesthetic agents and surgical manipulation in the area may temporarily depress bladder tone and response causing urinary retention.

a. Promote voiding by offering bedpan/bedside commode, or assistance to bathroom at regular intervals, noting the frequency, amount, and if any burning or urgency symptoms.

Frequency, burning, or urgency may indicate possible urinary tract abnormality.

b. Monitor urinary catheter drainage if present.

Communicate with the health care team if the patient's urinary output is less than 30 mL/hr or 240 mL/8-hr period.

c. Measure intake and output.

Intake and output are good indicators of fluid balance.

ACTION	**RATIONALE**
22. Promote optimal gastrointestinal function and meet nutritional needs:	Anesthetic agents and opioids depress peristalsis and normal functioning of the gastrointestinal tract (Karch, 2020). Flatus indicates return of peristalsis.
a. Assess abdomen for distention and firmness. Ask if patient feels nauseated, any vomiting, and if passing flatus.	
b. Auscultate for bowel sounds.	Presence of bowel sounds indicates return of peristalsis.
c. Assist with diet progression; encourage fluid intake; monitor intake.	Patients may experience nausea after surgery and are encouraged to resume diet slowly, starting with clear liquids and advancing as tolerated.
d. Medicate for nausea and vomiting, as prescribed. Institute nonpharmacologic interventions as appropriate and indicated.	Antiemetics are frequently prescribed to alleviate postoperative nausea. Complementary interventions may be effective in decreasing nausea and vomiting.
23. Promote optimal wound healing.	Alterations in nutritional, circulatory, and metabolic status may predispose the patient to infection and delayed healing.
a. Assess condition of wound for presence of drains and any drainage.	
b. Use surgical asepsis for dressing changes and drain care. Refer to Skills 8-2 and 8-6 to 8-10 in Chapter 8.	Surgical asepsis reduces the risk of infection.
c. Inspect all skin surfaces for beginning signs of pressure injury and use pressure-relieving supports to minimize potential skin breakdown.	Lying on the OR table in the same position can predispose some patients to pressure injury formation, especially in patients who have undergone lengthy procedures.
24. Promote optimal comfort and relief from pain.	This shortens recovery period and facilitates return to normal function.
a. Assess for pain (location and intensity using pain scale).	Control of postoperative pain promotes patient comfort and recovery.
b. Provide for rest and comfort; provide extra blankets, as needed, for warmth.	Patients may experience chills in the postoperative period.
c. Administer analgesics, as needed, and/or initiate non-pharmacologic methods, as appropriate.	Multimodal analgesia, combining analgesic drugs from different classes, is recommended to reduce the risk of adverse drug effects (Polomano et al., 2017; Poulsen et al, 2019).
25. Promote optimal outcomes related to psychosocial needs:	This facilitates individualized care, anxiety reduction, and patient's return to normal health.
a. Provide emotional support to patient and family/caregivers, as needed.	
b. Explain procedures and offer explanations regarding postoperative recovery, as needed, to both patient and family members/caregivers.	

EVALUATION

The expected outcomes have been met when the patient has recovered from surgery, the patient's temperature remained between 97.7°F and 99.5°F (36.5°C and 37.5°C), the patient's vital signs remained stable, the patient remained free from infection, the patient did not experience alterations in skin integrity, the patient regained mobility, the patient experienced adequate pain control, and the patient was comfortable with their body image. Specific expected outcomes are individualized based on risk factors, the surgical procedure, and the patient's unique needs.

DOCUMENTATION

Guidelines

Document the time that the patient returns from PACU to the surgical unit. Record the patient's level of consciousness, vital signs, all assessments, and condition of dressing. If patient has oxygen in place, an IV, or any other equipment, record this information. Document pain assessment, interventions that were instituted to alleviate pain, and the patient's response to the interventions. Document any patient teaching that is reviewed with the patient, such as use of incentive spirometer.

(continued on page 380)

Skill 6-5 ▶ Providing Postoperative Care *(continued)*

Sample Documentation

> 4/10/25 1330 Patient returned to room at 1315, drowsy but easily aroused; answers to name. Patient's temperature 98.8°F, pulse 78, BP 122/84, O_2 sat 96% on O_2 2 L/min. Right lower abdominal dressing dry and intact. Rates pain at a "4" on a scale of 1 to 10, was medicated in PACU with 4-mg morphine sulfate IV at 1030. Incentive spirometry completed × 10 cycles, 750 mL each. Patient deep breathing and coughing without production and turned to right side with HOB elevated. See EHR for additional system assessments.
>
> *—J. Grabbs, RN*

DEVELOPING CLINICAL REASONING AND CLINICAL JUDGMENT

UNEXPECTED SITUATIONS AND ASSOCIATED INTERVENTIONS

- *Vital signs are progressively increasing or decreasing from baseline:* Collaborate with the health care team. A continued decrease in blood pressure or an increase in heart rate could indicate internal bleeding or **hemorrhage**.
- *Dressing was clean before but now has large amount of fresh blood:* Do not remove dressing. Reinforce dressing with more bandages. Removing the bandage could dislodge any clot that is forming and lead to further blood loss. Consult with the health care team.
- *Patient reports pain that is not relieved by prescribed medication:* After fully assessing pain, consult with the health care team. Pain can be a clue to other problems, such as hemorrhage.
- *Patient is febrile within 12 hours of surgery:* Assist patient with coughing and deep breathing. If prescribed, encourage incentive spirometry. Continue to monitor vital signs and laboratory values such as complete blood count (CBC).
- *Adult patient has a urine output of less than 30 mL/hr:* Unless this is expected, consult with the health care team. Urine output is a good indicator of tissue perfusion. Patient may need more fluid or may need medication to increase blood pressure if blood pressure is low.

SPECIAL CONSIDERATIONS

General Considerations

- Be aware of baseline sensory deficits. Ensure appropriate aids are in place, such as glasses or hearing aids. Lack of appropriate aids may impact postoperative assessments, such as level of consciousness.
- For patients undergoing throat surgery, such as a tonsillectomy, evaluate swallowing pattern. A patient who has had throat surgery and swallows frequently may be bleeding from the incision site.
- Multimodal analgesia, which combines analgesic drugs from different classes and employs analgesic techniques that target different mechanisms of pain, is recommended in the treatment of acute postoperative pain. The synergistic effects maximize pain relief at lower analgesic doses, reducing the risk of adverse drug effects (Polomano et al., 2017, p. S12).
- Consider the need for a bariatric mattress or bariatric bed for a patient who is obese because this patient is at greater risk for alterations in skin integrity due to the poor vascular supply of adipose tissue and restrictions in movement (Hinkle et al., 2022).
- Intermittent manual vital sign measurement as single data points may provide an incomplete picture of patients' postoperative physiologic status (Downey et al., 2018; Verrillo et al., 2019). Wearable sensor packs using wireless technology are being used in some settings for continuous measurement of vital signs. This monitoring provides trending of vital signs (such as heart rate, respiratory rate, noninvasive blood pressure, temperature, and pulse oximetry) and may help in early detection of patient deterioration and improve patient outcomes (Verrillo et al., 2019).
- Aromatherapy has been used successfully to decrease postoperative nausea and vomiting. Inhalers using essential oils, including peppermint, ginger, lavender, rose and spearmint oils, or a blend of these oils, have been shown to be effective (Abril et al, 2019; Karaman et al., 2019; Spruce, 2020b).
- Ensure that written postoperative instructions specific to the patient and follow-up appointments with the surgeon or other health care professionals are provided to each patient upon discharge from the hospital or outpatient center. Information, such as signs and symptoms to report to the health care team, as well as restrictions in activity and diet, are addressed. In addition, patients discharged the same day as their surgery are required to have a responsible person accompany them home, and a contact telephone number is to be provided in case of emergency. The patient should be alert and oriented, or mental status should be at the patient's baseline. The vital signs of the patient should be stable. Have the patient "teach back" important information/instructions in their own words.

Infant and Child Considerations

- Postoperative complications are often related to the respiratory system in this age group. After receiving general anesthesia, premature infants are at greater risk for apnea (Subramaniam, 2019).
- Infants and children are at great risk for temperature-related complications because their body temperature can change rapidly. It is essential to have warmed blankets and other warming equipment available to avoid this complication.

Older Adult Considerations

- Older adults may take longer to return to normothermia and their baseline level of orientation. Drugs and anesthetics may delay this return.
- Forced-air warming systems are suggested as the most effective means of rewarming older patients with postoperative hypothermia (Xu et al., 2019).

EVIDENCE FOR PRACTICE ▶

PREVENTION OF DEEP VEIN THROMBOSIS

American Association of Critical Care Nurses. (2016). AACN practice alert: Preventing venous thromboembolism in adults. *Critical Care Nurse*, *36*(5), e20–e23.

Association of periOperative Registered Nurses (AORN). (2018). Guideline summary: Prevention of venous thromboembolism. *AORN Journal*, *107*(6), 750–754. http://doi.org/10.1002/aorn.12147

Refer to details in Skill 6-2, Evidence for Practice.

EVIDENCE FOR PRACTICE ▶

OPIOID-RELATED SEDATION AND THE PASERO OPIOID SEDATION SCALE

Hall, K. R., & Stanley, A. Y. (2019). Literature review: Assessment of opioid-related sedation and the Pasero Opioid Sedation Scale. *Journal of PeriAnesthesia Nursing*, *34*(1), 132–142. https://doi.org/10.1016/j.jopan.2017.12.009

This review of the literature examined sedation scales and monitoring practices, specifically evaluating utilization of the Pasero Opioid Sedation Scale (POSS) in the clinical setting. A literature search was performed from January 2009 to June 2016 using PubMed, CINAHL, and Goggle Scholar databases. Search terms included monitor, monitoring, opioid-induced, Pasero Opioid Sedation Scale, respiratory depression, and sedation. MeSH terms included monitoring, physiologic, analgesics, opioid, respiratory insufficiency/complications/nursing, and prevention and control. Six articles were selected for review, including three descriptive surveys, two quasi-experimental studies, and one evidence-based practice project. The studies and project were completed in a variety of settings, including general/non-critical care, postanesthesia care (PACU), postsurgical care, pediatric clinical care, and pediatric intensive care settings. Findings indicated that there is limited research regarding implementation of the POSS. The literature does support the goal of the POSS, citing the potential for fewer opioid-related adverse events and increase confidence among nursing staff.

Skill 6-6 ▶ Applying a Forced-Air Warming Device

Patients are at risk for altered body temperature related to the surgical procedure, length of the procedure, anesthetic agents, a cool surgical environment, age, and use of cool irrigating or infusion fluids. Inadvertent hypothermia (temperature below 96°F [36°C]) can lead to complications of poor wound healing, hemodynamic stress, cardiac disturbances, coagulopathy, delayed emergence from anesthesia, and shivering and its associated discomfort (AORN, 2019). Warming methods intra- and postoperatively are tailored to the individual patient and may include a combination of modalities (Link, 2020). Warmed blankets and forced-air warming devices are used for rewarming

(continued on page 382)

Skill 6-6   Applying a Forced-Air Warming Device   *(continued)*

postoperatively. Forced-air warming devices are placed over the patient and circulate warm air around the patient. Covering the patient with the device acts to reduce heat loss from the skin (through convective and radiant loss) and in combination with the transfer of heat to the patient's body from the forced-air acts to raise the patient's body temperature and/or prevent hypothermia (Spruce, 2020c). It is important to monitor the patient's body temperature and circulatory status during use of these devices. Follow the manufacturer's directions and facility policies for use.

DELEGATION CONSIDERATIONS

Application of a forced-air warming device is not delegated to assistive personnel (AP). Application of a forced-warm air device may be delegated to licensed practical/vocational nurses (LPN/LVNs). The decision to delegate must be based on careful analysis of the patient's needs and circumstances as well as the qualifications of the person to whom the task is being delegated. Refer to the Delegation Guidelines in Appendix A.

EQUIPMENT

- Forced-air warming device
- Forced-air blanket
- Electronic thermometer
- PPE, as indicated

ASSESSMENT

Assess the patient's temperature and skin color and perfusion. Patients who are hypothermic are generally pale to dusky and cool to the touch and have decreased peripheral perfusion. Inspect nail beds and mucous membranes of patients with darker skin tones for signs of decreased perfusion. Measure the patient's body temperature and assess the patient's vital signs.

ACTUAL OR POTENTIAL HEALTH PROBLEMS AND NEEDS

Many actual or potential health problems or issues may require the use of this skill as part of related interventions. An appropriate health problem or issue may include:
- Impaired thermoregulation
- Perioperative injury risk
- Thermal injury risk

OUTCOME IDENTIFICATION AND PLANNING

The expected outcome to achieve when applying a forced-air warming device is that the patient will return to and maintain a temperature of 97.7° to 99.5°F (36.5° to 37.5°C). Other outcomes that may be appropriate include the following: the skin will become warm, capillary refill will be less than 2 to 3 seconds, and the patient will not experience shivering.

IMPLEMENTATION

ACTION	RATIONALE
1. Check the patient's health record for the prescribed use of a forced-air warming device. Gather the necessary supplies.	Reviewing the order validates the correct patient and correct procedure. Organization facilitates performance of the task. Preparation promotes efficient time management and an organized approach to the task.
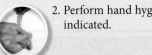 2. Perform hand hygiene and put on PPE, if indicated.	Hand hygiene and PPE prevent the spread of microorganisms. PPE is required based on transmission precautions.
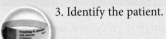 3. Identify the patient.	Identifying the patient ensures the right patient receives the intervention and helps prevent errors.
4. Close the curtains around the bed and close the door to the room, if possible. Explain what you are going to do and why you are going to do it to the patient or significant other. Place necessary supplies on the bedside stand, over-bed table, or other surface within easy reach.	Closing the curtains and door ensures the patient's privacy. Explanation relieves anxiety and facilitates engagement. Bringing everything to the bedside conserves time and energy. Arranging items nearby is convenient, saves time, and avoids unnecessary stretching and twisting of muscles on the part of the nurse.

ACTION

5. **Assess the patient's temperature.** Temperature measurement should be obtained using the same site and method of measurement (AORN, 2019).

6. Plug forced-air warming device into electrical outlet. Place forced-air blanket over the patient, with plastic side up (Figure 1). Keep air-hose inlet at foot of bed.

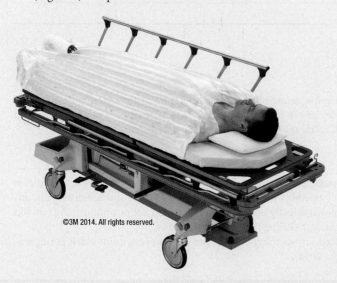

FIGURE 1. Forced-air blanket on patient, plastic side up, with air hose inlet at foot of bed. (The photograph is reproduced herein with permission. © 3M 2014. All rights reserved.)

7. Securely insert the air hose into the inlet. Place a lightweight fabric blanket over the forced-air blanket, according to the manufacturer's instructions. Turn the machine on and adjust temperature of air to desired effect.

 8. Remove PPE, if used. Perform hand hygiene.

9. **Monitor the patient's temperature at least every 30 minutes while using the forced-air device.**

10. Discontinue use of the forced-air device once the patient's temperature is adequate and the patient can maintain the temperature without assistance.

11. Remove device and clean according to facility policy and manufacturer's instructions.

RATIONALE

Baseline temperature validates the need for use of the device and provides baseline information for future comparison. Temperature measurement can vary significantly when temperatures are measured at different sites or by different methods; the same site and method of temperature measurement should be used throughout the perioperative phases when clinically feasible (AORN, 2019).

Blanket should always be used with the device. To avoid causing burns, do not place air hose under lightweight blankets with airflow blanket.

The air hose must be properly inserted to ensure that it will not fall out. The blanket will help keep warmed air near the patient. Adjust air temperature, depending on desired patient temperature. If the blanket is being used to maintain an already stable temperature, it may be turned down lower than if needed to raise patient's temperature.

Proper removal of PPE reduces the risk for infection transmission and contamination of other items. Hand hygiene prevents transmission of microorganisms.

Monitoring the patient's temperature ensures that the patient does not experience too rapid a rise in body temperature, resulting in vasodilation.

The forced-air device is not needed once the patient is warm and stable enough to maintain temperature.

Proper care of equipment helps to maintain function of the device.

EVALUATION

The expected outcomes have been met when the patient's temperature returned to the normal range of 97.7° to 99.5°F (36.5° to 37.5°C), the patient maintained this temperature, the patient's skin was warm, and patient was free from shivering.

(continued on page 384)

Skill 6-6 ▶ Applying a Forced-Air Warming Device *(continued)*

DOCUMENTATION

Guidelines

Document the patient's temperature and the route used for measurement. Record that the forced-air warming device was applied to the patient. Document appearance of the skin and that the patient did not experience any adverse effects from the warming device. Record that the patient's temperature was monitored every 30 minutes, as well as the actual temperature measurements.

Sample Documentation

<u>4/23/25</u> 1440 Patient's temperature 96.6° F (35.9°C) tympanically. Forced-air warming device applied to patient due to decreased temperature. Device temperature set on medium. Patient's temperature after first 30 minutes 97.5°F (36.4°C) tympanically. Device temperature setting decreased to low and continued. Will recheck temperature in 30 minutes.

—J. Grabbs, RN

DEVELOPING CLINICAL REASONING AND CLINICAL JUDGMENT

UNEXPECTED SITUATIONS AND ASSOCIATED INTERVENTIONS

- *Patient's temperature is increasing too quickly:* Decrease temperature of air-warming device. If air is down to lowest setting, turn device off. If patient's temperature increases too rapidly, it can lead to a vasodilation effect that will cause the patient to become hypotensive.

SPECIAL CONSIDERATIONS

- Use of forced-air warming devices has been associated with thermal injuries (Feil, 2017; John et al., 2014). Monitor for correct assembly of warmer hose to the blanket and accidental disconnection to avoid hot air being blown directly on the patient's skin; do not position patients on top of blankets designed to cover patients (Feil, 2017; John et al., 2014).
- Preoperative warming with forced-air warming blanket can help prevent unintended perioperative hypothermia (Broback et al., 2018).

Enhance Your Understanding

Focusing on Patient Care: Developing Clinical Reasoning and Clinical Judgment

Consider the case scenarios at the beginning of the chapter as you answer the following questions to enhance your understanding and apply what you have learned.

QUESTIONS

1. In Josie's health record there is a prescription for a prophylactic antibiotic to be given "on call to the OR," which means the nurse is to administer the prescribed medication after receiving the phone call to send Josie to the OR. However, the phone call comes during a busy period, and the nurse realizes that Josie has been transported down to the preoperative holding area without receiving her dose of prophylactic antibiotics. What should the nurse do?

2. After her surgery, Ms. Kelly rates her pain as 8 of 10. The nurse administers the prescribed pain medication.

Fifteen minutes later, Ms. Kelly is now rating her pain as 9 of 10 and is beginning to writhe with pain. She has no more prescribed pain medication for another hour. What should the nurse do?

3. Dorothy Gibbs returns from surgery with a core temperature of 95.4°F (35.2°C), blood pressure of 128/72 mm Hg, and pulse of 60 beats per minute. Her skin is pale and cool to the touch. A forced-air warming device is placed on Ms. Gibbs, and the nurse turns the warmer to the highest heat setting. An hour later, the nurse takes Ms. Gibbs' vital signs. Her tympanic temperature is 100.0°F (37.8°C), her blood pressure is 82/48 mm Hg, and her pulse is 100 beats per minute. What should the nurse do?

You can find suggested answers after the Bibliography at the end of this chapter.

Enhance Your Understanding (Continued)

Integrated Case Study Connection

The case studies in the back of the book focus on integrating concepts. Refer to the following case studies to enhance your understanding of the concepts and skills in this chapter.

- Basic Case Studies: Tiffany Jones, page 1195; Kate Townsend, page 1205.
- Intermediate Case Studies: Jason Brown, page 1215.
- Advanced Case Studies: Robert Espinoza, page 1230.

Bibliography

Abril, K., Diaz, S., Yasui, T., Collins, K., & Elsabrout, K. (2019). Inhaled peppermint aromatherapy for treatment of postoperative nausea and vomiting: A complement to traditional pharmacologic treatments. *MEDSURG Nursing, 28*(6), 375–380.

American Association of Critical Care Nurses. (2016). AACN practice alert: Preventing venous thromboembolism in adults. *Critical Care Nurse, 36*(5), e20–e23.

American Society of Anesthesiologists. (2017). Practice guidelines for preoperative fasting and the use of pharmacologic agents to reduce the risk of pulmonary aspiration: Application to healthy patients undergoing elective procedures. An updated report by the American Society of Anesthesiologists Task Force on Preoperative Fasting and the use of Pharmacologic Agents to Reduce the Risk of Pulmonary Aspiration. *Anesthesiology, 126*(3), 376–393. https://doi.org/10.1097/ALN.0000000000001452

Apfelbaum, J. L., Silverstein, J. H., Chung, F. F., Connis, R. T., Fillmore, R. B., Hunt, S. E., Nickinovich, D. G., Schreiner, M. S., Silverstein, J. H., Apfelbaum, J. L., Barlow, J. C., Chung, F. F., Connis, R. T., Fillmore, R. B., Hunt, S. E., Joas, T. A., Nickinovich, D. G., & American Society of Anesthesiologists Task Force on Postanesthetic Care. (2013). Practice guidelines for postanesthetic care: A report by the American Society of Anesthesiologists Task Force on Postanesthetic Care. *Anesthesiology, 118*(2), 291–307. https://doi.org/10.1097/ALN.0b013e31827773e9

Aranha, P. R., & Dsouza, S. N. (2019). Preoperative information needs of parents: A descriptive survey. *Journal of Research in Nursing, 24*(5), 305–314. DOI: 10.1177/1744987118821708

Association of periOperative Registered Nurses (AORN). (2017). *Guidelines for perioperative practice.* Denver, CO: AORN, Inc.

Association of periOperative Registered Nurses (AORN). (2018). Guideline summary: Prevention of venous thromboembolism. *AORN Journal, 107*(6), 750–754. http://doi.org/10.1002/aorn.12147

Association of periOperative Registered Nurses (AORN). (2019). Guideline quick overview: Hypothermia. *AORN Journal, 110*(4), 463–465. https://doi.org/10.1002/aorn.12843

Association of periOperative Registered Nurses (AORN). (2020). *Guidelines for perioperative practice.* https://www.aorn.org/guidelines

Bastable, S. B. (2017). *Essentials of patient education* (2nd ed.). Jones & Bartlett Learning.

Borczynski, E., & Worobel-Luk, P. (2019). Capnography monitoring of patients with obstructive sleep apnea in the post-anesthesia care unit: A best practice implementation project. *JBI Database of Systematic Reviews and Implementation Projects, 17*(7), 1532–1547. https://doi.org/10.11124/JBISRIR-2017-003939

Boston Medical Center and Boston University School of Medicine. (n.d.). *I COUGH.* Retrieved October 20, 2020, from https://www.bumc.bu.edu/surgery/quality-safety/i-cough/

Branson, R. D. (2013). The scientific basis for postoperative respiratory care. *Respiratory Care, 58*(11), 1974–1984. https://doi.org/10.4187/respcare.02832

Broback, B. E., Skutle, G. Ø., Dysvik, E., & Eskeland, A. (2018). Preoperative warming with a forced-air warming blanket prevents hypothermia during surgery. *Norwegian Journal of Clinical Nursing, 13*, e65819. https://doi.org/10.4220/Sykepleienf.2018.65819

Burns, S. M., & Delgado, S. A. (2019). *AACN essentials of critical care nursing* (4th ed.). McGraw Hill Education.

Cassidy, M. R., Rosenkranz, P., Macht, R. D., Talutis, S., & McAneny, D. (2020). The I COUGH multidisciplinary perioperative pulmonary care program: One decade of experience. *The Joint Commission Journal on Quality and Patient Safety, 46*(5), 241–249. https://doi.org/10.1016/j.jcjq.2020.01.005

Cassidy, M. R., Rosenkranz, P., McCabe, K., Rosen, J. E., & McAneny, D. (2013). I COUGH: Reducing postoperative pulmonary complications with a multidisciplinary patient care program. *JAMA Surgery, 148*(8), 740–745. https://doi.org/10.1001/jamasurg.2013.358

Chou, R., Gordon, D. B., de Leon-Casasola, O. A., Rosenberg, J. M., Bickler, S., Brennan, T., Carter, T., Cassidy, C. L., Chittenden, E. H., Dengenhardt, E., Griffith, S., Manworren, R., McCarberg, B., Montgomery, R., Murphy, J., Perkal, M. F., Suresh, S., Sluka, K., Strassels, S., … Wu, C. L. (2016). Management of postoperative pain: A clinical practice guideline from the American Pain Society, the American Society of Regional Anesthesia and Pain Medicine, and the American Society of Anesthesiologists' Committee on Regional Anesthesia, Executive Committee, and Administrative Council. *The Journal of Pain, 17*(2), 131–157. http://dx.doi.org/10.1016/j.jpain.2015.12.008

Croke, L. (2020a). Open communication and empathy during perioperative stage can ease patient anxiety. *AORN Journal, 111*(2), P5. http://dx.doi.org/10.1002/aorn.12968

Croke, L. (2020b). Nonpharmacologic strategies to help reduce preoperative patient anxiety. *AORN Journal, 111*(2), P8–P10. http://dx.doi.org/10.1002/aorn.12970

de la Vega, J., Gilliand, C., Martinez, L., Nardi, B., & Pierce, N. L. (2019). Aromatherapy in the PACU. *Journal of Perianesthesia Nursing, 34*(4), E51.

Downey, C., Randell, R., Brown, J., & Jayne, D. G. (2018). Continuous versus intermittent vital signs monitoring using a wearable, wireless patch in patients admitted to surgical wards: Pilot cluster randomized controlled trial. *Journal of Medical Internet Research, 20*(12), e10802. http://dx.doi.org/10.2196/10802.10.2196/10802

Eliopoulos, C. (2018). *Gerontological nursing* (9th ed.). Wolters Kluwer.

Fan, C., Jia, L., Fang, F., Zhang, Y., Faramand, A., Chong, W., & Hai, Y. (2020). Adjunctive intermittent pneumatic compression in hospitalized patients receiving pharmacologic prophylaxis for venous thromboprophylaxis: A systematic review and meta-analysis. *Journal of Nursing Scholarship, 52*(4), 397–405. http://dx.doi.org/10.1111/jnu.12566

Feil, M. (2017). Warming blankets and patient harm. *PA Patient Safety Advisory, 14*(4), 1–5. http://patientsafety.pa.gov/ADVISORIES/documents/201712_warmingdevices.pdf

Fischbach, F. T., & Fischbach, M. A. (2018). *A manual of laboratory and diagnostic tests* (10th ed.). Wolters Kluwer.

Hall, K. R., & Stanley, A. Y. (2019). Literature review: Assessment of opioid-related sedation and the Pasero Opioid Sedation Scale. *Journal of PeriAnesthesia Nursing, 34*(1), 132–142. https://doi.org/10.1016/j.jopan.2017.12.009

Hess, D. R., MacIntyre, N. R., Galvin, W. F., & Mishoe, S. C. (2021). *Respiratory care: Principles and practice* (4th ed.). Jones & Bartlett Learning.

Hinkle, J. L., Cheever, K. H., & Overbaugh, K. J. (2022). *Brunner & Suddarth's Textbook of medical-surgical nursing* (15th ed.). Wolters Kluwer.

International Council of Nurses (ICN). (2019). *Nursing diagnosis and outcome statements.* https://www.icn.ch/sites/default/files/inline-files/ICNP2019-DC.pdf

Jarvis, C., & Echkardt, A. (2020). *Physical examination & health assessment* (8th ed.). Elsevier.

Jensen, S. (2019). *Nursing health assessment. A best practice approach* (3rd ed.). Wolters Kluwer.

John, M., Ford, J., & Harper, M. (2014). Perioperative warming devices: performance and clinical application. *Anaesthesia, 69*(6), 623–638. https://doi.org/10.1111/anae.12626

The Joint Commission. (2020, July 1). *National patient safety goals.* https://www.jointcommission.org/standards/national-patient-safety-goals/hospital-2020-national-patient-safety-goals/

The Joint Commission. (n.d.). *The Universal Protocol for Preventing Wrong Site, Wrong Procedure, and Wrong Person Surgery™.* Retrieved October 18, 2020, from https://www.jointcommission.org/standards/universal-protocol/

Jungquist, C. R., Smith, K., Wiltse Nicely, K. L., & Polomano, R. C. (2017). Monitoring hospitalized adult patients for opioid-induced sedation and respiratory depression. *American Journal of Nursing, 117*(3 Suppl 1), S27–S35. https://doi.org/10.1097/01.NAJ.0000513528.79557.33

Karaman, S., Karaman, T., Tapar, H., Dogru, S., & Suren, M. (2019). A randomized placebo-controlled study of aromatherapy for the treatment of postoperative nausea and vomiting. *Complementary Therapies in Medicine, 42*, 417–421. https://doi.org/10.1016/j.ctim.2018.12.019

Karch, A. M. (2020). *Focus on nursing pharmacology* (8th ed.). Wolters Kluwer.

Koyuncu, O., Urfali, S., Hakimoğlu, S., & Taşdoğan, A. M. (2020). Strategies to prevent postoperative nausea and vomiting. *Turkish Journal of Oncology, 35*(3), 349–355. https://doi.org/10.5505/tjo.2020.2270

Kyle, T., & Carman, S. (2021). *Essentials of pediatric nursing* (4th ed.). Wolters Kluwer.

Link, T. (2020). Guidelines in practice: Hypothermia prevention. *AORN Journal, 111*(6), 654–663. https://doi.org/10.1002/aorn.13038

Lumb, A. B. (2019). Pre-operative respiratory optimisation: An expert review. *Anaesthesia, 74*(Suppl 1), 43–48. https://doi.org/10.1111/anae.14508

Milotte, H., Carroll, D. L., & Coakley, A. (2018). The effect of a therapeutic pillow on pain following a nephrectomy: A randomized clinical trial. *Urologic Nursing, 38*(3), 137–143. https://doi.org/10.7257/1053-816X.2018.38.3.137

Mok, W. Q., Ullal, M. J., Su, S., Yiap, P. L., Yu, L. H., Lim, S. M. M., Ker, S. Y. J., & Wang, J. (2019). An integrative care bundle to prevent surgical site infections among surgical hip patients: A retrospective cohort study. *American Journal of Infection Control, 47*(5), 540–544. https://doi.org/10.1016/j.ajic.2018.10.011

Nieh, H. C., & Su, S. F. (2018). Force-air warming for rewarming and comfort following laparoscopy: A randomized controlled trial. *Clinical Nursing Research, 27*(5), 540–559. https://doi.org/10.1177/1054773817708082 journals.sagepub.com/home/cnr

Norris, T. L. (2019). *Porth's essentials of pathophysiology* (5th ed.). Wolters Kluwer.

Parry, A. (2018). Preventing infection in surgical patients. *British Journal of Nursing, 27*(21), 1218–1220.

Polomano, R. C., Fillman, M., Giordano, N. A., Vallerand, A. H., Wiltse Nicely, K. L., & Jungquist, C. R. (2017). Multimodal analgesia for acute postoperative and trauma-related pain. *American Journal of Nursing, 117*(3 Suppl 1), S12–S26. https://doi.org/10.1097/01.NAJ.0000513527.71934.73

Poulsen, M. J., Coto, J., & Cooney, M. F. (2019). Music as a postoperative pain management intervention. *Journal of PeriAnesthesia Nursing, 34*(3), 662–666. https://doi.org/10.1016/j.jopan.2019.01.003

Restrepo, R. D., Wettstein, R., Wittnebel, L., & Tracy, M. (2011). AARC clinical practice guideline: Incentive spirometry. *Respiratory Care, 56*(10), 1600–1604.

Riddle, D., & Stannard, D. (2014). Evidence in perioperative care. *Nursing Clinics of North America, 49*(4), 485–492. https://doi.org/10.1016/j.cnur.2014.08.004

Robertson, M., & Ford, C. (2020). Care of the surgical patient: Part 1. *British Journal of Nursing, 29*(16), 934–939. DOI: 10.12968/bjon.2020.29.16.934

Silbert-Flagg, J., & Pillitteri, A. (2018). *Maternal and child health nursing* (8th ed.). Wolters Kluwer.

Spruce, L. (2020a). Reducing the risk of surgical site infections with effective preoperative patient skin antisepsis. *AORN Journal, 112*(1), 82–83. https://doi.org/10.1002/aorn.13089

Spruce, L. (2020b). Using a complementary intervention to decrease postoperative nausea and vomiting. *AORN Journal, 112*(4), 417–418. http://doi.org/10.1002/aorn.13193

Spruce, L. (2020c). Perioperative warming methods prevent unintended hypothermia. *AORN Journal, 112*(2), 174–175. https://doi.org/10.1002/aorn.13119

Strickland, S. L., Rubin, B. K., Drescher, G. S., Haas, C. F., O'Malley, C. A., Volsko, T. A., Branson, R. D., Hess, D. R., & American Association for Respiratory Care, Irving, Texas. (2013). AARC clinical practice guideline: Effectiveness of nonpharmacologic airway clearance therapies in hospitalized patients. *Respiratory Care, 58*(12), 2187–2193. https://doi.org/10.4187/respcare.02925

Subramaniam, R. (2019). Anaesthetic concerns in preterm and term neonates. *Indian Journal of Anaesthesia, 63*(9), 771–779. https://doi.org/10.4103/ija.IJA_591_19

Taylor, C., Lynn, P., & Bartlett, J. L. (2020). *Fundamentals of nursing: The art and science of person-centered care* (10th ed.). Wolters Kluwer.

Tubog, T. D. (2019). Combined intermittent pneumatic leg compression and pharmacological prophylaxis for prevention of venous thromboembolism. *Orthopaedic Nursing, 38*(4), 270–272. https://doi.org/10.1097/NOR.0000000000000574

Turunen, E., Miettinen, M., Setälä, L., & Vehviläinen-Julkunen, K. (2017). An integrative review of a preoperative nursing care structure. *Journal of Clinical Nursing, 26*(7–8), 915–930. https://doi.org/10.1111/jocn.13448

Verrillo, S. C., Cvach, M., Hudson, K. W., & Winters, B. D. (2019). Using continuous vital sign monitoring to detect early deterioration in adult postoperative inpatients. *Journal of Nursing Care Quality, 34*(2), 107–113. https://doi.org/10.1097/NCQ.0000000000000350

VHA Center for Engineering & Occupational Safety and Health (CEOSH). (2016). *Safe patient handling and mobility guidebook*. http://www.tnpatientsafety.com/pubfiles/Initiatives/workplace-violence/sphm-pdf.pdf

Weber, J. R., & Kelley, J. H. (2018). *Health assessment in nursing* (6th ed.). Wolters Kluwer.

Wolters Kluwer. (2022). Problem-based care plans. In *Lippincott Advisor*. Wolters Kluwer.

Xu, H., Xu, G., Ren, C, Liu, L., & Wei, L. (2019). Effect of forced-air warming system in prevention of postoperative hypothermia in elderly patients. A prospective controlled trial. *Medicine, 98*(22), 1–6. http://dx.doi.org/10.1097/MD.0000000000015895

SUGGESTED ANSWERS FOR FOCUSING ON PATIENT CARE: DEVELOPING CLINICAL REASONING AND CLINICAL JUDGMENT

1. Preoperative medications may be prescribed for administration before transfer to the preoperative holding area or for administration in the preoperative holding area. The nurse needs to call the nursing staff in the preoperative holding area. The nurse should explain the circumstances, identify the prescribed medication, and state that the medication was not administered. Depending on facility policy and procedure, the nurse should also notify the health care team, in this case the surgeon, of the missed medication dose. It is important that the appropriate health care personnel are aware of the missing dose of medication, so that appropriate action can be taken to ensure the patient receives the required medication to prevent intraoperative or postoperative complications.

2. The nurse needs to consider the onset of action and peak effect of the administered medication. If the appropriate time has not lapsed for the medication to take effect, the nurse should provide further explanation and reassurance to the patient. The nurse should initiate additional nonpharmacologic interventions to aid in pain management (refer to Chapter 10, Comfort). If the pain persists, the nurse should perform a complete pain assessment (refer to Chapter 10, Comfort). In addition, the nurse should assess for other postoperative complications. Pain can be a clue to other problems, such as hemorrhage. The nurse should notify the primary care provider of the initial assessment findings, information regarding analgesics administered, nonpharmacologic interventions, and the patient's response to interventions. In addition, some patients do not obtain adequate relief from the initial analgesic prescribed and require a change in analgesics to achieve adequate pain management.

3. Monitor the patient's temperature at least every 30 minutes while using the forced-air device. If rewarming a patient with hypothermia, do not raise temperature too quickly to prevent a rapid vasodilation effect. The nurse should not have waited 60 minutes to recheck the patient's temperature. Ms. Gibbs is experiencing the effects of rapid vasodilation, resulting in lowered blood pressure and increased heart rate. The nurse should discontinue the forced-air warming device. Assess the patient's cardiovascular and respiratory status. Notify the primary care provider of the assessment findings. Provide for the patient's safety; make sure the call bell is within reach and instruct the patient to remain in bed, to avoid a fall or other injury related to hypotension. Monitor the patient's vital signs at least every 30 minutes. Be prepared to reapply the forced-air heating device if the patient's temperature drops below prescribed limits.

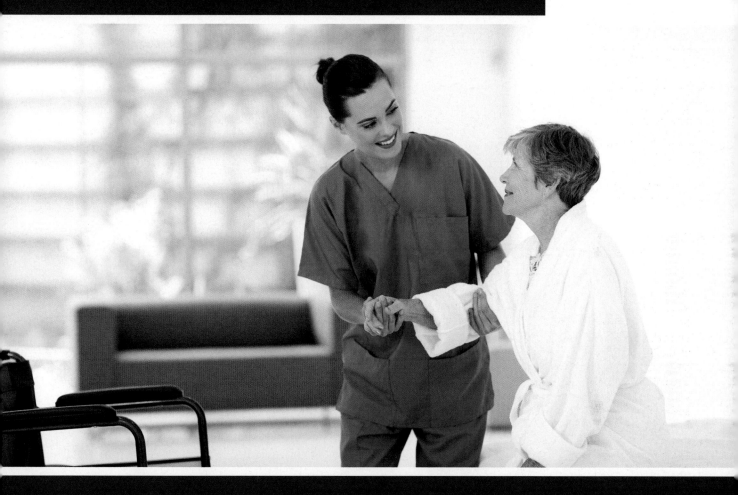

Promoting Healthy Physiologic Responses

7

Hygiene

Focusing on Patient Care

This chapter will help you develop some of the skills related to hygiene that may be necessary to care for the following patients:

Denasia Kerr, age 6, who lives in a pediatric long-term care facility, has limited mobility, and needs her hair washed.

Cindy Vortex, age 34, who is in a coma after a car accident and needs her contact lenses removed.

Carl Sheen, age 76, who needs help cleaning his dentures.

Refer to Focusing on Patient Care: Developing Clinical Reasoning and Clinical Judgment at the end of the chapter to apply what you learn.

Learning Outcomes

After completing the chapter, you will be able to accomplish the following:

1. Assist with a shower or tub bath.
2. Provide a bed bath.
3. Assist with oral care.
4. Provide oral care for a dependent patient.
5. Provide denture care.
6. Remove contact lenses.
7. Shampoo a patient's hair in bed.
8. Assist with shaving.
9. Provide nail care.
10. Make an unoccupied bed.
11. Make an occupied bed.

Nursing Concepts

- Assessment
- Clinical decision making/clinical judgment
- Comfort
- Functional ability
- Safety

Personal hygiene involves measures for maintaining a minimal level of personal cleanliness and grooming that promotes physical and psychological well-being. Personal hygiene practices vary widely among people. The time of day one bathes, how often a person shampoos his or her hair, and how often a person changes their bed linens are very individualized choices.

People who are well ordinarily are responsible for their own hygiene. In some cases, the nurse may provide teaching to assist a well person to develop personal hygiene habits they may lack. Acute and chronic illness, hospitalization, and institutionalization may make it necessary to modify hygiene practices. In these situations, the nurse helps the patient to continue sound hygiene practices and can teach the patient and family members/caregivers, when necessary, about hygiene. When assisting with basic hygiene, it is important to respect individual patient preferences and provide only the care those patients cannot, or should not, provide for themselves. Patient care flow sheets are documentation tools used to record routine aspects of nursing care and are often used to document hygiene-related interventions. Figure 7-1 shows an example of a patient care flow sheet that is part of an electronic health record.

This chapter covers skills that the nurse needs to promote hygiene, including bathing, skin care, oral care, removing dentures and contact lenses, shampooing hair, shaving, and changing bed linens. Fundamentals Review 7-1 outlines general skin care principles.

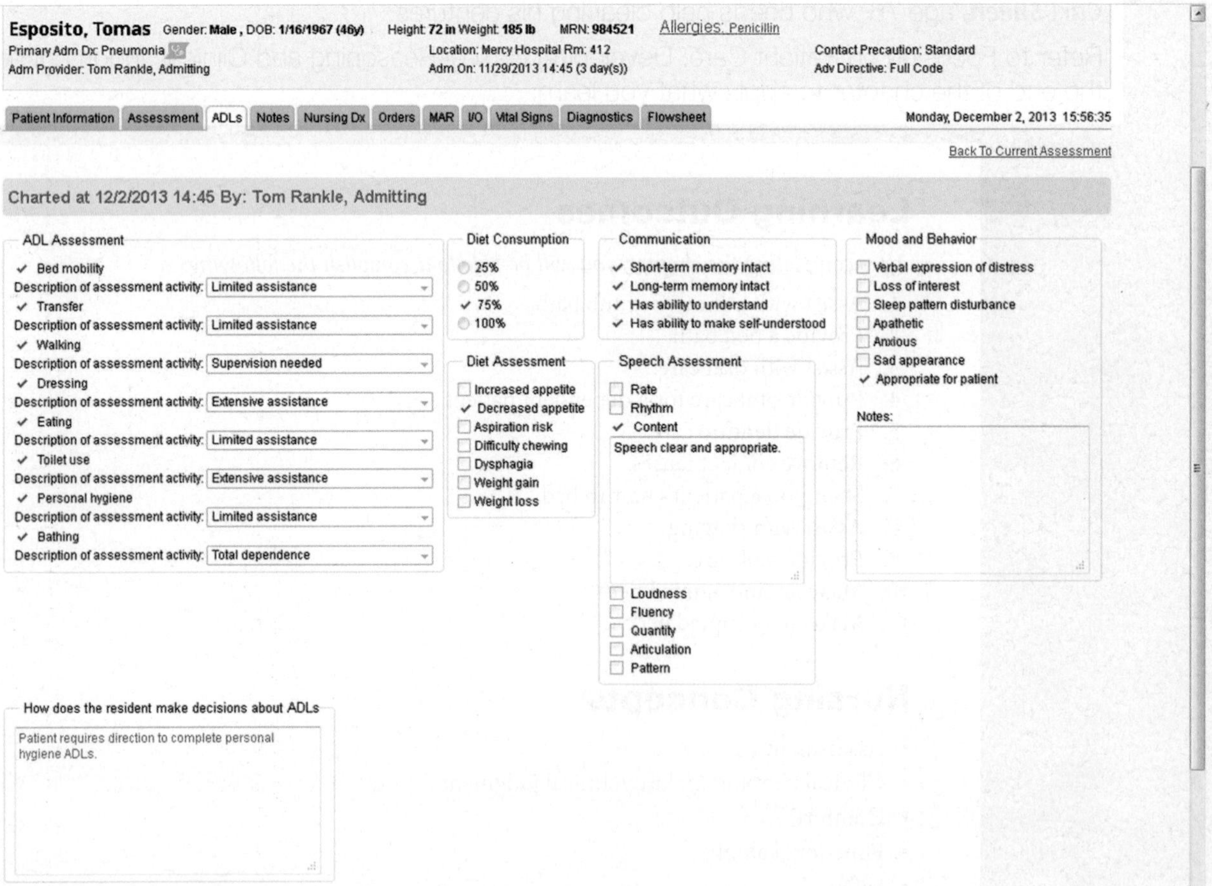

Esposito, Tomas Gender: Male, DOB: 1/16/1967 (46y) Height: 72 in Weight: 185 lb MRN: 984521 Allergies: Penicillin
Primary Adm Dx: Pneumonia
Adm Provider: Tom Rankle, Admitting
Location: Mercy Hospital Rm: 412
Adm On: 11/29/2013 14:45 (3 day(s))
Contact Precaution: Standard
Adv Directive: Full Code

Patient Information | Assessment | ADLs | Notes | Nursing Dx | Orders | MAR | I/O | Vital Signs | Diagnostics | Flowsheet

Monday, December 2, 2013 15:56:35

Back To Current Assessment

Charted at 12/2/2013 14:45 By: Tom Rankle, Admitting

ADL Assessment
✓ Bed mobility
Description of assessment activity: Limited assistance
✓ Transfer
Description of assessment activity: Limited assistance
✓ Walking
Description of assessment activity: Supervision needed
✓ Dressing
Description of assessment activity: Extensive assistance
✓ Eating
Description of assessment activity: Limited assistance
✓ Toilet use
Description of assessment activity: Extensive assistance
✓ Personal hygiene
Description of assessment activity: Limited assistance
✓ Bathing
Description of assessment activity: Total dependence

Diet Consumption
25%
50%
✓ 75%
100%

Diet Assessment
☐ Increased appetite
✓ Decreased appetite
☐ Aspiration risk
☐ Difficulty chewing
☐ Dysphagia
☐ Weight gain
☐ Weight loss

Communication
✓ Short-term memory intact
✓ Long-term memory intact
✓ Has ability to understand
✓ Has ability to make self-understood

Speech Assessment
☐ Rate
☐ Rhythm
✓ Content
Speech clear and appropriate.
☐ Loudness
☐ Fluency
☐ Quantity
☐ Articulation
☐ Pattern

Mood and Behavior
☐ Verbal expression of distress
☐ Loss of interest
☐ Sleep pattern disturbance
☐ Apathetic
☐ Anxious
☐ Sad appearance
✓ Appropriate for patient
Notes:

How does the resident make decisions about ADLs
Patient requires direction to complete personal hygiene ADLs.

FIGURE 7-1. Patient Care Flow Sheet as part of an electronic health record.

Fundamentals Review 7-1

GENERAL SKIN CARE PRINCIPLES

- Assess the patient's skin at least daily and after every episode of incontinence.
- Cleanse the skin, when indicated, such as when soiled, using a no-rinse, pH-balanced cleanser.
- Avoid using soap and hot water; avoid excessive friction and scrubbing.

- Minimize skin exposure to moisture (incontinence, wound leakage); use a skin barrier product as necessary.
- Use skin emollients after bathing and as needed.

Source: Adapted from Lichterfeld, A., Hauss, A., Surber, C., Peters, T., Blume-Peytavi, U., & Lottner, J. (2015). Evidence-based skin care: A systematic literature review and the development of a basic skin care algorithm. *Journal of Wound, Ostomy, and Continence Nursing,* *42*(5), 501–524. https://doi.org/10.1097/WON.0000000000000162; Wounds UK. (2018). *Best practice statement. Maintaining skin integrity.* https://www.wounds-uk.com/resources/details/maintaining-skin-integrity

Skill 7-1 ▶ Assisting With a Shower or Tub Bath

A shower may be the preferred method of bathing for patients who are ambulatory and able to tolerate the activity. Tub baths may be an option, particularly in long-term care or other community-based settings, depending on facility policy, as well as in a patient's home environment. Tub, or immersion, bathing can provide positive physical and mental effects, including mental and physical relaxation, decreased stress, and relief of menstrual cramps and labor contractions (Benfield et al., 2018; Goto et al., 2018).

Bathing is performed in a matter-of-fact and dignified manner. Make any necessary adaptations for individual patients to achieve person-centered bathing (Gozalo et al., 2014; Scales et al., 2018; Whitehead & Golding-Day, 2018). For example, if the patient is confused and becomes agitated as a result of overstimulation when bathing, reduce the stimuli. Turn down the lights and play soft music and/or warm the room before taking the patient into it (Konno et al., 2014). Box 7-1 outlines possible measures to implement to meet the bathing needs of patients with dementia.

Box 7-1 Meeting the Bathing Needs of Patients With Dementia

- Shift the focus of the interaction from the "task of bathing" to the needs and abilities of the patient. Focus on comfort, safety, autonomy, and self-esteem, in addition to cleanliness.
- Individualize patient care. Consult the patient, the patient's record, family members, and other caregivers to determine patient preferences.
- Consider what can be learned from the behaviors associated with dementia about the needs and preferences of the patient. A patient's behavior may be an expression of unmet needs; unwillingness to participate may be a response to uncomfortable water temperatures or levels of sound or light in the room.
- Ensure privacy and warmth.
- Consider the use of music to soothe anxiety and agitation.
- Consider other methods for bathing. Showers and tub baths are not the only options in bathing. Towel baths,

washing under clothes, and bathing "body sections" one day at a time are other possible options.
- Maintain a relaxed demeanor. Use calming language. Use one-step commands. Try to determine phrases and terms the patient understands in relation to bathing and make use of them. Offer frequent reassurance.
- Encourage independence. Use hand-over-hand or a guided hand technique to cue the patient regarding the purpose of the interaction and allow the patient to perform some of the activities independently.
- Explore the need for routine analgesia before bathing. Move limbs carefully and be aware of signs of discomfort during bathing.
- Wash the face and hair at the end of the bath or at a separate time. Water dripping in the face and having a wet head are often the most upsetting parts of the bathing process for people with dementia.

Source: Adapted from Gallagher, M., Hall, G. R., & Butcher H. K. (2014). Bathing persons with Alzheimer's disease and related dementias. *Journal of Gerontological Nursing, 40*(2), 14–20; Konno, R., Kang, H. S., & Makimoto, K. (2014). A best-evidence review of intervention studies for minimizing resistance-to-care behaviours for older adults with dementia in nursing homes. *Journal of Advanced Nursing, 70*(10), 2167–2180; and Toughy, T. A., & Jett, K. (2018). *Ebersol and Hess' gerontological nursing & healthy aging* (5th ed.). Elsevier.

(continued on page 392)

Skill 7-1 ▶ Assisting With a Shower or Tub Bath *(continued)*

DELEGATION CONSIDERATIONS	The implementation of a shower or tub bath may be delegated to assistive personnel (AP) as well as to licensed practical/vocational nurses (LPN/LVNs). The decision to delegate must be based on careful analysis of the patient's needs and circumstances as well as the qualifications of the person to whom the task is being delegated. Refer to the Delegation Guidelines in Appendix A.

EQUIPMENT

- Personal hygiene supplies (deodorant, lotion, and others)
- Skin-cleaning agent
- Emollient and skin barrier, as indicated
- Towels and washcloths
- Robe (as indicated) and slippers or nonskid socks
- Gown or pajamas, or clothing (as indicated)
- Laundry bag
- Shower or tub chair, as needed
- Nonsterile gloves, as indicated
- Additional PPE, as indicated

ASSESSMENT

Assess the patient's knowledge of hygiene practices and bathing preferences: frequency, time of day, and type of hygiene products. Assess for any physical activity limitations. Assess the patient's ability to perform and participate with bathing activities. Assess the patient's skin for dryness, redness, or areas of breakdown, and gather any other appropriate supplies that may be needed as a result of the assessment.

ACTUAL OR POTENTIAL HEALTH PROBLEMS AND NEEDS

Many actual or potential health problems or issues may require the use of this skill as part of related interventions. An appropriate health problem or issue may include:
- Impaired ability to bath
- Injury risk
- Activity intolerance

OUTCOME IDENTIFICATION AND PLANNING

The expected outcome to achieve when assisting with a shower or tub bath is that the patient will be clean and fresh and without injury. Other outcomes that may be appropriate include the following: the patient regains feelings of control by assisting with the bath, the patient verbalizes a positive body image, and the patient demonstrates understanding about the need for hygiene measures.

IMPLEMENTATION

ACTION	RATIONALE
1. Review the patient's health record for any limitations in physical activity. Check prescribed interventions for clearing the patient to shower, if required by facility policy.	Identifying limitations prevents patient discomfort and injury. In some settings, a prescribed intervention is required for showering.
2. Check to see that the bathroom is available, clean, and safe. Make sure showers and tubs have mats or nonskid strips to prevent patients from falling. Place a mat or towel on the floor in front of the shower or tub. Put a shower or tub chair in place, as appropriate. Place "occupied" sign on door of room, as appropriate for setting.	A clean bathroom prevents transmission of microorganisms. Mats and nonskid materials prevent patients from slipping and falling. Having a place for a weak or physically disabled patient to sit in a shower prevents falls; warm water could cause vasodilation and pooling of blood in lower extremities, contributing to lightheadedness or dizziness. Use of a sign allows others to be aware of use of the room and ensures patient privacy.
3. Gather necessary hygienic and toiletry items and linens. Place within easy reach of shower or tub.	Bringing everything to the bathing location conserves time and energy. Arranging items nearby is convenient, saves time, and avoids unnecessary reaching and possible falls.
4. Perform hand hygiene.	Hand hygiene prevents the spread of microorganisms.

ACTION

5. Identify the patient. Discuss the procedure with the patient and assess the patient's ability to assist in the bathing process, as well as personal hygiene preferences.

6. Assist the patient to bathroom to void or defecate, if appropriate.

7. Assist the patient to put on a robe and slippers or nonskid socks. Cover IV access site(s) according to facility policy.

8. Assist the patient to the shower or tub, as indicated.

9. Close the curtains around the shower or tub, as appropriate, and close the door to the bathroom. Adjust the room temperature, if necessary.

    Shower: Turn shower on. Check to see that the water temperature is safe and comfortable.

    Tub: Fill tub halfway with water. Check to see that the water temperature is safe and comfortable.

    Adjust water temperature, if appropriate, based on patient preference (Figure 1). **Water temperature should be adjusted to no more than 120°F to decrease the risk of burns and drying of the skin** (International Association of Fire Fighters [IAFF], n.d.).

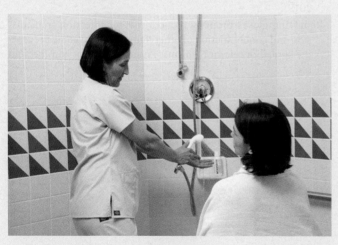

RATIONALE

Identifying the patient ensures the right patient receives the intervention and helps prevent errors. Discussion promotes reassurance and provides knowledge about the procedure. Dialogue encourages patient participation and allows for individualized nursing care.

Voiding or defecating before the bath lessens the likelihood that the bath will be interrupted, because warm bath water may stimulate the urge to void.

This ensures the patient's privacy, prevents chilling, and decreases the risk for slipping and fallings. Coverage of IV site prevents loosening of dressings from exposure to moisture, protects the site, and maintains integrity of IV access (Gorski et al., 2021).

This prevents accidental falls.

This ensures the patient's privacy and lessens the risk for loss of body heat during the bath. Warm water is relaxing, stimulates circulation, and provides for more effective cleansing. Adjusting the water temperature to no more than 120°F (49°C) decreases risk of burns and drying of the skin (IAFF, n.d.).

FIGURE 1. Adjusting water temperature.

10. Explain the use of the call device and ensure that it is within the reach of the shower or tub.

11. Put on gloves, as indicated. Help the patient get in and out of the shower or tub, as necessary. Use safety bars in and next to the shower, as needed. For a tub: Have the patient grasp the handrails at the side of the tub, or place a chair at the side of the tub. The patient sits on the chair and eases to the edge of the tub. After putting both feet into the tub, have the patient reach to the opposite side and ease down into the tub. The patient may kneel first in the tub and then sit in it.

Use of the call device allows the patient to call for help if necessary.

Gloves are required if contact with blood or body fluids is anticipated. Gloves prevent the transmission of microorganisms. The use of safety bars prevents slipping and falling.

(continued on page 394)

Skill 7-1 ▶ Assisting With a Shower or Tub Bath   *(continued)*

ACTION	RATIONALE
12. If necessary, use a hydraulic lift, when available, to lower patients who are unable to maneuver safely or completely bear their own weight. Some community-based settings have walk-in tubs available.	This prevents slipping and falling and prevents strain and injury to patients and nurses.
13. Keep room door unlocked. Remain in room with the patient to offer assistance, as appropriate. If assistance is needed with bathing, put on gloves. Otherwise, check on the patient every 5 minutes. **Never leave young children or confused patients alone in the bathroom.**	These actions promote safety. Health personnel should be able to enter with ease if the patient needs help. Gloves are required if contact with blood or body fluids is anticipated. Gloves prevent the transmission of microorganisms.
14. Assist the patient out of the shower or tub when bathing is complete. Obtain the assistance of additional personnel, as appropriate. Use safety bars. For a tub: Drain the water from the tub. Have the patient grasp the handrails at the side of the tub. Assist the patient to the edge of the tub. Have the patient ease to a chair placed at the side of the tub, then remove feet out of tub. The patient may kneel first in the tub and then move to the side of the tub.	This prevents slipping and falling. Use of additional personnel prevents strain and injury to patients and nurses.
15. If necessary, use a hydraulic lift, when available, to raise patients who are unable to maneuver safely or completely bear their own weight.	This prevents slipping and falling and prevents strain and injury to patients and nurses.
16. Put on gloves, as indicated. Assist the patient with drying, application of emollients, and dressing, as appropriate or necessary. Remove cover from IV access site.	Gloves are required if contact with blood or body fluids is anticipated. Gloves prevent the transmission of microorganisms.
	Drying prevents chilling and promotes patient comfort. Use of emollients is recommended to restore and maintain skin integrity (Haesler et al., 2018; Lichterfeld et al., 2015; Voegeli, 2019).
17. Remove gloves, if used. Perform hand hygiene. Assist the patient to the room (Figure 2) and into a position of comfort.	Removing gloves properly reduces risk for infection transmission and contamination of other items. Hand hygiene prevents the spread of microorganisms. Promotes patient comfort and safety.

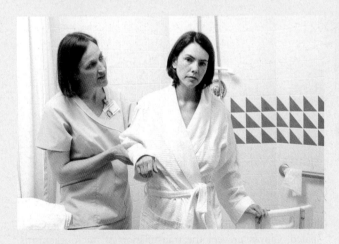

FIGURE 2. Assisting patient to room.

18. Clean shower or tub according to facility policy. Dispose of soiled linens according to facility policy. Remove "occupied" sign from door of bathroom.	Reduces risk for infection transmission and contamination of other items. Allows others to make use of room.
19. Perform hand hygiene.	Hand hygiene prevents the spread of microorganisms.

EVALUATION

The expected outcomes have been met when the patient is clean, the patient has demonstrated some feeling of control in their care, the patient has verbalized an improved body image, and the patient has verbalized understanding of the need for hygiene measures.

DOCUMENTATION

Guidelines

Record any significant observations and communication. Document the condition of the patient's skin. Record the procedure, amount of assistance given, and patient participation. Document the application of skin care products, such as an emollient.

Sample Documentation

> 7/14/25 1030 Shower provided with minimal assistance. Skin intact. Patient states improved sense of cleanliness and increased comfort.
> —C. Stone, RN

DEVELOPING CLINICAL REASONING AND CLINICAL JUDGMENT

UNEXPECTED SITUATIONS AND ASSOCIATED INTERVENTIONS

- *Patient becomes chilled during the bath:* If the room temperature is adjustable, increase temperature. Provide additional assistance to dry and dress quickly, to decrease chilling.
- *Patient becomes excessively fatigued during the bath process:* Allow for rest period sitting down after walking to bathing room and/or completion of bath, before returning to room. Assist the patient to and from bath in wheelchair, to conserve energy. Schedule bath after rest period or nap.

SPECIAL CONSIDERATIONS

General Considerations

- Patients with bariatric needs are at increased risk for skin integrity issues, including increased risk for alterations in skin integrity and therefore require focused nursing care to prevent skin issues (Earlam & Woods, 2020; Williamson, 2020). Assess the skin of bariatric inpatients twice a day, lifting and separating folds of skin to assess the area, utilizing extra help as necessary (Black & Hotaling, 2015). Nonsoap cleansers should be used, and the skin should be dried to prevent retained moisture (Black & Hotaling, 2015; Williamson, 2020).
- Incontinent patients require special attention to perineal care. Patients with urinary or fecal incontinence are at risk for incontinence-associated dermatitis (perineal dermatitis), one type of moisture-associated skin damage (MASD) (Voegeli, 2019). This damage is related to moisture, changes in the pH of the skin, overgrowth of bacteria and infection of the skin, and erosion of perineal skin from friction on moist skin. Remove soil and irritants from the skin during routine hygiene, and clean the area when the skin becomes exposed to irritants (Voegeli, 2019). Avoid using soap and excessive force for cleaning (Wounds UK, 2018). The use of perineal skin cleansers, moisturizers, and moisture barriers is recommended for skin care for the incontinent patient to help promote healing and prevent further skin damage (Voegeli, 2019).
- Basic wound care used for body piercings is usually called "aftercare." Aftercare techniques are used for the new piercing and whenever the piercing fistula has become disrupted through injury or exhibits signs of infection or inflammation (Association of Professional Piercers [APP], 2020; Mayo Foundation for Medical Education and Research [MFMER], 2020b). Clean the site with mild soap and warm water or normal saline solution (American Academy of Family Physicians [AAFP], 2019). Use a cotton swab to gently remove any crusting. Rinse well.

Infant and Child Considerations

- When bathing an infant or young child, have supplies within easy reach, and support or hold the child securely at all times to ensure safety.
- Never leave the child alone.

Older Adult Considerations

- Check the temperature of the water carefully before bathing an older adult, because their sensitivity to temperature may be impaired.
- An older continent adult may not require a bath every day. If dry skin is a problem, water and skin lotion or bath oil may be used on alternate days. Do not use bath oil in tub water, as it can cause tub surfaces to become slippery.

(continued on page 396)

Skill 7-1 ▶ Assisting With a Shower or Tub Bath (continued)

Community-Based Care Considerations

- Evaluate the safety of the bathing area in the home. Tub mats, adhesive strips, grab bars, and shower stools can help prevent falls.
- Instruct patients to apply emollients, lotions, or oils after leaving tub or shower to prevent slipping and falling.

EVIDENCE FOR PRACTICE ▶

EFFECTS OF BATHING

Bathing provides a means to cleanse the skin but also serves a variety of other purposes. Tub (immersion) bathing may provide for mental and physical relaxation and decreased stress (Goto et al., 2018).

Related Research

Goto, Y., Hayasaka, S., Kurihara, S., & Nakamura, Y. (2018). Physical and mental effects of bathing: A randomized intervention study. *Evidence-Based Complementary and Alternative Medicine*, 2018:9521086. https://doi.org/10.1155/2018/9521086

This randomized controlled trial compared the effects on health of immersion bathing and shower bathing. Participants ($n = 38$) were randomized to two groups ($n = 19$ each group). One group bathed for 2 weeks using tub (immersion) bathing (warm water for 10 minutes) and then using showering for 2 weeks. The other group first bathed using shower bathing for the 2 weeks and then tub bathing (warm water for 10 minutes) for the second 2 weeks. Perceived health status was self-reported using a visual analog scale after bathing every day during the intervention periods. The Short Form Health Survey (SF-8) and short form Profile of Mood States (POMS) were used to assess health and mood states after each 2-week intervention period. Paired t-test was used to compare subjective health status before and after bathing every day and between the 2-week bathing intervention and the 2-week showering intervention periods. Visual analog scale scores were significantly lower for fatigue, stress, and pain ($p < .05$) and significantly higher for self-reported health and skin condition ($p < .10$) during the bathing intervention than during showering intervention. The SF-8 Health Survey showed significantly higher general health, mental health, social functioning scores, and Mental Component Summary scores ($p < .05$). Profile of Mood State scores were significantly lower for tension-anxiety, anger–hostility, and depression–dejection ($p < .05$) after the bathing intervention. The researchers concluded that routine tub (immersion) bathing appears to be more beneficial to mental and physical health than routine shower bathing without immersion.

Relevance for Nursing Practice

The results of this study suggest that implementing tub (immersion) bathing procedures are effective in providing positive effects outside of personal hygiene. Nurses should consider implementing tub bathing and encourage patients to consider tub bathing to assist with improving the physical and emotional aspects of quality of life.

Skill 7-2 ▶ Providing a Bed Bath

Skill Variation: *Performing Perineal Cleansing*

Skill Variation: *Giving a Bath Using a Disposable Bathing System*

Some patients must remain in bed as a part of their therapeutic regimen but can still bathe themselves. Physical or mental deficits, such as fatigue or limited range of motion, may make total or partial assistance with bathing in bed the most appropriate intervention to complete personal hygiene. A bed bath may be considered a partial bed bath if the patient is well enough to perform most of the bath, and the nurse needs to assist with washing areas that the patient cannot reach easily. A partial bath may also refer to bathing only those body parts that absolutely have to be cleaned, such as the perineal area, and any soiled body parts. Perform bathing in a matter-of-fact and dignified manner. Many of the bedside skin-cleaning products available today do not require rinsing. After cleaning the body part, dry it thoroughly. See Table 7-1 for a summary of common cleaning and skincare products.

Table 7-1 Cleaning and Skin Care Products

PRODUCT	DESCRIPTION
Bathing cloths	Premoistened, pH-balanced, microwaveable, disposable cloths for rinse-free skin cleaning and moisturizing. Each package provides one complete bath using 8–10 cloths.
Bathing wipes	Packaged dry cloths. Adding water to the cloths causes them to foam, providing rinse-free skin pH-balanced cleaning. Cloths are in a resealable package for multiple uses.
No-rinse body wash and shampoo	No-rinse, concentrated skin cleanser and moisturizer. Mix with water, apply with a cloth, lather, and dry.
Body foam	Foam cleanser and moisturizer to be used as a body wash, no-rinse shampoo, and perineal cleanser. Pump bottle dispenses foam to be applied with a cloth.
Chlorhexidine gluconate	Reduces colonization of skin with pathogens (Hines et al., 2015). Bathing with chlorhexidine may be used to reduce the incidence of hospital-acquired infections, such as central line–associated bloodstream infections (CLABSI) and surgical site infections, and to decrease rates of transmission and infection of resistant microorganisms, as well as to reduce the acquisition of or decolonization with multidrug-resistant organisms (Cassir et al., 2015; Martinez et al., 2020; Musuuza et al., 2019; Reynolds et al., 2019; Shah et al., 2016; Urias et al., 2018). Daily bathing with chlorhexidine has also been shown to decrease the incidence of the risk of ventilator-associated pneumonia (Chen et al., 2015). Chlorhexidine can be added to bath water, but is also available, and easier to use, in prepackaged impregnated cloths.

The use of disposable bath products is an alternative to the traditional use of soap and water. Disposable bath products are prepackaged in single-use units, heated before use, do not require rinsing, and are equally effective at reducing skin bacteria (Matsumoto et al., 2019; Nøddeskou et al., 2015; Veje et al., 2020). Disposable baths eliminate cross-infection (Sturgeon et al., 2019) and may save time (Nøddeskou et al., 2015). Single-use disposable bath products are often more convenient and may be preferred by patients (Nøddeskou et al., 2015; Veje et al., 2019).

Make any necessary adaptations for individual patients to achieve person-centered bathing (Gozalo et al., 2014; Scales et al., 2018; Whitehead & Golding-Day, 2018). For example, if the patient is confused and becomes agitated as a result of overstimulation when bathing, reduce the stimuli. Turn down the lights and play soft music and/or warm the room before giving the patient a bath (Konno et al., 2014). Box 7-1 in Skill 7-1 outlines possible measures to implement to meet the bathing needs of patients with dementia.

This skill reviews providing a bed bath using water, skin cleanser, and a minimal number of wash cloths. An alternative approach is to use multiple cloth washcloths, using a new washcloth for each body area. The Skill Variation at the end of the skill offers guidelines to provide a bath using a disposable bathing system.

DELEGATION CONSIDERATIONS

The implementation of a bed bath may be delegated to assistive personnel (AP) as well as to licensed practical/vocational nurses (LPN/LVNs). The decision to delegate must be based on careful analysis of the patient's needs and circumstances as well as the qualifications of the person to whom the task is being delegated. Refer to the Delegation Guidelines in Appendix A.

EQUIPMENT

- Washbasin and warm water
- Personal hygiene supplies (deodorant, lotion, and others)
- Skin-cleaning agent
- Emollient and skin barrier, as indicated
- Towels (2)
- Washcloths (2)
- Bath blanket
- Gown, pajamas, or appropriate clothing
- Bedpan or urinal
- Laundry bag
- Nonsterile gloves; other PPE, as indicated

(continued on page 398)

Skill 7-2 ▶ Providing a Bed Bath *(continued)*

ASSESSMENT

Assess the patient's knowledge of hygiene practices and bathing preferences: frequency, time of day, and type of hygiene products. Assess for any physical activity limitations. Assess the patient's ability to bathe independently. Allow the patient to do any part of the bath that they can do. For example, the patient may be able to wash the face, while the nurse does the rest. Assess the patient's skin for dryness, redness, or areas of breakdown, and gather any other appropriate supplies that may be needed as a result of the assessment.

ACTUAL OR POTENTIAL HEALTH PROBLEMS AND NEEDS

Many actual or potential health problems or issues may require the use of this skill as part of related interventions. An appropriate health problem or issue may include:
- Impaired ability to bath
- Injury risk
- Activity intolerance

OUTCOME IDENTIFICATION AND PLANNING

The expected outcome to achieve when giving a bed bath is that the patient will be clean and fresh. Other outcomes that may be appropriate include the following: the patient regains feelings of control by assisting with the bath, the patient verbalizes a positive body image, and the patient demonstrates understanding about the need for hygiene measures.

IMPLEMENTATION

ACTION	RATIONALE
1. Review the patient's health record for any limitations in physical activity.	Identifying limitations prevents patient discomfort and injury.
2. Perform hand hygiene and put on gloves and/or other PPE, if indicated.	Hand hygiene and PPE prevent the spread of microorganisms. PPE is required based on transmission precautions.
3. Identify the patient. Discuss the procedure with the patient and assess the patient's ability to assist in the bathing process, as well as personal hygiene preferences.	Identifying the patient ensures the right patient receives the intervention and helps prevent errors. Discussion promotes reassurance and provides knowledge about the procedure. Dialogue encourages patient participation and allows for individualized nursing care.
4. Assemble equipment on the overbed table or other surface within reach.	Organization facilitates performance of the task.
5. Close the curtains around the bed and close the door to the room, if possible. Adjust the room temperature, if necessary.	This ensures the patient's privacy and lessens the risk for loss of body heat during the bath.
6. Adjust the bed to a comfortable working height (VHA Center for Engineering & Occupational Safety and Health [VHACEOSH], 2016).	Having the bed at the proper height prevents back and muscle strain.
7. Remove sequential compression devices (refer to Skill 9-11) and graduated compression (antiembolism) stockings (refer to Skill 9-10) from lower extremities according to facility protocol.	Most manufacturers and facilities recommend removal of these devices before the bath to allow for assessment.
8. Put on gloves. Offer the patient a bedpan or urinal.	Gloves are necessary for potential contact with blood or body fluids. Voiding or defecating before the bath lessens the likelihood that the bath will be interrupted, because warm bath water may stimulate the urge to void.
9. Remove gloves and perform hand hygiene.	Hand hygiene deters the spread of microorganisms.
10. Put on a clean pair of gloves. Lower the side rail nearest to you and assist the patient to the side of bed where you will work. Have the patient lie on their back.	Gloves prevent transmission of microorganisms. Having the patient positioned near the nurse and lowering the side rail prevent unnecessary stretching and twisting of muscles on the part of the nurse.

ACTION

11. Loosen top covers and remove all except the top sheet. Place a bath blanket over the patient and then remove the top sheet while the patient holds the bath blanket in place. If linen is to be reused, fold it over a chair. Place soiled linen in laundry bag. Take care to prevent linen from coming in contact with your clothing.

12. Remove the patient's gown or clothing and keep the bath blanket in place. If the patient has an IV line and is not wearing a gown with snap sleeves, remove gown from the other arm first. Pause the infusion pump and remove the tubing from the pump. Lower the IV container and pass the gown over the tubing and the container. **Rehang the IV container and insert the tubing into the infusion pump. Check the rate on the infusion pump and restart.**

13. **Raise side rails and lower the bed.** Fill basin with a sufficient amount of comfortably warm water (no more than 120°F [49°C]). Add the skin cleanser, if appropriate, according to the manufacturer's directions. Change, as necessary, throughout the bath.

14. Raise the bed to a comfortable working height and lower the side rail nearest to you when you return to the bedside to begin the bath. Put on gloves, if indicated. Lay a towel across the patient's chest and on top of bath blanket.

15. With no cleanser on the washcloth, wipe one eye from the inner part of the eye, near the nose, to the outer part (Figure 1). Rinse or turn the cloth before washing the other eye.

16. Bathe the patient's face, neck, and ears. Apply appropriate emollient.

17. Expose the patient's far arm and place towel lengthwise under it. Using firm strokes, wash hand, arm, and axilla, lifting the arm as necessary to access axillary region (Figure 2). Rinse, if necessary, and dry. Apply appropriate emollient. Cover the area with the bath blanket.

RATIONALE

This ensures that the patient is not exposed unnecessarily, and warmth is maintained. If a bath blanket is unavailable, the top sheet may be used in its place.

This provides uncluttered access during the bath and maintains warmth of the patient. IV fluids must be maintained at the prescribed rate.

Side rails and lower bed height maintain patient safety. Adjusting the water temperature to no more than 120°F (49°C) decreases risk of burns and drying of the skin (International Association of Fire Fighters [IAFF], n.d.). Warm water is comfortable and relaxing for the patient. It also stimulates circulation and provides for more effective cleansing.

Having the bed at the proper height prevents back and muscle strain. Gloves are necessary if there is potential contact with blood or body fluids. The towel prevents chilling and keeps the bath blanket dry.

Cleanser may be irritating to the eyes. Moving from the inner to the outer aspect of the eye prevents carrying debris toward the nasolacrimal duct. Rinsing or turning the washcloth prevents spreading organisms from one eye to the other.

Use of emollients is recommended to restore and maintain skin integrity (Haesler et al., 2018; Lichterfeld et al., 2015; Voegeli, 2019).

The towel helps to keep the bed dry. Washing the far side first eliminates contaminating a clean area once it is washed. Gentle friction stimulates circulation and muscles and helps remove dirt, oil, and organisms. Long, firm strokes are relaxing and more comfortable than short, uneven strokes. Rinsing is necessary when using some cleansing products. Use of emollients is recommended to restore and maintain skin integrity (Haesler et al., 2018; Lichterfeld et al., 2015; Voegeli, 2019). Re-covering the body maintains warmth.

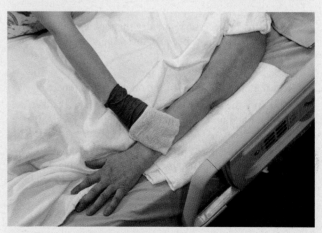

FIGURE 1. Washing from the inner corner of the eye outward.

FIGURE 2. Exposing the far arm and washing it.

(*continued on page 400*)

Skill 7-2 ▶ Providing a Bed Bath *(continued)*

ACTION	RATIONALE
18. Repeat Step 17 for the arm nearest you. Another option might be to bathe one side of the patient first and then move to the other side of the bed to complete the bath.	
19. Spread a towel across the patient's chest. Lower the bath blanket to the patient's umbilical area. Wash, rinse, if necessary, and dry chest. Keep chest covered with towel between the wash and rinse. Pay special attention to the folds of skin under the breasts. Apply appropriate emollient.	Exposing, washing, rinsing, and drying one part of the body at a time avoids unnecessary exposure and chilling. Areas of skin folds may be sources of odor and skin breakdown if not cleaned and dried properly. Use of emollients is recommended to restore and maintain skin integrity (Haesler et al., 2018; Lichterfeld et al., 2015; Voegeli, 2019).
20. Lower the bath blanket to the perineal area. Place a towel over the patient's chest.	Keeping the bath blanket and towel in place avoids exposure and chilling.
21. Wash, rinse, if necessary, and dry abdomen (Figure 3). Carefully inspect and clean umbilical area and any abdominal folds or creases. Apply appropriate emollient.	Skin-fold areas may be sources of odor and skin breakdown if not cleaned and dried properly. Use of emollients is recommended to restore and maintain skin integrity (Haesler et al., 2018; Lichterfeld et al., 2015; Voegeli, 2019).
22. Return bath blanket to original position and expose far leg. Place towel under far leg. Using firm strokes, wash, rinse, if necessary, and dry leg from ankle to knee and knee to groin (Figure 4). Apply appropriate emollient.	The towel protects linens and prevents the patient from feeling uncomfortable from a damp or wet bed. Washing from ankle to groin with firm strokes promotes venous return. Use of emollients is recommended to restore and maintain skin integrity (Haesler et al., 2018; Lichterfeld et al., 2015; Voegeli, 2019).

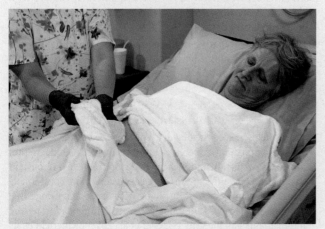

FIGURE 3. Washing the abdomen, with perineal and chest areas covered.

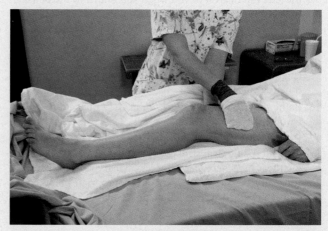

FIGURE 4. Washing and drying far leg, keeping the other leg covered.

ACTION	RATIONALE
23. Wash, rinse if necessary, and dry the foot. Pay particular attention to the areas between toes. Apply appropriate emollient.	Drying of the feet is important to prevent irritation, possible skin breakdown, and infections (Beuscher, 2019). Use of emollients is recommended to restore and maintain skin integrity (Haesler et al., 2018; Lichterfeld et al., 2015; Voegeli, 2019).
24. Repeat Steps 22 and 23 for the other leg and foot.	
25. Make sure the patient is covered with the bath blanket. Change water and washcloth at this point or earlier, if necessary.	The bath blanket maintains warmth and privacy. Clean, warm water prevents chilling and maintains patient comfort.
26. Assist the patient to a prone or side-lying position. Put on gloves, if not applied earlier. Position bath blanket and towel to expose only the back and buttocks.	Positioning the towel and bath blanket protects the patient's privacy and provides warmth. Gloves prevent contact with body fluids.

ACTION

27. Wash, rinse, if necessary, and dry back and buttocks area (Figure 5). **Pay particular attention to cleansing between gluteal folds and observe for any redness or skin breakdown in the sacral area.**

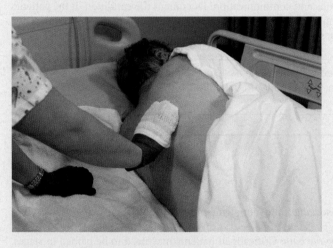

28. If not contraindicated, give the patient a backrub, as described in Skill 10-2, Chapter 10. Alternatively, back massage may be given after perineal care. Apply appropriate emollient and/or skin barrier product.

29. Remove gloves. Raise the side rail. Refill basin with clean water. Discard washcloth and towel. Put on clean gloves.

30. Set the patient up so they can complete perineal self-care. If the patient is unable to complete self-care, lower the side rail and complete perineal care. Follow the guidelines in the accompanying Skill Variation at the end of the skill. Apply skin barrier, as indicated. Raise the side rail, remove gloves, and perform hand hygiene.

31. Help the patient put on a clean gown or clothing and assist with the use of other personal toiletries, such as deodorant or cosmetics. If the gown does not have snap sleeves and the patient has an IV, follow the steps in Action 12 to replace the gown.

32. Protect pillow with towel, and groom the patient's hair.

33. **When finished, make sure the patient is comfortable, with the side rails up and the bed in the lowest position.**

 34. Change bed linens, as described in Skills 7-10 and 7-11. Dispose of soiled linens according to facility policy. Clean bath basin according to facility policy before returning to storage at bedside. Remove gloves and any other PPE, if used. Perform hand hygiene.

RATIONALE

Fecal material near the anus may be a source of microorganisms. Prolonged pressure on the sacral area or other bony prominences may compromise circulation and lead to development of decubitus ulcer.

FIGURE 5. Washing the back.

A backrub improves circulation to the tissues and is an aid to relaxation. A backrub may be contraindicated in patients with cardiovascular disease or musculoskeletal injuries. Use of emollients is recommended to restore and maintain skin integrity (Haesler et al., 2018; Lichterfeld et al., 2015; Voegeli, 2019). Skin barriers protect the skin from damage caused by excessive exposure to water and irritants, such as urine and feces (Williamson, 2020; Voegeli, 2019).

The washcloth, towel, and water are contaminated after washing the patient's gluteal area. Changing to clean supplies decreases the spread of organisms from the anal area to the genitals.

Providing perineal self-care may decrease embarrassment for the patient. Effective perineal care reduces odor and decreases the risk for infection through contamination. Skin barriers protect the skin from damage caused by excessive exposure to water and irritants, such as urine and feces.

This provides for the patient's warmth and comfort.

Proper positioning with raised side rails and proper bed height provides for patient comfort and safety.

Proper disposal of linens and cleaning of bath basin reduce the risk for transmission of microorganisms. Proper removal of PPE reduces the risk for infection transmission and contamination of other items. Hand hygiene prevents the spread of microorganisms.

(continued on page 402)

Skill 7-2 ▶ Providing a Bed Bath *(continued)*

EVALUATION

The expected outcomes have been met when the patient is clean, the patient has demonstrated some feeling of control in their care, the patient has verbalized an improved body image, and the patient has verbalized the importance of cleanliness.

DOCUMENTATION

Guidelines

Record any significant observations and communication. Document the condition of the patient's skin. Record the procedure, amount of assistance given, and patient participation. Document the application of skin care products, such as a skin barrier.

Sample Documentation

> 07/06/2025 2130 Bath provided with complete assistance; reddened area (3 cm × 3 cm) noted on patient's sacral area; skin-care team consultation made.
> —C. Stone, RN

DEVELOPING CLINICAL REASONING AND CLINICAL JUDGMENT

UNEXPECTED SITUATIONS AND ASSOCIATED INTERVENTIONS

- *Patient becomes chilled during the bath:* If the room temperature is adjustable, increase it. Another bath blanket may be needed.
- *Patient becomes unstable during the bath:* Critically ill patients may need to be bathed in stages. For instance, the right arm is bathed, and then the patient is allowed to rest for a short period before the left arm is bathed. The amount of rest time needed depends on how unstable the patient is and which parameter is being monitored. For example, the nurse may watch the blood pressure while bathing an unstable patient and stop when it begins to decrease. Once the blood pressure returns to the previous level, the nurse can begin to bathe the patient again.

SPECIAL CONSIDERATIONS

General Considerations

- To remove the gown without snap sleeves from a patient with an IV line, take the gown off the uninvolved arm first, then pause the infusion pump and remove the tubing from the pump. Lower the IV container and pass the gown over the tubing and the container. **Rehang the IV container and insert the tubing into the infusion pump. Check the rate on the infusion pump and restart.** To replace the gown, follow the same steps, placing the clean gown on the unaffected arm first. **Never disconnect IV tubing to change a gown, because this causes a break in a sterile system and could introduce microorganisms.**
- Patients with bariatric care needs are at increased risk for skin integrity issues, including increased risk for alterations in skin integrity (Earlam & Woods, 2020; Williamson, 2020). Assess the skin of bariatric inpatients twice a day, lifting and separating the folds of skin to assess the area, utilizing extra help as necessary (Black & Hotaling, 2015). Nonsoap cleansers should be used, and the skin should be dried to prevent retained moisture (Black & Hotaling, 2015; Williamson, 2020).
- When bathing a patient, the wipe or washcloth removes some of the outermost skin layer. This sloughed skin may be evident on the wipe or washcloth and in the bathwater and will vary in color depending on the ethnic group of the patient (Andrews et al., 2020). This is important to note, as this does not mean that the patient was dirty—the normal sloughing of the skin is more evident in darkly pigmented people compared with patients with lighter pigmentation (Andrews et al., 2020).
- Lying flat in bed during the bed bath may be contraindicated for certain patients. The position may have to be modified to accommodate their needs.
- Incontinent patients require special attention to perineal care. Patients with urinary or fecal incontinence are at risk for incontinence-associated dermatitis (perineal dermatitis), one type of moisture-associated skin damage (MASD) (Voegeli, 2019). Remove soil and irritants from the skin during routine hygiene as well as cleansing when the skin becomes exposed to irritants (Voegeli, 2019). Avoid using soap and excessive force for cleaning (Wounds UK, 2018). Use perineal skin cleansers, moisturizers, and moisture barriers for skin care for these patients to promote healing and prevent further skin damage (Voegeli, 2019).

- If the patient has an indwelling catheter, use mild soap and water or a perineal cleanser to clean the perineal area; rinse the area well. Do not clean the periurethral area with antiseptics to prevent CAUTI while the catheter is in place (Gould et al., 2019). Routine hygiene (cleansing of the meatal surface during daily bathing or showering) is appropriate (Gould et al., 2019). Inspect the meatus for drainage and note the characteristics of the urine. Do not use powders and lotions after cleaning.
- The use of chlorhexidine gluconate (CHG) for bathing has been shown to reduce colonization of skin with pathogens and is an important measure utilized by institutions in an attempt to decrease health care–associated infections (HAIs), such as central line–associated bloodstream infections and surgical site infections (Hines et al., 2015; Martinez et al., 2020; Musuuza et al., 2019; Urias et al., 2018). Some facilities' policies include the use of CHG for all inpatient bathing, expect for patients with a history of CHG allergy or intolerance or those age less than 2 months (Hines et al., 2015). Chlorhexidine can be added to bath water but is also available in prepackaged impregnated cloths.
- If applying lotion, warm the lotion in your hands before applying it to the patient to prevent chilling.
- Soaking the patient's hands in a basin of water is an additional comfort measure for the patient. It facilitates thorough washing of the hands and between the fingers and aids in removing debris from under the nails. If appropriate and as indicated, place a folded towel on the bed next to the patient's hand and put the basin of water on it. Wash, rinse if necessary, and dry hand. Apply appropriate emollient. Use of emollients is recommended to restore and maintain skin integrity (Haesler et al., 2018; Lichterfeld et al., 2015; Voegeli, 2019).
- Basic wound care used for body piercings is usually called "aftercare." Aftercare techniques are used for the new piercing and whenever the piercing fistula has become disrupted through injury or exhibits signs of infection or inflammation (Association of Professional Piercers [APP], 2020; MFMER, 2020b). Clean the site with mild soap and warm water or normal saline solution (AAFP, 2019). Use a cotton swab to gently remove any crusting. Rinse well.

Infant and Child Considerations

- When bathing an infant or young child, have supplies within easy reach, and support or hold the child securely at all times to ensure safety.
- Never leave the child alone.
- Consider bathing a newborn using a reverse-order procedure, from "trunk to head," wetting the infant's head last to reduce the amount of time the infant's head is wet. The method supports a more rapid recovery of body temperature and decreased heat loss from evaporation during bathing (So et al., 2014).
- Delaying the newborn bath for 24 hours has been associated with multiple benefits, including increased likelihood of exclusive breastfeeding at discharge and decreased incidence of hypothermia and hypoglycemia in healthy newborns (Warren et al., 2020).

Older Adult Considerations

- Check the temperature of the water carefully before bathing an older adult, because sensitivity to temperature may be impaired in older adults.
- An older continent patient may not require a full bed bath with soap and water every day. If dry skin is a problem, water and skin lotion or bath oil may be used on alternate days.

Community-Based Care Considerations

- Use plastic trash bags or a plastic shower-curtain liner to protect the mattress when bathing or shampooing a patient in bed. Disposable washcloths may also be an option to consider. A large plastic container or baby bathtub can effectively serve as a shampoo basin.
- If linens are soiled with blood or body fluids, instruct family members/caregivers to wear gloves when handling them. The linens should be rinsed first in cold water and then washed separately from other household wash, using hot water, laundry detergent, and bleach.
- Teach a family member or caregivers how to perform comfort measures, such as a backrub.
- If patients are home with an indwelling catheter, instruct them or their caregivers to wash the urinary meatus and perineal area with mild soap and water.

EVIDENCE FOR PRACTICE ▶

CONTAMINATION OF HEALTH CARE PROVIDER CLOTHING

Health care–acquired infections (HAIs) continue to be an issue in health care settings. Pathogens responsible for HAIs are typically spread from patient to patient in the health care setting through the hands and attire of health care providers (Thom et al., 2018). What factors are associated with contamination of health care providers' clothing?

(continued on page 404)

Skill 7-2 ▶ Providing a Bed Bath *(continued)*

Related Research

Thom, K. A., Escobar, D., Boutin, M. A., Zhan, M., Harris, A. D., & Johnson, K. (2018). Frequent contamination of nursing scrubs is associated with specific care activities. *American Journal of Infection Control, 46*(5), 503–506. https://doi.org/10.1016/j.ajic.2017.11.016

This cohort study examined patient care factors associated with bacterial contamination of the scrubs of health care workers. Participants included nurses and patient care technicians (*n* = 90; 79 nurses and 11 patient care technicians) in adult intensive and intermediate care units at two facilities, a medical center, and a trauma center. Participants were given four new, study-issued scrubs and a randomized schedule of wear; the wear schedule specified which scrub set should be worn on which working shift. Participants laundered the scrubs at home after wearing, using their normal laundry procedure. Each scrub set was sampled twice over an 8-month period (total of 8 samples per health care worker) on random days to identify the presence and amount of scrub bacterial contamination. Sampling of the scrubs was performed during the last 4 hours of a 12-hour shift; participants were not aware of the timing of the sampling. At the time of sampling, participants reported information related to scrub laundering habits, the number and quality of patient interactions, and patient care activities performed during the sampling shift. Of the 720 samples obtained, 30% were contaminated with pathogenic bacteria. Patient care activities associated with higher odds of scrub contamination included providing care for patients with wounds (*p* < .01) and providing the patient with a bath (*p* = .07). The researchers concluded health care worker attire was frequently contaminated with bacteria and providing care for patients with wounds or giving a bath were associated with scrub contamination by pathogenic bacteria. The researchers suggested contamination of health care worker attire associated with the identified patient care activities has the potential to contribute to transmission of bacteria to other patients.

Relevance for Nursing Practice

The results of this study suggest that nurses and other health care workers need to consider contamination of their work attire as a potential source of transmission of potential pathogens. Nurses should be conscious of this possible situation and take precautions to reduce contamination of their attire and evaluate each patient care situation for the need for personal protective equipment.

Skill Variation ▶ Performing Perineal Cleansing

Perineal cleaning should be performed in a matter-of-fact and dignified manner. When performing perineal care, follow these guidelines:

1. Perform hand hygiene and put on PPE, if indicated.

2. Identify the patient.

3. Explain what you are going to do and the reason for doing it to the patient.
4. Assemble necessary equipment on the bedside stand or overbed table.

5. Close curtains around the bed and close the door to the room, if possible.
6. Put on gloves. Cover the patient with a bath blanket and remove top linens to expose only the perineal area. Wash and rinse the groin area (both male and female patients):
   - For a female patient, spread the labia and move the washcloth from the pubic area toward the anal area to prevent carrying organisms from the anal area back over the genital area (Figure A). Always proceed from the least contaminated area to the most contaminated area. Use a clean portion of the washcloth for each stroke. Rinse the washed areas well with plain water.
   - For a male patient, clean the tip of the penis first, moving the washcloth in a circular motion from the meatus outward. Wash the shaft of the penis using downward strokes toward the pubic area (Figure B). Always proceed

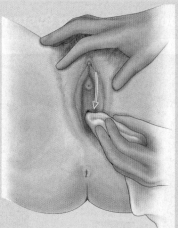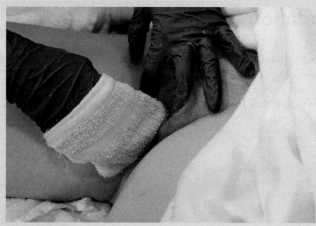

FIGURE A. Performing female perineal care.

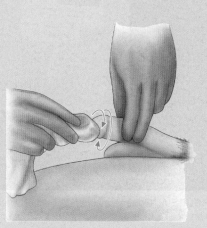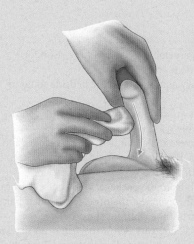

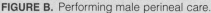

FIGURE B. Performing male perineal care.

from the least contaminated area to the most contaminated area. Rinse the washed areas well with plain water. In an uncircumcised male patient (teenage or older), retract the foreskin (prepuce) while washing the penis. **It is not recommended to retract the foreskin for cleaning during infancy and childhood, because injury and scarring could occur** (MedlinePlus, 2020).

- Pull the uncircumcised male patient's (teenage or older) foreskin back into place over the glans penis to prevent constriction of the penis, which may result in edema and tissue injury (MedlinePlus, 2020). Wash and rinse the male patient's scrotum. Handle the scrotum, which houses the testicles, with care because the area is sensitive.

7. Dry the cleaned areas and apply an emollient, as indicated. Apply skin barrier (protectant) to area, as indicated. Avoid the use of powder. Powder may become a medium for bacteria growth.
8. Turn the patient on their side and continue cleansing the anal area. Continue in the direction of least contaminated to most contaminated area. In the female, cleanse from the vagina toward the anus. In both female and male patients, change the washcloth with each stroke until the area is clean. Rinse and dry the area. Apply skin barrier (protectant) to area, as indicated.
9. Remove gloves and perform hand hygiene. Continue with additional care as necessary.

(*continued on page 406*)

Skill 7-2 ▶ Providing a Bed Bath *(continued)*

Skill Variation ▶ Giving a Bath Using a Disposable Bathing System

A disposable bathing system is packaged with premoistened disposable washcloths. If more than eight cloths are available in the package, use a separate cloth for hands and feet. When giving a bath with a disposable system, follow these guidelines:

1. Warm the unopened package in the microwave, according to the manufacturer's directions or remove package from storage warmer (Figure A).

2. Perform hand hygiene and put on PPE, if indicated.

3. Identify the patient.

4. Explain what you are going to do and the reason for doing it to the patient.
5. Assemble necessary equipment on the bedside stand or overbed table.
6. Close the curtains around the bed and close the door to the room, if possible.
7. Put on gloves. Cover the patient with a bath blanket and remove top linens. Remove the patient's gown and keep the bath blanket in place.
8. Remove first cloth from the package. Wipe one eye from the inner part of the eye, near the nose, to the outer part. Use a different part of the cloth for the other eye.
9. Bathe the face, neck, and ears. Allow the skin to air dry for approximately 30 seconds, according to the manufacturer's directions. Air drying allows the emollient ingredient of the cleanser to remain on the skin. Alternatively, dry the skin with a towel, based on the product used. Apply appropriate emollient. Dispose of cloth in trash receptacle.
10. Expose the patient's far arm. Remove another cloth. Using firm strokes, wash hand, arm, and axilla. Allow the skin to air dry for approximately 30 seconds, according to the manufacturer's directions. Air drying allows the emollient ingredient of the cleanser to remain on the skin. Alternatively, dry the skin with a towel, based on the product used. Apply appropriate emollient. Dispose of cloth in trash receptacle. Cover arm with blanket.
11. Repeat for nearer arm with a new cloth. Cover arm with blanket.
12. Expose the patient's chest. Remove new cloth and cleanse chest. Allow the skin to air dry for approximately 30 seconds, according to the manufacturer's directions. Cover chest with a towel. Expose the patient's abdomen. Cleanse abdomen. Allow the skin to air dry for approximately 30 seconds, according to the manufacturer's directions. Air drying allows the emollient ingredient of the cleanser to remain on the skin. Alternatively, dry the skin with a towel, based on the product used. Apply appropriate

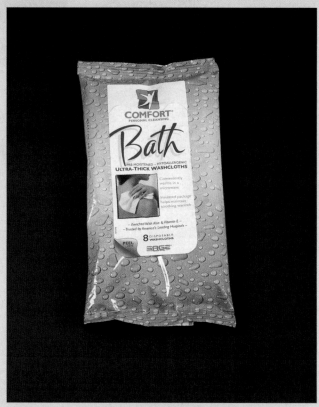

FIGURE A. Commercial self-contained bathing system. (Used with permission from Shutterstock. *Photo by B. Proud.*)

emollient. Dispose of cloth in trash receptacle. Cover the patient's body with blanket.

13. Expose far leg. Remove new cloth and cleanse leg and foot. Allow the skin to air dry for approximately 30 seconds, according to the manufacturer's directions. Air drying allows the emollient ingredient of the cleanser to remain on the skin. Alternatively, dry the skin with a towel, based on the product used. Apply appropriate emollient. Dispose of cloth in trash receptacle. Cover the patient's leg with blanket.
14. Repeat for nearer leg with a new cloth. Cover leg with blanket.
15. Assist the patient to prone or side-lying position. Put on gloves, if not applied earlier. Position blanket to expose back and buttocks. Remove a new cloth and cleanse back and buttocks area. Allow the skin to air dry for approximately 30 seconds, according to the manufacturer's directions. Air drying allows the emollient ingredient of the cleanser to remain on the skin. Alternatively, dry the skin with a towel, based on the product used. Apply appropriate emollient. Dispose of cloth in trash receptacle. If not contraindicated, give the patient a back massage. Apply skin barrier, as indicated. Cover the patient with blanket.

16. Remove gloves and perform hand hygiene. Put on clean gloves. Remove last cloth and cleanse the perineal area. Refer to the guidelines in the previous Skill Variation. Dispose of cloth in trash receptacle. Apply skin barrier, as indicated.

17. Remove gloves. Perform hand hygiene. Assist the patient to put on a clean gown or appropriate clothing. Assist with the use of other personal toiletries.

18. Change bed linens as described in Skills 7-10 and 7-11. Dispose of soiled linens according to facility policy.

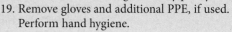

19. Remove gloves and additional PPE, if used. Perform hand hygiene.

EVIDENCE FOR PRACTICE ▶

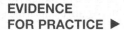

TWO BATH METHOD AND MICROORGANISMS

The use of disposable bath products is an alternative to traditional use of skin cleanser and water. Use of these disposable products has increased. Is washing with disposable wipes as effective in removing microorganisms on the skin as washing with soap/skin cleanser and water?

Related Research

Veje, P. L., Chen, M., Jensen, C. S., Sørensen, J., & Primdahl, J. (2020). Effectiveness of two bed bath methods in removing microorganisms from hospitalized patients: A prospective randomized crossover study. *American Journal of Infection Control, 48*(6), 638–643. https://doi.org/10.1016/j.ajic.2019.10.011

This study examined the use of prepackaged disposable wet wipes (DWW) versus the traditional bed bath using soap and water (SAW) and a bath basin to provide perineal hygiene to reduce microorganisms in the groin and perineum (intimate hygiene) of hospitalized patients. The study took place over 15 months and used a randomized crossover design involving 72 patients from an intensive care unit, a medical unit, and a surgical unit. Participants were randomized to a random sequence of the two washing methods. One group had intimate hygiene with SAW on day 1 and with DWW on day 2; the other group had intimate hygiene with DWW on day 1 and with SAW on day 2. Skin swabs from each participant were obtained before and after washing with SAW or DWW from one side of the groin and perineum; the same side of the groin was used on both days and the same person obtained all of the skin swabs. The same staff washed the participants in 31 of 58 patients. A total of 58 paired skin swabs were ultimately acquired. The swabs were then cultured; blinded cultivation, inspection, and qualitative classical microbiologic analyses were performed. Both washing methods resulted in a statistically significant reduction in the amount of all microorganisms (after SAW, $p = .0001$; after DWW, $p = .0148$), including microorganisms with the potential to cause urinary tract infections. No statistically significant difference ($p = .84$) in the removal of microorganisms was observed between the two washing methods. The researchers concluded both methods seem to be equally effective in removing microorganisms from the skin in the groin and perineum areas.

Relevance for Nursing Practice

This study suggests that implementing bathing procedures utilizing alternatives to traditional cleanser and water are effective in providing personal hygiene. Nurses and nursing staff are the primary providers of bathing activities in many health care settings, and should consider implementing efficient interventions, such as disposable wet wipes, to enhance patient experiences related to personal hygiene and improve skin health.

Skill 7-3 ▶ Assisting the Patient With Oral Care

Adequate oral hygiene care is imperative to promote the patient's sense of well-being and comfort, and prevent deterioration of the oral cavity (Kisely, 2016; Riley, 2018). Poor oral hygiene contributes to the colonization of the oropharyngeal secretions by respiratory pathogens. Diligent oral hygiene care can improve oral health and limit the growth of pathogens in the oropharyngeal secretions, decreasing the incidence of aspiration pneumonia, community-acquired pneumonia, nonventilator health care–associated pneumonia (NV-HAP), and ventilator-associated pneumonia (VAP) (American Association of Critical-Care Nurses [AACN], 2017; Chick & Wynne, 2020; Jenson et al., 2018; Quinn et al., 2020). Comprehensive oral care that includes thorough mechanical cleaning is an important part of care to achieve oral health outcomes for patients in all settings (Barbe et al., 2020; Chick & Wynne, 2020; Chicote, 2019; Gibney et al., 2019; Kisey, 2016).

The mouth requires care particularly during illness, but sometimes care must be modified to meet a patient's needs. If the patient can assist with mouth care, provide the necessary materials. Oral care is important not only to prevent dental **gingivitis** and **caries**, but also to improve the patient's self-image. Teeth should be brushed and flossed twice a day; the mouth should be rinsed after meals. If the patient is unable to perform oral hygiene, make certain that the mouth receives care as often as necessary to keep it clean and moist, as often as every 1 or 2 hours if necessary. This is especially important for patients who cannot drink or are not permitted fluids by mouth. Refer to Box 7-2 for suggestions to meet the oral hygiene needs for patients with cognitive impairments.

Box 7-2 Meeting the Oral Hygiene Needs of Patients With Cognitive Impairments

- Choose a time of day when the patient is most calm and accepting of care.
- Enlist the aid of a family member/caregiver or significant other.
- Break the task into small steps and provide short, simple instructions.
- Provide distraction, such as playing favorite music, while providing care.

- Allow the patient to participate. The nurse can put a hand over the patient's hand to guide the activity.
- Start the activity, showing the patient what to do, then let the patient take over.
- Withdraw and try again later if the patient strongly refuses care.
- Document effective and ineffective interventions to provide appropriate information for staff to give consistent, person-centered care.

Source: Adapted from Alzheimer's Association. (2020). *Dental care.* https://www.alz.org/help-support/caregiving/daily-care/dental-care; Eliopoulos, C. (2018). *Gerontological nursing* (9th ed.). Wolters Kluwer; and Konno, R., Kang, H. S., & Makimoto, K. (2014). A best-evidence review of intervention studies for minimizing resistance-to-care behaviours for older adults with dementia in nursing homes. *Journal of Advanced Nursing, 70*(10), 2167–2180.

DELEGATION CONSIDERATIONS	The implementation of oral care may be delegated to assistive personnel (AP) as well as to licensed practical/vocational nurses (LPN/LVNs). The decision to delegate must be based on careful analysis of the patient's needs and circumstances as well as the qualifications of the person to whom the task is being delegated. Refer to the Delegation Guidelines in Appendix A.
EQUIPMENT	• Toothbrush • Toothpaste • Emesis basin • Glass with cool water • Disposable gloves • Additional PPE, as indicated • Towel • Mouth rinse • Washcloth or paper towel • Lip lubricant (optional) • Dental floss or other interdental cleaner • Oral assessment tool, as indicated (Figure 1)
ASSESSMENT	Assess the patient's oral hygiene preferences: frequency, time of day, and type of hygiene products. Assess for any physical activity limitations. An oral assessment tool can assist with assessment of the status of the oral cavity, as well as help to determine the frequency and procedure for oral care (Figure 1). Assess the patient's oral cavity and dentition. Look for any inflammation or bleeding of the gums. Look for ulcers, lesions, and yellow or white patches. The yellow or white patches may indicate a fungal infection called thrush. Assess for signs of dehydration (dry mucosa) and dental decay. Look at the lips for dryness or cracking. Ask the patient if they are having pain, dryness, soreness, or difficulty chewing or swallowing. Assess the patient's ability to perform own care.

Oral Health Assessment Tool (OHAT) - Modified
Mouth Care Without a Battle©

Person Assessed:_____ Assessed by:_____ Date:_____

*For each category, circle the one best description. Then, in the column marked score, write the points for the assessment. Add the points in the bottom row. Problems **underlined and in bold** are indications for immediate referral to a dentist, as they may represent a serious condition. For nursing home residents, problems in **bold** may require documentation on the MDS 3.0 and may trigger the Dental Care CAA, regardless of the total score.*

Category	0 = Healthy	1 = Minor Problems	2 = Major Problems	Score*
Lips	Smooth, pink, moist	Dry, chapped, or red at corners	New or growing lump, ulcer, or lesion; white, red, and/or ulcerated patch; bleeding and/or ulcer at corners	
Gums, palate, and insides of cheeks	Pink, moist, smooth, no bleeding	Dry, shiny, rough, red, and/or swollen area; **one small ulcer, lesion, and/or sore spot under dentures**	<u>Swollen, tender area around a tooth or tooth root (suspected abscess);</u> swollen and/or bleeding ulcer; white, red and/or ulcerated patch; small pimple-like area with pus; widespread redness under dentures	
Natural teeth	No decay or broken or worn down teeth	1-3 decayed or broken and/or very worn down teeth	<u>One or more very loose teeth;</u> 4 or more decayed or broken or very worn down teeth; fewer than 4 teeth	
Dentures	No broken areas; teeth, dentures are regularly worn, and dentures are labeled with name	**1 broken area or tooth; denture loose, but adhesive not needed; denture uncleanable; denture not labeled with name;** dentures only worn for 1-2 hrs daily	**More than 1 broken area or tooth; denture so loose adhesive needed;** denture missing or not worn	
Quality of tooth hygiene	Clean and no food particles or tartar in mouth or on dentures	Food particles, tartar, and/or plaque in 1-2 areas of the mouth or on small area of dentures; bad breath (halitosis)	Food particles, tartar, and/or plaque in most areas of the mouth or on most of dentures; severe bad breath (halitosis)	
Tooth pain	No behavioral, verbal, or physical signs of dental pain	**Nonspecific verbal and/or behavioral signs of pain such as pulling at face, chewing lips, or not eating; unexplained aggression**	**Physical signs of pain (swelling of cheek or gum, broken teeth, ulcers); verbal and/or behavioral signs of pain specific to the mouth**	
Saliva / dry mouth	Moist tissues, watery and free flowing saliva	Dry, sticky tissues, little saliva present; person complains of dry mouth	Tissues parched and red; very little/no saliva present; saliva is thick	
Tongue	Normal, moist, roughness, pink	Patchy, fissured, red, coated	Patch that is red and/or white, ulcerated, and/or swollen	
			Total Score	

FIGURE 1. Oral Health Assessment Tool (OHAT). (Mouth Care Without a Battle, UNC Cecil G. Sheps Center for Health Services Research. Used by Permission.) (*continued*)

(*continued on page 410*)

Skill 7-3 ▶ Assisting the Patient With Oral Care *(continued)*

Oral Health Assessment Tool (OHAT)

Patient: _____   Scores at admission and regular reviews (date): _____

Completed by: _____

Category	0 = healthy	1 = changes*	2 = unhealthy*	Dates					
Lips	Smooth, pink, moist	Dry, chapped, or red at corners*	Swelling or lump, white/red/ulcerated patch: bleeding/ulcerated at corners						
Tongue	Normal, moist roughness, pink	Patchy, fissured, red, coated	Patch that is red &/or white, ulcerated, swollen						
Gums and tissues	Pink, moist, smooth, no bleeding	Dry, shiny, rough, red, swollen, one ulcer/sore spot under dentures	Swollen, bleeding, ulcers/white/red patches, generalized redness under dentures						
Saliva	Moist tissues, watery and free flowing saliva	Dry, sticky tissues, little saliva present, resident thinks they have dry mouth	Tissues parched and red, very little/no saliva present, saliva is thick, resident thinks they have a dry mouth						
Natural teeth Yes/No	No decayed or broken teeth/roots	1–3 decayed or broken teeth/roots or very worn down teeth	4+ decayed or broken teeth/roots, or very worn down teeth, or less than 4 teeth						
Dentures Yes/No	No broken areas or teeth, dentures regularly worn and labeled with name of resident	1 broken area/tooth or dentures only worn for 1-2 hours daily, or dentures not labeled with name, or loose	More than 1 broken area/tooth, denture missing or not worn, loose and needs denture adhesive or not labeled with name						
Oral cleanliness	Clean and no food particles or tartar in mouth or dentures	Food particles/tartar/plaque in 1–2 areas of the mouth or on small area of dentures or **halitosis** (bad breath)	Food particles/tartar/plaque in most areas of the mouth or on most of dentures or severe halitosis (bad breath)						
Dental pain	No behavioral, verbal, or physical signs of dental pain	Verbal &/or behavioral signs of pain such as pulling at face, chewing lips, not eating, aggression	Physical pain signs (swelling of cheek or gum, broken teeth, ulcers), as well as verbal &/or behavioral signs (pulling at face, not eating, aggression)						
Total Score: _____				16	16	16	16	16	16

_____ Arrange for resident to have a dental examination by a dentist   _____ Resident and/or family/guardian refused dental treatment

_____ Complete Oral Hygiene Care Plan and start oral hygiene care interventions for resident   _____ Review this resident's oral health again on:_____

*If 1 or 2 scored for any category, please arrange for a dentist to examine the resident
Modified from Kayser-Jones et al., (1995) by Chalmers (2000b); Chalmers, King et al., (2005); Chalmers et al., (2004)

FIGURE 1. *(Continued)*

ACTUAL OR POTENTIAL HEALTH PROBLEMS AND NEEDS	Many actual or potential health problems or issues may require the use of this skill as part of related interventions. An appropriate health problem or issue may include: • ADL deficit • Impaired dentition • Aspiration risk
OUTCOME IDENTIFICATION AND PLANNING	The expected outcome to achieve is that the patient's mouth and teeth will be clean, the patient will exhibit a positive body image, and the patient will verbalize the importance of oral care and demonstrate appropriate oral care skills.

IMPLEMENTATION

ACTION	RATIONALE
1. Perform hand hygiene and put on gloves if assisting with oral care, and/or other PPE, if indicated.	Hand hygiene and PPE prevent the spread of microorganisms. PPE is required based on transmission precautions.
2. Identify the patient. Explain the procedure to the patient.	Identifying the patient ensures the right patient receives the intervention and helps prevent errors. Explanation facilitates engagement in care.
3. Assemble equipment on the overbed table or other surface within the patient's reach.	Organization facilitates performance of the task.
4. Close the room door or curtains. Place the bed at an appropriate and comfortable working height (VHACEOSH, 2016).	Closing the door or curtains provides privacy. Proper bed height helps reduce back strain while performing the procedure.
5. Lower the side rail and assist the patient to a sitting position, if permitted, or turn the patient onto their side. Place a towel across the patient's chest.	The sitting or side-lying position prevents aspiration of fluids into the lungs. The towel protects the patient from dampness.
6. Encourage the patient to brush their own teeth according to the following guidelines. Assist, if necessary.	
a. Moisten the toothbrush and apply toothpaste to bristles.	Water softens the bristles.
b. Place the brush at a 45-degree angle to gum line (Figure 2) and brush from gum line to crown of each tooth (Figure 3). Brush outer and inner surfaces. Brush back and forth across the biting surface of each tooth.	Facilitates removal of **plaque** and **tartar**. The 45-degree angle of brushing permits cleansing of all tooth surface areas.

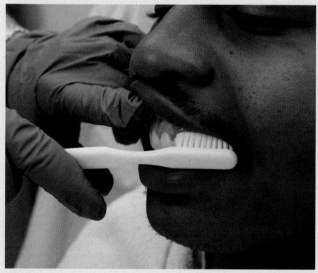

FIGURE 2. Placing brush at a 45-degree angle to gum line.

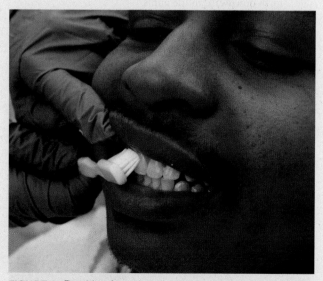

FIGURE 3. Brushing from gum line to the crown of each tooth.

(*continued on page 412*)

Skill 7-3 ▶ Assisting the Patient With Oral Care *(continued)*

ACTION

c. Brush the tongue gently with toothbrush or tongue scraper (Mayo Foundation for Medical Education and Research [MFMER], 2019a) (Figure 4).

d. Have the patient rinse vigorously with water and spit into emesis basin (Figure 5). Repeat until clear. Suction may be used as an alternative for removal of fluid and secretions from the mouth.

RATIONALE

This removes coating on the tongue. Gentle motion does not stimulate the gag reflex.

The vigorous swishing motion helps to remove debris. Suction is appropriate if the patient is unable to expectorate well.

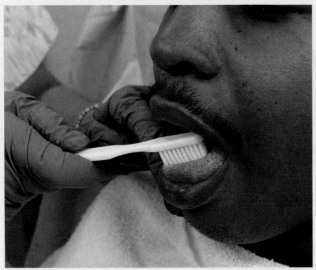

FIGURE 4. Brushing tongue.

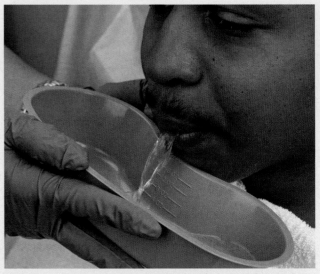

FIGURE 5. Holding emesis basin for patient to rinse and spit.

7. Assist the patient to floss their teeth, if appropriate:

a. Remove approximately 18 inches of dental floss from container or use a plastic floss holder. Wrap most of the floss around one of the middle fingers. Wind the remaining floss around the same finger of the opposite hand, keeping about 1 to 1.5 inches of floss taut between the fingers.

b. Insert floss gently between teeth, moving it back and forth downward to the gums.

c. Move the floss up and down, first on one side of a tooth and then on the side of the other tooth, until the surfaces are clean (Figure 6). Repeat in the spaces between all teeth and the backside of the last teeth.

Flossing aids in removal of food and plaque and promotes healthy gum tissue (American Dental Association [ADA], n.d.b).

The floss must be held taut to get between the teeth.

Trauma to the gums can occur if floss is forced between teeth.

This ensures that the sides of both teeth are cleaned.

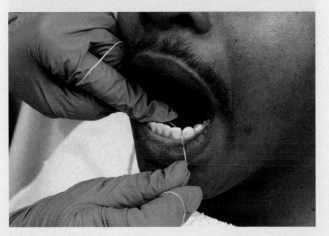

FIGURE 6. Flossing teeth.

ACTION	**RATIONALE**
d. Instruct the patient to rinse mouth well with water after flossing.	Vigorous rinsing helps to remove food particles and plaque that have been loosened by flossing.
8. Offer a mouth rinse if the patient prefers or if use has been recommended.	Use of a mouth rinse can reduce bacteria and can help reduce plaque, gingivitis, tartar (hardened plaque) and also freshen breath. Anticavity rinses with fluoride help protect tooth enamel to help prevent or control tooth decay (ADA, 2019).
9. Offer lip balm or petroleum jelly.	Lip balm lubricates lips and prevents drying.
10. Remove equipment. Remove gloves and discard. Perform hand hygiene. Raise the side rail and lower the bed. Assist the patient to a position of comfort.	Removing gloves properly reduces the risk for infection transmission and contamination of other items. These actions promote patient comfort and safety.
11. Remove any other PPE, if used. Perform hand hygiene.	Proper removal of PPE reduces the risk for infection transmission and contamination of other items. Hand hygiene prevents the spread of microorganisms.

EVALUATION

The expected outcomes have been met when the patient has received oral care, the patient has experienced little to no discomfort, the patient has reported their mouth feels refreshed, and the patient has demonstrated understanding of the reasons for proper oral care and appropriate oral care skills.

DOCUMENTATION

Guidelines

Record oral assessment, significant observations, and unusual findings, such as bleeding or inflammation. Document any teaching done. Document procedure and patient response.

Sample Documentation

> <u>10/2025</u> 0930 Patient performed oral care with minimal assistance. Oral cavity mucosa pink and moist. No evidence of bleeding or ulceration. Lips slightly dry; lip moisturizer applied. Reinforcement provided related to importance of flossing teeth every day. Patient demonstrates appropriate flossing technique.
>
> —*L. Schneider, RN*

DEVELOPING CLINICAL REASONING AND CLINICAL JUDGMENT

UNEXPECTED SITUATIONS AND ASSOCIATED INTERVENTIONS

- *While cleaning the teeth, you notice a large amount of bleeding from the gum line:* Stop brushing. Allow the patient to gently rinse mouth with water and spit into emesis basin. Before brushing again, check the patient's most recent platelet level. Consider the use of a softer toothbrush to provide oral hygiene.
- *Patient has braces on their teeth:* Braces collect food particles. Brush extra thoroughly. Reinforce the importance of using an appropriate interdental cleaner.

SPECIAL CONSIDERATIONS

General Considerations

- Use a soft-bristled toothbrush with a small head even when the patient has no or few teeth. It is the only effective way to remove plaque and debris from the teeth, gums, and tongue.
- Automatic toothbrushes, electric or battery operated, are simple to use and can be used to removing debris and plaque and clean the teeth effectively. Use of an electric toothbrush provide superior oral hygiene care when oral hygiene is provided by a caregiver (Vannah & Sammarco, 2019).

(*continued on page 414*)

Skill 7-3 ▶ Assisting the Patient With Oral Care *(continued)*

- The use of chlorhexidine gluconate (CHG) as part of oral hygiene has been integrated into oral hygiene regimens and is available as an oral rinse, oral spray, and dental gel (AACN, 2017; de Camargo et al., 2019). The use of CHG as part of protocols for systematic oral care for critically ill patients has been shown to reduce risk of VAP (AACN, 2017; Chen et al., 2015).

Infant and Child Considerations

- Begin brushing children's teeth as soon as they begin to come into the mouth and begin flossing when the child has two teeth that touch (American Dental Association [ADA], n.d.a).
- Clean an infant's gums by wiping with a clean, damp cloth (ADA, n.d.a).
- Young children should be supervised by an adult until they are between ages 7 and 10 years (Kyle & Carman, 2021); remind them not to swallow the toothpaste (ADA, n.d.a).
- Use smaller amounts of fluoride toothpaste on the toothbrush for children: a smear (size of a grain of rice) for children younger than age 3 years and a pea-sized amount for children ages 3 to 6 years (ADA, n.d.a).

Older Adults

- Physical limitations that may be associated with aging may interfere with the older adult's ability to perform adequate oral hygiene (Thomas, 2019). Pressurized water spray units (water flossing) are available to assist with oral hygiene to and can be a useful option for older adults and other patients who have trouble flossing by hand (American Dental Association [ADA], n.d.d).

EVIDENCE FOR PRACTICE ▶

ORAL HYGIENE AND OLDER ADULTS

Poor oral hygiene contributes to alterations in oral health and is associated with increased risk for aspiration pneumonia, community-acquired pneumonia, and other health concerns (Hata et al., 2019; Jenson et al., 2018; Müller, 2015; Quinn et al., 2020). Poor oral health in older adults compounds dental problems associated with aging. Adequate oral hygiene is essential to promote a sense of well-being and comfort and prevent deterioration of the oral cavity (Kisely, 2016; Riley, 2018).

Related Research

Red, A., & O'Neal, P. V. (2020). Implementation of an evidence-based oral care protocol to improve the delivery of mouth care in nursing home residents. *Journal of Gerontological Nursing, 46*(5), 33–39. https://doi.org/10.3928/00989134-20200316-01

This aims of quality improvement (QI) project were to determine if an evidence-based oral care protocol in addition to a staff oral care training program on a long-term care unit would increase staff knowledge of oral care in older adults and improve oral health outcomes in the long-term care residents. The Iowa Model of Evidence-Based Practice was used to guide this QI project. Staff knowledge, skills, and attitudes in oral care practices of older adults were assessed pre- and postintervention with a Likert scale questionnaire. Oral health status of the older adult residents ($n = 10$) was measured pre- and postintervention using the Oral Health Assessment Tool (OHAT). Nurses and certified nursing assistants ($n = 29$) attended four 30-minute oral health educational in-services centered on the significance of oral health in the older adult, basic mouth care, proper brushing techniques, denture care, oral care techniques, and standards of care. Caring for residents with disruptive behaviors and techniques to manage resistant care were also discussed. After completion of the educational sessions, an evidence-based Oral Care Protocol and daily oral care checklist were initiated, requiring oral care twice daily. Oral health outcomes of the residents were measured at three time points after 14 days of protocol use. Knowledge of oral health care improved significantly as evidenced by mean total pre-test score of 88.8 to mean total post-test score of 97.7 ($p = .021$). Statistically significant improvements ($p = .001$) were seen in oral health outcomes as measured by the OHAT. The authors concluded an oral health education intervention and evidence-based oral care protocol increases staff knowledge of oral care practices and improves oral health outcomes in older adults. The authors also suggested long-term care staff play an important role in improving oral hygiene of older adult residents through use of an evidence-based oral health protocol.

Relevance for Nursing Practice

Poor oral hygiene can contribute to poor oral health and oral diseases as well as other systemic health problems. By performing oral assessments, providing oral hygiene, and promoting tooth brushing and flossing, nurses and other health care providers can be instrumental in supporting optimal oral health outcomes and prevention of oral diseases in older adults.

Skill 7-4 ▶ Providing Oral Care for the Dependent Patient

Adequate oral hygiene care is imperative to promote the patient's sense of well-being and comfort, and prevent deterioration of the oral cavity (Kisely, 2016; Riley, 2018). Diligent oral hygiene care can improve oral health and limit the growth of pathogens in the oropharyngeal secretions, decreasing the incidence of aspiration pneumonia, community-acquired pneumonia, nonventilator health care–associated pneumonia (NV-HAP), and ventilator-associated pneumonia (VAP) (AACN, 2017; Chick & Wynne, 2020; Jenson et al., 2018; Quinn et al., 2020). Comprehensive oral care that includes thorough mechanical cleaning is an important part of care to achieve oral health outcomes for patients in all settings (Barbe et al., 2020; Chick & Wynne, 2020; Chicote, 2019; Gibney et al., 2019; Kisey, 2016).

Physical limitations, such as those associated with aging, often lead to less than adequate oral hygiene. The dexterity required for adequate brushing and flossing may decrease with age or illness. Older adults may be dependent on caregivers for oral hygiene. Patients with cognitive impairment, such as dementia and mental illness, are also at risk for inadequate oral hygiene (Brennan & Strauss, 2014; Jablonski et al., 2018; Kadia et al., 2014; Red & O'Neal, 2020). Refer to Box 7-2 in Skill 7-3 for suggestions to meet the oral hygiene needs for patients with cognitive impairments.

Teeth should be brushed and flossed twice a day; the mouth should be rinsed after meals. If the patient is unable to perform oral hygiene, make certain that the mouth receives care as often as necessary to keep it clean and moist, as often as every 1 or 2 hours, if necessary. This is especially important for patients who cannot drink or are not permitted fluids by mouth. Moisten the mouth with water, if allowed, and lubricate the lips often enough to keep the membranes well moistened.

DELEGATION CONSIDERATIONS

The implementation of oral care for a dependent patient may be delegated to assistive personnel (AP) after assessment by the registered nurse as well as to licensed practical/vocational nurses (LPN/LVNs). The decision to delegate must be based on careful analysis of the patient's needs and circumstances as well as the qualifications of the person to whom the task is being delegated. Refer to the Delegation Guidelines in Appendix A.

EQUIPMENT

- Suction toothbrush (see Figure 4) or soft toothbrush
- Suction swab
- Suction catheter with suction apparatus
- Toothpaste or other oral cleanser
- Emesis basin
- Glass with cool water
- Disposable gloves
- Additional PPE, as indicated
- Towel
- Mouth rinse (optional)

- Dental floss in holder or other interdental cleaner
- Mouth-prop or second toothbrush (Figure 1)
- Denture-cleaning equipment (if necessary)
- Denture cup
- Denture cleaner
- 4 × 4 gauze
- Washcloth or paper towel
- Lip lubricant (optional)
- Oral health assessment tool (see Figure 1 in Skill 7-3)
- Additional care giver, as indicated

ASSESSMENT

Assess the patient's oral hygiene preferences: frequency, time of day, and type of hygiene products. Assess for any physical activity limitations. Assess the patient's level of consciousness and overall ability to assist with oral care and respond to directions. Assess the patient's risk for oral hygiene problems. Alterations in cognitive function and/or consciousness increase the risk for alterations in oral tissue and structure integrity. Assess the patient's gag reflex. Decreased or absent gag reflex increases the risk for aspiration. An oral assessment tool can assist with assessment of the status of the oral cavity, as well as help to determine the frequency and procedure for oral care (see Figure 1 in Skill 7-3). Assess the patient's oral cavity and dentition. Look for any inflammation or bleeding of the gums. Look for ulcers, lesions, and yellow or white patches. The yellow or white patches may indicate a fungal infection called thrush. Assess for signs of dehydration (dry mucosa) and dental decay. Look at the lips for dryness or cracking. If the patient is conscious and/or cognitively able to respond, ask the patient if they are having pain, dryness, soreness, or difficulty chewing or swallowing.

(continued on page 416)

Skill 7-4 ▶ Providing Oral Care for the Dependent Patient *(continued)*

ACTUAL OR POTENTIAL HEALTH PROBLEMS AND NEEDS	Many actual or potential health problems or issues may require the use of this skill as part of related interventions. An appropriate health problem or issue may include: • Impaired ability to perform oral hygiene • Impaired oral mucous membrane • Aspiration risk
OUTCOME IDENTIFICATION AND PLANNING	The expected outcome to achieve when performing oral care is that the patient's mouth and teeth are clean; the patient does not experience impaired oral mucous membranes; and the patient verbalizes, if able, an understanding about the importance of oral care.

IMPLEMENTATION

ACTION	RATIONALE
1. Perform hand hygiene and put on PPE, if indicated.	Hand hygiene and PPE prevent the spread of microorganisms. PPE is required based on transmission precautions.
2. Identify the patient. Explain the procedure to the patient.	Identifying the patient ensures the right patient receives the intervention and helps prevent errors. Explanation facilitates engagement in care.
3. Assemble equipment on the overbed table or other surface within reach.	Organization facilitates performance of the task.
4. Close the room door or curtains. Place the bed at an appropriate and comfortable working height (VHACEOSH, 2016). Lower one side rail and position the patient on the side, with head tilted forward. Place towel across the patient's chest and emesis basin in position under chin. Depending on equipment in use, connect the suction toothbrush/swab or suction catheter to suction tubing and turn on suction. Put on gloves.	Closing the door or curtains provides privacy. Proper bed height helps reduce back strain while performing the procedure. The side-lying position with head forward prevents aspiration of fluid into lungs. Towel and emesis basin protect the patient from dampness. Suction provides means to remove oral hygiene products and saliva from oral cavity. Gloves prevent the spread of microorganisms.
5. Gently open the patient's mouth by applying pressure to the lower jaw at the front of the mouth. Do not use fingers to hold the patient's mouth open. Use another toothbrush or mouth prop (Figure 1) to keep the mouth open (Johnson, 2012). Remove dentures, if present. (Refer to Skill 7-5.)	Patients with altered cognition may inadvertently bite fingers inserted into the mouth. Removal of dentures allows for cleaning of dentures and oral cavity.

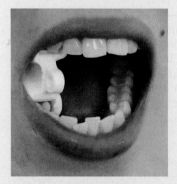

FIGURE 1. Example of a mouth prop. (Used with permission from Neo-Health Services, Inc. © 2011 OrofacialMyology.com. All rights reserved.)

6. If using a regular toothbrush and suction catheter, one care giver provides oral cleaning and the other removes secretions with the suction catheter.	This allows for efficient care to reduce the risk of aspiration.

ACTION

7. Brush the teeth and gums carefully with toothbrush and paste or other oral cleanser (Figure 2). Lightly brush the tongue.

8. Moisten toothbrush with water to rinse the oral cavity. **Position the patient's head to allow for return of water. If using regular toothbrush, use suction catheter to remove the water and cleanser from oral cavity** (Figure 3).

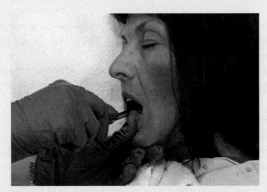

FIGURE 2. Carefully brushing patient's teeth.

9. Brush the tongue gently with toothbrush or tongue scraper (MFMER, 2019a).

10. Using the suction swab, apply a therapeutic antiseptic mouth rinse as indicated. Apply oral moisturizer as indicated.

11. Clean the dentures before replacing. (See Skill 7-5.)

12. Apply lubricant to the patient's lips.

13. Remove equipment and return the patient to a position of comfort. Remove gloves. Perform hand hygiene. Raise the side rail and lower the bed.

 14. Remove additional PPE, if used. Perform hand hygiene.

RATIONALE

The toothbrush provides friction necessary to clean areas where plaque and tartar accumulate.

Rinsing helps clean debris from the mouth. Suction toothbrush removes fluids and cleansers.

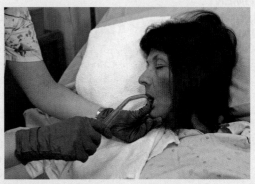

FIGURE 3. Using suction to remove excess fluid.

This removes coating on the tongue. Gentle motion does not stimulate the gag reflex.

Therapeutic and antiseptic mouth rinses reduce bacteria and reduce plaque, gingivitis, tartar, and reduce the incidence of health care–associated pneumonia (AACN, 2017; ADA, 2019; Chick & Wynne, 2020). Oral moisturizers provide moisture to the mucosa.

Cleaning maintains dentures and oral hygiene. Plaque can accumulate on dentures and promote oropharyngeal colonization of pathogens.

This prevents drying and cracking of lips.

Promotes patient comfort and safety. Removing gloves properly reduces the risk for infection transmission and contamination of other items. Hand hygiene prevents the spread of microorganisms.

Proper removal of PPE reduces the risk for infection transmission and contamination of other items. Hand hygiene prevents the spread of microorganisms.

EVALUATION

The expected outcomes have been met when the patient's oral cavity has been cleaned and is free from complications, and, the patient, if able, has verbalized a basic understanding of the need for oral care.

DOCUMENTATION

Guidelines   Record oral assessment, significant observations, and unusual findings, such as bleeding or inflammation. Document any teaching done. Document care provided and patient response.

(continued on page 418)

Skill 7-4 ▶ Providing Oral Care for the Dependent Patient *(continued)*

Sample Documentation

> <u>7/10/25</u> 0945 Oral care performed. Oral cavity mucosa pink and moist. Small amount of bleeding noted from gums after using soft-bristled toothbrush. Resolved spontaneously when brushing completed. No evidence of ulceration. Lips slightly dry; lip moisturizer applied.
> —C. Stone, RN

DEVELOPING CLINICAL REASONING AND CLINICAL JUDGMENT

UNEXPECTED SITUATIONS AND ASSOCIATED INTERVENTIONS

- *Patient begins to bite the toothbrush:* Do not jerk the toothbrush out. Wait for the patient to relax mouth before removing the toothbrush and continuing with care. Use distraction, gentle touch, or massage to divert the patient (Johnson, 2012).
- *Mouth is extremely dry with crusts that remain after oral care provided:* Increase frequency of oral hygiene. Apply mouth moisturizer to oral mucosa. Monitor fluid intake and output to ensure adequate intake of fluid.

SPECIAL CONSIDERATIONS

- Suction toothbrushes may be used with patients with **dysphagia** (Figure 4).
- Use a soft bristled toothbrush with a small head even when the patient has no or few teeth. It is the only effective way to remove plaque and debris from the teeth, gums, and tongue.
- Automatic toothbrushes, electric or battery operated, are simple to use and can be used to removing debris and plaque and clean the teeth effectively. Use of an electric toothbrush provide superior oral hygiene care when oral hygiene is provided by a caregiver (Vannah & Sammarco, 2019).
- The use of chlorhexidine gluconate (CHG) as part of oral hygiene has been integrated into oral hygiene regimens and is available as an oral rinse, oral spray, and dental gel (AACN, 2017; de Camargo et al., 2019). The use of CHG as part of protocols for systematic oral care for critically ill patients has been shown to reduce risk of VAP (AACN, 2017; Chen et al., 2015).

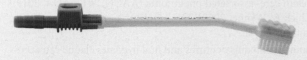

FIGURE 4. Example of a suction toothbrush. (Permission granted by Sage Products LLC.)

EVIDENCE FOR PRACTICE ▶

CAREGIVER-ASSISTED ORAL HYGIENE

Poor oral hygiene contributes to alterations in oral health, and is associated with increased risk for aspiration pneumonia, community-acquired pneumonia, and other health concerns (Hata et al., 2019; Jenson et al., 2018; Müller, 2015; Quinn et al., 2020). Poor oral health in older adults compounds dental problems associated with aging. Adequate oral hygiene is essential to promote a sense of well-being and comfort and prevent deterioration of the oral cavity (Kisely, 2016; Riley, 2018).

Related Research

Vannah, C. E., & Sammarco, V. R. (2019). Electric brushes improve outcomes in caregiver-assisted oral hygiene. *Nursing, 49*(8), 56–60. https://doi.org/10.1097/01.NURSE.0000569764.96290.70

This study investigated caregiver-assisted oral hygiene using an electric toothbrush compared with caregiver-assisted oral hygiene using manual brushing. The residents at a long-term care facility were divided into two groups, based on the side of the hallway in which they resided. Eight of the residents who were completely dependent on caregivers for oral hygiene were recruited for the study. An experienced registered dental hygienist measured the amount of plaque on participants' teeth pre- and postintervention using the Plaque Index, resulting in a PLI score; a score of 0 indicates no visible plaque and 3 indicates a large amount of plaque on the teeth and in the space between the tooth and surrounding gum tissue. Nursing staff received training in use of the electric toothbrush and in manual tooth brushing. Caregivers provided oral care to all hallway residents, using the electric toothbrush with one group (one side of the hallway, Group A) and manual brushing with the other group (other side of the hallway, (Group B) for 8 weeks. Caregivers were unaware of which residents were study participants. The intervention was implemented for a second time after a 2-week interval of regular oral care. After the 2 weeks, a second pre-intervention scoring of teeth was completed. Nursing staff then provided oral care to all hallway residents, this time providing care using the other type of toothbrush: manual brushing for Group A and oral care with the electric toothbrush for Group B. The mean pre- and postintervention PLI scores in both phases were compared to determine the difference. The mean differences between the electric and manual methods were compared. Electric brushing was associated with a decrease in PLI score, and manual brushing was associated with an increased PLI score, with a statistically significant difference between the scores ($p = .011$). The researchers concluded that, after proper training, electric brushing was superior to manual brushing for plaque control in residents in long-term care settings when oral care was provided by a caregiver.

Relevance for Nursing Practice
Poor oral hygiene can contribute to poor oral health and oral diseases, as well as other systemic health problems. Nurses should consider evidence-based interventions to improve patient outcomes. Use of an electric toothbrush as part of oral health protocols provides the potential to improve patient's oral care and support optimal oral health outcomes and prevention of oral diseases in older adults.

Skill 7-5 ▶ Providing Denture Care

Adequate oral hygiene care is imperative to promote the patient's sense of well-being and comfort, and prevent deterioration of the oral cavity (Kisely, 2016; Riley, 2018). Poor oral hygiene contributes to the colonization of the oropharyngeal secretions by respiratory pathogens. Plaque, which can accumulate on dentures, can promote oropharyngeal colonization of pathogens (American Dental Association [ADA], 2021). Diligent oral hygiene care can improve oral health and limit the growth of pathogens in the oropharyngeal secretions, decreasing the incidence of aspiration pneumonia, community-acquired pneumonia, nonventilator health care–associated pneumonia (NV-HAP), and ventilator-associated pneumonia (VAP) (AACN, 2017; Chick & Wynne, 2020; Jenson et al., 2018; Quinn et al., 2020). Comprehensive oral care that includes thorough mechanical cleaning is an important part of care to achieve oral health outcomes for patients in all settings (Barbe et al., 2020; Chick & Wynne, 2020; Chicote, 2019; Gibney et al., 2019; Kisey, 2016).

It is important to clean dentures daily and to remove and rinse dentures and mouth after meals. Dentures may be cleaned more often, based on need and the patient's personal preference. To reduce or minimize denture stomatitis (irritation of the oral tissues), it is recommended that dentures not be worn continuously (24 hours per day); dentures are often removed at night (American College of Prosthodontists [ACP], n.d.). Handle dentures with care to prevent breakage. Refer to Box 7-2 in Skill 7-3 for suggestions to meet the oral hygiene needs for patients with cognitive impairments.

DELEGATION CONSIDERATIONS

The implementation of denture care may be delegated to assistive personnel (AP) as well as to licensed practical/vocational nurses (LPN/LVNs). The decision to delegate must be based on careful analysis of the patient's needs and circumstances as well as the qualifications of the person to whom the task is being delegated. Refer to the Delegation Guidelines in Appendix A.

(continued on page 420)

Skill 7-5 ▶ Providing Denture Care *(continued)*

EQUIPMENT

- Denture brush
- Denture paste/cleanser
- Denture cleaner for soaking (optional)
- Denture adhesive (optional)
- Glass of cool water
- Emesis basin
- Denture cup (optional)

- Nonsterile gloves
- Additional PPE, as indicated
- Towel
- Oral hygiene supplies
- Washcloth or paper towel
- Lip lubricant
- Gauze

ASSESSMENT

Assess the patient's oral hygiene preferences: frequency, time of day, and type of hygiene products. Assess for any physical activity limitations. Assess for difficulty chewing, pain, tenderness, and discomfort. Assess the patient's gag reflex. Decreased or absent gag reflex increases the risk for aspiration. An oral assessment tool can assist with assessment of the status of the oral cavity as well as help to determine the frequency and procedure for oral care (Figure 1 in Skill 7-3). Assess the patient's oral cavity. Look for inflammation, edema, lesions, bleeding, or yellow/white patches. The patches may indicate a fungal infection called thrush. Assess for signs of dehydration (dry mucosa). Look at the lips for dryness or cracking. Assess the patient's ability to perform their own care.

ACTUAL OR POTENTIAL HEALTH PROBLEMS AND NEEDS

Many actual or potential health problems or issues may require the use of this skill as part of related interventions. An appropriate health problem or issue may include:
- ADL deficit
- Impaired oral mucous membrane
- Disturbed body image

OUTCOME IDENTIFICATION AND PLANNING

The expected outcome to achieve is that the patient's mouth and dentures will be clean, the patient will exhibit a positive body image, and the patient will verbalize the importance of oral and denture care and demonstrate appropriate oral and denture care skills.

IMPLEMENTATION

ACTION	RATIONALE
1. Perform hand hygiene and put on PPE, if indicated.	Hand hygiene and PPE prevent the spread of microorganisms. PPE is required based on transmission precautions.
2. Identify the patient. Explain the procedure to the patient.	Identifying the patient ensures the right patient receives the intervention and helps prevent errors. Explanation facilitates engagement in care.
3. Assemble equipment on the overbed table or other surface within reach.	Organization facilitates performance of the task.
4. Provide privacy for the patient.	The patient may be embarrassed by removal of dentures.
5. Lower the side rail and assist the patient to a sitting position, if permitted, or turn the patient onto the side. Place a towel across the patient's chest. Raise the bed to a comfortable working position (VHACEOSH, 2016). Put on gloves.	The sitting or side-lying position prevents aspiration of fluids into the lungs. The towel protects the patient from dampness. Proper bed height helps reduce back strain while performing the procedure. Gloves prevent the spread of microorganisms.
6. Apply gentle pressure with 4 × 4 gauze to grasp lower denture plate and remove it. If necessary, use a slight rocking motion to remove plate. Place it immediately in denture cup. Grasp upper denture with gauze and remove it (Figure 1). Place in the denture cup.	Remove bottom denture first, as it is easier to remove and minimizes bite risk (Jablonski, 2012). Rocking motion breaks suction between denture and gum. Using 4 × 4 gauze prevents slippage and discourages spread of microorganisms.

ACTION

7. Place paper towels or washcloth in sink while brushing. Using the denture brush and denture paste/cleanser, brush all denture surfaces gently but thoroughly (Figure 2). Be sure to completely remove any denture adhesive remaining on the denture. If the patient prefers, add denture cleaner to cup with water and follow directions on preparation. After denture soaks, brush denture as previously described.

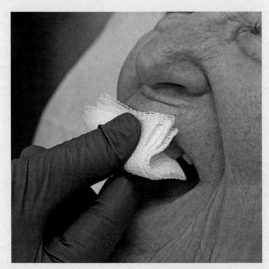

FIGURE 1. Removing dentures with a gauze sponge.

8. Rinse thoroughly with cool or lukewarm water. Apply denture adhesive, if appropriate, following product directions.

9. Use a toothbrush and toothpaste to gently clean gums, mucous membranes, and tongue. Offer water and/or mouth rinse so the patient can rinse mouth before replacing dentures. Refer to Skill 7-3 for additional details related to oral hygiene care.

10. Insert the upper denture in the mouth and press firmly. Insert the lower denture. If adhesive is used, ask the patient to bite firmly. Check that the dentures are securely in place and comfortable.

11. If the patient desires, dentures can be stored in the denture cup in cold water, instead of returning to the mouth. Label the cup and place it on the patient's bedside table.

12. Remove equipment. Remove your gloves. Perform hand hygiene. Assist the patient to a position of comfort. Raise the side rail and lower the bed.

13. Remove additional PPE, if used. Perform hand hygiene.

RATIONALE

Putting paper towels or a washcloth in the sink protects against breakage. Dentures collect food and microorganisms and require daily cleaning. Removal of any residual denture adhesive prevents buildup, plaque buildup, and potential problems with the fit of the denture. Do not use toothpaste as it can be too harsh for denture surfaces (ACP, n.d.).

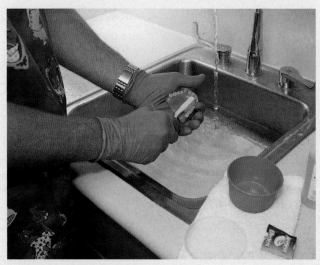

FIGURE 2. Brushing denture surfaces.

Water aids in removal of debris and acts as a cleaning agent. Denture adhesives, when properly used, can improve the retention and stability of dentures and help seal out the accumulation of food particles beneath the dentures (ADA, 2021).

Cleaning removes food particles and plaque, permitting proper fit and preventing infection (American Dental Association [ADA], n.d.c). Therapeutic and antiseptic mouth rinses reduce bacteria and reduce plaque, gingivitis, tartar, and reduce the incidence of health care–associated pneumonia (AACN, 2017; ADA, 2019; Chick & Wynne, 2020).

This ensures patient comfort. Biting firmly after insertion spreads the adhesive to the entire tissue-contacting surface (ADA, 2021).

Storing in water helps the denture retain its shape and keeps it from drying out (ADA, 2021). Proper storage prevents loss and damage.

Removing gloves properly reduces the risk for infection transmission and contamination of other items. Hand hygiene prevents transmission of microorganisms. This promotes patient comfort and safety.

Proper removal of PPE reduces the risk for infection transmission and contamination of other items. Hand hygiene prevents transmission of microorganisms.

(continued on page 422)

Skill 7-5 ▶ Providing Denture Care   *(continued)*

EVALUATION

The expected outcomes have been met when the patient's oral cavity and dentures have been cleaned and are free from complications, and the patient has verbalized or demonstrated improved body image. In addition, the patient has verbalized a basic understanding of the need for oral care and has demonstrated appropriate oral and denture care skills.

DOCUMENTATION

Guidelines

Record oral assessment, significant observations, and unusual findings, such as bleeding or inflammation. Document any teaching done. Document care provided and patient response.

Sample Documentation

> 7/10/25 0945 Oral care performed. Oral cavity mucosa pink and moist. Denture and oral care given. No evidence of bleeding, ulceration, or inflammation.
>
> —C. Stone, RN

DEVELOPING CLINICAL REASONING AND CLINICAL JUDGMENT

UNEXPECTED SITUATIONS AND ASSOCIATED INTERVENTIONS

- *Food or other material does not come off denture with brushing*: Place denture in a cup with cool water and soak. After soaking, use a toothbrush and denture paste to clean again. If necessary, use commercial denture cleaner added to water in the cup to soak, then brush clean.

SPECIAL CONSIDERATIONS

- Encourage the patient to wear their dentures, if not contraindicated. Dentures enhance appearance, assist in eating, facilitate speech, and maintain the gum line. Denture fit may be altered with long periods of nonuse.
- Encourage the patient to refrain from wrapping the denture in paper towels or napkins because they could be mistaken for trash.
- Encourage the patient to refrain from placing the dentures in the bedclothes because they can be lost in the laundry.
- Store dentures in cold water when not in the patient's mouth. Storing in water helps the denture retain its shape and keeps it from drying out (ADA, 2021).

EVIDENCE FOR PRACTICE ▶

CLINICAL PRACTICE GUIDELINE

Optimal Care and Maintenance of Full Dentures

Bartlett, D., Carter, N., de Baat, C., Duyck, J., Goffin, G., Müller, F., & Kawai, Y. (2018). *White Paper on optimal care and maintenance of full dentures for oral and general health*. Global Task Force for Care of Full Dentures. Oral Health Foundation. https://www.gskhealthpartner.com/content/dam/cf-consumer-healthcare/health-professionals/en_US/pdf/SM12378+OHF+Cleaning+Guideline+-+White+Paper+-+Refresh+-+Print+Version+4+RGB.pdf

This evidence-based guideline provides information to guide the care and maintenance of removable complete denture prostheses.

Skill 7-6 ▶ Removing Contact Lenses

Skill Variation: *Removing Different Types of Contact Lens*

If a patient wears contact lenses but cannot remove them, the nurse may be responsible for removing them. This may occur, for example, when the nurse is caring for an unconscious patient. Whenever an unconscious patient is admitted without any family/caregivers present, assess the patient to determine whether they wear contact lenses. Leaving contact lenses in place for long periods could result in permanent eye damage. However, if an eye injury is present, do not try to remove lenses because of the danger of causing an additional injury. Lenses should be cleaned and stored as prescribed. Different types of lenses require special care and certain types of products. Sleeping in any contact lens is not recommended as the incidence of serious eye infections is greatly increased (Cleveland Clinic, 2020).

DELEGATION CONSIDERATIONS

The removal of contact lenses may be delegated to assistive personnel (AP) as well as to licensed practical/vocational nurses (LPN/LVNs). The decision to delegate must be based on careful analysis of the patient's needs and circumstances as well as the qualifications of the person to whom the task is being delegated. Refer to the Delegation Guidelines in Appendix A.

EQUIPMENT

- Disposable gloves
- Additional PPE, if indicated
- Container for contact lenses (if unavailable, two small sterile containers marked "L" and "R" will suffice)
- Sterile normal saline solution and/or appropriate contact disinfecting solution, based on particular contact lenses
- Rubber pincer, if available (for removal of soft lenses)
- Suction-cup remover, if available (for removal of rigid lenses)

ASSESSMENT

Assess both eyes for contact lenses; some people wear them in only one eye. Assess eyes for any redness or drainage, which may indicate an eye infection or an allergic response. Assess for any eye injury. If an injury is present, notify the health care team about the presence of the contact lens. Do not try to remove the contact lens in this situation due to the risk for additional eye injury.

ACTUAL OR POTENTIAL HEALTH PROBLEMS AND NEEDS

Many actual or potential health problems or issues may require the use of this skill as part of related interventions. An appropriate diagnosis or patient problem may include:

- ADL deficit
- Risk for injury
- Knowledge deficiency

OUTCOME IDENTIFICATION AND PLANNING

The expected outcomes to achieve when removing contact lenses is that the lenses are removed without trauma to the eye and are stored safely, and the patient demonstrates appropriate contact lens care skills.

IMPLEMENTATION

ACTION	RATIONALE
1. Perform hand hygiene and put on PPE, if indicated.	Hand hygiene and PPE prevent the spread of microorganisms. PPE is required based on transmission precautions.
2. Identify the patient. Explain the procedure to the patient.	Patient identification validates the correct patient and correct procedure. Discussion and explanation help allay anxiety and prepare the patient for what to expect.
3. Assemble equipment on the overbed table or other surface within reach.	Organization facilitates performance of the task.

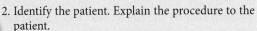

(continued on page 424)

Skill 7-6 ▶ Removing Contact Lenses *(continued)*

ACTION	**RATIONALE**
4. Close the curtains around the bed and close the door to the room, if possible.	This ensures the patient's privacy.
5. Assist the patient to a supine position. Raise the bed to a comfortable working position (VHACEOSH, 2016). Lower the side rail closest to you.	The supine position with the bed raised and the side rail down is the least stressful position for removing a contact lens. Proper bed height helps reduce back strain while performing the procedure.
6. If containers are not already labeled, do so now. Place 5 mL of normal saline or appropriate contact disinfecting solution in each container.	Many patients have different prescription strengths for each eye. The saline will prevent the contact from drying out.
7. Put on gloves. Remove soft contact lens:	Gloves prevent the spread of microorganisms.
a. Have the patient look forward. Retract the lower lid with one hand. Using the pad of the index finger of the other hand, move the lens down to the sclera (Figure 1).	
b. Using the pads of the thumb and index finger, grasp the lens with a gentle pinching motion and remove it (Figure 2).	

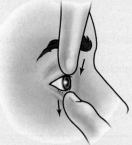

FIGURE 1. Retracting lower lid with one hand and using pad of index finger of other hand to move lens down to the sclera.

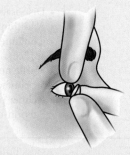

FIGURE 2. Using the pads of thumb and index finger to grasp lens with a gentle pinching motion to remove it.

See the accompanying Skill Variation figures for other techniques for removing both rigid and soft lenses.

ACTION	**RATIONALE**
8. Place the first lens in its designated cup in the storage case before removing the second lens (Figure 3).	Lenses may be different for each eye; this action avoids mixing them up.

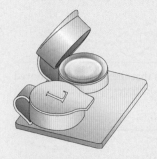

FIGURE 3. Storage cases are marked L and R, designating left and right lenses. Placing first lens in its designated cup before removing second lens avoids mixing them up.

ACTION	**RATIONALE**
9. Repeat actions to remove other contact lens.	
10. Remove gloves. Perform hand hygiene. If the patient is awake and has glasses at bedside, offer the patient glasses.	Proper removal of gloves reduces the risk for microorganism transmission and contamination of other items. Hand hygiene prevents transmission of microorganisms. Not being able to see clearly may create anxiety.
11. Remove equipment and return the patient to a position of comfort. Raise the side rail and lower the bed.	This promotes patient comfort and safety. Removing gloves properly reduces the risk for infection transmission and contamination of other items.
12. Remove additional PPE, if used. Perform hand hygiene.	Proper removal of PPE reduces the risk for infection transmission and contamination of other items. Hand hygiene prevents transmission of microorganisms.

EVALUATION

The expected outcomes have been met when the patient remains free of injury as the contact lenses are removed; the eyes have exhibited no signs and symptoms of trauma, irritation, or redness; contacts have been stored safely; and the patient has demonstrated appropriate contact lens care skills.

DOCUMENTATION

Guidelines

Record your assessment, significant observations, and unusual findings, such as drainage or pain. Document any teaching done. Document the removal of the contact lenses, their storage, any teaching provided, and patient response.

Sample Documentation

> <u>7/15/25</u> 1045 Soft contacts removed from eyes without trauma. Stored in patient's lens case in contact solution. Sclera white with no drainage from eye. Glasses placed at bedside.
> —*C. Stone, RN*

DEVELOPING CLINICAL REASONING AND CLINICAL JUDGMENT

UNEXPECTED SITUATIONS AND ASSOCIATED INTERVENTIONS

- *Contact lens cannot be removed:* Use a tool to remove the lens. For hard lenses, the tool has a small suction cup that is placed over the contact lens. For soft lenses, the tool is a small pair of rubber grippers that can be placed over the contact lens to aid in removal.
- *Hard contact is not over the cornea:* Place a cotton-tipped applicator over the upper eyelid and grasp the lid, inverting the lid over the applicator. Examine the eye for the lens. If the lens is not in the upper portion, place a finger below the eye and gently pull down on the lid while having the patient look up. When the lens is found, gently slide it over the cornea. Soft contacts may be removed from other areas of the eye.

Skill Variation ▶ Removing Different Types of Contact Lens

1. Perform hand hygiene and put on PPE, if indicated.

2. Identify the patient.

3. Explain to the patient what you are going to do and why you are doing it.
4. Assemble necessary equipment on the bedside stand or overbed table or other surface within reach.
5. Close the curtains around the bed and close the door to the room, if possible.
6. Assist the patient to a supine position. Raise bed to a comfortable working height (VHACEOSH, 2016). Lower the side rail closest to you.
7. If containers are not already labeled, do so now. Place 5 mL of normal saline or appropriate contact solution in each container.
8. Put on clean gloves.

To Remove Hard Contact Lenses—Patient Is Able to Blink

a. If the lens is not centered over the cornea, apply gentle pressure on the lower eyelid to center the lens (Figure A).
b. Gently pull the outer corner of the eye toward the ear (Figure B).
c. Position the other hand below the lens to catch it and ask the patient to blink (Figure C).

To Remove Hard Contact Lenses—Patient Is Unable to Blink

a. Gently spread the eyelids beyond the top and bottom edges of the lens (Figure D).
b. Gently press the lower eyelid up against the bottom of the lens (Figure E).
c. After the lens is tipped slightly, move the eyelids toward one another to cause the lens to slide out between the eyelids (Figure F).

(continued on page 426)

Skill 7-6 ▶ Removing Contact Lenses *(continued)*

Skill Variation ▶ Removing Different Types of Contact Lens *(continued)*

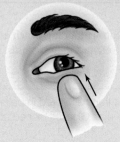

FIGURE A. Centering lens.

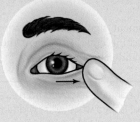

FIGURE B. Gently pulling outer corner of eye toward ear.

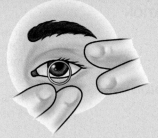

FIGURE C. Receiving lens as patient blinks.

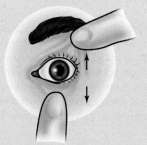

FIGURE D. Spreading eyelids.

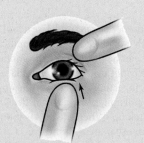

FIGURE E. Pressing lower lid up against bottom of lens.

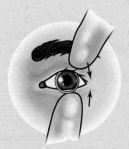

FIGURE F. Sliding lens out between lids.

To Remove Hard Contact Lenses With a Suction Cup—Patient Is Unable to Blink

a. Ensure that contact lens is centered on the cornea. Place a drop of sterile saline on the suction cup.

b. Place the suction cup in the center of the contact lens and gently pull the contact lens off the eye.

c. To remove the suction cup from the lens, slide the lens off sideways.

To Remove Soft Contact Lenses With a Rubber Pincer

a. Locate the contact lens and place the rubber pincers in the center of the lens.

b. Gently squeeze the pincers and remove the lens from the eye.

9. Place the first lens in its designated cup in the storage case before removing the second lens.

10. Repeat actions to remove other contact lens. Remove gloves. Perform hand hygiene.

11. If the patient is awake and has glasses at bedside, offer the patient glasses. Lower the bed. Assist the patient to a comfortable position.

12. Remove additional PPE, if used. Perform hand hygiene.

Skill 7-7 ▶ Shampooing a Patient's Hair in Bed

Skill Variation: *Shampooing a Patient's Hair With a Shampoo Cap*

The easiest way to wash a patient's hair may be to assist them in the shower or the tub. If the patient's hair needs to be washed but the patient is unable or not allowed to get out of bed, a bed shampoo can be performed. Shampoo caps are available and are being used with increasing frequency. These commercially prepared, disposable caps contain a rinseless shampoo product. Refer to the accompanying Skill Variation at the end of the skill. Other hair cleansing products are also available for use at the bedside and include foams, concentrates, and dry powders. Follow product directions for use.

DELEGATION CONSIDERATIONS	The shampooing of a patient's hair may be delegated to assistive personnel (AP) as well as to licensed practical/vocational nurses (LPN/LVNs). The decision to delegate must be based on careful analysis of the patient's needs and circumstances as well as the qualifications of the person to whom the task is being delegated. Refer to the Delegation Guidelines in Appendix A.
EQUIPMENT	• Water pitcher • Warm water • Shampoo • Conditioner (optional) • Disposable gloves • Additional PPE, as indicated • Protective pad for bed • Shampoo board or tray • Bucket • Towels • Gown • Comb or brush • Blow dryer (optional)
ASSESSMENT	Assess the patient's hygiene preferences: frequency, time of day, and type of hygiene products. Assess for any physical activity limitations. Assess the patient's ability to get out of bed to have their hair washed. If the prescribed interventions allow it and the patient is physically able to wash their hair in the shower, the patient may prefer to do so. If the patient cannot tolerate being out of bed or is not allowed to do so, perform a bed shampoo. Assess for any activity or positioning limitations. Inspect the patient's scalp for any cuts, lesions, or bumps. Note any flaking, drying, or excessive oiliness, or evidence of problems, such as **pediculosis**.
ACTUAL OR POTENTIAL HEALTH PROBLEMS AND NEEDS	Many actual or potential health problems or issues may require the use of this skill as part of related interventions. An appropriate diagnosis or patient problem may include: • Impaired ability to perform hygiene • Fatigue • Impaired ability to transfer
OUTCOME IDENTIFICATION AND PLANNING	The expected outcome to achieve is that the patient's hair will be clean. Other outcomes that may be appropriate include the following: the patient will tolerate the shampoo with little to no difficulty, the patient will demonstrate an improved body image, and the patient will verbalize an increase in comfort.

IMPLEMENTATION

ACTION	**RATIONALE**
1. Review the health record for any limitations in physical activity, or contraindications to the procedure. Confirm the presence of a prescribed intervention for shampooing the patient's hair, if required by facility policy.	Identifying limitations prevents patient discomfort and injury. In some settings, a prescribed intervention is required for shampooing a patient's hair.
2. Perform hand hygiene. Put on PPE, as indicated.	Hand hygiene and PPE prevent the spread of microorganisms. PPE is required based on transmission precautions.

(continued on page 428)

Skill 7-7 ▶ Shampooing a Patient's Hair in Bed *(continued)*

ACTION	RATIONALE

3. Identify the patient. Explain the procedure to the patient.

Patient identification validates the correct patient and correct procedure. Discussion and explanation help allay anxiety and prepare the patient for what to expect.

4. Assemble equipment on the overbed table or other surface within reach.

Organization facilitates performance of the task.

5. Close the curtains around the bed and close the door to the room, if possible.

This provides for patient privacy.

6. Lower the head of the bed. Raise the bed to a comfortable working height (VHACEOSH, 2016). Lower the side rail. Remove the pillow and place a protective pad under the patient's head and shoulders (Figure 1).

Proper bed height helps reduce back strain while performing the procedure. A protective pad keeps the sheets from getting wet.

7. **Fill the pitcher with comfortably warm water (no more than 120°F [49°C]).** Position the patient at the top of the bed, in a supine position. Have the patient lift their head and place the shampoo board underneath the patient's head (Figure 2). If necessary, pad the edge of the board with a small towel.

Warm water is comfortable and relaxing for the patient. It also stimulates circulation and provides for more effective cleaning. Adjusting the water temperature to no more than 120°F (49°C) decreases risk of burns and drying of the skin (IAFF, n.d.). Padding the edge of the shampoo board may help increase patient comfort.

8. Place a drain container underneath the drain of the shampoo board (Figure 3).

The container will catch the runoff water, preventing a mess on the floor.

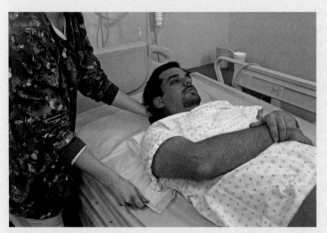

FIGURE 1. Placing protective pad under patient's head.

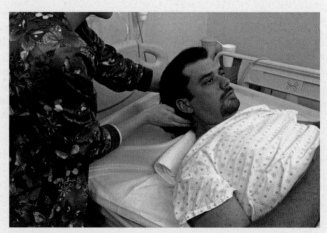

FIGURE 2. Placing patient's head on shampoo board.

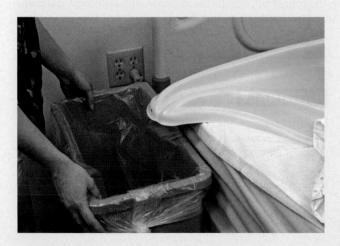

FIGURE 3. Positioning drain container for shampoo board.

ACTION

9. Put on gloves. If the patient is able, have them hold a folded washcloth at the forehead. Pour a pitcher of warm water slowly over the patient's head, making sure that all hair is saturated (Figure 4). Refill pitcher, if needed.

10. Apply a small amount of shampoo to the patient's hair. Lather shampoo. Massage deep into the scalp, avoiding any cuts, lesions, or sore spots.

11. Rinse with comfortably warm water until all shampoo is out of hair (Figure 5). Repeat shampoo, if necessary.

12. If the patient has thick hair or requests it, apply a small amount of conditioner to the hair and massage throughout. Avoid any cuts, lesions, or sore spots.

13. If drain container is small, empty before rinsing hair. Rinse with comfortably warm water until all conditioner is out of hair.

14. Remove shampoo board. Place towel around the patient's hair.

15. Pat hair dry, avoiding any cuts, lesions, or sore spots (Figure 6). Remove protective padding but keep one dry protective pad under the patient's hair.

RATIONALE

Gloves prevent the spread of microorganisms. A washcloth prevents water from running into the patient's eyes. By pouring slowly, more hair will become wet, and it is more soothing for the patient.

Shampoo will help to remove dirt or oil.

Shampoo left in hair may cause pruritus. If hair is still dirty, another shampoo treatment may be needed.

Conditioner eases tangles and moisturizes hair and scalp.

Container may overflow if not emptied. Conditioner left in hair may cause pruritus.

This prevents the patient from getting cold.

Patting dry removes any excess water without damaging hair or scalp.

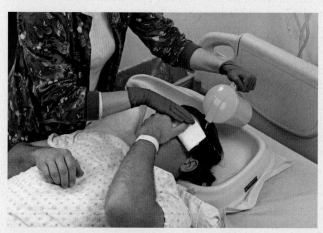

FIGURE 4. Pouring warm water over patient's head.

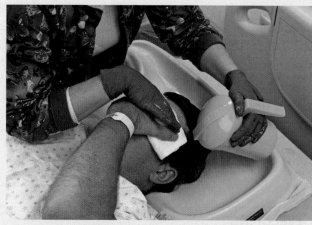

FIGURE 5. Rinsing shampoo from patient's head.

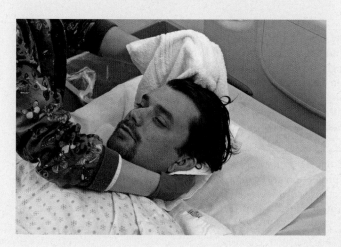

FIGURE 6. Patting patient's hair dry.

(*continued on page 430*)

Skill 7-7 ▶ Shampooing a Patient's Hair in Bed *(continued)*

ACTION	RATIONALE
16. Gently brush or comb hair, removing tangles, as needed. Apply additional hair product, such as leave-in conditioner, oil, or pomade, based on patient preferences. Style the hair according to the patient's preference.	Removing tangles helps hair to dry faster. Brushing and styling hair improves the patient's self-image.
17. Blow-dry hair on a cool setting, if allowed and if the patient wishes. If not, consider covering the patient's head with a dry towel, until hair is dry.	Blow-drying hair helps hair to dry faster and prevents the patient from becoming chilled. Keeping the head covered prevents chilling while hair is drying.
18. Change the patient's gown and remove protective pad. Replace pillow. Remove gloves. Perform hand hygiene.	If the patient's gown is damp, the patient will become chilled. Protective pad is no longer needed once hair is dry. Removing gloves properly reduces the risk for infection transmission and contamination of other items. Hand hygiene deters spread of microorganisms.
19. Remove the equipment and return the patient to a position of comfort. Raise the side rail and lower the bed.	Promotes patient comfort and safety. Removing gloves properly reduces the risk for infection transmission and contamination of other items.
20. Remove additional PPE, if used. Perform hand hygiene.	Proper removal of PPE reduces the risk for infection transmission and contamination of other items. Hand hygiene deters spread of microorganisms.

EVALUATION

The expected outcomes have been met when the patient's hair has been cleaned, the patient has verbalized a positive body image, and the patient has reported an increase in comfort level.

DOCUMENTATION

Guidelines

Record your assessment, significant observations, and unusual findings, such as bleeding or inflammation. Document any teaching done. Document care provided and patient response.

Sample Documentation

> 7/4/25 1130 Hair washed. Moderate amount of dried blood in hair noted. A 3-cm laceration noted over left parietal area. Edges well approximated, slight redness of wound, surrounding skin consistent with rest of skin tone, sutures intact, and no drainage noted.
>
> —C. Stone, RN

DEVELOPING CLINICAL REASONING AND CLINICAL JUDGMENT

UNEXPECTED SITUATIONS AND ASSOCIATED INTERVENTIONS

- *Glass is found in hair:* Carefully comb through hair before washing to remove as much glass as possible. Discard the glass in an appropriate container. When massaging the scalp, be alert to signs of pain from the patient; glass could be cutting the patient's head.
- *Nits (lice eggs) are noted on hair shafts:* Consult with the health care team regarding prescribed intervention to treat pediculosis. Follow facility policy regarding implementation of transmission precautions pending treatment. Depending on the patient's circumstances, follow up with the family/caregivers regarding possible infection.

SPECIAL CONSIDERATIONS

If the patient has a spinal cord or neck injury, use of the shampoo board may be contraindicated. In this case, a makeshift protection area can be created to wash the patient's hair without using the board. Place a protective pad underneath the patient's head and shoulders. Roll a towel into the bottom of the protective pad and direct the roll into one area so that water will drain into the container.

Skill Variation ▶ Shampooing a Patient's Hair With a Shampoo Cap

Shampoo caps are available and are being used with increasing frequency. These commercially prepared, disposable caps contain a rinseless shampoo product.

1. Review chart for any limitations in physical activity, or contraindications to the procedure. Confirm presence of prescribed intervention for shampooing the patient's hair, if required by facility policy.
2. Warm the cap in the microwave, according to the manufacturer's directions, or remove it from the storage warmer.

3. Perform hand hygiene and put on PPE, if indicated.

4. Identify the patient.

5. Explain what you are going to do and the reason for doing it to the patient.
6. Assemble necessary equipment on the bedside stand, overbed table, or other surface within reach.

7. Close the curtains around the bed and close the door to the room, if possible.
8. Put on gloves. Raise bed to a comfortable working height (VHACEOSH, 2016). Place a towel across the patient's chest. Place the shampoo cap on the patient's head (Figure A).
9. Massage the scalp and hair through the cap to lather the shampoo. Continue to massage according to the time frame specified by the manufacturer's directions (Figure B).
10. Remove and discard the shampoo cap.
11. Dry the patient's hair with a towel.
12. Remove the towel from the patient's chest.
13. Comb and style the hair. It may be appropriate to keep the head covered with a towel until the hair dries, to help minimize chilling of the patient.

14. Remove gloves. Perform hand hygiene.

15. Lower the bed. Assist the patient to a comfortable position.

16. Remove additional PPE, if used. Perform hand hygiene.

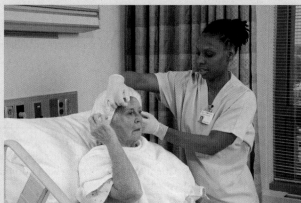

FIGURE A. Placing warmed shampoo cap on the patient's head.

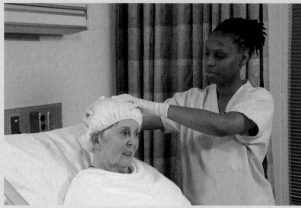

FIGURE B. Massaging the hair and scalp.

Skill 7-8 ▶ Assisting the Patient to Shave

For many patients, shaving is a daily hygiene ritual. They may feel disheveled and unclean without shaving. Some patients may need help with shaving when using a standard razor or may require that the nurse perform the shaving procedure for them completely. Patients with beards or mustaches may require nursing assistance to keep the beard and mustache clean. However, never trim or shave a patient's beard or mustache without the patient's consent. Female patients may require assistance with shaving underarm and leg hair, depending on the patient's personal preference and abilities. If available and permitted by the facility, electric shavers are usually recommended when the patient is receiving anticoagulant therapy or has a bleeding disorder (Hartford HealthCare, 2019). Electric shavers are especially convenient for ill and bedridden patients. This skill outlines one technique for shaving with a standard razor.

DELEGATION CONSIDERATIONS	The shaving of a patient's hair may be delegated to assistive personnel (AP) after assessment by the registered nurse as well as to licensed practical/vocational nurses (LPN/LVNs). The decision to delegate must be based on careful analysis of the patient's needs and circumstances as well as the qualifications of the person to whom the task is being delegated. Refer to the Delegation Guidelines Appendix A.

EQUIPMENT	• Shaving cream or gel • Disposable gloves • Safety razor • Additional PPE, as indicated • Towel • Waterproof pad • Washcloth • Aftershave or lotion (optional) • Bath basin

ASSESSMENT	Assess the patient's shaving preferences: frequency, time of day, and type of shaving products. Assess for any physical activity limitations. Assess the patient for any bleeding problems. If the patient is receiving any anticoagulant, such as heparin or warfarin, has received an antithrombolytic agent, or has a low platelet count, consider using an electric razor. Inspect the area to be shaved for any lesions or areas of altered skin integrity. Assess the patient's ability to shave independently or for the need of assistance with the procedure.

ACTUAL OR POTENTIAL HEALTH PROBLEMS AND NEEDS	Many actual or potential health problems or issues may require the use of this skill as part of related interventions. An appropriate health problem or issue may include: • Injury risk • Fatigue • Impaired ability to groom

OUTCOME IDENTIFICATION AND PLANNING	The expected outcome to achieve when assisting the patient with shaving is that the patient will be groomed with consideration to their preferences, without evidence of trauma to the skin. Other outcomes that may be appropriate include the following: the patient tolerates shaving with minimal to no difficulty, and the patient verbalizes feelings of improved self-esteem.

IMPLEMENTATION

ACTION	**RATIONALE**
1. Review the health record for any limitations in physical activity, or contraindications to the procedure. Confirm the presence of a prescribed intervention for shaving the patient, if required by facility policy.	Identifying limitations prevents patient discomfort and injury. In some settings, a prescribed intervention is required for shaving a patient with certain health problems or taking medications that affect coagulation.
2. Perform hand hygiene. Put on PPE, as indicated.	Hand hygiene and PPE prevent the spread of microorganisms. PPE is required based on transmission precautions.

ACTION

3. Identify the patient. Explain the procedure to the patient.

4. Assemble equipment on the overbed table or other surface within reach.

5. Close the curtains around the bed and close the door to the room, if possible.

6. Raise the bed to a comfortable working height (VHACEOSH, 2016). Lower the side rail. Cover the patient's chest with a towel or waterproof pad. Fill bath basin with comfortably warm (no more than 120°F [49°C]) water. Put on gloves. Wet a washcloth in the basin of water. Press the warm washcloth on the area to be shaved.

7. Dispense shaving cream or gel into the palm of the hand. Apply cream to the area to be shaved in a layer about 0.5 inch thick (Figure 1). Allow to remain on the skin for a few minutes.

8. With one hand, hold the skin steady at the area to be shaved. Using a smooth stroke, begin shaving. If shaving the face, shave with the direction of hair growth in short strokes (Figure 2). If shaving a leg, shave against the hair in upward, short strokes. If shaving an underarm, hold skin steady and use short, upward strokes.

9. Remove residual shaving cream with wet washcloth (Figure 3).

RATIONALE

Identifying the patient ensures the right patient receives the intervention and helps prevent errors. Explanation facilitates engagement in care.

Organization facilitates performance of the task.

This provides for patient privacy.

Proper bed height helps reduce back strain while performing the procedure. Adjusting the water temperature to no more than 120°F (49°C) decreases risk of burns and drying of the skin (IAFF, n.d.). Warm water is comfortable and relaxing for the patient. Moistens skin and softens hair. Gloves prevent the spread of microorganisms. Warm water softens the hair, making the process easier.

Using shaving cream or gel helps to prevent skin irritation and prevents hair from pulling. Applying cream or gel a few minutes before shaving softens the hair (MFMER, 2020a).

Holding the skin steady prevents the razor from pulling on the skin. Do not pull the skin taut while shaving to reduce the risk for ingrown hairs (MFMER, 2020a). The skin on the face is more sensitive and needs to be shaved with the direction of hair growth to prevent discomfort and ingrown hairs (MFMER, 2020a).

Shaving cream can lead to irritation if left on the skin.

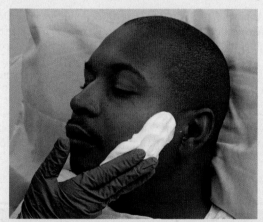
FIGURE 1. Applying shaving cream to face.

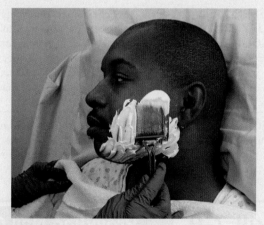
FIGURE 2. Shaving face.

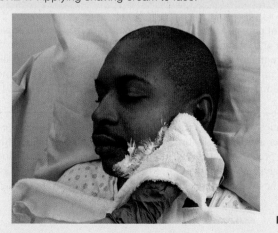

FIGURE 3. Using a wet washcloth to remove remaining shaving cream.

(continued on page 434)

Skill 7-8 ▶ Assisting the Patient to Shave *(continued)*

ACTION	RATIONALE
10. If the patient requests, apply aftershave or lotion to the area shaved. Remove gloves. Perform hand hygiene.	Aftershave and lotion can reduce skin irritation. Removing gloves properly reduces the risk for infection transmission and contamination of other items. Hand hygiene deters spread of microorganisms.
11. Remove equipment and return the patient to a position of comfort. Raise the side rail and lower the bed.	This promotes patient comfort and safety.
12. Remove additional PPE, if used. Perform hand hygiene.	Proper removal of PPE reduces the risk for infection transmission and contamination of other items. Hand hygiene deters spread of microorganisms.

EVALUATION

The expected outcome has been met when the patient has been groomed without evidence of trauma, irritation, or redness. In addition, the patient has verbalized feeling refreshed and has demonstrated improved self-esteem.

DOCUMENTATION

Shaving a patient does not usually require documentation. However, if your skin assessment reveals any unusual findings, document your assessment and the procedure. If the patient or nurse breaks the skin while shaving, document the occurrence and your assessment of the patient.

DEVELOPING CLINICAL REASONING AND CLINICAL JUDGMENT

UNEXPECTED SITUATIONS AND ASSOCIATED INTERVENTIONS

- *Patient is cut and bleeds during shave:* Apply pressure with gauze or towel to injured area. Do not release pressure for 2 to 3 minutes. After bleeding has stopped, resume shaving. The water basin may need to be rewarmed before washing off the shaving cream. Document the occurrence and assessment of area after the shave.
- *Patient has a large amount of hair to be shaved:* If the hair is longer, it may need to be trimmed with scissors before shaving to prevent pulling of hair when shaving.

SPECIAL CONSIDERATIONS

- *Patient is wearing a beard:* Do not shave the patient's beard without consent unless it is an emergency situation, such as insertion of an endotracheal tube. For this procedure, shave only the area needed and leave the rest of the beard.

Skill 7-9 ▶ Providing Nail Care

Care of the nails is important to prevent pain and infection. Poor toenail care may lead to impaired mobility. The nurse should document and communicate findings with the health care team: findings such as discoloration of the entire nail or a dark streak under the nail; changes in nail shape, such as curled nails; thinning or thickening of the nails; separation of the nail from the surrounding skin; bleeding around the nails; and redness, swelling, or pain around the nails (MFMER, 2019b).

DELEGATION CONSIDERATIONS

Depending on the organization's policies and procedures, the care of a patient's nails may be delegated to assistive personnel (AP) after assessment by the registered nurse. The care of a patient's nails may be delegated to licensed practical/vocational nurses (LPN/LVNs). The decision to delegate must be based on careful analysis of the patient's needs and circumstances as well as the qualifications of the person to whom the task is being delegated. Refer to the Delegation Guidelines in Appendix A.

EQUIPMENT	• Nail file	• Towel
	• Nail clipper	• Wash basin and skin cleanser, or commercially prepared bathing system
	• Cuticle scissors	
	• Orangewood stick or cuticle stick	• Disposable gloves
	• Emollient	• Additional PPE, if indicated
	• Disposable waterproof pad	

ASSESSMENT

Assess the patient's nail care preferences: frequency, time of day, and type of products. Assess for any physical activity limitations. Assess for conditions that may put the patient at high risk for nail problems, such as diabetes and peripheral vascular disease. Assess the color and temperature of fingers and toes. Assess adequacy of pulses to area and capillary refill. Assess the skin of fingers and toes for dryness, cracking, or inflammation. Assess the nails and surrounding skin for changes in nail color, changes in nail shape, thinning or thickening of the nails, separation of the nail from the surrounding skin, bleeding around the nails, and redness, swelling, or pain around the nails. Nails should appear intact, smooth, firmly attached to the nail bed, and pink in color, with a white crescent visible at the base. Dark streaks running lengthwise in nails and freckles are a normal variation for patients with darker skin tones (Jarvis & Echkhardt, 2020). Assess the patient's ability for self-care of nails or assist with the procedure.

ACTUAL OR POTENTIAL HEALTH PROBLEMS AND NEEDS

Many actual or potential health problems or issues may require the use of this skill as part of related interventions. An appropriate health problem or issue may include:
• Injury risk
• Fatigue
• Impaired ability to groom

OUTCOME IDENTIFICATION AND PLANNING

The expected outcome to achieve when assisting the patient with care of the nails is that the nails are trimmed and clean with smooth edges and intact cuticles, without evidence of trauma to nails or surrounding skin. Other outcomes that may be appropriate include the patient verbalizing feelings of improved self-esteem.

IMPLEMENTATION

ACTION	**RATIONALE**
1. Review the patient's health record for any limitations in physical activity, or contraindications to the procedure. Confirm presence of prescribed intervention for nail care, if required by facility policy.	Identifying limitations prevents patient discomfort and injury. In some settings, a prescribed intervention is required for nail care, particularly for a patient with certain health problems.
2. Perform hand hygiene. Put on PPE, as indicated.	Hand hygiene and PPE prevent the spread of microorganisms. PPE is required based on transmission precautions.
3. Identify the patient. Explain the procedure to the patient.	Identifying the patient ensures the right patient receives the intervention and helps prevent errors. Explanation facilitates engagement in care.
4. Assemble equipment on the overbed table or other surface within reach.	Organization facilitates performance of the task.
5. Close the curtains around the bed and close the door to the room, if possible.	This provides for patient privacy.
6. Raise the bed to a comfortable working position (VHACEOSH, 2016). Lower the side rail. Place a towel or waterproof pad under the patient's hand or foot.	Proper bed height helps reduce back strain while performing the procedure. Waterproof pad protects bed linens and surrounding surfaces.

(continued on page 436)

Skill 7-9 ▶ Providing Nail Care *(continued)*

ACTION	**RATIONALE**
7. Put on gloves. Wash the patient's hands or feet, depending on the care to be given.	Gloves prevent the spread of microorganisms. Washing removes surface dirt and softens nails and skin, making it easier to trim and care for cuticles.
8. Gently clean under the nails using the cuticle or orange-wood stick (Figure 1). Wash hand or foot.	Washing removes debris and dirt dislodged from under nails.
9. Clip nails, if necessary. Avoid cutting the whole nail in one attempt. Use the tip of the nail clipper and take small cuts (Beuscher, 2019). Cut the nail straight across (Figure 2). Do not trim so far down on the sides that the skin and cuticle are injured. This is particularly important for people with diabetes or circulatory problems (American College of Foot and Ankle Surgeons, n.d.b; Mayo Foundation for Medical Education and Research [MFMER], 2017).	Cutting the entire nail in one attempt may lead to splitting the nail. Cutting straight across prevents injury to nail, cuticle, and finger or toe and reduces risk for in-growing nails (American College of Foot and Ankle Surgeons, n.d.b; MFMER, 2019b).

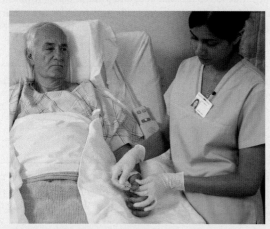

FIGURE 1. Gently cleaning under nails.

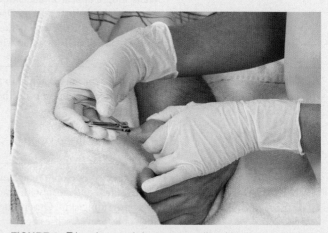

FIGURE 2. Trimming straight across nails with clipper.

10. File the nail straight across, then round the tips in a gentle curve, to shape the nail. Do not trim so far down on the sides that the skin and cuticle are injured. This is particularly important for people with diabetes or circulatory problems (American College of Foot and Ankle Surgeons [ACFAS], n.d.a; American College of Foot and Ankle Surgeons [ACFAS], n.d.b; MFMER, 2017).	This smooths the nail; prevents injury to the nail, cuticle, and finger or toe; and reduces the risk for ingrowing nails (American College of Foot and Ankle Surgeons, n.d.b; ACFAS, n.d.b; MFMER, 2019b).
11. Remove hangnails, which are broken pieces of cuticle, by carefully trimming them off with cuticle scissors. **Do not pull or rip off hangnails.** Avoid injury to tissue with the cuticle scissors.	This removes dead cuticle and reduces hangnail formation. Tearing of a hangnail can cause injury to live tissue (MFMER, 2019b).
12. Gently push cuticles back off the nail using the orangewood or cuticle stick or towel (Figure 3).	This keeps cuticles and nails neat and prevents cracking and drying of cuticles.
13. Dry hand or foot thoroughly, taking care to be sure to dry between fingers or toes (Figure 4). Apply an emollient to the hand or foot, rubbing it into the nails and cuticles. **Do not moisturize between the toes of patients with diabetes or peripheral artery disease** (ACFAS, n.d.b; MFMER, 2017).	Thorough drying reduces risk of maceration, damage from overly and consistently wet skin. Maceration increases risk for injury from rubbing or friction, and risk for fungal and bacterial infections. Moisturizing between the toes of patients with peripheral artery disease can encourage fungal growth (ACFAS, n.d.a).
14. Repeat Steps 7–13 for other extremity or extremities.	
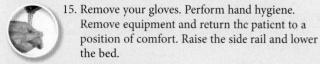 15. Remove your gloves. Perform hand hygiene. Remove equipment and return the patient to a position of comfort. Raise the side rail and lower the bed.	Removing gloves properly reduces the risk for infection transmission and contamination of other items. Hand hygiene deters spread of microorganisms. Promotes patient comfort and safety.

ACTION

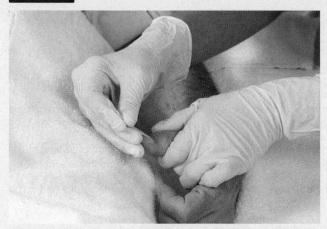

FIGURE 3. Gently pushing cuticles back off nail.

RATIONALE

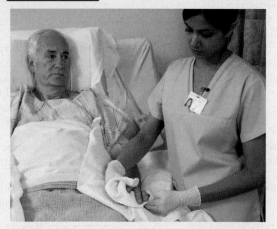

FIGURE 4. Drying hand thoroughly.

 16. Remove additional PPE, if used. Perform hand hygiene.

Proper removal of PPE reduces the risk for infection transmission and contamination of other items. Hand hygiene deters spread of microorganisms.

EVALUATION

The expected outcome has been met when the patient's nails have been trimmed and cleaned with smooth edges and intact cuticles, without evidence of trauma to nails or surrounding skin. In addition, the patient has verbalized feeling refreshed and has demonstrated improved self-esteem.

DOCUMENTATION

Guidelines

Record your assessment, significant observations, and unusual findings, such as broken nails or inflammation. Document any teaching done. Document care provided and patient response. Nail care is often recorded on routine flow sheet.

Sample Documentation

7/17/25 2030 Nail care performed for fingernails. Nails intact, supple, nail bed pink in color, with white crescent visible at the base. Significant amount of old food removed from under nails. Skin on fingers and hands dry and cracked; emollient applied.
—*J. Lyman, RN*

DEVELOPING CLINICAL REASONING AND CLINICAL JUDGMENT

UNEXPECTED SITUATIONS AND ASSOCIATED INTERVENTIONS

- *Patient is cut and bleeds during nail care:* Apply pressure with gauze or towel to the injured area. Do not release pressure for 2 to 3 minutes. Assess the area. Document the occurrence and assessment of area; communicate incident and findings with the health care team according to facility policy. Continue to monitor the area for bleeding and inflammation.
- *Cuticles, fingers, or toes are inflamed and tender:* Assess the area. Document findings. Communicate findings with the health care team. Resume care as appropriate after consultation with the health care team and based on facility policy.
- *Calluses, corns, or bunions are present:* Assess area and document findings. Do not cut or file. Communicate findings with the health care team and/or podiatrist for treatment.

(continued on page 438)

Skill 7-9 ▶ Providing Nail Care *(continued)*

SPECIAL CONSIDERATIONS

General Considerations

- Advise the patient to avoid using fingernails as tools to pick, poke, or pry things to prevent nail damage.
- Discourage biting of nails or picking at cuticles. These habits can damage the nail bed. Even a minor cut alongside a fingernail can allow bacteria or fungi to enter and cause an infection (MFMER, 2019b).
- Advise patients to avoid pulling off hangnails. This can cause injury to live tissue that is pulled off along with the hangnail. Instead, carefully clip off hangnails (MFMER, 2019b).
- Advise patients to wear appropriate footwear. Break in new shoes gradually. Improperly fitting shoes can lead to corns, calluses, bunions, and blisters.

Infant and Child Considerations

- A newborn's nail beds may be cyanotic (blue) for the first few hours of life, and then turn pink.
- Infants' nails should be carefully trimmed on a regular basis to prevent scratching.

Older Adult Considerations

- Nails may have lengthwise ridges, due to decreased nail growth rate and injury to the nail bed.
- Nails may be brittle or peeling. Toenails may be thickened.

Community-Based Care Considerations

- Advise patients with diabetes or peripheral vascular disease to inspect feet daily for blisters, cuts, cracks, sores, redness, tenderness, or swelling. Encourage patients to communicate problems to their health care team for early intervention.
- Encourage patients with diabetes and peripheral vascular disease to schedule annual foot checks with their healthcare provider or podiatrist; these patients should consult with an advance practice provider or podiatrist for treatment related to bunions, corns, or calluses (ACFAS, n.d.b; Beuscher, 2019; MFMER, 2017).
- Instruct patients with diabetes and/or peripheral vascular disease to trim nails carefully and, if necessary, ask for assistance from a caregiver as necessary (MFMER, 2017).

Skill 7-10 ▶ Making an Unoccupied Bed
Skill Variation: *Making a Bed With a Flat Bottom Sheet*

A comfortable bed and appropriate bedding contribute to a patient's sense of well-being. Bed linens are changed after the bath if the patient is bathed in the bed. Otherwise, many facilities change linens only when soiled. If the patient can get out of bed, the nurse should make the bed while it is unoccupied to decrease stress on the patient and the nurse. The following procedure explains how to make the bed using a fitted bottom sheet. Some facilities do not provide fitted bottom sheets, or sometimes a fitted bottom sheet may not be available. If this is the case, refer to the Skill Variation at the end of this skill for using a flat bottom sheet, instead of a fitted sheet.

DELEGATION CONSIDERATIONS

The making of an unoccupied bed may be delegated to assistive personnel (AP) as well as to licensed practical/vocational nurses (LPN/LVNs). The decision to delegate must be based on careful analysis of the patient's needs and circumstances as well as the qualifications of the person to whom the task is being delegated. Refer to the Delegation Guidelines in Appendix A.

EQUIPMENT

- One large flat sheet
- One fitted sheet
- Lifting/repositioning sheet or friction-reducing sheet (optional)
- Blankets
- Bedspread
- Pillowcases
- Linen hamper or bag
- Bedside chair
- Waterproof protective pad (optional)
- Disposable gloves
- Additional PPE, as indicated

ASSESSMENT

Assess facility policies and patient preferences regarding linen changes. Assess for any physical activity limitations. Check for any patient belongings that may have accidentally been placed in the bed linens, such as eyeglasses or prayer cloths. Assess the need for a lifting/repositioning or friction-reducing sheet and waterproof protective pad based on patient circumstances.

ACTUAL OR POTENTIAL HEALTH PROBLEMS AND NEEDS	Many actual or potential health problems or issues may require the use of this skill as part of related interventions. An appropriate health problem or issue may include: • Impaired comfort • Altered skin integrity risk • Activity intolerance
OUTCOME IDENTIFICATION AND PLANNING	The expected outcome to achieve when making an unoccupied bed is that the bed linens will be changed without injury to the patient or nurse.

IMPLEMENTATION

ACTION	**RATIONALE**
1. Perform hand hygiene. Put on PPE, as indicated.	Hand hygiene and PPE prevent the spread of microorganisms. PPE is required based on transmission precautions.
2. Explain to the patient what you are going to do and the reason for doing it, if the patient is present in the room.	Explanation facilitates engagement in care.
3. Assemble necessary equipment on the bedside stand, over-bed table, or other surface within reach.	Arranging items nearby is convenient, saves time, and avoids unnecessary stretching and twisting of muscles on the part of the nurse.
4. Adjust the bed to a comfortable working height (VHACEOSH, 2016). Drop the side rails.	Having the bed at the proper height prevents back and muscle strain. Having the side rails down reduces strain on the nurse while working.
5. Disconnect the call bell or any tubes from bed linens.	Disconnecting devices prevents damage to the devices.
6. Put on gloves. Loosen all linen as you move around the bed, from the head of the bed on the far side to the head of the bed on the near side.	Gloves prevent the spread of microorganisms. Loosening the linen helps prevent tugging and tearing on linen. Loosening the linen and moving around the bed systematically reduce strain caused by reaching across the bed.
7. Fold reusable linens, such as sheets, blankets, or spread, in place on the bed in fourths and hang them over a clean chair.	Folding saves time and energy when reusable linen is replaced on the bed. Folding linens while they are on the bed reduces strain on the nurse's arms. Some facilities change linens only when soiled.
8. Snugly roll all the soiled linen inside the bottom sheet. Hold linen away from your body and place directly into the laundry hamper (Figure 1). **Do not place on floor or furniture. Do not hold soiled linens against your clothing.**	Rolling soiled linens snugly and placing them directly into the hamper helps prevent the spread of microorganisms. The floor is heavily contaminated; soiled linen will further contaminate furniture. Soiled linen contaminates the nurse's clothing, and this may spread organisms to another patient.

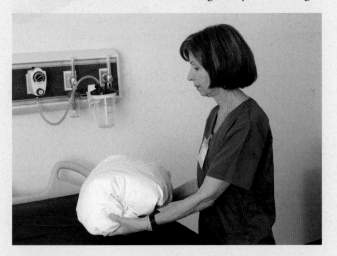

FIGURE 1. Bundling soiled linens in bottom sheet and holding them away from clothing.

(continued on page 440)

Skill 7-10 ▶ Making an Unoccupied Bed   *(continued)*

ACTION	**RATIONALE**

ACTION

9. If possible, shift the mattress up to the head of the bed. If the mattress is soiled, clean and dry according to facility policy before applying new sheets.

10. Remove your gloves, unless indicated for transmission-based precautions. Perform hand hygiene. Place the bottom sheet on the mattress and secure the bottom sheet over the corners at the head and foot of the mattress.

11. Push the sheet open to the center of the mattress, pulling the sheet taut from the secured corners (Figure 2). (See the Skill Variation at the end of this skill for using a flat bottom sheet, instead of a fitted sheet.)

12. If using, place the lifting/repositioning or friction-reducing sheet with its centerfold in the center of the bed and positioned so it will be located under the patient's midsection; open it and fanfold to the center of the mattress (Figure 3). If a protective pad is used, place it over the lifting/repositioning or friction-reducing sheet in the proper area and open to the centerfold. Not all facilities use lifting/repositioning sheets routinely. The nurse may decide to use one or a friction-reducing sheet based on patient circumstances. In some institutions, the protective pad doubles as a lifting/repositioning sheet. Tuck the lifting/repositioning or friction-reducing sheet securely under the mattress.

RATIONALE

This allows more foot room for the patient.

Gloves are not necessary to handle clean linen. Hand hygiene prevents the spread of microorganisms. Secures bottom sheet on one side of the bed.

Making the bed on one side and then completing the bedmaking on the other side saves time. Pulling the sheet taut keeps it in place on the mattress. Having bottom linens free of wrinkles reduces patient discomfort.

If the patient soils the bed, lifting/repositioning or friction-reducing sheet and pad can be changed without changing the bottom and top linens. Having all bottom linens in place before tucking them under the mattress avoids unnecessary moving about the bed. A lifting/repositioning or friction-reducing sheet can aid moving the patient in bed.

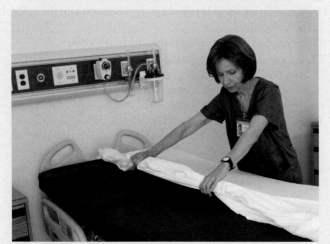

FIGURE 2. Pushing the bottom sheet open to the center of the mattress.

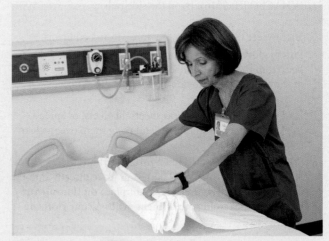

FIGURE 3. Placing lifting/repositioning sheet on bed.

13. Move to the other side of the bed to secure bottom linens. Pull the bottom sheet tightly and secure over the corners at the head and foot of the mattress. Pull the lifting/repositioning or friction-reducing sheet tightly and tuck it securely under the mattress.

This removes wrinkles from the bottom linens, which can cause patient discomfort and promote skin breakdown.

14. Place the top sheet on the bed with its centerfold in the center of the bed and with the hem even with the head of the mattress. Unfold the top sheet. Follow same procedure with top blanket or spread, placing the upper edge about 6 inches below the top of the sheet.

Opening linens by shaking them spreads organisms into the air. Holding linens overhead to open causes strain on the nurse's arms.

ACTION

15. Tuck the top sheet and blanket under the foot of the bed on the near side. Miter the corners (Figure 4). (See the Skill Variation at the end of this skill for information to miter a corner.)
16. Fold the upper 6 inches of the top sheet down over the spread and make a cuff.
17. Move to the other side of the bed and follow the same procedure for securing top sheets under the foot of the bed and making a cuff (Figure 5).

RATIONALE

This saves time and energy and keeps the top linen in place.

This makes it easier for the patient to get into bed and pull up the covers.

Working on one side of the bed at a time saves energy and is more efficient.

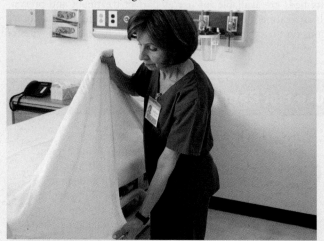

FIGURE 4. Mitering corner of top sheet and blanket.

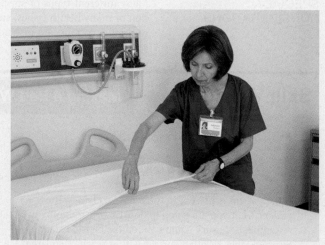

FIGURE 5. Cuffing top linens.

18. Place the pillows on the bed. Open each pillowcase in the same manner as you opened other linens. Gather the pillowcase over one hand toward the closed end. Grasp the pillow with the hand inside the pillowcase. Keep a firm hold on the top of the pillow and pull the cover onto the pillow. Place the pillow at the head of the bed.
19. Fan-fold or pie-fold the top linens.

20. Secure the signal device on the bed, according to facility policy.
21. Raise the side rail and lower the bed.
22. Dispose of soiled linen according to facility policy.

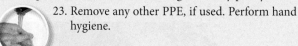 23. Remove any other PPE, if used. Perform hand hygiene.

Opening linens by shaking causes organisms to be carried on air currents. Covering the pillow while it rests on the bed reduces strain on the nurse's arms and back.

Having linens opened makes it more convenient for the patient to get into bed.

The patient will be able to call for assistance as necessary. Promotes patient comfort and safety.

This promotes patient comfort and safety.

This deters the spread of microorganisms.

Proper removal of PPE reduces the risk for infection transmission and contamination of other items. Hand hygiene prevents the spread of microorganisms.

EVALUATION   The expected outcome is met when the bed linens have been changed without any injury to the patient or nurse.

DOCUMENTATION   Changing of bed linens does not require documentation. The use of a specialty bed or bed equipment should be documented.

(continued on page 442)

Skill 7-10 ▶ Making an Unoccupied Bed *(continued)*

DEVELOPING CLINICAL REASONING AND CLINICAL JUDGMENT

UNEXPECTED SITUATIONS AND ASSOCIATED INTERVENTIONS

- *Lifting/repositioning sheet is not available:* A flat sheet can be folded in half to substitute for a lifting/repositioning sheet, but extra care must be taken to avoid wrinkles in the bed.
- *Patient is frequently incontinent of stool or urine:* More than one protective pad can be placed under the patient to protect the bed, but take care to ensure that the patient is not lying on wrinkles from linens.

SPECIAL CONSIDERATIONS

- Many different types of specialty beds are available for use as part of treatment and prevention of many health issues, such as treatment of pressure injuries. Refer to the manufacturer's recommendations and instructions on use of specialty linens and products with these types of equipment.

Skill Variation ▶ Making a Bed With a Flat Bottom Sheet

1. Perform hand hygiene and put on PPE, if indicated.

2. If the patient is present in the room, explain to the patient what you are going to do why you are doing it.
3. Assemble necessary equipment on the bedside stand, overbed table, or other surface within reach. Two large flat sheets are needed.
4. Raise the bed to a comfortable working position (VHACEOSH, 2016). Disconnect the call bell or any other equipment from bed linens.
5. Put on gloves. Loosen all linen as you move around the bed, from the head of the bed on the far side to the head of the bed on the near side.
6. Fold reusable linens, such as sheets, blankets, or spread, in place on the bed in fourths and hang them over a clean chair.
7. Snugly roll all the soiled linen inside the bottom sheet and place directly into the laundry hamper. Do not place on floor or furniture. Do not hold soiled linens against your clothing.

8. If possible, shift mattress up to head of bed.

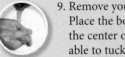

9. Remove your gloves. Perform hand hygiene. Place the bottom sheet with its centerfold in the center of the bed and high enough to be able to tuck it under the head of the mattress. Open the sheet and fan-fold it to the center.
10. If using, place the lifting/repositioning or friction-reducing sheet with its centerfold in the center of the bed and positioned so it will be located under the patient's midsection. Open it and fan-fold it to the center of the mattress. If a protective pad is used, place it over the lifting/repositioning or friction-reducing sheet in the proper area and open it to the centerfold.
11. Tuck the bottom sheet securely under the head of the mattress on one side of the bed, making a corner. Corners are usually mitered. Grasp the side edge of the sheet about 18 inches down from the mattress top (Figure A). Lay the sheet on top of the mattress to form a triangular, flat fold (Figure B). Tuck the portion of the sheet that is hanging loose below the mattress under the mattress without pulling on the triangular fold (Figure C). Pick the top of the triangle fold and place it over the side of

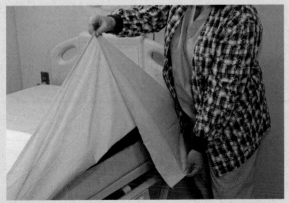

FIGURE A. Grasping side edge of sheet and lifting off the bed.

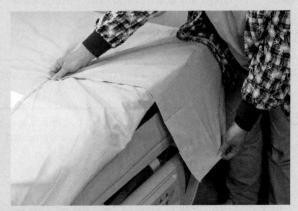

FIGURE B. Laying sheet on top of bed to make triangular, flat fold.

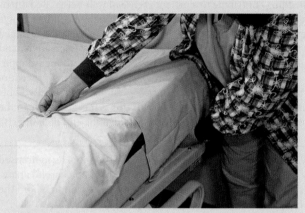

FIGURE C. Tucking the loose part of the sheet under the mattress.

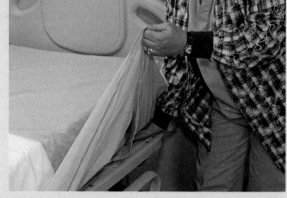

FIGURE D. Picking up the top of the triangular fold to place down over the side of the mattress.

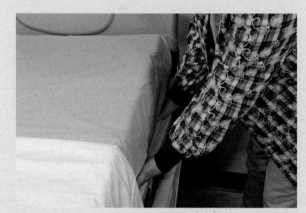

FIGURE E. Tucking the loose portion of triangular fold under mattress.

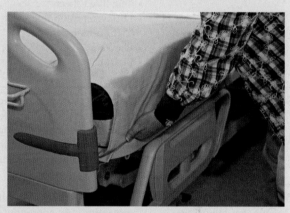

FIGURE F. Tucking remaining sheet snugly under mattress.

the mattress (Figure D). Tuck this loose portion of the sheet under the mattress (Figure E). Continue tucking the remaining bottom sheet and lifting/repositioning or friction-reducing sheet securely under the mattress. Move to the other side of the bed to secure the bottom linen. Pull the sheets across the mattress from the centerfold. Secure the bottom of the sheet under the head of the bed and miter the corner. Pull the remainder of the sheet and the lifting/repositioning or friction-reducing sheet tightly and tuck under the mattress, starting at the head of the bed and moving toward the foot (Figure F).

12. Place the top sheet on the bed with its centerfold in the center of the bed and with the hem even with the head of the mattress. Unfold the top sheet. Follow the same procedure with the top blanket or spread, placing the upper edge about 6 inches below the top of the sheet.

13. Tuck the top sheet and blanket under the foot of the bed on the near side. Miter the corners.

14. Fold the upper 6 inches of the top sheet down over the spread and make a cuff.

15. Move to the other side of the bed and follow the same procedure for securing the top sheet under the foot of the bed and making a cuff.

16. Place the pillows on the bed. Open each pillowcase in the same manner as you opened other linens. Gather the pillowcase over one hand toward the closed end. Grasp the pillow with the hand inside the pillowcase. Keep a firm hold on the top of the pillow and pull the cover onto the pillow. Place the pillow at the head of the bed.

17. Fan-fold or pie-fold the top linen.

18. Secure the signal device on the bed according to facility policy.

19. Adjust the bed to the low position. Raise the rail.

 20. Dispose of soiled linens according to facility policy. Remove any other PPE, if used. Perform hand hygiene.

Skill 7-11 ▶ Making an Occupied Bed

A comfortable bed and appropriate bedding contribute to a patient's sense of well-being. Bed linens are changed after the bath if the patient is bathed in the bed. Otherwise, many facilities change linens only when soiled. If the patient cannot get out of bed, the linens may need to be changed with the patient still in the bed. This is termed an "occupied" bed. In some instances, creativity and flexibility are necessary when changing linens because of the patient's condition, orthopedic appliances or other equipment in use, or treatments that may be in progress. The following procedure explains how to make the bed using a fitted bottom sheet. Some facilities do not provide fitted bottom sheets, or sometimes a fitted bottom sheet may not be available. If this is the case, refer to the Skill Variation for using a flat bottom sheet instead of a fitted sheet, located at the end of Skill 7-10.

DELEGATION CONSIDERATIONS	The making of an occupied bed may be delegated to assistive personnel (AP) as well as to licensed practical/vocational nurses (LPN/LVNs). The decision to delegate must be based on careful analysis of the patient's needs and circumstances as well as the qualifications of the person to whom the task is being delegated. Refer to the Delegation Guidelines in Appendix A.

EQUIPMENT

- One large flat sheet
- One fitted sheet
- Lifting/repositioning sheet (optional) or friction-reducing sheet
- Blankets
- Bedspread
- Pillowcases
- Linen hamper or bag
- Bedside chair
- Protective pad (optional)
- Disposable gloves
- Additional PPE, as indicated

ASSESSMENT	Assess the facility policies and patient's preferences regarding linen changes. Assess for any precautions or activity restrictions for the patient. Check the bed for any patient belongings that may have accidentally been placed or fallen there, such as eyeglasses or prayer cloths. Note the presence and position of any tubes or drains that the patient may have. Assess the need for a lifting/repositioning or friction-reducing sheet and waterproof protective pad based on patient circumstances.
ACTUAL OR POTENTIAL HEALTH PROBLEMS AND NEEDS	Many actual or potential health problems or issues may require the use of this skill as part of related interventions. An appropriate health problem or issue may include: • Impaired comfort • Impaired mobility in bed • Activity intolerance
OUTCOME IDENTIFICATION AND PLANNING	The expected outcome to achieve when making an occupied bed is that the bed linens are applied without injury to the patient or nurse. Other possible outcomes may include the patient participating in moving from side to side, and the patient verbalizes feelings of increased comfort.

IMPLEMENTATION

ACTION	**RATIONALE**
1. Check the health care record for limitations on the patient's physical activity.	This facilitates patient engagement in care, determines level of activity, and promotes patient safety.
2. Perform hand hygiene. Put on PPE, as indicated.	Hand hygiene and PPE prevent the spread of microorganisms. PPE is required based on transmission precautions.
3. Identify the patient. Explain what you are going to do.	Patient identification validates the correct patient and correct procedure. Discussion and explanation allay anxiety and prepare the patient for what to expect.
4. Assemble equipment on the overbed table or other surface within reach.	Organization facilitates performance of the task.

ACTION

5. Close the curtains around the bed and close the door to the room, if possible.

6. Adjust the bed to a comfortable working height (VHACEOSH, 2016).

7. Lower the side rail nearest you, leaving the opposite side rail up. Place the bed in a flat position unless contraindicated.

8. Put on gloves. Check bed linens for the patient's personal items. **Disconnect the call bell or any tubes/drains from bed linens.**

9. Place a bath blanket over the patient. Have the patient hold on to the bath blanket while you reach under it and remove the top linen (Figure 1). Leave the top sheet in place if a bath blanket is not used and loosen from bottom of bed. Fold linen that is to be reused over the back of a chair. Discard soiled linen in a laundry bag or hamper. **Do not place on floor or furniture. Do not hold soiled linens against your clothing.**

10. If possible, and another person is available to assist, grasp the mattress securely and shift it up to head of bed.

11. Assist the patient to turn toward the opposite side of the bed, and reposition the pillow under the patient's head. If the patient is partially able or unable to assist, friction-reducing devices, lifting/repositioning sheets, lateral transfer devices, and a full-body sling are potential equipment to consider, based on screening and assessment. Consider available bed features (turning, pressure release, rotation) to assist with the action (VA Mobile Health, n.d.).

12. Loosen all bottom linens from the head, foot, and side of the bed.

13. Fan-fold or roll soiled linens as close to the patient as possible (Figure 2).

RATIONALE

This ensures the patient's privacy.

Having the bed at the proper height prevents back and muscle strain.

Having the mattress flat makes it easier to prepare a wrinkle-free bed.

Gloves prevent the spread of microorganisms. It is costly and inconvenient when personal items are lost. Disconnecting tubes from linens prevents discomfort and accidental dislodging of the tubes.

The blanket provides warmth and privacy. Placing linens directly into the hamper helps prevent the spread of microorganisms. The floor is heavily contaminated; soiled linen will further contaminate furniture. Soiled linen contaminates the nurse's clothing, and this may spread organisms to another patient.

This allows more foot room for the patient.

This allows the bed to be made on the vacant side. Use of safe patient handling and mobility devices are best practice to prevent patient and health care provider injury (VA Mobile Health, n.d.; VHACEOSH, 2016).

This facilitates removal of linens.

This makes it easier to remove linens when the patient turns to the other side.

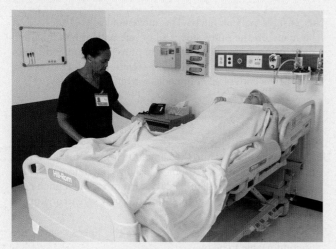

FIGURE 1. Removing top linens from under bath blanket.

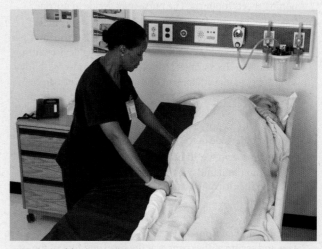

FIGURE 2. Moving soiled linen as close to patient as possible.

(continued on page 446)

Skill 7-11 ▶ Making an Occupied Bed *(continued)*

ACTION	RATIONALE

ACTION

14. Use clean linen and make the near side of the bed. Place the bottom sheet in the center of the bed. Open the sheet and pull the bottom sheet over the corners at the head and foot of the mattress (Figure 3). Push the sheet toward the center of the bed, pulling it taut and positioning it under the old linens (Figure 4). (See the Skill Variation at the end of Skill 7-10 for information on using a flat bottom sheet, instead of a fitted sheet.)

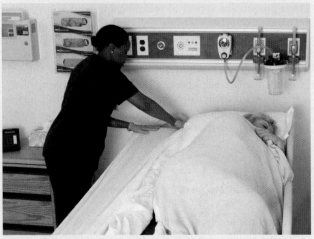

FIGURE 3. Pulling the bottom sheet over the corners at the head and foot of the mattress.

15. If using, place the lifting/repositioning or friction-reducing sheet with its centerfold in the center of the bed and positioned so it will be located under the patient's midsection. Open the lifting/repositioning or friction-reducing sheet and fan-fold it to the center of the mattress. Tuck it securely under the mattress (Figure 5). If a protective pad is used, place it over the lifting/repositioning or friction-reducing sheet in the proper area and open to the centerfold. Not all facilities use lifting/repositioning sheets routinely. The nurse may decide to use one.

16. Raise the side rail. Assist the patient to roll over the folded linen in the middle of the bed toward you. If the patient is partially able or unable to assist, friction-reducing devices, lifting/repositioning sheets, lateral transfer devices, and a full-body sling are potential equipment to consider, based on screening and assessment. Consider available bed features (turning, pressure release, rotation) to assist with the action (VA Mobile Health, n.d.). Reposition pillow and bath blanket or top sheet. Move to other side of the bed and lower the side rail.

17. Loosen and remove all bottom linen (Figure 6). Discard soiled linen in laundry bag or hamper. **Do not place on floor or furniture. Do not hold soiled linens against your clothing.**

18. Ease clean linen from under the patient. Pull the bottom sheet taut and secure at the corners at the head and foot of the mattress. Pull the lifting/repositioning or friction-reducing sheet tight and smooth. Tuck it securely under the mattress. (See the Skill Variation at the end of Skill 7-10 for information on using a flat bottom sheet, instead of a fitted sheet.)

RATIONALE

Opening linens on the bed reduces strain on the nurse's arms and diminishes the spread of microorganisms. Centering the sheet ensures sufficient coverage for both sides of the mattress. Positioning under the old linens makes it easier to remove linens.

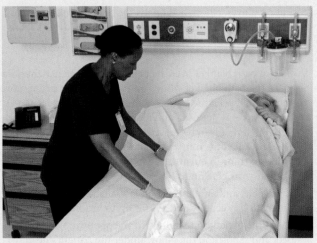

FIGURE 4. Pushing the bottom sheet toward the center of the bed, positioning it under old linens.

If the patient soils the bed, lifting/repositioning or friction-reducing sheet and pad can be changed without the bottom and top linens on the bed. A lifting/repositioning or friction-reducing sheet can aid in moving the patient in bed.

This ensures patient safety. The movement allows the bed to be made on the other side. Use of safe patient handling and mobility devices is best practice to prevent patient and health care provider injury (VA Mobile Health, n.d.; VHACEOSH, 2016). The bath blanket provides warmth and privacy.

Placing linens directly into the hamper helps prevent the spread of microorganisms. The floor is heavily contaminated; soiled linen will further contaminate the furniture. Soiled linen contaminates the nurse's clothing, and this may spread organisms to another patient.

This removes wrinkles and creases in the linens, which are uncomfortable to lie on.

ACTION

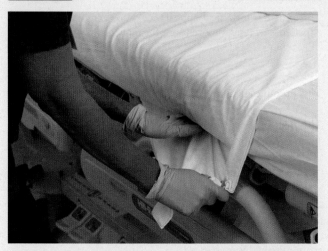

FIGURE 5. Tucking lifting/repositioning or friction-reducing sheet tightly.

19. Assist the patient to turn back to the center of bed. If the patient is partially able or unable to assist, friction-reducing devices, lifting/repositioning sheets, lateral transfer devices, and a full-body sling are potential equipment to consider, based on screening and assessment. Consider available bed features (turning, pressure release, rotation) to assist with the action (VA Mobile Health, n.d.). Remove the pillow and change the pillowcase. Open each pillowcase in the same manner as you opened other linens. Gather the pillowcase over one hand toward the closed end. Grasp the pillow with the hand inside the pillowcase. Keep a firm hold on the top of the pillow and pull the cover onto the pillow. Place the pillow under the patient's head.

20. Apply top linen, sheet, and blanket, if desired, so that it is centered. Fold the top linens over at the patient's shoulders to make a cuff. Have the patient hold on to top linen and remove the bath blanket from underneath (Figure 7). Discard soiled linen in laundry bag or hamper. **Do not place on floor or furniture. Do not hold soiled linens against your clothing.** Remove gloves. Perform hand hygiene.

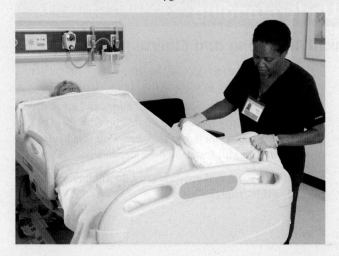

FIGURE 7. Removing bath blanket from under top linens.

RATIONALE

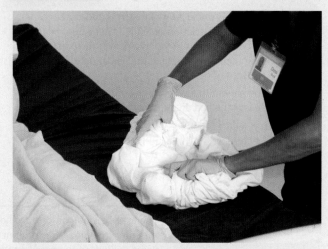

FIGURE 6. Removing soiled bottom linens from other side of bed.

Use of safe patient handling and mobility devices is best practice to prevent patient and health care provider injury (VA Mobile Health, n.d.; VHACEOSH, 2016). Opening linens by shaking causes organisms to be carried on air currents.

This allows bottom hems to be tucked securely under the mattress and provides for privacy. Placing linens directly into the hamper helps prevent the spread of microorganisms. The floor is heavily contaminated; soiled linen will further contaminate the furniture. Soiled linen contaminates the nurse's clothing, and this may spread organisms to another patient. Removing gloves properly reduces the risk for infection transmission and contamination of other items. Hand hygiene prevents the spread of microorganisms.

(continued on page 448)

Skill 7-11 ▶ Making an Occupied Bed   *(continued)*

ACTION	**RATIONALE**
21. Secure top linens under foot of mattress and miter corners. (Refer to the Skill Variation in Skill 7-10 for information to miter a corner.) Loosen top linens over the patient's feet by grasping them in the area of the feet and pulling gently toward the foot of bed.	This provides for a neat appearance. Loosening linens over the patient's feet gives more room for movement.
22. Return the patient to a position of comfort. Raise the side rail and lower the bed. Reattach call bell.	This promotes patient comfort and safety.
23. Dispose of soiled linens according to facility policy.	This deters the spread of microorganisms.
24. Remove any other PPE, if used. Perform hand hygiene.	Proper removal of PPE reduces the risk for infection transmission and contamination of other items. Hand hygiene prevents the spread of microorganisms.

EVALUATION

The expected outcomes have been met when the bed linens have been changed, and the patient and nurse remained free of injury. In addition, the patient assisted in moving from side to side and stated feelings of increased comfort after the bed was changed.

DOCUMENTATION

Changing of bed linens does not require documentation. The use of a specialty bed or bed equipment should be documented. Document any significant observations and communication.

DEVELOPING CLINICAL REASONING AND CLINICAL JUDGMENT

UNEXPECTED SITUATIONS AND ASSOCIATED INTERVENTIONS

- *Dirty linens are grossly contaminated with urinary or fecal drainage:* Obtain an extra towel or protective pad. Place the pad under and over the soiled linens so that new linens will not be in contact with soiled linens. Clean and dry the mattress according to facility policy before applying new sheets.

SPECIAL CONSIDERATIONS

Older Adult Considerations

- Using a soft bath blanket or a flannelette blanket as a bottom sheet may solve the problem of "coldness" for older adult patients with vascular problems or arthritis.

Enhance Your Understanding

Focusing on Patient Care: Developing Clinical Reasoning and Clinical Judgment

Consider the case scenarios at the beginning of the chapter as you answer the following questions to enhance your understanding and apply what you have learned.

QUESTIONS

1. Denasia Kerr, the 6-year-old with limited mobility, needs her hair shampooed. How would you accomplish this task?

2. Cindy Vortex, the 34-year-old woman who is now in a coma after a car accident, is wearing contact lenses.

What information would be important to gather before attempting to remove the contact lenses?

3. Carl Sheen, 76 years of age, asks, "How can I clean my dentures with my right hand all tied up with this IV?" How best could you help Mr. Sheen with this hygiene activity while still fostering his independence?

You can find suggested answers after the Bibliography at the end of this chapter.

Enhance Your Understanding (Continued)

Integrated Case Study Connection

The case studies in the back of the book focus on integrating concepts. Refer to the following case studies to enhance your understanding of the concepts and skills in this chapter.

- Basic Case Studies: Joe LeRoy, page 1203.
- Intermediate Case Studies: Victoria Holly, page 1211.

Bibliography

Alzheimer's Association. (2020). *Dental care.* https://www.alz.org/help-support/caregiving/daily-care/dental-care

American Academy of Family Physicians (AAFP). (2019, July 19). *Body piercing.* https://familydoctor.org/body-piercing/?adfree=true

American Association of Critical-Care Nurses (AACN). (2017). AACN Practice alert: Oral care for acutely and critically ill patients. *Critical Care Nurse, 37*(3), e19–e21.

American College of Foot and Ankle Surgeons (ACFAS). (n.d.a). *Diabetes foot care guidelines.* Retrieved August 25, 2020, from https://www.foothealthfacts.org/conditions/diabetic-foot-care-guidelines

American College of Foot and Ankle Surgeons (ACFAS). (n.d.b). *Peripheral arterial disease (PAD).* Retrieved August 25, 2020, from https://www.foothealthfacts.org/conditions/peripheral-arterial-disease-(p-a-d-)

American College of Prosthodontists (ACP). (n.d.). *Denture FAQs. Can I sleep in my dentures?* Retrieved July 31, 2020, from https://www.gotoapro.org/dentures-faq/#346

American Dental Association (ADA). (2019, August 29). *Oral health topics. Mouthwash (Mouthrinse).* https://www.ada.org/resources/research/science-and-research-institute/oral-health-topics/mouthrinse-mouthwash

American Dental Association (ADA). (2021, September 14). *Denture care and maintenance.* https://www.ada.org/resources/research/science-and-research-institute/oral-health-topics/dentures

American Dental Association (ADA). (n.d.a). *Babies and kids. Health habits.* Retrieved August 30, 2020, from https://www.mouthhealthy.org/en/babies-and-kids/healthy-habits

American Dental Association (ADA). (n.d.b). *Flossing.* Retrieved August 15, 2020, from https://www.mouthhealthy.org/en/az-topics/f/flossing

American Dental Association (ADA). (n.d.c). *Removable partial dentures.* Retrieved July 31, 2020, from https://www.mouthhealthy.org/en/az-topics/d/dentures-partial

American Dental Association (ADA). (n.d.d) *Water flossing.* Retrieved July 31, 2020, from https://www.mouthhealthy.org/en/az-topics/w/water-flossers

Andrews, M., Boyle, J. S., & Collins, J. (2020). *Transcultural concepts in nursing care* (8th ed.). Wolters Kluwer.

Association of Professional Piercers (APP). (2020). *Aftercare.* https://safepiercing.org/aftercare/

Barbe, A. G., Küpeli, L. S., Hamacher, S., & Hoack, M. J. (2020). Impact of regular professional toothbrushing on oral health, related quality of life, and nutritional and cognitive status in nursing home residents. *International Journal of Dental Hygiene, 18*(3), 238–250. DOI: 10.1111/idh.12439

Bartlett, D., Carter, N., de Baat, C., Duyck, J., Goffin, G., Müller, F., & Kawai, Y. (2018). *White paper on optimal care and maintenance of full dentures for oral and general health.* Global Task Force for Care of Full Dentures. Oral Health Foundation. https://www.gskhealthpartner.com/content/dam/cf-consumer-healthcare/health-professionals/en_US/pdf/SM12378+OHF+Cleaning+Guideline+-+White+Paper+-+Refresh+-+Print+Version+4+RGB.pdf

Bausch + Lomb. (2020). *Inserting and removing soft contact lenses.* https://www.bausch.com/reference/inserting-and-removing-contact-lenses#:~:text=Removing%20contact%20lenses%201%20Wash%2C%20rinse%2C%20and%20dry,the%20other%20lens%20by%20following%20the%20same%20procedure

Benfield, R., Heitkemper, M., & Newton, E. R. (2018). Culture, bathing and hydrotherapy in labor: An exploratory descriptive pilot study. *Midwifery, 64,* 110–114. DOI: 10.1016/j.midw.2018.06.005

Beuscher, T. L. (2019). Guidelines for diabetic foot care. A template for the care of all feet. *Journal of Wound, Ostomy, and Continence Nursing, 46*(3), 241–245. https://doi.org/10.1097/WON.0000000000000532

Black, J., & Hotaling, T. (2015). Ten top tips: Bariatric skin care. *Wounds International, 6*(3), 17–21.

Brennan, L. J., & Strauss, J. (2014). Cognitive impairment in older adults and oral health considerations: Treatment and management. *Dental Clinics of North America, 58*(4), 815–828. https://doi.org/10.1016/j.cden.2014.07.001

Cadavona, J. J. P., Rimtepathip, P. P., & Jacob, S. E. (2018). Moisturization. *Journal of the Dermatology Nurses' Association, 10*(3), 158–160. https://doi.org/10.1097/JDN.0000000000000401

Cassir, N., Thomas, G., Hraiech, S., et al. (2015). Chlorhexidine daily bathing: Impact on health care-associated infections caused by gram-negative bacteria. *American Journal of Infection Control, 43*(6), 640–643. https://doi.org/10.1016/j.ajic.2015.02.010

Chen, W., Cao, Q, Li, S., Li, H., & Zhang, W. (2015). Impact of daily bathing with chlorhexidine gluconate on ventilator associated pneumonia in intensive care units: A meta-analysis. *Journal of Thoracic Disease, 7*(4), 746–753. https://doi.org/10.3978/j.issn.2072-1439.2015.04.21

Chick, A., & Wynne, A. (2020). Introducing an oral care assessment tool with advanced cleaning products into a high-risk clinical setting. *British Journal of Nursing, 29*(5), 290–296.

Chicote, A. (2019). Care aide abilities in oral care delivery and seniors' oral health outcomes. *Canadian Journal of Dental Hygiene, 53*(3), 178–181.

Cleveland Clinic. (2020, June 16). *6 do's and don'ts for contact lens wearers.* https://health.clevelandclinic.org/dos-and-donts-for-contact-lens-wearers/

Croney, S. (2018). Choosing an emollient. *British Journal of Nursing, 27*(11), 597–598.

Davis, C. (2014). Caring for…patients with tattoos and body piercings. *Nursing Made Incredibly Easy, 12*(6), 48–51. https://doi.org/10.1097/01.NME.0000454748.95582.1e

de Camargo, L., Nunes da Silva, S., & Chambrone, L. (2019). Efficacy of toothbrushing procedures performed in intensive care units in reducing risk of ventilator-associated pneumonia: A systematic review. *Journal of Periodontal Research, 54*(6), 601–611. https://doi.org/10.1111/jre.12668

Dementia Care Central. (2019, September 23). *How to safely and effectively assist an individual with dementia with bathing.* https://www.dementiacarecentral.com/caregiverinfo/handsoncare/bathtime/

DePrez, B., Schreeder, C., & Davidson, S. (2019). Implementation of chlorhexidine gluconate bathing to reduce HAIs. *Nursing Management, 50*(11), 13–17. https://doi.org/10.1097/01.NUMA.0000602824.95678.0a

Earlam, A. S., & Woods, L. (2020). Obesity: Skin issues and skinfold management. *American Nurse Journal, 15*(6), 42–45.

Eliopoulos, C. (2018). *Gerontological nursing* (9th ed.). Wolters Kluwer.

Emery, K. P., & Guido-Sanz, F. (2019). Oral care practices in non-mechanically ventilated intensive care unit patients: An integrative review. *Journal of Clinical Nursing, 28*(13/14), 2462–2471. https://doi.org/10.1111/jocn.14829

Fisher, P., & Himan, C. (2020). Moisture-associated skin damage: A skin issue more prevalent than pressure ulcers. *Wounds UK, 16*(1), 58–63.

Gallagher, M., & Hall, G. R. (2014). Bathing persons with Alzheimer's disease and related dementias. *Journal of Gerontological nursing, 40*(2), 14–20. https://doi.org/10.3928/00989134-20131220-01

Gibney, J. M., Wright, F. A., D'Souza, M., & Naganathan, V. (2019). Improving the oral health of older people in hospital. *Australasian Journal on Ageing, 38*(1), 33–38. DOI: 10.1111/ajag.12588

Gorski, L. A., Hadaway, L., Hagle, M. E., Broadhurst, D., Clare, S., Kleidon, T., Meyer, B. M., Nickel, B., Rowley, S., Sharpe, E., & Alexander, M. Infusion Nurses Society. (2021). Infusion therapy. *Standards of practice.* (8th ed.). *Journal of Infusion Nursing, 44*(Suppl 1), S1–S224. doi: 10.1097/NAN.0000000000000396

Goto, Y., Hayasaka, S., Kurihara, S., & Nakamura, Y. (2018). Physical and mental effects of bathing: A randomized intervention study. *Evidence-Based Complementary and Alternative Medicine, 2018,* 9521086. https://doi.org/10.1155/2018/9521086

Gould, C. V., Umscheid, C. A., Agarwal, R. K., Kuntz, G., & Pegues, D. A.; Healthcare Infection Control Practices Advisory Committee (HICPAC). (2019, June 6). *Guideline for prevention of catheter-associated urinary tract infections 2009.* Centers for Disease Control and Prevention. https://www.cdc.gov/infectioncontrol/pdf/guidelines/cauti-guidelines-H.pdf

Gozalo, P., Prakash, S., Qato, D. M., Sloane, P. D., & Mor, V. (2014). Effect of the bathing without a battle training intervention on bathing-associated physical and verbal outcomes in nursing home residents with dementia: A randomized crossover diffusion study. *Journal of the American Geriatrics Society, 62*(5), 797–804. https://doi.org/10.1111/jgs.12777

Greene, L. R. (2020). Non-ventilator health care-associated pneumonia (NV-HAP): Putting it all together. *American Journal of Infection Control, 48*(5), A36–A38. https://doi.org/10.1016/j.ajic.2020.03.003

Griffiths, J., Jones, V., Leeman, I., Lewis, D., Patel, K., Wilson, K., & Blankenstein, R. (2020). *Oral health care for people with mental health problems. Guidelines and recommendations.* British Society for Disability and Oral Health. http://www.bsdh.org/documents/mental.pdf

Haesler, E., Frescos, N., & Rayner, R. (2018). The fundamental goal of wound prevention: Recent best evidence. *Wound Practice and Research, 26*(1), 14–22.

Hartford HealthCare. (2019, December 9). *Caregiving: Shaving an adult.* Hartford Hospital. https://hartfordhospital.org/health-wellness/health-resources/health-library/detail?id=abq1752

Hata, R., Noguchi, S., Kawanami, T., Yamasaki, K., Akata, K., Ikegami, H., Fukuda, K., Hirashima, S., Miyawaki, A., Fujino, Y., Oya, R., Yatera, K., & Mukae, H. (2019). Poor oral hygiene is associated with the detection of obligate anaerobes in pneumonia. *Journal of Periodontology, 91*(1), NP. https://doi.org/10.1002/JPER.19-0043

Herter, R., & Kazer, M. W. (2010). Best practices in urinary catheter. *Home Healthcare Nurse, 28*(6), 342–349.

Hines, A. G., Nuss, S., Rupp, M. E., Lyden, E., Tyner, K., & Hewlett, A. (2015). Chlorhexidine bathing of hospitalized patients: Beliefs and practices of nurses and patient care technicians, and potential barriers to compliance. *Infection Control & Hospital Epidemiology, 36*(8), 993–994. https://doi.org/10.1017/ice.2015.92

Hinkle, J. L., Cheever, K. H., & Overbaugh, K. J. (2022). *Brunner & Suddarths's Textbook of medical-surgical nursing* (15th ed.). Wolters Kluwer.

International Association of Fire Fighters (IAFF). (n.d.). *The epidemic of liquid and steam burns.* National Scald Prevention Campaign. Retrieved August 22, 2020, from https://flashsplash.org/

International Council of Nurses (ICN). (2019). *Nursing diagnosis and outcome statements.* https://www.icn.ch/sites/default/files/inline-files/ICNP2019-DC.pdf

Jablonski, R. A. (2012). Oral health and hygiene content in nursing fundamentals textbooks. *Nursing Research and Practice, 2012,* 372617. http://www.hindawi.com/journals/nrp/2012/372617

Jablonski, R. A., Kolanowski, A. M., Azuero, A., Winstead, V., Jones-Townsend, C., & Geisinger, M. L. (2018). Randomised clinical trial: Efficacy of strategies to provide oral hygiene activities to nursing home residents with dementia who resist mouth care. *Gerontology, 35*(4), 365–375. https://doi.org/10.1111/ger.12357

Jablonski, R., Mertz, E., Featherstone, J. D., & Fulmer, T. (2014). Maintaining oral health across the life span. *Nurse Practitioner, 39*(6), 39–48. https://doi.org/10.1097/01.NPR.0000446872.76779.56

Jarvis, C., & Echkardt, A. (2020). *Physical examination & health assessment* (8th ed.). Elsevier.

Jensen, S. (2019). *Nursing health assessment. A best practice approach* (3rd ed.). Wolters Kluwer.

Jenson, H., Maddux, S., & Waldo, M. (2018). Improving oral care in hospitalized non-ventilated patients: Standardizing products and protocol. *MEDSURG Nursing, 27*(1), 38–45.

Johnson, J., Suwantarat, N., Colantuoni, E., Ross, T. L., Aucott, S. W., Carroll, K. C., & Milstone, A. M. (2019). The impact of chlorhexidine gluconate bathing on skin bacterial burden of neonates admitted to the neonatal intensive care unit. *Journal of Perinatology, 39*(1), 63–71. https://doi.org/10.1038/s41372-018-0231-7

Johnson, V. B. (2012). Oral hygiene care for functionally dependent and cognitively impaired older adults. *Journal of Gerontological Nursing, 38*(11), 11–19. https://doi.org/10.3928/00989134-20121003-02

Jusino-Leon, G. N., Matheson, L., & Forsythe, L. (2019). Chlorhexidine gluconate baths. *Clinical Journal of Oncology Nursing, 23*(2), E32–E38. https://doi.org/10.1188/19.CJON.E32-E38

Kadia, S., Bawas, R., Shah, H., Narang, P., & Lippmann, S. (2014). Poor oral hygiene in the mentally ill: Be aware of the problem, and intervene. *Current Psychiatry, 13*(7), 47–48.

Kisely, S. (2016). No mental health without oral health. *The Canadian Journal of Psychiatry, 61*(5), 277–282. https://doi.org/10.1177/0706743716632523

Konno, R., Kang, H. S., & Makimoto, K. (2014). A best-evidence review of intervention studies for minimizing resistance-to-care behaviours for older adults with dementia in nursing homes. *Journal of Advanced Nursing, 70*(10), 2167–2180. https://doi.org/10.1111/jan.12432

Kyle, T., & Carman, S. (2021). *Essentials of pediatric nursing* (4th ed.). Wolters Kluwer.

Lichterfeld, A., Hauss, A., Surber, C., Peters, T., Blume-Peytavi, U., & Lottner, J. (2015). Evidence-based skin care: A systematic literature review and the development of a basic skin care algorithm. *Journal of Wound, Ostomy, and Continence Nursing, 42*(5), 501–524. https://doi.org/10.1016/j.ijnurstu.2019.103509

Lichterfeld-Kottner, A., El Genedy, M., Lahmann, N., Blume-Peytavi, U., Büscher, A., & Kottner, J. (2020). Maintaining skin integrity in the aged: A systematic review. *International Journal of Nursing Studies, 103,* 103509. https://doi.org/10.1016/j.ijnurstu.2019.103509

Magnani, C., Mastroianni, C., Giannarelli D., Stefanelli, M. C., Di Cienzo, V., Valerioti, T., & Casale,

G. (2019). Oral hygiene care in patients with advance disease: An essential measure to improve oral cavity conditions and symptom management. *American Journal of Hospice & Palliative Medicine, 36*(9), 815–819. https://doi.org/10.1177/1049909119829411

Martinez, T., Baugnon, T., Vergnaud, E., Duracher, C., Perie, A. C., Bustarret, O., Jugie, M., Rubinsztajn, R., Frange, P., Meyer, P., Orliaguet, G., & Blanot, S. (2020). Central-line-associated bloodstream infections in a surgical paediatric intensive care unit: Risk factors and prevention with chlorhexidine bathing. *Journal of Paediatrics and Child Health, 56*(6), 936–942. https://doi.org/10.1111/jpc.14780

Matsumoto, C., Nanke, K., Furumura, S., Arimatsu, M., Fukuyama, M., & Maeda, H. (2019). Effects of disposable bath and towel bath on the transition of resident skin bacteria, water content of the stratum corneum, and relaxation. *American Journal of Infection Control, 47*(7), 811–815. https://doi.org/10.1016/j.ajic.2018.12.008

Mayo Foundation for Medical Education and Research (MFMER). (2017, August 8). *Amputation and diabetes: How to protect your feet.* https://www.mayoclinic.org/diseases-conditions/diabetes/in-depth/amputation-and-diabetes/art-20048262

Mayo Foundation for Medical Education and Research (MFMER). (2019a, June 6). *Adult health. Oral health: Brush up on dental care basics.* https://www.mayoclinic.org/healthy-lifestyle/adult-health/in-depth/dental/art-20045536

Mayo Foundation for Medical Education and Research (MFMER). (2019b, March 27). *Contact lenses: What to know before you buy.* https://www.mayoclinic.org/healthy-lifestyle/adult-health/in-depth/contact-lenses/art-20046293

Mayo Foundation for Medical Education and Research (MFMER). (2019c, October 16). *Fingernails: Do's and don'ts for healthy nails.* https://www.mayoclinic.org/healthy-lifestyle/adult-health/in-depth/nails/art-20044954

Mayo Foundation for Medical Education and Research (MFMER). (2020a, March 31). *Ingrown hair.* https://www.mayoclinic.org/diseases-conditions/ingrown-hair/symptoms-causes/syc-20373893

Mayo Foundation for Medical Education and Research (MFMER). (2020b, July 18). *Piercings: How to prevent complications.* https://www.mayoclinic.org/healthy-lifestyle/adult-health/in-depth/piercings/art-20047317

McCormick, R., Robin, A. T., Gluch, J., & Lipman, T. H. (2019). Oral health assessment in acute care pediatric nursing. *Pediatric Nursing, 45*(6), 299–309.

MedlinePlus. (2020, July 2). *Penis care (uncircumcised).* National Library of Medicine. https://medlineplus.gov/ency/article/001917.htm

Mitchell, A., & Hill, B. (2020). Moisture-associated skin damage: An overview of its diagnosis and management. *Community Wound Care, 25*(3), S12–S18.

Musuuza, J. S., Guru, P. K., O'Horo, J. C., Bongiorno, C. M., Korobkin, M. A., Gangnon, R. E., & Safdar, N. (2019). The impact of chlorhexidine bathing on hospital-acquired bloodstream infections: A systematic review and meta-analysis. *BMC Infectious Diseases, 19*(1), 416. https://doi.org/10.1186/s12879-019-4002-7

Müller, F. (2015). Oral hygiene reduces the mortality from aspiration pneumonia in frail elders. *Journal of Dental Research, 94*(3 Suppl), 14S–16S. https://doi.org/10.1177/0022034514552494

National Institute on Aging. (2020). *Taking care of your teeth and mouth.* https://www.nia.nih.gov/health/taking-care-your-teeth-and-mouth

National Institutes of Health (NIH). (2015, October). *Keep your mouth healthy. Oral care for older adults.* NIH News in Health. https://newsinhealth.nih.gov/2015/10/keep-your-mouth-healthy

Nøddeskou, L. H., Hemmingsen, L. E., & Hørdam, B. (2015). Elderly patients' and nurses' assessment of traditional bed bath compared to prepacked single units—randomised controlled trial. *Scandinavian Journal of Caring Sciences, 29*(2), 347–352. https://doi.org/10.1111/scs.12170

Parnham, A., Copson, D., & Loban, T. (2020). Moisture-associated skin damage: Causes and an overview of assessment, classification and management. *British Journal of Nursing, 29*(12), S30–S37.

Quinn, B., Giuliano, K. K., & Baker, D. (2020). Non-ventilator health care-associated pneumonia

(NV-HAP): Best practices for prevention of NV-HAP. *American Journal of Infection Control, 48*(5), A23–A27. https://doi.org/10.1016/j.ajic.2020.03.006

Red, A., & O'Neal, P. V. (2020). Implementation of an evidence-based oral care protocol to improve the delivery of mouth care in nursing home residents. *Journal of Gerontological Nursing, 46*(5), 33–39. https://doi.org/10.3928/00989134-20200316-01

Reynolds, S. S., Sova, C., McNalty, B., Lambert, S., & Granger, B. (2019). Implementation strategies to improve evidence-based bathing practices in a neuro ICU. *Journal of Nursing Care Quality, 34*(2), 133–138. https://doi.org/10.1097/NCQ.0000000000000347

Riley, E. (2018). The importance of oral health in palliative care patients. *Journal of Community Nursing, 32*(3), 57–61.

Scales, K., Zimmerman, S., & Miller, S. J. (2018). Evidence-based nonpharmacological practices to address behavioral and psychological symptoms of dementia. *The Gerontologist, 58*(1), S88–S102. https://doi.org/10.1093/geront/gnx167

Schreiber, M. L. (2019). Tattoos and piercings: Considerations for nursing practice. *MEDSURG Nursing, 28*(2), 130–134.

Shah, H. N., Schwartz, J. L., & Cullen, D. L. (2016). Bathing with 2% chlorhexidine gluconate. Evidence and costs associated with central line-associated blood stream infections. *Critical Care Nursing Quarterly, 39*(1), 42–50. https://doi.org/10.1097/CNQ.0000000000000096

Silbert-Flagg, J., & Pillitteri, A. (2018). *Maternal and child health nursing* (8th ed.). Wolters Kluwer.

So, H. S., You, M. A., Mun, J. Y., et al. (2014). Effect of trunk to head bathing on physiological responses in newborns. *Journal of Obstetric, Gynecological, & Neonatal Nursing, 43*(6), 742–751. https://doi.org/10.1111/1552-6909.12496

Sturgeon, L. P., Garrett-Wright, D., Lartey, G., Jones, M. S., Bormann, L., & House, S. (2019). A descriptive study of bathing practices in acute care facilities in the United States. *American Journal of Infection Control, 47*(1), 23–26. https://doi.org/10.1016/j.ajic.2018.07.007

Taylor, C., Lynn, P., & Bartlett, J. (2023). *Fundamentals of nursing: The art and science of person-centered care* (10th ed.). Wolters Kluwer.

Thom, K. A., Escobar, D., Boutin, M. A., Zhan, M., Harris, A. D., & Johnson, K. (2018). Frequent contamination of nursing scrubs is associated with specific care activities. *American Journal of Infection Control, 46*(5), 503–506. https://doi.org/10.1016/j.ajic.2017.11.016

Thomas, C. (2019). Dental care in older adults. *British Journal of Community Nursing, 24*(5), 233–235.

Toughy, T. A., & Jett, K. (2018). *Ebersol and Hess' gerontological nursing & healthy aging* (5th ed.). Elsevier.

U.S. Food and Drug Administration (FDA). (2017a, December 11). *A guide to bed safety bed rails in hospitals, nursing homes and home health care: The facts.* https://www.fda.gov/medical-devices/hospital-beds/guide-bed-safety-bed-rails-hospitals-nursing-homes-and-home-health-care-facts

U.S. Food and Drug Administration (FDA). (2018a, August 30). *Bed rail safety.* https://www.fda.gov/medical-devices/consumer-products/bed-rail-safety?source=govdelivery&utm_medium=email&utm_source=govdelivery

Underwood, L. (2015). The effect of implementing a comprehensive unit-based safety program on urinary catheter use. *Urologic Nursing, 35*(6), 271–279. https://doi.org/10.7257/1053-816X.2015.35.6.271

Urias, D. S., Varghese, M., Simunich, T., Morrissey, S., & Dumire, R. (2018). Preoperative decolonization to reduce infections in urgent lower extremity repairs. *European Journal of Truama and Emergency Surgery, 44*(5), 787–793. https://doi.org/10.1007/s00068-017-0896-1

VA Mobile Health. (n.d.). *Safe patient handling.* (Version 1.3.3). [Mobile app]. U. S. Department of Veteran Affairs. https://mobile.va.gov/app/safe-patient-handling

Vannah, C. E., & Sammarco, V. R. (2019). Electric brushes improve outcomes in caregiver-assisted oral hygiene. *Nursing, 49*(8), 56–60. https://doi.org/10.1097/01.NURSE.0000569764.96290.70

Veje, P. L., Chen, M., Jensen, C. S., Sørenen, J., & Primdahl, J. (2019). Bed bath with soap and water or disposable wet wipes: Patients' experiences and preferences. *Journal of Clinical Nursing, 28*(11/12), 2235–2244. https://doi.org/10.1111/jocn.14825

Veje, P. L., Chen, M., Jensen, C. S., Sørenen, J., & Primdahl, J. (2020). Effectiveness of two bed bath methods in removing microorganisms from hospitalized patients: A prospective randomized crossover study. *American Journal of Infection Control, 48*(6), 638–643. https://doi.org/10.1016/j.ajic.2019.10.011

VHA Center for Engineering & Occupational Safety and Health (CEOSH). (2016). *Safe patient handling and mobility guidebook.* http://www.tnpatientsafety.com/pubfiles/Initiatives/workplace-violence/sphm-pdf.pdf

Voegeli, D. (2019). Prevention and management of moisture-associated skin damage. *Nursing Standard, 34*(2), 77–82. https://doi.org/10.7748/ns.2019.e11314

Warren, S., Midodzi, W. K., Newhook, L. A. A., Murphy, P., & Twells, L. (2020). Effects of delayed newborn bathing on breastfeeding, hypothermia, and hypoglycemia. *Journal of Obstetric, Gynecologic & Neonatal Nursing, 49*(2), 181–189. https://doi.org/10.1016/j.jogn.2019.12.004

Weber, J. R., & Kelley, J. H. (2018). *Health assessment in nursing* (6th ed.). Wolters Kluwer.

Whitehead, P. J., & Golding-Day, M. R. (2018). The lived experience of bathing adaptations in the homes of older adults and their carers (BATH-OUT): A qualitative interview study. *Health and Social Care in the Community, 27*(6), 1534–1543. https://doi.org/10.1111/hsc.12824

Williamson, K. (2020). Nursing people with bariatric care needs: More questions than answers. *Wounds UK, 16*(1), 64–71. https://www.wounds-uk.com/journals/issue/608/article-details/nursing-people-with-bariatric-care-needs-more-questions-than-answers

Wolters Kluwer. (2022). Problem-based care plans. In *Lippincott Advisor.* Wolters Kluwer.

Woon, C. (2019). Brushing up on oral care. *Kai Tiaki Nursing New Zealand, 25*(6), 18–19.

Woon, C. (2020). Improving oral care for hospitalised patients: Choosing appropriate products. *British Journal of Nursing, 29*(9), 520–525.

Wounds UK. (2018). *Best practice statement. Maintaining skin integrity.* https://www.wounds-uk.com/resources/details/maintaining-skin-integrity

SUGGESTED ANSWERS FOR FOCUSING ON PATIENT CARE: DEVELOPING CLINICAL REASONING AND CLINICAL JUDGMENT

1. Before Denasia's hair is washed, assess the situation. Assess the patient's hygiene preferences: frequency, time of day, and type of shampoo products. Assess for any physical activity limitations. Assess the patient's ability to get out of bed to have her hair washed. If the prescribed interventions allow it and the patient is physically able to wash her hair in the shower, the patient may prefer to do so. Otherwise, the shampoo could take place at the sink, if available. If the patient cannot tolerate being out of bed or is not allowed to do so, or a sink is not available, perform a bed shampoo. Assess for any activity or positioning limitations. Inspect the patient's scalp for any cuts, lesions, or bumps. Note any flaking, drying, or excessive oiliness. Find out if Denasia would prefer a family member/caregiver to shampoo her hair. If shampooing in bed, a shampoo cap can be used. Otherwise, use a shampoo board or tray, shampoo, and water.

2. Before removing Ms. Vortex's contacts assess the following: Assess both eyes for contact lenses, because some people wear them in only one eye. Determine the type of contact lenses worn. Assess eyes for any redness or drainage, which may indicate an eye infection or an allergic response. Assess for any eye injury. If an injury is present, notify the health care team about the presence of the contact lens. Do not try to remove the contact lens in this situation due to the risk for additional eye injury.

3. Assess the patient's oral hygiene preferences: frequency, time of day, and type of hygiene products. Assess for any physical activity limitations. Assess the patient's ability to perform own care. Determine if the IV site can be covered with water-protecting material, such as a glove or plastic wrap, to allow Mr. Sheen the ability to care for his dentures. Explore the possibility of discontinuing the IV infusion for a short period of time to keep the IV tubing from interfering with oral hygiene. If this is a possibility, review facility policy and determine the need for clearance from the health care team to implement this option. Encourage Mr. Sheen to do as much as he can; offer assistance, as needed. Patients are often afraid they will damage the IV or hurt themselves. Reinforce the fact that normal range of motion and activity are acceptable and should not interfere with the IV infusion.

8

Skin Integrity and Wound Care

Focusing on Patient Care

This chapter will help you develop some of the skills related to skin integrity and wound care necessary to care for the following patients:

Lori Downs, a patient with diabetes mellitus, is being treated in the outpatient wound center for a chronic wound on her left foot.

Tran Nguyen, diagnosed with breast cancer, has had a modified radical mastectomy and is 3 days post-op.

Arthur Lowes, has an appointment with his surgeon today for a follow-up examination and removal of surgical staples following a colon resection.

Refer to Focusing on Patient Care: Developing Clinical Reasoning and Clinical Judgment at the end of the chapter to apply what you learn.

Learning Outcomes

After completing the chapter, you will be able to accomplish the following:

1. Provide interventions to prevent pressure injury.
2. Clean a wound and apply a dry, sterile dressing.
3. Perform wound irrigation.
4. Collect a wound culture.
5. Provide care to a Penrose drain.
6. Provide care to a Jackson-Pratt drain.
7. Provide care to a Hemovac drain.
8. Apply negative-pressure wound therapy.
9. Remove sutures.
10. Remove surgical staples.
11. Apply an external heating pad.
12. Apply a warm compress.
13. Assist with a sitz bath.
14. Apply cold therapy.

Nursing Concepts

- Assessment
- Clinical Decision Making/Clinical Judgment
- Infection
- Safety
- Tissue integrity

T he skin is the body's first line of defense, protecting the underlying structures, tissues, and organs. Alteration in skin integrity, disruption in the normal integrity and function of the skin and underlying tissues, is a potentially dangerous and possibly life-threatening situation. Disruptions in skin and tissue integrity are called wounds. Patients with a wound and/or pressure injury are at risk for complications such as infection, hemorrhage, **dehiscence**, evisceration, and delayed wound healing.

The nurse plays a major role in maintaining the patient's skin integrity, identifying risk factors that predispose a patient to a break in integrity, intervening to prevent or reduce a patient's risk for impaired skin integrity, and providing specific wound care when breaks in integrity occur. Nursing responsibilities related to skin integrity and wound care involve assessment of the patient and the wound and staging of pressure injuries (Fundamentals Review 8-1, 8-2, and 8-3), followed by the development of a plan of care, including the identification of appropriate outcomes, nursing interventions, and evaluation of the nursing care. Depending upon the patient's individualized care plan, specific wound care skills may be needed. Refer to Chapter 3 for additional information related to assessment of the skin and integumentary system.

It is important to use appropriate aseptic technique when caring for wounds and pressure injuries to prevent introduction of microorganisms. Hand hygiene before and after dressing changes is imperative; follow *Standard Precautions* and, if needed, *Transmission-Based Precautions* when providing wound care. Pressure injuries and chronic wounds may be treated using clean technique (Baranoski & Ayello, 2020; EPUAP, NPIAP, & PPPIA, 2019a; WOCN, 2012). Fundamentals Review 8-4 identifies basic principles related to the use of clean technique and wound care. Refer to Chapter 1 for a discussion of infection control precautions and additional information related to sterile technique, medical asepsis, and clean technique.

Ongoing assessment for possible skin or wound complications is required. An ideal dressing/product is one that provides an environment that promotes wound healing maintains a moist environment to promote healing, manages wound exudate, provides thermal insulation, acts as a barrier to microorganisms, reduces or eliminates pain, and allows for pain-free removal (Baranoski & Ayello, 2020; McNichol et al., 2022; Ousey et al., 2016; WOCN, 2016). There are hundreds of products available for use, each with distinctive actions as well as indications, contraindications, advantages, and disadvantages (see Fundamentals Review 8-5). As a result, inclusion of skills related to the use of each type of product is not possible. It is extremely important for the nurse to be familiar with the indications for and correct application of each type of dressing and wound care product in use. Fundamentals Review 8-5 outlines the characteristics, purposes, and the use of some of these wound dressing products.

Nurses must also be skilled in assessing the patient for pain and employing strategies to minimize the patient's pain experience. Some patients may experience both physiologic and psychological pain related to dressing changes and wound care. Perform a pain assessment prior to and during wound procedures (EPUAP, NPIAP, & PPPIA, 2019a). Ask the patient about pain from the wound and determine if the pain is a one-time episode, occurs with dressing changes, at rest, or is constant pain (Baranoski & Ayello, 2020). If the patient experiences increased or constant pain from the wound, perform further assessments. Increasing pain, especially when accompanied by an increased or purulent flow of drainage, may indicate delayed healing or an infection (Baranoski & Ayello, 2020; EPUAP, NPIAP, & PPPIAa, 2019a). Surgical incisional pain is usually most severe for the first 2 to 3 days and then progressively diminishes. Refer to Chapter 10 for additional information related to patient comfort and pain management.

It is often appropriate and necessary to consult with a wound care specialist, often a wound certified nurse specialist, to plan and coordinate the most effective care for a patient.

This chapter covers general guidelines to assist the nurse in providing care related to skin integrity and wounds. The nurse must be familiar with the indications for and correct application of the prescribed dressing and/or wound care and refer to the policies and procedures for the individual facility.

Fundamentals Review 8-1

GENERAL WOUND ASSESSMENT

Wounds are assessed for appearance, size, drainage, pain, presence of sutures, drains, and tubes, and evidence of complications. Refer to Chapter 3 for additional information related to assessment of the skin and integumentary system.

PERFORMING GENERAL WOUND ASSESSMENT

- Note the location of the wound. Location is described in relation to the nearest anatomic landmark, such as bony prominences (Taylor et al., 2023). Assess the wound's appearance by inspecting and palpating. Look for the approximation of the edges of a healing surgical wound and the color of the wound and surrounding area. The edges should be clean and well **approximated**. Edges may be reddened and slightly swollen for about a week, then closer to normal in appearance. Skin around the wound may be bruised initially.
- Observe for signs of infection: redness, **erythema**, warmth, pain, **edema**/swelling, presence of purulent drainage (WOCN, 2016).
- Observe for these additional signs of infection in chronic wounds, as the classic symptoms of infection may be diminished or altered: serous drainage with concurrent inflammation, delayed healing, discolored and/or friable

granulation tissue, pocketing at the base of the wound, foul odor, wound breakdown (WOCN, 2016).
- Note the presence of any sutures, drains, and tubes. These areas are assessed in the same manner as the incision. Make sure they are intact and functioning.
- Assess the amount, color, odor, and consistency of any wound drainage.
- Assess the patient's pain, using an objective scale. Incisional pain is usually most severe for the first 2 to 3 days, after which it progressively diminishes. Increased or constant pain, especially an acute change in pain, requires further assessment. It can be a sign of delayed healing, infection, or other complication.
- Assess the patient's general condition for signs and symptoms of infection and hemorrhage.
- Consider use of photography to document the appearance of the wound, based on access and facility policy (Baranoski & Ayello, 2020).
- Consider use of a tool to monitor and document patient symptoms and wound healing, such as the Pressure Ulcer Scale for Healing (PUSH), the Bates-Jensen Wound Assessment Tool (BWAT), and the Toronto Symptom Assessment System for Wounds (TSAS-W) (Baranoski & Ayello, 2016; Harris et al., 2010; Maida et al., 2009; McNichol et al., 2022).

Fundamentals Review 8-2

MEASURING WOUNDS AND PRESSURE INJURIES

Wounds are assessed for appearance, size, drainage, pain, presence of sutures, drains, and tubes, and the evidence of complications. Refer to Chapter 3 for additional information related to assessment of the skin and integumentary system.

SIZE OF THE WOUND

- Draw the shape and describe it.
- Measure the head-to-toe length, side-to-side width, and depth—use the greatest measurement for length, width, and depth (Taylor et al., 2023).

DEPTH OF THE WOUND

- Perform hand hygiene. Put on gloves.
- Moisten a sterile, flexible cotton-tipped applicator with saline and insert it gently into the wound at a 90-degree angle, with the tip down (Figure A).
- Mark the point on the swab that is even with the surrounding skin surface or grasp the applicator with

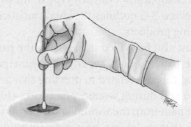

FIGURE A.

the thumb and forefinger at the point corresponding to the wound's margin (Figure B).

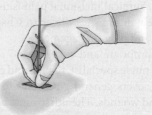

FIGURE B.

Fundamentals Review 8-2 continued

MEASURING WOUNDS AND PRESSURE INJURIES

- Remove the swab and measure the depth with a ruler (Figure C).

WOUND TUNNELING

- Perform hand hygiene. Put on gloves.
- Determine direction: Moisten a sterile, flexible cotton-tipped applicator with saline and gently insert a sterile applicator into the site where **tunneling** occurs. View the direction of the applicator as if it were the hand of a clock (Figure D). The direction of the patient's head represents 12 o'clock.

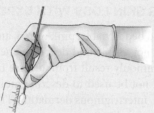

FIGURE C.

Moving in a clockwise direction, document the deepest sites where the wound tunnels.

- Determine the depth: While the applicator is inserted into the tunneling, mark the point on the swab that is even with the wound's edge, or grasp the applicator with the thumb and forefinger at the point corresponding to the wound's margin. Remove the swab and measure the depth with a ruler (see Figure C).
- Document both the direction and depth of tunneling.

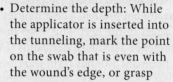
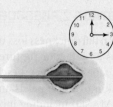

FIGURE D.

Source: Adapted from Baranoski, S., & Ayello, E. A. (2020). *Wound care essentials: Practice principles* (5th ed.). Wolters Kluwer.

Fundamentals Review 8-3

PRESSURE INJURY STAGES

PRESSURE INJURY

A pressure injury is localized damage to the skin and underlying soft tissue usually over a bony prominence or related to a medical or other device. The injury can present as intact skin or an open ulcer and may be painful. The injury occurs as a result of intense and/or prolonged pressure or pressure in combination with shear. The tolerance of soft tissue for pressure and shear may also be affected by microclimate, nutrition, perfusion, comorbidities, and condition of the soft tissue.

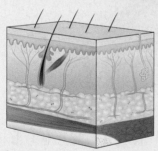

Healthy skin, lightly pigmented.

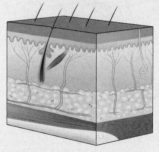

Healthy skin, darkly pigmented.

STAGE 1 PRESSURE INJURY: NONBLANCHABLE ERYTHEMA OF INTACT SKIN

Intact skin with a localized area of nonblanchable erythema, which may appear differently in darkly pigmented skin. Presence of blanchable erythema or changes in sensation, temperature, or firmness may precede visual changes. Color changes do not include purple or maroon discoloration; these may indicate deep tissue pressure injury.

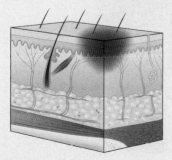

Stage 1 pressure injury, lightly pigmented.

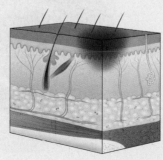

Stage 1 pressure injury, darkly pigmented.

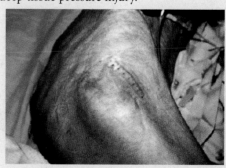

(continued)

Fundamentals Review 8-3   continued

PRESSURE INJURY STAGES

STAGE 2 PRESSURE INJURY: PARTIAL-THICKNESS SKIN LOSS WITH EXPOSED DERMIS

Partial-thickness loss of skin with exposed dermis. The wound bed is viable, pink or red, and moist and may also present as an intact or ruptured serum-filled blister. Adipose (fat) is not visible and deeper tissues are not visible. Granulation tissue, slough, and **eschar** are not present. These injuries commonly result from adverse microclimate and shear in the skin over the pelvis and shear in the heel. This stage should not be used to describe moisture-associated skin damage (MASD) including incontinence-associated dermatitis (IAD), intertriginous dermatitis (ITD), medical adhesive–related skin injury (MARSI), or traumatic wounds (skin tears, burns, abrasions).

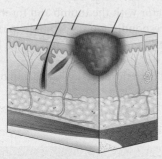
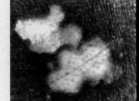
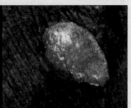

Stage 2 pressure injury.

STAGE 3 PRESSURE INJURY: FULL-THICKNESS SKIN LOSS

Full-thickness loss of skin, in which adipose (fat) is visible in the ulcer and granulation tissue and epibole (rolled wound edges) are often present. Slough and/or eschar may be visible. The depth of tissue damage varies by anatomical location; areas of significant adiposity can develop deep wounds. **Undermining** and tunneling may occur. Fascia, muscle, tendon, ligament, cartilage, and/or bone are not exposed. If slough or eschar obscures the extent of tissue loss, this is an Unstageable Pressure Injury.

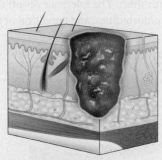
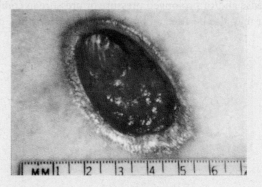

Stage 3 pressure injury.

STAGE 4 PRESSURE INJURY: FULL-THICKNESS SKIN AND TISSUE LOSS

Full-thickness skin and tissue loss with exposed or directly palpable fascia, muscle, tendon, ligament, cartilage, or bone in the ulcer. Slough and/or eschar may be visible. **Epibole** (rolled edges), undermining, and/or tunneling often occur. Depth varies by anatomical location. If slough or eschar obscures the extent of tissue loss, this is an Unstageable Pressure Injury.

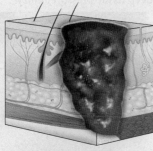
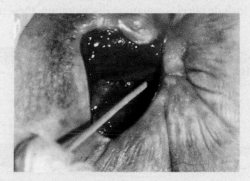

Stage 4 pressure injury.

Fundamentals Review 8-3   continued

PRESSURE INJURY STAGES

UNSTAGEABLE PRESSURE INJURY: OBSCURED FULL-THICKNESS SKIN AND TISSUE LOSS

Full-thickness skin and tissue loss in which the extent of tissue damage within the ulcer cannot be confirmed because it is obscured by slough or eschar. If slough or eschar is removed, a stage 3 or stage 4 pressure injury will be revealed. Stable eschar (i.e., dry, adherent, intact without erythema or fluctuance) on the heel or ischemic limb should not be softened or removed.

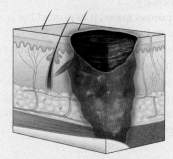

Unstageable pressure injury, dark eschar.

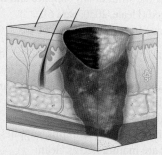

Unstageable pressure injury, slough and eschar.

DEEP TISSUE PRESSURE INJURY: PERSISTENT NONBLANCHABLE DEEP RED, MAROON, OR PURPLE DISCOLORATION

Intact or nonintact skin with localized area of persistent nonblanchable deep red, maroon, or purple discoloration or epidermal separation revealing a dark wound bed or blood-filled blister. The process leading to deep tissue pressure injury (DTPI) begins 48 hours prior to any color changes. Pain and temperature change often precede skin color changes. Discoloration may appear differently in darkly pigmented skin. This injury results from intense and/or prolonged pressure and shear forces at the bone–muscle interface. The wound may evolve rapidly to reveal the actual extent of tissue injury or may resolve without tissue loss. If necrotic tissue, subcutaneous tissue, granulation tissue, fascia, muscle, or other underlying structures are visible, this indicates a full-thickness pressure injury (unstageable, stage 3, or stage 4). Do not use DTPI to describe vascular, traumatic, neuropathic, or dermatologic conditions.

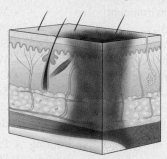

Deep tissue pressure injury.

Source: Reprinted with permission from National Pressure Injury Advisory Panel (NPIAP). (2016a). *NPIAP Pressure injury stages.* https://npiap.com/page/PressureInjuryStages; National Pressure Injury Advisory Panel (NPIAP). (2021). *Evolution of deep tissue pressure injury.* https://npiap.com/news/546664/Evolution-of-Deep-Tissue-Pressure-Injury.htm

Fundamentals Review 8-4

CLEAN (NONSTERILE) TECHNIQUE AND WOUND CARE

Clean technique involves strategies to reduce the overall number of microorganisms or to prevent or reduce the risk of transmission of microorganisms from one person to another or from one place to another (WOCN, 2012, p. S30). The aim of the use of clean technique in wound care is to ensure that contamination of the wound, any supplies and the environment is minimized (Heale, 2020, para 6).

Clean technique in wound care involves:

- Consideration of patient and wound factors, care environment, and likelihood of exposure to microorganisms
- Meticulous hand hygiene before initiating care and before/after glove changes
- Use of clean gloves
- Use of sterile instruments, solutions, supplies, and dressings that are maintained as clean

- Preventing direct contamination of materials and supplies
- Avoiding direct touching of the wound or any surface that might come in contact with the wound
- Sterile gloves should be worn if direct contact with the wound is necessary
- Use of a nonporous material to protect the surface under the wound
- Change gloves after removal of old dressing and after cleaning of the wound
- Cutting dressing materials with sterile scissors and storing dry and uncontaminated cut dressing materials in the original package, sealed and labeled in a clean, plastic storage bag

Source: Adapted from Heale, M. (2020, December 11). *What you need to know about clean and sterile techniques.* Wound Source. [Blog]. https://www.woundsource.com/blog/what-you-need-know-about-clean-and-sterile-techniques; Wound, Ostomy and Continence Nurses Society (WOCN). (2012). Clean vs. sterile dressing techniques for management of chronic wounds. A fact sheet. *Journal of Wound, Ostomy, and Continence Nursing, 39*(Suppl 2), S30–S34.

Fundamentals Review 8-5

EXAMPLES OF WOUND DRESSINGS/PRODUCTS

Type	Purposes	Use

Transparent films, such as:
    3M™ Tegaderm™
    BIOCLUSIVE™ Plus
       Transparent Film
       Dressing
    DermaView
    OPSITE™
	• Allow exchange of oxygen between wound and environment
	• Are self-adhesive
	• Protect against contamination; waterproof
	• Prevent loss of wound fluid
	• Maintain a moist wound environment
	• Facilitate autolytic debridement
	• No absorption of drainage
	• Allow visualization of wound
		• Wounds that are small; partial thickness
		• May remain in place for 4 to 7 days, resulting in less interference with healing
		• Stage 1 pressure injuries
		• Wounds with minimal drainage
		• Cover dressings for gels, foams, and gauze
		• Secure intravenous catheters, nasal cannulas, chest tube dressing, central venous access devices

Hydrocolloid dressings, such as:
    Comfeel® Plus Sacral
       Dressing
    DermaFilm Thin
    DuoDERM® CGF
       Dressing
    Hydrocolloid Dressing
       3M™
    Restore™ Hydrocolloid
       Dressing
	• Are occlusive or semiocclusive, limiting exchange of oxygen between wound and environment
	• Inner layer is self-adherent, gel forming, and composed of colloid particles
	• Outer layer seals and protects the wound from contamination
	• Minimal to moderate absorption of drainage
	• Maintain a moist wound environment
	• Thermal insulation
	• Provide cushioning
	• Facilitate autolytic debridement
	• May remain in place for 3 to 7 days, depending on exudate
		• Partial- and full-thickness wounds
		• Stage 2 and stage 3 pressure injuries
		• Prevention at high-risk friction areas
		• Wounds with light to moderate drainage
		• Wounds with necrosis or slough
		• First- and second-degree burns
		• Not for use with wounds that are infected

Fundamentals Review 8-5   continued

EXAMPLES OF WOUND DRESSINGS/PRODUCTS

Type	Purposes	Use
Hydrogels, such as: AquaDerm DermaGauze Elasto-Gel™ Island Hydrogel INTRASITE Gel Hydrogel Wound Dressing	• Polymer gels comprised of an 80% to 99% water base • Available in many sizes and forms (gels, sheets, gauze, strips) • Maintain a moist wound environment • Minimal absorption of drainage • Facilitate autolytic debridement • Thermal insulation • Do not adhere to wound • Less effective barrier than occlusive dressings • Reduce pain • Most require a secondary dressing to secure • May remain in place for 24 to 72 hours, depending on the gel form	• Partial- and full-thickness wounds • Stages 2–4 pressure injuries • Necrotic wounds • First- and second-degree burns • Dry wounds • Wounds with minimal exudate • Infected wounds • Radiation tissue damage
Alginates, such as: AQUACEL® EXTRA Wound Dressing Eclypse® Super Absorbent Dressing KALTOSTAT® Wound Dressing Melgisorb® Plus Alginate Dressing	• Contain alginic acid from brown seaweed; covered in calcium–sodium salts • Absorb exudate • Maintain a moist wound environment • Facilitate autolytic debridement • Require secondary dressing to secure	• Partial- and full-thickness wounds • May remain in place for 1 to 3 days • Stage 3 and stage 4 pressure injuries • Infected and noninfected wounds • Wounds with moderate to heavy exudate • Tunneling wounds; undermining • Moist red and yellow wounds • Not for use with wounds with minimal drainage or dry eschar
Foams, such as: 3M™ Tegaderm™ Foam Adhesive Dressing Advazorb® Heel Hydrophilic Foam Dressings Mepilex® Absorbent Foam Dressing Optifoam Gentle POLYDERM Plus Barrier Foam Dressing PolyMem® Dressing	• Foam covered by hydrophilic polyurethane or gel • Maintain a moist wound environment • Do not adhere to wound • Insulate wound • Highly absorbent • May require a secondary dressing to secure	• Partial- and full-thickness wounds • May remain in place 3 to 5 days (7 days for foams with silver), depending on exudate • Stages 2–4 pressure injuries • Surgical wounds • Absorb light to heavy amounts of drainage • Use around tubes and drains • Not for use with wounds with dry eschar
Antimicrobials, such as: AQUACEL™ Ag Surgical Wound Dressing Mepilex® Ag Antimicrobial Foam Dressing Optifoam Ag+ Post-Op PolyMem® Silver™ Dressing	• Antimicrobial or antibacterial action (reduce and/or prevent infection) • Do not adhere to wound • Can be highly absorbent • May require a secondary dressing to secure • Antimicrobial action may last 7 days	• Partial- and full-thickness wounds • Stages 2–4 pressure injuries • Burns • Primary dressing over skin graft(s) and donor sites • Draining, exuding, and nonhealing wounds of any kind (pressure injury, venous/arterial, diabetic, surgical) • Acute and chronic wounds

(*continued*)

Fundamentals Review 8-5   continued

EXAMPLES OF WOUND DRESSINGS/PRODUCTS

Type	Purposes	Use
Collagens, such as: DermaCOL PROMOGRAN™ Matrix Wound Dressing Stimulen™	• Protein (collagen derived from bovine, porcine, or avian sources) stimulates cellular migration and fosters new tissue development • Highly absorbent • Maintain a moist wound environment • Do not adhere to wound • Compatible with topical agents • Conform well to the wound surface • Require secondary dressing to secure • May remain in place 3 to 5 days (7 days for foams with silver), depending on exudate	• Partial- or full-thickness wounds • Stage 3 pressure injuries • Infected and noninfected wounds • Primary dressing over skin graft(s) and donor sites • Tunneling wounds • Moist red and yellow wounds
Contact layers, such as: ADAPTIC TOUCH™ Non-Adhering Silicone Dressing Profore WCL Silflex® Silicone Contact Layer	• Placed in contact with base of wound, protecting base from trauma during dressing change • Allow exudate to pass to a secondary dressing • Not intended to be changed with every dressing change • May be used with topical medication, wound filler, or gauze dressings	• Partial- and full-thickness wounds • Require secondary dressing to secure • Shallow, dehydrated wounds • Wounds with eschar • Wounds with viscous exudate
Composites, such as: 3M™ Tegaderm™ Absorbant Clear Acrylic Dressing Covaderm Plus Stratasorb	• Combine two or more physically distinct products in a single dressing with several functions • Allow exchange of oxygen between wound and environment • May facilitate autolytic debridement • Provide physical bacterial barrier and absorptive layer • Semiadherent or nonadherent	• Partial- and full-thickness wounds • Primary or secondary dressing • Stages 1–4 pressure injures • Wounds with minimal to heavy exudate • Necrotic tissue • Mixed (granulation and necrotic tissue) wounds • Infected wounds
Cellular and tissue-based products (CPTs) AlloSkin™ Grafix CORE®	• Nonviable or viable human or animal cells, tissue-based from humans and animals	• Partial- and full-thickness wounds • Venous and diabetic ulcers • Burns • Chronic wounds

Source: Adapted from Baranoski, S., & Ayello, E. A. (2020). *Wound care essentials: Practice principles* (5th ed.). Wolters Kluwer; Hess, C. (2019). *Product guide to skin & wound care* (8th ed.). Wolters Kluwer; Hurd, T., Rossington, A., Trueman, P., & Smith, J. (2017). A retrospective comparison of the performance of two negative pressure wound therapy systems in the management of wounds of mixed etiology. *Advances in Wound Care, 6*(1), 33–37. https://doi.org/10.1089/wound.2015.0679; and Norman, G., Goh, E. L., Dumville, J. C., Shi, C., Liu, Z., Chiverton, L., Stankiewicz, M., & Reid, A. (2020). Negative pressure wound therapy for surgical wounds healing by primary closure. *The Cochrane Database of Systematic Reviews, 6*(6), CD009261. https://doi.org/10.1002/14651858.CD009261.pub6

Skill 8-1 ▶ Preventing Pressure Injury

Localized damage to the skin and/or underlying tissue, as a result of pressure or pressure in combination with sheer is termed **pressure injury** (EPUAP, NPIAP, & PPPIA, 2019a, p. 16). Pressure injuries usually occur over a boney prominence but may also be related to a medical device or other object (EPUAP, NPIAP, & PPPIA, 2019a, p. 16; Joint Commission, 2018). Any tube, electrode, sensor or other rigid or stiff device element under pressure can create pressure damage; examples of devices associated with pressure injuries include device securements, surgical drains, chest tubes, blood pressure cuffs, objects left in the bed or chair (mobile phone, call bell, hearing aid, needle caps, toiletry items, toys), respiratory devices (oxygen tubing, nasotracheal tubes, nasogastric tubes, continuous positive airway pressure masks), cervical collars, casts, urinary catheters, restraints, graduated compression stockings (Baranoski & Ayello, 2020; EPUAP, NPIAP, & PPPIAa, 2019a).

Factors contributing to development of pressure injuries are identified in Box 8-1. Assessment of pressure injury risk informs the development and implementation of an individualized plan to reduce risk and prevent development of pressure injury (EPUAP, NPIAP, & PPPIA, 2019a). A risk assessment tool may be used as part of the assessment of risk; although no one risk assessment tool is universally recommended, these tools are part of an assessment that must be structured, comprehensive, and based on clinical judgment (Baranoski & Ayello, 2020; Black, 2018; EPUAP, NPIAP, & PPPIA, 2019a). Several different scales are available to assess risk, such as the Norton Scale, Waterlow Scale, Braden Scale, and the Braden QD scale (for use with children) (Black, 2018; Braden, 2005; McNichol et al., 2022; Mitchell, 2018; Waterlow, 1985). Patients may have additional risk factors and/or other health problems not measured by the chosen assessment scale. Therefore, good nursing judgment may reveal the need for a higher intensity of preventive intervention than what may be identified by the scale alone (Braden, 2012). Note that the development of a pressure injury may be unavoidable, even with preventative measures and provision of evidence-based care by the health care team (Alvarez et al., 2016; NPIAP, 2017).

These risk factors are incorporated into pressure injury prevention plans, which are based on knowledge and assessment data related to the patient's clinical condition, current skin condition overall pressure injury risk status and specific risk factors, and resource availability (McNichol et al., 2022; Taylor et al., 2023). Interdisciplinary collaboration and communication are also essential to pressure injury prevention in high-risk patient populations (Bergstrom et al., 2018).

The following skill identifies potential interventions related to prevention of pressure injuries. The interventions are listed sequentially for teaching purposes; after completion of appropriate assessments, the order in which the interventions are completed is not sequential and should be adjusted based on the individual patient assessment, health status and situation, as well as nursing judgment and facility policies. Not every intervention discussed will be appropriate for every patient. Additional interventions related to prevention of pressure injuries are discussed in other chapters. Refer to Chapter 5 for nursing skills related to administering medications for pain relief. Chapter 7 provides skills addressing hygiene and skin care. Interventions related to mobility and repositioning are discussed in Chapter 9.

Box 8-1 Risk Factors Contributing to Development of Pressure Injuries

- Mobility and activity limitations
- Skin status: existing pressure injury, alterations in skin integrity, previous pressure injury
- Perfusion, circulation, and oxygenation factors: diabetes, vascular disease, alterations in blood pressure, smoking, edema, mechanical ventilation, oxygen use, respiratory disease
- Nutrition indicators: Altered nutritional and/or hydration status, significant obesity, or thinness
- Moisture: urinary and/or bowel incontinence, excessive skin moisture, diaphoresis
- Increased body temperature
- Older age (age >65 years)
- Sensory perception limitations
- Altered mental health status
- Trauma and/or surgery
- Critically ill individuals
- Neonates and children

Source: Adapted from Alvarez, O. M., Brindle, C. T., Langemo, D., Kennedy-Evans, K. L., Krasner, D. L., Brennan, M. R., & Levine, J. M. (2016). The VCU Pressure Ulcer Summit: The search for a clearer understanding and more precise clinical definition of the unavoidable pressure injury. *Journal of Wound, Ostomy, and Continence Nursing, 43*(5), 455–463; McNichol, L. L., Ratliff, C. R., & Yates, S. S (Eds.). (2022). *Wound, Ostomy and Continence Nurses Society™. Core curriculum. Wound management.* Wolters Kluwer; and European Pressure Ulcer Advisory Panel (EPUAP), National Pressure Injury Advisory Panel (NPIAP), and Pan Pacific Pressure Injury Alliance (PPPIA). (2019). *Prevention and treatment of pressure ulcers/injuries: Clinical Practice guideline. The international guideline.* E. Haesler (Ed.). http://www.internationalguideline.com/

(continued on page 462)

Skill 8-1 ▶ Preventing Pressure Injury *(continued)*

DELEGATION CONSIDERATIONS

The assessment of a patient's skin is not delegated to assistive personnel (AP). Depending on the state's nurse practice act and the organization's policies and procedures, the licensed practical/vocational nurses (LPN/LVNs) may perform some or all of the parts of assessment of the patient's skin. The use of interventions related to prevention of pressure injuries may be delegated to assistive personnel (AP) as well as to LPN/LVNs. The decision to delegate must be based on careful analysis of the patient's needs and circumstances as well as the qualifications of the person to whom the task is being delegated. Refer to the Delegation Guidelines in Appendix A.

EQUIPMENT

- Pressure injury assessment form and/or risk assessment tool
- Functional assessment tool, as indicated
- Support surfaces, such as integrated bed systems, specialized and/or low-pressure mattresses and overlays, seating surfaces and cushions, heel elevation devices, and foam positioning wedges, as indicated
- Safe patient handling and movement devices, as indicated
- Protective dressings, such as polyurethane foam dressing, as indicated
- Low-friction patient care textiles, such as bed linens and patient gowns
- Personal hygiene and skin barrier products, as indicated
- PPE, as indicated

ASSESSMENT

Review the patient's health record and care plan for information about the patient's status and contraindications to any of the potential interventions. Assess the patient's skin at least daily, paying special attention to the skin over bony prominences and the skin in contact with medical devices (Baranoski & Ayello, 2020; McNichol et al., 2022). A full pressure injury risk assessment should be conducted as soon as possible after admission to the care service (including community-based care); after admission, a full pressure injury risk assessment should be conducted as often as required based on the patient's acuity and guided by the screening outcome (EPUAP, NPIAP, & PPPIA, 2019a). A full pressure assessment should also be conducted as a result of any change in the patient's status (EPUAP, NPIAP, & PPPIA, 2019a). Assess the patient's response to a particular intervention to evaluate effectiveness, presence of adverse effects, and indication for continuation.

ACTUAL OR POTENTIAL HEALTH PROBLEMS AND NEEDS

Many actual or potential health problems or issues may require the use of this skill as part of related interventions. An appropriate health problem or issue may include:
- Altered skin integrity risk
- Altered skin integrity
- Knowledge deficiency

OUTCOME IDENTIFICATION AND PLANNING

The expected outcome to achieve is that the patient does not experience pressure injury and/or alterations in skin integrity. Other outcomes that may be appropriate include the patient and/or caregivers are able to participate in prevention activities, and the patient and caregivers verbalize an understanding of the pressure injury prevention plan.

IMPLEMENTATION

ACTION	RATIONALE
1. Perform hand hygiene and put on PPE, if indicated.	Hand hygiene and PPE prevent the spread of microorganisms. PPE is required based on transmission precautions.
2. Identify the patient.	Identifying the patient ensures the right patient receives the intervention and helps prevent errors.

ACTION

3. Discuss pressure injury prevention with the patient and/or patient family/caregivers. Explain what pressure injury is, the causes of pressure injuries, and the importance of a pressure injury prevention plan (McNichol et al., 2022).

4. Assess the patient's skin at least daily, paying special attention to the skin over bony prominences and the skin in contact and under medical devices (Camacho-Del Rio, 2018; McNichol et al., 2022; EPUAP, NPIAP, & PPPIA, 2019a). Briefly assess the patient's skin at the pressure points during repositioning of the patient (EPUAP, NPIAP, & PPPIA, 2019a). Refer to Chapter 3 for additional skin assessment information.

5. Assess the patient's risk for pressure injury upon entry to a health care setting and on a regularly scheduled basis or when there is a significant change in the patient's condition, incorporating appropriate assessment tools and scales, based on facility policy (WOCN, 2016). Refer to Box 8-1.

6. Utilize appropriate support surfaces to redistribute tissue loads, both while in bed and when seated, based on individual patient assessment and needs, facility policy, and availability (Baranoski & Ayello, 2020; Haesler, 2018). Appropriate support surfaces may include, but are not limited to, integrated bed systems, specialized and/or low-pressure mattresses and overlays, seating surfaces and cushions, heel elevation devices, and foam positioning wedges. Note: Pressure redistribution devices should serve as adjuncts and not replacements for repositioning of patients (WOCN, 2016). **Do not use foam rings, foam cut-outs, or donut-type devices.** The Wound, Ostomy and Continence Nurses Society (WOCN, 2016) has developed a content-validated algorithm for support surface selection. Refer to the General Considerations below.

7. Routinely reposition the patient: determine frequency with consideration to the patient's level of activity, physical, cognitive and psychological condition; ability to independently reposition; the type of support surface in use; general health condition; patient comfort and pain (EPUAP, NPIAP, & PPPIA, 2019a; McNichol et al., 2022).

8. Implement early mobilization to increase the patient's activity and mobility as tolerated. Develop a schedule for progressive sitting and ambulation as rapidly as tolerated by the individual patient. Collaborate with the physical and occupational therapists to develop an individualized intervention plan. Refer to Chapter 9 for additional discussion related to early mobilization and ambulation of patients.

RATIONALE

These measures promote a collaborative relationship in which the patient is treated with respect. Explanation encourages patient understanding and reduces apprehension. Patient and caregiver education support engagement in care and assist patients to implement behaviors to meet goals for care (Joint Commission, 2018; Mitchell, 2018).

Skin assessment provides information related to the patient's current status and detects impending or actual alterations in skin integrity (McNichol et al., 2022). Skin assessment provides information needed to develop an appropriate care plan (Taylor et al., 2023). For patients at risk for pressure injury, the skin should be inspected as soon as possible upon admission to a health care service, as part of every pressure injury risk assessment, and additionally based on the individual's degree of pressure injury risk (EPUAP, NPIAP, & PPPIA, 2019a). Assessment of pressure points allows for identification of alterations in status and evaluation of the effectiveness of repositioning regimen; presence of persistent erythema may indicate the need to increase frequency of repositioning; pressure points onto which the patient will be repositioned should appear fully recovered from previous loading (EPUAP, NPIAP, & PPPIA, 2019a).

Risk for pressure injury development should be determined on admission, as often as required based on the patient's acuity, and as a result of any change in the patient's status (EPUAP, NPIAP, & PPPIA, 2019a). Identification of people at risk for developing pressure injury is a critical component of prevention (Baranoski & Ayello, 2020).

Support surfaces help prevent pressure injury by redistributing pressure and manage tissue loads, sequentially altering the parts of the body that bear load (to reduce the duration of loading on individual anatomical sites), managing the microclimate (moisture and temperature control), and friction and shear control (Baranoski & Ayello, 2020; Kalowes, 2018). Support surfaces also provide for proper body alignment and comfort (Baranoski & Ayello, 2020). Foam rings, foam cut-outs, or donut-type devices concentrate pressure on the surrounding tissue and should be avoided (WOCN, 2016).

Repositioning reduces or relieves pressure and limits the amount of time tissues are exposed to pressure and contributes to the patient's functional abilities (EPUAP, NPIAP, & PPPIA, 2019a; McNichol et al., 2022; WOCN, 2016).

Mobilization and ambulation relieve pressure, contributes to the patient's functional abilities, and may reduce risk for deterioration related to prolonged immobility (EPUAP, NPIAP, & PPPIA, 2019a; Taylor et al., 2023). Early mobility plays an important role in the patient's physical and psychological well-being (Arnold et al., 2018). Physical and occupational therapists are important resources for maximizing patient mobility (Baranoski & Ayello, 2020).

(continued on page 464)

Skill 8-1 ▶ Preventing Pressure Injury *(continued)*

ACTION	RATIONALE
9. Use a 20- to 30-degree side-lying position or flat in bed (if not contraindicated) when positioning patients at risk for pressure injury in side-lying positions (EPUAP, NPIAP, & PPPIA, 2019a; WOCN, 2016).	Avoid lying positions that increase pressure, such as the 90-degree position (EPUAP, NPIAP, & PPPIA, 2019a).
10. Maintain the head-of-bed elevation at or below 30 degrees, or at the lowest degree of elevation appropriate for the patient's medical condition.	Head-of-bed elevation at or below 30 degrees prevents shear-related injury (WOCN, 2016).
11. Consider the use of a prophylactic (preventative) dressing, such as a polyurethane foam dressing, on bony prominences, such as heels, hips, and the sacrum (Kalowes, 2018). Assess skin under a prophylactic dressing at least daily; replace prophylactic dressings that are damaged, loosened, displaced, excessively moist, or if the dressing or skin under the dressing becomes soiled and according to the manufacturer's directions (EPUAP, NPIAP, & PPPIA, 2019a).	Prophylactic dressings reduce friction, pressure and shear, protect fragile skin, and influence microclimate (Cornish, 2017; Kalowes, 2018; Lovegrove et al., 2020; EPUAP, NPIAP, & PPPIA, 2019a; WOCN, 2016).
12. Consider the use of low-friction patient care textiles, such as bed linens and patient gowns. Refer to Chapter 9 for additional information related to safe patient handling and the use of patient handling and mobility devices.	Low-friction textiles reduce shear, minimize skin irritation and dry quickly (EPUAP, NPIAP, & PPPIA, 2019a; WOCN, 2016).
13. Utilize safe patient handling interventions when moving a patient. Collaborate with the physical and occupational therapists to develop an individualized intervention plan. Refer to Chapter 9 for additional information related to safe patient handling and the use of patient handling and mobility devices.	Proper lifting, positioning, and repositioning techniques are critical to prevent injury from shearing forces (McNichol et al., 2022). Physical and occupational therapists are important resources for maximizing patient mobility (Baranoski & Ayello, 2020).
14. Provide appropriate skin and personal hygiene (Kalowes, 2018; Mitchell, 2018; Yilmazer et al., 2019). Utilize interventions to protect the skin from excessive exposure to moisture from wound exudate, perspiration, mucous, saliva, fistula or stoma effluent, and urinary and fecal incontinence. Refer to Chapters 7, 12, and 13 for additional information related to these interventions.	Exposure to excessive moisture contributes to skin damage and pressure injury development due to decreased tissue tolerance and increases susceptibility to friction, pressure, and shear (Baranoski & Ayello, 2020; Gray & Guiliano, 2018; Voegili, 2019; WOCN, 2016).
15. Provide appropriate interventions to support the patient's nutritional status and ensure adequate nutritional and fluid intake (Kalowes, 2018). Interventions may include strategies to enhance oral intake, high-calorie/high-protein nutritional supplements, fortified foods, and/or enteral or parenteral nutritional support (Baranoski & Ayello, 2020; Munoz et al., 2020). Collaborate with the registered dietician and dietary staff to develop an individualized nutrition intervention plan (Kawoles, 2018; EPUAP, NPIAP, & Pan Pacific Pressure Injury Alliance, 2019a).	Adequate calories, protein, fluids, vitamins, and minerals are required for health and tissue maintenance (Kalowes, 2018; McNichol et al., 2022). Nutritional management is an important aspect of a comprehensive care plan for pressure injury prevention (Bergstrom et al., 2018; EPUAP, NPIAP, & PPPIA, 2019a; Lovegrove et al., 2020; Munoz et al., 2020; WOCN, 2016).
16. Implement interventions to prevent pressure injury related to the use of medical devices, based on the individual patient's situation.	Interventions are necessary to prevent pressure injury related to the use of medical devices (Camacho-Del Rio, 2018; Joint Commission, 2018; EPUAP, NPIAP, & PPPIA, 2019a; WOCN, 2016).
a. Ensure correctness for patient size and application of devices in use.	Correct size and accurate application minimize pressure and shear.
b. Use prophylactic dressings under the device, as appropriate to the individual patient and clinical use (EPUAP, NPIAP, & PPPIA, 2019a).	Appropriate use of prophylactic dressing manages moisture and provides cushioning to reduce pressure (EPUAP, NPIAP, & PPPIA, 2019a).
c. Inspect the skin under the devices and observe for edema under the devices more than twice daily or more often, as indicated.	Presence of edema increases risk for alterations in skin integrity (EPUAP, NPIAP, & PPPIA, 2019a).
d. Remove device as soon as medically feasible. Routinely reposition or rotate any medical device daily when possible.	Removal prevents pressure injury. Repositioning or rotating redistributes pressure and decreases shear (EPUAP, NPIAP, & PPPIA, 2019a).

ACTION	**RATIONALE**
e. Keep the skin clean and dry under medical devices.	Moisture underneath medical device increases risk of alterations in skin integrity (Camacho-Del Rio, 2018).
17. Provide education to the patient and caregiver(s) about the prevention plan and ways to minimize the risk of pressure injury.	These measures promote a collaborative relationship in which the patient is treated with respect. Explanation encourages patient understanding and engagement and reduces apprehension. Patient and caregiver education assist patients to implement behaviors to meet goals for care (EPUAP, NPIAP, & PPPIA, 2019a; McNichol et al., 2022; Taylor et al., 2023; WOCN, 2016).
18. Remove gloves and additional PPE, if used. Perform hand hygiene.	Removing gloves and PPE properly reduces the risk for infection transmission and contamination of other items. Hand hygiene prevents the transmission of microorganisms.
19. Evaluate the patient's response to interventions. Reassess and alter care plan as indicated by facility policies and procedures, as appropriate.	Evaluation allows for individualization of care plan and promotes optimal patient comfort.

EVALUATION

The expected outcomes have been met when the patient has not experienced pressure injury and/or alterations in skin integrity, the patient and/or caregivers have participated in prevention activities, and the patient and caregivers have verbalized and demonstrated an understanding of the pressure injury prevention plan and interventions.

DOCUMENTATION

Guidelines

Document risk and skin assessments, as well as other appropriate assessments, based on individual patient circumstances. Document interventions provided and patient responses. Record alternative treatments to consider, if appropriate. Document reassessment after interventions, at an appropriate interval, based on specific interventions used. Documentation related to pressure injury prevention is often completed on checklists or other tools on the patient's health record. Include any pertinent patient and family/caregiver education provided.

DEVELOPING CLINICAL REASONING AND CLINICAL JUDGMENT

UNEXPECTED SITUATIONS AND ASSOCIATED INTERVENTIONS

- *Patient develops a pressure injury:* Reassess the patient's condition. Perform assessment to differentiate pressure injuries from wounds and/or injuries due to other causes (WOCN, 2016). Consult with the patient's health care team regarding the injury and collaborate on a revised plan of care. Review and revise the current care plan to reflect the change in the patient's status and ensure implementation of appropriate nursing interventions. Implement appropriate wound care as prescribed and indicated in facility policy. Continue vigilant preventive interventions to avoid further pressure injury.

SPECIAL CONSIDERATIONS

General Considerations

- Preventive interventions related to pressure injury prevention should be based on nursing clinical judgment, the use of a reliable risk assessment tool, and assessment of individual patient extrinsic and intrinsic risk factors (EPUAP, NPIAP, & PPPIA, 2019a; WOCN, 2016). Interdisciplinary collaboration and communication are essential to pressure injury prevention in high-risk patient populations (Bergwtrom et al., 2018).
- Extended use of prone-positioning should be avoided unless required for management of the patient's medical condition; special consideration must be given to offloading of pressure points on the face, breast region, knees, toes, penis, clavicles, iliac crest and symphysis pubis, as well as

(continued on page 466)

Skill 8-1 ▶ Preventing Pressure Injury *(continued)*

the potential for uneven distribution of pressure and positioning of medical devices (EPUAP, NPIAP, & PPPIA, 2019a).

- Nurses must participate in continued pressure injury prevention and treatment education to ensure provision of evidence-based nursing care, achieve desired outcomes, and provide patients the best possible care (EPUAP, NPIAP, & PPPIA, 2019a).
- WOCN (2016) has developed a content-validated algorithm for support surface selection. This evidence- and consensus-based algorithm for support surface selection had a Content Validity Index (CVI) of 0.95 with an overall mean score of 3.72, indicating strong content validity and steps that are appropriate to the purpose of the algorithm (McNichol et al., 2015). Visit the WOCN website at https://www.wocn.org/learning-center/clinical-tools/ to access evidence for practice describing the Support Surface Algorithm, including the algorithm (McNichol et al., 2015); the interactive Support Surface Algorithm tool; and additional Support Surface Algorithm resources (WOCN, n.d.).

Infant and Child Considerations

- An age-appropriate risk assessment for pediatric, adolescent, and neonate populations considers risk factors of specific concern, including activity and mobility levels, skin texture and maturity, perfusion and oxygenation measures, presence of an external device, sensory perception, humidity, nutrition, friction and sheer, severity of illness, and duration of hospitalization (EPUAP, NPIAP, & PPPIA, 2019a; Ferreira et al., 2018).

Community-Based Care Considerations

- Pressure injury prevention in home settings can be challenging and may be compromised by access to resources and devices. Assessment of the patient and individual risk factors, as well as implementation of pressure injury prevention interventions in the home are critical in meeting patients' needs (Ellis, 2017; McGraw, 2018).
- Education of the patient, family, and caregivers is critical to ensure successful implementation of the pressure injury prevention care plan (Payne, 2016).

EVIDENCE FOR PRACTICE ▶

BEDSIDE TECHNOLOGIES AND EARLY DETECTION OF PRESSURE INJURIES

Pressure injuries are painful, costly, negatively impact a patient's quality of life, and are often preventable (EPUAP, NPIAP, & PPPIA, 2019a; Scafide et al., 2020). Early detection and prevention of pressure injuries is critical for improving patient outcomes and decreasing associated economic burden on patients and the health care system (Scafide et al., 2020). Pressure injury risk and skin assessments rely on visual assessment of the patient's skin to identify signs of damage. Early detection may be limited due to the challenges with visual assessment, particularly in patients with darker skin tones (Scafide et al., 2020). Are there technologies to aid in early detection of pressure injuries?

Related Research

Scafide, K. N., Narayan, M. C., & Arundel, L. (2020). Bedside technologies to enhance the early detection of pressure injuries. A systematic review. *Journal of Wound, Ostomy, and Continence Nursing, 47*(2), 128–136. https://doi.org/10.1097/WON.0000000000000626

The purpose of this systematic review was to determine whether sufficient research evidence exists to support the use of bedside technologies for early detection of pressure injuries. A search of Medline, CINAHL, Web of Science, and Cochrane databases was performed. Quantitative studies were included that investigated whether accessible technologies could indicate the presence of pressure-related blanchable erythema, pressure-related nonblanchable erythema, and deep tissue pressure injury. Evidence quality was evaluated using the Johns Hopkins Nursing Evidence-Based Practice (JHNEBP) Rating Scale. Identified studies ($n = 18$) established five technologies that have been studied for their potential to provide early detection of pressure injury, including ultrasound ($n = 5$), thermography ($n = 7$), subepidermal moisture (SEM) ($n = 5$), reflectance spectrometry ($n = 2$), and laser Doppler flowmetry ($n = 1$). The multiple studies that investigated SEM measures were of high quality, increasing the reliability of the findings. The methodologic rigor in study quality was variable. Based on assessment using the JHNEBP

Rating Scale, methodologic rigor was consistently higher across the SEM measurement studies compared to the other technologies. The researchers concluded these devices may help identify early pressure–related skin damage before clinical manifestations, potentially benefiting patients of all skin tones. The researchers suggested SEM measurement can be used for early identification of pressure injury, specifically blanchable erythema and nonblanchable erythema.

Relevance to Nursing Practice

Nurses need to identify patients at risk for pressure injuries due to predisposing factors and recognize when there is evidence of actual pressure injuries. Use of technologies such as subepidermal moisture (SEM) technology as part of comprehensive nursing assessments, combined with clinical judgment, can help nurses with early identification of alterations in skin and tissue integrity, enabling implementation of appropriate interventions and therefore should be part of evidence-based practice nursing care.

Skill 8-2 ▶ Cleaning a Wound and Applying a Dressing (General Guidelines)

The goal of wound care is to promote tissue repair and regeneration to restore skin integrity. Often, wound care includes cleaning of the wound and the use of a dressing to maintain an environment to promote healing, absorb excess wound fluid, decrease or eliminate pain, and as a protective covering, a barrier to microorganisms (Baranoski & Ayello, 2020; Brown, 2018). Wound cleansing is indicated to remove debris, bacteria, contaminants, and inflammatory exudate from the wound surface, making the wound less conducive to microbial growth (Baranoski & Ayello, 2020, p. 150; Brown, 2018). Routine cleaning of a granulating, healthy wound, particularly acute wounds, if often not necessary and may damage fragile new tissue formation and can contribute to a delay in wound healing (Brown, 2018).

When cleaning of a wound is indicated, normal saline (0.9% sodium chloride) is traditionally recommended (Taylor et al., 2023). However, tap water of drinkable quality has been suggested as a safe alternative to normal saline, with data showing no difference in infection rates with cleansing with tap water versus normal saline (Cornish & Douglas, 2016; Fernandez & Griffiths, 2012). Home prepared saline solution has also been suggested as an inexpensive alternative (Baranoski & Ayello, 2020). Use of saline has also been identified as common for surgical wounds and tap water for chronic wounds (Annesley, 2019). Commercially prepared wound cleansing solutions, many of which contain antimicrobials and surfactants, are available, and may be considered for use with open wounds with exudate or debris (Baranoski & Ayello, 2020; Mahoney, 2020b; EPUAP, NPIAP, & PPPIA, 2019a). Sterile saline is recommended for cleaning surgical wounds up to 48 hours post surgery (NICE, 2013, as cited in Brown, 2018). Skin cleansers are harmful if used to cleanse wounds and should not be used (Baranoski & Ayello, 2020). Sterile equipment and solutions are required for irrigating an open wound, even in the presence of an existing infection (Taylor et al., 2023). Nonsterile solutions are generally used to clean the skin surface if the wound edges are approximated (Taylor et al., 2023). Clean, not sterile, dressings and gloves can usually be used in the home for care of chronic wounds, based on agency policy (Baranoski & Ayello, 2020).

There is no standard frequency for how often dressings should be changed; advances in dressing composition have resulted in the need for less frequent dressing changes (Baranoski & Ayello, 2020; Brown, 2018). Frequency of dressing changes depends on the wound characteristics, amount of drainage, and the particular wound care product being used. It is customary for the surgeon or other advanced practice provider to perform the first dressing change on a surgical wound, usually within 24 to 48 hours after surgery (Taylor et al., 2023).

There are many commercially prepared wound care products; primary dressings come in contact with the wound bed and are intended to maintain adequate moisture, absorb excess moisture, or add moisture. Secondary dressings cover a primary dressing or secure a dressing in place. The cleaning of a wound and application of many of these products is completed using similar

(continued on page 468)

Skill 8-2 ▶ Cleaning a Wound and Applying a Dressing (General Guidelines) *(continued)*

underlying principles. It is very important for the nurse to be aware of the products available in a particular facility and be knowledgeable of the indications for and correct use of each type of dressing and wound care product in use. Refer to Fundamentals Review 8-4 and 8-5 for additional information.

This skill provides general guidelines and focuses on application of a sterile dressing; specifics may change based on the particular dressing and/or wound care product in use.

DELEGATION CONSIDERATIONS

Wound care and procedures requiring the use of a sterile field and other sterile items are not delegated to assistive personnel (AP). Depending on the state's nurse practice act and the organization's policies and procedures, these procedures may be delegated to licensed practical/vocational nurses (LPN/LVNs). The decision to delegate must be based on careful analysis of the patient's needs and circumstances as well as the qualifications of the person to whom the task is being delegated. Refer to the Delegation Guidelines in Appendix A.

EQUIPMENT

- Sterile gloves, as indicated
- Gloves
- Additional PPE, as indicated
- Primary and secondary dressings (if indicated) as prescribed
- Sterile dressing set or suture set (for the sterile scissors and forceps)
- Sterile cleaning solution as prescribed (commonly 0.9% normal saline solution, or a commercially prepared wound cleanser)
- Skin protectant/barrier wipes

- Sterile basin (may be optional)
- Sterile drape (may be optional)
- Plastic bag or other appropriate waste container for soiled dressings
- Waterproof pad and bath blanket
- Bath blanket or other linens for draping patient
- Additional dressings and supplies needed or required based on the wound dressing/care prescribed for the patient

ASSESSMENT

Assess the situation to determine the need for wound cleaning and a dressing change. Confirm any prescribed interventions relevant to wound care and wound care included in the plan of care. Assess the patient's level of comfort and the need for analgesics before wound care. Assess if the patient experienced any pain related to prior dressing changes and the effectiveness of interventions employed to minimize the patient's pain. Assess the current dressing to determine if it is intact. Assess for excess drainage, bleeding, or saturation of the dressing. Inspect the wound and the surrounding tissue. Assess the appearance of the wound for the approximation of wound edges, the color of the wound and surrounding area, and signs of dehiscence. Assess for the presence of sutures, staples, or adhesive closure strips. Note the stage of the healing process and characteristics of any drainage. Also assess the surrounding skin for color, temperature, and edema, **ecchymosis**, or **maceration**.

ACTUAL OR POTENTIAL HEALTH PROBLEMS AND NEEDS

Many actual or potential health problems or issues may require the use of this skill as part of related interventions. An appropriate health problem or issue may include:
- Altered skin integrity risk
- Altered skin integrity
- Infection risk

OUTCOME IDENTIFICATION AND PLANNING

The expected outcome to achieve when cleaning a wound and applying a sterile dressing is that the wound is cleaned and dressed without contaminating the wound area, causing trauma to the wound, or causing the patient to experience pain or discomfort. Other outcomes that are appropriate include the following: the wound continues to show signs of progression of healing, and the patient demonstrates an understanding of the wound care and dressing.

IMPLEMENTATION

ACTION	RATIONALE
1. Review the patient's health record for prescribed wound care or the care plan related to wound care. Gather necessary supplies.	Reviewing the health record and care plan validates the correct patient and correct procedure. Preparation promotes efficient time management and an organized approach to the task.
2. Perform hand hygiene and put on PPE, if indicated.	Hand hygiene and PPE prevent the spread of microorganisms. PPE is required based on transmission precautions.
3. Identify the patient.	Identifying the patient ensures the right patient receives the intervention and helps prevent errors.
4. Assemble equipment on the overbed table or other surface within reach.	Organization facilitates performance of the task.
5. Close the curtains around the bed and close the door to the room, if possible. Explain to the patient what you are going to do and why you are going to do it.	This ensures the patient's privacy. Explanation relieves anxiety and facilitates engagement.
6. Assess the patient for the possible need for nonpharmacologic pain-reducing interventions or analgesic medication before wound care dressing change. Administer appropriate prescribed analgesic. Allow enough time for the analgesic to achieve its effectiveness.	Pain is a subjective experience influenced by past experience. Wound care and dressing changes may cause pain for some patients.
7. Place a waste receptacle or bag at a convenient location for use during the procedure.	Having a waste container handy means the soiled dressing may be discarded easily, without the spread of microorganisms.
8. Adjust the bed to a comfortable working height (VHA Center for Engineering & Occupational Safety and Health [CEOSH], 2016).	Having the bed at the proper height prevents back and muscle strain.
9. Assist the patient to a comfortable position that provides easy access to the wound area. Use the bath blanket to cover any exposed area other than the wound. Place a waterproof pad under the wound site.	Patient positioning and the use of a bath blanket provide for comfort and warmth. Waterproof pad protects underlying surfaces.
10. Check the position of drains, tubes, or other adjuncts before removing the dressing. Put on gloves and loosen the tape or adhesive edge on the old dressings by removing in the direction of hair growth and the use of a push–pull method (Fumarola et al., 2020) (Figure 1). Push–pull method: lift a corner of the dressing away from the skin, and then gently push the skin down and away from the dressing/adhesive (Fumarola et al., 2020). Continue moving fingers of the opposite hand to support the skin as the product is removed (Fumarola et al., 2020). Once all adhesive is loosened from the skin, carefully lift dressing from the surrounding skin to prevent medical adhesive–related skin injury (MARSI). Remove the sides/edges first, then the center. If the patient is at increased risk for MARSI (see Box 8-2), requires repeated application or removal of adhesive devices, or there is resistance, use an adhesive remover (Barton, 2020; Fumarola et al., 2020; Kelly-O'Flynn et al., 2020).	Checking ensures that a drain is not removed accidentally if one is present. Gloves protect the nurse from contaminated dressings and prevent the spread of microorganisms. Removal of the tape in the direction of hair growth minimizes trauma to the skin (Fumarola et al., 2020). Pushing the skin down and away from the adhesive reduces the risk for MARSI (Fumarola et al., 2020). The use of adhesive remover allows for the easy, rapid, and painless removal without the associated problems of skin stripping and helps reduce patient discomfort (Barton, 2020; Fumarola et al., 2020; Kelly-O'Flynn et al., 2020).

(continued on page 470)

Skill 8-2 ▶ Cleaning a Wound and Applying a Dressing (General Guidelines) *(continued)*

ACTION

RATIONALE

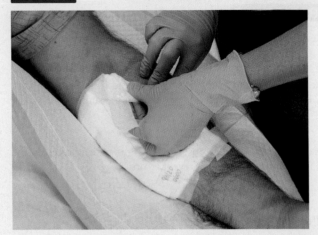

FIGURE 1. Loosening dressing tape or adhesive edge.

Box 8-2	Risk Factors for Medical Adhesive–Related Skin Injury

Intrinsic

- Extremes of age: older adults, infants
- Comorbidities: diabetes, venous insufficiency, dermatologic conditions (e.g., eczema), renal insufficiency, immunosuppression
- Underlying health issues: dehydration, malnutrition, edema

Extrinsic

- Prolonged moisture exposure or drying of the skin
- Radiation treatment
- Use of medications that prolong epidermal barrier recovery (e.g., corticosteroids, chemotherapeutic agents, anti-inflammatory agents, and anticoagulants)
- Photodamage or exposure to ultraviolet light
- Repeated taping or dressing removal
- Use of harsh, non-pH balanced skin cleansers

Source: Fumarola, S., Allaway, R., Callaghan, R., Collier, M., Downie, F., Geraghty, J., Kiernan, S., & Spratt, F. (2020). Overlooked and underestimated: Medical adhesive-related skin injuries. Best practice consensus document on prevention. *Journal of Wound Care, 29*(Suppl 3c), S1–S24. https://doi.org/10.12968/jowc.2020.29.Sup3c.S1; Kelly-O'Flynn, S., Mohamud, L., & Copson, D. (2020). Medical adhesive-related skin injury. *British Journal of Nursing, 29*(6), S20–S26. https://doi.org/10.12968/bjon.2020.29.6.S20.

11. Carefully remove the soiled dressings. If any part of the dressing sticks to the underlying skin, use small amounts of sterile saline to help loosen and remove it.

   Cautious removal of the dressing is more comfortable for the patient and ensures that any drain present is not removed. Sterile saline moistens the dressing for easier removal and minimizes damage and pain.

12. After removing the dressing, note the presence, amount, type, color, and odor of any drainage on the dressings (Figure 2). Place soiled dressings in the appropriate waste receptacle. Remove your gloves and perform hand hygiene.

   The presence of drainage should be documented. Proper disposal of soiled dressings and used gloves prevents the spread of microorganisms. Hand hygiene prevents the transmission of microorganisms.

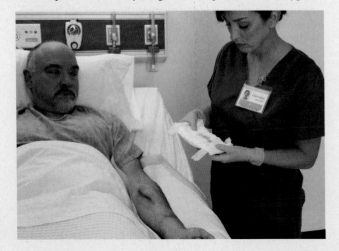

FIGURE 2. Noting characteristics of drainage on dressing that has been removed.

ACTION

13. Inspect the wound site for size, appearance, and drainage (Refer to Fundamentals Review 8-2). Assess if any pain is present. Check the status of sutures, adhesive closure strips, staples, and drains or tubes, if present. Note any problems to include in your documentation.

14. **Using sterile technique, prepare a sterile work area and open the needed supplies.**

15. Open the sterile cleaning solution. Moisten gauze for cleaning the periwound skin. Depending on the amount of cleaning needed, the solution might be poured directly over gauze sponges over a container for small cleaning jobs, or into a basin for more complex or larger cleaning.

16. Put on sterile gloves. Alternatively, clean gloves (clean technique) may be used when cleaning a chronic wound or pressure injury.

17. Clean the wound. Pour the cleaning solution over the wound from top to bottom. Alternatively, spray the wound from top to bottom with a commercially prepared wound cleanser. Wound irrigation is often used to clean open wounds and may also be used for other types of wounds. Refer to Skill 8-3.

18. Clean the skin surrounding the wound. Clean from top to bottom and/or from the center to the outside, beginning at the wound edges. Refer to Box 8-3 (Figure 3). Use new gauze for each wipe, placing the used gauze in the waste receptacle.

19. Once the wound and surrounding skin are cleaned, dry the surrounding skin area using a gauze sponge in the same manner.

20. If a drain is in use at the wound location, clean around the drain. Refer to Skills 8-5, 8-6, and 8-7.

RATIONALE

Wound healing or the presence of irritation or infection should be documented.

Supplies are within easy reach and sterility is maintained.

Sterility of dressings and solution is maintained.

The use of sterile gloves maintains surgical asepsis and sterile technique and reduces the risk for spreading microorganisms. Aseptic technique should be used to change dressings for surgical wounds and in the acute clinical setting, to reduce the risk of transfer of pathogens, likely to be present in an acute care setting, to the wound (Brown, 2018). Clean technique is appropriate for cleaning chronic wounds, wounds in the home, or pressure injuries (Baranoski & Ayello, 2020; EPUAP, NPIAP, & PPPIA, 2019a; Taylor et al., 2023).

Cleaning from top to bottom and center to outside ensures that cleaning occurs from the least to most contaminated area and a previously cleaned area is not contaminated again. Using a single gauze for each wipe ensures that the previously cleaned area is not contaminated again.

Cleaning from top to bottom and center to outside ensures that cleaning occurs from the least to most contaminated area and a previously cleaned area is not contaminated again. Using a single gauze for each wipe ensures that the previously cleaned area is not contaminated again.

Excess moisture on healthy skin increases risk for moisture-associated skin damage and interferes with proper adhesion of securement of dressings.

Cleaning the insertion site helps prevent infection.

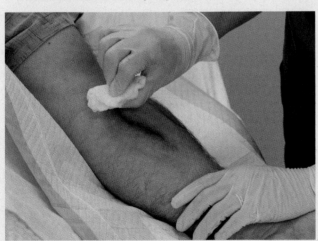

FIGURE 3. Cleaning the skin surrounding the wound.

(continued on page 472)

Skill 8-2 ▶ Cleaning a Wound and Applying a Dressing (General Guidelines) *(continued)*

ACTION	RATIONALE

Box 8-3 | Cleaning a Wound

Cleaning a Wound With Approximated Edges

- Use standard precautions; use appropriate transmission-based precautions when indicated.
- Moisten a sterile gauze pad or swab with the prescribed cleansing agent.
- Use a new swab or gauze for each downward stroke.
- Clean from top to bottom.
- Work outward from the incision in lines parallel to it (Figure A).
- Wipe from the clean area (at wound edges) toward the less clean area.

Cleaning a Wound With Unapproximated Edges

- Use standard precautions; use appropriate transmission-based precautions when indicated.
- Moisten a sterile gauze pad or swab with the prescribed cleansing agent and squeeze out excess solution.
- Use a new swab or gauze for each circle.
- Clean the wound in full or half circles, beginning at the wound edges and working outward (Figure B).
- Clean to at least 1 inch beyond the end of the new dressing.
- If a dressing is not being applied, clean to at least 2 inches beyond the wound margins.

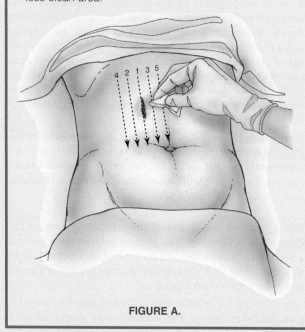

FIGURE A.

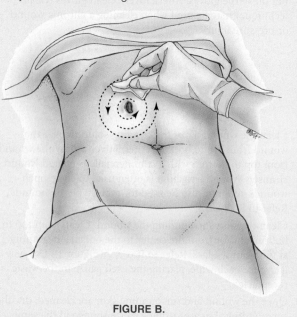

FIGURE B.

Source: Hess, C. (2013). *Clinical guide to skin & wound care* (7th ed.). Wolters Kluwer.

21. Remove gloves and place in the waste receptacle. Perform hand hygiene.

Proper disposal of used gloves and hand hygiene prevent the spread of microorganisms.

22. Put on sterile gloves. Alternatively, clean gloves (clean technique) may be used when cleaning a chronic wound or pressure injury. Apply a skin protectant or barrier to the healthy skin around the wound where the dressing adhesive or tape will be placed and where wound drainage may come in contact with the skin (Figure 4).

The use of sterile gloves maintains surgical asepsis and sterile technique and reduces the risk for spreading microorganisms. Clean technique is appropriate for cleaning chronic wounds, wounds in the home, or pressure injuries (Baranoski & Ayello, 2020; EPUAP, NPIAP, & PPPIA, 2019a; Taylor et al., 2023). Skin barrier/protectant prevents skin irritation and excoriation from tape, adhesives, and wound drainage (Fumarola et al., 2020; Kelly-O'Flynn et al., 2020).

ACTION

23. Apply any topical medications, foams, gels, and/or dressing product to the wound as prescribed; ensure products stay confined to the wound and do not impact on intact surrounding tissue/skin (Figure 5).

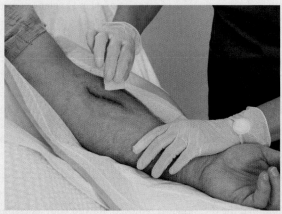

FIGURE 4. Applying skin protectant to skin surrounding the wound.

24. Gently place the prescribed cover dressing at the wound center and extend it at least 1 inch beyond the wound in all directions. Alternatively, follow the manufacturer's directions for application (Figure 6).

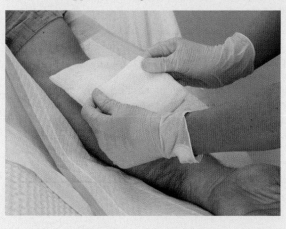

FIGURE 6. Applying cover dressing to site.

25. As necessary, apply a secondary dressing, based on products in use, prescribed interventions, and facility policy. Note: May not be necessary or appropriate, based on the cover dressing used in Step 23. Some dressings act as both primary and secondary dressings (Baranoski & Ayello, 2020).

26. Apply additional materials, such as roller gauze, to secure the dressings as needed. Alternatively, many commercial wound products are self-adhesive and do not require additional tape. Remove gloves and perform hand hygiene.

RATIONALE

The growth of microorganisms may be inhibited and the healing process improved with the use of prescribed medications, foams, gels, and/or other wound care product.

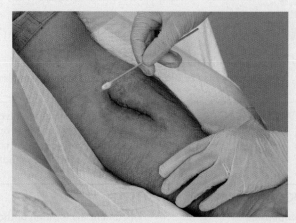

FIGURE 5. Applying prescribed wound care product.

Extending the dressing at least 1 inch past the wound edges ensures the dressing covers and protects the wound.

Secondary dressings cover the primary dressing or secure the dressing (Baranoski & Ayello, 2020).

Additional securing products keep the dressing in place. Proper disposal of gloves and hand hygiene prevent the spread of microorganisms.

(continued on page 474)

Skill 8-2 ▶ Cleaning a Wound and Applying a Dressing (General Guidelines) *(continued)*

ACTION	RATIONALE
27. Label the dressing with date and time. Remove all remaining equipment; place the patient in a comfortable position, with side rails up as indicated and bed in the lowest position.	Recording date and time provides communication and demonstrates adherence to care plan. Proper patient and bed positioning promotes safety and comfort.
28. Remove PPE, if used. Perform hand hygiene.	Proper removal of PPE reduces the risk for infection transmission and contamination of other items. Hand hygiene prevents the spread of microorganisms.
29. Check all wound dressings at least every shift. More frequent checks may be needed if the wound is more complex.	Checking dressings ensures the assessment of changes in patient condition and timely intervention to prevent complications.

EVALUATION

The expected outcomes have been met when the wound was cleaned and dressed without contaminating the wound area or causing trauma to the wound, the patient did not experience pain or discomfort, the wound has continued to show signs of progression of healing, and the patient has demonstrated an understanding of the wound care and dressing.

DOCUMENTATION

Guidelines

Document the location of the wound and that the dressing was removed. Record your assessment of the wound: size; approximation of wound edges; presence of sutures, staples, or adhesive closure strips if wound edges are approximated; record size and wound assessment if wound edges are not approximated; and the condition of the surrounding skin. Note if redness, edema, or drainage is observed and document characteristics if present. Document cleansing of wound and application of topical medications, foams, gels, and/or gauze to the wound as prescribed. Record the type of dressing that was reapplied. Note pertinent patient and family/caregiver education and any patient reaction to the procedure, including patient's pain level and effectiveness of nonpharmacologic interventions or analgesia if administered.

Sample Documentation

Lippincott DocuCare

Practice documenting wound care in *Lippincott DocuCare*.

> 9/8/25 0600 Dressing removed from left lateral calf incision. Scant purulent secretions noted on dressing. Incision edges approximately 1 mm apart, red, with ecchymosis and edema present. Small amount of purulent drainage from wound noted. Area cleansed with normal saline; antibiotic ointment applied as prescribed. Surrounding tissue red and ecchymotic. Redressed with nonadhering dressing and wrapped with stretch gauze. Patient reports adequate pain control after preprocedure analgesic; states pain is dull ache, 1/10 on pain scale.
> —N. Joiner, RN

DEVELOPING CLINICAL REASONING AND CLINICAL JUDGMENT

UNEXPECTED SITUATIONS AND ASSOCIATED INTERVENTIONS

- *The previous wound assessment states that the incision was clean and dry, and the wound edges were approximated, with the staples and surgical drain intact. The surrounding tissue was without inflammation, edema, or erythema. After the dressing is removed, the nurse notes the incision edges are not approximated at the distal end, multiple staples are evident in the old dressing, the surrounding skin tissue is red and swollen, and purulent drainage is on the dressing and leaking from the wound:* Assess the patient for any other signs and symptoms, such as pain, malaise, fever, and paresthesias. Place a dry sterile dressing over the wound site. Report the findings to the health care team and document the event in the patient's record. Be prepared to obtain a wound culture and implement any changes in wound care as prescribed.
- *When removing a patient's dressing, the assessment reveals deterioration or significant improvement in the wound:* Notify the health care team or wound care specialist, as a different treatment modality and/or dressing product may be necessary.

SPECIAL CONSIDERATIONS

General Considerations

- Instruct the patient, if appropriate, and other members of the health care team to observe for excessive drainage that may overwhelm the dressing. They should also report when dressings become soiled or loosened from the skin.
- There are many dressing types and manufacturers—the nurse needs to collaborate with the health care team to ensure the correct dressing type is chosen, ongoing assessment occurs, and updates to the treatment plan (dressing choice) are made as the wound evolves (Taylor et al., 2023). The choice of wound dressing will change during the healing period, based on a minimum of once-a-week wound assessment (more often with notable changes) (Baranoski & Ayello, 2020). The type of wound and status/characteristics of the wound influence the choice of the wound dressing, and several different types of products may be needed as the wound progresses through the stages of healing (Baranoski & Ayello, 2020, p. 191).
- Products designed to assist with dressing removal can reduce pain, avoid damaging the peri-wound skin and resulting skin stripping and MARSI and result in time savings (Fumarola et al., 2020; Kelly-O'Flynn et al., 2020; Reevell et al., 2016).
- When using adherent dressings, such as a hydrocolloid dressing, cut the dressing to size, allowing at least a 1-inch margin of healthy skin around the wound to be covered with the dressing (Baranoski & Ayello, 2020). Apply the dressing to the wound without stretching the dressing.
- Optimum and timely wound healing are supported by adequate nutrition and hydration (Dudek, 2018; Stuart, 2020). Collaborate with the registered dietician and dietary staff to develop an individualized nutrition intervention plan for the patient.

Infant and Child Considerations

- The skin of neonates is more fragile as a result of incomplete epidermal-to-dermal cohesion; use skin barrier products and adhesive removers, paper tape, or nonadherent dressings to prevent tearing of the skin (Baranoski et al., 2016; Fumarola et al., 2020; Kelly-O'Flynn et al., 2020).

Older Adult Considerations

- The skin of older adults is less elastic and more fragile as a result of age-related changes; use skin barrier products and adhesive removers, paper tape, nonadherent dressings, or roller gauze (on extremities) to prevent tearing of the skin (Baranoski et al., 2016; Fumarola et al., 2020; Kelly-O'Flynn et al., 2020).

Community-Based Care Considerations

- Patients may shower to clean the wound before dressing changes in the community; patients should avoid using perfumed soaps, body wash, or antiseptics or soaps and instead use pH neutral shower and bath skin cleansers/emollients (Brown, 2018; Milne, 2019).
- Saline solution can be prepared at home by combining 1 teaspoon of noniodized salt with 1 quart of distilled water and stirring until the salt is completely dissolved (Baranoski & Ayello, 2020). This solution can be kept in a tightly covered glass or plastic container for up to 1 week at room temperature (Baranoski & Ayello, 2020).

EVIDENCE FOR PRACTICE ▶

PREVENTION OF MEDICAL ADHESIVE–RELATED SKIN INJURIES
Fumarola, S., Allaway, R., Callaghan, R., Collier, M., Downie, F., Geraghty, J., Kiernan, S., & Spratt, F. (2020). Overlooked and underestimated: Medical adhesive-related skin injuries. Best practice consensus document on prevention. *Journal of Wound Care, 29*(Suppl 3c), S1–S24. https://doi.org/10.12968/jowc.2020.29.Sup3c.S1

This consensus document is the result of a review of the literature on medical adhesive-related skin injury (MARSI) by a panel of wound care experts, educators, and researchers. This best practice guideline provides recommendations for the assessment and prevention of MARSI, with the goal of standardizing care across all health care settings.

Skill 8-3 ▶ Performing Irrigation of a Wound

Irrigation is a directed flow of solution over tissues. Wound irrigations are prescribed to clean the area of **pathogens** and other debris and to promote wound healing. Irrigation procedures may also be prescribed to apply heat or antiseptics locally. An ideal pressure for wound cleansing is 5 to 15 psi (Baranoski & Ayello, 2020). A needle or angiocath and syringe are often used to deliver fluid for irrigation of a wound. The size of the syringe and the needle/angiocath gauge determine the amount of pressure of the fluid stream, with larger syringes providing less force and needles/angiocaths with larger lumen diameters providing greater flow and greater pressures (Baranoski & Ayello, 2020). An 18- to 19-gauge needle/angiocath and a 30- to 35-mL syringe is an inexpensive and easy-to-use method for irrigation (Baranoski & Ayello, 2020, p. 152; McLain et al., 2021). If the wound edges are approximated, nonsterile solutions and clean technique may be used; if the wound edges are not approximated, sterile equipment and solutions are used for irrigation (Taylor et al., 2023). Normal saline (0.9% sodium chloride) is often the solution of choice when irrigating wounds, but sterile water, commercially prepared wound cleansers containing an antimicrobial, or potable tap water may be used (Baranoski & Ayello, 2020; Mahoney, 2020b; Taylor et al., 2023; WOCN, 2016).

DELEGATION CONSIDERATIONS

Irrigation of a wound and procedures requiring the use of a sterile field and other sterile items are not delegated to assistive personnel (AP). Depending on the state's nurse practice act and the organization's policies and procedures, these procedures may be delegated to licensed practical/vocational nurses (LPN/LVNs). The decision to delegate must be based on careful analysis of the patient's needs and circumstances as well as the qualifications of the person to whom the task is being delegated. Refer to the Delegation Guidelines in Appendix A.

EQUIPMENT

- An 18- to 19-gauge needle/angiocath and 30- to 35-mL syringe or a commercial cleanser packaged in a pressurized container (Baranoski & Ayello, 2020, p. 152; McLain et al., 2021; WOCN, 2016)
- Sterile irrigation solution as prescribed, warmed to body temperature, commonly 0.9% normal saline solution or other solution as prescribed
- Alternatively, irrigation solution may be packaged in individual, single-use syringe
- Plastic bag or other waste container to dispose of soiled dressings
- Sterile gloves
- Sterile drape (may be optional)
- Clean, disposable gloves
- Moisture-proof gown; mask, and eye protection or face shield
- Waterproof pad and bath blanket
- Bath blanket or other linens for draping patient
- Additional PPE, as indicated
- Additional dressings and supplies needed or required based on the wound dressing/care prescribed for the patient

ASSESSMENT

Assess the situation to determine the need for wound irrigation. Confirm any prescribed interventions relevant to wound care and any wound care included in the plan of care. Assess the current dressing to determine if it is intact. Assess the patient's level of comfort and the need for analgesics before wound care. Assess if the patient experienced any pain related to previous dressing changes and the effectiveness of interventions employed to minimize the patient's pain. Assess for excess drainage or bleeding or saturation of the dressing. Inspect the wound and the surrounding tissue. Assess the location, appearance of the wound, stage (if appropriate), drainage, and types of tissue present in the wound. Measure the wound. Note the stage of the healing process and characteristics of any drainage. Also assess the surrounding skin for color, temperature, and edema, ecchymosis, or maceration.

ACTUAL OR POTENTIAL HEALTH PROBLEMS AND NEEDS

Many actual or potential health problems or issues may require the use of this skill as part of related interventions. An appropriate health problem or issue may include:
- Altered skin integrity
- Infection risk
- Knowledge deficiency

OUTCOME
IDENTIFICATION
AND PLANNING

The expected outcome to achieve when irrigating a wound is that the irrigation is performed without contamination or trauma, without damaging proliferative cells and newly formed tissues, and without causing the patient to experience pain or discomfort. Other outcomes that might be appropriate include: the wound continues to show signs of progression of healing, and the patient demonstrates an understanding of the wound care.

IMPLEMENTATION

ACTION	RATIONALE
1. Review the patient's health record for prescribed wound care or the plan of care related to wound care. Gather necessary supplies.	Reviewing the health record and care plan validates the correct patient and correct procedure. Preparation promotes efficient time management and an organized approach to the task.
2. Perform hand hygiene and put on PPE, if indicated.	Hand hygiene and PPE prevent the spread of microorganisms. PPE is required based on transmission precautions.
3. Identify the patient.	Identifying the patient ensures the right patient receives the intervention and helps prevent errors.
4. Assemble equipment on the overbed table or other surface within reach.	Organization facilitates performance of the task.
5. Close the curtains around the bed and close the door to the room if possible. Explain what you are going to do and why you are going to do it to the patient.	This ensures the patient's privacy. Explanation relieves anxiety and facilitates engagement.
6. Assess the patient for possible need for nonpharmacologic pain-reducing interventions or analgesic medication before wound care and/or dressing change. Administer appropriate prescribed analgesic. Allow enough time for the analgesic to achieve its effectiveness before beginning the procedure.	Pain is a subjective experience influenced by past experience. Wound care and dressing changes may cause pain for some patients.
7. Place a waste receptacle or bag at a convenient location for use during the procedure.	Having a waste container handy means the soiled dressing may be discarded easily, without the spread of microorganisms.
8. Adjust the bed to a comfortable working height (VHACEOSH, 2016).	Having the bed at the proper height prevents back and muscle strain.
9. Assist the patient to a comfortable position that provides easy access to the wound area. Position the patient so the irrigation solution will flow from the clean end of the wound toward the dirtier end or top to bottom. Use the bath blanket to cover any exposed area other than the wound. Place a waterproof pad under the wound site.	Patient positioning and the use of a bath blanket provide for comfort and warmth. Gravity directs the flow of liquid from the least contaminated to the most contaminated area. Waterproof pad protects underlying surfaces.
10. Put on a gown, mask, and eye protection or face shield.	Using PPE, such as gowns, masks, and eye protection, is part of *Standard Precautions*. A gown protects clothes from contamination should splashing occur. Appropriate personal protective equipment, including a mask and eye protection or face shield is essential when irrigating a wound with any degree of pressure (WOCN, 2016).

(continued on page 478)

Skill 8-3 ▶ Performing Irrigation of a Wound *(continued)*

ACTION	RATIONALE
11. Check the position of drains, tubes, or other adjuncts before removing the dressing. Put on clean, disposable gloves and loosen the tape on the old dressings by removing in the direction of hair growth and the use of a push–pull method (see Figure 1, Skill 8-2) (Fumarola et al., 2020). Push–pull method: lift a corner of the dressing away from the skin, then gently push the skin away from the dressing/adhesive (Fumarola et al., 2020). Continue moving the fingers of the opposite hand to support the skin as the product is removed (Fumarola et al., 2020). Once all adhesive is loosened from the skin, carefully lift the dressing from the surrounding skin to prevent medical adhesive–related skin injury (MARSI). Remove the sides/edges first, then the center. If the patient is at increased risk for MARSI (see Box 8-2 in Skill 8-2), requires repeated application or removal of adhesive devices, or there is resistance, use an adhesive remover (Barton, 2020; Fumarola et al., 2020; Kelly-O'Flynn et al., 2020).	Checking ensures that a drain is not removed accidentally if one is present. Gloves protect the nurse from contaminated dressings and prevent the spread of microorganisms. Removal of the tape in the direction of hair growth minimizes trauma to the skin (Fumarola et al., 2020). The use of adhesive remover allows for the easy, rapid, and painless removal without the associated problems of skin stripping and helps reduce patient discomfort (Barton, 2020; Fumarola et al., 2020; Kelly-O'Flynn et al., 2020).
12. Carefully remove the soiled dressings. If any part of the dressing sticks to the underlying skin, use small amounts of sterile saline to help loosen and remove it.	Cautious removal of the dressing is more comfortable for the patient and ensures that any drain present is not removed. Sterile saline moistens the dressing for easier removal and minimizes damage and pain.
13. After removing the dressing, note the presence, amount, type, color, and odor of any drainage on the dressings. Place soiled dressings in the appropriate waste receptacle.	The presence of drainage should be documented. Proper disposal of soiled dressings and used gloves prevents the spread of microorganisms.
14. Assess the wound for appearance, stage, presence of eschar, granulation tissue, **epithelialization**, undermining, tunneling, necrosis, **sinus tract**, and drainage. Assess the appearance of the surrounding tissue. Measure the wound. Refer to Fundamentals Review 8-2.	This information provides evidence about the wound healing process and/or the presence of infection.
15. Remove your gloves and put them in the receptacle. Perform hand hygiene.	Discarding gloves prevents the spread of microorganisms. Hand hygiene prevents the spread of microorganisms.
16. Set up a sterile field, if indicated, and wound cleaning and irrigation supplies. Pour warmed sterile irrigating solution into the sterile container (based on supplies in use). Moisten gauze for cleaning the periwound skin. Put on the sterile gloves. Alternatively, clean gloves (clean technique) may be used when cleaning a chronic wound or pressure injury.	Using warmed solution prevents chilling the patient and may minimize patient discomfort. Aseptic technique should be used to change dressings for surgical wounds and in the acute clinical setting, to reduce the risk of transfer of pathogens, likely to be present in an acute care setting, to the wound (Brown, 2018). Clean technique is appropriate for cleaning chronic wounds, wounds in the home, or pressure injuries (Baranoski & Ayello, 2020; EPUAP, NPIAP, & PPPIA, 2019a; Taylor et al., 2023).
17. Position the sterile basin below the wound to collect the irrigation fluid.	Patient and bed linens are protected from contaminated fluid.
18. Fill the irrigation syringe with solution (Figure 1). Alternatively, irrigation solution may be packaged in individual, single-use syringe; remove cap on syringe. Using your nondominant hand, gently apply pressure to the basin against the skin below the wound to form a seal with the skin (Figure 2).	The solution will collect in the basin and prevent the irrigant from running down the skin. Patient and bed linens are protected from contaminated fluid.

ACTION

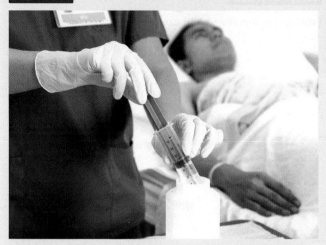

FIGURE 1. Drawing up solution into irrigation syringe.

19. Using either a pulsatile or continuous flow pattern, direct a stream of solution into the wound from top to bottom (Figure 3). Flush all wound areas.

20. Watch for the solution to flow smoothly and evenly. When the solution from the wound flows out clear, discontinue irrigation.

21. Once the wound is cleaned, clean the skin surrounding the wound and then dry the skin surrounding the wound (Figure 4). (Refer to Steps 18 and 19, Skill 8-2).

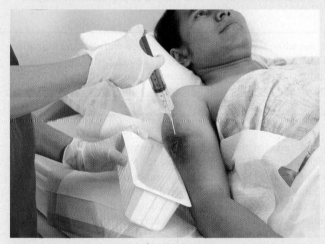

FIGURE 3. Irrigating wound with a stream of solution. Solution drains into collection container.

22. If a drain is in use at the wound location, clean around the drain. Refer to Skills 8-6, 8-7, 8-8, and 8-9.

23. Remove gloves and perform hand hygiene.

RATIONALE

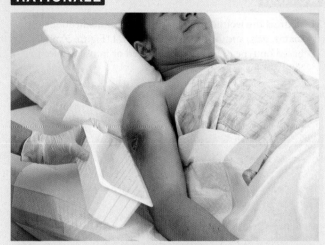

FIGURE 2. Applying pressure to basin to form seal.

The wound irrigating fluid stream can be delivered in either a pulsatile or continuous flow pattern (Baranoski & Ayello, 2020). Directing flow from top to bottom ensures that a previously cleaned area is not contaminated again.

Irrigation removes exudate and debris.

Excess moisture on healthy skin increases risk for moisture-associated skin damage and interferes with proper adhesion of securement of dressings.

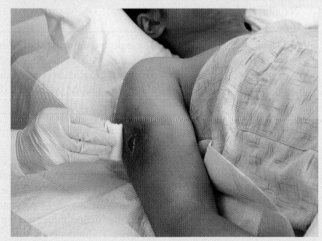

FIGURE 4. Drying around wound, not in wound, with gauze pad.

Cleaning the insertion site helps prevent infection.

Proper disposal of used gloves and hand hygiene prevent the spread of microorganisms.

(continued on page 480)

Skill 8-3 ▶ Performing Irrigation of a Wound *(continued)*

ACTION

24. Redress the wound, applying any topical medications, foams, gels, and/or gauze to the wound (Figure 5) and based on type of dressing prescribed or in use. (Refer to Skill 8-2 for general guidelines.)

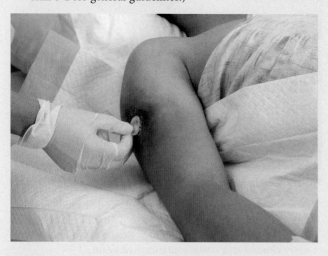

FIGURE 5. Applying wound contact material.

25. Remove PPE, if used. Perform hand hygiene.

26. Check all wound dressings at least every shift. More frequent checks may be needed if the wound is more complex.

RATIONALE

Provides appropriate wound care to support plan of care.

Proper removal of PPE reduces the risk for infection transmission and contamination of other items. Hand hygiene prevents the spread of microorganisms.

Checking dressings ensures the assessment of changes in patient condition and timely intervention to prevent complications.

EVALUATION

The expected outcomes have been met when the irrigation was completed without contamination or trauma, without damaging proliferative cells and newly formed tissues, and without causing the patient to experience pain or discomfort; the wound has continued to show signs of progression of healing; and the patient has demonstrated an understanding of the wound care and dressing.

DOCUMENTATION

Guidelines

Document the location of the wound and that the dressing was removed. Record your assessment of the wound, including evidence of granulation tissue, presence of necrotic tissue, stage (if pressure injury), and characteristics of drainage. Include the appearance of the surrounding skin. Document the irrigation of the wound and solution used. Record the type of dressing that was applied. Note pertinent patient and family/caregiver education and any patient reaction to this procedure, including patient's pain level and effectiveness of nonpharmacologic interventions or analgesia if administered.

Sample Documentation

> 3/5/25 1700 Dressing removed from left outer heel area. Minimal serosanguineous drainage noted on dressings. Wound 4 cm × 5 cm × 2 cm, pink, with granulation tissue evident. Surrounding skin tone consistent with patient's skin, no edema or redness noted. Irrigated with normal saline and hydrogel dressing applied.
>
> —J. Lark, RN

DEVELOPING CLINICAL REASONING AND CLINICAL JUDGMENT

UNEXPECTED SITUATIONS AND ASSOCIATED INTERVENTIONS

- *Patient experiences pain when the wound irrigation is begun:* Stop the procedure and administer an analgesic, as prescribed. Obtain new sterile supplies and begin the procedure after an appropriate amount of time has elapsed to allow the analgesic to begin working. Note the patient's pain on the plan of care so that pain medication can be given before future wound treatments.
- *During the wound irrigation, the nurse notes bleeding from the wound. This has not been documented as happening with previous irrigations:* Stop the procedure. Assess the patient for other symptoms. Obtain vital signs. Report the findings to the health care team and document the event in the patient's record.

SPECIAL CONSIDERATIONS

- Optimum and timely wound healing are supported by adequate nutrition and hydration (Dudek, 2018; EPUAP, NPIAP, & PPPIA, 2019a; Stuart, 2020). Collaborate with the registered dietician and dietary staff to develop an individualized nutrition intervention plan for the patient.
- A whirlpool bath may be prescribed as an alternative to irrigation for some chronic wounds (Baranoski & Ayello, 2020). The wound should not come in close contact with the water jets in the whirlpool to avoid tissue injury.

EVIDENCE FOR PRACTICE ▶

PREVENTION OF MEDICAL ADHESIVE–RELATED SKIN INJURIES

Fumarola, S., Allaway, R., Callaghan, R., Collier, M., Downie, F., Geraghty, J., Kiernan, S., & Spratt, F. (2020). Overlooked and underestimated: Medical adhesive-related skin injuries. Best practice consensus document on prevention. *Journal of Wound Care, 29*(Suppl 3c), S1–S24. https://doi.org/10.12968/jowc.2020.29.Sup3c.S1

This consensus document is the result of a review of the literature on medical adhesive–related skin injury (MARSI) by a panel of wound care experts, educators, and researchers. This best practice guideline provides recommendations for the assessment and prevention of MARSI, with the goal of standardizing care across all health care settings.

Skill 8-4 ▶ Collecting a Wound Culture

A wound culture may be prescribed to identify the causative organism(s) of an infected wound. Identifying the invading microorganism will provide useful information for selecting the most appropriate therapy. A wound culture involves collecting a specimen of exudate, drainage or tissue by swab, aspiration, or tissue removal. Nurses generally perform collection of a culture by swab; wound cultures collected by aspiration and tissue removal are performed by advanced practice professionals and physicians. The collection of a wound culture by swab is addressed in the following skill.

Maintaining strict asepsis is crucial so that only the pathogen present in the wound is isolated. It is essential to use optimal technique and the correct collection device based on the tests prescribed for the collection of a specimen to isolate aerobic and/or anaerobic organisms (WOCN, 2016).

DELEGATION CONSIDERATIONS

The collection of a wound culture is not delegated to assistive personnel (AP). Depending on the state's nurse practice act and the organization's policies and procedures, the collection of a wound culture may be delegated to licensed practical/vocational nurses (LPN/LVNs). The decision to delegate must be based on careful analysis of the patient's needs and circumstances as well as the qualifications of the person to whom the task is being delegated. Refer to the Delegation Guidelines in Appendix A.

(continued on page 482)

Skill 8-4 ▶ Collecting a Wound Culture *(continued)*

EQUIPMENT

- A sterile culture kit (aerobic and/or anaerobic) with swab, or a culture tube with individual sterile swabs
- Sterile gloves
- Clean, disposable gloves
- Additional PPE, as indicated
- Plastic bag or appropriate waste receptacle

- Patient label for the sample tube
- Biohazard specimen bag
- Bath blanket (if necessary to drape the patient)
- Supplies to clean the wound with saline without preservatives (Baranoski & Ayello, 2020) and reapply the prescribed dressing after obtaining the culture. (Refer to Skills 8-2 and 8-3.)

ASSESSMENT

Assess the situation to determine the need for wound culture. Confirm any prescribed interventions relevant to obtaining a wound culture as well as wound care and/or any wound care included in the plan of care. Assess the patient's level of comfort and the need for analgesics before obtaining the wound culture. Inspect the wound and the surrounding tissue. Assess the location, appearance of the wound, stage (if appropriate), drainage, and types of tissue present in the wound. Measure the wound. Note the stage of the healing process and characteristics of any drainage. Also assess the surrounding skin for color, temperature, and edema, ecchymosis, or maceration.

ACTUAL OR POTENTIAL HEALTH PROBLEMS AND NEEDS

Many actual or potential health problems or issues may require the use of this skill as part of related interventions. An appropriate health problem or issue may include:
- Altered skin integrity
- Infection risk
- Knowledge deficiency

OUTCOME IDENTIFICATION AND PLANNING

The expected outcomes to achieve when collecting a wound culture are that the culture is obtained without contamination, exposing the patient to additional pathogens or causing discomfort for the patient, and the patient demonstrates understanding of the reason for the wound culture.

IMPLEMENTATION

ACTION	RATIONALE
1. Review the patient's health record for prescribed intervention for obtaining a wound culture. Gather necessary supplies. If possible, obtain the wound culture prior to the start of antimicrobial therapy.	Reviewing the health record and care plan validates the correct patient and correct procedure. Preparation promotes efficient time management and an organized approach to the task. Antimicrobial therapy interferes with microorganism growth, so it is important to obtain the wound culture prior to the start of antimicrobial therapy, if possible (Huddleston Cross, 2014; Fischbach & Fischbach, 2018). If obtained after the initiation of antimicrobial therapy, provide information about the name of the antimicrobial, dose, and the date the therapy was initiated to the lab to aid in accurate interpretation of the culture findings (Baranoski & Ayello, 2020).
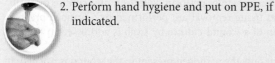 2. Perform hand hygiene and put on PPE, if indicated.	Hand hygiene and PPE prevent the spread of microorganisms. PPE is required based on transmission precautions.
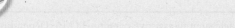 3. Identify the patient.	Identifying the patient ensures the right patient receives the intervention and helps prevent errors.
4. Assemble equipment on the overbed table or other surface within reach.	Organization facilitates performance of the task.
5. Close the curtains around the bed and close the door to the room, if possible. Explain to the patient what you are going to do and why you are going to do it.	This ensures the patient's privacy. Explanation relieves anxiety and facilitates engagement.

ACTION

6. Assess the patient for possible need for nonpharmacologic pain-reducing interventions or analgesic medication before obtaining the wound culture. Administer appropriate prescribed analgesic. Allow enough time for the analgesic to achieve its effectiveness before beginning the procedure.

7. Place an appropriate waste receptacle within easy reach for use during the procedure.

8. Adjust the bed to a comfortable working height (VHACEOSH, 2016).

9. Assist the patient to a comfortable position that provides easy access to the wound. If necessary, drape the patient with the bath blanket to expose only the wound area. Place a waterproof pad under the wound site. Check the culture label against the patient's identification bracelet (Figure 1).

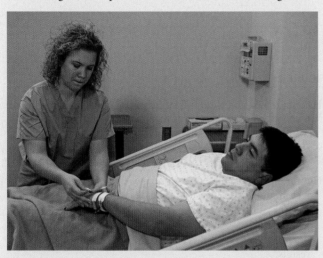

FIGURE 1. Checking culture label with the patient's identification band.

10. If there is a dressing in place on the wound, put on clean gloves and carefully remove the dressing. Refer to Skill 8-2. Note the presence, amount, type, color, and odor of any drainage on the dressings. Place soiled dressings in the appropriate waste receptacle.

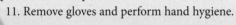 11. Remove gloves and perform hand hygiene.

12. Put on gloves. Assess and clean the wound, **using saline that has no preservative** (Baranoski & Ayello, 2020), as outlined in Skills 8-2 and 8-3. Refer also to Fundamentals Review 8-1, 8-2, 8-3, and 8-4.

13. Dry the skin surrounding the wound with gauze. Put on clean gloves.

RATIONALE

Pain is a subjective experience influenced by past experience. Wound care and dressing changes may cause pain for some patients.

Having the waste container handy means that soiled materials may be discarded easily, without the spread of microorganisms.

Having the bed at the proper height prevents back and muscle strain.

Patient positioning and the use of a bath blanket provide for comfort and warmth. Checking the culture label with the patient's identification ensures the correct patient and the correct procedure.

Gloves protect the nurse from handling contaminated dressings. The dressing must be removed to allow access to the wound.

Hand hygiene prevents the transmission of microorganisms.

Gloves prevent contact with blood and/or body fluids. This information provides evidence about the wound healing process and/or the presence of infection. Cleaning the wound removes wound exudate, topical therapies and wound debris, which could introduce extraneous organisms into the collected specimen, resulting in inaccurate results (Baranoski & Ayello, 2020).

Excess moisture can contribute to skin irritation and breakdown. The use of a culture swab does not require immediate contact with the skin or wound, so clean gloves are appropriate to protect the nurse from contact with blood and/or body fluids.

(*continued on page 484*)

Skill 8-4 ▶ Collecting a Wound Culture *(continued)*

ACTION	RATIONALE

ACTION

14. Twist the cap to loosen the swab on the culture tube or open the separate swab(s) and remove the cap from the culture tube. **Keep the swab and inside of the culture tube(s) sterile (Figure 2).**

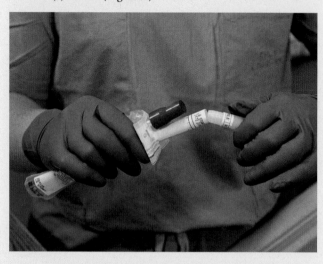

15. If contact with the wound is necessary to separate wound margins to permit insertion of the swab deep into the wound, put a sterile glove on one hand to manipulate the wound margins. Clean gloves may be appropriate for contact with pressure injuries and chronic wounds.

16. **Identify a 1-cm area of the wound that is free from necrotic tissue.** Carefully insert the swab into this area of clean viable tissue. **Press the swab to apply sufficient pressure to express fluid from the wound tissue and rotate the swab for 5 seconds** (Baranoski & Ayello, 2020). **Avoid touching the swab to intact skin at the wound edges (Figure 3).**

17. Place the swab back in the culture tube (Figure 4). **Do not touch the outside of the tube with the swab.** Secure the cap. Some swab containers have an ampule of medium at the bottom of the tube. It might be necessary to crush this ampule to activate. Follow the manufacturer's instructions for use.

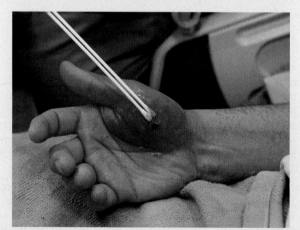

FIGURE 3. Rotating swab several times over wound surface.

RATIONALE

Supplies are ready to use and within easy reach, and aseptic technique is maintained.

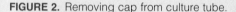

FIGURE 2. Removing cap from culture tube.

If contact with the wound is necessary to collect the specimen, a sterile glove is necessary to prevent contamination of the wound. Clean technique may be appropriate for cleaning chronic wounds or pressure injuries (Baranoski & Ayello, 2020; EPUAP, NPIAP, & PPPIA, 2019a; Taylor et al., 2023).

Cotton tip absorbs wound drainage. This technique (Levine technique) is considered to provide more accurate results and best practice for swab cultures (Baranoski & Ayello, 2020; WOCN, 2016). Contact with skin could introduce extraneous organisms into the collected specimen, resulting in inaccurate results.

The outside of the container is protected from contamination with microorganisms, and the sample is not contaminated with organisms not in the wound. Surrounding the swab with culture medium is necessary for accurate culture results.

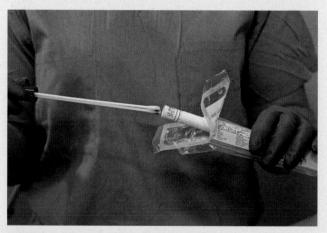

FIGURE 4. Placing swab in culture tube.

ACTION

RATIONALE

18. Use another swab if collecting a specimen from another area of the wound or site and repeat the procedure.

Using another swab at a different site prevents cross-contamination of the wound.

19. Remove gloves and discard them accordingly. Perform hand hygiene.

Removing gloves properly reduces the risk for infection transmission and contamination of other items. Hand hygiene prevents the transmission of microorganisms.

20. Put on gloves. Place a dressing on the wound, as appropriate, based on prescribed interventions and/or the plan of care. Refer to Skill 8-2. Remove gloves. Perform hand hygiene.

Wound dressings protect, absorb drainage, provide a moist environment, and promote wound healing. Removing gloves and performing hand hygiene reduce the risk for transmission of microorganisms and contamination of other items.

21. After securing the dressing, label dressing with date and time. Remove all remaining equipment; place the patient in a comfortable position, with side rails up as indicated and bed in the lowest position.

Recording date and time provides communication and demonstrates adherence to care plan. Proper patient and bed positioning promotes safety and comfort.

22. Label the specimen according to your institution's guidelines. Information included in addition to the patient's identification may include wound site, time the specimen was collected, any antimicrobials the patient is receiving, and the identity of the person who obtained the specimen (Baranoski & Ayello, 2020). Send or transport specimen to the laboratory in a biohazard bag immediately or within the optimal time from for transport as indicated by facility policy and guidelines (Figure 5).

Proper labeling ensures proper identification of the specimen. Specimens must be sent to the laboratory immediately or within the optimal time from for transport as indicated by facility policy and guidelines to ensure accurate results (Baranoski & Ayello, 2020; Fischbach & Fischbach, 2018; WOCN, 2016).

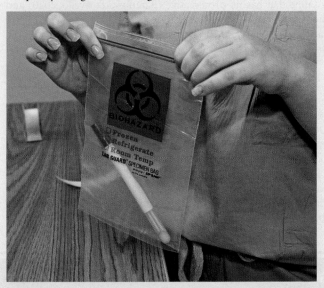

FIGURE 5. Labeled culture tube in biohazard bag.

23. Remove PPE, if used. Perform hand hygiene.

Proper removal of PPE reduces the risk for infection transmission and contamination of other items. Hand hygiene prevents the spread of microorganisms.

EVALUATION

The expected outcomes have been met when the culture was obtained without contamination, the patient was not exposed to additional pathogens, the patient did not experience discomfort, and the patient has demonstrated understanding of the reason for the wound culture.

(*continued on page 486*)

Skill 8-4 ▶ Collecting a Wound Culture *(continued)*

DOCUMENTATION

Guidelines

Document the location of the wound, the assessment of the wound, including the type of tissue present, presence of necrotic tissue, stage (if appropriate), and characteristics of drainage. Include the appearance of the surrounding skin. Document cleansing of the wound and the obtained culture. Record any skin care and/or dressing applied. Note pertinent patient and family/caregiver education and any patient reaction to this procedure, including patient's pain level and effectiveness of nonpharmacologic interventions or analgesia, if administered.

Sample Documentation

> 6/22/25 2100 Wound noted on patient's hand: 2 cm × 3 cm × 1 cm, red, tender, with purulent drainage present. Edges macerated, without erythema and tenderness. Wound cleaned with normal saline, culture obtained. Skin protectant/barrier applied to surrounding area, wound redressed with alginate, cover dressing, and roller gauze. Hand elevated. Culture labeled and sent to lab.
>
> —J. Wentz, RN

DEVELOPING CLINICAL REASONING AND CLINICAL JUDGMENT

UNEXPECTED SITUATIONS AND ASSOCIATED INTERVENTIONS

- *The nurse has inserted the culture swab into the patient's wound to obtain the specimen and realizes that the wound was not cleaned:* Discard this swab. Obtain the additional supplies needed to clean the wound according to facility policy and a new culture swab. Cleaning the wound removes wound exudate, topical therapies, and wound debris, which could introduce extraneous organisms into the collected specimen, resulting in inaccurate results (Baranoski & Ayello, 2020). Clean the wound using a using saline that has no preservative (Baranoski & Ayello, 2020) and then proceed to obtain the culture specimen.
- *As the nurse prepares to insert the culture swab into the wound, the nurse inadvertently touches the swab to the patient's bedclothes or other surface:* Discard this swab, obtain a new culture swab, and collect the specimen.

GENERAL CONSIDERATIONS

- Tissue biopsy is considered the "gold standard" of wound cultures; however, it and the aspiration technique are invasive and are performed by physicians and advanced practice professionals (Baranoski & Ayello, 2020; WOCN, 2016). Swab specimens are more commonly used because they are most easily collected, readily available, and may be collected by nurses in general practice (Baranoski & Ayello, 2020).
- Final culture results may take 24 to 72 hours depending on the method used and organism suspected; antimicrobial therapy based on the pathogens most commonly involved in a particular type of wound may be started immediately and changed if indicated when culture and sensitivity results are available (WOCN, 2016).

Skill 8-5 ▶ Caring for a Penrose Drain

Wound drainage devices (drains) are inserted into or near a wound when it is anticipated that a collection of fluid in a closed area would delay healing and increase the potential for infection (Morton & Fontaine, 2018); removal of excess fluid decreases pressure in the wound area, promoting healing and decreasing complications (Bauldoff et al., 2020). A Penrose drain is a hollow, soft, flexible, open-ended rubber tube. It does not have a collection device and allows fluid to drain passively, with the drainage moving from the area of greater pressure (in the wound) to the area of less pressure (the dressing) (Orth, 2018). Penrose drains are commonly used after a surgical procedure or for drainage of an abscess. After a surgical procedure, the surgeon places one end of the drain in or near the area to be drained. The other end passes through the skin, directly through the incision or through a separate opening referred to as a stab wound. A Penrose drain is not sutured. A large safety pin or small tab is usually placed in the end of the drain outside the wound to prevent the drain from slipping into the wound (Memorial Sloan Kettering Cancer Center, 2019). The patency and placement of the drain are included in the wound assessment.

DELEGATION CONSIDERATIONS	Care for a Penrose drain insertion site and wound care is not delegated to assistive personnel (AP). Depending on the state's nurse practice act and the organization's policies and procedures, these procedures may be delegated to licensed practical/vocational nurses (LPN/LVNs). The decision to delegate must be based on careful analysis of the patient's needs and circumstances as well as the qualifications of the person to whom the task is being delegated. Refer to the Delegation Guidelines in Appendix A.

EQUIPMENT

- Sterile gloves
- Gauze dressings
- Sterile cotton-tipped applicators, if appropriate
- Sterile drain sponges
- Surgical or abdominal pads
- Sterile dressing set or suture set (for the sterile scissors and forceps)
- Sterile cleaning solution as prescribed (commonly 0.9% normal saline solution)

- Sterile container to hold cleaning solution
- Clean safety pin
- Clean, disposable gloves
- Plastic bag or other appropriate waste container for soiled dressings
- Waterproof pad and bath blanket
- Skin protectant/barrier wipes
- Additional dressings and supplies needed or as required for prescribed wound care

ASSESSMENT	Assess the situation to determine the necessity for wound cleaning and a dressing change. Confirm any prescribed interventions relevant to drain care and any drain care included in the plan of care. Assess the patient's level of comfort and the need for analgesics before wound care. Assess if the patient experienced any pain related to prior dressing changes and the effectiveness of interventions employed to minimize the patient's pain. Assess the current dressing to determine if it is intact, and assess for the presence of excess drainage, bleeding, or saturation of the dressing. Assess the patency of the Penrose drain. Inspect the drain site and characteristics of the drainage.
	Inspect the wound and the surrounding tissue. Assess the appearance of the surgical site for the approximation of wound edges, the color of the wound and surrounding area, and signs of dehiscence. Note the stage of the healing process and the characteristics of any drainage.
	Assess the surrounding skin for color, temperature, and the presence of edema, ecchymosis, or maceration.

ACTUAL OR POTENTIAL HEALTH PROBLEMS AND NEEDS	Many actual or potential health problems or issues may require the use of this skill as part of related interventions. An appropriate health problem or issue may include: • Infection risk • Altered body image perception • Knowledge deficiency

OUTCOME IDENTIFICATION AND PLANNING	The expected outcomes to achieve when performing care for a Penrose drain are that the Penrose drain remains patent and intact, and the site care is accomplished without contaminating the area or causing trauma and without causing the patient to experience pain or discomfort. Other outcomes that are appropriate may include the following: the surgical wound shows signs of progressive healing without evidence of complications, and the patient demonstrates understanding of drain care.

IMPLEMENTATION

 ACTION

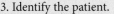 **RATIONALE**

1. Review the patient's health record for prescribed wound care or the plan of care related to wound/drain care. Gather necessary supplies.

Reviewing the health record and plan of care validates the correct patient and correct procedure. Preparation promotes efficient time management and an organized approach to the task.

 2. Perform hand hygiene and put on PPE, if indicated.

Hand hygiene and PPE prevent the spread of microorganisms. PPE is required based on transmission precautions.

3. Identify the patient.

Identifying the patient ensures the right patient receives the intervention and helps prevent errors.

(continued on page 488)

Skill 8-5 ▶ Caring for a Penrose Drain *(continued)*

ACTION	RATIONALE
4. Assemble equipment on the overbed table or other surface within reach.	Organization facilitates performance of the task.
5. Close the curtains around the bed and close the door to the room, if possible. Explain what you are going to do and why you are going to do it to the patient.	This ensures the patient's privacy. Explanation relieves anxiety and facilitates engagement.
6. Assess the patient for possible need for nonpharmacologic pain-reducing interventions or analgesic medication before wound care dressing change. Administer appropriate prescribed analgesic. Allow enough time for the analgesic to achieve its effectiveness before beginning the procedure.	Pain is a subjective experience influenced by past experience. Wound care and dressing changes may cause pain for some patients.
7. Place a waste receptacle at a convenient location for use during the procedure.	Having a waste container handy means that the soiled dressing may be discarded easily, without the spread of microorganisms.
8. Adjust the bed to a comfortable working height (VHACEOSH, 2016).	Having the bed at the proper height prevents back and muscle strain.
9. Assist the patient to a comfortable position that provides easy access to the drain and/or wound area. Use a bath blanket to cover any exposed area other than the wound. Place a waterproof pad under the wound site.	Patient positioning and the use of a bath blanket provide for comfort and warmth. Waterproof pad protects underlying surfaces.
10. Put on gloves; put on mask or face shield, as indicated. Check the position of the drain or drains before removing the dressing. Loosen the tape on the old dressings by removing in the direction of hair growth and the use of a push–pull method (Fumarola et al., 2020). Push–pull method: lift a corner of the dressing away from the skin, and then gently push the skin down and away from the dressing/adhesive (Fumarola et al., 2020). Continue moving fingers of the opposite hand to support the skin as the product is removed (Fumarola et al., 2020). Once all adhesive is loosened from the skin, carefully lift dressing from the surrounding skin to prevent medical adhesive–related skin injury (MARSI). Remove the sides/edges first, then the center. If the patient is at increased risk for MARSI (see Box 8-2 in Skill 8-2), requires repeated application or removal of adhesive devices, or there is resistance, use an adhesive remover (Barton, 2020; Fumarola et al., 2020; Kelly-O'Flynn et al., 2020).	Gloves protect the nurse from contaminated dressings and prevent the spread of microorganisms; mask reduces the risk of transmission should splashing occur. Checking ensures that a drain is not removed accidentally if one is present. Gloves protect the nurse from contaminated dressings and prevent the spread of microorganisms. Removal of the tape in the direction of hair growth minimizes trauma to the skin (Fumarola et al., 2020). Pushing the skin down and away from the adhesive reduces the risk for medical adhesive–related skin injury (MARSI) (Fumarola et al., 2020). The use of adhesive remover allows for the easy, rapid, and painless removal without the associated problems of skin stripping and helps reduce patient discomfort (Barton, 2020; Fumarola et al., 2020; Kelly-O'Flynn et al., 2020).
11. Carefully remove the soiled dressings. If any part of the dressing sticks to the underlying skin, use small amounts of sterile saline to help loosen and remove it. Note the presence, amount, type, color, and odor of any drainage on the dressings. Place soiled dressings in the appropriate waste receptacle.	Cautious removal of the dressing is more comfortable for the patient and ensures that any drain present is not removed. Sterile saline moistens the dressing for easier removal and minimizes damage and pain. The presence of drainage should be documented. Discarding dressings appropriately prevents the spread of microorganisms.
12. Inspect the drain site for appearance and drainage. Assess if any pain is present.	The wound healing process and/or the presence of irritation or infection must be documented.
13. Remove gloves and perform hand hygiene.	Removal of gloves and performance of hand hygiene prevent the transmission of microorganisms.
14. Using sterile technique, prepare a sterile work area and open the needed supplies.	Supplies are within easy reach and sterility is maintained.
15. Open the sterile cleaning solution. Pour it into the basin. Add the gauze sponges.	Sterility of dressings and solution is maintained.
16. Put on sterile gloves.	Sterile gloves help to maintain surgical asepsis and sterile technique and prevent the spread of microorganisms.

ACTION

17. Cleanse the drain site with the cleaning solution. Use the forceps and the moistened gauze or cotton-tipped applicators. **Start at the drain insertion site, moving in a circular motion toward the periphery (Figure 1). Use each gauze sponge or applicator only once.** Discard and use new gauze if additional cleansing is needed.

18. Dry the skin with a new gauze pad in the same manner. Apply skin protectant/barrier to the skin around the drain; extend out to include the area of skin that will be taped. Place a pre-split drain sponge under and around the drain (Figure 2). Assess the status of the safety pin or tab in the drain. If the pin/tab or drain is crusted, replace the pin with a new sterile pin. **Take care not to dislodge the drain.**

RATIONALE

Using a circular motion ensures that cleaning occurs from the least to most contaminated area and a previously cleaned area is not contaminated again.

Drying prevents skin irritation. Skin barrier/protectant prevents skin irritation and excoriation from tape, adhesives, and wound drainage (Fumarola et al., 2020; Kelly-O'Flynn et al., 2020). The gauze absorbs drainage and prevents the drainage from accumulating on the patient's skin.

Microorganisms grow more easily in a soiled environment. A large safety pin or small tab is usually placed in the end of the drain outside the wound to prevent the drain from slipping into the wound because the drain is not sutured in place (Memorial Sloan Kettering Cancer Center, 2019).

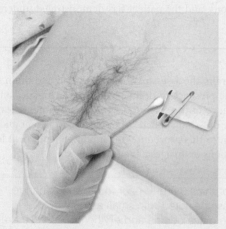

FIGURE 1. Cleaning drain site in circular motion toward periphery.

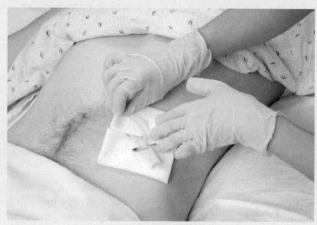

FIGURE 2. Placing pre-split dressing around Penrose drain.

19. Apply gauze pads over the drain (Figure 3). Apply surgical pad, ABD, or other cover dressing over the gauze.

The gauze absorbs drainage. Pads provide both extra absorption for excess drainage and a moisture barrier.

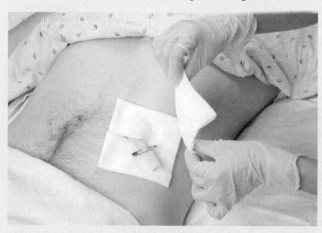

FIGURE 3. Applying gauze pads over drain.

20. Apply additional materials, such as a transparent dressing or tape, to secure the dressings. Remove gloves and perform hand hygiene.

Tape or other securing products keep the dressing in place. Proper disposal of gloves and hand hygiene prevent the spread of microorganisms.

(continued on page 490)

Skill 8-5 ▶ Caring for a Penrose Drain *(continued)*

ACTION

21. After securing the dressing, label dressing with date and time. Remove all remaining equipment; place the patient in a comfortable position, with side rails up as indicated and bed in the lowest position.

22. Remove additional PPE, if used. Perform hand hygiene.

23. Check all wound dressings at least every shift. More frequent checks may be needed if the wound is more complex, or dressings become saturated quickly.

RATIONALE

Recording date and time provides communication and demonstrates adherence to care plan. Proper patient and bed positioning promotes safety and comfort.

Proper removal of PPE reduces the risk for infection transmission and contamination of other items. Hand hygiene prevents the spread of microorganisms.

Checking dressings ensures the assessment of changes in patient condition and timely intervention to prevent complications.

EVALUATION

The expected outcomes have been met when the Penrose drain has remained patent and intact, wound care was accomplished without contaminating the wound area or causing trauma to the wound, the patient did not experience pain or discomfort, the wound has showed signs of progressive healing without evidence of complications, and the patient has demonstrated understanding of drain care.

DOCUMENTATION

Guidelines

Document the location of the wound and drain, the assessment of the wound and drain site, and patency of the Penrose drain. Document the presence of drainage and characteristics on the old dressing upon removal. Include the appearance of the surrounding skin. Document cleansing of the drain site. Record any skin care and the dressing applied. Note pertinent patient and family/caregiver education and any patient reaction to this procedure, including patient's pain level and effectiveness of nonpharmacologic interventions or analgesia if administered.

Sample Documentation

3/13/25 1400 Patient medicated with morphine 3 mg IV prior to dressing change. Dressing to right forearm removed. Dressings noted with small amount of serosanguineous drainage. Forearm with gross edema and erythema. Penrose drain intact, with safety pin in place. Incision edges approximated, staples intact. Area cleansed with normal saline, dried, and redressed with nonadherent gauze, ABD pads, and roller gauze. Reinforced the importance of keeping arm elevated on pillows, with patient verbalizing understanding.

—*P. Towns, RN*

DEVELOPING CLINICAL REASONING AND CLINICAL JUDGMENT

UNEXPECTED SITUATIONS AND ASSOCIATED INTERVENTIONS

- *Assessment of the drain site reveals significantly increased edema, erythema, and drainage from the site, in addition to drainage via the drain:* Cleanse the site, as prescribed, or per the plan of care. Obtain vital signs, including the patient's temperature. Document care and assessments. Notify the health care team of the findings.
- *Assessment of the drain site reveals that the drain has slipped back into the incision:* Follow facility policy and the prescribed interventions related to advancing Penrose drains. Document assessments and interventions. Notify the health care team of the findings and interventions.
- *When preparing to change a dressing on a Penrose drain site, the nurse's assessment reveals that the drain is completely out, lying in the dressing material:* Assess the site and the patient for symptoms of pain, increased edema/erythema/drainage. Provide site care, as prescribed. Notify the health care team of situation. Often, depending on the patient's stage of recovery, the drain is left out. Document the findings and interventions.

SPECIAL CONSIDERATIONS

- Evaluate a sudden increase in the amount of drainage or bright-red drainage and notify the health care team of these findings.
- Wound care is often uncomfortable, and patients may experience significant pain. Assess the patient's comfort level and past experiences with wound care. Offer analgesics, as prescribed, and nonpharmacologic comfort/pain interventions to maintain the patient's level of comfort.
- Appropriate nutritional support is critical in achieving successful wound healing and may be overlooked (Quain & Khardori, 2015). Collaborate with the registered dietician and dietary staff to develop an individualized nutrition intervention plan for the patient (Baranoski & Ayello, 2020).

Community-Based Care Considerations

- Drain site care in the community setting is a clean, not sterile, procedure. Patients will use soap and water to clean the skin around the drain site (Memorial Sloan Kettering Cancer Center (2019).

EVIDENCE FOR PRACTICE ▶

PREVENTION OF MEDICAL ADHESIVE–RELATED SKIN INJURIES

Fumarola, S., Allaway, R., Callaghan, R., Collier, M., Downie, F., Geraghty, J., Kiernan, S., & Spratt, F. (2020). Overlooked and underestimated: Medical adhesive-related skin injuries. Best practice consensus document on prevention. *Journal of Wound Care, 29*(Suppl 3c), S1–S24. https://doi.org/10.12968/jowc.2020.29.Sup3c.S1

This consensus document is the result of a review of the literature on medical adhesive–related skin injury (MARSI) by a panel of wound care experts, educators, and researchers. This best practice guideline provides recommendations for the assessment and prevention of MARSI, with the goal of standardizing care across all health care settings.

Skill 8-6 ▶ Caring for a Jackson-Pratt Drain

Wound drainage devices (drains) are inserted into or near a wound when it is anticipated that a collection of fluid in a closed area would delay healing and increase the potential for infection (Morton & Fontaine, 2018); removal of excess fluid decreases pressure in the wound area, promoting healing and decreasing complications (Bauldoff et al., 2020).

A Jackson-Pratt (JP) or grenade drain collects wound drainage in a bulblike device that is compressed to create low suction (negative) pressure (Figure 1). It consists of perforated tubing connected to a portable vacuum unit. After a surgical procedure, the surgeon places one end of the drain in or near the area to be drained. The other end passes through the skin via a separate

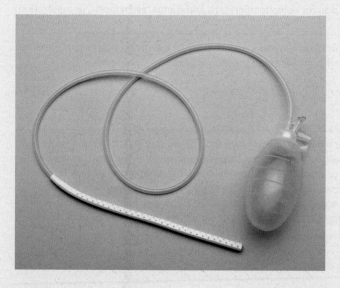

FIGURE 1. Jackson-Pratt drain.

(*continued on page 492*)

Skill 8-6 ▶ Caring for a Jackson-Pratt Drain *(continued)*

incision. These drains are usually sutured in place. A sterile dressing is usually maintained for 24 to 48 hours; the use of a dressing after this time depends on the site assessment and amount of drainage (Orth, 2018). The site may be treated as an additional surgical wound, but often these sites are left open to air 24 hours after surgery. This type of drain is typically used with breast and abdominal surgery.

As the drainage accumulates in the bulb, the bulb expands and suction is lost, requiring recompression. These drains should be emptied and recompressed when the bulb is approximately 25% to 50% full for optimal accuracy and maintenance of adequate suction (Mamuyac et al., 2019; Yue et al., 2015). However, based on nursing assessment and judgment, the drain could be emptied and recompressed more frequently.

DELEGATION CONSIDERATIONS

Care for a JP drain insertion site is not delegated to assistive personnel (AP). Depending on the organization's policies and procedures, the drain may be emptied and reconstituted by AP. Depending on the state's nurse practice act and the organization's policies and procedures, these procedures may be delegated to licensed practical/vocational nurses (LPN/LVNs). The decision to delegate must be based on careful analysis of the patient's needs and circumstances as well as the qualifications of the person to whom the task is being delegated. Refer to the Delegation Guidelines in Appendix A.

EQUIPMENT

- Graduated container for measuring drainage
- Clean, disposable gloves
- Additional PPE, as indicated
- Cleansing solution, usually sterile normal saline
- Sterile gauze pads
- Skin protectant/barrier wipes
- Sterile drain sponges
- Sterile gloves
- Sterile cotton-tipped applicators, if appropriate
- Sterile container to hold cleaning solution
- Plastic bag or other appropriate waste container for soiled dressings
- Waterproof pad and bath blanket
- Additional dressings and supplies needed or as required for prescribed wound care

ASSESSMENT

Assess the situation to determine the need for site care, a dressing change, and/or emptying of the drain. Assess the patient's level of comfort and the need for analgesics before care. Assess if the patient experienced any pain related to prior dressing changes and the effectiveness of interventions employed to minimize the patient's pain. Assess the current dressing. Assess for the presence of excess drainage or bleeding or saturation of the dressing. Assess the patency of the JP drain and the drain site. Note the characteristics of the drainage in the collection bag.

If a surgical wound is present, inspect the wound and the surrounding tissue. Assess the appearance of the incision for the approximation of wound edges, the color of the wound and surrounding area, and signs of dehiscence. Note the stage of the healing process and characteristics of any drainage. Also assess the surrounding skin for color, temperature, and edema, ecchymosis, or maceration.

ACTUAL OR POTENTIAL HEALTH PROBLEMS AND NEEDS

Many actual or potential health problems or issues may require the use of this skill as part of related interventions. An appropriate health problem or issue may include:
- Infection risk
- Altered body image perception
- Knowledge deficiency

OUTCOME IDENTIFICATION AND PLANNING

The expected outcome to achieve when performing care for a JP drain is that the drain remains patent and intact, site care is accomplished without contaminating the area or causing trauma, and the patient does not experience pain or discomfort. Other outcomes that are appropriate may include the following: the surgical wound shows signs of progressive healing without evidence of complications, drainage amounts are measured accurately at the frequency required by facility policy and recorded as part of the intake and output record, and the patient demonstrates understanding of drain care.

IMPLEMENTATION

ACTION	RATIONALE
1. Review the patient's health record for prescribed wound care or the plan of care related to wound/drain care. Gather necessary supplies.	Reviewing the health record and care plan validates the correct patient and correct procedure. Preparation promotes efficient time management and organized approach to the task.
2. Perform hand hygiene and put on PPE, if indicated.	Hand hygiene and PPE prevent the spread of microorganisms. PPE is required based on transmission precautions.
3. Identify the patient.	Identifying the patient ensures the right patient receives the intervention and helps prevent errors.
4. Assemble equipment on the overbed table or other surface within reach.	Organization facilitates performance of the task.
5. Close the curtains around the bed and close the door to the room, if possible. Explain what you are going to do and why you are going to do it to the patient.	This ensures the patient's privacy. Explanation relieves anxiety and facilitates engagement.
6. Assess the patient for possible need for nonpharmacologic pain-reducing interventions or analgesic medication before wound care dressing change. Administer appropriate pre-scribed analgesic. Allow enough time for the analgesic to achieve its effectiveness before beginning the procedure.	Pain is a subjective experience influenced by past experience. Wound care and dressing changes may cause pain for some patients.
7. Place a waste receptacle at a convenient location for use during the procedure.	Having a waste container handy means that the soiled dressing may be discarded easily, without the spread of microorganisms.
8. Adjust the bed to a comfortable working height (VHACEOSH, 2016).	Having the bed at the proper height prevents back and muscle strain.
9. Assist the patient to a comfortable position that provides easy access to the drain and/or wound area. Use a bath blanket to cover any exposed area other than the drain. Place a waterproof pad under the drain site.	Patient positioning and the use of a bath blanket provide for comfort and warmth. Waterproof pad protects underlying surfaces.

Emptying Drainage

ACTION	RATIONALE
10. Put on gloves; put on mask or face shield, as indicated.	Gloves prevent the spread of microorganisms; mask reduces the risk of transmission should splashing occur.
11. Using sterile technique, open a gauze pad, making a sterile field with the outer wrapper.	Using sterile technique deters the spread of microorganisms.
12. Place the graduated collection container under the drain outlet. Without contaminating the outlet valve, pull off the cap. The chamber will expand completely as it draws in air. **Empty the chamber's contents completely into the container (Figure 2). Use the gauze pad to wipe the outlet. With one hand, fully compress the chamber along the long axis, side to side (Mamuyac et al., 2019), and replace the cap with your other hand (Figure 3).**	Emptying the drainage allows for accurate measurement. Cleaning the outlet reduces the risk of contamination and helps prevent the spread of microorganisms. Compressing the chamber along the long axis, side to side, reestablishes the suction. And generates higher negative pressure compared to the bottom-up methods (Mamuyac et al., 2019). Refer to the Evidence for Practice at the end of this Skill.

(continued on page 494)

Skill 8-6 ▶ Caring for a Jackson-Pratt Drain *(continued)*

ACTION

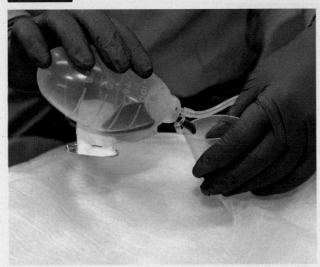

FIGURE 2. Emptying contents of Jackson-Pratt drain into collection container.

13. Check the patency of the equipment. Bulb should remain compressed (Figure 4). **Check that the tubing is free from twists and kinks.**

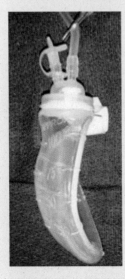

FIGURE 4. Compressed drain bulb.

 14. Carefully measure and record the character, color, and amount of the drainage. Discard the drainage according to facility policy.

15. Remove gloves. Perform hand hygiene.

RATIONALE

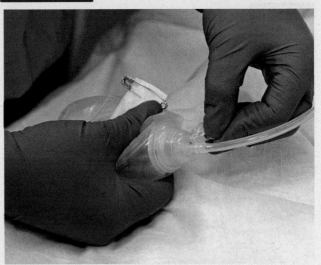

FIGURE 3. Compressing Jackson-Pratt drain and replacing cap.

Compressed chamber establishes suction. Patent, untwisted, or unkinked tubing promotes appropriate wound drainage.

Documentation promotes continuity of care and communication. Appropriate disposal of biohazard material reduces the risk for microorganism transmission.

Removal of gloves and hand hygiene prevents the transmission of microorganisms.

ACTION	**RATIONALE**

Cleaning the Drain Site

16. Put on gloves. Check the position of the drain or drains before removing the dressing. Loosen the tape on the old dressings by removing in the direction of hair growth and the use of a push–pull method (Fumarola et al., 2020). Push–pull method: lift a corner of the dressing away from the skin, and then gently push the skin down and away from the dressing/adhesive (Fumarola et al., 2020). Continue moving the fingers of the opposite hand to support the skin as the product is removed (Fumarola et al., 2020). Once all adhesive is loosened from the skin, carefully lift dressing from the surrounding skin to prevent medical adhesive–related skin injury (MARSI). Remove the sides/edges first, then the center. If the patient is at increased risk for MARSI (see Box 8-2 in Skill 8-2), requires repeated application or removal of adhesive devices, or there is resistance, use an adhesive remover (Barton, 2020; Fumarola et al., 2020; Kelly-O'Flynn et al., 2020).

Gloves protect the nurse from contaminated dressings and prevent the spread of microorganisms. Dressing protects the site. Checking ensures that a drain is not removed accidentally. Removal of the tape in the direction of hair growth minimizes trauma to the skin (Fumarola et al., 2020). Pushing the skin down and away from the adhesive reduces the risk for medical adhesive–related skin injury (MARSI) (Fumarola et al., 2020). The use of adhesive remover allows for the easy, rapid, and painless removal without the associated problems of skin stripping and helps reduce patient discomfort (Barton, 2020; Fumarola et al., 2020; Kelly-O'Flynn et al., 2020).

17. Carefully remove the soiled dressings. If any part of the dressing sticks to the underlying skin, use small amounts of sterile saline to help loosen and remove it.

Cautious removal of the dressing is more comfortable for the patient and ensures that any drain present is not removed. Sterile saline moistens the dressing for easier removal and minimizes damage and pain.

18. Note the presence, amount, type, color, and odor of any drainage on the dressings. Place soiled dressings in the appropriate waste receptacle. Remove your gloves and perform hand hygiene.

The presence of drainage should be documented. Proper disposal of soiled dressings and used gloves prevents the spread of microorganisms. Hand hygiene prevents the transmission of microorganisms.

19. Inspect the drain site for appearance and drainage. Assess if any pain is present. Check the status of sutures, adhesive closure strips, and staples, if present. Note any problems to include in your documentation.

The wound healing process and/or the presence of irritation or infection must be documented.

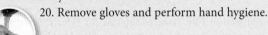

20. Remove gloves and perform hand hygiene.

Removal of gloves and performance of hand hygiene prevent transmission of microorganisms.

21. **Using sterile technique, prepare a sterile work area and open the needed supplies.** Refer to facility policy and prescribed interventions regarding use of a sterile approach to site care.

Supplies are within easy reach and sterility is maintained. A sterile dressing is usually maintained for 24 to 48 hours; the use of a dressing after this time depends on the site assessment and amount of drainage (Orth, 2018). The site may be treated as an additional surgical wound, but often these sites are left open to air 24 hours after surgery. Refer to facility policy and prescribed interventions regarding need for sterile approach to site care and use of dressing.

22. Open the sterile cleaning solution. Pour it into the basin. Add the gauze sponges.

Sterility of dressings and solution is maintained.

23. Put on sterile gloves. Alternatively, clean gloves (clean technique) may be used based on facility policy and care setting.

The use of sterile gloves maintains surgical asepsis and sterile technique and reduces the risk of microorganism transmission. Clean technique is appropriate for cleaning chronic wounds, wounds in the home, or pressure injuries (Baranoski & Ayello, 2020; EPUAP, NPIAP, & PPPIA, 2019a; Taylor et al., 2023).

(continued on page 496)

Skill 8-6 ▸ Caring for a Jackson-Pratt Drain *(continued)*

ACTION	**RATIONALE**
24. Cleanse the drain site with the cleaning solution. Use the forceps and the moistened gauze or cotton-tipped applicators. **Start at the drain insertion site, moving in a circular motion toward the periphery. Use each gauze sponge or applicator only once.** Discard and use new gauze/applicator if additional cleansing is needed. (Refer to Figure 1 in Skill 8-5.)	Cleaning is done from the least to most contaminated area so that a previously cleaned area is not contaminated again.
25. Dry with new sterile gauze in the same manner. Apply skin protectant/barrier to the skin around the drain; extend out to include the area of skin that will be taped.	Drying prevents skin irritation. Skin barrier/protectant prevents skin irritation and excoriation from tape, adhesives, and wound drainage (Fumarola et al., 2020; Kelly-O'Flynn et al., 2020).
26. Place a pre-split drain sponge under the drain. (Refer to Figure 2 in Skill 8-5.) Apply gauze pads or other cover dressing, such as a transparent dressing, as indicated by facility policy, over the drain. Secure the dressings with tape, as needed. Remove and discard gloves. Perform hand hygiene.	The gauze absorbs drainage and prevents the drainage from accumulating on the patient's skin. Transparent dressing, tape or other securing products keep the dressing in place. Proper disposal of gloves prevents the spread of microorganisms. Hand hygiene prevents the transmission of microorganisms.
27. Secure the drain tubing to the patient's skin using a tape or a commercial securement/stabilization device, allowing slack in the tubing to avoid excessive tension. **Be careful not to kink the tubing and ensure the collection bag remains below the drain site.** Label the dressing with date and time.	Securing the tubing prevents accidental dislodgement or movement and avoids excessive tension on tube. Kinked tubing could block drainage. Maintaining the drain collection bag remains below the drain site facilitates proper drainage. Recording date and time provides communication and demonstrates adherence to plan of care.
28. Alternatively, if the drain site is open to air, observe the sutures that secure the drain to the skin. Look for signs of pulling, tearing, swelling, or infection of the surrounding skin. Gently clean the sutures with the gauze pad moistened with normal saline. Dry with a new gauze pad. Apply skin protectant/barrier to the surrounding skin. Remove and discard gloves. Perform hand hygiene.	Early detection of problems leads to prompt intervention and prevents complications. Gentle cleaning and drying prevent the growth of microorganisms. Skin barrier/protectant prevents skin irritation and excoriation from tape, adhesives, and wound drainage (Fumarola et al., 2020; Kelly-O'Flynn et al., 2020). Proper removal of gloves prevents the spread of microorganisms. Hand hygiene prevents the transmission of microorganisms.
29. Remove all remaining equipment; place the patient in a comfortable position, with side rails up as indicated and bed in the lowest position.	Proper patient and bed positioning promotes safety and comfort.
30. Remove additional PPE, if used. Perform hand hygiene.	Proper removal of PPE reduces the risk for infection transmission and contamination of other items. Hand hygiene prevents the spread of microorganisms.
31. Check drain status at least every 4 hours. Empty and reengage suction (compress device) when device is approximately 25% to 50% full (Mamuyac et al., 2019). Check all wound dressings at least every shift. More frequent checks may be needed if the wound is more complex, or dressings become saturated quickly.	Checking drain ensures proper functioning and early detection of problems. Emptying and compression ensure appropriate suction. Adequate suction pressure declines as bulb volume increases; bulb emptying should occur when the bulb is approximately 25% to 50% full for optimal accuracy and maintenance of adequate suction (Mamuyac et al., 2019; Yue et al., 2015). Checking dressings ensures the assessment of changes in patient condition and timely intervention to prevent complications.

EVALUATION The expected outcome has been met when the drain has remained patent and intact, site care was accomplished without contaminating the area or without causing trauma to the wound, the patient did not experience pain or discomfort, the drainage amounts were measured accurately at the frequency required by facility policy and recorded as part of the intake and output record, and the patient has demonstrated understanding of drain care.

DOCUMENTATION

Guidelines

Document the location of the drain, the assessment of the drain site, and patency of the drain. Note if sutures are intact. Document the presence and characteristics of drainage on the old dressing upon removal. Include the appearance of the surrounding skin. Document cleansing the drain site. Record any skin care and the dressing applied. Note that the drain was emptied and recompressed. Note pertinent patient and family/caregiver education and any patient reaction to this procedure, including patient's pain level and effectiveness of nonpharmacologic interventions or analgesia, if administered. Document the amount and characteristics of drainage obtained on the appropriate intake and output record.

Sample Documentation

> 2/7/25 2400 Right chest incision and drain open to air. Wound edges approximated, slight ecchymosis, no edema, redness, or drainage. Steri-Strips intact. JP drain patent and secured with suture. Exit site without edema, drainage, or redness; drain site cleaned with normal saline, and skin barrier applied. Drain emptied and recompressed. 40-mL sanguineous drainage recorded.
>
> —C. White, RN

DEVELOPING CLINICAL REASONING AND CLINICAL JUDGMENT

UNEXPECTED SITUATIONS AND ASSOCIATED INTERVENTIONS

- *Patient has a JP drain in the right lower quadrant following abdominal surgery. The record indicates it has been draining serosanguineous fluid, 40 to 50 mL every shift. While performing your initial assessment, you note that the dressing around the drain site is saturated with serosanguineous secretions and there is minimal drainage in the collection chamber:* Inspect the tubing for kinks or obstruction. Assess the patient for changes in condition. Remove the dressing and assess the site. Often, if the tubing becomes blocked with a blood clot or drainage particles, the wound drainage will leak around the exit site of the drain. Cleanse the area and redress the site. Notify the health care team of the findings and document the event in the patient's record.
- *Patient calls you to the room and says, "I found this in the bed when I went to get up." He has his JP drain in his hand. It is completely removed from the patient:* Assess the patient for any new and abnormal signs or symptoms and assess the surgical site and drain site. Apply a sterile dressing the drain site. Notify the health care team of the findings and document the event in the patient's record.

SPECIAL CONSIDERATIONS

- A sterile dressing is usually maintained for 24 to 48 hours; the use of a dressing after this time depends on the site assessment and amount of drainage (Orth, 2018). The site may be treated as an additional surgical wound, but often these sites are left open to air 24 hours after surgery. Refer to facility policy and prescribed interventions regarding need for sterile approach to site care and use of dressing.
- Often patients have more than one JP drain. Number or letter the drains for easy identification. Record the drainage from each drain separately, identified by the number or letter, on the intake and output record.
- When the patient with a drain is ready to ambulate, empty and compress the drain before activity. Secure the drain to the patient's gown below the wound, making sure there is no tension on the drainage tubing. This removes excess drainage, maintains maximum suction, and avoids strain on the drain's suture line.
- Appropriate nutritional support is critical in achieving successful wound healing and may be overlooked (Quain & Khardori, 2015). Collaborate with the registered dietician and dietary staff to develop an individualized nutrition intervention plan for the patient (Baranoski & Ayello, 2020).

Community-Based Care Considerations

- Drain site care in the community setting is a clean, not sterile, procedure. Patients will use soap and water to clean the skin around the drain site (Memorial Sloan Kettering Cancer Center (2019).

(continued on page 498)

Skill 8-6 ▶ Caring for a Jackson-Pratt Drain *(continued)*

EVIDENCE FOR PRACTICE ▶

MAINTAINING ADEQUATE PRESSURE IN A JACKSON-PRATT DRAIN

Surgical drains, such as the Jackson-Pratt (JP) drain, are used to prevent fluid accumulation in surgical sites and promote wound healing. The JP drain must be emptied and recompressed to maintain the negative pressure as the bulb fills. How can optimal functioning of the device be supported?

Related Research

Mamuyac, E. M., Pappa, A. K., Thorp, B. D., Ebert, C. S. Jr, Senior, B. A., Zanation, A. M., Lin, F. C., & Kimple, A. J. (2019). How much blood could a JP suck if a JP could suck blood? *The Laryngoscope*, *129*(8), 1806–1809. https://doi.org/10.1002/lary.27710

The purpose of this study was to determine whether two methods for compression of the JP bulb resulted in similar amounts of negative pressure and to examine the effect of various baseline reservoir volumes on bulb suction. Three separate JP bulbs of the same brand, type, and volume were compressed, and pressure recordings were measured with a digital manometer. The JP bulbs were randomly compressed either by squeezing them perpendicular to the long axis (side to side; side-in) or perpendicular to the short axis (bottom-up), and pressure was recorded; random compressions were continued until triplicate values from the three separate bulbs using each compression technique were achieved. Negative pressure was also tested by compressing a bulb in the side-in manner while the bulb contained specific measurements of water (25 mL, 50 mL, 75 mL, 100 mL). The volumes of water were placed into the bulb, air was evacuated, and the pressure was recorded.

The average pressure after a side-in compression of the JP bulb was 87.4 cm H_2O versus 17.7 cm H_2O for the bottom-up compression ($p < .0001$). The average pressure in the empty bulb using the side-in compression was 87.4 cm H_2O. Upon addition of the four volumes of water, the pressure generated using the side-in compression dropped to 72.6 cm H_2O (25 mL), 41.3 cm H_2O (50 mL), 37 cm H_2O (75 mL), and 35.6 cm H_2O (100 mL). The researchers concluded the specific method for evacuating the bulb (side-in) and the amount of fluid in the bulb significantly affect the performance of the JP drain. The researchers suggested emptying and recompression of a JP drain should occur when the bulb is approximately 25% full, and the drain should be compressed using the side-in method to generate higher negative pressure to support optimal functioning of the vacuum and optimal drainage of the wound bed, supporting improved postoperative healing.

Relevance for Nursing Practice

Nurses must make use of evidence-based interventions to support excellence in nursing care and achieve the best patient outcomes possible. Nurses should be proactive in assessing current practice and policy and procedures to ensure care interventions align with evidence for practice.

EVIDENCE FOR PRACTICE ▶

PREVENTION OF MEDICAL ADHESIVE–RELATED SKIN INJURIES

Fumarola, S., Allaway, R., Callaghan, R., Collier, M., Downie, F., Geraghty, J., Kiernan, S., & Spratt, F. (2020). Overlooked and underestimated: Medical adhesive-related skin injuries. Best practice consensus document on prevention. *Journal of Wound Care*, *29*(Suppl 3c), S1–S24. https://doi.org/10.12968/jowc.2020.29.Sup3c.S1

This consensus document is the result of a review of the literature on medical adhesive–related skin injury (MARSI) by a panel of wound care experts, educators, and researchers. This best practice guideline provides recommendations for the assessment and prevention of MARSI, with the goal of standardizing care across all health care settings.

Skill 8-7 ▶ Caring for a Hemovac Drain

Wound drainage devices (drains) are inserted into or near a wound when it is anticipated that a collection of fluid in a closed area would delay healing and increase the potential for infection (Morton & Fontaine, 2018); removal of excess fluid decreases pressure in the wound area, promoting healing and decreasing complications (Bauldoff et al., 2020).

A Hemovac drain is placed into a vascular cavity where blood drainage is expected after surgery, such as with abdominal and orthopedic surgery. The drain consists of perforated tubing connected to a portable suction (vacuum) unit (Figure 1). Suction is maintained by compressing a spring-like device in the collection unit. After a surgical procedure, the surgeon places one end of the drain in or near the area to be drained. The other end passes through the skin via a separate incision. These drains are usually sutured in place. A sterile dressing is usually maintained for 24 to 48 hours; the use of a dressing after this time depends on the site assessment and amount of drainage (Orth, 2018). The site may be treated as an additional surgical wound, but often these sites are left open to air 24 hours after surgery.

As the drainage accumulates in the collection unit, it expands and suction is lost, requiring recompression. Typically, the drain is emptied every 2 to 4 hours (Bauldoff et al., 2020) and when it is half full of drainage or air. However, based on the prescribed interventions and nursing assessment and judgment, it could be emptied and recompressed more frequently.

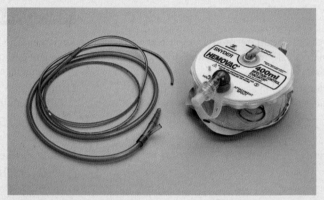

FIGURE 1. Hemovac drain.

DELEGATION CONSIDERATIONS

Care for a Hemovac drain insertion site is not delegated to assistive personnel (AP). Depending on the organization's policies and procedures, the drain may be emptied and reconstituted by AP. Depending on the state's nurse practice act and the organization's policies and procedures, these procedures may be delegated to licensed practical/vocational nurses (LPN/LVNs). The decision to delegate must be based on careful analysis of the patient's needs and circumstances as well as the qualifications of the person to whom the task is being delegated. Refer to the Delegation Guidelines in Appendix A.

EQUIPMENT

- Graduated container for measuring drainage
- Clean, disposable gloves
- Additional PPE, as indicated
- Cleansing solution, usually sterile normal saline
- Sterile gauze pads
- Skin protectant/barrier wipes
- Sterile gloves
- Sterile cotton-tipped applicators, if appropriate
- Sterile container to hold cleaning solution
- Plastic bag or other appropriate waste container for soiled dressings
- Waterproof pad and bath blanket
- Additional dressings and supplies needed or as required for prescribed wound care

ASSESSMENT

Assess the situation to determine the need for site care, a dressing change, or emptying of the drain. Assess the patient's level of comfort and the need for analgesics before care. Assess if the patient experienced any pain related to prior dressing changes and the effectiveness of interventions employed to minimize the patient's pain. Assess the current dressing. Assess for the presence of excess drainage or bleeding or saturation of the dressing. Assess the patency of the Hemovac drain and the drain site. Note the characteristics of the drainage in the collection bag.

If a surgical wound is present, inspect the wound and the surrounding tissue. Assess the appearance of the incision for the approximation of wound edges, the color of the wound and surrounding area, and signs of dehiscence. Note the stage of the healing process and characteristics of any drainage. Also assess the surrounding skin for color, temperature, and edema, ecchymosis, or maceration.

(*continued on page 500*)

Skill 8-7 ▶ Caring for a Hemovac Drain *(continued)*

ACTUAL OR POTENTIAL HEALTH PROBLEMS AND NEEDS	Many actual or potential health problems or issues may require the use of this skill as part of related interventions. An appropriate health problem or issue may include: • Infection risk • Altered body image perception • Knowledge deficiency
OUTCOME IDENTIFICATION AND PLANNING	The expected outcomes to achieve when performing care for a Hemovac drain are that the drain remains patent and intact, drain care is accomplished without contaminating the area and without causing trauma, and the patient does not experience pain or discomfort. Other outcomes that are appropriate may include the following: if there is a surgical wound, it shows signs of progressive healing without evidence of complications; the drainage amounts are measured accurately at the frequency required by facility policy and recorded as part of the intake and output record; and the patient demonstrates understanding of drain care.

IMPLEMENTATION

ACTION

1. Review the patient's health record for prescribed wound care or the plan of care related to wound/drain care. Gather necessary supplies.

2. Perform hand hygiene and put on PPE, if indicated.

3. Identify the patient.

4. Assemble equipment on the overbed table or other surface within reach.

5. Close the curtains around the bed and close the door to the room, if possible. Explain what you are going to do and why you are going to do it to the patient.

6. Assess the patient for possible need for nonpharmacologic pain-reducing interventions or analgesic medication before wound care dressing change. Administer appropriate prescribed analgesic. Allow enough time for analgesic to achieve its effectiveness before beginning the procedure.

7. Place a waste receptacle at a convenient location for use during the procedure.

8. Adjust the bed to a comfortable working height (VHACEOSH, 2016).

9. Assist the patient to a comfortable position that provides easy access to the drain and/or wound area. Use a bath blanket to cover any exposed area other than the drain. Place a waterproof pad under the drain site.

Emptying Drainage

10. Put on gloves; put on mask or face shield, as indicated.

11. Using sterile technique, open a gauze pad, making a sterile field with the outer wrapper.

RATIONALE

Reviewing the health record and care plan validates the correct patient and correct procedure. Preparation promotes efficient time management and an organized approach to the task.

Hand hygiene and PPE prevent the spread of microorganisms. PPE is required based on transmission precautions.

Identifying the patient ensures the right patient receives the intervention and helps prevent errors.

Organization facilitates performance of the task.

This ensures the patient's privacy. Explanation relieves anxiety and facilitates engagement.

Pain is a subjective experience influenced by past experience. Wound care and dressing changes may cause pain for some patients.

Having a waste container handy means that the soiled dressing may be discarded easily, without the spread of microorganisms.

Having the bed at the proper height prevents back and muscle strain.

Patient positioning and the use of a bath blanket provide for comfort and warmth. Waterproof pad protects underlying surfaces.

Gloves prevent the spread of microorganisms; mask reduces the risk of transmission should splashing occur.

Using sterile technique deters the spread of microorganisms.

ACTION

RATIONALE

12. Place the graduated collection container under the drain outlet. **Without contaminating the outlet, pull off the cap.** The chamber will expand completely as it draws in air. **Empty the chamber's contents completely into the container (Figure 2). Use the gauze pad to wipe the outlet. Place the container or a clean, flat surface. Fully compress the chamber by pushing down on the top until it meets the bottom and is flat (Wechter, 2020b). Keep the device tightly compressed while you apply the cap (Figure 3).**

Emptying the drainage allows for accurate measurement. Cleaning the outlet reduces the risk of contamination and helps prevent the spread of microorganisms. Compressing the chamber reestablishes the suction.

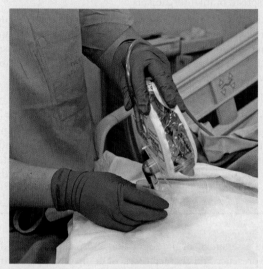

FIGURE 2. Emptying Hemovac drain into collection container.

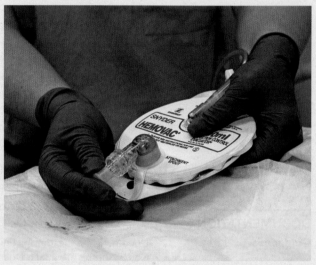

FIGURE 3. Compressing Hemovac and securing cap.

13. The device should remain compressed. Check the patency of the equipment. **Make sure the tubing is free from twists and kinks.**

Compressed device establishes suction. Patent, untwisted, or unkinked tubing promotes appropriate drainage from the wound.

14. Carefully measure and record the character, color, and amount of the drainage. Discard the drainage according to facility policy. Remove gloves. Perform hand hygiene.

Documentation promotes continuity of care and communication. Appropriate disposal of biohazard material reduces the risk for microorganism transmission. Proper disposal of gloves deters transmission of microorganisms. Hand hygiene prevents the transmission of microorganisms.

Cleaning the Drain Site

15. Put on gloves. If the drain site has a dressing, remove the dressing, assess and clean the site, and replace the dressing as outlined in Skill 8-6, Steps 16–26.

Dressing protects the site. Cleaning and drying sutures deters the growth of microorganisms.

16. Secure the drain tubing to the patient's skin using a tape or a commercial securement/stabilization device, allowing slack in the tubing to avoid excessive tension. **Be careful not to kink the tubing and ensure the collection bag remains below the drain site.** Label the dressing with date and time.

Securing the tubing prevents accidental dislodgement or movement and avoids excessive tension on tube. Kinked tubing could block drainage. Maintaining the drain collection bag remains below the drain site facilitates proper drainage. Recording date and time provides communication and demonstrates adherence to plan of care.

17. Alternatively, if the drain site is open to air, observe the sutures that secure the drain to the skin. Look for signs of pulling, tearing, swelling, or infection of the surrounding skin. Gently clean the sutures with the gauze pad moistened with normal saline. Dry with a new gauze pad. Apply skin protectant/barrier to the surrounding skin.

Early detection of problems leads to prompt intervention and prevents complications. Gentle cleaning and drying prevent the growth of microorganisms. Skin barrier/protectant prevents skin irritation and excoriation from tape, adhesives, and wound drainage (Fumarola et al., 2020; Kelly-O'Flynn et al., 2020).

(*continued on page 502*)

Skill 8-7 ▶ Caring for a Hemovac Drain *(continued)*

ACTION	RATIONALE
18. Remove and discard gloves. Perform hand hygiene.	Proper removal of gloves prevents the spread of microorganisms. Hand hygiene prevents the transmission of microorganisms.
19. Remove all remaining equipment; place the patient in a comfortable position, with side rails up as indicated and bed in the lowest position.	Proper patient and bed positioning promotes safety and comfort.
20. Remove additional PPE, if used. Perform hand hygiene.	Proper removal of PPE reduces the risk for infection transmission and contamination of other items. Hand hygiene prevents the spread of microorganisms.
21. Check drain status at least every 4 hours. Empty and reengage suction (compress device) every 2 to 4 hours (Bauldoff et al., 2020) and when it is half full of drainage or air. Check all wound dressings at least every shift. More frequent checks may be needed if the wound is more complex, or dressings become saturated quickly.	Checking the drain ensures proper functioning and early detection of problems. Emptying and compression ensure appropriate suction. Checking dressings ensures the assessment of changes in patient condition and timely intervention to prevent complications.

EVALUATION

The expected outcomes have been met when the drain has remained patent and intact, drain care was accomplished without contaminating the area and without causing trauma to the wound, the patient did not experience pain or discomfort, the drainage amounts were measured accurately at the frequency required by facility policy and recorded as part of the intake and output record, and the patient has demonstrated understanding of drain care.

DOCUMENTATION

Guidelines

Document the location of the drain, the assessment of the drain site, and patency of the drain. Note if sutures are intact. Document the presence and characteristics of drainage on the old dressing upon removal. Include the appearance of the surrounding skin. Document cleansing of the drain site. Record any skin care and any dressing applied. Note that the drain was emptied and recompressed. Note pertinent patient and family/caregiver education and any patient reaction to this procedure, including patient's pain level and effectiveness of nonpharmacologic interventions or analgesia, if administered. Document the amount and characteristics of drainage obtained on the appropriate intake and output record.

Sample Documentation

> <u>1/18/25</u> 1000 Hemovac drain in place at lateral aspect of left knee. Gauze dressing removed; no drainage noted on dressing. Suture intact; exit site slightly pink, without redness, edema, or drainage. Surrounding skin without edema, ecchymosis, or redness. Exit site and suture cleansed with normal saline and redressed with dry gauze dressing. Hemovac emptied of 90-mL sanguineous secretions and recompressed.
>
> —A. Smith, RN

DEVELOPING CLINICAL REASONING AND CLINICAL JUDGMENT

UNEXPECTED SITUATIONS AND ASSOCIATED INTERVENTIONS

- *Patient has a Hemovac drain placed in the left knee following surgery. The record indicates it has been draining serosanguineous secretions, 40 to 50 mL every shift. While performing your initial assessment, you note that the collection chamber is completely expanded. The nurse empties the device and compresses to resume suction. A short time later, the nurse observes that the chamber is completely expanded again:* Inspect the tubing for kinks or obstruction. Inspect the device, looking for breaks in the integrity of the chamber. Make sure the cap is in place and closed. Assess the patient for changes in condition. Remove the dressing and assess the site. Make sure the drainage tubing has not advanced out of the wound, exposing any of the perforations in the tubing. If you are not successful in maintaining the suction, notify the health care team of the findings and interventions and document the event in the patient's record.

**SPECIAL
CONSIDERATIONS**

- A sterile dressing is usually maintained for 24 to 48 hours; the use of a dressing after this time depends on the site assessment and amount of drainage (Orth, 2018). The site may be treated as an additional surgical wound, but often these sites are left open to air 24 hours after surgery. Refer to facility policy and prescribed interventions regarding need for sterile approach to site care and use of dressing.
- When the patient with a drain is ready to ambulate, empty and compress the drain before activity. Secure the drain to the patient's gown below the wound, making sure there is no tension on the drainage tubing. This removes excess drainage, maintains maximum suction, and avoids strain on the drain's suture line.
- Appropriate nutritional support is critical in achieving successful wound healing and may be overlooked (Quain & Khardori, 2015). Collaborate with the registered dietician and dietary staff to develop an individualized nutrition intervention plan for the patient (Baranoski & Ayello, 2020).

**Community-Based Care
Considerations**

- Drain site care in the community setting is a clean, not sterile, procedure. Patients will use soap and water to clean the skin around the drain site (Memorial Sloan Kettering Cancer Center, 2019).

**EVIDENCE
FOR PRACTICE ▶**

PREVENTION OF MEDICAL ADHESIVE–RELATED SKIN INJURIES
Fumarola, S., Allaway, R., Callaghan, R., Collier, M., Downie, F., Geraghty, J., Kiernan, S., & Spratt, F. (2020). Overlooked and underestimated: Medical adhesive-related skin injuries. Best practice consensus document on prevention. *Journal of Wound Care*, 29(Suppl 3c), S1–S24. https://doi.org/10.12968/jowc.2020.29.Sup3c.S1

This consensus document is the result of a review of the literature on medical adhesive–related skin injury (MARSI) by a panel of wound care experts, educators, and researchers. This best practice guideline provides recommendations for the assessment and prevention of MARSI, with the goal of standardizing care across all health care settings.

Skin 8-8 ▶ Applying Negative-Pressure Wound Therapy

Skill Variation: *Applying a Single-Use Negative-Pressure Wound Therapy System*

Negative-pressure wound therapy (NPWT), also known as topical negative pressure, vacuum therapy, and vacuum-assisted closure (VAC), promotes wound healing and wound closure through the application of controlled, uniform suction (vacuum) to the wound surface (Apelqvist et al., 2017; Baranoski & Ayello, 2020; Hurd et al., 2017; Taylor et al., 2023). NPWT results in reduction in bacteria in the wound and the removal of excess wound fluid, while providing a moist wound healing environment (Taylor et al., 2023). The negative pressure results in mechanical tension on the wound tissues, stimulating cell proliferation, blood flow to wounds, and the growth of new blood vessels (Lalezari et al., 2017). NPWT also acts to pull the wound edges together. Refer to Figure 1 for an illustration of the principles of NPWT.

A wound contact material is applied to fit the contours of the wound. There are various wound contact materials, including open-cell foam dressings or fillers and open-weave gauze dressing fillers (Milne, 2015). An airtight adhesive polyurethane drape that is permeable to water vapor, transparent, and bacteria proof or thin hydrocolloid is used to seal the wound and dressing (Apelqvist et al., 2017; Baranoski & Ayello, 2020). A small hole is made in the drape and a connection pad is applied over the hole, sealing the opening, and is connected to tubing and a vacuum source (Apelqvist et al., 2017). This system prevents air from entering the system from the external environment and provides for the application of the negative pressure. Excess wound fluid, small tissue debris, and infectious materials are removed through tubing into a collection container (Apelqvist et al., 2017; Benbow, 2016). A cycle of continuous, intermittent, or variable pressure (75 to 125 mm Hg) is used, depending on the particular device, the patient's condition, the location and type of wound, type of filler material, and the amount of drainage (Apelqvist et al., 2017; EPUAP, NPIAP, & PPPIA, 2019a; Schreiber, 2016). Refer to Figure 2 for examples of components of an NPWT system.

(continued on page 504)

Skill 8-8 ▶ Applying Negative-Pressure Wound Therapy *(continued)*

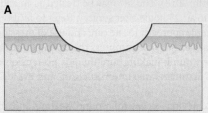
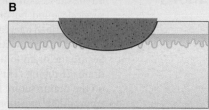

The wound (A) and a foam, cut to fit to the wound geometry, which is placed inside the wound (B).

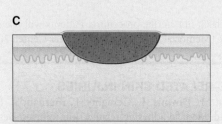
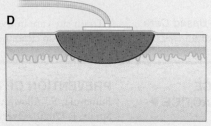

The wound is sealed airtight with a thin adhesive drape (C) with the attached "suction pad" (connecting pad) including the drainage tube (D).

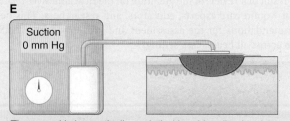
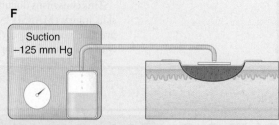

The wound is hermetically sealed with a thin adhesive drape and connected to the vacuum source by means of the attached "suction pad" (suction strength 0 mm Hg) (E). At suction strength –125 mm Hg, the foam has collapsed and the exudate collection reservoir is already partly filled (F).

FIGURE 1. Principles of negative pressure wound therapy.

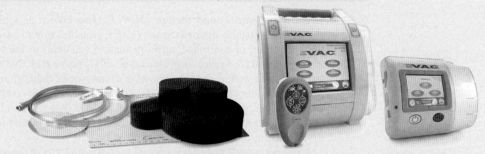

FIGURE 2. Examples of components of an NPWT system. (*Source:* From Hess, C. [2013]. *Clinical guide to skin & wound care* [7th ed.]. Wolters Kluwer, pp. 482, 484.)

NPWT is used in the management of complex and nonhealing wounds, including stage 3 and 4 pressure injuries as well as to prevent surgical-site infections in patients who are high risk for surgical-site infections (Baranoski & Ayello, 2020; EPUAP, NPIAP, & PPPIA, 2019a; Gantz et al., 2020; Lindsay, 2019).

There are several modifications of conventional NPWT in use as well. Instillation and dwell-time therapy (NPWTi-d) is a modification of NPWT that involves retrograde instillation of a topical solution into the sealed wound using a computer-controlled programmable therapy unit with a period of dwell, followed by removal of the solution via the negative pressure cycles (Apelqvist et al., 2017; Kanapathy et al., 2020; Ludolph et al., 2018). Solutions used include normal saline, hypochlorous acid, and antimicrobials to enhance wound irrigation and cleansing and decrease bacterial colonization on the surface of the wound, potentially contributing to decreased time taken to complete wound healing (Baranoski & Ayello, 2020; Ludolph et al., 2018). Single-use NPWTs (sNPWTs) are cannister-free, battery-powered, disposable, and portable systems. The sNPWT dressing may integrate multiple layers within the dressing, including a silicone adhesive wound contact layer, foam layer, absorbent layer, and outer film layer as well as integrated tubing and tubing port/connector pad (Lindsay, 2019; Smith & Nephew, 2018). sNPWT systems handle fluid mainly through evaporation from the outer layer of the dressing and are therefore appropriate for smaller wounds and wounds with low-to-moderate exudate levels (Banasiewicz et al., 2019) (Figure 3). sNPWTs may be used for treatment of a wide variety of wounds, such as postoperatively on closed surgical incisions to reduce surgical-site complications, chronic wounds, chronic ulcers on the lower extremities, plastic surgery wounds, and skin grafts (Banasiewicz et al., 2019; Edwards et al., 2018; Kirsner et al., 2019; Lindsay, 2019). Refer to the Skill Variation Applying a Single-Use Negative-Pressure Wound Therapy System at the end of this skill.

NPWT dressings are ideally changed based on the characteristics of the individual patient and the wound (EPUAP, NPIAP, & PPPIA, 2019a). Initial dressing changes may be necessary every 12 hours (wounds with heavy exudate) to 48 hours, then two to three times a week as indicated by the wound's response to the therapy, the manufacturer's specifications, and prescribed intervention (Baranoski & Ayello, 2020; EPUAP, NPIAP, & PPPIA, 2019a).

The following skill outlines one procedure for one example of NPWT. The Skill Variation at the end of this skill outlines the procedure for one example of sNPWT. There are many manufacturers of NPWT systems. **The nurse must be familiar with the components of and procedures related to the particular system in use for an individual patient.**

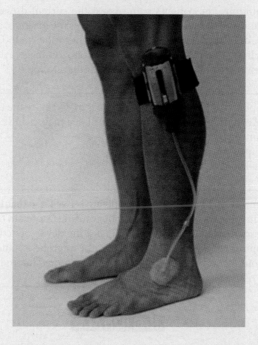

FIGURE 3. Single-use NPWT (sNPWT).

DELEGATION CONSIDERATIONS

The application of NPWT is not delegated to assistive personnel (AP). Depending on the state's nurse practice act and the organization's policies and procedures, the application of NPWT may be delegated to licensed practical/vocational nurses (LPN/LVNs). The decision to delegate must be based on careful analysis of the patient's needs and circumstances as well as the qualifications of the person to whom the task is being delegated. Refer to the Delegation Guidelines in Appendix A.

(continued on page 506)

Skill 8-8 ▶ Applying Negative-Pressure Wound Therapy *(continued)*

EQUIPMENT

- Negative pressure unit
- Evacuation/collection canister (depending on specific system in use)
- Wound contact material, as indicated by wound care plan and device/materials in use
- Transparent adhesive drape
- Connection pad/tubing port
- Drainage tubing
- Skin protectant/barrier wipes
- Sterile gauze sponge
- An 18- to 19-gauge needle/angiocath and 30- to 35-mL syringe or a commercial cleanser packaged in a pressurized container (Baranoski & Ayello, 2020, p. 152; McLain et al., 2021; WOCN, 2016)

- Sterile irrigation solution as prescribed, warmed to body temperature, commonly 0.9% normal saline solution or other solution as prescribed
- Waste receptacle to dispose of contaminated materials
- Sterile gloves (two pairs)
- Sterile scissors
- Clean, disposable gloves
- Gown, mask, eye protection
- Additional PPE, as indicated
- Sterile scissors
- Waterproof pad and bath blanket

ASSESSMENT

Confirm the prescribed intervention for the application of NPWT. Check the patient's chart and question the patient about current treatments and medications that may make the application contraindicated. Assess the situation to determine the need for a dressing change. Confirm any prescribed interventions relevant to wound care and any wound care included in the plan of care. Assess the patient's level of comfort and the need for analgesics before wound care. Assess if the patient experienced any pain related to prior dressing changes and the effectiveness of interventions employed to minimize the patient's pain. Assess the current dressing to determine if it is intact. Inspect the wound and the surrounding tissue. Assess the location, appearance of the wound, stage (if appropriate), drainage, and types of tissue present in the wound. Measure the wound. Note the stage of the healing process and characteristics of any drainage. Also assess the surrounding skin for color, temperature, and edema, ecchymosis, or maceration.

ACTUAL OR POTENTIAL HEALTH PROBLEMS AND NEEDS

Many actual or potential health problems or issues may require the use of this skill as part of related interventions. An appropriate health problem or issue may include:

- Altered skin integrity
- Altered body image perception
- Knowledge deficiency

OUTCOME IDENTIFICATION AND PLANNING

The expected outcomes to achieve when applying NPWT are that the application is accomplished without contaminating the wound area, without causing trauma to the wound, and without causing the patient to experience pain or discomfort, and the device functions correctly. Other outcomes that may be appropriate include the following: the appropriate and prescribed pressure is maintained throughout therapy, and the wound exhibits progression in healing.

IMPLEMENTATION

ACTION	RATIONALE
1. Review the patient's health record for prescribed application of NPWT therapy, including the prescribed pressure setting for the device. Gather necessary supplies.	Reviewing the health record validates the correct patient and correct procedure. Preparation promotes efficient time management and an organized approach to the task.
2. Perform hand hygiene and put on PPE, if indicated.	Hand hygiene and PPE prevent the spread of microorganisms. PPE is required based on transmission precautions.

ACTION	**RATIONALE**
3. Identify the patient.	Identifying the patient ensures the right patient receives the intervention and helps prevent errors.
4. Assemble equipment on the overbed table or other surface within reach.	Organization facilitates performance of task.
5. Close the curtains around the bed and close the door to the room, if possible. Explain what you are going to do and why you are going to do it to the patient.	This ensures the patient's privacy. Explanation relieves anxiety and facilitates engagement.
6. Assess the patient for possible need for nonpharmacologic pain-reducing interventions or analgesic medication before wound care dressing change. Administer appropriate prescribed analgesic. Allow enough time for the analgesic to achieve its effectiveness before beginning the procedure.	Pain is a subjective experience influenced by past experience. Wound care and dressing changes may cause pain for some patients.
7. Adjust the bed to a comfortable working height (VHACEOSH, 2016).	Having the bed at the proper height prevents back and muscle strain.
8. Assist the patient to a comfortable position that provides easy access to the wound area. Position the patient so the cleaning/irrigation solution will flow from the clean end of the wound toward the dirty end. Expose the area and drape the patient with a bath blanket, if needed. Put a waterproof pad under the wound area.	Patient positioning and draping provide for comfort and warmth. Gravity directs the flow of liquid from the least contaminated to the most contaminated area. Waterproof pad protects the patient and the bed linens.
9. Have the disposal bag or waste receptacle within easy reach for use during the procedure.	Having a waste container handy allows for easy disposal of the soiled dressings and supplies, without the spread of microorganisms.
10. Using sterile technique, prepare a sterile field and add all the sterile supplies needed for the procedure to the field. Pour warmed, sterile irrigating solution into the sterile container, as indicated.	Proper preparation ensures that supplies are within easy reach and sterility is maintained. Warmed solution may result in less discomfort.
11. Put on a gown, mask, and eye protection.	The use of PPE is part of *Standard Precautions*. A gown protects your clothes from contamination if splashing should occur. Goggles protect mucous membranes of your eyes from contact with irrigant fluid.
12. If NPWT is currently in use, turn off the negative pressure unit. Consider turning off suction 5 to 10 minutes before dressing change to reduce pressure (Banasiewicz et al., 2019) Put on gloves. Loosen the tape on the old dressings by removing in the direction of hair growth and the use of a push–pull method (Fumarola et al., 2020). Push–pull method: lift a corner of the dressing away from the skin, and then gently push the skin down and away from the dressing/adhesive (Fumarola et al., 2020). Continue moving fingers of the opposite hand to support the skin as the product is removed (Fumarola et al., 2020). Once all adhesive is loosened from the skin, carefully lift dressing from the surrounding skin to prevent medical adhesive–related skin injury (MARSI). Remove the sides/edges first, then the center. If the patient is at increased risk for MARSI (see Box 8-2 in Skill 8-2), requires repeated application or removal of adhesive devices, or there is resistance, use an adhesive remover (Banasiewicz et al., 2019; Barton, 2020; Fumarola et al., 2020; Kelly-O'Flynn et al., 2020).	Reduction in pressure reduces risk of pain associated with dressing removal (Banasiewicz et al., 2019). Gloves protect the nurse from contaminated dressings and prevent the spread of microorganisms. Removal of the tape in the direction of hair growth minimizes trauma to the skin (Fumarola et al., 2020). Pushing the skin down and away from the adhesive reduces the risk for MARSI (Fumarola et al., 2020). The use of adhesive remover allows for the easy, rapid, and painless removal without the associated problems of skin stripping and helps reduce patient discomfort (Banasiewicz et al., 2019; Barton, 2020; Fumarola et al., 2020; Kelly-O'Flynn et al., 2020).

(continued on page 508)

Skill 8-8 Applying Negative-Pressure Wound Therapy (continued)

ACTION	RATIONALE
13. Carefully remove the soiled dressings. If any part of the dressing sticks to the underlying skin, use small amounts of sterile saline to help loosen and remove it.	Cautious removal of the dressing is more comfortable for the patient and ensures that any drain present is not removed. Sterile saline moistens the dressing for easier removal and minimizes damage and pain.
14. Note the presence, amount, type, color, and odor of any drainage on the dressings. **Note the number of pieces of wound contact material removed from the wound. Compare with the documented number from the previous dressing change.**	The presence and characteristics of drainage should be documented. All dressing materials must be removed from the wound bed during NPWT dressing changes (Baranoski & Ayello, 2020). Counting the number of pieces of wound contact material assures the removal of all foam that was placed during the previous dressing change (Schreiber, 2016).
15. Discard the dressings in the receptacle. Remove your gloves and put them in the receptacle. Perform hand hygiene.	Proper disposal of dressings and used gloves prevents the spread of microorganisms. Hand hygiene prevents the transmission of microorganisms.
16. Put on sterile gloves. Using sterile technique, clean or irrigate the wound, based on wound care plan and prescribed wound care (see Skill 8-3). Alternatively, clean gloves (clean technique) may be used when cleaning a chronic wound or pressure injury.	Aseptic technique maintains sterility of items to come in contact with wound. Cleaning and/or irrigation remove exudate and debris. Clean technique is appropriate for cleaning chronic wounds, wounds in the home, or pressure injuries (Baranoski & Ayello, 2020; EPUAP, NPIAP, & PPPIA, 2019a; Taylor et al., 2023).
17. Clean the area around the wound with normal saline or prescribed skin cleanser. Dry the surrounding skin with a sterile gauze sponge.	Cleaning of skin removes debris and aids in adherence of dressing materials. Moisture provides a medium for the growth of microorganisms.
18. Assess the wound for appearance, stage, presence of eschar, granulation tissue, epithelialization, undermining, tunneling, necrosis, sinus tract, and drainage. Assess the appearance of the surrounding tissue. Measure the wound. Refer to Fundamentals Review 8-2 and 8-3.	This information provides evidence about the wound healing process and/or the presence of infection.
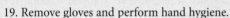 19. Remove gloves and perform hand hygiene.	Hand hygiene prevents the transmission of microorganisms.
20. Put on sterile gloves. **Wipe intact skin around the wound with a skin protectant/barrier wipe and allow it to dry.** Alternatively, clean gloves (clean technique) may be used when cleaning a chronic wound or pressure injury.	Aseptic technique maintains sterility of items to come in contact with wound. Skin barrier/protectant prevents skin irritation and excoriation from tape, adhesives, and wound drainage (Fumarola et al., 2020; Kelly-O'Flynn et al., 2020). Clean technique is appropriate for cleaning chronic wounds, wounds in the home, or pressure injuries (Baranoski & Ayello, 2020; EPUAP, NPIAP, & PPPIA, 2019a; Taylor et al., 2023).
21. If the use of a wound contact layer (impregnated porous gauze or silicone adhesive contact layer) is indicated, use sterile scissors to cut the wound contact layer to fit the wound bed. Apply wound contact layer to the wound bed.	Impregnated porous gauze or silicone adhesive contact layer may be indicated, depending on wound filler material in use, to prevent adherence of wound filler to wound be to protect the wound bed (McNichol et al., 2022).
22. Fit the wound contact material to the shape of the wound. • If using foam wound contact material, use sterile scissors to cut the foam to the shape and measurement of the wound. **Do not cut foam over the wound.** More than one piece of foam may be necessary if the first piece is cut too small. Carefully place the foam in the wound (Figure 4). **Ensure foam-to-foam contact if more than one piece is required.** • **Note the number of pieces of wound filler placed in the wound.** • **Do not under- or overfill.**	Wound contact material should fill the wound, but not cover intact surrounding skin. Foam fragments may fall into the wound if cutting is performed over the wound. Foam-to foam contact allows for even distribution of negative pressure. Recording the number of pieces of wound contact material aids in assuring the removal of all dressing material with next dressing change (Schreiber, 2016). Appropriate filling of wound is necessary to ensure safe and effective application of NPWT (Apelqvist et al., 2017; Schreiber, 2016).

ACTION

23. Trim and place the transparent adhesive drape or hydrocolloid to cover the wound contact material and an additional 3- to 5-cm border of intact periwound tissue (Figure 5). **Avoid stretching the transparent adhesive drape tight over the wound.**

RATIONALE

The occlusive air-permeable adhesive drape or hydrocolloid provides a seal, allowing the application of the negative pressure. Tight stretching of transparent adhesive drape during application may cause periwound damage (Schreiber, 2016).

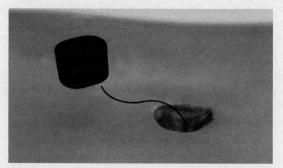

FIGURE 4. Cutting wound contact material (foam) to shape and measurement of wound. (Used with permission. Courtesy of KCI, an Acelity Company.)

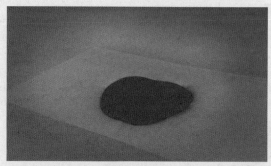

FIGURE 5. Placing transparent adhesive drape to cover the wound. (Used with permission. Courtesy of KCI, an Acelity Company.)

24. Apply the connector pad/tubing port, if necessary, depending on the device and dressing materials in use. Choose an appropriate site to apply the connector pad/tubing port. Pinch the transparent adhesive drape and cut a hole through it (Figure 6). Apply the connector pad/tubing port and connective tubing over the hole (Figure 7). Position tubing away from the periwound area and anchor (Schreiber, 2016). Some devices, such as sNPWT, have integrated tubing, tubing port/connector pad and dressing, which do not require separate connection to the dressing. Refer to the Skill Variation: Applying a Single-Use Negative-Pressure Wound Therapy System at the end of this skill.

Position the connector pad/tubing port and tubing to avoid placement over pressure areas, bony prominences, or skin creases to avoid excess pressure on the underlying skin and tissues (Schreiber, 2016). A hole in the drape and application of connector pad/tubing port and connective tubing are necessary for the application of negative pressure and removal of fluid and/or exudate. Securing the tubing prevents accidental excessive tension on the dressing (Schreiber, 2016).

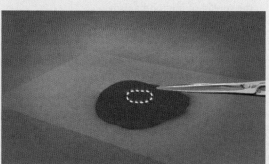

FIGURE 6. Cutting a hole in the drape.

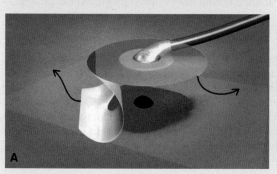

A

B

FIGURE 7. Applying the connecting pad over the hole.

(continued on page 510)

Skill 8-8 ▶ Applying Negative-Pressure Wound Therapy *(continued)*

ACTION	**RATIONALE**

25. Attach the drainage cannister, depending on the device in use. Remove the drainage collection canister from the package and insert into the negative pressure unit until it locks into place. Attach the connective tubing to the canister and check that the clamps on the tubing are open, if present.

The tubing and canister provide means for the collection of drainage. Clamps must be open for the device to work properly.

26. Remove gloves and discard. Perform hand hygiene. Turn on the power to the negative pressure unit. Select the prescribed therapy settings (suction and cycle type) and start the device.

Removal of gloves, proper disposal, and hand hygiene prevent transmission of microorganisms.

27. **Assess the dressing to ensure seal integrity. The dressing should be collapsed, shrinking to the wound contact material and skin (Figure 8). Observe drainage in tubing.**

Shrinkage confirms a good seal, allowing for accurate application of pressure and treatment. Observation of drainage in device tubing ensures proper flow (Schreiber, 2016).

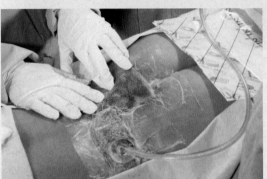

FIGURE 8. Dressing is collapsed, shrinking to wound contact material and skin. (Used with permission. Courtesy of KCI, an Acelity Company.)

28. Label dressing with date and time. Remove all remaining equipment; place the patient in a comfortable position, with side rails up as indicated and bed in the lowest position.

Recording the date and time provides communication and demonstrates adherence to the care plan. Proper patient and bed positioning promotes safety and comfort.

29. Remove PPE, if used. Perform hand hygiene.

Proper removal of PPE reduces the risk for infection transmission and contamination of other items. Hand hygiene prevents the spread of microorganisms.

30. Check all wound dressings at least every shift. More frequent checks may be needed if the wound is more. Check negative pressure settings at least every shift. Assess the patient's tolerance of and response to the therapy at least every shift.

Checking dressings, the device, and patient response ensures the assessment of changes in patient condition and timely intervention to prevent complications.

EVALUATION

The expected outcomes have been met when the application of NPWT was accomplished without contaminating the wound area, causing trauma to the wound, or causing the patient to experience pain or discomfort; the device functions correctly; the appropriate and prescribed pressure was maintained throughout therapy; and the wound has exhibited progression in healing.

DOCUMENTATION

Guidelines

Record your assessment of the wound, including evidence of granulation tissue, stage (if appropriate), and characteristics of drainage. Include the appearance of the surrounding skin. Document the cleansing or irrigation of the wound and solution used. Document the application of the NPWT, noting the pressure setting, patency, and seal of the dressing. Describe the color and characteristics of the drainage in the collection chamber. Record pertinent patient and family/caregiver education and any patient reaction to this procedure, including the presence of pain and effectiveness or ineffectiveness of pain interventions.

Sample Documentation

> 4/5/25 0800 NPWT dressing intact with good seal maintained, system patent, pressure setting 80 mm Hg. Purulent, sanguineous drainage noted in collection chamber and tubing. Surrounding tissue without edema, redness, ecchymosis, or signs of irritation. Patient verbalizes an understanding of use of the device and movement limitations related to the system.
>
> —*B. Clark, RN*

DEVELOPING CLINICAL REASONING AND CLINICAL JUDGMENT

UNEXPECTED SITUATIONS AND ASSOCIATED INTERVENTIONS

- *While assessing the patient, the nurse notes that the seal between the transparent adhesive drape and the wound contact material and skin is not tight:* Check the dressing seals, tubing connections, and canister insertion, and ensure the clamps are open. If a leak in the transparent drape is identified, the appropriate pressure is not being applied to the wound. Apply additional transparent dressing to reseal. If this application does not correct the break, change the dressing.
- *Patient reports acute pain while NPWT is operating:* Assess the patient for other symptoms, obtain vital signs, assess the wound, and assess the vacuum device for proper functioning. Report your findings to the health care team and document the event in the patient's health record. Administer analgesics, as prescribed. Continue or change the wound therapy, as prescribed. Some patients may be unable to tolerate NPWT and may require a change in the type of wound contact material used, addition of a wound contact layer, intermittent therapy cycling, a reduction in suction pressure, or discontinuation of the therapy (Apelqvist et al., 2017; Milne, 2015; Schreiber, 2016).

SPECIAL CONSIDERATIONS

- The wound should be debrided of as much necrotic tissue as possible before using NPWT; it is best to have the wound bed free of necrotic tissue (Baranoski & Ayello, 2020).
- Time dressing changes to allow for wound assessment by other members of the health care team.
- Dressings may need to be changed more often than 48 to 72 hours for wounds with heavy exudate (Baranoski & Ayello, 2020; EPUAP, NPIAP, & PPPIA, 2019a).
- Measure and record the amount of drainage each shift as part of the intake and output record.
- Check the fluid level in the canister periodically. Depending on the particular device in use, replace the canister whenever full or nearly full.
- The battery pack for sNPWT devices may contain a magnet; these devices should be kept at least 4 inches away from other medical devices to avoid disruption of nearby medical devices (Smith & Nephew, Inc., 2018; Watret et al., 2020).
- Be alert for audible and visual alarms on the vacuum device to alert you to problems, such as tipping of the device greater than 45 degrees, a full collection canister, an air leak in the dressing, or dislodgment of the canister.
- NPWT should operate for 24 hours a day. It should not be shut off for more than 2 hours in a 24-hour period. Remove the dressing any time therapy cannot be reestablished within the 2-hour time period (McNichol et al., 2022). When suction is lost, there is no mechanism for exudate control and allowing the dressing to remain in place without suction significantly increases the risk of wound infection (McNichol et al., 2022, p. 226). When NPWT is restarted, clean/irrigate the wound as prescribed or per facility policy and apply a new NPWT dressing.
- When maceration of the surrounding skin beneath the occlusive dressing occurs, this may be treated by placing a barrier/wafer dressing beneath the transparent dressing to protect the skin. Verify with facility policy, as needed.
- Approaches to NPWT continue to change, including the size of the vacuum pumps, types of wound contact materials, and length of time recommended for the use of NPWT (Benbow, 2016).
- Appropriate nutritional support is critical in achieving successful wound healing and may be overlooked (Quain & Khardori, 2015). Collaborate with the registered dietician and dietary staff to develop an individualized nutrition intervention plan for the patient (Baranoski & Ayello, 2020).

(continued on page 512)

Skill 8-8 ▶ Applying Negative-Pressure Wound Therapy *(continued)*

Community-Based Care Considerations

- NPWT can be used in outpatient and home and other community settings (Edwards et al., 2018; EPUAP, NPIAP, & PPPIA, 2019a).
- Patients and caregivers must be educated about NPWT: how NPWT works, the risks and benefits of NPWT, device operation, signs of and actions for possible complications, response to alarms and emergencies, and when to seek and whom to contact for assistance (Benbow, 2016; Schreiber, 2016).

Skill Variation ▶ Applying a Single-Use Negative-Pressure Wound Therapy System

Single-use negative-pressure wound therapy (sNPWT) systems have a multi-layered wound dressing with integrated tubing and tubing port/connector pad (Figure 3 on p. 505). sNPWT systems are cannister-free, battery-powered, disposable, and portable. sNPWT systems manage fluid through evaporation from the outer layer of the dressing and are therefore appropriate for smaller wounds and wounds with low-to-moderate exudate levels (Banasiewicz et al., 2019). This Skill Variation outlines the general procedure for one example of sNPWT. There are many manufacturers of NPWT systems. **The nurse must be familiar with the components of and procedures related to the particular system in use for an individual patient.**

1. Review the patient's health record for prescribed application of sNPWT. Gather the necessary supplies.

2. Perform hand hygiene and put on PPE, if indicated.

3. Identify the patient.

4. Assemble equipment on the overbed table or other surface within reach.
5. Close the curtains around the bed and close the door to the room, if possible. Explain to the patient what you are going to do and why you are going to do it.
6. Assess the patient for the possible need of nonpharmacologic pain-reducing interventions or analgesic medication before wound care dressing change. Administer the appropriate prescribed analgesic. Allow enough time for the analgesic to achieve its effectiveness before beginning the procedure.
7. Adjust the bed to a comfortable working height (VHACEOSH, 2016).

8. Remove the current sNPWT dressing (if present), clean the wound, and apply skin protectant as outlined in Steps 8–20 in Skill 8-8.
9. Remove the paper backing from the adhesive on one side of the outer film layer of the dressing. Orient and place the dressing centrally over the wound with the tubing port located uppermost from the wound (Smith & Nephew, 2018).
10. Remove the paper backing from the remaining edges of the outer film layer of the dressing. Smooth the dressing around the wound to prevent creasing (Smith & Nephew, 2018).
11. Attach the device to the dressing by twisting together the tubing connector from the device and the dressing.

12. Remove gloves and perform hand hygiene.

13. If not already in place, insert the batteries into the device.
14. Turn the device on to start the application of negative pressure.
15. Apply the fixation strips to each of the sides of the dressing to reduce the risk of the dressing edges curling.
16. **Assess the dressing to ensure seal integrity. The dressing should be collapsed, shrinking to the wound contact material and skin.**
17. Label the dressing with date and time. Remove all remaining equipment; place the patient in a comfortable position, with side rails up as indicated and the bed in the lowest position.

18. Remove PPE, if used. Perform hand hygiene.

19. Check all wound dressings at least every shift. Check the device display status to monitor system functioning at least every shift. Assess the patient's tolerance of and response to the therapy at least every shift.

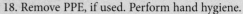

EVIDENCE FOR PRACTICE ▶

NEGATIVE PRESSURE WOUND THERAPY AND QUALITY OF LIFE

Because the skin is a sensory organ and plays a major role in communication with others and self-image, wounds and pressure injuries require emotional as well as physical adaptation. Although stress and adaptation vary greatly among people, actual and potential emotional stressors are common in all patients with wounds. Therapies related to wound care may also be a source of stress and could impact the quality of life (QoL) of the patient and caregivers

Related Research

Janssen, A. H., Wegdam, J. A., de Vries Rellingh, T. S., Eskes, A. M., & Vermeulen, H. (2020). Negative pressure wound therapy for patients with hard-to-heal wounds: A systematic review. *Journal of Wound Care, 29*(4), 206–212. https://doi.org/10.12968/jowc.2020.29.4.206

This systematic review examined the effect of negative pressure wound therapy (NPWT) on QoL. Eight databases were searched from 2000 to 2019 for qualitative studies that addressed patients' experiences with NPWT in relation to QoL. The primary reason for study exclusion was that it did not focus on QoL or had a nonqualitative research design. Studies were selected by two independent reviewers and evaluated for methodologic quality using the Critical Appraisal Skills Programme (CASP) for Qualitative Research. Of the 43 studies identified, 5 matched the eligibility criteria in which 51 individual patients shared their personal experiences with NPWT. Content analysis was used to extract and define central themes in patients' personal experiences. Four major themes emerged: reduced freedom of movement caused by an electric device, decreased self-esteem, increased social and professional dependency, and gaining self-control. The authors concluded that NPWT is associated with major effects on the physical, psychological, and social domains of QoL. The researchers suggested health care professionals should be aware of the strong effects of NPWT on patient QoL and assess the ability of a patient to cope with the device and potential associated limitations as well as the possible gains in self-control. Decisions to use NPWT must be tailored to the patient and involve shared decision making with regard to use of NPWT or standard wound care.

Relevance for Nursing Practice

Using the best treatment for a wound or pressure injury is important. However, the best treatment may not produce the best patient experience, if the patient's physical, psychological, and emotional needs are not met. Nurses need to be holistic in their approach to patients receiving wound care and be aware of patient experiences related to any prescribed treatments for wounds and pressure injuries. Interventions, including patient education; support; collaboration; and a thoughtful, person-centered approach, can foster use of the best treatment choice for patients.

EVIDENCE FOR PRACTICE ▶

PREVENTION OF MEDICAL ADHESIVE–RELATED SKIN INJURIES

Fumarola, S., Allaway, R., Callaghan, R., Collier, M., Downie, F., Geraghty, J., Kiernan, S., & Spratt, F. (2020). Overlooked and underestimated: Medical adhesive-related skin injuries. Best practice consensus document on prevention. *Journal of Wound Care, 29*(Suppl 3c), S1–S24. https://doi.org/10.12968/jowc.2020.29.Sup3c.S1

This consensus document is the result of a review of the literature on medical adhesive–related skin injury (MARSI) by a panel of wound care experts, educators, and researchers. This best practice guideline provides recommendations for the assessment and prevention of MARSI, with the goal of standardizing care across all health care settings.

Skill 8-9 ▶ Removing Sutures

Skin sutures are used to hold the tissue and skin together. Sutures may be made from several natural or synthetic materials, such as silk, cotton, linen, or fine wire. **Surgical sutures** are removed when enough tensile strength has developed to hold the wound edges together during healing. Sutures should be removed within 1 to 2 weeks of placement, depending on the anatomic location, to reduce the risk of suture marks, infection, and tissue reaction (Ratner, 2020a). The removal of sutures may be done by the primary health care provider and an advanced practice professional, or by the nurse, as indicated in facility policy. Adhesive wound closure strips may be applied across the wound after suture removal to provide continued wound support as it continues to heal. Some sutures are buried sutures, placed with absorbable material, which are not removed but left in place because they dissolve (Ratner, 2020a).

DELEGATION CONSIDERATIONS	The removal of surgical sutures is not delegated to assistive personnel (AP). Depending on the state's nurse practice act and the organization's policies and procedures, the removal of surgical sutures may be delegated to licensed practical/vocational nurses (LPN/LVNs). The decision to delegate must be based on careful analysis of the patient's needs and circumstances as well as the qualifications of the person to whom the task is being delegated. Refer to the Delegation Guidelines in Appendix A.
EQUIPMENT	• Suture removal kit or forceps and scissors • Gauze • Wound cleansing agent, according to facility policy • Disposable gloves • Additional PPE, as indicated • Adhesive wound closure strips, as indicated • Skin protectant/barrier wipes
ASSESSMENT	Inspect the surgical incision and the surrounding tissue. Assess the appearance of the wound for the approximation of wound edges, the color of the wound and surrounding area, presence of wound drainage noting color, volume, and odor, and for signs of dehiscence. Note the stage of the healing process and characteristics of any drainage. Assess the surrounding skin for color, temperature, and the presence of edema, maceration, or ecchymosis.
ACTUAL OR POTENTIAL HEALTH PROBLEMS AND NEEDS	Many actual or potential health problems or issues may require the use of this skill as part of related interventions. An appropriate health problem or issue may include: • Altered skin integrity • Infection risk • Knowledge deficiency
OUTCOME IDENTIFICATION AND PLANNING	The expected outcome to achieve when removing surgical sutures is that the sutures are removed without causing trauma to the wound or causing the patient to experience pain or discomfort.

IMPLEMENTATION

ACTION	**RATIONALE**
1. Review the patient's health record for prescribed intervention for suture removal. Gather necessary supplies.	Reviewing the health record and care plan validates the correct patient and correct procedure. Preparation promotes efficient time management and an organized approach to the task.
2. Perform hand hygiene and put on PPE, if indicated.	Hand hygiene and PPE prevent the spread of microorganisms. PPE is required based on transmission precautions.

ACTION

3. Identify the patient.

4. Assemble equipment on the overbed table or other surface within reach.

5. Close the curtains around the bed and close the door to the room, if possible. Explain what you are going to do and why you are going to do it to the patient. Describe the sensation of suture removal as a pulling or slightly uncomfortable experience.

6. Assess the patient for possible need for nonpharmacologic pain-reducing interventions or analgesic medication before beginning the procedure. Administer appropriate prescribed analgesic. Allow enough time for the analgesic to achieve its effectiveness before beginning the procedure.

7. Place a waste receptacle at a convenient location for use during the procedure.

8. Adjust the bed to a comfortable working height (VHACEOSH, 2016).

9. Assist the patient to a comfortable position that provides easy access to the incision area. Use a bath blanket to cover any exposed area other than the incision. Place a waterproof pad under the incision site.

10. Put on clean gloves. Carefully and gently remove any dressings that may be in place. Refer to Skill 8-2.

11. Clean the incision, according to prescribed wound care or facility policy and procedure. Refer to Skill 8-2. Assess the wound (Refer to Assessment section of skill and Fundamentals Review 8-1) (Figure 1).

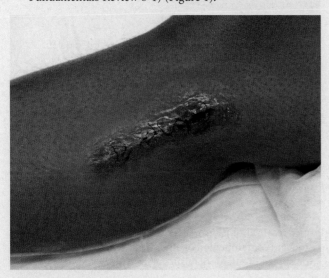

FIGURE 1. Incision with sutures.

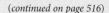

12. Perform hand hygiene. Open the suture removal kit. Put on gloves.

RATIONALE

Identifying the patient ensures the right patient receives the intervention and helps prevent errors.

Organization facilitates performance of task.

This ensures the patient's privacy. Explanation relieves anxiety and facilitates engagement.

Pain is a subjective experience influenced by past experience. Wound care and dressing changes may cause pain for some patients.

Having a waste container handy means that the soiled dressing may be discarded easily, without the spread of microorganisms.

Having the bed at the proper height prevents back and muscle strain.

Patient positioning and the use of a bath blanket provide for comfort and warmth. Waterproof pad protects underlying surfaces.

Gloves protect the nurse from handling contaminated dressings. Appropriate removal of the dressing is more comfortable for the patient and prevents medical adhesive–related skin injury (MARSI) (Fumarola et al., 2020).

Incision cleaning prevents the spread of microorganisms and contamination of the wound. Assessment provides validation of healing related to timing of suture removal.

Hand hygiene prevents the transmission of microorganisms. Gloves prevent contact with blood and body fluids.

(continued on page 516)

Skill 8-9 ▶ Removing Sutures *(continued)*

ACTION

13. Using the forceps, grasp the first suture and gently lift the suture up off the skin.

14. Using the scissors, cut one side of the suture below the knot, close to the skin (Figure 2). Grasp the knot with the forceps and gently pull the suture toward the wound or suture line until the suture material is completely removed. **Avoid pulling the suture away from the suture line.**

15. Remove every other suture to be sure the wound edges are healed. If the wound edges remain approximated, remove the remaining sutures, as prescribed. Dispose of sutures according to facility policy.

16. If wound closure strips are to be used, apply skin protectant/barrier to skin around incision. **Do not apply to incision.** Apply adhesive closure strips (Figure 3). Take care to handle the strips by the paper backing.

RATIONALE

Raising the suture knot prevents accidental injury to the wound or skin when cutting.

Cutting close to the skin results in minimal exposed suture to pull through skin, reducing the risk for contamination of the incision area. Pulling the cut suture toward the wound or suture line reduces the risk the wound edges will separate; pulling the suture away from the suture line increases the risk the wound edges may separate (Ratner, 2020a).

Removing every other suture allows for inspection of the wound, while leaving adequate suture in place to promote continued healing if the edges are not totally approximated. Follow Standard Precautions in disposing of sutures.

Skin protectant helps adherence of closure strips and prevents skin irritation and excoriation from tape, adhesives, and wound drainage (Fumarola et al., 2020). Adhesive wound closure strips provide additional support to the wound as it continues to heal. Handling by the paper backing avoids contamination.

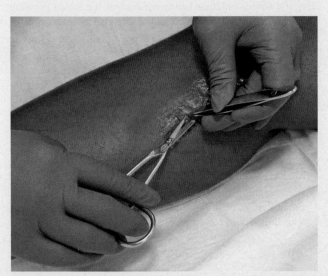

FIGURE 2. Using forceps to pull up on a suture and cutting suture with sterile scissors.

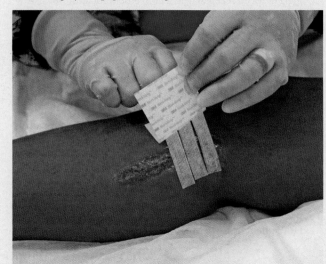

FIGURE 3. Applying adhesive closure strips on incision.

17. Reapply the dressing, based on the prescribed interventions and facility policy. Refer to Skill 8-2.

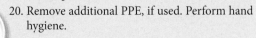 18. Remove and discard gloves. Perform hand hygiene.

19. Remove all remaining equipment; place the patient in a comfortable position, with side rails up as indicated and bed in the lowest position.

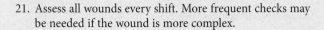 20. Remove additional PPE, if used. Perform hand hygiene.

21. Assess all wounds every shift. More frequent checks may be needed if the wound is more complex.

A new dressing protects the wound. Some policies advise leaving the area uncovered.

Proper removal of gloves prevents the spread of microorganisms. Hand hygiene prevents the transmission of microorganisms.

Proper patient and bed positioning promotes safety and comfort.

Proper removal of PPE reduces the risk for infection transmission and contamination of other items. Hand hygiene prevents the spread of microorganisms.

Checking wound and dressings ensures the assessment of changes in patient condition and timely intervention to prevent complications.

EVALUATION

The expected outcomes have been met when the sutures were removed without causing trauma to the wound or causing the patient to experience pain or discomfort.

DOCUMENTATION

Guidelines

Document the location of the incision and the assessment of the site. Include the appearance of the surrounding skin. Document cleansing of the site and suture removal. Record any skin care, application of wound closure strips, and the dressing applied, if appropriate. Note pertinent patient and family/caregiver education and any patient reaction to this procedure, including the patient's pain level and effectiveness of nonpharmacologic interventions or analgesia if administered.

Sample Documentation

> 3/4/25 1800 Right lower lateral leg surgical wound appears healed. Incision edges are approximated, without erythema, edema, ecchymosis, or drainage. Skin warm with consistent tone. Sutures removed without difficulty; skin protectant/barrier applied to skin surrounding incision and adhesive wound closure strips applied. Patient instructed on how to care for wound and expectations regarding wound closure strips; patient and wife verbalized an understanding of information and asked appropriate questions.
> —L. Downs, RN

DEVELOPING CLINICAL REASONING AND CLINICAL JUDGMENT

UNEXPECTED SITUATIONS AND ASSOCIATED INTERVENTIONS

- *Sutures are crusted with dried blood or secretions, making them difficult to remove:* Moisten sterile gauze with sterile saline and gently loosen crusts before removing sutures.
- *Resistance is met when attempting to pull suture through the tissue:* Use a gentle, continuous pulling motion to remove the suture. If the suture still does not come out, do not use excessive force. Report findings to the health care team and document the event in the patient's record.

SPECIAL CONSIDERATIONS

- After suture removal, continue to encourage the patient to splint chest and abdominal wounds during activity, such as changing position, ambulating, coughing, and sneezing. This provides increased support for the skin and underlying tissues and can decrease discomfort.

Skill 8-10 ▶ Removing Surgical Staples

Skin staples made of stainless steel are used to hold the tissue and skin together and are frequently used in wounds under high tension (Ratner, 2020b). Staples are made of stainless steel and are quicker to place, are associated with minimal tissue reaction, decreased risk of infection, and strong wound closure but are also associated with less precise wound edge alignment and higher cost (Ratner, 2020b). **Surgical staples** are removed when enough tensile strength has developed to hold the wound edges together during healing. The time frame for removal varies depending on the anatomic location of the wound. The removal of sutures may be done by the primary health care provider and an advanced practice professional, or by the nurse, as indicated in facility policy. Adhesive wound closure strips may be applied across the wound after staple removal to provide continued wound support as it continues to heal.

DELEGATION CONSIDERATIONS

The removal of surgical staples is not delegated to assistive personnel (AP). Depending on the state's nurse practice act and the organization's policies and procedures, the removal of surgical staples may be delegated to licensed practical/vocational nurses (LPN/LVNs). The decision to delegate must be based on careful analysis of the patient's needs and circumstances as well as the qualifications of the person to whom the task is being delegated. Refer to the Delegation Guidelines in Appendix A.

(continued on page 518)

Skill 8-10 ▶ Removing Surgical Staples (continued)

EQUIPMENT	
• Staple remover	• Disposable gloves
• Gauze	• Additional PPE, as indicated
• Wound cleansing agent, according to facility policy	• Adhesive wound closure strips, as indicated
	• Skin protectant/barrier wipes

ASSESSMENT

Inspect the surgical incision and the surrounding tissue. Assess the appearance of the wound for the approximation of wound edges, the color of the wound and surrounding area, and signs of dehiscence. Note the stage of the healing process and the characteristics of any drainage. Assess the surrounding skin for color, temperature, and the presence of edema or ecchymosis.

ACTUAL OR POTENTIAL HEALTH PROBLEMS AND NEEDS

Many actual or potential health problems or issues may require the use of this skill as part of related interventions. An appropriate health problem or issue may include:
• Altered skin integrity
• Infection risk
• Knowledge deficiency

OUTCOME IDENTIFICATION AND PLANNING

The expected outcome to achieve when removing surgical staples is that the staples are removed without causing trauma to the wound or causing the patient to experience pain or discomfort.

IMPLEMENTATION

ACTION	RATIONALE
1. Review the patient's health record for prescribed intervention for staple removal. Gather necessary supplies.	Reviewing the health record and care plan validates the correct patient and correct procedure. Preparation promotes efficient time management and an organized approach to the task.
2. Perform hand hygiene and put on PPE, if indicated.	Hand hygiene and PPE prevent the spread of microorganisms. PPE is required based on transmission precautions.
3. Identify the patient.	Identifying the patient ensures the right patient receives the intervention and helps prevent errors.
4. Assemble equipment on the overbed table or other surface within reach.	Organization facilitates the performance of the task.
5. Close the curtains around the bed and close the door to the room, if possible. Explain what you are going to do and why you are going to do it to the patient. Describe the sensation of staple removal as a pulling experience.	This ensures the patient's privacy. Explanation relieves anxiety and facilitates engagement.
6. Assess the patient for possible need for nonpharmacologic pain-reducing interventions or analgesic medication before beginning the procedure. Administer the appropriate prescribed analgesic. Allow enough time for the analgesic to achieve its effectiveness before beginning the procedure.	Pain is a subjective experience influenced by past experience. Wound care and dressing changes may cause pain for some patients.
7. Place a waste receptacle at a convenient location for use during the procedure.	Having a waste container handy means that the soiled dressing may be discarded easily, without the spread of microorganisms.
8. Adjust the bed to a comfortable working height (VHACEOSH, 2016).	Having the bed at the proper height prevents back and muscle strain.

ACTION

9. Assist the patient to a comfortable position that provides easy access to the incision area. Use a bath blanket to cover any exposed area other than the incision. Place a waterproof pad under the incision site.

10. Put on clean gloves. Carefully remove any dressings that may be in place. Refer to Skill 8-2.

11. Clean the incision, according to prescribed wound care or facility policy and procedure. Refer to Skill 8-2. Assess the wound (Figure 1). Refer to assessment section of this skill.

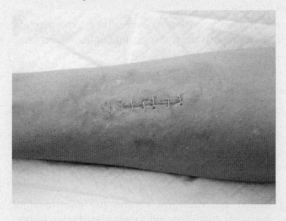

RATIONALE

Patient positioning and the use of a bath blanket provide for comfort and warmth. Waterproof pad protects underlying surfaces.

Gloves protect the nurse from handling contaminated dressings. Appropriate removal of the dressing is more comfortable for the patient and prevents medical adhesive–related skin injury (MARSI) (Fumarola et al., 2020).

Incision cleaning prevents the spread of microorganisms and contamination of the wound. Assessment provides validation of healing related to timing of suture removal.

FIGURE 1. Incision with surgical staples.

 12. Perform hand hygiene. Open the staple remover kit. Put on clean disposable gloves.

Hand hygiene prevents the transmission of microorganisms. Gloves prevent contact with blood and body fluids.

13. Grasp the staple remover (Figure 2). **Position the staple remover under the staple to be removed. Firmly close the staple remover.** The staple will bend in the middle and the edges will pull up out of the skin (Figure 3).

Correct use of the staple remover prevents accidental injury to the wound and contamination of the incision area and resulting infection.

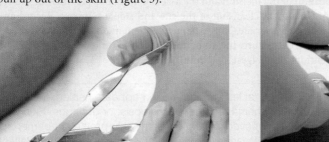

FIGURE 2. Grasping staple remover.

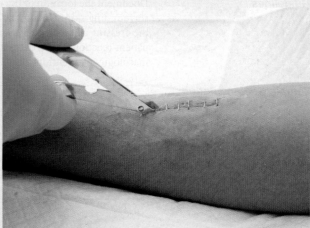

FIGURE 3. Firmly closing the staple remover, bending the staple in the middle, pulling the edges up out of the skin.

(continued on page 520)

Skill 8-10 ▶ Removing Surgical Staples *(continued)*

ACTION	RATIONALE
14. Remove every other staple to be sure the wound edges are healed. If the wound edges remain approximated, remove the remaining staples, as prescribed. Dispose of staples in the sharps container.	Removing every other staple allows for inspection of the wound, while leaving an adequate number of staples in place to promote continued healing if the edges are not totally approximated.
15. If wound closure strips are to be used, apply skin protectant to the skin around the incision. **Do not apply to the incision.** Apply adhesive closure strips. Take care to handle the strips by the paper backing (refer to Skill 8-9, Step 16).	Skin protectant helps adherence of closure strips and prevents skin irritation and excoriation from tape, adhesives, and wound drainage (Fumarola et al., 2020). Adhesive wound closure strips provide additional support to the wound as it continues to heal. Handling by the paper backing avoids contamination.
16. Reapply the dressing, based on the prescribed interventions and facility policy. Refer to Skill 8-2.	A new dressing protects the wound. Some policies advise leaving the area uncovered.
17. Remove and discard gloves. Perform hand hygiene.	Proper removal of gloves prevents the spread of microorganisms. Hand hygiene prevents the transmission of microorganisms.
18. Remove all remaining equipment; place the patient in a comfortable position, with side rails up as indicated and bed in the lowest position.	Proper patient and bed positioning promotes safety and comfort.
19. Remove additional PPE, if used. Perform hand hygiene.	Proper removal of PPE reduces the risk for infection transmission and contamination of other items. Hand hygiene prevents the spread of microorganisms.
20. Assess all wounds every shift. More frequent checks may be needed if the wound is more complex.	Checking wound and dressings ensures the assessment of changes in patient condition and timely intervention to prevent complications.

EVALUATION

The expected outcomes have been met when the staples were removed without causing trauma to the wound or causing the patient to experience pain or discomfort.

DOCUMENTATION

Guidelines

Document the location of the incision and the assessment of the site. Include the appearance of the surrounding skin. Document cleansing of the site and staple removal. Record any skin care and the dressing applied, if appropriate. Note pertinent patient and family/caregiver education and any patient reaction to this procedure, including the patient's pain level and effectiveness of nonpharmacologic interventions or analgesia if administered.

Sample Documentation

3/4/25 1800 Left upper lateral leg surgical wound appears healed. Incision edges are approximated, without erythema, edema, ecchymosis, or drainage. Skin warm with consistent tone. Staples removed without difficulty; skin protectant/barrier applied to skin surrounding incision and adhesive wound closure strips applied. Patient instructed in how to care for wound and expectations regarding wound closure strips; patient and wife verbalized an understanding of information and asked appropriate questions.

—S. Hoffman, RN

DEVELOPING CLINICAL REASONING AND CLINICAL JUDGMENT

UNEXPECTED SITUATIONS AND ASSOCIATED INTERVENTIONS

- *Wound edges appear approximated before staple removal but pull apart afterward:* Report the findings to the health care team and document the event in the patient's record. Apply adhesive wound closure strips and/or further wound care according to facility policy or prescribed intervention.
- *Staples are stuck to the wound because of dried blood or secretions:* Per facility policy or prescribed intervention, apply moist saline compresses to loosen crusts before attempting to remove the staples.

SPECIAL CONSIDERATIONS

- Encourage the patient to splint chest and abdominal wounds (before and after surgical staple removal) during activity, such as changing position, ambulating, coughing, and sneezing. This provides increased support for the skin and underlying tissues and can help decrease patient discomfort.

Skin 8-11 ▶ Applying an External Heating Pad

Heat applications accelerate the inflammatory response, promoting healing. Heat is also used to reduce muscle tension, and to relieve muscle spasm, joint stiffness, and relieve pain (Bauldoff et al., 2020). It is used to treat muscle strain and sprains, muscle spasms, menstrual cramps, arthritis, joint pain, superficial thrombophlebitis, and chronic pain (Cleveland Clinic, 2020; Klein, 2019).

Heat may be applied by moist and dry methods. The prescribed intervention should include information addressing the type of application, the body area to be treated, the frequency of application, and the length of time for the applications. Water used for heat applications needs to be at the appropriate temperature to avoid skin damage: set the temperature of the water within a range of 105° to 109°F (40.5° to 43°C), which is considered to be physiologically effective and comfortable for the patient (Taylor et al., 2023). **Water temperature should not exceed 120°F (49°C)** (International Association of Fire Fighters, n.d.).

Common types of external heating devices include aquathermia pads (e.g., Aqua-K), microwaveable hot packs, and air-activated heat therapy patches. Aquathermia pads are used in health care facilities and are safer to use than heating pads. Microwaveable packs are easy and inexpensive to use but have several disadvantages. They may leak and pose a danger from burns related to improper use. Microwaveable packs and air-activated heat therapy patches are used most often in the home setting.

DELEGATION CONSIDERATIONS

The application of an external heating pad may be delegated to assistive personnel (AP) as well as to licensed practical/vocational nurses (LPN/LVNs). The decision to delegate must be based on careful analysis of the patient's needs and circumstances as well as the qualifications of the person to whom the task is being delegated. Refer to the Delegation Guidelines in Appendix A.

EQUIPMENT

- Aquathermia heating pad with electronic unit
- Distilled water
- Cover for the pad, if not part of pad
- Gauze bandage or tape to secure the pad
- Bath blanket
- PPE, as indicated

ASSESSMENT

Assess the situation to determine the appropriateness for the application of heat. Identify patients at risk for burns, including older adults, young children, cognitively and physically impaired persons (Field, 2018). Assess the patient's physical and mental status and the condition of the body area to be treated with heat. Assess for circulatory compromise in the area where the heat will be applied, including skin color, pulses distal to the site, evidence of edema, and the presence of sensation. Check the equipment to be used, including the condition of cords, plugs, and heating elements. Look for fluid leaks. Once the equipment is turned on, make sure there is a consistent distribution of heat and the temperature is within safe limits. Assess the application site frequently during the treatment, as tissue damage can occur.

(continued on page 522)

Skill 8-11 ▶ Applying an External Heating Pad   *(continued)*

ACTUAL OR POTENTIAL HEALTH PROBLEMS AND NEEDS	Many actual or potential health problems or issues may require the use of this skill as part of related interventions. An appropriate health problem or issue may include: • Chronic pain • Acute pain • Altered skin integrity risk
OUTCOME IDENTIFICATION AND PLANNING	The expected outcome to achieve when applying an external heat source depends on the patient's health problem or need and the rationale for application. Outcomes that may be appropriate include the following: the patient experiences increased comfort, the patient experiences decreased muscle spasms, the patient experiences a reduction in inflammation, the patient remains free from injury, and the patient demonstrates knowledge of safe application of the external heat source.

IMPLEMENTATION

ACTION	RATIONALE
1. Review the patient's health record for prescribed intervention for the application of heat therapy, including frequency, type of therapy, body area to be treated, and length of time for the application. Gather necessary supplies.	Reviewing the health record and care plan validates the correct patient and correct procedure. Preparation promotes efficient time management and an organized approach to the task.
2. Perform hand hygiene and put on PPE, if indicated.	Hand hygiene and PPE prevent the spread of microorganisms. PPE is required based on transmission precautions.
3. Identify the patient.	Identifying the patient ensures the right patient receives the intervention and helps prevent errors.
4. Assemble equipment on the overbed table or other surface within reach.	Organization facilitates performance of task.
5. Close the curtains around the bed and close the door to the room if possible. Explain what you are going to do and why you are going to do it to the patient.	This ensures the patient's privacy. Explanation relieves anxiety and facilitates engagement.
6. Adjust the bed to a comfortable working height (VHACEOSH, 2016).	Having the bed at the proper height prevents back and muscle strain.
7. Assist the patient to a comfortable position that provides easy access to the area where the heat will be applied; use a bath blanket to cover any other exposed area.	Patient positioning and the use of a bath blanket provide for comfort and warmth.
8. Assess the condition of the skin where the heat is to be applied.	Assessment supplies baseline data for post-treatment comparison and identifies conditions that may contraindicate the application.
9. Check that the water in the electronic unit (Figure 1) is at the appropriate level. Fill the unit two thirds full or to the fill mark, with distilled water, if necessary. Check the temperature setting on the unit to ensure it is within the safe range.	Sufficient water in the unit is necessary to ensure proper function of the unit. Tap water leaves mineral deposits in the unit. Checking the temperature setting helps to prevent skin or tissue damage.
10. Attach pad tubing to the electronic unit tubing (Figure 2).	Allows flow of warmed water through the heating pad.
11. Plug in the unit and warm the pad before use. Apply the aquathermia pad to the prescribed area (Figure 3). Secure with roller gauze or tape.	Plugging in the pad readies it for use. Heat travels by conduction from one object to another. Gauze bandage or tape holds the pad in position; **do not use pins, as they may puncture and damage the pad.**
12. Remove PPE, if used, and perform hand hygiene.	Proper removal of PPE reduces the risk for infection transmission and contamination of other items. Hand hygiene prevents the spread of microorganisms.

ACTION

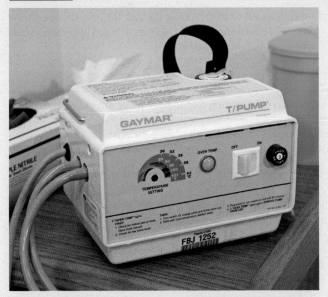

FIGURE 1. External heating pad electronic unit.

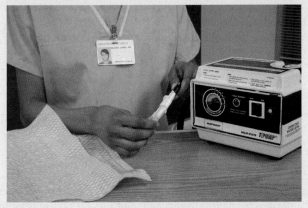

FIGURE 2. Attaching pad tubing to electronic unit tubing.

13. **Monitor the condition of the skin and the patient's response to the heat at frequent intervals, according to facility policy. Do not exceed the prescribed length of time for the application of heat.**

14. After the prescribed time for the treatment (up to 20 to 30 minutes) (Cleveland Clinic, 2020; Klein, 2019) remove the aquathermia pad. **Do not exceed the prescribed amount of time.** Reassess the patient and area of application, noting the effect and presence of any adverse effects.

15. Remove all remaining equipment; place the patient in a comfortable position, with side rails up as indicated and bed in the lowest position.

RATIONALE

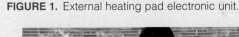

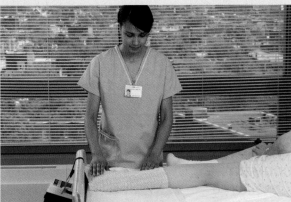

FIGURE 3. Applying heating pad to the prescribed area.

Maximum **vasodilation** and therapeutic effects from the application of heat occur within 20 to 30 minutes. Using heat for more than this amount of time results in tissue congestion and **vasoconstriction**, known as the rebound phenomenon (Taylor et al., 2023). Prolonged heat application may also result in an increased risk of burns and tissue damage (Taylor et al., 2023). Assessment of the patient's skin is necessary for early detection of adverse effects, thereby allowing prompt intervention to avoid complications.

Using heat for more than this amount of time results in tissue congestion and vasoconstriction, known as the rebound phenomenon. Prolonged heat application may also result in an increased risk of burns and tissue damage (Taylor et al., 2023). Assessment provides input as to the effectiveness of the treatment.

Proper patient and bed positioning promotes safety and comfort.

(continued on page 524)

Skill 8-11 ▶ Applying an External Heating Pad *(continued)*

ACTION

16. Remove additional PPE, if used. Perform hand hygiene.

RATIONALE

Proper removal of PPE reduces the risk for infection transmission and contamination of other items. Hand hygiene prevents the spread of microorganisms.

EVALUATION

The expected outcomes have been met when (depending on the patient's health problem or need) the patient has experienced increased comfort, the patient has experienced decreased muscle spasms, the patient has experienced a reduction in inflammation, the patient has remained free from injury, and the patient has demonstrated knowledge of safe application of the external heat source.

DOCUMENTATION

Guidelines

Document the rationale for application of heat therapy. If the patient is receiving heat therapy for pain, document the assessment of pain pre- and post-intervention. Specify the type of heat therapy and location where it is applied as well as the length of time applied. Record the condition of the skin, noting any redness or irritation before the heat application and after the application. Document the patient's reaction to the heat therapy. Record any appropriate patient or family/caregiver education.

Sample Documentation

> <u>9/13/25</u> 2300 Patient states he has lower back pain, rating it 5 of 10, constant and aching. Aquathermia pad applied to patient's lower back for 30 minutes; patient now rating pain as 2 of 10 and intermittent. Skin without signs of redness or irritation before and after application.
>
> —M. Martinez, RN

DEVELOPING CLINICAL REASONING AND CLINICAL JUDGMENT

UNEXPECTED SITUATIONS AND ASSOCIATED INTERVENTIONS

- *When performing a periodic assessment of the site during the application of heat, the nurse notes excessive swelling and redness at the site and the patient reports pain that was not present prior to the application of heat:* Remove the heat source. Assess the patient for other symptoms and obtain vital signs. Report your findings to the health care team and document the assessment and related interventions in the patient's record. Complete a variance or occurrence report, based on facility policy and procedures, to document the occurrence of an event that is out of the ordinary that has the potential to result in harm (Taylor et al., 2023).

SPECIAL CONSIDERATIONS

General Considerations

- Direct heat treatment may be contraindicated for patients at risk for bleeding, patients with a sprained limb in the acute stage, or patients with a condition associated with acute inflammation (Klein, 2019). Use cautiously with children and older adults. Patients with diabetes, stroke, spinal cord injury, and peripheral neuropathy are at risk for thermal injury, as are patients with very thin or damaged skin. Be extremely careful when applying to heat-sensitive areas, such as scar tissue and stomas.
- Instruct the patient not to lean or lie directly on the heating device, as this reduces air space and increases the risk of burns.
- Check the water level in the aquathermia unit periodically. Evaporation may occur. If the unit runs dry, it could become damaged. Refill with distilled water periodically.

Older Adult Considerations

- Older adults are more at risk for skin and tissue damage because of their thin skin, loss of heat sensation, decreased subcutaneous tissue, and changes in the body's ability to regulate temperature (Eliopoulos, 2018). Check these patients more frequently during therapy.

Community-Based Care Considerations

- A hot water bag or commercially prepared hot pack may be used in the home to apply heat. If using a hot water bag, fill with hot tap water to warm the bag, then empty it to detect any leaks. Check the temperature of the water with a thermometer or test on your inner wrist, adjusting the temperature as prescribed. (Water used for heat applications needs to be at the appropriate temperature to avoid skin damage: set the temperature of the water within a range of 105° to 109°F (40.5° to 43°C), which is considered to be physiologically effective and comfortable for the patient (Taylor et al., 2023). **Water temperature should not exceed 120°F (49°C)** (International Association of Fire Fighters, n.d.). Fill the bag one half to two thirds full. Partial filling keeps the bag lightweight and flexible so that it can be molded to the treatment area. Squeeze the bag until the water reaches the neck; this expels air, which would make the bag inflexible and would reduce heat conduction. Fasten the top and cover the bag with an absorbent cloth. The covering protects the skin from direct contact with the bag. If using a commercially prepared hot pack, follow manufacturer's directions and carefully assess skin before and after heat application.
- Electric heating pads may be used in the home to apply heat. Avoid the use of pins to prevent electric shocks. Use a dry covering over the pad to protect skin. Place a heating pad anteriorly or laterally to, not under, the body part. If the heating pad is between the patient and the mattress, heat dissipation may be inadequate, leading to burning of the patient or the bed linens. Caution the patient to use a heating pad with a selector switch that cannot be turned up beyond a safe temperature. The patient's receptors adapt to the initial application of heat, the patient may attempt to inappropriately increase the heat because the pad does not seem sufficiently warm, with the potential for burns (Taylor et al., 2023).

Skill 8-12 ▶ Applying a Warm Compress

Warm, moist compresses are used to help promote circulation, encourage healing, decrease edema, promote consolidation of exudate, and decrease pain and discomfort. Moist heat softens crusted material and is less drying to the skin. Moist heat also penetrates tissues more deeply than dry heat.

The prescribed intervention should include information addressing the type of application, the body area to be treated, the frequency of application, and the length of time for the applications. Water used for heat applications needs to be at the appropriate temperature to avoid skin damage: set the temperature of the water within a range of 105° to 109°F (40.5° to 43°C), which is considered to be physiologically effective and comfortable for the patient (Taylor et al., 2023). **Water temperature should not exceed 120°F (49°C)** (International Association of Fire Fighters, n.d.). Many facilities have warming devices to heat the dressing package to an appropriate temperature for the compress. These devices help reduce the risk of burning or skin damage.

The heat of a warm compress dissipates quickly, so the compresses must be changed frequently. If a constant warm temperature is required, a heating device such as an aquathermia pad (refer to Skill 8-11) is applied over the compress. However, **because moisture conducts heat, a low temperature setting is needed on the heating device.**

DELEGATION CONSIDERATIONS

The application of a warm compress may be delegated to assistive personnel (AP) as well as to licensed practical/vocational nurses (LPN/LVNs). The decision to delegate must be based on careful analysis of the patient's needs and circumstances as well as the qualifications of the person to whom the task is being delegated. Refer to the Delegation Guidelines in Appendix A.

EQUIPMENT

- Prescribed solution to moisten the compress material, warmed to 105° to 109°F (40.5° to 43°C) (Taylor et al., 2023
- Container for solution
- Gauze dressings or compresses
- Alternatively, obtain the appropriate number of commercially packaged, prewarmed dressings from the warming device
- Clean, disposable gloves
- Additional PPE, as indicated
- Waterproof pad and bath blanket
- Dry bath towel
- Tape or ties
- Aquathermia or other external heating device, if prescribed required to maintain the temperature of the compress

(continued on page 526)

Skill 8-12 ▶ Applying a Warm Compress *(continued)*

ASSESSMENT	Assess the situation to determine the appropriateness for the application of heat. Identify patients at risk for burns, including older adults, young children, cognitively and physically impaired persons (Field, 2018). Assess the patient's physical and mental status and the condition of the body area to be treated with heat. Assess for circulatory compromise in the area where the compress will be applied, including skin color, pulses distal to the site, evidence of edema, and the presence of sensation. Assess the equipment to be used, if necessary, including the condition of cords, plugs, and heating elements. Look for fluid leaks. Once the equipment is turned on, make sure there is a consistent distribution of heat and the temperature is within safe limits. Assess the application site frequently during the treatment, as tissue damage can occur.
ACTUAL OR POTENTIAL HEALTH PROBLEMS AND NEEDS	Many actual or potential health problems or issues may require the use of this skill as part of related interventions. An appropriate health problem or issue may include: • Chronic pain • Acute pain • Altered skin integrity risk
OUTCOME IDENTIFICATION AND PLANNING	The expected outcome to achieve when applying a warm compress depends on the patient's health problem or need and the rationale for application. Outcomes that may be appropriate include the following: the patient experiences increased comfort, the patient experiences decreased muscle spasms, the patient experiences a reduction in inflammation, the patient remains free from injury, and the patient demonstrates knowledge of safe application of the external heat source.

IMPLEMENTATION

ACTION	RATIONALE
1. Review the patient's health record for prescribed intervention for the application of a moist warm compress, including the frequency and length of time for the application. Gather necessary supplies.	Reviewing the health record and care plan validates the correct patient and correct procedure. Preparation promotes efficient time management and an organized approach to the task.
2. Perform hand hygiene and put on PPE, if indicated.	Hand hygiene and PPE prevent the spread of microorganisms. PPE is required based on transmission precautions.
3. Identify the patient.	Identifying the patient ensures the right patient receives the intervention and helps prevent errors.
4. Assemble equipment on the overbed table or other surface within reach.	Organization facilitates performance of task.
5. Assess the patient for possible need for nonpharmacologic pain-reducing interventions or analgesic medication before beginning the procedure. Administer appropriate analgesic, as prescribed, and allow enough time for the analgesic to achieve its effectiveness before beginning the procedure.	Pain is a subjective experience influenced by past experience. Depending on the site of application, manipulation of the area may cause pain for some patients.
6. Close the curtains around the bed and close the door to the room, if possible. Explain what you are going to do and why you are going to do it to the patient.	This ensures the patient's privacy. Explanation relieves anxiety and facilitates engagement.
7. If using an electronic heating device with the compress, check that the water in the unit is at the appropriate level. Fill the unit two thirds full with distilled water, or to the fill mark, if necessary. Check the temperature setting on the unit to ensure it is within the safe range (refer to Skill 8-11).	Sufficient water in the unit is necessary to ensure proper function of the unit. Tap water leaves mineral deposits in the unit. Checking the temperature setting helps to prevent skin or tissue damage.

ACTION	**RATIONALE**
8. Assist the patient to a comfortable position that provides easy access to the area. Use a bath blanket to cover any exposed area other than the intended site. Place a waterproof pad under the site.	Patient positioning and the use of a bath blanket provide for comfort and warmth. Waterproof pad protects underlying surfaces.
9. Place a waste receptacle at a convenient location for use during the procedure.	Having a waste container handy means that the used materials may be discarded easily, without the spread of microorganisms.
10. Pour the warmed solution into the container and drop the gauze for the compress into the solution. Alternatively, if commercially packaged, prewarmed gauze is used, open packaging.	Prepares compress for application.
11. Put on gloves. Assess the application site for inflammation, skin color, and ecchymosis.	Gloves protect the nurse from potential contact with microorganisms. Assessment provides information about the area, the healing process, and the presence of infection, and allows for documentation of the condition of the area before the compress is applied.
12. Retrieve the compress from the warmed solution, squeezing out any excess moisture. Alternatively, remove pre-warmed gauze from open package. **Apply the compress by gently and carefully molding it to the intended area (Figure 1). Ask the patient if the application feels too hot.**	Excess moisture may contaminate the surrounding area and is uncomfortable for the patient. Molding the compress to the skin promotes retention of warmth around the site.
13. Cover the site with a clean dry bath towel (Figure 2); secure in place with a tape or roller gauze, if necessary.	The towel provides extra insulation.

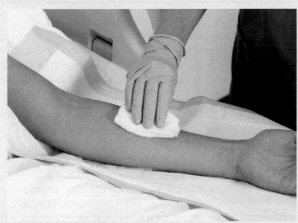

FIGURE 1. Applying compress to the intended area.

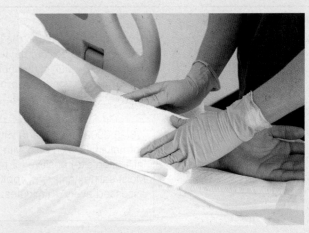

FIGURE 2. Covering site with clean dry bath towel.

ACTION	**RATIONALE**
14. Place the aquathermia or heating device, if used, over the towel. Refer to Skill 8-11.	The use of a heating device maintains the temperature of the compress and extends the therapeutic effect.
15. Remove gloves and discard them appropriately. Perform hand hygiene and remove additional PPE, if used.	Hand hygiene prevents the spread of microorganisms. Proper removal of PPE reduces the risk for infection transmission and contamination of other items.
16. **Monitor the time the compress is in place to prevent burns and skin/tissue damage. Monitor the condition of the patient's skin and the patient's response at frequent intervals.**	Extended use of heat results in an increased risk for burns from the heat. Impaired circulation may affect the patient's sensitivity to heat. Assessment of the patient's skin is necessary for early detection of adverse effects, thereby allowing prompt intervention to avoid complications.
17. After the prescribed time for the treatment (up to 20 to 30 minutes) (Cleveland Clinic, 2020; Klein, 2019) remove the aquathermia pad. **Do not exceed the prescribed amount of time.** Reassess the patient and area of application, noting the effect and presence of any adverse effects. Put on gloves.	Using heat for more than this amount of time results in tissue congestion and vasoconstriction, known as the "rebound phenomenon." Prolonged heat application may also result in an increased risk of burns and tissue damage (Taylor et al., 2023). Gloves protect the nurse from potential contact with microorganisms.

(continued on page 528)

Skill 8-12 ▶ Applying a Warm Compress *(continued)*

ACTION	**RATIONALE**
18. Carefully remove the compress while assessing the skin condition around the site and observing the patient's response to the heat application. Note any changes in the application area.	Assessment provides information about the healing process; the presence of irritation or infection should be documented.
19. Remove gloves. Perform hand hygiene.	Proper removal of gloves prevents the spread of microorganisms. Hand hygiene prevents the transmission of microorganisms.
20. Place the patient in a comfortable position. Lower the bed. Dispose of any other supplies appropriately.	Repositioning promotes patient comfort and safety.
21. Remove additional PPE, if used. Perform hand hygiene.	Proper removal of PPE reduces the risk for infection transmission and contamination of other items. Hand hygiene prevents the spread of microorganisms.

EVALUATION

The expected outcomes have been met when (depending on the patient's health problem or need) the patient has experienced increased comfort, the patient has experienced decreased muscle spasms, the patient has experienced a reduction in inflammation, the patient has remained free from injury, and the patient has demonstrated knowledge of safe application of the external heat source.

DOCUMENTATION

Guidelines

Document the procedure, the length of time the compress was applied, including any use of an aquathermia pad. Record the temperature of the aquathermia pad and length of application time. Include a description of the application area, noting any edema, redness, or ecchymosis. Document the patient's reaction to the procedure including pain assessment. Record any patient and family/caregiver education provided.

Sample Documentation

> 7/6/25 0900 Left forearm with positive radial pulse, sensation and movement within normal limits, skin pale with brisk capillary refill. Left medial forearm (IV access infiltration site) positive for redness, edema; no evidence of maceration or drainage. Moist saline compress applied with aquathermia pad set at 100°F for 30 minutes. Site assessed every 10 minutes; no evidence of injury noted. Left arm elevated on pillows.
> —S. Tran, RN

DEVELOPING CLINICAL REASONING AND CLINICAL JUDGMENT

UNEXPECTED SITUATIONS AND ASSOCIATED INTERVENTIONS

- *The nurse is monitoring a patient with a warm compress. Procedure requires that the nurse check the area of application every 5 minutes for tissue tolerance. The nurse notes excessive redness and slight maceration of the surrounding skin, and the patient verbalizes increased discomfort:* Stop the heat application. Remove the compress. Assess the patient for other symptoms and obtain vital signs. Report your findings to the health care team and document the assessment and related interventions in the patient's record. Complete a variance or occurrence report, based on facility policy and procedures to document the occurrence of an event that is out of the ordinary that has the potential to result in harm (Taylor et al., 2023).

SPECIAL CONSIDERATIONS

General Considerations
- Use warm moist compresses cautiously with children and older adults.
- Patients with diabetes, stroke, spinal cord injury, and peripheral neuropathy are at increased risk for thermal injury, as are patients with very thin or damaged skin.
- Be extremely careful when applying to heat-sensitive areas, such as scar tissue and stomas.

Older Adult Considerations
- Older adults are more at risk for skin and tissue damage because of their thin skin, loss of heat sensation, decreased subcutaneous tissue, and changes in the body's ability to regulate temperature (Eliopoulos, 2018). Check these patients more frequently during therapy.

Skill 8-13 ▶ Assisting With a Sitz Bath

A sitz bath is a method of applying tepid or warm water to the perineal, pelvic, or anal areas by sitting in a basin filled with this water. A sitz bath can help relieve itching, pain, and discomfort in the perineal area, such as after childbirth or surgery or from hemorrhoids, and can increase circulation to the tissues, promoting healing.

DELEGATION CONSIDERATIONS

Assisting with a sitz bath may be delegated to assistive personnel (AP) as well as to licensed practical/vocational nurses (LPN/LVNs). The decision to delegate must be based on careful analysis of the patient's needs and circumstances as well as the qualifications of the person to whom the task is being delegated. Refer to the Delegation Guidelines in Appendix A.

EQUIPMENT

- Clean gloves
- Additional PPE, as indicated
- Towel
- Adjustable IV pole
- Disposable sitz bath bowl with water bag

ASSESSMENT

Assess the situation to determine the appropriateness for the application of heat. Assess the patient's physical and mental status and the condition of the body area to be treated with heat. Determine the patient's ability to ambulate to the bathroom and maintain a sitting position for 15 to 20 minutes. Prior to the sitz bath, inspect perineal/rectal area for swelling, drainage, redness, warmth, and tenderness. Assess bladder fullness and encourage the patient to void before sitz bath. Confirm the prescribed intervention for the sitz bath, including frequency and length of time for the application. Assess the application site frequently during the treatment, as tissue damage can occur.

ACTUAL OR POTENTIAL HEALTH PROBLEMS AND NEEDS

Many actual or potential health problems or issues may require the use of this skill as part of related interventions. An appropriate health problem or issue may include:
- Infection risk
- Acute pain
- Altered skin integrity

OUTCOME IDENTIFICATION AND PLANNING

The expected outcome to achieve when administering a sitz bath is that the patient verbalizes an increase in comfort. Other outcomes that may be appropriate include the following: the patient remains free of any signs and symptoms of infection and exhibits signs and symptoms of healing.

IMPLEMENTATION

ACTION	RATIONALE
1. Review the patient's health record for prescribed intervention for the application of a sitz bath, including the frequency and length of time for the application. Gather necessary supplies.	Reviewing the health record and care plan validates the correct patient and correct procedure. Preparation promotes efficient time management and an organized approach to the task.

(continued on page 530)

Skill 8-13 ▶ Assisting With a Sitz Bath *(continued)*

ACTION	RATIONALE
2. Perform hand hygiene and put on PPE, if indicated.	Hand hygiene and PPE prevent the spread of microorganisms. PPE is required based on transmission precautions.
3. Identify the patient.	Identifying the patient ensures the right patient receives the intervention and helps prevent errors.
4. Close the curtains around the bed and close the door to the room, if possible.	This ensures the patient's privacy.
5. Put on gloves. Assemble equipment either at the bedside if using a bedside commode or in the bathroom.	Gloves prevent exposure to blood and body fluids. Organization facilitates performance of task.
6. Raise the lid of the toilet or commode. Place the bowl of the sitz bath, with drainage ports to the rear and infusion port in front, in the toilet (Figure 1). Fill the bowl of the sitz bath about halfway full with tepid to warm water (within a range of 105° to 109°F (40.5° to 43°C) (Taylor et al., 2023). **Water temperature should not exceed 120°F (49°C)** (International Association of Fire Fighters, n.d.). Add salt or medicine to the water if prescribed (Saint Luke's, n.d.).	Sitz bath will not drain appropriately if placed in the toilet backward. Tepid water can promote relaxation and help with edema; warm water can help with circulation. Water used for heat applications needs to be at the appropriate temperature to avoid skin damage: set the temperature of the water within a range of 105° to 109°F (40.5° to 43°C), which is considered to be physiologically effective and comfortable for the patient (Taylor et al., 2023). **Water temperature should not exceed 120°F (49°C)** (International Association of Fire Fighters, n.d.).

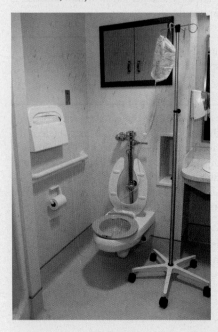

FIGURE 1. Disposable sitz bath in place in toilet.

ACTION	RATIONALE
7. Clamp tubing on the bag. Fill the bag with same temperature water as mentioned above. Hang the bag above the patient's shoulder height on the IV pole.	If the bag is hung lower, the flow rate will not be sufficient, and water may cool too quickly.
8. Assist the patient to sit on the toilet or commode. The patient should be able to sit in the basin or tub with the feet flat on the floor without any pressure on the sacrum or thighs. Wrap a blanket around the shoulders and provide extra draping, if needed. Insert tubing into the infusion port of the sitz bath. Slowly unclamp tubing and allow the sitz bath to fill.	Excessive pressure on the sacrum or thighs could cause tissue injury. Blanket and draping protect from chilling and exposure. If tubing is placed into the sitz bath before the patient sits on the toilet, the patient may trip over tubing. Filling the sitz bath ensures that the tissue is submerged in water.

ACTION

9. Clamp tubing once the sitz bath is full. Instruct the patient to open clamp when water in bowl becomes cool. **Ensure that the call bell is within reach. Instruct the patient to call if he or she feels light-headed or dizzy or has any problems. Instruct the patient not to try standing without assistance.**

10. Remove gloves and perform hand hygiene.

11. When the patient is finished (in about 10 to 20 minutes, or prescribed time), put on gloves. Assist the patient to stand and gently pat the perineal area dry. Remove gloves. Perform hand hygiene.

12. Assist the patient to bed or chair. Ensure that the call bell is within reach.

13. Put on gloves. Empty and disinfect sitz bath bowl according to facility policy.

14. Remove gloves and any additional PPE, if used. Perform hand hygiene.

RATIONALE

Cool water may produce hypothermia. The patient may become light-headed due to vasodilation, so call bell should be within reach.

Hand hygiene deters the spread of microorganisms.

Gloves prevent contact with blood and body fluids. The patient may be light-headed or dizzy due to vasodilation. The patient should not stand alone and bending over to dry self may cause the patient to fall.

The patient should not stand or walk alone. Having call bell within reach ensures the patient is able to ring for assistance as needed.

Proper equipment cleaning deters the spread of microorganisms.

Proper removal of PPE reduces the risk for infection transmission and contamination of other items. Hand hygiene prevents the spread of microorganisms.

EVALUATION

The expected outcomes have been met when the patient has verbalized an increase in comfort, the patient has remained free of any signs and symptoms of infection, and the patient exhibits signs and symptoms of healing.

DOCUMENTATION

Guidelines

Document administration of the sitz bath, including water temperature and duration. Document patient response and assessment of perineum, pelvic, and/or rectal areas before and after administration.

Sample Documentation

7/30/25 1620 Perineum assessed. Episiotomy edges well approximated, no drainage noted. Patient assisted to sitz bath. Patient took warm water sitz bath (temperature 99°F) for 20 minutes. Denies feeling light-headed or dizzy. Assisted back to bed after bath. Patient states pain level has dropped "from a 5 to a 2."

—C. Stone, RN

DEVELOPING CLINICAL REASONING AND CLINICAL JUDGMENT

UNEXPECTED SITUATIONS AND ASSOCIATED INTERVENTIONS

- *Patient reports feeling light-headed or dizzy during sitz bath:* Stop sitz bath. Do not attempt to ambulate the patient alone. Use the call bell to summon help. Let the patient sit on the toilet until feeling subsides or help has arrived to assist the patient back to bed.
- *Temperature of water is uncomfortable:* The water may be too warm or cold, depending on the patient's preference. If this happens, clamp the tubing, disconnect the water bag, and refill it with water that is comfortable for the patient, but no warmer than 120°F (49°C) (International Association of Fire Fighters, n.d.).

(continued on page 532)

Skill 8-13 ▶ Assisting With a Sitz Bath   (continued)

SPECIAL CONSIDERATIONS

Community-Based Care Considerations

- A sitz bath can be accomplished in a bathtub as well. Fill a clean bathtub with 3 to 4 inches of warm water. The patient may add salt or medicine as prescribed, and sits on the bottom of the tub, with the area to be treated submerged in the water (Saint Luke's, n.d.).

Skill 8-14 ▶ Applying Cold Therapy

Skill Variation: *Applying an Electronically Controlled Cooling Device*

Cold constricts the peripheral blood vessels, reducing blood flow to the tissues and decreasing the local release of pain-producing substances (Cleveland Clinic, 2020). Cold reduces the formation of edema and inflammation, reduces muscle spasm, and promotes comfort by slowing the transmission of pain stimuli. The application of cold therapy reduces bleeding and hematoma formation. The application of cold is appropriate after direct trauma, for dental pain, for muscle spasms, after muscle sprains, and for the treatment of chronic pain (Klein, 2019). Ice can be used to apply cold therapy, usually in the form of an ice bag or ice collar, or in a glove. Commercially prepared cold packs are also available. For electronically controlled cooling devices, see the accompanying Skill Variation.

DELEGATION CONSIDERATIONS

The application of cold therapy may be delegated to assistive personnel (AP) as well as to licensed practical/vocational nurses (LPN/LVNs). The decision to delegate must be based on careful analysis of the patient's needs and circumstances, as well as the qualifications of the person to whom the task is being delegated. Refer to the Delegation Guidelines in Appendix A.

EQUIPMENT

- Ice bag, ice collar, glove, and ice
- Commercially prepared cold packs
- Small towel or washcloth
- PPE, as indicated
- Disposable waterproof pad
- Gauze wrap or tape
- Bath blanket

ASSESSMENT

Assess the situation to determine the appropriateness for the application of cold therapy. Assess the patient's physical and mental status and the condition of the body area to be treated with the cold therapy. Assess for circulatory compromise in the area where the compress will be applied, including skin color, pulses distal to the site, evidence of edema, and the presence of sensation. Confirm the prescribed intervention for the application of cold, including frequency, type of therapy, body area to be treated, and length of time for the application. Assess the equipment to be used to make sure it will function properly. Assess the application site frequently during the treatment, as tissue damage can occur.

ACTUAL OR POTENTIAL HEALTH PROBLEMS AND NEEDS

Many actual or potential health problems or issues may require the use of this skill as part of related interventions. An appropriate health problem or issue may include:
- Chronic pain
- Acute pain
- Injury risk

OUTCOME IDENTIFICATION AND PLANNING

The expected outcome to achieve when applying cold therapy depends on the patient's health problem or need and the rationale for application. Outcomes that may be appropriate include the following: the patient experiences increased comfort, the patient experiences decreased muscle spasms, the patient experiences decreased inflammation, the patient remains free from injury, and the patient demonstrates knowledge of safe application of the external cold source.

IMPLEMENTATION

ACTION	RATIONALE
1. Review the patient's health record for prescribed intervention or plan of care for the application of cold therapy, including frequency, type of therapy, body area to be treated, and length of time for the application. Gather necessary supplies.	Reviewing the health record validates the correct patient and correct procedure. Preparation promotes efficient time management and an organized approach to the task.
2. Perform hand hygiene and put on PPE, if indicated.	Hand hygiene and PPE prevent the spread of microorganisms. PPE is required based on transmission precautions.
3. Identify the patient. Determine if the patient has had any previous adverse reaction to cold therapy.	Identifying the patient ensures the right patient receives the intervention and helps prevent errors. Individual differences exist in tolerating specific therapies.
4. Assemble equipment on the overbed table or other surface within reach.	Organization facilitates performance of task.
5. Close the curtains around the bed and close the door to the room, if possible. Explain what you are going to do and why you are going to do it to the patient.	This ensures the patient's privacy. Explanation relieves anxiety and facilitates engagement.
6. Assess the condition of the skin where the cold is to be applied.	Assessment supplies baseline data for posttreatment comparison and identifies any conditions that may contraindicate the application.
7. Assist the patient to a comfortable position that provides easy access to the area to be treated. Expose the area and drape the patient with a bath blanket, if needed. Put the waterproof pad under the treatment area, if necessary.	Patient positioning and the use of a bath blanket provide for comfort and warmth. Waterproof pad protects the patient and the bed linens.
8. Prepare device: Fill the bag, collar, or glove about three fourths full with ice (Figure 1). Remove any excess air from the device. Securely fasten the end of the bag or collar; tie the glove closed, checking for holes and leakage of water. Prepare commercially prepared ice pack, according to the manufacturer's directions, if appropriate.	Ice provides a cold surface. Excess air interferes with cold conduction. Fastening the end prevents leaks.

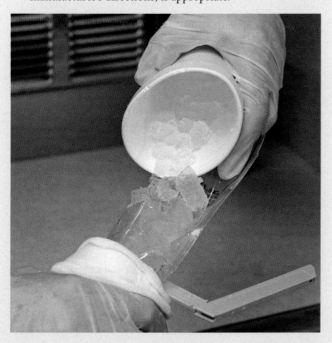

FIGURE 1. Filling ice bag with ice.

(*continued on page 534*)

Skill 8-14 ▶ Applying Cold Therapy *(continued)*

ACTION	RATIONALE
9. **Cover the device with a towel or washcloth; commercially prepared devices may come with a cover (Figure 2).** (If the device has a cloth exterior, this is not necessary.)	The cover protects the skin and absorbs condensation.
10. Positioning the ice bag on the intended area and lightly secure in place, as needed (Figure 3).	Proper positioning ensures the cold therapy to the specified body area.

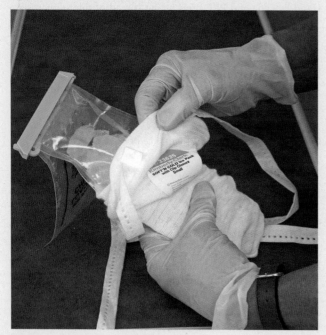

FIGURE 2. Covering ice bag with cover.

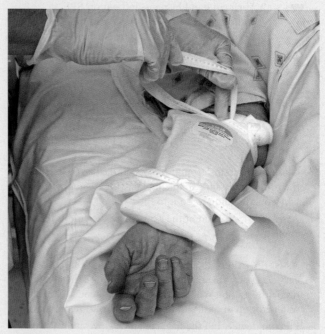

FIGURE 3. Positioning ice bag on the intended area and securing in place.

ACTION	RATIONALE
11. **Remove the ice and assess the site for redness after 30 seconds. Ask the patient about the presence of burning sensations.**	These actions prevent tissue injury.
12. Replace the device snugly against the site if no problems are evident. Secure it in place with gauze wrap, ties, or tape.	Wrapping or taping stabilizes the device in the proper location.
13. **Monitor the time the compress is in place to prevent burns and skin/tissue damage. Monitor the condition of the patient's skin and the patient's response at frequent intervals.**	Assessment of the patient's skin is necessary for early detection of adverse effects, thereby allowing prompt intervention to avoid complications.
14. After the prescribed time for the treatment (up to 20 minutes) (Cleveland Clinic, 2020; Klein, 2019), remove the cold therapy and dry the skin. **Do not exceed the prescribed amount of time.**	Limiting the time of application prevents injury due to overexposure to cold. Prolonged application of cold may result in decreased blood flow with resulting tissue **ischemia**. A compensatory vasodilation or rebound phenomenon may also occur as a means to provide warmth to the area.
15. Remove PPE, if used. Perform hand hygiene.	Proper removal of PPE reduces the risk for infection transmission and contamination of other items. Hand hygiene prevents the spread of microorganisms.
16. Place the patient in a comfortable position. Lower the bed. Dispose of any other supplies appropriately.	Repositioning promotes patient comfort and safety.
17. Remove additional PPE, if used. Perform hand hygiene.	Proper removal of PPE reduces the risk for infection transmission and contamination of other items. Hand hygiene prevents the spread of microorganisms.

EVALUATION	The expected outcomes have been met when (depending on the patient's health problem or need) the patient has reported increased comfort, the patient has verbalized a decrease in muscle spasms, the patient has exhibited a reduction in inflammation, the patient has remained free from injury, and the patient has demonstrated knowledge of safe application of the cold therapy.

DOCUMENTATION

Guidelines

Document the location of the application, time of placement, and time of removal of the cold therapy. Record the assessment of the area where the cold therapy was applied, including the patient's mobility, sensation, color, temperature, and any presence of numbness, tingling, or pain. Document the patient's response, such as any decrease in pain or change in sensation. Include any pertinent patient and family/caregiver education.

Sample Documentation

> 11/1/25 1430 Swelling noted on right lower extremity from mid-calf to foot. Toes warm, pink, positive sensation and movement, negative for numbness, tingling, and pain. Ice bags wrapped in cloth applied to right ankle and lower calf. Patient instructed to communicate any changes in sensation or pain; verbalizes an understanding of information.
> —L. Semet, RN
>
> 11/1/20 1450 Ice removed from right lower extremity; neurovascular assessment unchanged. Right lower extremity elevated on two pillows.
> —L. Semet, RN

DEVELOPING CLINICAL REASONING AND CLINICAL JUDGMENT

UNEXPECTED SITUATIONS AND ASSOCIATED INTERVENTIONS

- *When performing a skin assessment during therapy, the nurse notes increased pallor at the treatment site and sluggish capillary refill, and the patient reports alterations in sensation at the application site:* Discontinue therapy, obtain vital signs, assess for other symptoms, notify the health care team, and document the event in the patient's record.

SPECIAL CONSIDERATIONS

General Considerations

- Allow at least 20 to 30 minutes between episodes of application of cold therapy (Cleveland Clinic, 2020; Klein, 2019).

Older Adult Considerations

- Older adults are more at risk for skin and tissue damage because of their thin skin, loss of cold sensation, decreased subcutaneous tissue, and changes in the body's ability to regulate the temperature. Check these patients more frequently during therapy.

Community-Based Care Considerations

- A bag of frozen vegetables (such as peas or corn) or ice cubes in a baggie makes a good substitute for an ice pack (Cleveland Clinic, 2020).

(continued on page 536)

Skill 8-14 ▶ Applying Cold Therapy *(continued)*

Skill Variation ▶ Applying an Electronically Controlled Cooling Device

Electronically controlled cooling devices may be used in situations to deliver a constant cooling effect, such as after orthopedic surgery or for patients with acute musculoskeletal injuries. Use of this device is a prescribed intervention. Initial and ongoing assessment of the involved extremity or body area is necessary throughout the period of use. As with application of any electronic device, ongoing monitoring for proper functioning and temperature regulation is necessary.

1. Gather equipment and verify the prescribed intervention.

2. Perform hand hygiene. Put on PPE, as indicated.

3. Identify the patient and explain the procedure.
4. Assess the involved extremity or body part.
5. Set the correct temperature on the device.

6. Plug in the unit and cool the pad before use. Assess to ensure that the cooling pad is functioning properly.
7. Wrap the cooling water-flow pad around the involved body part.
8. Wrap roller gauze, Ace bandage, or tape around the water-flow pads to secure in place.

9. Remove PPE, if used. Perform hand hygiene.

10. Monitor frequently to ensure proper functioning of equipment.
11. Unwrap at intervals to assess skin integrity of the body part.
12. Remove device after the prescribed time for the treatment (up to 20 minutes) (Cleveland Clinic, 2020; Klein, 2019). Do not exceed the prescribed amount of time.

EVIDENCE FOR PRACTICE ▶

COLD APPLICATION AND PAIN RELIEF

Chest tube removal is a painful procedure for many, if not most, patients. Pharmacologic and nonpharmacologic interventions have been used to decrease patients' discomfort during this procedure.

Related Research

Özcan, N., & Karagözoğlu, Ş. (2020). Effects of progressive muscle relaxation exercise, cold application and local anesthesia performed before chest tube removal on pain and comfort levels and vital signs of the patient. *Turkiye Klinikleri Journal of Medical Sciences*, 40(3), 285–296. https://doi.org/10.5336/medsci.2019-72505

The objective of this randomized controlled experiment was to examine whether progressive muscle relaxation exercise, the application of cold to the chest wall, and local anesthesia had an effect on pain and comfort related to chest tube removal. The study was conducted with 160 adult patients admitted to the inpatient thoracic surgery department who had a chest tube. Participants were randomly assigned to one of the three intervention groups or the control group. Pain intensity, comfort level, and vital signs were measured within 5 minutes before the chest tube was removed. Participants in the progressive muscle relaxation exercise group ($n = 40$) performed progressive muscle relaxation exercises for 1 to 2 minutes prior to tube removal. Participants in the cold application group ($n = 40$) had a cold gel pack wrapped in gauze placed directly on the site of chest tube insertion for 20 minutes prior to tube removal. Participants in the local anesthesia group ($n = 40$) received an injection of a local anesthetic at the chest tube insertion site 1 to 2 minutes prior to tube removal. Patients in the control group ($n = 40$) did not receive any additional intervention prior to tube removal. Pain intensity, comfort level, and vital signs were again measured immediately after tube removal and 15 minutes after tube removal. The pain score in the relaxation exercise and control group increased and comfort decreased compared to before tube removal. Pain in the cold application and local anesthetic groups significantly decreased ($p < .001$, $p < .001$) and comfort increased in both the period immediately after and 15 minutes after tube removal. No significant changes in vital signs were observed between any of the groups during and after chest tube removal. The authors concluded the application of cold and the use of local anesthesia were effective in reducing pain and increasing comfort related to removal of chest tubes. The researchers suggested the use of cold application and local anesthetic as a strategy to implement related to chest tube removal.

Relevance for Nursing Practice

Nursing interventions related to decreasing pain and increasing patient comfort are an important nursing responsibility. Interventions should include the use of nonpharmacologic interventions, in addition to the administration of analgesics. The application of cold to the chest wall could significantly decrease the pain and discomfort experienced by a patient during removal of a chest tube. Nurses could easily incorporate this simple intervention as part of nursing care for these patients.

Enhance Your Understanding

Focusing on Patient Care: Developing Clinical Reasoning and Clinical Judgment

Consider the case scenarios at the beginning of the chapter as you answer the following questions to enhance your understanding and apply what you have learned.

QUESTIONS

1. While providing wound care for Lori Downs' foot wound, you note that the drainage, which was scant and yellow 2 days ago, is now green and has saturated the old dressing. Should you continue with the prescribed wound care?

2. Three days ago, Tran Nguyen underwent a modified radical mastectomy. She has three Jackson-Pratt drains at her surgical site. She has started asking questions about her surgery and has anticipated discharge home. Until this morning, she has avoided looking at her surgical site. You are helping her with her bathing and dressing. As you help her remove her gown, she becomes visibly upset and anxious and exclaims, "Oh no! What's wrong? I'm bleeding from the cuts!" You realize she is looking at her drains. How should you respond?

3. Arthur Lowes has come to his surgeon's office today for a follow-up examination after a colon resection. After he sees the health care provider, you, the treatment nurse, will remove the surgical staples from the incision and apply adhesive wound strips. As you prepare to remove the staples, Mr. Lowes comments, "I hope my stomach doesn't pop out now!" What should you tell him?

You can find suggested answers after the Bibliography at the end of this chapter.

Integrated Case Study Connection

The case studies in the back of the book focus on integrating concepts. Refer to the following case studies to enhance your understanding of the concepts and skills in this chapter.

Bibliography

Alderen, J., Cowan, L. J., Dimas, J. B., Chen, D., Zhang, Y., Cummins, M., & Ypa, T. L. (2020). Risk factors for hospital-acquired pressure injury in surgical critical care patients. *American Journal of Critical Care, 29*(6), e128–e134. https://doi.org/10.4037/ajcc2020810

Al-Qudah, G., & Tuma, F. (2020). T tube. *StatPearls.* National Center for Biotechnology Information (NCBI), U.S. National Library of Medicine (NLM). https://www.ncbi.nlm.nih.gov/books/NBK532867/

Alvarez, O. M., Brindle, C. T., Langemo, D., Kennedy-Evans, K. L., Krasner, D. L., Brennan, M. R., & Levine, J. M. (2016). The VCU Pressure Ulcer Summit: The search for a clearer understanding and more precise clinical definition of the unavoidable pressure injury. *Journal of Wound, Ostomy, and Continence Nursing, 43*(5), 455–463. https://doi.org/10.1097/WON.0000000000000255

American College of Surgeons; Division of Education. (2018). *Surgical patient education program:* Prepare for the *best recovery.* https://www.facs.org/~/media/files/education/patient%20ed/wound_surgical.ashx

Annesley, S. H. (2019). Current thinking on caring for patients with a wound: A practical approach. *British Journal of Nursing, 28*(5), 290–294.

Apelqvist, J., Willy, C., Fagerdah, A. M., Fraccalvieri, M., Malmsjö, M., Piaggesi, A., Probst, A., Vowden, P., & European Wound Management Association (EWMA). (2017). EWMA document: Negative pressure wound therapy. Overview, challenges and perspectives. *Journal of Wound Care, 26*(Suppl 3), S1–S154. https://doi.org/10.12968/jowc.2017.26.Sup3.S1

Arnold, M., Needham, D. M., & Nydahl, P. (2018). International round table discussion: Early Mobility. *International Journal of Safe Patient Handling & Mobility (SPHM), 8*(1), 57–64.

Association of periOperative Registered Nurses (AORN). (2018). AORN guideline quick view: Sterile technique. *AORN Journal, 108*(6), 705–710. https://doi.org/10.1002/aorn.12458

Atkin, L. (2019). Chronic wounds: The challenges of appropriate management. *Community Wound Care, 24*(Suppl 9), S26–S32. https://doi.org/10.12968/bjcn.2019.24.Sup9.S26

Banasiewicz, T., Banky, B., Karsenti, A., Sancho, J., Sekáč, J., & Walczak, D. (2019). Traditional and single use NPWT: When to use and how to decide on the appropriate use? Recommendations of an expert panel. *Wounds International, 10*(3), 56–62.

Baranoski, S., & Ayello, E. A. (2020). *Wound care essentials. Practice principles* (5th ed.). Wolters Kluwer.

Baranoski, S., LeBlanc, K., & Gloeckner, M. (2016). Preventing, assessing, and managing skin tears: A clinical review. *American Journal of Nursing, 116*(11), 24–30. http://doi.org/10.1097/01.NAJ.0000505581.01967.75

Barton, A. (2020). Medical adhesive-related skin injuries associated with vascular access: Minimising risk with Appeel Sterile. *British Journal of Nursing, 29*(8), S20–S27. http://doi.org/10.12968/bjon.2020.29.8.S20

Bates-Jensen, B. M., McCreath, H. E., Harputlu, D., & Patlan, A. (2019). Reliability of the Bates-Jensen wound assessment tool for pressure injury assessment: The pressure ulcer detection study. *Wound Repair and Regeneration, 27*(4), 386–395. https://doi.org/10.1111/wrr.12714

Bauldoff, G., Gubrud, P., & Carno, M. A. (2020). *LeMone and Burke's Medical-surgical nursing: Clinical reasoning in patient care* (7th ed.). Pearson.

Benbow, M. (2016). Understanding safe practice in the use of negative pressure wound therapy in the community. *British Journal of Community Nursing, 21*(Suppl 12), S32–S34. https://doi.org/10.12968/bjcn.2016.21.Sup12.S32

Bergstrom, A., O'Harra, P., & Foster, W. M. (2018). Collaborative interdisciplinary teams and pressure injury prevention: High-acuity patient skin care requires consistent communication between perioperative and critical-care staff. *American Nurse Today, Supplement Pressure Injuries,* 27–28.

Black, J. (2018). Take three steps forward to prevent pressure injury in medical-surgical patients: Nursing care is key to pressure injury prevention. *American Nurse Today, Supplement,* 10–39.

Bonifant, H., & Holloway, S. (2019). A review of the effects of ageing on skin integrity and wound healing. *Community Wound Care, 24*(Suppl 3), S28–S33. https://doi.org/10.12968/bjcn.2019.24.Sup3.S28

Braden, B. J. (2012). The Braden Scale for predicting pressure sore risk: Reflections after 25 years. *Advances in Skin & Wound Care, 25*(2), 61.

Braden, B., & Maklebust, J. (2005). Preventing pressure ulcers with the Braden scale. *American Journal of Nursing, 105*(6), 70–72.

Brown, A. (2018). Dispelling some myths and misconceptions in wound care. *Journal of Community Nursing, 32*(6), 24–32.

Burr, S. (2018). Assessment and management of skin conditions in older people. *British Journal of Community Nursing, 23*(8), 388–393. https://doi.org/10.12968/bjcn.2018.23.8.388

Camacho-Del Rio, G. (2018). Evidence-based practice: Medical device-related pressure injury prevention. *American Nurse Today, 13*(10), 50–52.

Centers for Disease Control and Prevention (CDC). (2016). *Healthcare-associated infections (HAIs).* https://www.cdc.gov/hai/

Centers for Disease Control and Prevention (CDC). (2019, May 9). *Healthcare-associated infections (HAIs).* Frequently asked questions about surgical site infections. https://www.cdc.gov/HAI/ssi/faq_ssi.html

Cleveland Clinic. (2020, December 8). *Here's how to choose between using ice or heat for pain.* https://health.clevelandclinic.org/should-you-use-ice-or-heat-for-pain-infographic/

Cornish, L. (2017). The use of prophylactic dressings in the prevention of pressure ulcers: A literature review. *British Journal of Community Nursing, 22*(Suppl 6), S26–S32. https://doi.org/10.12968/bjcn.2017.22.Sup6.S26

Cornish, L., & Douglas, H. E. (2016). Cleansing of acute traumatic wounds: Tap water or normal saline? *Wounds UK, 12*(4), 30–35.

Dudek, S. (2018). *Nutrition essentials for nursing practice* (8th ed.). Wolters Kluwer.

Edwards, D., Bourke, N., Murdoch, J., & Verma, S. (2018). Using portable, single-use, canister-free, negative-pressure wound therapy for plastic surgery wounds. *Wounds UK, 14*(3), 56–62.

Eliopoulos, C. (2018). *Gerontological nursing* (9th ed.). Wolters Kluwer Health.

Ellis, M. (2017). Pressure ulcer prevention in care home settings. *Nursing Older People, 29*(3), 29–35.

European Pressure Ulcer Advisory Panel (EPUAP), National Pressure Injury Advisory Panel (NPIAP), and Pan Pacific Pressure Injury Alliance (PPPIA). (2019a). *Prevention and treatment of pressure ulcers/injuries: Clinical Practice guideline. The international guideline.* E. Haesler (Ed.). http://www.internationalguideline.com/

European Pressure Ulcer Advisory Panel [EPUAP], National Pressure Injury Advisory Panel [NPIAP], & Pan Pacific Pressure Injury Alliance [PPPIA] (2019b). *Prevention and treatment of pressure ulcers/injuries: Quick reference guide* (3rd ed.). http://www.internationalguideline.com/static/pdfs/Quick_Reference_Guide-10Mar2019.pdf

Fernandez, R., & Griffiths, R. (2012). Water for wound cleansing. *Cochrane Database of Systematic Reviews,* (2), CD003861. https://doi.org/10.1002/14651858.CD003861.pub3

Ferreira, M., de Souza Gurgel, S., Lima, F., Cardoso, M., da Silva, V. (2018). Instruments for the care of pressure injury in pediatrics and hebiatrics: An integrative review of the literature. *Revista Latino-Americana de Enfermagem, 26,* e3034. https://doi.org/10.1590/1518-8345.2289.3034

Field, C. (2018). Hot topic: Nonsurgical, healthcare-associated burn injuries. *PA Patient Safety Advisory, 15*(1). http://patientsafety.pa.gov/ADVISORIES/Pages/201803_BurnInjuries.aspx

Fischbach, F. T., & Fischbach, M. A. (2018). *A manual of laboratory and diagnostic tests* (10th ed.). Wolters Kluwer.

Fumarola, S., Allaway, R., Callaghan, R., Collier, M., Downie, F., Geraghty, J., Kiernan, S., & Spratt, F. (2020). Overlooked and underestimated: Medical adhesive-related skin injuries. Best practice consensus document

on prevention. *Journal of Wound Care, 29*(Suppl 3c), S1–S24. https://doi.org/10.12968/jowc.2020.29.Sup3c.S1

Gantz, O. B., Rynecki, N. D., Para, A., Levidy, M., & Beebe, K. S. (2020). Postoperative negative pressure wound therapy is associated with decreased surgical site infections in all lower extremity amputations. *Journal of Orthopaedics, 21,* 507–511. https://doi.org/10.1016/j.jor.2020.09.005

Gray, M., & Guiliano, K. K. (2018). Incontinence-associated dermatitis, characteristics and relationship to pressure injury: A multisite epidemiologic analysis. *Journal of Wound, Ostomy & Continence Nursing, 45*(10), 63–67. https://doi.org/10.1097/WON.0000000000000390

Haesler, E. (2018). Evidence summary. Pressure injuries: Active support surfaces for preventing and treating pressure injuries. *Wound Practice and Research, 26*(1), 50–51. https://journals.cambridgemedia.com.au/application/files/3015/8518/8556/summary.pdf

Harris, C., Bates-Jensen, B., Parslow, N., Raizman, R., Singh, M., & Ketchen, R. (2010). Bates-Jensen Wound Assessment Tool: Pictorial guide validation project. *Journal of Wound, Ostomy, and Continence Nursing, 37*(3), 253–259. https://doi.org/10.1097/WON.0b013e3181d73aab

Heale, M. (2020, December 11). *What you need to know about clean and sterile techniques.* Wound Source. [Blog]. https://www.woundsource.com/blog/what-you-need-know-about-clean-and-sterile-techniques

Hess, C. (2013). *Clinical guide to skin & wound care* (7th ed.). Wolters Kluwer.

Hess, C. (2019). *Product guide to skin & wound care* (8th ed.). Wolters Kluwer.

Hogan-Quigley, B., Palm, M. L., & Bickley, L. (2017). *Bates' nursing guide to physical examination and history taking* (2nd ed.). Wolters Kluwer.

Huddleston Cross, H. (2014). Obtaining a wound swab culture specimen. *Nursing, 44*(7), 68–69.

Hurd, T., Rossington, A., Trueman, P., & Smith, J. (2017). A retrospective comparison of the performance of two negative pressure wound therapy systems in the management of wounds of mixed etiology. *Advances in Wound Care, 6*(1), 33–37. https://doi.org/10.1089/wound.2015.0679

Intermountain Healthcare. (2018, February). *Using a suction drain.*Fact sheet for patients and families. https://intermountainhealthcare.org/ckr-ext/Dcmnt?ncid=521066388

International Association of Fire Fighters. (n.d.). *The epidemic of liquid and steam burns.* National Scald Prevention Campaign. Retrieved August 22, 2020, http://flashsplash.org/

International Council of Nurses (ICN). (2019). *Nursing diagnosis and outcome statements.* https://www.icn.ch/sites/default/files/inline-files/ICNP2019-DC.pdf

Janssen, A. H., Wegdam, J. A., de Vries Rellingh, T. S., Eskes, A. M., & Vermeulen, H. (2020). Negative pressure wound therapy for patients with hard-to-heal wounds: A systematic review. *Journal of Wound Care, 29*(4), 206–212. https://doi.org/10.12968/jowc.2020.29.4.206

Jarvis, C., & Echkardt, A. (2020). *Physical examination & health assessment* (8th ed.). Elsevier.

Jensen, S. (2019). *Nursing health assessment. A best practice approach* (3rd ed.). Wolters Kluwer.

The Joint Commission. (2018, July 23). *Quick safety 43: Managing medical device-related pressure injuries.* https://www.jointcommission.org/resources/news-and-multimedia/newsletters/newsletters/quick-safety/quick-safety-43-managing-medical-devicerelated-pressure-injuries/

Kaiser Permanente. (2020, February 26). *Surgical drain care: Care instructions.* https://healthy.kaiserpermanente.org/health-wellness/health-encyclopedia/he.surgical-drain-care-care-instructions.ug6099

Kalowes, P. (2018). Preventing pressure injuries in critically ill patients. *American Nurse Today, Supplement Pressure Injuries,* 14–40.

Kanapathy, M., Matelakis, A., Khan, N., Younis, I., & Mosahebi, A. (2020). Clinical application and efficacy of negative pressure wound therapy with instillation and dwell time (NPWTi-d): A systematic review and meta-analysis. *International Wound Journal, 17*(6), 1948–1959. https://doi.org/10.1111/iwj.13487

Kelly-O'Flynn, S., Mohamud, L., & Copson, D. (2020). Medical adhesive-related skin injury. *British Journal of Nursing, 29*(6), S20–S26. https://doi.org/10.12968/bjon.2020.29.6.S20

Kent, D. J., Scardillo, J. N., Dale, B., & Pike, C. (2018). Does the use of clean or sterile dressing technique affect the incidence of wound infection? *Journal of Wound, Ostomy and Continence Nursing, 45*(3), 265–269. https://doi.org/10.1097/WON.0000000000000425

Kirsner, R., Dove, C., Reyzelman, A., Vayser, D., & Jaimes, H. (2019). A prospective, randomized, controlled clinical trial on the efficacy of a single-use negative pressure wound therapy system, compared to traditional negative pressure wound therapy in the treatment of chronic ulcers of the lower extremities. *Wound Repair and Regeneration, 27*(5), 519–529. https://doi.org/10.1111/wrr.12727

Klein, M. J. (2019, September 3). *Superficial heat and cold.* Medscape. https://emedicine.medscape.com/article/1833084-overview

Kyle, T., & Carman, S. (2021). *Essentials of pediatric nursing* (4th ed.). Wolters Kluwer.

Lalezari, S., Lee, C. J., Borovikova, A. A., Banyard, D. A., Paydar, K. Z., Wirth, G. A., & Widgerow, A. D. (2017). Deconstructing negative pressure wound therapy. *International Wound Journal, 14*(4), 649–657. https://doi.org/10.1111/iwj.12658

LeBlanc, K., Langemo, D., Woo, K., Campos, H. M. H., Santos, V., & Holloway, S. (2019). Skin tears: Prevention and management. *British Journal of Community Nursing, 24*(Suppl 9), S12–S18. https://doi.org/10.12968/bjcn.2019.24.Sup9.S12

Lindsay, C. (2019). Use of the PICO™ single use NPWT system in the prevention of surgical site infections. *Wounds International, 10*(4), 57–61.

Lovegrove, J., Fulbrook, P., & Miles, S. (2020). International consensus on pressure injury preventative interventions by risk level for critically ill patients: A modified Delphi study. *International Wound Journal, 17*(5), 1112–1127. https://doi.org/10.1111/iwj.13461

Ludolph, I., Fried, F. W., Kneppe, K., Arkudas, A., Schmitz, M., & Horch, R. E. (2018). Negative pressure wound treatment with computer-controlled irrigation/instillation decreases bacterial load in contaminated wounds and facilitates wound closure. *International Wound Journal, 15*(6), 978–984. https://doi.org/10.1111/iwj.12958

Mahoney, K. (2020a). Part 1: Wound assessment. *Journal of Community Nursing, 34*(2), 28–35.

Mahoney, K. (2020b). Part 2: Wound cleansing and debridement. *Journal of Community Nursing, 34*(3), 26–32.

Mahoney, K. (2020c). Part 3: Wound infection. *Journal of Community Nursing, 34*(4), 36–44.

Mahoney, K. (2020d). Part 4: Dressing selection. *Journal of Community Nursing, 34*(5), 28–35.

Maida, V., Ennis, M., & Kuziemsky, C. (2009). The Toronto symptom assessment system for wounds: A new clinical and research tool. *Advances in Skin & Wound Care, 22*(10), 468–474. https://doi.org/10.1097/01.ASW.0000361383.12737.a9

Mamuyac, E. M., Pappa, A. K., Thorp, B. D., Ebert, C. S. Jr, Senior, B. A., Zanation, A. M., Lin, F. C., & Kimple, A. J. (2019). How much blood could a JP suck if a JP could suck blood? *The Laryngoscope, 129*(8), 1806–1809. https://doi.org/10.1002/lary.27710

McCluskey, P., Brennan, K., Mullan, J., Costello, M., McDonagh, D., Meagher, H., McLoughlin, G., Moloney, H., Styche, T., & Murdoch, J. (2020). Impact of a single-use negative pressure wound therapy system on healing. *Journal of Community Nursing, 34*(1), 36–43.

McGraw, C. A. (2018). Nurses' perceptions of the root causes of community-acquired pressure ulcers: Application of the model for examining safety and quality concerns in home health care. *Journal of Clinical Nursing, 28*(3–4), 575–588. https://doi.org/10.1111/jocn.14652

McLain, N. E. M., Moore, Z. E. H., & Avsar, P. (2021). Wound cleansing for treating venous leg ulcers. *Cochrane Database of Systematic Reviews, 3*(3), CD011675. https://doi.org/10.1002/14651858.CD011675

McNichol, L. L., Ratliff, C. R., & Yates, S. S. (Eds.). (2022). *Wound, Ostomy, and Continence Nurses Society™ (WOCN®). Core curriculum. Wound management* (2nd ed). Wolters Kluwer.

McNichol, L., Watts, C., Mackey, D., Beitz, J. M., & Gray, M. (2015). Identifying the right surface for the right patient at the right time: Generation and content validation of an Algorithm for Support Surface selection. *Journal of Wound, Ostomy, and Continence Nursing, 42*(1), 19–37. https://doi.org/10.1097/WON.0000000000000103

Memorial Sloan Kettering Cancer Center. (2019, October 8). *Caring for your Penrose drain.* https://www.mskcc.org/cancer-care/patient-education/caring-your-penrose-drain

Milne, J. (2015). Using disposable negative pressure wound therapy in the community. *Journal of Community Nursing,* Supplement Oct/Nov, 10–15.

Milne, J. (2019). The importance of skin cleansing in wound care. *British Journal of Nursing, 28*(12), S20–S22. https://doi.org/10.12968/bjon.2019.28.12.S20

Mitchell, A. (2018). Adult pressure area care: Preventing pressure ulcers. *British Journal of Nursing, 27*(18), 1050–1052. https://doi.org/10.12968/bjon.2018.27.18.1050

Morton, P. G., & Fontaine, D. K. (2018). *Critical care nursing. A holistic approach* (11th ed.). Wolters Kluwer.

Munoz, N., Posthauer, M. E., Cereda, E., Schols, J. M. G. A., & Haesler, E. (2020). The role of nutrition for pressure injury prevention and healing: the 2019 International Clinical Practice Guideline recommendations. *Advances in Skin & Wound Care, 33*(3), 123–136. https://doi.org/10.1097/01.ASW.0000653144.90739.ad

National Pressure Injury Advisory Panel (NPIAP). (2016a). *NPIAP pressure injury stages.* https://npiap.com/page/PressureInjuryStages</bib>

National Pressure Ulcer Advisory Panel (NPUAP) (2016b). *Pressure Ulcer Scale for Healing (PUSH). PUSH tool.* https://npiap.com/page/PUSHTool

National Pressure Injury Advisory Panel (NPIAP). (2017). *NPUAP position statement on staging – 2017 clarifications.* https://cdn.ymaws.com/npiap.com/resource/resmgr/npuap-position-statement-on-.pdf

National Pressure Injury Advisory Panel (NPIAP). (2020). *Pressure injury prevention points.* https://cdn.ymaws.com/npiap.com/resource/resmgr/online_store/1a._pressure-injury-preventi.pdf

Norman, G., Goh, E. L., Dumville, J. C., Shi, C., Liu, Z., Chiverton, L., Stankiewicz, M., & Reid, A. (2020). Negative pressure wound therapy for surgical wounds healing by primary closure. *The Cochrane Database of Systematic Reviews, 6*(6), CD009261. https://doi.org/10.1002/14651858.CD009261.pub6

Norris, T. L. (2020). *Porth's essentials of pathophysiology* (5th ed.). Wolters Kluwer.

Orth, K. (2018). Preventing surgical site infections related to abdominal drains in the intensive care unit. *Critical Care Nurse, 38*(4), 20–26. https://doi.org/10.4037/ccn2018254

Ousey, K., Rogers, A. A., & Rippon, M. G. (2016). Hydro-responsive wound dressings simplify T.I.M.E. wound management framework. *British Journal of Community Nursing, 21*(Suppl 12), S39–S49. https://doi.org/10.12968/bjcn.2016.21.Sup12.S39

Özcan, N., & Karagözoğlu, Ş. (2020). Effects of progressive muscle relaxation exercise, cold application and local anesthesia performed before chest tube removal on pain and comfort levels and vital signs of the patient. *Turkiye Klinikleri Journal of Medical Sciences, 40*(3), 285–296. https://doi.org/10.5336/medsci.2019-72505

Payne, D. (2016). Strategies to support prevention, identification and management of pressure ulcers in the community. *British Journal of Community Nursing, 21*(Suppl 6), S10–S18. https://doi.org/10.12968/bjcn.2016.21.Sup6.S10

Problem-based care plans. (2020). In *Lippincott Advisor.* Wolters Kluwer.

Prody, M. R. (2017, October 6). A better way to secure Jackson-Pratt drains. *American Nurse* [Online]. https://www.myamericannurse.com/better-way-secure-jackson-pratt-drains/

Quain, A. M., & Khardori, N. M. (2015). Nutrition in wound care management: A comprehensive overview. *Wounds, 27*(12), 327–335.

Ratner, D. (2020a, March 5). *Suturing techniques periprocedural care.* Medscape. https://emedicine.medscape.com/article/1824895-periprocedure#b6

Ratner, D. (2020b, March 5). Alternative methods of wound closure. Medscape. https://emedicine.medscape.com/article/1824895-technique#c4

Reevell, G., Anders, T., & Morgan, T. (2016). Improving patients' experience of dressing removal in practice. *Journal of Community Nursing, 30*(5), 44–49.

Saint Luke's. (n.d.). *Taking a Sitz bath.* Retrieved February 8, 2021, from https://www.saintlukeskc.org/health-library/taking-sitz-bath

Scafide, K. N., Narayan, M. C., & Arundel, L. (2020). Bedside technologies to enhance the early detection of pressure injuries. A systematic review. *Journal of Wound, Ostomy, and Continence Nursing, 47*(2), 128–136. https://doi.org/10.1097/WON.0000000000000626

Schreiber, M. L. (2016). Negative pressure wound therapy. *Med Surg Nursing, 25*(6), 425–428.

Silbert-Flagg, J., & Pillitteri, A. (2018). *Maternal and child health nursing* (8th ed.). Wolters Kluwer.

Smith & Nephew, Inc. (2018). *PICO™ 7 system. Quick reference guide. PICO™ 7 single use negative pressure wound therapy system.* https://possiblewithpico.com/sites/default/files/picoImages/documents/resources/PCEE2-14182-0818PICO7QuickReferenceGuide.pdf

Sonoiki, T., Young, J., & Alexis, O. (2020). Challenges faced by nurses in complying with aseptic non-touch technique principles during wound care: A review. *British Journal of Nursing, 29*(5), S28–S35. https://doi.org/10.12968/bjon.2020.29.5.S28

Stone, A. (2020). Preventing pressure injuries in nursing home residents using a low-profile alternating pressure overlay: A point-of-care trial. *Advances in Skin & Wound Care, 33*(10), 533–539. https://doi.org/10.1097/01.ASW.0000695756.80461.64

Stuart, E. (2020). Nutrition and wound care: What community nurses should know. *Journal of Community Nursing, 34*(6), 58–62.

Taylor, C., Lynn, P., & Bartlett, J. (2023). *Fundamentals of nursing: The art and science of person-centered care* (10th ed.). Wolters Kluwer.

VHA Center for Engineering & Occupational Safety and Health (CEOSH). (2016). *Safe patient handling and mobility guidebook.* http://www.tnpatientsafety.com/pubfiles/Initiatives/workplace-violence/sphm-pdf.pdf

Voegeli, D. (2019). Prevention and management of moisture-associated skin damage. *Nursing Standard, 34*(2), 77–82. https://doi.org/10.7748/ns.2019.e11314

Waterlow, J. (1985). Pressure sores: A risk assessment card. *Nursing Times, 81*(48), 49–55.

Watret, L., Wright, S., Rodgers, A., Shankie, S., Macaskill, C., McShange, T., Potter, R., Hollis, A., & Farrell, E. (2020, August 19). *Clinical guideline. Single use negative pressure wound therapy (sNPWT).* National Health Service (NHS). Greater Glasgow and Clyde. https://ggcmedicines.org.uk/media/1maoodt2/single-use-negative-pressure-wound-therapy-snpwt-aug-2020.pdf

Wechter, D. G. (2020a, March 5). *Close suction drain with bulb.* U.S. National Library of Medicine. MedlinePlus. https://medlineplus.gov/ency/patientinstructions/000039.htm

Wechter, D. G. (2020b, March 5). Hemovac drain. U.S. National Library of Medicine. MedlinePlus. https://medlineplus.gov/ency/patientinstructions/000038.htm

Wolters Kluwer. (2022). Problem-based care plans. In *Lippincott Advisor.* Wolters Kluwer.

Wound, Ostomy and Continence Nurses Society (WOCN) Wound Committee; Association for Professionals in Infection Control and Epidemiology, Inc. (APIC) 2000 Guidelines Committee. (2012). Clean vs. sterile dressing techniques for management of chronic wounds. A fact sheet. *Journal of Wound, Ostomy, and Continence Nursing, 39*(Suppl 2), S30–S34. https://doi.org/10.1097/WON.0b013e3182478e06

Wound, Ostomy and Continence Nurses Society (WOCN). (n.d.). *Clinical tools. Support Surface Algorithm.* Retrieved January 23, 2021, from https://www.wocn.org/learning-center/clinical-tools/

Wound, Ostomy and Continence Nurses Society (WOCN). Wound Guidelines Task Force. (2016). WOCN 2016 guideline for prevention and management of pressure injuries (ulcers). *Journal of Wound Ostomy & Continence Nursing, 44*(3), 241–246. https://doi.org/10.1097/WON.0000000000000321

Yilmazer, T., Inkaya, B., & Tuzer, H. (2019). Care under the guidance of pressure injury prevention protocol: A nursing home sample. *Community Wound Care, 24*(Suppl 12), S26–S33. https://doi.org/10.12968/bjcn.2019.24.Sup12.S26

Yue, B., Nizzero, D., Zhang, C., van Zyl, N., & Ting, J. (2015). Accuracy of surgical wound drainage measurements: An analysis and comparison. *ANZ Journal of Surgery, 85*(5), 327–329. https://doi.org/10.1111/ans.12657

SUGGESTED ANSWERS FOR FOCUSING ON PATIENT CARE: DEVELOPING CLINICAL REASONING AND CLINICAL JUDGMENT

1. This is a significant change in the patient's assessment. Perform a thorough wound assessment and obtain vital signs. Assess the patient for any new symptoms, such as increased pain, chills, or abnormal sensation (e.g., numbness, tingling). Report findings to the health care team; a change in wound care, additional assessments (e.g., diagnostic tests, laboratory tests), or change/ addition of medication may be required.

2. Reassure the patient regarding her wound status. Explain what the drains are, how they work, and their intended purpose. Provide information regarding wound care, drain care, and recording of drainage amounts. Discuss anticipated care requirements at home and potential arrangements to ensure required care is performed, either by the patient or significant other.

3. Reassure the patient regarding his wound status. Explain the purpose of the staples, the process of wound healing, and the purpose of adhesive wound strips. Discuss the patient's responsibilities for wound care at this point in his healing.

9

Activity

Focusing on Patient Care

This chapter will help you develop some of the skills related to activity necessary to care for the following patients:

Bobby Rowden, age 8, was knocked down during soccer practice and has come to the emergency room with pain, swelling, and deformity of his right forearm. He is diagnosed with a fracture.

Esther Levitz, age 58, is receiving rehabilitation services at an extended-care facility after a recent surgery. She has been debilitated by nausea, anorexia, overwhelming fatigue, and weight loss. Her underlying diagnosis of lymphoma and inactivity put her at risk for thrombus formation.

Manuel Esposito, age 62, has a fractured femur and other health issues that must be resolved before he can have surgery to fix the fracture. His health care team has implemented skeletal traction to stabilize the position of the bones until Manuel can have the necessary surgery.

Refer to Focusing on Patient Care: Developing Clinical Reasoning and Clinical Judgment at the end of the chapter to apply what you learn.

Learning Outcomes

After completing the chapter, you will be able to accomplish the following:

1. Assist a patient with repositioning in bed.
2. Transfer a patient from the bed to a stretcher.
3. Transfer a patient from the bed to a chair.
4. Transfer a patient using a full-powered body sling lift.
5. Provide range-of-motion exercises.
6. Assist a patient with ambulation.
7. Assist a patient with ambulation using a walker.
8. Assist a patient with ambulation using crutches.
9. Assist a patient with ambulation using a cane.
10. Apply and remove graduated compression stockings.
11. Apply pneumatic compression devices.
12. Apply a continuous passive motion device.
13. Apply a sling.
14. Apply a figure-eight bandage.
15. Assist with a cast application.

16. Care for a patient with a cast.
17. Apply and care for a patient in skin traction.
18. Care for a patient in skeletal traction.
19. Care for a patient with an external fixation device.

Nursing Concepts

- Assessment
- Clinical Decision Making/Clinical Judgment
- Functional ability
- Health promotion
- Mobility

The ability to move is closely related to the fulfillment of other basic human needs. Regular exercise contributes to the healthy functioning of each body system. Conversely, lack of exercise and immobility affect each body system negatively. A summary of the effects of immobility on the body is outlined in Fundamentals Review 9-1. An important nursing role is to encourage activity and exercise to promote wellness, prevent illness, and restore health.

Nursing interventions are directed at preventing potential problems and treating actual problems related to a patient's activity and mobility status. Strategies designed to promote correct body alignment, mobility, and fitness are important parts of nursing care. Nurses use knowledge of **safe patient handling and mobility (SPHM)** along with specific nursing interventions to promote fitness and to address mobility problems.

An effective approach to safe patient transfers includes patient assessment criteria; screening and algorithms for patient handling and mobility decisions; specialized patient handling equipment used properly and operated using proper ergonomics; and the use of lift teams. The proper use of assistive devices to lift, move, reposition, and transport patients is key to SPHM (Fragala et al., 2016). In addition, the use of assistive patient handling equipment contributes to patient comfort and protects patient dignity, while increasing safety. The National Institute for Occupational Safety and Health (NIOSH, 2013) and the Occupational Safety and Health Administration and the Joint Commission recommend a no-lift policy in conjunction with technology, assistive devices, education, and a culture of safety for all health care facilities (Fragala et al., 2016; OSHA and Joint Commission Resources Alliance, 2017). Many devices and equipment are available to aid in transferring, repositioning, lifting and/or moving patients. It is important to use the right equipment and appropriate device based on patient assessment and desired movement and to use the equipment in the proper manner (Arnold, 2019; Fragala et al., 2016).

Always check facility practices and guidelines and available equipment related to safe patient handling and movement. Samples of algorithms to aid decision making to prevent injury to staff and patients during patient movement and handling are provided in the appropriate skills. When using any equipment, check for proper functioning before using with the patient. Fundamentals Review 9-2 presents guidelines for safe patient handling and mobility. Fundamentals Review 9-3 discusses examples of equipment and assistive devices that are available to aid with safe patient mobility and handling. Fundamentals Review 9-4 provides an example of a mobility assessment tool to aid in patient assessment and associated SPHM equipment to consider. See also Figure 1 in Skill 9-1 for an example of an algorithm (assessment tool) to aid in decision making regarding safe patient handling and mobility to reposition a patient in bed.

This chapter covers skills to assist the nurse in providing care related to activity and inactivity, and health care problems related to the musculoskeletal system.

Fundamentals Review 9-1

EFFECTS OF IMMOBILITY ON THE BODY

- Decreased muscle strength and tone, decreased muscle size
- Decreased joint mobility and flexibility
- Limited endurance and activity intolerance
- Bone demineralization
- Decreased coordination and altered gait
- Decreased ventilatory effort and pooling of respiratory secretions, respiratory congestion, increased risk for atelectasis

- Increased cardiac workload, increased risk for orthostatic hypotension and venous thrombosis
- Altered circulation and increased risk for alterations in skin integrity
- Altered appetite, constipation
- Urinary stasis, increased risk for infection
- Altered sleep patterns, pain, increased risk for depression

Fundamentals Review 9-2

GUIDELINES FOR SAFE PATIENT HANDLING AND MOVEMENT

Keep the patient in good alignment and protect from injury while being moved. The use of safe patient handling devices and techniques is critical in the prevention of patient care–related injuries.

Follow these recommended guidelines when moving and transferring patients:

- Assess the patient. Know the patient's medical diagnosis and health issues, capabilities, and any movement not allowed. Apply braces or any device the patient wears before helping the patient from the bed.
- Assess the patient's ability to assist with the planned movement. Encourage the patient to assist in own transfers. Encouraging the patient to perform tasks that are within their capabilities promotes independence. Eliminating or reducing unnecessary tasks by the nurse reduces the risk of injury.
- Assess the patient's ability to understand instructions and collaborate with the staff to achieve the movement (see Box 9-1 in Skill 9-1 for general guidelines related to mobility and safe handling of people with dementia).
- Ensure sufficient staff is available and present to move the patient safely.
- Assess the area for clutter, accessibility to the patient, and availability of devices. Remove any obstacles that may make moving and transferring inconvenient.
- Use a screening or assessment tool to aid in patient assessment and decision making regarding safe patient handling and mobility (Arnold, 2019; VA Mobile Health, n.d.). Use of a standardized tool supports consistency and appropriate use of Safe Patient Handling and Mobility (SPHM) equipment to assist patients with the appropriate level of mobility (Arnold, 2019; Boynton et al., 2020).
- Decide which equipment to use. Protocols and algorithms are available to aid decision making to prevent injury to staff and patients.

- Plan carefully what you will do before moving or lifting a patient. Assess the mobility of attached equipment. You may injure the patient or yourself if you have not planned well. Communicate the plan with staff and the patient to ensure coordinated movement.
- Explain to the patient what you plan to do. Then, use what abilities the patient has to assist you. This technique often decreases the effort required and the possibility of injury to you.
- If the patient is in pain, administer the prescribed analgesic sufficiently in advance of the transfer to allow the patient to participate in the move comfortably.
- Elevate the bed, as necessary, so that you are working at a height that is comfortable and safe for you.
- Lock the wheels of the bed, wheelchair, or stretcher so that they do not slide while you are moving the patient.
- Be sure the patient is in good body alignment while being moved and lifted, to protect the patient from strain and muscle injury.
- Support the patient's body properly. Avoid grabbing and holding an extremity by its muscles.
- Use friction-reducing devices, whenever possible, especially during lateral transfers.
- Move your body and the patient in a smooth, rhythmic motion. Jerky movements tend to put extra strain on muscles and joints and are uncomfortable for the patient.
- Use SPHM equipment/devices when moving patients. Be sure that you understand how the device operates and that the patient is properly secured and informed of what will occur. If you are not comfortable with the operation of the equipment, obtain assistance from a caregiver who is.
- Assure equipment used meets weight requirements. Institute Bariatric Algorithms for any patient that weights more than 300 lb, or 100 lb over ideal weight, or who has a BMI over 40 (VHA CEOSH, 2015).

Fundamentals Review 9-3

SPHM EQUIPMENT AND DEVICES

Many devices and equipment are available to aid in transferring, repositioning, and lifting patients. It is important to use the right equipment and appropriate device based on patient assessment and desired movement.

GAIT BELTS

A gait belt is a belt, often with handles, used for transferring patients and assisting with ambulation. It is placed around the patient's waist and secured. The handles can be placed in a variety of configurations so the caregiver can have better access to, improved grasp, and control of the patient. Some belts are hand-held slings that go around the patient, providing a firm grasp for the caregiver and facilitating the transfer. The gait belt is used to steady the patient and provide stabilization during pivoting, not to pull the patient up or as a lifting device. Gait belts also allow the nurse to assist in ambulating patients who have leg strength, can cooperate, and require minimal assistance. Do not use gait belts on patients with abdominal or thoracic incisions or chest trauma. Gait belts should also not be used with patients exhibiting behavioral aggression, as the belt might be used as a weapon and for patients at risk for suicide, as the belt might be used for self-harm (Wintersgill, 2019). See Figure A for an example of a gait belt.

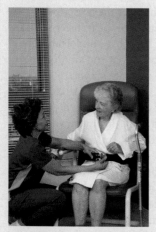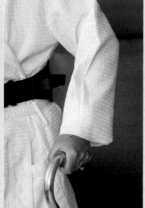

FIGURE A. Using a gait belt.

STANDING ASSIST AND REPOSITIONING AIDS

Some patients need minimal assistance to stand up. With an appropriate support to grasp, they can lift themselves. Many types of nonpowered standing assist and repositioning devices can provide leverage and help a patient to stand (VHACEOSH, 2016). These devices are freestanding or attach to the bed or wheelchair. One type of stand-assist aid attaches to the bed. Other aids have a pull bar to assist the patient to stand, and then a seat unfolds under the patient. After sitting on the seat, the device can

be wheeled to the toilet, chair, shower, or bed. Sliding assists are useful for patients who are cooperative, partially dependent but have some weight-bearing capability, and have upper body mobility and strength sufficient to grip device handles.

LATERAL-ASSIST DEVICES

Lateral-assist devices reduce patient-surface friction during lateral transfers. Roller boards, slide boards, transfer boards, inflatable mattresses, and friction-reducing, lateral-assist devices are examples of these devices that make transfers safer and more comfortable for the patient. An inflatable lateral-assist device is a flexible mattress that is placed under the patient. An attached, portable air supply inflates the mattress, which provides a layer of air under the patient. This air cushion allows nursing staff to perform the move with much less effort, but may place the care providers at an increased risk of injury because of the horizontal reach required, posture adopted during transfer, and lack of handles. Transfer boards are placed under the patient. They provide a slick surface for the patient during transfers, reducing friction and the force required to move the patient. Transfer boards are made of smooth, rigid, low-friction material, such as coated wood or plastic. In order to use a board for transfers to or from a chair, the chair must have retractable or removable arm rests (Smith et al., 2015). Another lateral-sliding aid is made of a special fabric that reduces friction. Some devices have long handles that reduce reaching by staff, to improve safety and make the transfer easier (Figure B).

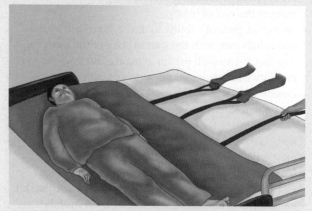

FIGURE B. Lateral-assist device with long handles to reduce reaching by staff.

FRICTION-REDUCING SHEETS

Friction-reducing sheets can be used under patients to prevent skin shearing when moving a patient in the bed and to assist with lateral transfers. The use of these sheets when moving the patient up in bed, turning, and repositioning

Fundamentals Review 9-3   continued

SPHM EQUIPMENT AND DEVICES

reduces friction and the force required to move the patient. They can also be used to assist patients to perform range-of-motion exercises in bed (Smith et al., 2015). However, use of these sheets may require excessive force and overexertion by the caregiver and increase the risk of musculoskeletal injuries for health care personnel (Battiste-McKinney & Halvorson, 2018; VHACEOSH, 2016).

MECHANICAL LATERAL-ASSIST DEVICES

Mechanical lateral-assist devices eliminate the need to slide the patient manually. Some devices are motorized, and some use a hand crank (Figure C). A portion of the device moves from the stretcher to the bed, sliding under the patient, bridging the bed and stretcher. The device is then returned to the stretcher, effectively moving the patient without pulling by staff members.

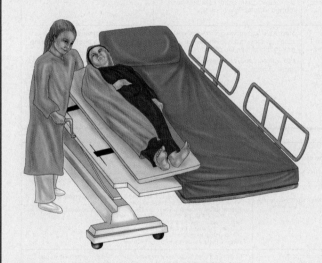

FIGURE C. Mechanical lateral-assist device.

TRANSFER CHAIRS

Chairs that can convert into stretchers are available. These are useful with patients who have no weight-bearing capacity, cannot follow directions, and/or cannot cooperate. The back of the chair bends back and the leg supports elevate to form a stretcher configuration, eliminating the need for lifting the patient. Some of these chairs have built-in mechanical aids to perform the patient transfer, as detailed above.

POWERED STAND-ASSIST AND REPOSITIONING LIFTS

Powered stand-assist and repositioning devices can be used with patients who have some weight-bearing ability, can follow directions, and are cooperative. A simple sling is placed around the patient's back and under the arms (see Figure 2 in Skill 9-3). Standing/ambulation vests may be used instead of a sling (Boynton et al., 2020); a vest may provide additional stability and security in the upper body area, distributing pressure over a larger area, often with extra padding at potential pressure areas and/or leg straps (Enos, 2019). Once in the sling or vest, the patient's feet rest on the device's footrest and then the patient places their hands on the handle. The device mechanically assists the patient to stand, without any lifting by the nurse. Once the patient is standing, the device can be wheeled to a chair, the toilet, or bed. Some devices have removable footrests and can be used as a walker. Some have scales incorporated into the device that can be used to weigh the patient. The duration of time spent in slings should be limited to reduce risks for pressure injuries, especially for vulnerable populations (Peterson et al., 2015).

POWERED FULL-BODY LIFTS

Powered full-body lifts are used with patients who cannot bear any weight to move them out of bed, into and out of a chair, and to a commode or stretcher. A full-body sling is placed under the patient's body, including head and torso, and then the sling is attached to the lift. The device slowly lifts the patient. Some devices can be lowered to the floor to pick up a patient who has fallen. These devices are available on portable bases and ceiling-mounted tracks (see Figure 6 in Skill 9-4). Note: For safe operation, a mobile lifts' wheels must be positioned under the patient, which makes them unsuitable for use with platform beds used typically in psychiatric units (Smith et al., 2015). The duration of time spent in slings should be limited to reduce risks for pressure injuries, especially for vulnerable populations (Peterson et al., 2015).

Fundamentals Review 9-4

BEDSIDE MOBILITY ASSESSMENT TOOL (BMAT 2.0)

Test/Assessment Level	Description of Test	Pass Response	PASS =
Assessment Level 1 Assessment of: • sitting balance • upper extremity and core strength • ability to sit upright without getting tachycardic, diaphoretic or lightheaded; i.e. sitting tolerance.	**Sit and Shake:** From semi-reclined position or at EOB, ask patient to sit upright for up to 1 minute (if there is any concern regarding orthostatic hypotension or postural intolerance); then reach across midline and shake hands with caregiver – repeat with other hand. (Patient's feet may either be flat on floor or dangling.) **Safe Mode:** Use sling and lift to assist to side of bed (e.g., sternal precautions, abdominal incision) or bed in chair position, then complete "Sit and Shake."	**Sit:** Able to follow commands and sit unsupported (i.e., unsupported by sling or bed surface) for up to 1 minute. **Shake:** Able to maintain seated balance while challenged by reaching across midline of trunk with one or both hands and shaking caregiver's hand.	**Pass** Assessment Level 1 "Sit and Shake" = **Proceed to Assessment Level 2, "Stretch"** **Fail = Mobility Level 1 Patient** As appropriate, follow Critical Care Early/Progressive Mobility Program protocol to advance through BMAT Assessment Levels.
Assessment Level 2 Assessment of: • leg strength in preparation for weight bearing • control and strength of leg muscles, including quadriceps and lower leg muscles • foot drop	**Stretch:** While sitting upright unsupported, extend one leg and straighten knee (knee remains below hip level) and point toes/pump ankle between dorsiflexion/plantar flexion x 3 repetitions. (Patient's feet may either be flat on floor or dangling.) **Safe Mode:** Continue to use sling and lift (mobile or overhead/ceiling), bed in Fowler's or chair position to complete "Stretch."	**Stretch:** Able to extend leg and straighten knee = engage quadriceps; then able to pump ankle for 3 repetitions = AROM/move ankle between dorsiflexion/plantar flexion = engage calf muscles/skeletal muscle pump and assist with venous return/fluid shifts.	**Pass** Assessment Level 2 "Stretch" = **Proceed to Assessment Level 3, "Stand"** **Fail = Mobility Level 2 Patient**
Assessment Level 3 Assessment of: • ability to shift forward, raise buttocks and rise smoothly; balance and strength to rise • standing tolerance for up to 1 minute, which allows for fluid shifts and other compensatory changes to occur • static standing balance	**Stand:** With feet flat on floor about shoulder width apart, shift forward, raise buttocks/rise and stand upright for up to 1 minute (if there is any concern regarding orthostatic hypotension, postural intolerance or syncope). **Safe Mode:** Use sit-to-stand lift and vest/sling, or ambulation vest/pants and lift. Always default to using Safe Mode if concerned regarding orthostatic hypotension/syncopal event or other compensatory changes.	**Stand:** Able to rise, maintain balance and upright standing position for up to 1 minute. The majority of patients who exhibit orthostatic hypotension do so within the first minute of standing, which is the rationale for 1 minute. Use walker, cane, crutches or prosthetic leg(s) as appropriate to assist.	**Pass** Assessment Level 3 "Stand" = **Proceed to Assessment Level 4, "Step"** **Fail = Mobility Level 3 Patient**
Assessment Level 4 Assessment of: • pre-ambulation weight shift abilities • further assessment of leg strength • dynamic standing balance, which further allows for fluid shifts and other compensatory changes to occur • cognitive ability to follow directions	**Step:** 1) March- or step-in-place taking small steps (not high-marching steps) x 3 repetitions; if able to pass then 2) Step forward with one foot, weight-bear/shift weight onto foot and return foot to starting position; repeat with other foot. **Safe Mode:** Use ambulation vest/pants and lift; consider use of bed in chair position and egress from end-of-bed. Always default to using Safe Mode if concerned regarding orthostatic hypotension/syncopal event, other compensatory changes or falls.	**Step:** Able to perform both marching-in-place and forward step and return with one foot and then the other. Use walker, cane, crutches or prosthetic leg(s) as appropriate.	**Pass** Assessment Level 4 "Step" = **Progress through Discharge Planning** Continue to complete BMAT per protocol; address medical issues and stability; use multidisciplinary approach: work on discharge goals for best destination/placement; consider functional status, ongoing equipment needs and ADL's **Fail = Remain a Mobility Level 4 Patient**

Patient's BMAT Mobility Level	Assessment Level 1. Sit & Shake*	2. Stretch*	3. Stand*	4. Step*	Test Options in SAFE MODE (See Figure A, page one for Description of Basic Test)	Patient Care and Strengthening in SAFE MODE SPHM Equipment to Consider for patient care/strengthening NOTE: Consult with PT/OT per facility protocol
Mobility Level 1 = Fails/unable to "Sit and Shake" As appropriate, follow Critical Care Early/ Progressive Mobility Program protocol	FAIL	NA	NA	NA	1) Perform with patient sitting upright in bed 2) Using lift and sling help patient sit at Edge of Bed (EOB) As appropriate, follow Critical Care Early/Progressive Mobility Program protocol to advance through BMAT Assessment Levels.	**Goals:** Avoid complications of immobility, engage and strengthen postural muscles and progress to Level 2. 1) Edge of Bed (EOB) dangling with sling and lift; work on sitting balance and reaching across midline; perform calf pump exercises 2) Bed in Fowler's or chair position: sitting supported or unsupported to cross midline and shake hands; also perform calf pump exercises 3) Lift and repo sheet: for boosting and turning 4) Lift and multistraps: for turning and limb holding 5) Lift and sling: for bed to chair/commode transfer 6) Friction Reducing Device (FRD): for PROM/AROM exercises
Mobility Level 2 = Passes "Sit and Shake;" Fails/unable to "Stretch"	PASS	FAIL	NA	NA	1) Perform with patient sitting upright in chair position 2) While at EOB dangling and secured by sling and lift	**Goals:** Avoid complications of immobility, engage and strengthen postural and lower extremity muscles, assist with fluid shifts and progress to Level 3. 1) FRD: partial squats and leg AROM exercises – bed flat or tilt position 2) Lift and repo sheet: boosting and turning 3) Lift and multistraps: limb holding or turning 4) Lift and sling: bed to chair/toilet transfer 5) In bed: perform additional calf pump exercises
Mobility Level 3 = Passes" Sit and Shake," and "Stretch;" Fails/unable to "Stand"	PASS	PASS	FAIL	NA	1) Using sit-to-stand lift with vest: evaluate patient's tolerance for standing upright and weight bearing; monitor patient's BP and HR; maintain balance for up to 1 minute. 2) Using standing/ambulation vest or pants and floor-based or ceiling lift: starting with patient's feet flat on floor, instruct patient to rise and stand; monitor patient's BP, HR, balance and tolerance for up to 1 minute. As appropriate, after testing in Safe Mode, use walker, cane, crutches, prosthetic leg(s) to evaluate standing tolerance and to progress to "Step."	**Goals:** Strengthen muscles in upright position, assist fluid shifts, avoid falls and progress to Level 4. 1) Sit-to-stand lift with vest/sling: stand for 1-2 minutes; shift weight from one foot/leg to the other, 2 – 3 deep breaths 2) Squats using FRD with bed in tilt position 3) Lift and multistraps: limb holding 4) Powered or non-powered sit-to-stand lift for bed to chair/toilet transfers (e.g., quick night-time transfer to and from toilet) 5) If using aid (walker, cane, crutches, prosthetic), after standing with sit-to-stand lift, work on standing with aid.
Mobility Level 4 = Passes "Sit and Shake," "Stretch" and "Stand;" Fails/unable to "Step"	PASS	PASS	PASS	FAIL	1) If a sit-to-stand lift with vest was used and patient passed "Stand:" evaluate first portion of "Step," march-in-place while patient is still secure in vest attached to sit-to-stand lift. 2) Using ambulation vest or pants attached to lift: evaluate "Step" by instructing patient to march-in-place. If able to perform march-in-place, instruct patient to advance step with one foot and return foot to starting position. If able to pass, repeat with other foot. Use walker, cane, crutches or prosthetic leg(s) as appropriate.	**Goals:** Improve standing tolerance and endurance with stepping and weight-shifts, balance and ambulation; avoid falls; consider mobility, functional status, and discharge goals. 1) Lift and ambulation vest/pants for standing, stepping-in-place, weight-shifting/balance activities, and walking 2) Set distance goals to improve endurance and confidence with lift and without lift after passing "Step." 3) If using aid (walker, cane, crutches, prosthetic) to pass "Step," assure that aid is always easily accessible and used for transfers in-room and during hallway ambulation.
Progress through Discharge Planning = Passes all 4 Assessments Review Discharge Goals; Post-acute Discharge Planning	PASS	PASS	PASS	PASS	• Continue to complete BMAT per protocol; with any change in status adjust Mobility Level and goals as needed. • While improving/maintaining mobility, continue to address medical issues and stability as needed; evaluate other medical conditions/treatment plan prior to physician release. • Mobility goals may include: independence with bed mobility and transfers; improve balance, standing tolerance, endurance with walking; independence with aid(s) - walker, cane, crutches, prosthetic(s).	**Multidisciplinary approach:** • Compare pre-admit status, including ability to perform ADLs, to discharge status; i.e., previous level of function (PLOF) compared to post-acute functional status; review rehabilitation goals – have they been met? • Review discharge goals and guide discharge recommendations: appropriate post-acute discharge destination and equipment needs.

NOTE: Always default to the safest testing/lifting/transfer method (e.g., total lift and sling) if there is any doubt in the patient's ability to perform the task.

Skill 9-1 ▶ Assisting a Patient With Repositioning in Bed

Skill Variation: *Using a Full-Body Sling to Reposition a Patient*

Patients experiencing decreased mobility as a result of illness or injury may be unable to reposition themselves. The patient is at risk for injuries from **friction** and **shearing forces** while being moved. Knowledge of correct body alignment, SPHM, and assistive devices to turn the patient in bed are crucial to achieve patient movement and avoid injury. Use a decision-making tool to help make decisions about SPHM. One suggested decision-making strategy is outlined in Fundamentals Review 9-4. This tool includes suggestions for associated SPHM equipment. Another example of a decision-making tool is provided in Figure 1. If the patient is fully able to assist in turning, allow the patient to complete the movement independently, with safe supervision. If the patient is partially able or unable to assist, friction-reducing devices, lifting/repositioning sheets, lateral transfer devices, and a full-body sling are potential equipment to consider, based on screening and assessment. Consider available bed features (turning, pressure release, rotation) to assist with the action (VA Mobile Health, n.d.).

Fundamentals Review 9-3 reviews examples of equipment and assistive devices that are available to aid in patient movement and handling. Refer to Box 9-1 (on page 548) for additional considerations related to mobility and safe handling of people with dementia. The procedure below describes general guidelines for repositioning a patient; the Skill Variation at the end of the skill discusses using a full-body sling to reposition the patient. Refer to facility policy and procedures and specific manufacturer guidelines related to other available devices and equipment.

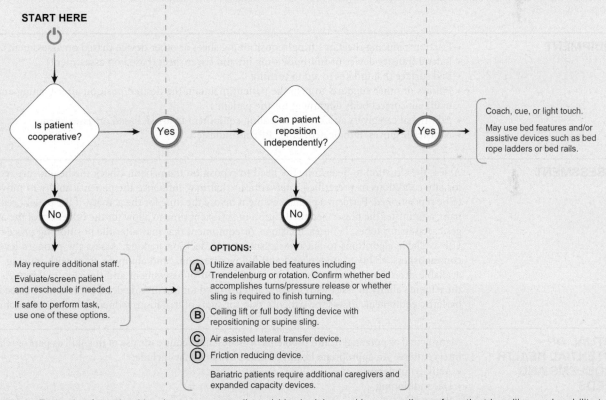

FIGURE 1. Example of an algorithm (assessment tool) to aid in decision making regarding safe patient handling and mobility to reposition a patient in bed. (*Source:* VA Mobile Health. [n.d.]. *Safe patient handling.* [Version 1.3.3]. Algorithm 3. [Mobile app]. U. S. Department of Veteran Affairs. https://mobile.va.gov/app/safe-patient-handling.)

DELEGATION CONSIDERATIONS

Assisting a patient to turn in bed may be delegated to assistive personnel (AP) as well as to licensed practical/vocational nurses (LPN/LVNs). The decision to delegate must be based on careful analysis of the patient's needs and circumstances as well as the qualifications of the person to whom the task is being delegated. Refer to the Delegation Guidelines in Appendix A.

(continued on page 548)

Skill 9-1 ▶ Assisting a Patient With Repositioning in Bed   *(continued)*

Box 9-1 Safe Handling of Patients With Dementia

- Be aware that communication problems and weakness can make the handling of patients with dementia challenging.
- Face the patient when speaking. Speak slowly.
- Use clear, short sentences.
- Call patient by name.
- Use calm, reassuring tone of voice.
- Allow time for response.
- Offer simple, one-step instructions.
- Repeat verbal cues and prompts, as necessary. This assists when thought processes are delayed.
- Determine if the patient experiencing dementia has receptive aphasia. This inability to understand what is being said results in noncompliance with verbal instructions.
- Phrase instructions positively. For example, remind the patient to "Stand up" until the chair is correctly positioned, instead of saying "Don't sit down." The patient may not register the "Don't" and will try to sit too early. Positive instructions are more likely to result in successful maneuvers.
- Ask one question at a time, allow the patient to answer, and repeat the question, if necessary.
- Allow the patient to focus on the task; avoid correcting the process of the action unless it would be dangerous to the patient not to do so.
- Identify the patient's established patterns of behavior, customs, traits, and everyday habits and try to incorporate these habits into desired activities. For instance, a patient with dementia may resist or become frightened when a morning shower is attempted if the patient was accustomed to evening baths. Another person may have difficulty getting out of bed in the morning for the simple reason that he is being asked to get out on what he considers the wrong side of the bed.

Source: Adapted from Eliopoulos, C. (2018). *Gerontological nursing* (9th ed.). Wolters Kluwer; Jootun, D., & Pryde, A. (2013). Moving and handling of patients with dementia. *Journal of Nursing Education and Practice, 3*(2), 126–131; Toughy, T. A., & Jett, K. (2018). *Ebersol and Hess' gerontological nursing & healthy aging* (5th ed.). Elsevier; and Varnam, W. (2011). How to mobilise patients with dementia to a standing position. *Nursing Older People, 23*(8), 31–36.

EQUIPMENT	• Friction-reducing sheet or lifting/repositioning sheet or other device (based on assessment) • Lateral transfer device or full-body sling lift and cover sheet (based on assessment) • Bed surface that inflates to aid in turning • Pillows or other supports to help the patient maintain the desired position after turning and to maintain correct body alignment for the patient • Additional caregivers and/or safe handling equipment to assist, based on assessment • Nonsterile gloves, if indicated; other PPE as indicated
ASSESSMENT	Assess the situation to determine the need to reposition the patient. Check the health care record for any conditions or prescribed interventions that may influence the patient's ability to move or to be repositioned. Perform a pain assessment before the time for the activity. If the patient reports pain, administer the prescribed medication in sufficient time to allow for the full effect of the analgesic. Assess for tubes, IV lines, incisions, or equipment that may alter the positioning procedure. Use available algorithms to aid in assessment and decision making. Assess the patient's level of consciousness, ability to understand and follow directions, and ability to assist with moving. Use available decision-making tools or algorithms to aid in assessment and decision making. Assess the patient's ability to assist with moving and the need for assistive devices. Determine the need for bariatric equipment. Assess the patient's skin for signs of irritation, redness, edema, or blanching.
ACTUAL OR POTENTIAL HEALTH PROBLEMS AND NEEDS	Many actual or potential health problems or issues may require the use of this skill as part of related interventions. An appropriate health problem or issue may include: • Activity intolerance • Deconditioning • Injury risk
OUTCOME IDENTIFICATION AND PLANNING	The expected outcome to achieve when repositioning a patient in bed is that the patient is repositioned without injury to patient or nurse. Additional outcomes may include the following: the patient reports improved comfort, and the patient maintains proper body alignment.

IMPLEMENTATION

ACTION

1. Review the health record for prescribed interventions and plan of care for patient activity. Identify any movement limitations, conditions that may influence the patient's ability to move or be positioned, and the ability of the patient to assist with turning. **Consult a patient handling algorithm or other decision-making tool to plan an appropriate approach to moving the patient.**

2. Gather any positioning aids or supports, if necessary.

3. Perform hand hygiene. Put on PPE, as indicated.

4. Identify the patient. Explain the procedure to the patient.

5. Close the curtains around the bed and close the door to the room, if possible. Position at least one nurse on either side of the bed. Place pillows, wedges, or any other support to be used for positioning within easy reach. Place the bed at an appropriate and comfortable working height (VHACEOSH, 2016). Lower both side rails.

6. If not already in place, position a friction-reducing sheet or lifting/repositioning sheet or other transfer device under the patient, based on assessment.

7. Remove all pillows from under the patient's head, back, or legs. If moving the patient up in the bed, leave one pillow at the head of the bed, leaning upright against the headboard.

8. Based on the screening and assessment information, position at least one nurse or other health care provider on either side of the bed, and lower both side rails.

9. If the patient is fully able to assist in repositioning, allow the patient to complete the move independently, with supervision.

10. If the patient is partially able or unable to assist, make use of friction-reducing devices, lifting/repositioning sheets (Figure 2), lateral transfer devices, full-body sling lift and/or engage the turning or rotation to assist with the action (VA Mobile Health, n.d.).

11. If turning, activate the bed-turn mechanism to inflate the side of the bed behind the patient's back.

12. Alternatively, follow manufacturer's directions to utilize the ceiling lift or full-body lifting device with the repositioning or supine sling or air-assisted transfer device. Refer to the Skill Variation at the end of the skill for guidelines related to use of a full-body sling lift.

RATIONALE

Checking the health care record validates the correct patient and correct procedure. Identification of limitations and ability along with use of an algorithm helps to prevent injury and aids in determining the best plan for patient movement.

Having aids readily available promotes efficient time management.

Hand hygiene and PPE prevent the spread of microorganisms. PPE is required based on transmission precautions.

Patient identification validates the correct patient and correct procedure. Discussion and explanation help allay anxiety and prepare the patient for what to expect.

Closing the door or curtains provides for privacy. Proper bed height helps reduce back strain while performing the procedure. Proper positioning and lowering of the side rails facilitate moving the patient and minimizes strain on the nurses.

Friction-reducing/lifting/repositioning sheets and other transfer devices aid in preventing shearing and in reducing friction and the force required to move the patient.

Removing pillows from under the patient facilitates movement; placing a pillow at the head of the bed prevents accidental head injury against the top of the bed.

Proper positioning and lowering the side rails facilitate moving the patient and minimize strain on the care providers.

Safe supervision allows for intervention by care giver if necessary and reduces the risk for injury.

Use of SPHM equipment is necessary to reduce risk of injury to patient and care providers (Fragala et al., 2016; OSHA and Joint Commission Resources Alliance, 2017; VA Mobile Health, n.d.).

Activating the turn mechanism inflates the side of the bed for approximately 10 seconds, aiding in propelling the patient to turn, and reducing the work required by the nurse. This helps avoid injury to the nurse or other care provider.

Use of SPHM equipment is necessary to reduce risk of injury to patient and care providers (Fragala et al., 2016; OSHA and Joint Commission Resources Alliance, 2017; VA Mobile Health, n.d.).

(continued on page 550)

Skill 9-1 ▶ Assisting a Patient With Repositioning in Bed *(continued)*

ACTION

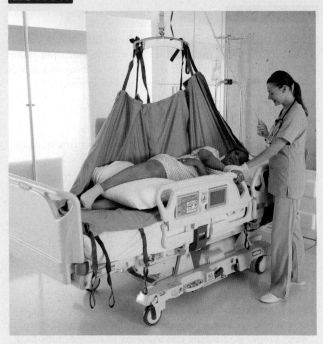

FIGURE 2. Example of a repositioning sheet for use with a lift.

13. Once the patient has been repositioned, make the patient comfortable and position in proper alignment, using pillows or other supports behind the patient's back (pull the shoulder blade forward and out from under the patient), under the leg and arm, as needed. Readjust the pillow under the patient's head. Elevate the head of the bed as needed for comfort.

14. Place the bed in the lowest position, with the side rails up, as indicated. Make sure the call bell and other necessary items are within easy reach.

15. Clean transfer aids, per facility policy, if not indicated for single-patient use. Remove gloves and other PPE, if used. Perform hand hygiene.

RATIONALE

Positioning in proper alignment with supports ensures that the patient will be able to maintain the desired position and will be comfortable. Positioning the shoulder blade removes pressure from the bony prominence.

Adjusting the bed height ensures patient safety. Having the call bell and essential items readily available helps promote safety.

Proper cleaning of equipment between patient use prevents the spread of microorganisms. Proper removal of PPE reduces the risk for infection transmission and contamination of other items. Hand hygiene prevents the spread of microorganisms.

EVALUATION

The expected outcomes have been achieved when the patient has been repositioned without injury to patient or nurse, the patient has reported improved comfort, and the patient has maintained proper body alignment.

DOCUMENTATION

Guidelines

Many facilities provide areas on the bedside flow sheet to document repositioning. Be sure to document the time the patient's position was changed, use of supports, and any pertinent observations, including skin assessment. Document the patient's tolerance of the position change. Document completed assessment algorithm for patient handling and movement decision and SPHM aids used to facilitate movement.

Sample Documentation

> 11/10/25 1130 Patient repositioned from right side to left side; alignment maintained with wedge support behind back and pillow between legs. Skin on pressure points on right side without signs of irritation, edema, or redness. Patient reported no pain with movement. Bed-turn mechanism and friction-reducing sheet used to facilitate transfer; sheet left in place under patient. Patient partially able to assist with turn by pulling on bed rail.
>
> —B. Clapp, RN

DEVELOPING CLINICAL REASONING AND CLINICAL JUDGMENT

UNEXPECTED SITUATIONS AND ASSOCIATED INTERVENTIONS

- *You are attempting to move a patient up in the bed when you realize your initial assessment was inaccurate and the patient is not able to participate with repositioning to the extent you thought*: Cover the patient, make sure all rails are up, lower the bed to the lowest position, and take a moment to reassess the situation using SPHM decision-making tool. Obtain the necessary equipment and number of personnel as indicated. Document the assessment and necessary equipment in the plan of care for continuity of care.

SPECIAL CONSIDERATIONS

- Institute Bariatric Algorithms for any patient who weighs more than 300 lb, or is 100 lb over ideal weight, or who has a body mass index (BMI) over 40 (VHA CEOSH, 2015).
- When moving a patient with a leg or foot problem, such as a cast, wound, or **fracture**, one caregiver should be assigned to monitor movement of that extremity to reduce risk of further injury.

Skill Variation ▶ Using a Full-Body Sling to Reposition a Patient

1. Review the health care record for prescribed interventions and plan of care for patient activity. Identify any movement limitations, conditions that may influence the patient's ability to move or be positioned, and the ability of the patient to assist with repositioning. **Consult the patient handling algorithm to plan an appropriate approach to moving the patient** (see Figure 1 in Skill 9-1).
2. Gather any positioning aids or supports, if necessary.

3. Perform hand hygiene and put on gloves and/or other PPE, as indicated.

4. Identify the patient. Explain the procedure to the patient.

5. Close the curtains around the bed and close the door to the room, if possible. Place the bed at an appropriate and comfortable working height. Adjust the head of the bed to a flat position or as low as the patient can tolerate.
6. Remove all pillows from under the patient. If moving the patient up in the bed, leave one at the head of the bed, leaning upright against the headboard.
7. Position at least one nurse on either side of the bed, and lower both side rails.
8. Place the cover sheet on the sling surface. Place the sling under the patient.

9. Roll the base of the lift under the side of the bed nearest to the chair. **Center the frame over the patient. Lock the wheels of the lift.**
10. **Using the base-adjustment lever, widen the stance of the base of the device.**
11. Position yourself and the other caregiver at the patient's midsection. If necessary, additional staff can support the patient's legs.
12. Crank or engage the mechanism to raise the sling, with the patient, up off the bed. Raise the patient just high enough to clear the bed surface.
13. Guide the sling and relocate the patient to the appropriate place at the head of the bed.
14. Release the sling slowly or activate the lowering device on the lift and slowly lower the patient to the bed surface.
15. Remove the sling or leave in place for future use, based on facility policy.
16. Assist the patient to a comfortable position and readjust the pillows and supports, as needed.
17. Raise the side rails. Place the bed in the lowest position. Make sure the call bell and other necessary items are within easy reach.

18. Clean transfer aids, per facility policy, if not indicated for single-patient use. Remove gloves and any other PPE, if used, and perform hand hygiene.

(continued on page 552)

Skill 9-1 ▶ Assisting a Patient With Repositioning in Bed *(continued)*

EVIDENCE FOR PRACTICE ▶

SAFE PATIENT HANDLING AND MOBILITY

VA Mobile Health. (n.d.). Safe patient handling. (Version 1.3.3). [Mobile app]. U. S. Department of Veteran Affairs. https://mobile.va.gov/app/safe-patient-handling

VHA Center for Engineering & Occupational Safety and Health (CEOSH). (2015). *Bariatric safe patient handling and mobility guidebook: A resource guide for care of persons of size.* https://www.asphp.org/wp-content/uploads/2011/05/Baraiatrice-SPHM-guidebook-care-of-Person-of-Size.pdf

These tools incorporate patient assessment guidelines, scoring tools, algorithms, and equipment guides to provide best-practice guidance in addressing the safe handling and mobility needs of patients, including bariatric patients, their families, and caregivers. These tools and information enable health care providers to plan and implement safe care of patients and promote caregiver safety.

Skill 9-2 ▶ Transferring a Patient From the Bed to a Stretcher

Considerable care must be taken when moving someone from one surface to another, such as from a bed to a stretcher or from a stretcher to a bed, to prevent injury to the patient or caregivers. The patient is at risk for injuries from **friction** and shearing forces while being moved. Knowledge of correct body alignment, SPHM, and assistive devices to transfer the patient are crucial to achieve patient movement and avoid injury. Use a decision-making tool to help make decisions about SPHM. One suggested decision-making strategy is outlined in Fundamentals Review 9-4 and includes suggestions for associated SPHM equipment. Another example of a decision-making tool is provided in Figure 1. Be familiar with the proper way to use lateral-assist devices, based on the manufacturer's directions. Refer to facility policy and procedures and specific manufacturer guidelines related to other available devices and equipment. Fundamentals Review 9-3 reviews examples of equipment and assistive devices that are available to aid in patient movement and handling. Refer to Box 9-1 in Skill 9-1 for additional considerations related to mobility and safe handling of people with dementia.

DELEGATION CONSIDERATIONS

The transfer of a patient from bed to stretcher may be delegated to assistive personnel (AP) as well as to licensed practical/vocational nurses (LPN/LVNs). The decision to delegate must be based on careful analysis of the patient's needs and circumstances as well as the qualifications of the person to whom the task is being delegated. Refer to the Delegation Guidelines in Appendix A.

EQUIPMENT

- Transport stretcher
- Ceiling lift or full-body lift
- Lateral-assist device, such as a transfer board, roller board, or air or mechanical lateral-assist device and cover sheet
- Bath blanket
- Regular blanket
- At least two assistants, depending on assessment and data
- Nonsterile gloves and/or other PPE, as indicated

ASSESSMENT

Assess the situation to determine the need to transfer the patient. Check the health record for any conditions or prescribed interventions that may influence the patient's ability to move or to be transferred. Perform a pain assessment before the time for the activity. If the patient reports pain, administer the prescribed medication in sufficient time to allow for the full effect of the analgesic.

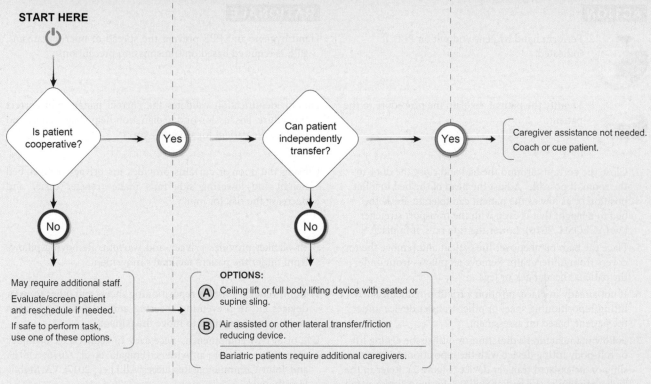

FIGURE 1. Example of an algorithm to aid in decision making regarding safe patient handling and mobility to transfer a patient from bed to stretcher. (*Source:* VA Mobile Health. [n.d.]. Safe patient handling. [Version 1.3.3]. Algorithm 2. [Mobile app]. U. S. Department of Veteran Affairs. https://mobile.va.gov/app/safe-patient-handling.)

Assess for tubes, IV lines, incisions, or equipment that may alter the positioning procedure. Assess the patient's level of consciousness, ability to understand and follow directions, and ability to assist with the transfer. Use available decision-making tools or algorithms to aid in assessment and decision making. Assess the patient's ability to assist with moving and the need for assistive devices. Determine the need for bariatric equipment.

ACTUAL OR POTENTIAL HEALTH PROBLEMS AND NEEDS	Many actual or potential health problems or issues may require the use of this skill as part of related interventions. An appropriate health problem or issue may include: • Activity intolerance • Deconditioning • Injury risk
OUTCOME IDENTIFICATION AND PLANNING	The expected outcome to achieve when transferring a patient from the bed to a stretcher is that the patient is transferred without injury to the patient or nurse.

IMPLEMENTATION

ACTION	**RATIONALE**
1. Identify any movement limitations, conditions that may influence the patient's ability to move or be positioned, and the ability of the patient to assist with the transfer. **Consult a patient handling algorithm, if available, to plan an appropriate approach to moving the patient.** Assess for tubes, IV lines, incisions, or equipment that may alter the positioning procedure. Gather transfer aids or supports as necessary.	Reviewing the health record and plan of care validates the correct patient and correct procedure. Checking for interfering equipment helps reduce the risk for injury. Identification of limitations and ability along with use of an algorithm helps to prevent injury and aids in determining the best plan for patient movement. Having aids readily available promotes efficient time management.

(*continued on page 554*)

Skill 9-2 ▶ Transferring a Patient From the Bed to a Stretcher *(continued)*

ACTION	RATIONALE

 2. Perform hand hygiene and put on PPE, if indicated.

Hand hygiene and PPE prevent the spread of microorganisms. PPE is required based on transmission precautions.

 3. Identify the patient. Explain the procedure to the patient.

Patient identification validates the correct patient and correct procedure. Discussion and explanation help allay anxiety and prepare the patient for what to expect.

4. Close the curtains around the bed and close the door to the room, if possible. Adjust the head of the bed to a flat position or as low as the patient can tolerate. Raise the bed to a height that is even with the transport stretcher (VHACEOSH, 2016). Lower the side rails, if in place.

Closing the door or curtains provides for privacy. Proper bed height and lowering side rails make transfer easier and decrease the risk for injury.

5. Place the bath blanket over the patient and remove the top covers from underneath. Remove all pillows from under the patient's head, back or legs.

Bath blanket provides privacy and warmth. Removing pillows from under the patient facilitates movement.

6. If not already in place, position a friction-reducing sheet or lifting/repositioning sheet or other transfer device under the patient, based on assessment.

Friction-reducing/lifting/repositioning sheets and other transfer devices aid in preventing shearing and in reducing friction and the force required to move the patient.

7. Follow manufacturer's directions to utilize the ceiling lift or full-body lifting device with the repositioning or supine sling or air-assisted transfer device (Figure 2). Refer to the Skill Variation at the end of Skill 9-1 for guidelines related to use of a full-body sling lift.

Use of SPHM equipment is necessary to reduce risk of injury to patient and care providers (Fragala et al., 2016; OSHA and Joint Commission Resources Alliance, 2017; VA Mobile Health, n.d.).

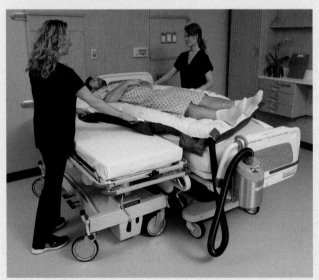

FIGURE 2. Example of an air-assisted transfer device. (HoverTech International, HoverSling® Repositioning Sheet.)

8. Position the stretcher next (and parallel) to the bed. **Lock the wheels on the stretcher and the bed.**

Positioning equipment makes the transfer easier and decreases the risk for injury. Locking the wheels keeps the bed and stretcher from moving.

9. At a minimum, one caregiver should be positioned on the stretcher side of the bed, and another should stand on the side of the bed without the stretcher. Depending on the transfer device, other care givers should be positioned accordingly.

Team coordination provides for patient safety during transfer.

ACTION

10. Use the friction-reducing sheet to roll the patient away from the stretcher (Figure 3). Place the transfer device under the patient (Figure 4).

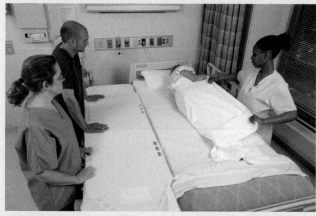

FIGURE 3. Using sheet to roll patient away from stretcher.

11. **At a signal given by one of the caregivers and based on the manufacturer's directions for use of the device, move the patient from the bed to the stretcher (Figure 5).**

12. Once the patient is transferred to the stretcher (Figure 6), remove the SPHM device or leave in place for future use, based on device type and facility policy. Provide a pillow and other supports as indicated. Secure the patient and raise the side rails. To ensure the patient's comfort, cover the patient with blanket and remove the bath blanket from underneath.

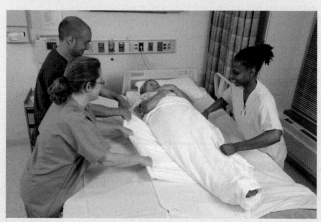

FIGURE 5. Transferring patient onto stretcher.

13. Clean transfer aids, per facility policy, if not indicated for single-patient use. Remove gloves and any other PPE, if used. Perform hand hygiene.

RATIONALE

The transfer board or other lateral-assist device reduces friction, easing the workload to move patient.

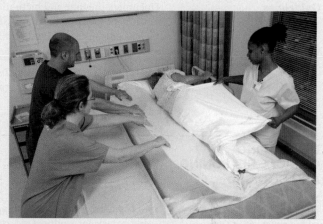

FIGURE 4. Positioning transfer device under patient.

Working in unison distributes the work of moving the patient and facilitates the transfer.

Positioning in proper alignment with supports ensures that the patient will be able to maintain the desired position and will be comfortable. Side rails promote safety. Blanket promotes comfort and warmth.

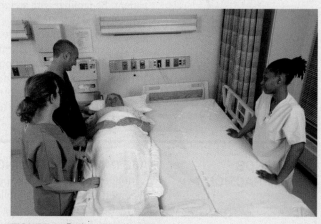

FIGURE 6. Patient on stretcher.

Proper cleaning of equipment between patient use prevents the spread of microorganisms. Proper removal of PPE reduces the risk for infection transmission and contamination of other items. Hand hygiene prevents the spread of microorganisms.

(*continued on page 556*)

Skill 9-2 ▶ Transferring a Patient From the Bed to a Stretcher   *(continued)*

EVALUATION

The expected outcome has been met when the patient has been transferred to the stretcher without injury to the patient or nurse.

DOCUMENTATION

Guidelines

Document the time and method of transport, and patient's destination, according to facility policy. Document the completed assessment algorithm for patient handling and movement decision and the use of transfer aids and number of staff required for transfer.

Sample Documentation

> 5/12/25 1005 Patient transferred to stretcher via air-assisted lateral transfer device. Three caregivers required. Transported to radiology for chest x-ray.
>
> —M. Joliet, RN

DEVELOPING CLINICAL REASONING AND CLINICAL JUDGMENT

UNEXPECTED SITUATIONS AND ASSOCIATED INTERVENTIONS

- *Your patient needs to be transported to another department by stretcher. The patient is very heavy and somewhat confused, so you are concerned about his ability to cooperate with the transfer:* Consult a Bariatric Algorithm. Confirm that the patient handling equipment and stretcher meet weight, width, and height requirements of the patient (VHA CEOSH, 2015). Obtain the assistance of additional caregivers; bariatric patients and use of expanded capacity equipment requires more caregivers (VHA CEOSH, 2015). Use bariatric equipment and devices to move the patient (VHA CEOSH, 2015).

SPECIAL CONSIDERATIONS

- If the patient is unconscious or weakened, additional caregivers are needed to support the extremities and the head to reduce risk of further injury.
- Some mechanical lateral-transfer aids are motorized, and others use a hand crank. If a mechanical lateral-assist device is used, follow the manufacturer's directions for safe movement of the patient. Be familiar with weight restrictions for individual pieces of equipment.
- Keep in mind that the transfer of patients is often delegated to assistive personnel. Before moving patients, all personnel need to complete instructions about this skill and must be able to provide return demonstrations of transfer skills. When a patient is being transferred, communicate clearly any mobility restrictions or special care needs.
- Bariatric patients require additional caregivers and expanded capacity devices (VA Mobile Health, n.d.; VHACEOSH, 2016). Institute Bariatric Algorithms for any patient who weighs more than 300 lb, or is 100 lb over ideal weight, or who has a BMI over 40 (VHA CEOSH, 2015).

EVIDENCE FOR PRACTICE ▶

SAFE PATIENT HANDLING AND MOBILITY

VA Mobile Health. (n.d.). Safe patient handling. (Version 1.3.3). [Mobile app]. U. S. Department of Veteran Affairs. https://mobile.va.gov/app/safe-patient-handling

VHA Center for Engineering & Occupational Safety and Health (CEOSH). (2015). *Bariatric safe patient handling and mobility guidebook: A resource guide for care of persons of size.* https://www.asphp.org/wp-content/uploads/2011/05/Baraiatrice-SPHM-guidebook-care-of-Person-of-Size.pdf

Refer to details in Skill 9-1, Evidence for Practice.

Skill 9-3 ▶ Transferring a Patient From the Bed to a Chair

Moving a patient from the bed to a chair helps them begin engaging in physical activity. Changing a patient's position will also help prevent complications related to immobility. Safety and comfort are key concerns when assisting the patient out of bed. Before performing the transfer, identify any restrictions related to the patient's condition and determine how activity levels may be affected. Knowledge of correct body alignment, SPHM, and assistive devices to transfer the patient are crucial to achieve patient movement and avoid injury. Use a decision-making tool to help make decisions about SPHM. One suggested decision-making strategy is outlined in Fundamentals Review 9-4 and includes suggestions for associated SPHM equipment. Another example of a decision-making tool is provided in Figure 1. If the patient is fully able to assist in getting out of bed, allow the patient to complete the movement independently, with safe supervision. If the patient is partially able to assist and has upper extremity strength, sitting balance, and the ability to grasp with at least one hand, use a seated transfer aid, nonpowered standing aid, or powered standing assist device (Figure 2). If the patient is unable to assist, friction-reducing devices, lifting/repositioning sheets, lateral transfer devices, and a full-body sling are potential equipment to consider, based on screening and assessment. Fundamentals Review 9-3 reviews examples of equipment and assistive devices that are available to aid in patient movement and handling. Refer to Box 9-1 in Skill 9-1 for additional considerations related to mobility and safe handling of people with dementia. The procedure below describes general guidelines for transferring a patient out of bed to a chair. Refer to facility policy and procedures and specific manufacturer guidelines related to other available devices and equipment. Skill 9-4 describes the use of a powered full-body sling lift.

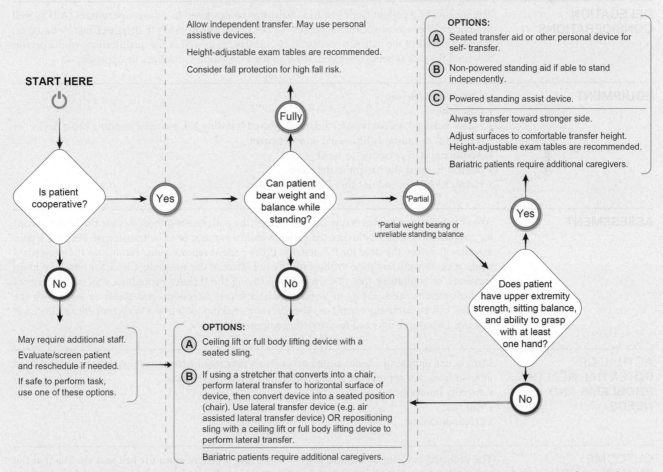

FIGURE 1. Example of an algorithm to aid in decision making regarding safe patient handling and mobility to transfer a patient from bed to a chair. (*Source:* VA Mobile Health. [n.d.]. Safe patient handling. [Version 1.3.3]. Algorithm 1. [Mobile app]. U. S. Department of Veteran Affairs. https://mobile.va.gov/app/safe-patient-handling.)

(continued on page 558)

Skill 9-3 ▶ Transferring a Patient From the Bed to a Chair *(continued)*

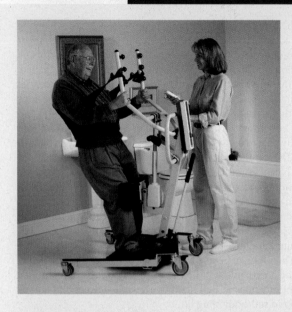

FIGURE 2. Powered stand-assist device. (© Invacare Corporation. Used with permission)

DELEGATION CONSIDERATIONS

The transfer of a patient from bed to a chair may be delegated to assistive personnel (AP) as well as to licensed practical/vocational nurses (LPN/LVNs). The decision to delegate must be based on careful analysis of the patient's needs and circumstances as well as the qualifications of the person to whom the task is being delegated. Refer to the Delegation Guidelines in Appendix A.

EQUIPMENT

- Chair or wheelchair
- Gait belt
- Stand-assist aid, seated transfer aid, nonpowered standing aid, powered standing assist device, or ceiling lift or full-body lift, based on assessment
- Additional staff person(s) to assist
- Blanket to cover the patient in the chair
- Nonsterile gloves and/or other PPE, as indicated

ASSESSMENT

Assess the situation to determine the need to get the patient out of bed. Review the health record for conditions that may influence the patient's ability to move or to be transferred. Perform a pain assessment before the time for the activity. If the patient reports pain, administer the prescribed medication in sufficient time to allow for the full effect of the analgesic. Check for tubes, IV lines, incisions, or equipment that may require modifying the transfer procedure. Assess the patient's level of consciousness, ability to understand and follow directions, and ability to assist with the transfer. Use available algorithms or other decision-making tools to aid in assessment and decision making. Determine the need for bariatric equipment.

ACTUAL OR POTENTIAL HEALTH PROBLEMS AND NEEDS

Many actual or potential health problems or issues may require the use of this skill as part of related interventions. An appropriate health problem or issue may include:
- Activity intolerance
- Fall risk
- Deconditioning

OUTCOME IDENTIFICATION AND PLANNING

The expected outcome to achieve when transferring a patient from the bed to a chair is that the transfer is accomplished without injury to the patient or nurse.

IMPLEMENTATION

ACTION	RATIONALE
1. Review the health record for prescribed interventions and plan of care for patient activity. Identify any movement limitations, conditions that may influence the patient's ability to move or be positioned, and the ability of the patient to assist with the transfer. Assess for tubes, IV lines, incisions, or equipment that may alter the positioning procedure. **Consult a patient handling algorithm or other decision-making tool to plan an appropriate approach to moving the patient.** Gather transport aids or supports as necessary.	Reviewing the health record and care plan validates the correct patient and correct procedure. Identification of limitations and ability and use of an algorithm help to prevent injury and aid in determining best plan for patient movement. Having aids readily available promotes efficient time management.

ACTION	RATIONALE
2. Perform hand hygiene and put on PPE, as indicated.	Hand hygiene and PPE prevent spread of microorganisms. PPE is required based on transmission precautions.

ACTION	RATIONALE
3. Identify the patient. Explain the procedure to the patient.	Patient identification validates the correct patient and correct procedure. Discussion and explanation help allay anxiety and prepare the patient for what to expect.
4. If needed, move equipment to make room for the chair. Close the curtains around the bed and close the door to the room, if possible.	A clear pathway from the bed to the chair facilitates the transfer. Closing the door or curtains provides for privacy.
5. Place the bed in a position that allows the patient's feet to reach the floor. Raise the head of the bed to a sitting position, or as high as the patient can tolerate.	Proper bed height and positioning facilitate the transfer. The amount of energy needed to move from a sitting position or elevated position to a sitting position is decreased.
6. **Make sure the bed brakes are locked. Put the chair next to the bed. If available, lock the brakes of the chair. If the chair does not have brakes, brace the chair against a secure object.**	Locking brakes or bracing the chair prevents movement during transfer and increases stability and patient safety.
7. Encourage the patient to make use of a stand-assist aid, either freestanding or attached to the side of the bed, if available, to move to the side of the bed and to a side-lying position, facing the side of the bed on which the patient will sit.	Encourages independence, reduces strain for staff, and decreases risk for patient injury.
8. Lower the side rail, if necessary, and stand near the patient's hips. Stand with your legs shoulder width apart with one foot near the head of the bed, slightly in front of the other foot.	The nurse's center of gravity is placed near the patient's greatest weight to assist the patient to a sitting position safely.
9. Encourage the patient to make use of the stand-assist device (Figure 3). Assist the patient to sit up on the side of the bed; ask the patient to swing their legs over the side of the bed. At the same time, the patient should use the stand-assist device to sit upright at the side of the bed.	Gravity lowers the patient's legs over the bed.
10. **Stand in front of the patient, and assess for any balance problems or complaints of dizziness. Allow the patient's legs to dangle a few minutes before continuing.**	Standing in front of the patient prevents falls or injuries from orthostatic hypotension. The sitting position facilitates transfer to the chair and allows the circulatory system to adjust to a change in position.
11. Assist the patient to put on a robe, as necessary and skid-proof footwear.	Robe provides warmth and privacy. Nonskid soles reduce the risk for falling.

(continued on page 560)

Skill 9-3 ▶ Transferring a Patient From the Bed to a Chair *(continued)*

ACTION

12. Wrap the gait belt around the patient's waist, based on assessed need and facility policy (Figure 4).

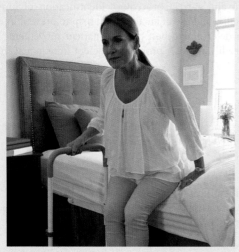

FIGURE 3. Example of a stand-assist aid. (Photo courtesy of HealthCraft Products Inc.)

13. Encourage the patient to make use of the stand-assist device. Cue the patient to stand. Assess the patient's balance and leg strength. If the patient is weak or unsteady, return the patient to the bed.

14. Assist the patient to pivot and turn until the patient feels the chair against their legs.

15. Ask the patient to use their arm to steady themselves on the arm of the chair while slowly lowering to a sitting position.

16. Assess the patient's alignment in the chair. Remove the gait belt, if desired. Depending on patient comfort, it could be left in place to use when returning to bed. Cover with a blanket, if needed. Make sure call bell and other essential items are within easy reach.

 17. Clean transfer aids, per facility policy, if not indicated for single-patient use. Remove gloves and any other PPE, if used. Perform hand hygiene.

RATIONALE

Gait belts improve the caregiver's grasp, reducing the risk of musculoskeletal injuries to staff and the patient. The belt also provides a firmer grasp for the caregiver if the patient should lose their balance. A gait belt is used to steady the patient, not a lifting device (Wintersgill, 2019).

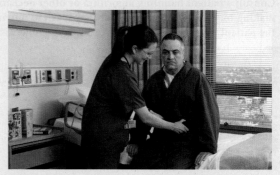

FIGURE 4. Wrapping gait belt around patient's waist.

Use of a stand-assist device decreases the risk of injury to the nurse and to the patient. Assessing balance and strength helps to identify the need for additional assistance to prevent falling.

This action ensures proper positioning before sitting.

The patient uses their own arm for support and stability.

Assessment promotes comfort; blanket provides warmth and privacy; having the call bell and other essential items readily available helps promote safety.

Proper cleaning of equipment between patient use prevents the spread of microorganisms. Proper removal of PPE reduces the risk for infection transmission and contamination of other items. Hand hygiene prevents the spread of microorganisms.

EVALUATION

The expected outcome has been met when the patient has transferred from the bed to the chair without injury to the patient or nurse.

DOCUMENTATION

Guidelines

Document the activity, including the length of time the patient sat in the chair, any other pertinent observations, and the patient's tolerance of and reaction to the activity. Document the completed assessment algorithm for patient handling and movement decision and the use of transfer aids and number of staff required for transfer.

Sample Documentation

5/13/25 1135 Patient dangled at side of bed for 5 minutes without complaints of dizziness or lightheadedness. Patient assisted out of bed to chair with minimal difficulty; gait belt in place. Tolerated sitting in chair for 30 minutes. Assisted back to bed. Resting in semi-Fowler position. Both upper side rails up.

—*J. Minkins, RN*

DEVELOPING CLINICAL REASONING AND CLINICAL JUDGMENT

UNEXPECTED SITUATIONS AND ASSOCIATED INTERVENTIONS

- *You are assisting a patient out of bed. The previous times the patient has gotten up, you have not had any difficulty helping him by yourself, so you are working alone at this time. The patient is positioned on the side of the bed and uses the stand-assist device to stand. As you move to pivot to the chair, the patient becomes very lightheaded and weak and his knees buckle:* Do not continue the move to the chair. Lower the patient back to the side of the bed. Pivot him back into bed, cover him, and raise the side rails. Check vital signs and assess for any other symptoms. After his symptoms have subsided and you are ready to get him up again, arrange for the assistance of another staff member. Have the patient dangle his legs for a longer period of time before standing. Assess for lightheadedness or dizziness before helping him to stand. Notify the health care team if there are any significant findings or if his symptoms persist.

SPECIAL CONSIDERATIONS

- Transfer of a patient to a chair or toilet can be accomplished using a powered stand-assist and repositioning lift, if available. These devices can be used with patients who have weight-bearing ability on at least one leg and who can follow directions and are cooperative. A simple sling is placed around the patient's back and under the arms. The patient rests feet on the device's foot-rest and places their hands on the handle. The device mechanically assists the patient to stand, without any lifting by the nurse (see Fundamentals Review 9-3). Once the patient is standing, the device can be wheeled to a chair, the toilet, or bed. Some devices have removable footrests and can be used as a walker. Some have scales incorporated into the device that can be used to weigh the patient.
- Patients who are unable to bear partial weight or full weight or who are uncooperative, as well as bariatric patients, should be transferred using a full-body sling lift (VHACEOSH, 2016) (refer to Skill 9-4). Use of SPHM equipment is necessary to reduce risk of injury to patient and care providers (Fragala et al., 2016; OSHA and Joint Commission Resources Alliance, 2017; VA Mobile Health, n.d.).
- Consider use of a gait belt for any patient who is not independent to promote safety (Wintersgill, 2019). A gait belt is used to steady the patient, not a lifting device (Wintersgill, 2019).
- Gait belts should also not be used with patients exhibiting behavioral aggression, as the belt might be used as a weapon and for patients at risk for suicide, as the belt might be used for self-harm (Wintersgill, 2019).
- Keep in mind that the transfer of patients is often delegated to assistive personnel. Before moving patients, all personnel need to complete instructions about this skill and must be able to provide return demonstrations of transfer skills. When a patient is being transferred, communicate clearly any mobility restrictions or special care needs.
- Bariatric patients require additional caregivers and expanded capacity devices (VA Mobile Health, n.d; VHACEOSH, 2016). Institute Bariatric Algorithms for any patient who weighs more than 300 lb, or is 100 lb over ideal weight, or who has a BMI over 40 (VHA CEOSH, 2015).

EVIDENCE FOR PRACTICE ▶

SAFE PATIENT HANDLING AND MOBILITY

VA Mobile Health. (n.d.). Safe patient handling. (Version 1.3.3). [Mobile app]. U. S. Department of Veteran Affairs. https://mobile.va.gov/app/safe-patient-handling

VHA Center for Engineering & Occupational Safety and Health (CEOSH). (2015). *Bariatric safe patient handling and mobility guidebook: A resource guide for care of persons of size.* https://www.asphp.org/wp-content/uploads/2011/05/Baraiatrice-SPHM-guidebook-care-of-Person-of-Size.pdf

Refer to details in Skill 9-1, Evidence for Practice.

Skill 9-4 ▶ Transferring a Patient Using a Powered Full-Body Sling Lift

A powered full-body sling lift may be used to reposition and transfer patients based on results of assessment through screening or use of an assessment tool to assess the patient's status and the need for SPHM devices (VA Mobile Health, n.d.; VHACDOSH, 2016). One suggested decision-making strategy is outlined in Fundamentals Review 9-4; this tool includes suggestions for associated SPHM equipment. A powered full-body sling lift may be used to reposition a patient in bed and/or move a patient in or out of bed, into and out of a chair, and to a commode or stretcher (refer to Fundamentals Review 9-3). A full-body sling is placed under the patient's body, including head and torso, and then the sling is attached to the lift. The device slowly lifts the patient. Some devices can be lowered to the floor to pick up a patient who has fallen. These devices are available on portable bases and ceiling-mounted tracks. Each manufacturer's device is slightly different, so review the instructions for your particular device. Refer to facility policy and procedures and specific manufacturer guidelines related to other available devices and equipment. Box 9-1 in Skill 9-1 outlines general guidelines related to mobility and safe handling of people with dementia.

DELEGATION CONSIDERATIONS	The transfer of a patient from bed to a chair may be delegated to assistive personnel (AP) as well as to licensed practical/vocational nurses (LPN/LVNs). The decision to delegate must be based on careful analysis of the patient's needs and circumstances as well as the qualifications of the person to whom the task is being delegated. Refer to the Delegation Guidelines in Appendix A.
EQUIPMENT	• Powered full-body sling lift • Sheet or pad to cover the sling, if sling is not dedicated to only one patient • Chair or wheelchair • One or more caregivers for assistance, based on assessment • Nonsterile gloves and/or other PPE, as indicated
ASSESSMENT	Assess the situation to determine the need to use the lift. Review the health record and care plan for conditions that may influence the patient's ability to move or to be transferred. Use available algorithms to aid in assessment and decision making. Determine the need for bariatric equipment. Assess for tubes, IV lines, incisions, or equipment that may alter the transfer procedure. Assess the patient's level of consciousness and ability to understand and follow directions. Assess the patient's comfort level; if needed, medicate, as prescribed, with analgesics. Assess the condition of the equipment to ensure proper functioning before using with the patient. Determine the need for bariatric equipment.
ACTUAL OR POTENTIAL HEALTH PROBLEMS AND NEEDS	Many actual or potential health problems or issues may require the use of this skill as part of related interventions. An appropriate health problem or issue may include: • Injury risk • Deconditioning • Fall risk
OUTCOME IDENTIFICATION AND PLANNING	The expected outcome to achieve when transferring a patient using a powered full-body sling lift is that the transfer is accomplished without injury to the patient or nurse.

IMPLEMENTATION

ACTION

RATIONALE

1. Review the health record and care plan for conditions that may influence the patient's ability to move or to be positioned. Identify any movement limitations, conditions that may influence the patient's ability to move or be positioned, and the ability of the patient to assist with the transfer. **Consult a patient handling algorithm, if available, to plan an appropriate approach to moving the patient.** Assess for tubes, IV lines, incisions, or equipment that may alter the positioning procedure. Gather transfer aids or supports as necessary.

Reviewing the health record and care plan validates the correct patient and correct procedure. Checking for equipment and limitations reduces the risk for injury during the transfer. Identification of limitations and ability along with use of an algorithm helps to prevent injury and aids in determining the best plan for patient movement. Having aids readily available promotes efficient time management.

2. Perform hand hygiene and put on PPE, if indicated.

Hand hygiene and PPE prevent the spread of microorganisms. PPE is required based on transmission precautions.

3. Identify the patient. Explain the procedure to the patient.

Patient identification validates the correct patient and correct procedure. Discussion and explanation allay anxiety and prepare the patient for what to expect.

4. If needed, move the equipment to make room for the chair. Close the curtains around the bed and close the door to the room, if possible.

Moving equipment out of the way provides a clear path and facilitates the transfer. Closing the door or curtains provides for privacy.

5. Adjust the bed to a comfortable working height (VHACEOSH, 2016). **Lock the bed brakes.**

Having the bed at the proper height prevents back and muscle strain. Locking the brakes prevents bed movement and ensures patient safety.

6. Lower the side rail, if in use, on the side of the bed you are working. If the sling is for use with more than one patient, place a cover or pad on the sling. Place the sling evenly under the patient. Roll the patient to one side and place half of the sling with the sheet or pad on it under the patient from shoulders to mid-thigh (Figure 1). Raise the rail and move to the other side. Lower the rail, if necessary. Roll the patient to the other side and pull the sling under the patient (Figure 2). Raise the side rail.

Lowering the side rail prevents strain on the nurse's back. Covering the sling prevents transmission of microorganisms. Some facilities, such as long-term care institutions, provide each patient with own transport sling. Rolling the patient positions the patient on the sling with minimal movement. Even distribution of the patient's weight in the sling provides for patient comfort and safety.

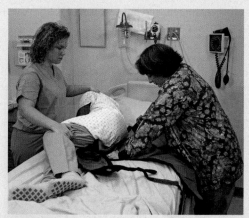

FIGURE 1. Rolling patient to one side and placing rolled sling underneath patient.

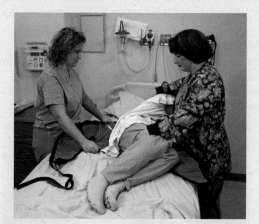

FIGURE 2. Rolling patient to opposite side and pulling sling under patient.

7. Bring the chair to the side of the bed. **Lock the wheels, if present.**

Bringing the chair close to the bed minimizes the distance needed for transfer. Locking the wheels prevents chair movement and ensures patient safety.

(continued on page 564)

Skill 9-4 ▶ Transferring a Patient Using a Powered Full-Body Sling Lift *(continued)*

ACTION

8. Lower the side rail on the chair side of the bed. Roll the base of the lift under the side of the bed nearest to the chair. **Center the frame over the patient. Lock the wheels of the lift.**

9. **Using the base-adjustment lever, widen the stance of the base** (Figure 3).

10. Lower the arms on the lift frame close enough to attach the sling to the frame (Figure 4).

RATIONALE

Lowering the rail allows for ease of transfer. Use of SPHM equipment is necessary to reduce risk of injury to patient and care providers (Fragala et al., 2016; OSHA and Joint Commission Resources Alliance, 2017; VA Mobile Health, n.d.). Positioning on the side of the bed close to the chair reduces the distance necessary for transfer. Centering the frame helps maintain the balance of the lift. Locking the lift's wheels prevents the lift from rolling.

A wider stance provides greater stability and prevents tipping.

Lowering the arms is necessary to allow for the attachment of the sling's hooks.

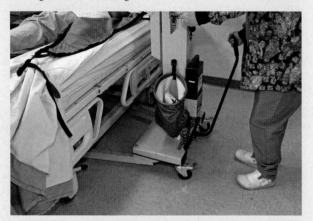

FIGURE 3. Widening stance of lift base.

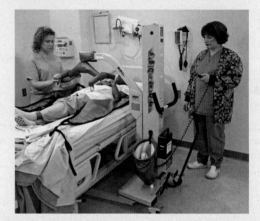

FIGURE 4. Lowering lift arms.

11. Attach the straps on the sling to the hooks on the frame (Figure 5). Short straps attach behind the patient's back and long straps attach at the other end of the sling. Check the patient to make sure the straps are not pressing into the skin. Some lifts have straps or chains with hooks that attach to holes in the sling. Check the manufacturer's instructions for each lift.

12. Check all equipment, lines, and drains attached to the patient so that they are not interfering with the device. Have the patient fold their arms across the chest.

13. With a person standing on each side of the lift, tell the patient that they will be lifted from the bed. Support injured limbs as necessary. Engage the pump to raise the patient about 6 inches above the bed (Figure 6).

Connecting the straps or chains permits attachment of the sling to the lift. Checking the patient's skin for pressure from the hooks prevents injury.

Ensuring that equipment and lines are free of the device prevents dislodgement and possible injury.

Having the necessary people available provides for safety. Supporting injured limbs helps maintain stability. Informing the patient about what will occur reassures the patient and reduces fear.

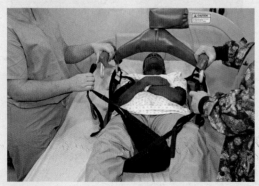

FIGURE 5. Connecting lift straps.

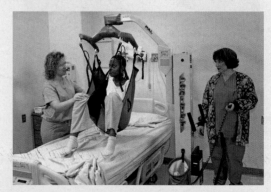

FIGURE 6. Raising patient 6 inches above bed.

ACTION

14. Unlock the wheels of the lift. **Carefully wheel the patient straight back and away from the bed. Support the patient's limbs, as needed.**

15. Position the patient over the chair with the base of the lift straddling the chair (Figure 7). Lock the wheels of the lift.

16. Gently lower the patient to the chair until the hooks or straps are slightly loosened from the sling or frame (Figure 8). Guide the patient into the chair with your hands as the sling lowers.

RATIONALE

Moving in this manner promotes stability and safety.

Proper positioning of the patient and device promotes stability and safety.

Gently lowering the patient in this manner places the patient fully in the chair and reduces the risk for injury.

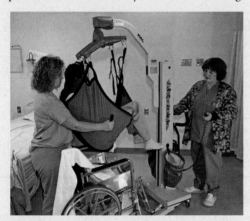

FIGURE 7. Positioning patient in sling over chair.

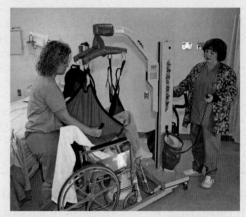

FIGURE 8. Lowering patient in sling into chair.

17. Disconnect the hooks or strap from the frame. Keep the sling in place under the patient.

18. Adjust the patient's position, using pillows, if necessary. Check the patient's alignment in the chair. Cover the patient with a blanket, if necessary. Make sure call bell and other essential items are within easy reach. When it is time for the patient to return to bed, reattach the hooks or straps and reverse the steps.

19. Clean transfer aids, per facility policy, if not indicated for single-patient use. Remove gloves and any other PPE, if used. Perform hand hygiene.

Disconnecting the hooks or straps allows the patient to be supported by the chair and promotes comfort. The sling will need to be reattached to the lift to move the patient back to bed.

Pillows and proper alignment provide for patient safety and comfort. Having the call bell and other essential items readily available helps promote safety. Reattaching the hooks or straps allows the lift to support the patient for transfer back to bed.

Proper cleaning of equipment between patient use prevents the spread of microorganisms. Proper removal of PPE reduces the risk for infection transmission and contamination of other items. Hand hygiene prevents the spread of microorganisms.

EVALUATION

The expected outcome has been met when the transfer was accomplished without injury to the patient or nurse.

DOCUMENTATION

Guidelines

Document the activity, transfer, any other pertinent observations, the patient's tolerance of the procedure, and the length of time in the chair. Document the completed assessment algorithm for patient handling and movement decision and the use of transfer aids and number of staff required for transfer.

Sample Documentation

5/13/25 1430 Patient transferred out of bed to chair using powered full-body sling lift. Tolerated sitting in chair for 25 minutes without complaints of dizziness or pain. Assisted back to bed via lift. Patient sitting in semi-Fowler position with upper two side rails up.
—P. Jefferson, RN

(continued on page 566)

Skill 9-4 ▶ Transferring a Patient Using a Powered Full-Body Sling Lift   *(continued)*

DEVELOPING CLINICAL REASONING AND CLINICAL JUDGMENT

UNEXPECTED SITUATIONS AND ASSOCIATED INTERVENTIONS

- *You are preparing to move a patient using a powered full-body sling lift. After you apply the sling and attach it to the frame, the patient becomes anxious and tells you they are afraid:* Acknowledge the patient's feelings and explain the procedure again. Reassure the patient about the safety of the device. Obtain an additional person to support the patient during the move by holding her hand or supporting her head. If possible, plan the transfer when a family member/caregiver or friend is present to offer support.

SPECIAL CONSIDERATIONS

- The duration of time spent in slings should be limited to reduce risk for pressure injuries, especially for vulnerable populations (Peterson et al., 2015).
- The transfer of patients is often delegated to assistive personnel. Before moving patients, all personnel need to complete instructions and must be able to provide return demonstrations of transfer skills. Before the transfer, communicate clearly any mobility restrictions or special care needs.
- Bariatric patients require additional caregivers and expanded capacity devices (VA Mobile Health, n.d; VHACEOSH, 2016). Institute Bariatric Algorithms for any patient who weighs more than 300 lb, or id 100 lb over ideal weight, or who has a BMI over 40 (VHA CEOSH, 2015).

EVIDENCE FOR PRACTICE ▶

SAFE PATIENT HANDLING AND MOBILITY

VA Mobile Health. (n.d.). Safe patient handling. (Version 1.3.3). [Mobile app]. U. S. Department of Veteran Affairs. https://mobile.va.gov/app/safe-patient-handling

VHA Center for Engineering & Occupational Safety and Health (CEOSH). (2015). Bariatric safe patient handling and mobility guidebook: A resource guide for care of persons of size. https://www.asphp.org/wp-content/uploads/2011/05/Baraiatrice-SPHM-guidebook-care-of-Person-of-Size.pdf

Refer to details in Skill 9-1, Evidence for Practice.

Skill 9-5 ▶ Providing Range-of-Motion Exercises

Range of motion (ROM) is the complete extent of movement of which a joint is normally capable. When a person performs routine activities of daily living (ADLs), they are using muscle groups that help to keep many joints in an effective ROM. When all or some of the normal ADLs are impossible due to illness or injury, it is important to give attention to the joints not being used or to those that have limited use. When the patient does the exercise themselves, it is referred to as *active ROM*. Exercises performed by the nurse or caregiver without participation by the patient are referred to as *passive ROM*. Exercises should be as active as the patient's physical condition permits. Allow the patient to do as much independent activity as their condition permits. Initiate ROM exercises as soon as possible; routine activity and mobilization of patients is an important activity and is appropriate for most patient populations (Arnold et al., 2018; Liu et al., 2018; Nack et al., 2019; Tasheva et al., 2020).

DELEGATION CONSIDERATIONS

Patient teaching regarding ROM exercises cannot be delegated to assistive personnel (AP). Reinforcement or implementation of ROM exercises may be delegated to AP as well as to licensed practical/vocational nurses (LPN/LVNs). The decision to delegate must be based on careful analysis of the patient's needs and circumstances as well as the qualifications of the person to whom the task is being delegated. Refer to the Delegation Guidelines in Appendix A.

EQUIPMENT

No special equipment or supplies are necessary to perform ROM exercises. Wear nonsterile gloves and/or other PPE, as appropriate.

ASSESSMENT

Review the health record and plan of care for any conditions or prescribed interventions that limit mobility. Perform a pain assessment before the time for the exercises. If the patient reports pain, administer the prescribed medication in sufficient time to allow for the full effect of the analgesic. Assess the patient's ability to perform ROM exercises. Inspect and palpate joints for redness, tenderness, pain, swelling, or deformities.

ACTUAL OR POTENTIAL HEALTH PROBLEMS AND NEEDS

Many actual or potential health problems or issues may require the use of this skill as part of related interventions. An appropriate health problem or issue may include:
- Impaired active range of motion
- Fatigue
- Deconditioning

OUTCOME IDENTIFICATION AND PLANNING

The expected outcome to achieve when performing ROM exercises is that the patient completes the exercises and maintains or improves joint mobility. Other outcomes include improving or maintaining muscle strength and preventing muscle atrophy and **contractures**.

IMPLEMENTATION

ACTION	RATIONALE
1. Review the prescribed interventions and plan of care for patient activity. Identify any movement limitations.	Reviewing the prescribed interventions and care plan validates the correct patient and correct procedure. Identification of limitations prevents injury.
2. Perform hand hygiene and put on PPE, if indicated.	Hand hygiene and PPE prevent the spread of microorganisms. PPE is required based on transmission precautions.
3. Identify the patient. Explain the procedure to the patient.	Patient identification validates the correct patient and correct procedure. Discussion and explanation help allay anxiety and prepare the patient for what to expect.
4. Close the curtains around the bed and close the door to the room, if possible. Place the bed at an appropriate and comfortable working height (VHACEOSH, 2016). Adjust the head of the bed to a flat position or as low as the patient can tolerate.	Closing the door or curtains provides for privacy. Proper bed height helps reduce back strain while performing the procedure.
5. Stand on the side of the bed where the joints are to be exercised. Lower side rail on that side, if in place. Uncover only the limb to be used during the exercise.	Standing on the side to be exercised and lowering the side rail prevent strain on the nurse's back. Proper draping provides for privacy and warmth.
6. Perform the exercises slowly and gently, providing support by holding the areas proximal and distal to the joint. Repeat each exercise two to five times, moving each joint in a smooth and rhythmic manner. **Stop movement if the patient reports of pain or if you meet resistance.**	Slow, gentle movements with support prevent discomfort and muscle spasms resulting from jerky movements. Repeated movement of muscles and joints improves flexibility and increases circulation to the body part. Pain may indicate the exercises are causing damage.
7. While performing the exercises, begin at the head and move down one side of the body at a time. **Encourage the patient to do as many of these exercises independently as possible.**	Proceeding from head to toe, one side at a time, promotes efficient time management and an organized approach to the task. Both active and passive exercises improve joint mobility and increase circulation to the affected part, but only active exercise increases muscle mass, tone, and strength and improves cardiac and respiratory functioning.

(continued on page 568)

Skill 9-5 ▶ Providing Range-of-Motion Exercises *(continued)*

ACTION	RATIONALE
8. Move the chin down to rest on the chest (Figure 1). Return the head to a normal upright position (Figure 2). Tilt the head as far as possible toward each shoulder (Figure 3).	These movements provide for **flexion**, **extension**, and lateral flexion of the head and neck.
9. Move the head from side to side, bringing the chin toward each shoulder (Figure 4).	These movements provide for **rotation** of neck.

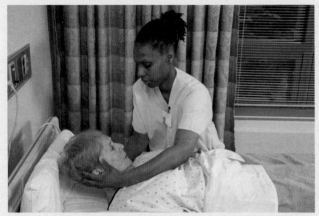

FIGURE 1. Moving patient's chin down to rest on chest.

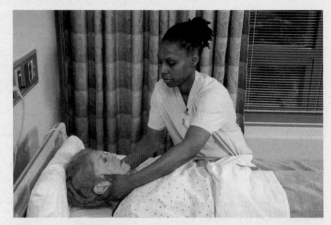

FIGURE 2. Holding patient's head upright and centered.

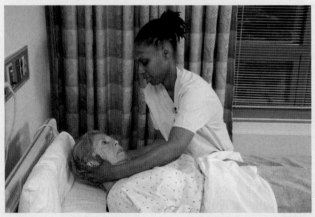

FIGURE 3. Moving patient's head to one shoulder.

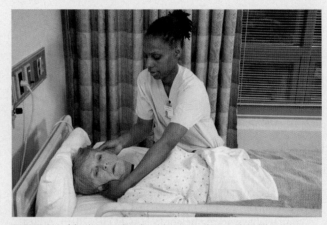

FIGURE 4. Moving patient's chin toward one shoulder.

10. Start with the arm at the patient's side (Figure 5) and lift the arm forward to above the head (Figure 6). Return the arm to the starting position at the side of the body.

These movements provide for flexion and extension of the shoulder.

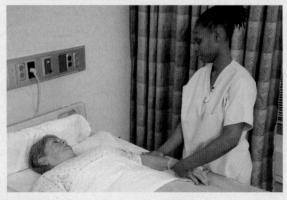

FIGURE 5. Holding patient's arm at side.

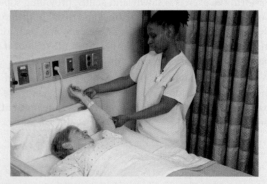

FIGURE 6. Lifting patient's arm above patient's head.

ACTION

11. With the arm back at the patient's side, move the arm laterally to an upright position above the head (Figure 7), and then return it to the original position. Move the arm across the body as far as possible (Figure 8).

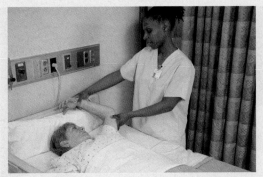

FIGURE 7. Moving patient's arm laterally to an upright position above patient's head.

12. Raise the arm at the side until the upper arm is in line with the shoulder. Bend the elbow at a 90-degree angle (Figure 9) and move the forearm upward and downward, then return the arm to the side.

13. Bend the elbow and move the lower arm and hand upward toward the shoulder (Figure 10). Return the lower arm and hand to the original position while straightening the elbow.

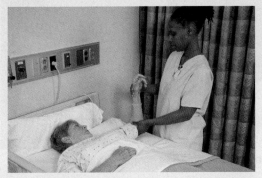

FIGURE 9. Raising patient's arm until upper arm is in line with patient's shoulder, with elbow bent.

14. Rotate the lower arm and hand so the palm is up (Figure 11). Rotate the lower arm and hand so the palm of the hand is down.

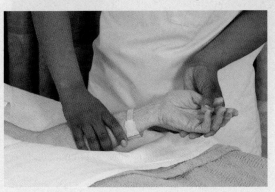

RATIONALE

These movements provide for **abduction** and **adduction** of the shoulder.

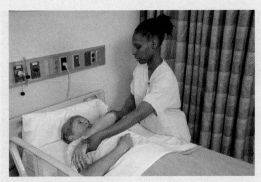

FIGURE 8. Moving arm across patient's body as far as possible.

These movements provide for internal and external rotation of the shoulder.

These movements provide for flexion and extension of the elbow.

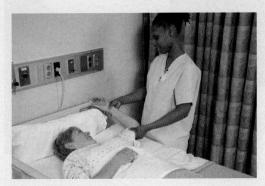

FIGURE 10. Bending patient's elbow, lower arm, and hand upward toward shoulder.

These movements provide for **supination** and **pronation** of the forearm.

FIGURE 11. Rotating patient's lower arm and hand so palm is up.

(*continued on page 570*)

Skill 9-5 ▶ Providing Range-of-Motion Exercises *(continued)*

ACTION	**RATIONALE**
15. Move the hand downward toward the inner aspect of the forearm (Figure 12). Return the hand to a neutral position even with the forearm (Figure 13). Then move the dorsal portion of the hand backward as far as possible.	These movements provide for flexion, extension, and hyperextension of the wrist.

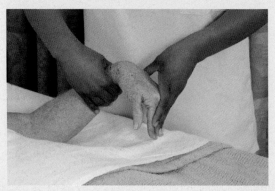

FIGURE 12. Moving patient's hand downward toward inner aspect of forearm.

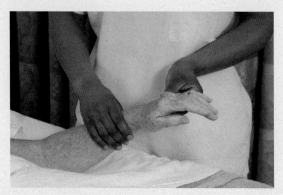

FIGURE 13. Returning hand to neutral position.

ACTION	**RATIONALE**
16. Bend the fingers to make a fist (Figure 14), and then straighten them out (Figure 15). Spread the fingers apart (Figure 16) and return them back together. Touch the thumb to each finger on the hand (Figure 17).	These movements provide for flexion, extension, abduction, and adduction of the fingers.

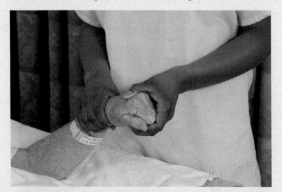

FIGURE 14. Bending patient's fingers to make a fist.

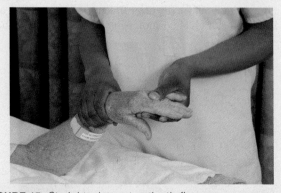

FIGURE 15. Straightening out patient's fingers.

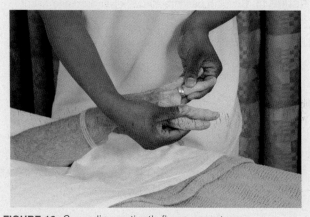

FIGURE 16. Spreading patient's fingers apart.

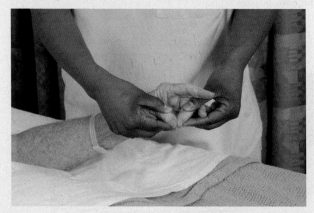

FIGURE 17. Assisting patient to touch thumb to each finger on hand.

ACTION

17. Extend the leg and lift it upward (Figure 18). Return the leg to the original position beside the other leg.

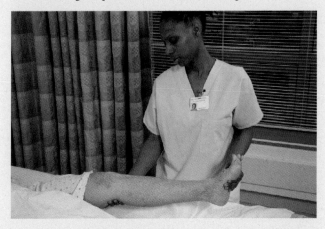

FIGURE 18. Extending and lifting patient's leg.

18. Lift the leg laterally away from the patient's body (Figure 19). Return the leg back toward the other leg and try to extend it beyond the midline (Figure 20).

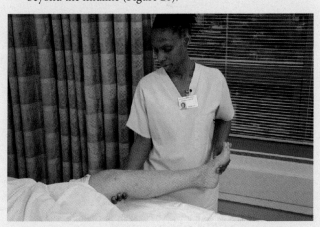

FIGURE 19. Lifting patient's leg laterally away from body (abduction).

19. Turn the foot and leg toward the opposite leg to rotate it internally (Figure 21). Turn the foot and leg outward away from the opposite leg to rotate it externally (Figure 22).

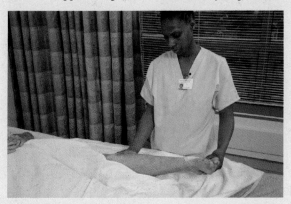

FIGURE 21. Turning patient's foot and leg toward opposite leg to rotate it internally.

RATIONALE

These movements provide for flexion and extension of the hip.

These movements provide for abduction and adduction of the hip.

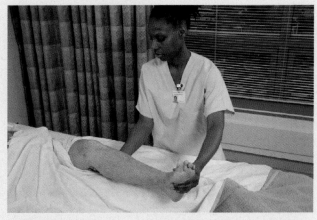

FIGURE 20. Returning leg back toward other leg and trying to extend it beyond midline, if possible.

These movements provide for internal and external rotation of the hip.

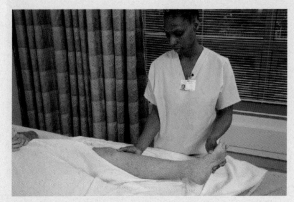

FIGURE 22. Turning patient's foot and leg outward, away from opposite leg, to rotate it externally.

(*continued on page 572*)

Skill 9-5 ▶ Providing Range-of-Motion Exercises *(continued)*

ACTION	RATIONALE
20. Bend the leg and bring the heel toward the back of the leg (Figure 23). Return the leg to a straight position (Figure 24).	These movements provide for flexion and extension of the knee.

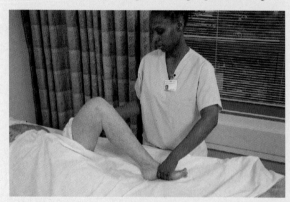

FIGURE 23. Bending patient's leg and bringing heel toward back of leg.

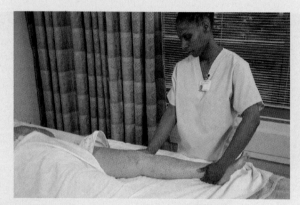

FIGURE 24. Returning leg to a straight position.

ACTION	RATIONALE
21. At the ankle, move the foot up and back until the toes are upright (Figure 25). Move the foot with the toes pointing downward (Figure 26).	These movements provide for dorsiflexion and plantar flexion of the ankle.

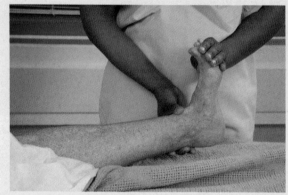

FIGURE 25. At the ankle, moving patient's foot up and back until toes are upright.

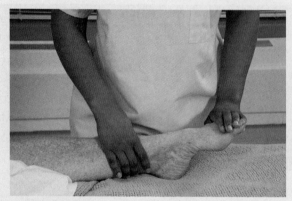

FIGURE 26. Moving patient's foot with toes pointing down.

ACTION	RATIONALE
22. Turn the sole of the foot toward the midline (Figure 27). Turn the sole of the foot outward (Figure 28).	These movements provide for inversion and eversion of the ankle.

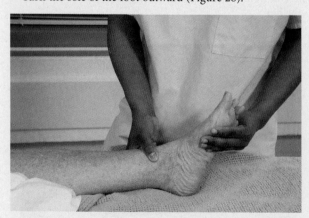

FIGURE 27. Turning sole toward midline.

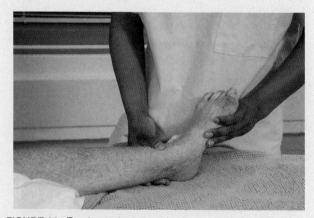

FIGURE 28. Turning sole outward.

ACTION

23. Curl the toes downward (Figure 29), and then straighten them out (Figure 30). Spread the toes apart (Figure 31) and bring them together (Figure 32).

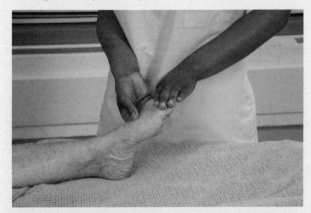

FIGURE 29. Curling patient's toes downward.

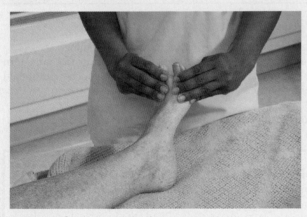

FIGURE 31. Spreading patient's toes apart.

24. Repeat these exercises on the other side of the body. Encourage the patient to do as many of these exercises independently as possible.

25. When finished, make sure the patient is comfortable, with the side rails up and the bed in the lowest position. Place the call bell and other essential items within reach.

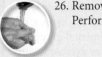
26. Remove gloves and any other PPE, if used. Perform hand hygiene.

RATIONALE

These movements provide for flexion, extension, abduction, and adduction of the toes.

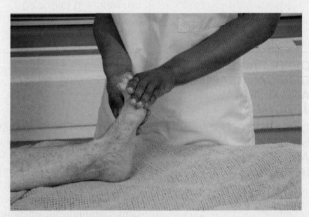

FIGURE 30. Straightening patient's toes.

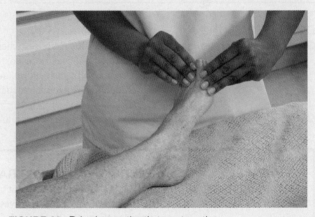

FIGURE 32. Bringing patient's toes together.

Repeating motions on the other side provides exercise for the entire body. Self-esteem, self-care, and independence are encouraged through the patient performing the exercises on their own.

Proper positioning with raised side rails and proper bed height provide for patient comfort and safety. Having the call bell and other essential items within reach promotes safety.

Proper removal of PPE reduces the risk for infection transmission and contamination of other items. Hand hygiene prevents the spread of microorganisms.

EVALUATION   The expected outcome has been met when the patient has completed the exercises and maintained or improved joint mobility and muscle strength, and muscle atrophy and contractures have been prevented.

DOCUMENTATION

Guidelines   Document the exercises performed, any significant observations, and the patient's reaction to the activities.

(*continued on page 574*)

Skill 9-5 ▶ Providing Range-of-Motion Exercises *(continued)*

Sample Documentation

> 5/1/25 0945 Range-of-motion exercises performed to all joints. Patient able to perform active ROM of head, neck, shoulders, and arms. Required moderate assistance with ROM to lower extremities. Denied any complaints of pain during exercises. Patient tolerated exercise session well. Sitting in semi-Fowler position with two upper side rails up, watching television.
>
> —J. Chrisp, RN

DEVELOPING CLINICAL REASONING AND CLINICAL JUDGMENT

UNEXPECTED SITUATIONS AND ASSOCIATED INTERVENTIONS

- *While you are performing ROM exercises, the patient reports feeling tired:* Stop the activity for that time. Reevaluate the nursing care plan. Space the exercises out at different times of the day. Schedule exercise times for the parts of the day the patient is typically feeling more rested.
- *While exercising your patient's leg, he reports sudden, sharp pain:* Stop the exercises. Assess the patient for other symptoms. Notify the health care team of the event, the patient's uncomfortable reaction, and your assessment findings. Joints should be moved until there is resistance, but not pain. Communicate uncomfortable reactions and halt exercises. Revise activity plan, if necessary.

SPECIAL CONSIDERATIONS

General Considerations

- Incorporate the exercises when possible into daily activities, such as during bathing.
- Prescribed interventions for ROM exercises for patients with acute arthritis, fractures, torn ligaments, joint dislocation, acute myocardial infarction, and bone tumors or metastases should include? Keep specific instructions for performance.

Older Adult Considerations

- Avoid neck hyperextension and attempts to achieve full ROM in all joints with older adults.

EVIDENCE FOR PRACTICE ▶

EXERCISE AND RESPIRATORY FUNCTION

ROM exercises improve joint mobility; increase circulation, muscle mass, muscle tone, and muscle strength; and improves cardiac and respiratory functioning. Exercises should be as active as the patient's physical condition permits. ROM exercises should be initiated as soon as possible as part of a patient's care plan, because body changes can occur after only a few days of impaired mobility.

Related Research

Cho, S. H., Lee, J. H., & Jang, S. H. (2015). Efficacy of pulmonary rehabilitation using cervical range of motion exercise in stroke patients with tracheostomy tubes. *Journal of Physical Therapy Science, 27*(5), 1329–1331. https://doi.org/10.1589/jpts.27.1329

This study examined the effect of cervical range-of-motion exercises on pulmonary and coughing function in poststroke patients with tracheostomy tubes who had no history of respiratory disease. Participants were randomly assigned to either an experimental group or a control group. The experimental group performed cervical range-of-motion exercises with a physical therapist five times a week for 8 weeks; the control group did not perform cervical range-of-motion exercises. Measurements of pulmonary function and coughing ability were obtained for both groups at the beginning and at the end of the 8 weeks. When the measurements were compared, the control group did not show any significant changes in pulmonary or coughing function. The experimental group showed a statistically significant increase in pulmonary and coughing function. The researchers concluded that cervical range-of-motion exercises can effectively improve the pulmonary function and coughing ability of stroke patients with tracheostomy tubes.

> **Relevance for Nursing Practice**
> An exercise program that includes ROM exercises can generate positive effects in enhancing physical function of stroke survivors. Methods to assist patients in maintaining or increasing physical activity should be a part of routine nursing care. Nurses are in ideal positions to discuss the effects of exercise with patients and include exercise programs in the care plan.

Skill 9-6 ▶ Assisting a Patient With Ambulation

Walking exercises most of the body's muscles and increases joint flexibility. It improves respiratory and gastrointestinal function. Ambulating also reduces the risk for complications of immobility. Early mobility plays an important role in the patient's physical and psychological well-being (Arnold et al., 2018). Use a screening or assessment tool to assess the patient's ability to walk and the need for SPHM devices and assistance to guide decision making (VA Mobile Health, n.d.; VHACDOSH, 2016). One example of a decision-making tool and associated SPHM equipment are outlined in Fundamentals Review 9-4. Figure 1 provides another example of a decision-making tool related to ambulation. Fundamentals Review 9-3 provides examples of assistive equipment and devices. Box 9-1 in Skill 9-1 outlines general guidelines related to mobility and safe handling of people with dementia. The procedure below describes general guidelines for ambulating a patient who is able to bear weight, balance, and raise and advance both feet while standing. Refer to facility policy and procedures and specific manufacturer guidelines related to other available devices and equipment.

DELEGATION CONSIDERATIONS	Assisting a patient with ambulation may be delegated to assistive personnel (AP) as well as to licensed practical/vocational nurses (LPN/LVNs). The decision to delegate must be based on careful analysis of the patient's needs and circumstances as well as the qualifications of the person to whom the task is being delegated. Refer to the Delegation Guidelines in Appendix A.
EQUIPMENT	• Gait belt, as necessary • Nonskid shoes or slippers • Nonsterile gloves and/or other PPE, as indicated • Stand-assist device, based on assessment • Additional staff for assistance, as needed
ASSESSMENT	Review the health record for conditions that may influence the patient's ability to walk. Assess the patient's ability to walk and the need for assistance (one nurse, two nurses, walker, cane, walking belt, or crutches). Check for tubes, IV lines, incisions, or equipment that may require modifying the transfer procedure. Perform a pain assessment before the time for the activity. If the patient reports pain, administer the prescribed medication in sufficient time to allow for the full effect of the analgesic. Take vital signs and assess the patient for dizziness or lightheadedness with position changes. Use available algorithms or other decision-making tools to aid in assessment and decision making.
ACTUAL OR POTENTIAL HEALTH PROBLEMS AND NEEDS	Many actual or potential health problems or issues may require the use of this skill as part of related interventions. An appropriate health problem or issue may include: • Activity intolerance • Fall risk • Impaired walking
OUTCOME IDENTIFICATION AND PLANNING	The expected outcome to achieve when assisting a patient with ambulation is that the patient ambulates safely, without falls or injury. Additional appropriate outcomes include the patient demonstrates improved muscle strength and joint mobility, and the patient's level of independence increases.

(continued on page 576)

Skill 9-6 ▶ Assisting a Patient With Ambulation *(continued)*

IMPLEMENTATION

ACTION	RATIONALE
1. Review the health record and plan of care for conditions that may influence the patient's ability to move and ambulate. Assess for tubes, IV lines, incisions, or equipment that may alter the procedure for ambulation. Identify any movement limitations. **Consult a patient handling algorithm or other decision-making tool to plan an appropriate approach to moving the patient** (refer to Figure 1 for an example).	Reviewing the medical record and care plan validates the correct patient and correct procedure. Checking for equipment and limitations reduces the risk for patient injury. Identification of limitations and ability and use of an algorithm help to prevent injury and aid in determining best plan for patient movement.

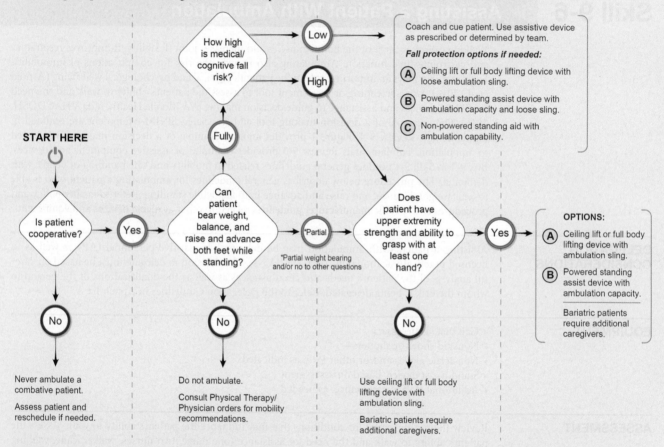

FIGURE 1. Example of an algorithm to aid in decision making regarding safe patient handling and mobility to assist a patient with ambulation. (*Source:* VA Mobile Health. [n.d.]. Safe patient handling. [Version 1.3.3]. Algorithm 10. [Mobile app]. U. S. Department of Veteran Affairs. https://mobile.va.gov/app/safe-patient-handling.)

ACTION	RATIONALE
2. Perform hand hygiene. Put on PPE, as indicated.	Hand hygiene and PPE prevent the spread of microorganisms. PPE is required based on transmission precautions.
3. Identify the patient. Explain the procedure to the patient. Ask the patient to report any feelings of dizziness, weakness, or shortness of breath while walking. Decide how far to walk.	Patient identification validates the correct patient and correct procedure. Discussion and explanation help allay anxiety and prepare the patient for what to expect.
4. Place the bed in a position that allows the patient's feet to reach the floor.	Proper bed height ensures safety when getting the patient out of bed.

ACTION

5. Encourage the patient to make use of a stand-assist aid, either freestanding or attached to the side of the bed, if available, to move to the side of the bed. Assist the patient to the side of the bed, if necessary.

6. Have the patient sit on the side of the bed for several minutes and assess for dizziness or lightheadedness. Have the patient stay sitting until they feel secure.

7. Assist the patient to put on skid-proof footwear and a robe, if desired.

8. Wrap the gait belt around the patient's waist, based on assessed need and facility policy.

9. Encourage the patient to make use of the stand-assist device. Cue the patient to stand. Assess the patient's balance and leg strength. If the patient is weak or unsteady, return the patient to the bed or assist to a chair.

10. If you are the only person assisting, position yourself to the side and slightly behind the patient. Steady the patient by the waist or gait belt (Figure 2).

    • When two caregivers assist, position yourself to the side and slightly behind the patient, supporting the patient by the waist or gait belt. Have the other caregiver carry or manage equipment or provide additional support from the other side.

    • Alternatively, when two caregivers assist, stand at the patient's sides (one nurse on each side) with near hands grasping the gait belt and far hands holding the patient's lower arm or hand.

RATIONALE

Encourages independence, reduces strain for staff, and decreases risk for patient injury.

Having the patient sit at the side of the bed minimizes the risk for blood pressure changes (orthostatic hypotension) that can occur with position change. Allowing the patient to sit until they feel secure reduces anxiety and helps prevent injury.

Doing so ensures safety and patient warmth. Skid-proof footwear decreases risk of falls.

Gait belts improve the caregiver's grasp, reducing the risk of musculoskeletal injuries to staff and the patient. The belt also provides a firmer grasp for the caregiver if the patient should lose their balance. A gait belt is used to steady the patient, not a lifting device (Wintersgill, 2019).

Use of a stand-assist device decreases the risk of injury to the nurse and to the patient. Assessing balance and strength helps to identify the need for additional assistance to prevent falling.

Positioning to the side and slightly behind the patient encourages the patient to stand and walk erect. It also places the nurse in a safe position if the patient should lose their balance or begin to fall.

Gait belts improve the caregiver's grasp, reducing the risk of musculoskeletal injuries to staff and the patient, and allow for a firmer grasp for the caregiver if the patient should lose their balance. A gait belt is used to steady the patient, not a lifting device (Wintersgill, 2019).

Gait belts improve the caregiver's grasp, reducing the risk of musculoskeletal injuries to staff and the patient, and allow for a firmer grasp for the caregiver if the patient should lose their balance. A gait belt is used to steady the patient, not a lifting device (Wintersgill, 2019).

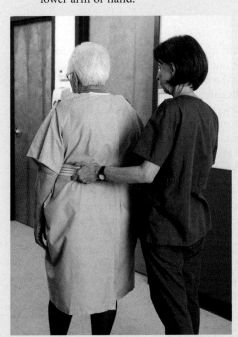

FIGURE 2. Nurse positioned to side and slightly behind patient while walking, supporting patient by gait belt or waist.

(continued on page 578)

Skill 9-6 ▶ Assisting a Patient With Ambulation *(continued)*

ACTION	RATIONALE
11. Take several steps forward with the patient. Continue to assess the patient's strength and balance. Remind the patient to stand erect.	Taking several steps with the patient and standing erect promote good balance and stability. Continued assessment helps maintain patient safety.
12. Continue with ambulation for the planned distance and time. Return the patient to the bed or chair based on the patient's tolerance and condition. Remove the gait belt.	Ambulation as prescribed promotes activity and prevents fatigue.
13. Ensure the patient is comfortable, with the side rails up and the bed in the lowest position, as necessary. Place the call bell and other essential items within reach.	Proper positioning with raised side rails and proper bed height provide for patient comfort and safety. Having the call bell and other essential items within reach promotes safety.
14. Clean transfer aids per facility policy, if not indicated for single-patient use. Remove gloves and any other PPE, if used. Perform hand hygiene.	Proper cleaning of equipment between patient use prevents the spread of microorganisms. Proper removal of PPE reduces the risk for infection transmission and contamination of other items. Hand hygiene prevents the spread of microorganisms.

EVALUATION

The expected outcome has been met when the patient has ambulated safely for the prescribed distance and time and has remained free from falls or injury, and the patient has exhibited increasing muscle strength, joint mobility, and independence.

DOCUMENTATION

Guidelines

Document the activity, any other pertinent observations, the patient's tolerance of the procedure, and the distance walked. Document the use of SPHM aids and number of staff required for ambulation.

Sample Documentation

> <u>5/14/25</u> 1720 Patient ambulated with assistance in hallway for a distance of approximately 15 ft. Patient tolerated ambulation well; denied any complaints of dizziness, pain, or fatigue. Ambulated back to room and sitting in chair listening to music.
>
> —*J. Minkins, RN*

DEVELOPING CLINICAL REASONING AND CLINICAL JUDGMENT

UNEXPECTED SITUATIONS AND ASSOCIATED INTERVENTIONS

- *You are walking with a patient in the hallway. She tells you she feels faint and begins to lean over as if she is going to fall:* Place your feet wide apart, with one foot in front. Rock your pelvis out on the side nearest the patient. This widens and stabilizes the base of support. Grasp the gait belt. This ensures a safe hold on the patient. While grasping the gait belt, guide the patient slowly to the floor, supporting them on your thigh and your large quadriceps muscle and protecting the patient's head (Wintersgill, 2019). This enables you to support the patient's weight with large muscle groups and protects you from back strain. Stay with the patient. Call for help. If another staff member was assisting you with ambulation, each of you should use one hand to grasp the gait belt and grasp the patient's hand or wrist with your other hand. Slowly lower them to the floor.

SPECIAL CONSIDERATIONS

- Secure all equipment, such as indwelling urinary catheters, drains, or IV infusions, to a pole for ambulation. Do not carry equipment while helping the patient. Your hands should be free to provide support.
- Consider use of a gait belt for any patient who is not independent to promote safety (Wintersgill, 2019). A gait belt is used to steady the patient, not a lifting device (Wintersgill, 2019).
- Gait belts should also not be used with patients exhibiting behavioral aggression, as the belt might be used as a weapon and for patients at risk for suicide, as the belt might be used for self-harm (Wintersgill, 2019).

EARLY AMBULATION AND PREVENTION OF THROMBOSIS

National Institute for Health and Care Excellence (NICE) (UK). (2019). *Venous thromboembolism in over 16s: Reducing the risk of hospital-acquired deep vein thrombosis or pulmonary embolism*. NICE Guideline. https://www.nice.org.uk/guidance/ng89

This evidence-based guideline outlines best practices for the prevention of venous thromboembolism (VTE). The implementation of early ambulation as part of prophylaxis is included in the discussion.

Skill 9-7 ▶ Assisting a Patient With Ambulation Using a Walker

A walker is a lightweight metal frame with four legs. Walkers improve balance by increasing the patient's base of support, enhancing stability during ambulation, and supporting the patient's weight (Eliopoulos, 2018). There are several kinds of walkers; the choice of which to use is based on the patient's arm strength and balance needs. Regardless of the type used, the patient stands between the back legs of the walker with arms relaxed at the side; the top of the walker should line up with the crease on the inside of the patient's wrist. When the patient's hands are placed on the grips, elbows should be slightly bent, flexed about 15 degrees (MFMER, 2019a). Usually, the legs of the walker can be adjusted to the appropriate height.

Early mobility plays an important role in the patient's physical and psychological well-being (Arnold et al., 2018). Use a screening or assessment tool to assess the patient's ability to walk and the need for SPHM devices and assistance to guide decision making (VA Mobile Health, n.d.; VHACDOSH, 2016). One example of a decision-making tool and associated SPHM equipment are outlined in Fundamentals Review 9-4. Figure 1 in Skill 9-6 provides an example of a decision-making tool related to ambulation. Box 9-1 in Skill 9-1 outlines general guidelines related to mobility and safe handling of people with dementia.

DELEGATION CONSIDERATIONS

Patient teaching regarding use of a walker cannot be delegated to assistive personnel (AP). Reinforcement or implementation of ambulation using a walker may be delegated to AP. Assisting a patient with ambulation using a walker may be delegated to licensed practical/vocational nurses (LPN/LVNs). The decision to delegate must be based on careful analysis of the patient's needs and circumstances as well as the qualifications of the person to whom the task is being delegated. Refer to the Delegation Guidelines in Appendix A.

EQUIPMENT

- Walker, adjusted to the appropriate height
- Nonskid shoes or slippers
- Nonsterile gloves and/or other PPE, as indicated
- Additional staff for assistance, as needed
- Stand-assist device, as necessary, if available
- Gait belt, based on assessment

ASSESSMENT

Assess the patient's ability to walk and the need for assistance. Review the patient's health record for conditions that may affect ambulation. Perform a pain assessment before the time for the activity. If the patient reports pain, administer the prescribed medication in sufficient time to allow for the full effect of the analgesic. Take vital signs and assess the patient for dizziness or lightheadedness with position changes. Assess the patient's knowledge regarding the use of a walker. Ensure that the walker is at the appropriate height for the patient.

(continued on page 580)

Skill 9-7 ▶ Assisting a Patient With Ambulation Using a Walker *(continued)*

ACTUAL OR POTENTIAL HEALTH PROBLEMS AND NEEDS	Many actual or potential health problems or issues may require the use of this skill as part of related interventions. An appropriate health problem or issue may include: • Fall risk • Impaired walking • Knowledge deficiency
OUTCOME IDENTIFICATION AND PLANNING	The expected outcomes to achieve are that the patient ambulates safely with the walker and is free from falls or injury. Additional outcomes may include: the patient demonstrates proper use of the walker and verbalizes an understanding of the rationale for use of the walker; and the patient demonstrates increasing muscle strength, joint mobility, and independence.

IMPLEMENTATION

ACTION	**RATIONALE**
1. Review the health record and plan of care for conditions that may influence the patient's ability to move and ambulate, and for specific instructions for ambulation, such as distance. Assess for tubes, IV lines, incisions, or equipment that may alter the procedure for ambulation. Assess the patient's knowledge and previous experience regarding the use of a walker. Identify any movement limitations.	Reviewing the medical record and care plan validates the correct patient and correct procedure. Checking for equipment and limitations helps minimize the risk for injury.
2. Perform hand hygiene. Put on PPE, if indicated.	Hand hygiene and PPE prevent the spread of microorganisms. PPE is required based on transmission precautions.
3. Identify the patient. Explain the procedure to the patient. Tell the patient to report any feelings of dizziness, weakness, or shortness of breath while walking. Decide how far to walk.	Patient identification validates the correct patient and correct procedure. Discussion and explanation help allay anxiety and prepare the patient for what to expect.
4. Place the bed in a position that allows the patient's feet to reach the floor, if the patient is in bed.	Proper bed height ensures safety when getting the patient out of bed.
5. Encourage the patient to make use of a stand-assist aid, either freestanding or attached to the side of the bed, if available, to move to the side of the bed.	Use of a stand-assist device encourages independence, reduces strain for staff, and decreases risk for patient injury.
6. Assist the patient to the side of the bed, if necessary. Have the patient sit on the side of the bed. Assess for dizziness or lightheadedness. Have the patient stay seated until they feel secure.	Having the patient sit on the side of the bed minimizes the risk for blood pressure changes (orthostatic hypotension) that can occur with position change. Assessing patient complaints helps prevent injury.
7. Assist the patient to put on skid-proof footwear and a robe, if desired.	Doing so ensures safety and warmth. Skid-proof footwear decreases the risk of falls.
8. Wrap the gait belt around the patient's waist, based on assessed need and facility policy.	Gait belts improve the caregiver's grasp, reducing the risk of musculoskeletal injuries to staff and the patient and provide for a firmer grasp if patient should lose their balance. A gait belt is used to steady the patient, not a lifting device (Wintersgill, 2019).
9. Place the walker directly in front of the patient (Figure 1). Ask the patient to push themselves off the bed or chair; make use of the stand-assist device to stand. Once the patient is standing, have them hold the walker's handgrips firmly and equally. Stand slightly behind the patient, on one side.	Proper positioning with the walker ensures balance. Standing within the walker and holding the handgrips firmly provide stability when moving the walker and help ensure safety. Positioning to the side and slightly behind the patient encourages the patient to stand and walk erect. It also places the nurse in a safe position if the patient should lose their balance or begin to fall.

ACTION

10. Remind the patient to keep their back upright, and then lift and position or push the walker forward, about one step ahead, and set it down or stop pushing, making sure all four feet of the walker stay on the floor. The patient should not hunch forward (MFMER, 2019a). Then, tell the patient to step forward with either foot into the walker, supporting themselves on their arms. The patient should not step all the way to the front of the space (AAOS, 2015). Remind the patient to keep the walker still and to push straight down on the grips of the walker and then step forward with the remaining leg into the walker.

11. Move the walker forward again, and continue the same pattern. Continue with ambulation for the planned distance and time (Figure 2). Return the patient to the bed or chair based on the patient's tolerance and condition, ensuring that the patient is comfortable. Remove the gait belt if used.

RATIONALE

Having all four feet of the walker on the floor provides a broad base of support. Moving the walker and stepping forward moves the center of gravity toward the walker, ensuring balance and preventing tipping of the walker.

Moving the walker promotes activity. Continuing for the planned distance and time prevents the patient from becoming fatigued.

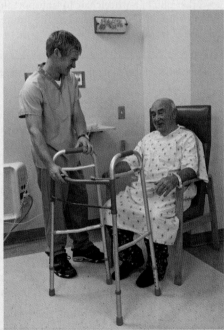

FIGURE 1. Setting walker in front of a seated patient.

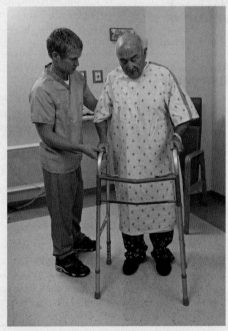

FIGURE 2. Assisting patient to walk with walker.

12. Ensure the patient is comfortable, with the side rails up and the bed in the lowest position, as necessary. Place the call bell and other essential items within reach.

13. Clean transfer aids per facility policy, if not indicated for single-patient use. Remove gloves and any other PPE, if used. Perform hand hygiene.

Proper positioning with raised side rails and proper bed height provides for patient comfort and safety. Having the call bell and other essential items within reach promotes safety.

Proper cleaning of equipment between patient use prevents the spread of microorganisms. Proper removal of PPE reduces the risk for infection transmission and contamination of other items. Hand hygiene prevents the spread of microorganisms.

EVALUATION

The expected outcome has been met when the patient has used the walker to ambulate safely and has remained free of injury, and the patient has exhibited increased muscle strength, joint mobility, and independence.

(continued on page 582)

Skill 9-7 ▶ Assisting a Patient With Ambulation Using a Walker *(continued)*

DOCUMENTATION

Guidelines

Document the activity, any other pertinent observations, the patient's ability to use the walker, the patient's tolerance of the procedure, and the distance walked. Document the use of transfer aids and number of staff required for transfer.

Sample Documentation

> <u>5/15/25</u> 0900 Patient ambulated with walker from bed to bathroom for morning care with minimal assistance; demonstrated proper steps in using walker. Able to ambulate back to bed using walker independently.
>
> —P. Collins, RN

DEVELOPING CLINICAL REASONING AND CLINICAL JUDGMENT

UNEXPECTED SITUATIONS AND ASSOCIATED INTERVENTIONS

- *You are assisting a patient ambulating in the hallway using a walker. She becomes extremely tired and says she cannot pick up the walker anymore ("it's too heavy"). However, she cannot walk without the walker:* Call for assistance. Have a coworker obtain a wheelchair to transport the patient back to her room. Assess the patient for other symptoms, if necessary. In the future, plan to ambulate for shorter distances to prevent the patient from becoming fatigued.

SPECIAL CONSIDERATIONS

- Never use a walker on the stairs or an escalator (American Academy of Orthopaedic Surgeons [AAOS], 2015).
- Ensure the patient wears nonskid shoes or slippers.
- If the patient has an injured or weaker leg, the injured/weaker leg should be moved into the walker first, followed by the stronger or unaffected leg (AAOS, 2015; MFMER, 2019a).
- Some walkers have wheels on the front legs. These walkers are best for patients with a gait that is too fast for a walker without wheels and for patients who have difficulty lifting a walker. This type of walker is rolled forward while the patient walks as normally as possible. Because lifting repeatedly is not required, energy expenditure and stress to the back and upper extremities are less than with a standard walker.
- Keep in mind, walkers often prove to be difficult to maneuver through doorways and congested areas.
- Advise the patient to check the walker before use for signs of damage, frame deformity, or loose or missing parts.
- Teach patients to use the arms of the chair or a stand-assist device for leverage when getting up from a chair. Explain to patients that they should not pull on the walker to get up; the walker could tip over or become unbalanced.

EVIDENCE FOR PRACTICE ▶

EARLY AMBULATION AND PREVENTION OF THROMBOSIS

National Institute for Health and Care Excellence (NICE) (UK). (2019). *Venous thromboembolism in over 16s: Reducing the risk of hospital-acquired deep vein thrombosis or pulmonary embolism.* NICE Guideline. https://www.nice.org.uk/guidance/ng89

Refer to the details in Skill 9-6, Evidence for Practice.

Skill 9-8 ▶ Assisting a Patient With Ambulation Using Crutches

Crutches enable a patient to walk and remove weight from one or both legs. The patient uses their arms to support the body weight. Crutches can be used for the short or the long term. This section will discuss short-term use of axillary crutches. Crutches must be fitted to each person. When standing up straight, the top of the crutches should be about 1 to 2 inches below the armpits (AAOS, 2015). When using crutches, the patient's weight should rest on the hands, not on the underarm supports (AAOS, 2015). Pressure placed on the axillae can cause damage to nerves and circulation. When using crutches, the elbow should be slightly bent at about 30 degrees and kept close to the sides. Fitting of and the procedure for crutch walking is usually the responsibility of a physical therapist, but it is important for the nurse to be knowledgeable about the patient's progress and the gait being taught. Be prepared to guide the patient at home or in the hospital after the initial teaching is completed. Remind the patient that the support of body weight should be primarily on the hands and arms while using the crutches. There are a number of different ways to walk using crutches, based on how much weight the patient is allowed to bear on one or both legs.

Early mobility plays an important role in the patient's physical and psychological well-being (Arnold et al., 2018). Use a screening or assessment tool to assess the patient's ability to walk and the need for SPHM devices and assistance to guide decision making (VA Mobile Health, n.d.; VHACDOSH, 2016). One example of a decision-making tool and associated SPHM equipment are outlined in Fundamentals Review 9-4. Figure 1 in Skill 9-6 provides an example of a decision-making tool related to ambulation.

DELEGATION CONSIDERATIONS	Patient teaching regarding use of crutches cannot be delegated to assistive personnel (AP). Reinforcement or implementation of the use of crutches may be delegated to AP. Assisting a patient with ambulation using crutches may be delegated to licensed practical/vocational nurses (LPN/LVNs). The decision to delegate must be based on careful analysis of the patient's needs and circumstances as well as the qualifications of the person to whom the task is being delegated. Refer to the Delegation Guidelines in Appendix A.
EQUIPMENT	• Crutches with axillary pads, handgrips, and rubber suction tips • Nonskid shoes or slippers • PPE, as indicated • Stand-assist device, as necessary, if available • Gait belt, based on assessment
ASSESSMENT	Review the patient's health record and plan of care to determine the reason for using crutches and instructions for weight bearing. Check for specific instructions from physical therapy. Perform a pain assessment before the time for the activity. If the patient reports pain, administer the prescribed medication in sufficient time to allow for the full effect of the analgesic. Determine the patient's knowledge regarding the use of crutches and assess the patient's ability to balance on the crutches. Assess for muscle strength in the legs and arms.
ACTUAL OR POTENTIAL HEALTH PROBLEMS AND NEEDS	Many actual or potential health problems or issues may require the use of this skill as part of related interventions. An appropriate health problem or issue may include: • Impaired walking • Knowledge deficiency • Fall risk
OUTCOME IDENTIFICATION AND PLANNING	The expected outcomes to achieve when assisting a patient with ambulation using crutches are that the patient ambulates safely without experiencing falls or injury, and the patient demonstrates proper crutch-walking technique.

(continued on page 584)

Skill 9-8 ▶ Assisting a Patient With Ambulation Using Crutches *(continued)*

IMPLEMENTATION

ACTION	**RATIONALE**
1. Review the health record and plan of care for conditions that may influence the patient's ability to move and ambulate. Assess for tubes, IV lines, incisions, or equipment that may alter the procedure for ambulation. Assess the patient's knowledge and previous experience regarding the use of crutches. Determine that the appropriate size crutch has been obtained.	Reviewing the health record and plan of care validates the correct patient and correct procedure. Assessment helps identify problem areas to minimize the risk for injury.
2. Perform hand hygiene. Put on PPE, if indicated.	Hand hygiene and PPE prevent the spread of microorganisms. PPE is required based on transmission precautions.
3. Identify the patient. Explain the procedure to the patient. Tell the patient to report any feelings of dizziness, weakness, or shortness of breath while walking. Decide how far to walk.	Patient identification validates the correct patient and correct procedure. Discussion and explanation help allay anxiety and prepare the patient for what to expect.
4. Place the bed in a position that allows the patient's feet to reach the floor, if the patient is in bed.	Proper bed height ensures safety when getting the patient out of bed.
5. Encourage the patient to make use of a stand-assist aid, either freestanding or attached to the side of the bed, if available, to move to the side of the bed.	Use of assistive devices encourages independence, reduces strain for staff, and decreases risk for patient injury.
6. Assist the patient to the side of the bed, if necessary. Have the patient sit on the side of the bed. Assess for dizziness or lightheadedness. Have the patient stay seated until they feel secure.	Having the patient sit on the side of the bed minimizes the risk for blood pressure changes (orthostatic hypotension) that can occur with position change. Assessing patient complaints helps prevent injury.
7. Assist the patient to put on skid-proof footwear and a robe, if desired.	Doing so ensures safety and warmth. Skid-proof footwear decreases the risk of falls.
8. Wrap the gait belt around the patient's waist, based on assessed need and facility policy.	Gait belts improve the caregiver's grasp, reducing the risk of musculoskeletal injuries to staff and the patient and provide for a firmer grasp if patient should lose their balance. A gait belt is used to steady the patient, not a lifting device (Wintersgill, 2019).
9. Assist the patient to stand erect, face forward in the tripod position (Figure 1). This means the patient holds the crutches 12 inches in front of, and 12 inches to the side of, each foot.	Positioning the crutches in this manner provides a wide base of support to increase stability and balance.
10. For the four-point gait:	This movement ensures stability and safety.
a. Have the patient move the right crutch forward 12 inches and then move the left foot forward to the level of the right crutch.	
b. Then have the patient move the left crutch forward 12 inches and then move the right foot forward to the level of the left crutch.	
11. For the three-point gait:	The patient bears weight on the stronger leg.
a. Have the patient move the affected leg and both crutches forward about 12 inches.	
b. Have the patient move the stronger leg forward to the level of the crutches.	
12. For the two-point gait:	The patient bears partial weight on both feet.
a. Have the patient move the left crutch and the right foot forward about 12 inches at the same time.	
b. Have the patient move the right crutch and left leg forward to the level of the left crutch at the same time.	

ACTION

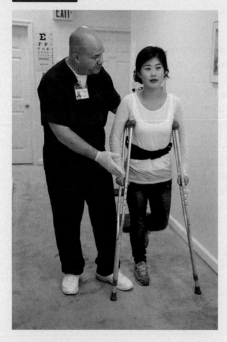

RATIONALE

FIGURE 1. Assisting patient to stand erect facing forward in tripod position.

13. For the swing-to gait:

    a. Have the patient move both crutches forward about 12 inches.

    b. Have the patient lift the legs and swing them to the crutches, supporting their body weight on the crutches.

14. Continue with ambulation for the planned distance and time. Return the patient to the bed or chair based on the patient's tolerance and condition. Remove the gait belt if used.

15. Ensure the patient is comfortable, with the side rails up and the bed in the lowest position, as necessary. Place the call bell and other essential items within reach.

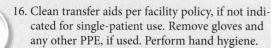 16. Clean transfer aids per facility policy, if not indicated for single-patient use. Remove gloves and any other PPE, if used. Perform hand hygiene.

The swing-to gait provides mobility for patients with weakness or paralysis of the hips or legs.

Continued ambulation promotes activity, and adhering to the planned distance and time prevents the patient from becoming fatigued.

Proper positioning with raised side rails and proper bed height provide for patient comfort and safety. Having the call bell and other essential items within reach promotes safety.

Proper cleaning of equipment between patient use prevents the spread of microorganisms. Proper removal of PPE reduces the risk for infection transmission and contamination of other items. Hand hygiene prevents the spread of microorganisms.

EVALUATION

The expected outcomes have been met when the patient has ambulated safely without experiencing falls or injury, and the patient has demonstrated proper crutch-walking technique.

DOCUMENTATION

Guidelines

Document the activity, any other pertinent observations, the patient's ability to use the crutches, the patient's tolerance of the procedure, and the distance walked. Document the use of transfer aids and number of staff required for transfer.

Sample Documentation

> 5/10/25 1830 Patient reviewed crutch walking using four-point gait. Patient return demonstrated gait, ambulating for approximately 15 ft in hallway, without difficulty.
> —H. Pointer, RN

(continued on page 586)

Skill 9-8 ▶ Assisting a Patient With Ambulation Using Crutches   *(continued)*

DEVELOPING CLINICAL REASONING AND CLINICAL JUDGMENT

UNEXPECTED SITUATIONS AND ASSOCIATED INTERVENTIONS

- *You are assisting a patient ambulating in the hallway using crutches when the patient reports fatigue. You notice that the patient is bearing weight on the axillary area:* Call for assistance and have a coworker obtain a wheelchair to transport the patient back to the room. Once the patient is back in bed, reinforce instructions about avoiding pressure on the axillary area. In the future, plan to ambulate for a shorter distance to prevent the patient from becoming fatigued. Talk with the multidisciplinary health care team about possible exercises for upper extremity strengthening.

SPECIAL CONSIDERATIONS

- Crutches can be used when climbing stairs. The patient grasps both crutches as one, on one side of the body and uses the stair railing. The patient transfers their weight to the crutches and holds the railing. The patient places the unaffected leg on the first stair tread past the crutches. The patient then transfers their weight to the unaffected leg, moving up onto the stair tread. The patient moves the affected leg then crutches up to the step. Continue with this sequence until top of stairs is reached. Using this process, the crutches always support the affected leg.
- Patients should not lean on the crutches. Prolonged pressure on the axillae can damage the brachial nerves, causing nerve palsy (Warees et al., 2020), with resulting loss of sensation and inability to move the upper extremities.
- Patients using crutches should perform arm- and shoulder-strengthening exercises to aid with crutch walking.

Skill 9-9 ▶ Assisting a Patient With Ambulation Using a Cane

Canes are useful for patients who can bear weight but need support for balance. They are also useful for patients who have decreased strength in one leg. Canes provide an additional point of support during ambulation. Canes should not be used for bearing weight (Eliopoulos, 2018). Canes are made of wood or metal and often have a rubberized cap on the tip to prevent slipping. Canes come in three variations: single-ended canes with half-circle handles (recommended for patients requiring minimal support and for those who will be using stairs frequently); single-ended canes with straight handles (recommended for patients with hand weakness because the handgrip is easier to hold, but not recommended for patients with poor balance); and canes with three (tripod) or four prongs (quad cane) or legs to provide a wide base of support (recommended for patients with poor balance). The cane should rise from the floor to the crease in the patient's wrist and the elbow should be bent slightly, flexed about 15 degrees when holding the cane (AAOS, 2015; MFMER, 2019b). The patient holds the cane in the hand opposite the side that needs support (AAOS, 2015; MFMER, 2019b). If the cane is used for stability, the patient may hold it in either hand.

Early mobility plays an important role in the patient's physical and psychological well-being (Arnold et al., 2018). Use a screening or assessment tool to assess the patient's ability to walk and the need for SPHM devices and assistance to guide decision making (VA Mobile Health, n.d.; VHACDOSH, 2016). One example of a decision-making tool and associated SPHM equipment are outlined in Fundamentals Review 9-4. Figure 1 in Skill 9-6 provides an example of a decision-making tool related to ambulation.

DELEGATION CONSIDERATIONS

Patient teaching regarding use of a cane cannot be delegated to assistive personnel (AP). Reinforcement or implementation of the use of a cane may be delegated to AP. Assisting a patient with ambulation using a cane may be delegated to licensed practical/vocational nurses (LPN/LVNs). The decision to delegate must be based on careful analysis of the patient's needs and circumstances as well as the qualifications of the person to whom the task is being delegated. Refer to the Delegation Guidelines in Appendix A.

EQUIPMENT

- Cane of appropriate size with rubber tip
- Nonskid shoes or slippers
- Nonsterile gloves and/or other PPE, as indicated
- Stand-assist aid, if necessary and available
- Gait belt, based on assessment

ASSESSMENT

Assess the patient's upper body strength, ability to bear weight and to walk, and the need for assistance. Review the patient's health record for conditions that may affect ambulation. Perform a pain assessment before the time for the activity. If the patient reports pain, administer the prescribed medication in sufficient time to allow for the full effect of the analgesic. Take vital signs and assess the patient for dizziness or lightheadedness with position changes. Assess the patient's knowledge regarding the use of a cane.

ACTUAL OR POTENTIAL HEALTH PROBLEMS AND NEEDS

Many actual or potential health problems or issues may require the use of this skill as part of related interventions. An appropriate health problem or issue may include:

- Fall risk
- Impaired walking
- Knowledge deficiency

OUTCOME IDENTIFICATION AND PLANNING

The expected outcome to achieve when assisting a patient with ambulation using a cane is that the patient ambulates safely without falls or injury. Additional appropriate outcomes include the following: the patient demonstrates proper use of the cane, and the patient demonstrates increased independence.

IMPLEMENTATION

ACTION	RATIONALE
1. Review the health record and plan of care for conditions that may influence the patient's ability to move and ambulate. Assess for tubes, IV lines, incisions, or equipment that may alter the procedure for ambulation.	Review of the health record and plan of care validates the correct patient and correct procedure. Identification of equipment and limitations helps reduce the risk for injury.
2. Perform hand hygiene. Put on PPE, as indicated.	Hand hygiene and PPE prevent the spread of microorganisms. PPE is required based on transmission precautions.
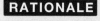 3. Identify the patient. Explain the procedure to the patient. Tell the patient to report any feelings of dizziness, weakness, or shortness of breath while walking. Decide how far to walk.	Patient identification validates the correct patient and correct procedure. Discussion and explanation help allay anxiety and prepare the patient for what to expect.
4. Place the bed in a position that allows the patient's feet to reach the floor, if the patient is in bed.	Proper bed height ensures safety when getting the patient out of bed.
5. Encourage the patient to make use of a stand-assist aid, either freestanding or attached to the side of the bed, if available, to move to the side of the bed.	Use of assistive devices encourages independence, reduces strain for staff, and decreases risk for patient injury.
6. Assist the patient to the side of the bed, if necessary. Have the patient sit on the side of the bed. Assess for dizziness or lightheadedness. Have the patient stay seated until they feel secure.	Having the patient sit on the side of the bed minimizes the risk for blood pressure changes (orthostatic hypotension) that can occur with position change. Assessing patient complaints helps prevent injury.
7. Assist the patient to put on skid-proof footwear and a robe, if desired.	Doing so ensures safety and warmth. Skid-proof footwear reduces risk of falls.

(continued on page 588)

Skill 9-9 ▶ Assisting a Patient With Ambulation Using a Cane *(continued)*

ACTION	RATIONALE
8. Wrap the gait belt around the patient's waist, based on assessed need and facility policy.	Gait belts improve the caregiver's grasp, reducing the risk of musculoskeletal injuries to staff and the patient and provide firmer grasp for the caregiver if patient should lose their balance. A gait belt is used to steady the patient, not a lifting device (Wintersgill, 2019).
9. Encourage the patient to make use of the stand-assist device to stand with weight evenly distributed between the feet and the cane.	A stand-assist device reduces strain for caregiver and decreases risk for patient injury. Evenly distributed weight provides a broad base of support and balance.
10. Have the patient hold the cane on their stronger side, close to the body, while the nurse stands to the side and slightly behind the patient (Figure 1).	Holding the cane on the stronger side helps to distribute the patient's weight away from the involved side and prevents leaning. Positioning to the side and slightly behind the patient encourages the patient to stand and walk erect. It also places the nurse in a safe position if the patient should lose their balance or begin to fall.

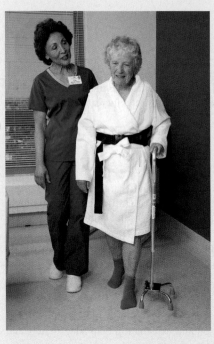

FIGURE 1. Nurse stands slightly behind patient. Cane is held on patient's stronger side, close to body.

ACTION	RATIONALE
11. Tell the patient to one small stride ahead (AAOS, 2015) and then, while supporting their weight on the stronger leg and the cane, advance the weaker foot forward, parallel with the cane.	Moving in this manner provides support and balance.
12. While supporting their weight on the weaker leg and the cane, have the patient advance the stronger leg forward to finish the step (AAOS, 2015).	Moving in this manner provides support and balance.
13. Continue with ambulation for the planned distance and time. Return the patient to the bed or chair based on the patient's tolerance and condition. Remove the gait belt if used.	Continued ambulation promotes activity. Adhering to the planned distance and time prevents the patient from becoming fatigued.
14. Ensure the patient is comfortable, with the side rails up and the bed in the lowest position, as necessary. Place the call bell and other essential items within reach.	Proper positioning with raised side rails and proper bed height provides for patient comfort and safety. Having the call bell and other essential items within reach promotes safety.
15. Clean transfer aids per facility policy, if not indicated for single-patient use. Remove gloves and any other PPE, if used. Perform hand hygiene.	Proper cleaning of equipment between patient use prevents the spread of microorganisms. Proper removal of PPE reduces the risk for infection transmission and contamination of other items. Hand hygiene prevents the spread of microorganisms.

EVALUATION

The expected outcomes have been met when the patient has used the cane to ambulate safely without falls or injury, the patient has demonstrated proper use of the cane, and the patient has demonstrated increased independence.

DOCUMENTATION

Guidelines

Document the activity, any other pertinent observations, the patient's ability to use the cane, the patient's tolerance of the procedure, and the distance walked. Document the use of transfer aids and the number of staff required for transfer.

Sample Documentation

> 5/14/25 1330 Patient reviewed instructions for cane use. Patient return demonstrated gait, ambulating approximately 10 ft in room. Patient needed continued reminders about leaning to one side. Requires continued instruction in cane use. Another teaching session planned for early evening.
>
> —*J. Phelps, RN*

DEVELOPING CLINICAL REASONING AND CLINICAL JUDGMENT

UNEXPECTED SITUATIONS AND ASSOCIATED INTERVENTIONS

- *You are assisting a patient ambulating in the hallway using a cane when the patient says she "can't walk any more":* Call for assistance. Have a coworker obtain a wheelchair to transport the patient back to her room. Assess the patient for possible causes, such as anxiety, fatigue, or a change in her condition. In the future, plan shorter distances to prevent the patient from becoming fatigued. Confer with the health care team regarding the need for referral to physical therapy for muscle strengthening.

SPECIAL CONSIDERATIONS

- Patients with bilateral weakness should not use a cane. Canes should not be used for bearing weight (Eliopoulos, 2018). Crutches or a walker would be more appropriate.
- To climb stairs, the patient should advance the stronger leg up the stair first, followed by the cane and weaker leg. To descend, reverse the process.
- When less support is required from the cane, the patient can advance the cane and weaker leg forward simultaneously, while the stronger leg supports the patient's weight.
- Teach patients to position their canes within easy reach when they sit down so that they can rise easily.
- While a cane might help with mobility, it can also make it more difficult for people to stabilize themselves during a fall.

Skill 9-10 ▶ Applying and Removing Graduated Compression Stockings

Graduated compression stockings are often used for patients at risk for venous stasis, thrombophlebitis, **deep vein thrombosis (DVT)** as a passive intervention to aid in the prevention of these complications (AACN, 2016; Sachdeva et al., 2018). Manufactured by several companies, graduated compression stockings are made of elastic material and are available in either knee- or thigh-high length. Graduated compression stockings apply pressure to increase the velocity of blood flow in the superficial and deep veins and improve venous valve function in the legs, promoting venous return to the heart. Pooling of blood is reduced, decreasing the risk of clot formation. Use of graduated compressions stockings is a prescribed intervention.

Be prepared to apply the stockings in the morning before the patient is out of bed and while the patient is supine. If the patient is sitting or has been up and about, have the patient lie down with their legs and feet elevated for at least 15 minutes before applying the stockings. Otherwise, the leg vessels are congested with blood, reducing the effectiveness of the stockings.

(continued on page 590)

Skill 9-10 ▶ Applying and Removing Graduated Compression Stockings *(continued)*

DELEGATION CONSIDERATIONS	The application and removal of graduated compression stockings may be delegated to assistive personnel (AP) as well as to licensed practical/vocational nurses (LPN/LVNs). The decision to delegate must be based on careful analysis of the patient's needs and circumstances as well as the qualifications of the person to whom the task is being delegated. Refer to the Delegation Guidelines in Appendix A.

EQUIPMENT

- Elastic graduated compression stockings in the prescribed length and correct size. See Assessment for appropriate measurement procedure.
- Measuring tape
- Talcum powder (optional)
- Skin cleanser, basin, towel
- PPE, as indicated

ASSESSMENT

Assess the skin condition and neurovascular status of the legs. Collaborate with the health care team regarding any abnormalities before continuing with the application of the stockings. Assess patient's legs for any redness, swelling, warmth, tenderness, or pain that may indicate DVT. If any of these symptoms are noted, confer with the health care team before applying stockings. Measure the patient's legs to obtain the correct size stocking. For knee-high length: Measure around the widest part of the calf and the leg length from the bottom of the heel to the back of the knee, at the bend. For thigh-high length: Measure around the widest part of the calf and the thigh. Measure the length from the bottom of the heel to the gluteal fold. Follow the manufacturer's specifications to select the correct-sized stockings. **Each leg should have a correctly fitted stocking; if measurements differ, then two different sizes of stocking need to be obtained to ensure correct fitting on each leg** (Muñoz-Figueroa & Ojo, 2015).

ACTUAL OR POTENTIAL HEALTH PROBLEMS AND NEEDS

Many actual or potential health problems or issues may require the use of this skill as part of related interventions. An appropriate health problem or issue may include:
- Venous thromboembolism risk
- Altered skin integrity risk
- Knowledge deficiency

OUTCOME IDENTIFICATION AND PLANNING

The expected outcome to achieve when applying and removing graduated compression stockings is that the stockings will be applied and removed with minimal discomfort to the patient. Other outcomes that may be appropriate include the following: edema will decrease in the lower extremities, the patient will understand the rationale for stocking application, and the patient will remain free from DVT.

IMPLEMENTATION

ACTION	**RATIONALE**
1. Review the health record and prescribed interventions to determine the need for graduated compression stockings.	Reviewing the health record and prescribed interventions validates the correct patient and correct procedure.
2. Perform hand hygiene. Put on PPE, as indicated.	Hand hygiene and PPE prevent the spread of microorganisms. PPE is required based on transmission precautions.
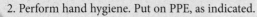 3. Identify the patient. Explain what you are going to do and the rationale for use of graduated compression stockings.	Patient identification validates the correct patient and correct procedure. Discussion and explanation allay anxiety and prepare the patient for what to expect.
4. Close the curtains around the bed and close the door to the room, if possible.	This ensures the patient's privacy.
5. Adjust the bed to a comfortable working height (VHACEOSH, 2016).	Having the bed at the proper height prevents back and muscle strain.

ACTION

6. Assist patient to supine position. If patient has been sitting or walking, have them lie down with legs and feet well elevated for at least 15 minutes before applying stockings.

7. Expose legs one at a time. Wash and dry legs, if necessary. Powder the leg lightly unless patient has a respiratory problem, dry skin, or sensitivity to the powder. If the skin is dry, a moisturizing lotion may be used. **Powders and lotions are not recommended by some manufacturers; check the package material for manufacturer specifications.**

8. Stand at the foot of the bed. Place your hand inside the stocking and grasp the heel area securely. Turn the stocking inside-out to the heel area, leaving the foot inside the stocking leg (Figure 1).

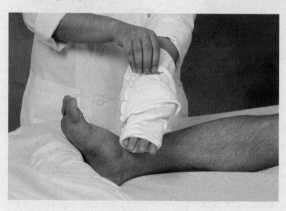

9. With the heel pocket down, ease the foot of the stocking foot over the patient's foot and heel (Figure 2). Check that the patient's heel is centered in the heel pocket of the stocking (Figure 3).

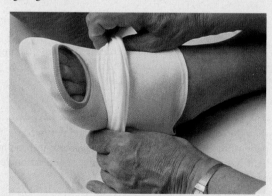

FIGURE 2. Putting foot of stocking onto patient.

10. Using your fingers and thumbs, carefully grasp the edge of the stocking and pull it up smoothly over the ankle and calf, toward the knee (Figure 4). Make sure it is distributed evenly.

11. Pull forward slightly on the toe section. If the stocking has a toe window, make sure it is properly positioned. Adjust if necessary to ensure the material is smooth.

RATIONALE

Dependent positioning of the legs encourages blood to pool in the veins, reducing the effectiveness of the stockings if they are applied to congested blood vessels.

Helps maintain patient's privacy. Powder and lotion reduce friction and make application of stockings easier.

The inside-out technique provides for easier application; bunched elastic material can compromise extremity circulation.

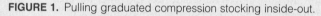

FIGURE 1. Pulling graduated compression stocking inside-out.

Wrinkles and improper fit interfere with circulation.

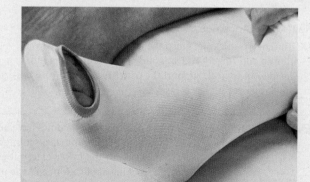

FIGURE 3. Ensuring heel is centered after stocking is on foot.

Easing the stocking carefully into position ensures proper fit of the stocking to the contour of the leg. Even distribution prevents interference with circulation.

This ensures toe comfort and prevents interference with circulation.

(continued on page 592)

Skill 9-10 ▶ Applying and Removing Graduated Compression Stockings *(continued)*

ACTION

12. If the stockings are knee-length, make sure each stocking top is 1 to 2 inches below the patella. Make sure the stocking does not roll down.

13. If applying a thigh-length stocking, continue the application. Flex the patient's leg. Stretch the stocking over the knee.

14. Pull the stocking over the thigh until the top is 1 to 3 inches below the gluteal fold (Figure 5). Adjust the stocking, as necessary, to distribute the fabric evenly. Make sure the stocking does not roll down.

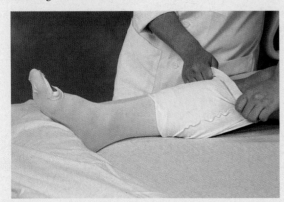

FIGURE 4. Pulling stocking up leg.

15. Remove equipment and return the patient to a position of comfort. Remove gloves. Raise side rails and lower the bed. Place the call bell and other essential items within reach.

 16. Remove any other PPE, if used. Perform hand hygiene.

Removing Stockings

17. To remove stocking, grasp the top of stocking with your thumb and fingers and smoothly pull the stocking off inside-out to heel. Support the patient's foot and ease the stocking over it.

RATIONALE

This prevents pressure and interference with circulation. Rolling stockings may have a constricting effect on veins.

This ensures even distribution.

This prevents excessive pressure and interference with circulation. Rolling stockings may have a constricting effect on veins.

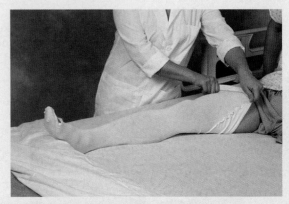

FIGURE 5. Pulling stocking up over thigh.

This promotes patient comfort and safety. Removing gloves properly reduces the risk for infection transmission and contamination of other items. Having the call bell and other essential items within reach promotes safety.

Proper removal of PPE reduces the risk for infection transmission and contamination of other items. Hand hygiene prevents the spread of microorganisms.

This preserves the elasticity and contour of the stocking. It allows assessment of circulatory status and condition of skin on lower extremity and for skin care.

EVALUATION

The expected outcomes have been met when the stockings have been applied and removed, as indicated, with minimal discomfort to the patient; the patient has exhibited a decrease in peripheral edema in the lower extremities; the patient has verbalized an understanding of the rationale for stocking application; and the patient has remained free from DVT.

DOCUMENTATION

Guidelines

Document the patient's leg measurements as a baseline. Document the application of the stockings, size stocking applied, skin and leg assessment, and neurovascular assessment.

Sample Documentation

7/22/25 0945 Leg measurements: calf 14½ in, length heel to knee 16 in. Measurements equal bilaterally. Knee-high graduated compression stockings (medium/regular) applied bilaterally. Posterior tibial and dorsalis pedis pulses + 2 bilaterally; capillary refill less than 2 seconds and skin on toes consistent with rest of skin and warm. Skin on lower extremities is intact bilaterally.

—*C. Stone, RN*

DEVELOPING CLINICAL REASONING AND CLINICAL JUDGMENT

UNEXPECTED SITUATIONS AND ASSOCIATED INTERVENTIONS

- *Patient's leg measurements are outside the guidelines for the available sizes:* Notify prescriber. Patient may require custom-fitted stockings.
- *Patient has a lot of pain with application of stockings:* If pain is expected (e.g., if the patient has a leg incision), it may be necessary to premedicate the patient and apply the stockings once the medication has had time to take effect. If the pain is unexpected, notify the health care team because the patient may be developing a deep vein thrombosis.
- *Patient has an incision on the leg:* When applying and removing stockings, be careful not to hit the incision. If the incision is draining, apply a small bandage to the incision so that it does not drain onto the stockings. If the stockings become soiled by drainage, wash and dry according to instructions.
- *Patient is to ambulate with stockings:* Place skid-proof socks or slippers on before patient attempts to ambulate.

SPECIAL CONSIDERATIONS

General Considerations

- Each leg should have a correct fitting stocking; if measurements are different, then two different sizes of stocking need to be obtained to ensure correct fitting on each leg (Muñoz-Figueroa & Ojo, 2015). The manufacturer whose stockings are being used provides directions for measuring. Some stockings fit either leg; others are designated right or left. An improperly fitting stocking is uncomfortable and ineffective and possibly even harmful (Muñoz-Figueroa & Ojo, 2015).
- Remove stockings daily and inspect and bathe legs and feet. Wash and air-dry the stockings, as necessary, according to the manufacturer's directions.
- Assess the patient's extremities at least every shift for skin color, temperature, sensation, swelling, and the ability to move. If complications are evident, remove the stockings and notify the health care team.
- Evaluate stockings to ensure the top or toe opening does not roll with movement. Rolled stocking edges can cause excessive pressure and interfere with circulation.
- Despite the use of elastic stockings, a patient may develop DVT or phlebitis. Unilateral swelling, redness, tenderness, pain, and warmth are possible indicators of these complications. Notify the health care team of the presence of any symptoms.

Community-Based Care Considerations

- Make sure that the patient has an extra pair of stockings during hospitalization before discharge (for payment and convenience purposes).
- In general, it is best to take time to wash stockings by hand; stockings may be laundered with other "white" clothing. Avoid excessive bleach. Remove from dryer as soon as "low-heat" cycle is complete to avoid shrinkage. Stockings may also be air-dried; lay on a flat surface to prevent stretching. Check the manufacturer's directions.
- Take all jewelry off before putting on stockings as rings and bracelets can snag on the compression hose, causing rips and tears.
- Instruct the patient to remove the stockings and contact their health care provider if they experience numbness, tingling, pins and needles, pain or soreness in the foot or leg, or a pale/cool/discolored foot or leg, as these indicate the stockings are too tight (Canterbury District Health Board, 2018).

(*continued on page 594*)

Skill 9-10 ▶ Applying and Removing Graduated Compression Stockings *(continued)*

• Instruct the patients to contact their health care provider if a rash develops on their toes or feet, as this could be the result of an allergy to the elastic fibers in the stockings (Canterbury District Health Board, 2018).

EVIDENCE FOR PRACTICE ▶

VENOUS THROMBOEMBOLISM PREVENTION

American Association of Critical-Care Nurses (AACN). (2016). *Practice alert. Preventing venous thromboembolism in adults.* https://www.aacn.org/clinical-resources/practice-alerts/venous-thromboembolism-prevention

The American Association of Critical-Care Nurses provides Practice Alerts. Practice Alerts are succinct, dynamic directives that are supported by authoritative evidence to ensure excellence in practice and a safe and humane work environment. Almost all hospitalized patients have at least one risk factor for venous thromboembolism (VTE). VTE, a common complication, contributes to excess length of stay, excess charges, and mortality. This Venous Thromboembolism Prevention Practice Alert supports the use of mechanical methods of prophylaxis, including graduated compression stockings, to reduce the risk of VTE. Nurses must select the correct size of stockings, properly apply them, and ensure that they are removed for only a short time each day.

EVIDENCE FOR PRACTICE ▶

GRADUATED COMPRESSION STOCKINGS AND VENOUS THROMBOEMBOLISM PREVENTION

Hospitalized patients are at increased risk of developing deep vein thrombosis (DVT) in the lower limb and pelvic veins related to prolonged immobilization, surgery, and other comorbidities (Sachdeva et al., 2018; Wilson et al., 2018). Patients with a DVT are at increased risk of developing a pulmonary embolism (Morton & Fontaine, 2018). Expected nursing practice includes interventions to prevent venous thromboembolism (AACN, 2016). Does the use of graduated compression stockings decrease the risk of DVT?

Related Evidence

Sachdeva, A., Dalton, M., & Lees, T. (2018). Graduated compression stockings for prevention of deep vein thrombosis. *Cochrane Database of Systematic Reviews, 11*(11), CD001484. https://doi.org/10.1002/14651858.CD001484.pub4

This systematic review aimed to evaluate the effectiveness and safety of graduated compression stockings in preventing deep vein thrombosis (DVT) in hospitalized patients. Multiple databases were searched for randomized controlled trials involving graduated compression stockings (GCS) alone, or GCS used along with any other DVT prophylactic method. Twenty randomized controlled trials were identified; 10 included patients undergoing general surgery; 6 included patients undergoing orthopedic surgery; 3 trials included patients undergoing neurosurgery, cardiac surgery, and gynecologic surgery; and 1 included medical patients. GCS were applied on the day before or on the day of surgery and were worn until discharge, or the participants were fully mobile. Analysis of the pooled data from the studies indicated GCS are effective in reducing the risk of DVT in hospitalized patients who have had general and orthopedic surgery, with or without other methods of thromboprophylaxis. Data also indicated that GCS probably reduce the risk of proximal DVT and may reduce the risk of pulmonary embolism. There were insufficient data to assess the effectiveness of GCS in reducing the risk of DVT in medical patients. The authors concluded wearing GCS reduced the overall risk of developing DVT and may reduce the risk of pulmonary embolism among surgical patients.

Relevance for Nursing Practice

Expected nursing practice includes incorporation of best practice evidence. Use of graduated compression stockings are indicated for the prevention of venous thromboembolism. Nurses must ensure safe and accurate implementation of use of these devices to support quality patient care and outcomes.

Skill 9-11 Applying Pneumatic Compression Devices

Pneumatic compression devices (PCDs), also known as intermittent pneumatic compression devices (IPCDs) and sequential compression devices (SCDs), consist of fabric sleeves containing air bladders that apply brief pressure to the legs. Intermittent compression pushes blood from the smaller blood vessels into the deeper vessels and into the femoral veins. This action enhances blood flow and venous return, stimulating the normal muscle-pumping action in the legs, and promotes fibrinolysis, deterring venous thrombosis (DVT). The sleeves are attached by tubing to an air pump. The sleeve may cover the entire leg or may extend from the foot to the knee.

PCDs may be used in combination with graduated compression stockings (antiembolism stockings) and anticoagulant therapy to prevent thrombosis formation. They can be used preoperatively and postoperatively with patients at risk for blood clot formation. They are also prescribed for patients with other risk factors for clot formation, including inactivity or immobilization, chronic venous disease, and malignancies. Use of a pneumatic compression device is a prescribed intervention and may be prescribed for high-risk surgical patients, those with decreased mobility or chronic venous disease, and patients at risk for deep vein disorders. PCDs/SCDs should be kept on at all times except when patients are walking (Wilson et al., 2018).

DELEGATION CONSIDERATIONS	The application and removal of PCDs may be delegated to assistive personnel (AP) as well as to licensed practical/vocational nurses (LPN/LVNs). The decision to delegate must be based on careful analysis of the patient's needs and circumstances as well as the qualifications of the person to whom the task is being delegated. Refer to the Delegation Guidelines in Appendix A.
EQUIPMENT	• Compression sleeves of appropriate size based on the manufacturer's guidelines • Inflation pump with connection tubing • PPE, as indicated
ASSESSMENT	Assess the patient's history, health record, and current condition and status to identify risk for development of deep vein thrombosis. Assess lower extremity skin integrity. Identify any leg conditions that would be exacerbated by the use of the pneumatic compression device or would contraindicate its use.
ACTUAL OR POTENTIAL HEALTH PROBLEMS AND NEEDS	Many actual or potential health problems or issues may require the use of this skill as part of related interventions. An appropriate health problem or issue may include: • Venous thromboembolism risk • Altered skin integrity risk • Risk for impaired peripheral neurovascular function
OUTCOME IDENTIFICATION AND PLANNING	The expected outcomes to achieve when applying a PCD are that the patient maintains adequate circulation in the extremities, and the patient understands the rationale for stocking application and is free from symptoms of neurovascular compromise and DVT.

IMPLEMENTATION

ACTION	RATIONALE
1. Review the health record and prescribed interventions to determine the need for a pneumatic compression device (PCD) and for conditions that may contraindicate its use.	Reviewing the health record and prescribed interventions validates the correct patient and correct procedure and minimizes the risk for injury.
2. Perform hand hygiene. Put on PPE, as indicated.	Hand hygiene and PPE prevent the spread of microorganisms. PPE is required based on transmission precautions.

(continued on page 596)

Skill 9-11 ▶ Applying Pneumatic Compression Devices *(continued)*

ACTION	RATIONALE

3. Identify the patient. Explain the procedure to the patient.

Patient identification validates the correct patient and correct procedure. Discussion and explanation help allay anxiety and prepare the patient for what to expect.

4. Close the curtains around the bed and close the door to the room, if possible. Place the bed at an appropriate and comfortable working height (VHACEOSH, 2016).

Closing the door or curtains provides for privacy. Proper bed height helps reduce back strain.

5. Hang the compression pump on the foot of the bed and plug it into an electrical outlet (Figure 1). Attach the connecting tubing to the pump.

Equipment preparation promotes efficient time management and provides an organized approach to the task.

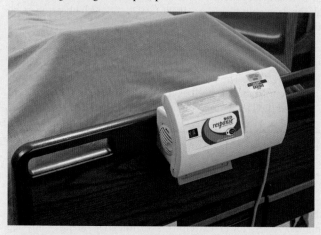

FIGURE 1. PCD machine at foot of bed.

6. Remove the compression sleeves from the package and unfold them. Lay the unfolded sleeves on the bed with the cotton lining facing up. **Note the markings indicating the correct placement for the ankle and popliteal areas.**

Proper placement of the sleeves prevents injury.

7. Apply graduated compression stockings. Place a sleeve under the patient's leg with the tubing toward the heel. Each one fits either leg. **For total leg sleeves, place the behind-the-knee opening at the popliteal space to prevent pressure there. For knee-high sleeves, make sure the back of the ankle is over the ankle marking.**

Proper placement prevents injury.

8. Wrap the sleeve snugly around the patient's leg so that two fingers fit between the leg and the sleeve. Secure the sleeve with the Velcro fasteners. Repeat for the second leg (Figure 2), if bilateral therapy is prescribed. Connect each sleeve to the tubing, following manufacturer's recommendations (Figure 3).

Correct placement ensures appropriate, but not excessive, compression of the extremity.

9. Set the pump to the prescribed maximal pressure (usually 35 to 55 mm Hg). Make sure the tubing is free from kinks. Check that the patient can move about without interrupting the airflow. Turn on the pump. Initiate cooling setting, if available.

Proper pressure setting ensures patient safety and prevents injury. Some devices have a cooling setting available to increase patient comfort.

10. **Observe the patient and the device during the first cycle. Check the audible alarms.**

Observation and frequent checking ensure proper fit and inflation and reduce the risk for injury from the device.

11. Place the bed in the lowest position. Make sure the call bell and other essential items are within easy reach.

Returning the bed to the lowest position and having the call bell and other essential items readily available promote patient safety.

ACTION

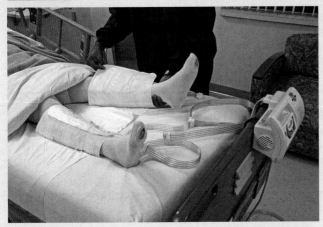

FIGURE 2. Wrap the PCD sleeve snugly around the patient's leg.

 12. Remove PPE, if used. Perform hand hygiene.

13. Assess the extremities for peripheral pulses, edema, changes in sensation, and movement. Check the sleeves and pump at least once per shift or per facility policy. Remove the sleeves and assess and document skin integrity every 8 hours.

RATIONALE

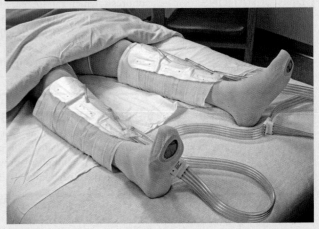

FIGURE 3. PCD sleeves around patient's legs with sleeve tubing connected to device.

Proper removal of PPE reduces the risk for infection transmission and contamination of other items. Hand hygiene prevents the spread of microorganisms.

Assessment provides for early detection and prompt intervention for possible complications, including skin irritation.

EVALUATION

The expected outcomes have met when the patient has exhibited adequate circulation in extremities without symptoms of neurovascular compromise and DVT, and the patient has verbalized an understanding of the rationale for stocking application.

DOCUMENTATION

Guidelines

Document the time and date of application of the PCD, the patient's response to the therapy, and the patient's understanding of the therapy. Document the status of the alarms and pressure settings. Note the use of the cooling setting, if appropriate. Document your assessment of the extremities.

Sample Documentation

4/27/25 1615 Patient instructed regarding reason for PCD therapy; verbalizes understanding of therapy. Knee-high PCD applied to both lower extremities; pressure set at 45 mm Hg. Patient denies any complaints of numbness or tingling. Feet and toes warm and pink; quick capillary refill; bilateral pedal pulses present and equal. Alarms and cooling settings as prescribed.

—J. Trotter, RN

DEVELOPING CLINICAL REASONING AND CLINICAL JUDGMENT

UNEXPECTED SITUATIONS AND ASSOCIATED INTERVENTIONS

• *Your postoperative patient is wearing PCD on both legs. While you are performing a routine assessment, he tells you that he has started to have pain in his left leg, along with tingling and numbness:* Remove the PCD and assess both lower extremities. Perform skin and neurovascular assessments. Assess the extremities for peripheral pulses, edema, changes in sensation, and movement. Communicate the patient's symptoms and assessment to the health care team.

(continued on page 598)

Skill 9-11 ▶ Applying Pneumatic Compression Devices *(continued)*

SPECIAL CONSIDERATIONS

- Use the cooling setting, if the unit has one. The skin under the sleeve can become wet with diaphoresis, which can increase the risk for impaired skin integrity.
- In general, the PCD should be worn continuously. It may be removed for bathing, walking, and physical therapy. Use is usually discontinued when the patient is ambulating consistently.
- The risk for DVT formation and injury as a result of excessive pressure on blood vessels and underlying tissues is greater if the sleeves are not applied correctly (Rabe et al., 2020).

EVIDENCE FOR PRACTICE ▶

VENOUS THROMBOEMBOLISM PREVENTION

American Association of Critical-Care Nurses (AACN). (2016). *Practice alert. Preventing venous thromboembolism in adults.* https://www.aacn.org/clinical-resources/practice-alerts/venous-thromboembolism-prevention
   Refer to details in Skill 9-10, Evidence for Practice.

EVIDENCE FOR PRACTICE ▶

PNEUMATIC COMPRESSION AND PREVENTION OF THROMBOSIS

National Institute for Health and Care Excellence (NICE) (UK). (2019). *Venous thromboembolism in over 16s: Reducing the risk of hospital-acquired deep vein thrombosis or pulmonary embolism.* NICE Guideline. https://www.nice.org.uk/guidance/ng89
   Refer to the details in Skill 9-6, Evidence for Practice.

Skill 9-12 ▶ Applying a Continuous Passive Motion Device

A continuous passive motion (CPM) is a motorized device that continuously passively moves a joint through a set degree of range of motion (Rex, 2018). The impact and benefit of CPM therapy is controversial, with studies providing conflicting evidence related to benefit of use (Chen et al., 2020; Wirries et al., 2020; Yang et al., 2019). However, CPM may be prescribed after total knee **arthroplasty** as well as after surgery on other joints, such as shoulders, elbows, or ankles. The degree of flexion and extension of the joint and the cycle rate (the number of revolutions per minute) are determined by the prescriber, but nurses place the patient in and out of the device and monitor the patient's response to the therapy.

DELEGATION CONSIDERATIONS

The application and removal of a CPM device is not delegated to assistive personnel (AP). The application and removal of a CPM device may be delegated to licensed practical/vocational nurses (LPN/LVNs). The decision to delegate must be based on careful analysis of the patient's needs and circumstances as well as the qualifications of the person to whom the task is being delegated. Refer to the Delegation Guidelines in Appendix A.

EQUIPMENT

- CPM device
- Single-patient-use soft-goods kit (sheepskin or padding)
- Tape measure
- Nonsterile gloves and/or other PPE, if indicated

ASSESSMENT	Review the health record and prescribed interventions for the prescribed degrees of flexion and extension. Assess the neurovascular status of the involved extremity. Perform a pain assessment. Administer the prescribed medication in sufficient time to allow for the full effect of the analgesic before starting the device. Assess for proper alignment of the joint in the CPM device. Assess the patient's ability to tolerate the prescribed treatment.
ACTUAL OR POTENTIAL HEALTH PROBLEMS AND NEEDS	Many actual or potential health problems or issues may require the use of this skill as part of related interventions. An appropriate health problem or issue may include: • Risk for impaired peripheral neurovascular function • Altered skin integrity risk • Knowledge deficiency
OUTCOME IDENTIFICATION AND PLANNING	The expected outcomes to achieve when applying a CPM device are that the patient experiences increased joint mobility and does not exhibit atrophy or contractures, alterations in skin integrity, or impaired peripheral neurovascular function.

IMPLEMENTATION

ACTION	**RATIONALE**
1. Review the health record and prescribed interventions for the appropriate degrees of flexion and extension, the cycle rate, and the length of time the CPM is to be used.	Reviewing the health record and prescribed interventions validates the correct patient and correct procedure and reduces the risk for injury.
2. Obtain equipment. Apply the soft goods to the CPM device.	Equipment preparation promotes efficient time management and provides an organized approach to the task. The soft goods help to protect the skin that is in contact with the CPM device from friction and pressure.
3. Perform hand hygiene. Put on PPE, as indicated.	Hand hygiene and PPE prevent the spread of microorganisms. PPE is required based on transmission precautions.
4. Identify the patient. Explain the procedure to the patient.	Patient identification validates the correct patient and correct procedure. Discussion and explanation help allay anxiety and prepare the patient for what to expect.
5. Close the curtains around the bed and close the door to the room, if possible. Place the bed at an appropriate and comfortable working height (VHACEOSH, 2016).	Closing the door or curtains provides for privacy. Proper bed height helps reduce back strain.
6. Position the patient in the middle of the bed, with the head of the bed between 30 and 45 degrees. Make sure the affected extremity is in a slightly abducted position.	Proper positioning promotes correct body alignment and prevents pressure on the unaffected extremity.
7. Support the affected extremity, lift it up, and place it in the padded CPM device (Figure 1).	Support and elevation assist in movement of the affected extremity without injury.
8. **Make sure the knee is aligned at the hinged joint of the CPM device.** Check to confirm the padding is protecting any skin that is in contact with the CPM.	Proper positioning in the device promotes patient comfort and prevents injury and complications.
9. Adjust the footplate to maintain the patient's foot in a neutral position (Figure 2). Assess the patient's position to make sure the leg is not internally or externally rotated.	Adjustment helps ensure proper positioning and prevents injury.

(continued on page 600)

Skill 9-12 ▶ Applying a Continuous Passive Motion Device *(continued)*

ACTION

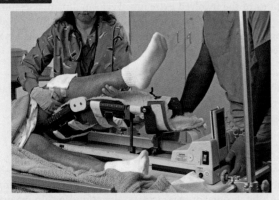

FIGURE 1. Placing patient's leg into CPM machine.

10. Apply the restraining straps under the CPM device and around the leg. **Check that two fingers fit between the strap and the leg (Figure 3).**

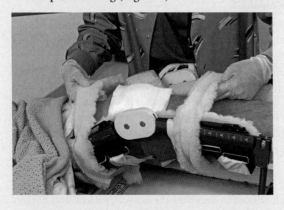

RATIONALE

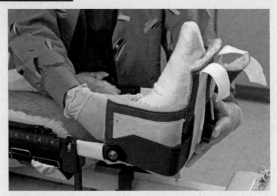

FIGURE 2. Adjusting footplate to maintain patient's foot in a neutral position.

Restraining straps maintain the leg in position. Leaving a space between the strap and leg prevents injury from excessive pressure from the strap.

FIGURE 3. Using two fingers to check fit between straps and leg.

11. Raise the bed rail closest to the CPM. Confirm that the foot of the bed is flat and the knee control option on the bed is locked. Place pillows if needed at the foot of the bed in front of the footboard on the CPM device to prevent the device from sliding away from the patient (Horse, 2010, as cited in Rex, 2018, p. 57).

12. Explain the use of the STOP/GO button to the patient. Set the controls to the prescribed levels of flexion and extension and cycles per minute. Turn on the power to the CPM.

13. Set the device to ON and start the therapy by pressing the GO button. Observe the patient and the device during the first three or four cycles; assess for any change in pain intensity rating or sudden breakthrough pain (Rex, 2018).

14. Place the bed in the lowest position, with the side rails up. Make sure the call bell and other essential items are within easy reach.

15. Remove PPE, if used. Perform hand hygiene.

A raised bed rail prevents the CPM device from falling off the bed. Locking the knee control prevents accidental raising of the lower part of the bed, displacing the CPM device and displacing the patient's knee (Horse, 2010, as cited in Rex, 2018, p. 57).

Explanation decreases anxiety by allowing the patient to participate in care.

Observation ensures that the device is working properly, thereby ensuring patient safety and evaluates the patient's tolerance of the intervention.

Having the bed at the proper height and having the call bell and other items handy ensure patient safety.

Proper removal of PPE reduces the risk for infection transmission and contamination of other items. Hand hygiene prevents the spread of microorganisms.

ACTION

16. Check the patient's level of comfort and perform skin and neurovascular assessments at least every 4 hours or per facility policy. Assess for pinching of the leg by the device and that the straps are not too tight (Rex, 2018).

RATIONALE

Frequent assessments provide for early detection and prompt intervention should problems arise.

EVALUATION

The expected outcomes have been met when the patient demonstrated increased joint mobility and did not exhibit atrophy or contractures, alterations in skin integrity, or impaired peripheral neurovascular function.

DOCUMENTATION

Guidelines

Document the time and date of application of the CPM, the extension and flexion settings, the speed of the device, the patient's response to the therapy, and your assessment of the extremity.

Sample Documentation

> 5/03/25 1430 Right knee incision clean and dry; dressing intact. Right toes pink and warm, with brisk capillary refill; equal to left. Pedal pulses present and equal bilaterally. CPM device applied with range of motion at 30 degrees of knee flexion, for 5 cycles/min for 30 minutes. Patient reports slight increase in pain from a rating of 4/10 to 5/10, but states, "I don't want anything for the pain right now." Plan to reassess in 15 minutes and offer analgesic as prescribed.
>
> —K. Dugas, RN

DEVELOPING CLINICAL REASONING AND CLINICAL JUDGMENT

UNEXPECTED SITUATIONS AND ASSOCIATED INTERVENTIONS

- *Patient is prescribed therapy with a CPM device. After you initiate the prescribed flexion and extension of the joint, the patient reports sudden pain in the joint:* Stop the CPM device. Check the settings to make sure the device is set correctly for the prescribed therapy. Assess the patient for other signs and symptoms and obtain vital signs. Perform a neurovascular assessment of the affected extremity. Notify the health care team of the patient's pain and any other findings. When therapy is resumed, evaluate the need for premedication with analgesics. Continue pain intervention with analgesics, as prescribed.

SPECIAL CONSIDERATIONS

General Considerations

- The physical therapist will usually fit the CPM device to the patient. The thigh length on the CPM device is adjusted based on the distance between the gluteal crease and the popliteal space. The position of the footplate is adjusted based on the measurement of the leg from the knee to 14 in beyond the bottom of the foot.
- Patient education should include the purpose, benefits, and possible complications of CPM therapy; the function of the device; and how to maintain safety precautions during CPM therapy (Rex, 2018).

Skill 9-13 ▶ Applying a Sling

A sling is a bandage that can provide support for an arm or immobilize an injured arm, wrist, or hand. Slings can be used to restrict movement of a fracture or dislocation and to support a muscle sprain. They may also be used to support a splint or secure dressings. Health care facilities usually use commercial slings. The sling should distribute the supported weight over a large area of the shoulders and trunk, not just the back of the neck, to prevent pressure on the cervical spinal nerves (Hinkle et al., 2022).

DELEGATION CONSIDERATIONS	The application of a sling may not be delegated to assistive personnel (AP). The application of a sling may be delegated to licensed practical/vocational nurses (LPN/LVNs). The decision to delegate must be based on careful analysis of the patient's needs and circumstances as well as the qualifications of the person to whom the task is being delegated. Refer to the Delegation Guidelines in Appendix A.
EQUIPMENT	• Commercial arm sling • ABD gauze pad (if the sling does not include padding for the neck strap) • Nonsterile gloves and/or other PPE, as indicated
ASSESSMENT	Assess the situation to determine the need for a sling. Assess the affected limb for pain and edema. Perform a neurovascular assessment of the affected extremity. Assess body parts distal to the site for cyanosis, pallor, coolness, numbness, tingling, swelling, and absent or diminished pulses.
ACTUAL OR POTENTIAL HEALTH PROBLEMS AND NEEDS	Many actual or potential health problems or issues may require the use of this skill as part of related interventions. An appropriate health problem or issue may include: • Acute pain • Altered skin integrity risk • Risk for impaired peripheral neurovascular function
OUTCOME IDENTIFICATION AND PLANNING	The expected outcomes to achieve when applying a sling are that the arm is immobilized in proper alignment; the patient shows no evidence of contractures, **venous stasis**, thrombus formation, or alterations in skin integrity; and the patient demonstrates proper use of the sling.

IMPLEMENTATION

ACTION	**RATIONALE**
1. Review the health record and prescribed interventions to determine the need for the use of a sling.	Reviewing the health record and prescribed interventions validates the correct patient and correct procedure and prevents injury.
2. Perform hand hygiene. Put on PPE, as indicated.	Hand hygiene and PPE prevent the spread of microorganisms. PPE is required based on transmission precautions.
3. Identify the patient. Explain the procedure to the patient.	Patient identification validates the correct patient and correct procedure. Discussion and explanation help allay anxiety and prepare the patient for what to expect.
4. Close the curtains around the bed and close the door to the room, if possible. Place the bed at an appropriate and comfortable working height (VHACEOSH, 2016).	Closing the door or curtains provides for privacy. Proper bed height helps reduce back strain.
5. Perform a pain assessment. If the patient reports pain, administer the prescribed medication in sufficient time to allow for the full effect of the analgesic.	Injury to the arm requiring the use of a sling may cause discomfort and/or pain. Allowing sufficient time for analgesic to take effect promotes optimal patient comfort.
6. Assist the patient to a sitting position. Place the patient's forearm across the chest with the elbow flexed and the palm against the chest. Measure the sleeve length, if indicated.	Proper positioning facilitates sling application. Measurement ensures proper sizing of the sling and proper placement of the arm.

ACTION

7. Enclose the arm in the sling, making sure the elbow fits into the corner of the fabric (Figure 1) and extends from the elbow to at least the palmar crease. Run the strap up the patient's back and across the shoulder opposite the injury, then down the chest to the fastener on the end of the sling (Figure 2).

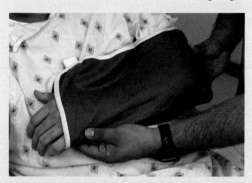

FIGURE 1. Placing patient's arm into canvas sling.

8. Place the ABD pad under the strap, between the strap and the patient's neck (Figure 3). **Ensure that the sling and forearm are slightly elevated and at a right angle to the body (Figure 4).**

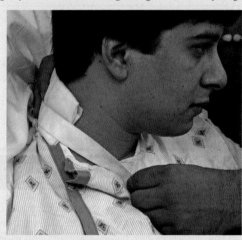

FIGURE 3. Placing padding between strap and patient's neck.

9. Place the bed in the lowest position, with the side rails up. Make sure the call bell and other essential items are within easy reach.

10. Remove PPE, if used. Perform hand hygiene.

11. Check the patient's level of comfort, pain, arm positioning, and neurovascular status of the affected limb every 4 hours or according to facility policy. Assess the axillary and cervical skin frequently for irritation or alterations in integrity.

RATIONALE

This position ensures adequate support and keeps the arm out of a dependent position, preventing edema.

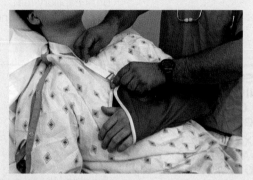

FIGURE 2. Fastening the strap to the sling.

Padding prevents skin irritation and reduces pressure on the neck. Proper positioning ensures alignment, provides support, and prevents edema.

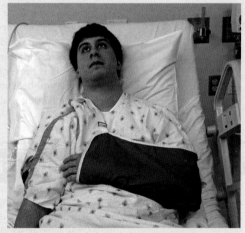

FIGURE 4. Patient with sling in place.

Having the bed at the proper height and leaving the call bell and other items within reach ensure patient safety.

Proper removal of PPE reduces the risk for infection transmission and contamination of other items. Hand hygiene prevents the spread of microorganisms.

Frequent assessment ensures patient safety, prevents injury, and provides early intervention for skin irritation and other complications.

EVALUATION

The expected outcomes have been met when the patient's arm has been immobilized in proper alignment. In addition, the patient has showed no evidence of contractures, venous stasis, thrombus formation, or alterations in skin integrity, and the patient has demonstrated proper use of the sling.

(*continued on page 604*)

Skill 9-13 ▶ Applying a Sling *(continued)*

DOCUMENTATION

Guidelines

Document the time and date the sling was applied. Document the patient's response to the sling and the neurovascular status of the extremity. Document the pain assessment and associated interventions, as well as patient response.

Sample Documentation

> 5/22/25 2015 Sling applied to left arm. Left hand and fingers warm to touch and pink. Brisk capillary refill. Left radial pulse present and equal to right. Patient denies any complaints of numbness, pain, or tingling of left upper extremity.
>
> —P. Peterson, RN

DEVELOPING CLINICAL REASONING AND CLINICAL JUDGMENT

UNEXPECTED SITUATIONS AND ASSOCIATED INTERVENTIONS

- *Patient needs a sling to support a wrist fracture, but you cannot obtain a commercially prepared sling:* Make a sling using a triangular bandage or cloth. Place the cloth or bandage on the chest with a corner of the cloth at the elbow. Place the affected arm across the chest with the elbow flexed and the palm on the chest. Wrap the end closest to the head around the neck, on the opposite side from the injured arm. Bring the end of the cloth that is farthest from the head up over the injured arm and tie it at the side of the neck. Make sure that the sling and forearm are slightly elevated and at a right angle to the body.

SPECIAL CONSIDERATIONS

- If the sling is used for a patient with a hand or wrist injury or after surgery to the hand or wrist, ensure the arm is supported in the sling with the hand elevated at the level of the heart to decrease the risk of swelling (Hinkle et al., 2022).
- Be sure that the patient's wrist is enclosed in the sling. Do not allow it to hang out and down over the edge. This prevents pressure on nerves and blood vessels and prevents muscle contractures, deformity, and discomfort.
- Assess circulation and comfort at regular intervals.

Skill 9-14 ▶ Applying a Figure-Eight Bandage

Bandages are used to apply pressure over an area, immobilize a body part, prevent or reduce edema, and secure splints and dressings. Bandages can be elasticized or made of gauze, flannel, or muslin. In general, narrow bandages are used to wrap feet, the lower legs, hands, and arms, and wider bandages are used for the thighs and trunk. A roller bandage is a continuous strip of material wound on itself to form a roll. The free end is anchored, and the roll is passed or rolled around the body part, maintaining equal tension with all turns. The bandage is unwound gradually and only as needed. The bandage should overlap itself evenly and by one half to two thirds the width of the bandage. The figure-eight turn consists of oblique overlapping turns that ascend and descend alternatively. It is used around the knee, elbow, ankle, and wrist.

DELEGATION CONSIDERATIONS

The application of a figure-eight bandage may not be delegated to assistive personnel (AP). The application of a figure-eight bandage may be delegated to licensed practical/vocational nurses (LPN/LVNs). The decision to delegate must be based on careful analysis of the patient's needs and circumstances as well as the qualifications of the person to whom the task is being delegated. Refer to the Delegation Guidelines in Appendix A.

EQUIPMENT

- Elastic or other bandage of the appropriate width
- Tape, pins, or self-closures
- Gauze pads
- Nonsterile gloves and/or other PPE, as indicated

ASSESSMENT

Review the health record and plan of care and assess the situation to determine the need for a bandage. Assess the affected limb for pain and edema. Perform a neurovascular assessment of the affected extremity. Assess body parts distal to the site for evidence of cyanosis, pallor, coolness, numbness, tingling, and swelling and absent or diminished pulses. Assess the distal circulation of the extremity after the bandage is in place and at least every 4 hours thereafter.

ACTUAL OR POTENTIAL HEALTH PROBLEMS AND NEEDS

Many actual or potential health problems or issues may require the use of this skill as part of related interventions. An appropriate health problem or issue may include:
- Acute pain
- Risk for impaired peripheral neurovascular function
- Altered skin integrity risk

OUTCOME IDENTIFICATION AND PLANNING

The expected outcomes to achieve when applying a figure-eight bandage are that the bandage is applied correctly, and the patient maintains adequate circulation to the affected body part and remains free of neurovascular complications.

IMPLEMENTATION

ACTION	RATIONALE
1. Review the health record and plan of care to determine the need for a figure-eight bandage.	Reviewing the health record and plan of care validates the correct patient and correct procedure and reduces risk for injury.
2. Perform hand hygiene. Put on PPE, as indicated.	Hand hygiene and PPE prevent the spread of microorganisms. PPE is required based on transmission precautions.
3. Identify the patient. Explain the procedure to the patient.	Patient identification validates the correct patient and correct procedure. Discussion and explanation help allay anxiety and prepare the patient for what to expect.
4. Close the curtains around the bed and close the door to the room, if possible. Place the bed at an appropriate and comfortable working height (VHACEOSH, 2016).	Closing the door or curtains provides for privacy. Proper bed height helps reduce back strain.
5. Assist the patient to a comfortable position, with the affected body part in a normal-functioning position.	Keeping the body part in a normal-functioning position promotes circulation and prevents deformity and discomfort.
6. Hold the bandage roll with the roll facing upward in one hand, while holding the free end of the roll in the other hand. Make sure to hold the bandage roll so it is close to the affected body part.	Proper handling of the bandage allows application of even tension and pressure.
7. Wrap the bandage around the limb twice, below the joint, to anchor it (Figure 1).	Anchoring the bandage ensures that it will stay in place.

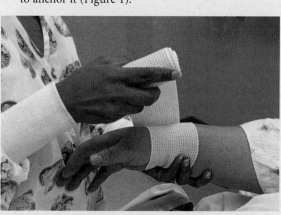

FIGURE 1. Wrapping bandage around patient's limb twice, below joint, to anchor it.

(*continued on page 606*)

Skill 9-14 ▶ Applying a Figure-Eight Bandage *(continued)*

ACTION

8. Use alternating ascending and descending turns to form a figure eight (Figure 2). Overlap each turn of the bandage by one half to two thirds the width of the strip (Figure 3).

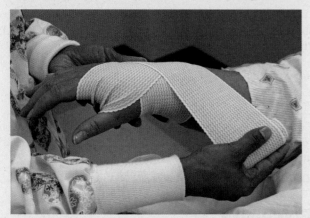

FIGURE 2. Using alternating ascending and descending turns to form a figure eight.

9. Unroll the bandage as you wrap, not before wrapping.

10. **Wrap firmly, but not tightly. Assess the patient's comfort as you wrap. If the patient reports tingling, itching, numbness, or pain, loosen the bandage.**

11. After the area is covered, wrap the bandage around the limb twice, above the joint, to anchor it (Figure 4). Secure the end of the bandage with tape, pins, or self-closures. Avoid metal clips.

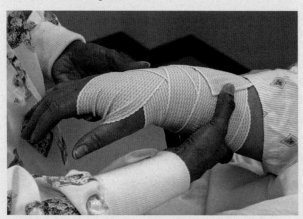

12. Place the bed in the lowest position, with the side rails up. Make sure the call bell and other necessary items are within easy reach.

13. Remove PPE, if used. Perform hand hygiene.

14. Elevate the wrapped extremity for 15 to 30 minutes after application of the bandage.

RATIONALE

Making alternating ascending and descending turns helps to ensure the bandage will stay in place on a moving body part.

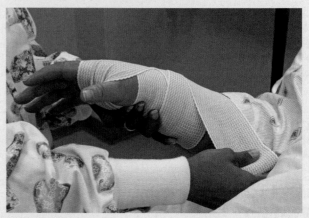

FIGURE 3. Overlapping each turn of bandage by one half to two thirds strip width.

Unrolling the bandage with wrapping prevents uneven pressure, which could interfere with blood circulation.

Firm wrapping is necessary to provide support and prevent injury, but wrapping too tightly interferes with circulation. Patient complaints are helpful indicators of possible circulatory compromise.

Anchoring at the end ensures the bandage will stay in place. Metal clips can cause injury.

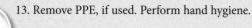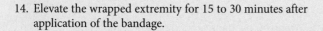
FIGURE 4. Wrapping bandage around patient's limb twice, above joint, to anchor it.

Repositioning the bed and having items nearby ensure patient safety.

Proper removal of PPE reduces the risk for infection transmission and contamination of other items. Hand hygiene prevents the spread of microorganisms.

Elevation promotes venous return and reduces edema.

ACTION

15. Assess the distal circulation after the bandage is in place.

16. Lift the distal end of the bandage and assess the skin for color, temperature, and integrity. Assess for pain and perform a neurovascular assessment of the affected extremity after applying the bandage and at least every 4 hours thereafter, or per facility policy.

RATIONALE

Elastic may tighten as it is wrapped. Frequent assessment of distal circulation ensures patient safety and prevents injury.

Assessment aids in prompt detection of compromised circulation and allows for early intervention for skin irritation and other complications.

EVALUATION

The expected outcomes have been met when the patient has exhibited a correctly applied bandage, and the patient has maintained adequate circulation to the affected body part and remained free of neurovascular complications.

DOCUMENTATION

Guidelines

Document the time, date, and site that the bandage was applied and the size of the bandage used. Include the skin assessment and care provided before application. Document the patient's response to the bandage and the neurovascular status of the extremity.

Sample Documentation

> 5/27/25 1615 3-inch bandage applied to right knee using figure-eight technique. Skin warm, consistent tone, and dry, with quick capillary refill; pedal and dorsalis pedis pulses present and equal bilaterally. Patient denies any complaints of pain, numbness, or tingling. Patient instructed to report any complaints immediately. Right lower extremity resting on two pillows at present.
>
> —J. Wilkins, RN

DEVELOPING CLINICAL REASONING AND CLINICAL JUDGMENT

UNEXPECTED SITUATIONS AND ASSOCIATED INTERVENTIONS

- *After you have applied a figure-eight bandage to a patient's elbow to hold dressings in place, the patient reports tingling, numbness, and pain in his hand during a routine assessment:* Remove the bandage, wait 30 minutes, and reapply the bandage with less tension. Continue to monitor the neurovascular status of the extremity. Symptoms should subside fairly quickly. If symptoms persist, notify the health care team.
- *You remove the bandage on a patient's ankle and note the bandage is limp and less elastic than when it was applied:* Obtain a new bandage and apply it to the ankle.

SPECIAL CONSIDERATIONS

- Keep in mind that a figure-eight bandage may be contraindicated if skin breakdown or lesions are present on the area to be wrapped.
- When wrapping an extremity, elevate it for 15 to 30 minutes before applying the bandage, if possible. This promotes venous return and prevents edema. Avoid applying the bandage to a dependent extremity.
- Place gauze pads or cotton between skin surfaces, such as toes and fingers, to prevent skin irritation. Skin surfaces should not touch after the bandage is applied.
- Include the heel when wrapping the foot, but do not wrap the toes or fingers unless necessary. Assess distal body parts to detect impaired circulation.
- Avoid leaving gaps in bandage layers or leaving skin exposed, because this may result in uneven pressure on the body part.
- Remove and change the bandage at least once a day, or per prescribed intervention or facility policy. Cleanse the skin and dry thoroughly before applying a new bandage. Assess the skin for irritation and breakdown.

Skill 9-15 ▶ Assisting With Cast Application

A cast is a rigid external immobilizing device that is molded to the contours of the body and encases a body part (Hinkle et al., 2022). Casts are used to immobilize a body part in a specific position and to apply uniform pressure on the encased soft tissue. They may be used to treat injuries, correct a deformity, stabilize weakened joints, or promote healing after surgery. Casts generally allow the patient mobility while restricting movement of the affected body part (Hinkle et al., 2022). Casts may be made of plaster or synthetic materials, such as fiberglass. Each material has advantages and disadvantages. Nonplaster casts set in 15 minutes and can sustain weight bearing or pressure in 15 to 30 minutes. Plaster casts can take 24 to 72 hours to dry, and weight bearing or pressure is contraindicated during this period. Patient safety is of utmost importance during the application of a cast. Typically, a physician, advanced practice nurse, or other advanced practice professional applies the cast. Nursing responsibilities include preparing the patient and equipment, assisting during the application, and patient education. The nurse provides skin care to the affected area before, during, and after the cast is applied.

DELEGATION CONSIDERATIONS

Assisting with the application of a cast may not be delegated to assistive personnel (AP). Depending on the state's nurse practice act and the organization's policies and procedures, assisting with the application of a cast may be delegated to licensed practical/vocational nurses (LPN/LVNs). The decision to delegate must be based on careful analysis of the patient's needs and circumstances as well as the qualifications of the person to whom the task is being delegated. Refer to the Delegation Guidelines in Appendix A.

EQUIPMENT

- Casting materials, such as plaster rolls or fiberglass, depending on the type of cast being applied
- Padding material, such as stockinette or sheet wadding, depending on the type of cast being applied
- Plastic bucket or basin filled with warm water
- Disposable, nonsterile gloves and aprons
- Scissors
- Waterproof, disposable pads
- PPE, as indicated

ASSESSMENT

Assess the skin condition in the affected area, noting redness, **contusions**, edema, or open wounds. Assess the neurovascular status of the affected extremity, including distal pulses, color, temperature, presence of edema, capillary refill to fingers or toes, weakness, sensation, and motion. Perform a pain assessment. If the patient reports pain, administer the prescribed analgesic in sufficient time to allow for the full effect of the medication. Assess for muscle spasms and administer the prescribed muscle relaxant in sufficient time to allow for the full effect of the medication. Assess for the presence of disease processes that may interfere with wound healing, including skin diseases, peripheral vascular disease, diabetes, and open or draining wounds.

ACTUAL OR POTENTIAL HEALTH PROBLEMS AND NEEDS

Many actual or potential health problems or issues may require the use of this skill as part of related interventions. An appropriate health problem or issue may include:
- Altered skin integrity risk
- Risk for impaired peripheral neurovascular function
- ADL deficit

OUTCOME IDENTIFICATION AND PLANNING

The expected outcome to achieve when assisting with a cast application is that the cast is applied without interfering with neurovascular function. Other outcomes that may be appropriate include that the patient is free from complications, verbalizes an understanding of cast care, and experiences increased comfort.

IMPLEMENTATION

ACTION

1. Review the health record and prescribed interventions to determine the need for the cast.

2. Perform hand hygiene. Put on gloves and/or other PPE, as indicated.

3. Identify the patient. Explain the procedure to the patient and verify area to be casted.

4. Perform a pain assessment and assess for muscle spasm. Administer prescribed medications in sufficient time to allow for the full effect of the analgesic and/or muscle relaxant.

5. Close the curtains around the bed and close the door to the room, if possible. Place the bed at an appropriate and comfortable working height (VHACEOSH, 2016).

6. Position the patient, as needed, depending on the type of cast being applied and the location of the injury. Support the extremity or body part to be casted. Remove any rings or other jewelry from area to be casted.

7. Drape the patient with the waterproof pads.

8. Cleanse and dry the affected body part.

9. Position and maintain the affected body part in the position indicated by the physician or advanced practice professional as the stockinette (Figure 1), sheet wadding, and padding are applied. The stockinette should extend beyond the ends of the cast. As the wadding is applied, check for wrinkles.

10. Continue to position and maintain the affected body part in the position indicated by the physician or advanced practice professional as the casting material is applied (Figure 2). Assist with finishing by folding the stockinette or other padding down over the outer edge of the cast.

RATIONALE

Reviewing the health record and prescribed interventions validates the correct patient and correct procedure.

Hand hygiene and PPE prevent the spread of microorganisms. PPE is required based on transmission precautions.

Patient identification validates the correct patient and correct procedure. Discussion and explanation help allay anxiety and prepare the patient for what to expect.

Assessment of pain and analgesic administration ensures patient comfort and enhances cooperation.

Closing the door or curtains provides for privacy. Proper bed height helps reduce back strain while you are performing the procedure.

Proper positioning minimizes movement, maintains alignment, and increases patient comfort. Rings or other jewelry could produce pressure points and contribute to alterations in circulation and perfusion.

Draping provides warmth and privacy and helps protect other body parts from contact with casting materials.

Skin care before cast application helps prevent skin breakdown.

Stockinette and other materials protect the skin from casting materials and create a smooth, padded edge, protecting the skin from abrasion. Padding protects the skin, tissues, and nerves from the pressure and raw edges of the cast.

Smooth edges lessen the risk for skin irritation and abrasion.

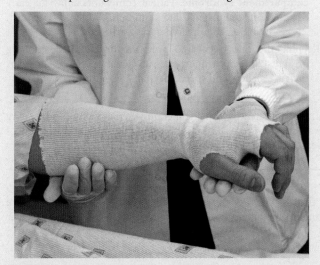

FIGURE 1. Stockinette in place.

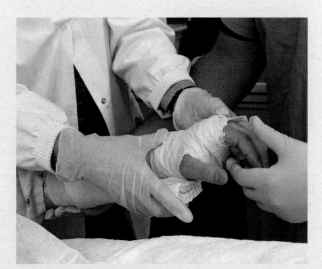

FIGURE 2. Casting material being applied.

(continued on page 610)

Skill 9-15 ▶ Assisting With Cast Application *(continued)*

ACTION	**RATIONALE**
11. **Support the cast during hardening.** Handle hardening plaster casts with the palms of hands, not fingers (Figure 3). Support the cast on a firm, smooth surface. Do not rest it on a hard surface or sharp edges. Avoid placing pressure on the cast. **Do not rest cast on pillows while drying.**	Proper handling avoids denting of the cast and development of pressure areas. Resting the cast on a pillow can increase the risk of thermal injury to the extremity as a result of the exothermic reactions during maturing and hardening of the cast materials (Sabeh et al., 2020).

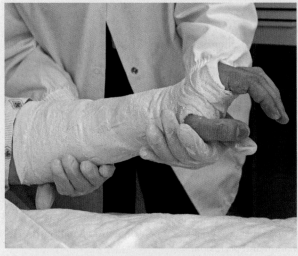

FIGURE 3. Using palms to handle casted limb.

12. **Elevate the affected area at heart level as prescribed, making sure pressure is evenly distributed under the cast.**	Elevation promotes venous return and reduces swelling. Evenly distributed pressure prevents molding and denting of the cast and development of pressure areas.
13. Place the bed in the lowest position, with the side rails up. Make sure the call bell and other essential items are within easy reach.	Having the bed at the proper height and leaving the call bell and other items within reach ensure patient safety.
14. Remove gloves and any other PPE, if used. Perform hand hygiene.	Proper removal of PPE reduces the risk for infection transmission and contamination of other items. Hand hygiene prevents the spread of microorganisms.
15. Obtain x-rays, as prescribed.	X-rays identify that the affected area is positioned properly.
16. Instruct the patient to report pain, odor, drainage, changes in sensation, abnormal sensation, or the inability to move fingers or toes of the affected extremity.	Pressure within a cast may increase with edema and lead to **compartment syndrome**. Patient complaints allow for early detection of, and prompt intervention for, complications such as skin irritation or impaired tissue perfusion.
17. Leave the cast uncovered and exposed to the air. Reposition the patient every 2 hours. Depending on facility policy, a fan may be used to dry the cast.	Keeping the cast uncovered promotes drying. Repositioning prevents development of pressure areas. Using a fan helps increase airflow and speeds drying.

EVALUATION

The expected outcomes have been met when neurovascular function was maintained and healing occurred. In addition, the patient was free from complications, has verbalized an understanding of cast care, and has experienced increased comfort.

DOCUMENTATION

Guidelines

Document the time, date, and site that the cast was applied. Include the skin assessment and care provided before application. Document the patient's response to the cast and the neurovascular status of the extremity.

Sample Documentation

> 6/1/25 1245 Fiberglass cast applied to right forearm from mid-upper arm to middle of hand. Cast clean and dry; edges padded. No signs of irritation noted. Patient able to move fingers freely. Fingers pale with consistent skin tone, warm, and dry. Capillary refill less than 2 seconds. Patient denies any numbness, tingling, or pain. Right forearm resting on two pillows. Patient verbalized an understanding of the need to report any complaints of pain, pressure, numbness, tingling, or decreased ability to move fingers.
>
> —*P. Collins, RN*

DEVELOPING CLINICAL REASONING AND CLINICAL JUDGMENT

UNEXPECTED SITUATIONS AND ASSOCIATED INTERVENTIONS

- *Patient, who has a cast on his hand and forearm, has been experiencing pain relief in the extremity with ice application and oral analgesics. He now reports pain unrelieved by the analgesic and a feeling of tightness in his arm. In addition, his fingers are cool, with sluggish capillary refill: Compartment syndrome may be developing. Adjust the position of the arm so that it is no higher than heart level. This enhances arterial perfusion and controls edema. Notify the health care team of the situation immediately. Prepare for bivalving of the cast (cutting of the cast in half longitudinally) to relieve pressure.*

SPECIAL CONSIDERATIONS

General Considerations

- Perform frequent, regular assessment of neurovascular status. Early recognition of diminished circulation and nerve function is essential to prevent loss of function. Be alert for the presence of compartment syndrome.
- If a fiberglass cast was applied, remove any fiberglass resin residue on the skin with alcohol or acetone.
- Synthetic casts are lightweight, easy to clean, and somewhat water resistant. A fiberglass cast with a waterproof liner may be immersed in water without affecting the cast integrity (MFMER, 2020).

Infant and Child Considerations

- Synthetic casts come in different colors and with designs, such as cartoons and stripes. These features may make the experience more pleasant for a child.

Skill 9-16 ▶ Caring for a Patient With a Cast

A cast is a rigid external immobilizing device that is molded to the contours of the body and encases a body part (Hinkle et al., 2022). Casts are used to immobilize a body part in a specific position and to apply uniform pressure on the encased soft tissue. They may be used to treat injuries, correct a deformity, stabilize weakened joints, or promote healing after surgery. Casts generally allow the patient mobility while restricting movement of the affected body part (Hinkle et al., 2022). Nursing responsibilities after the cast is in place include maintaining the cast, preventing complications, and providing patient teaching related to cast care.

DELEGATION CONSIDERATIONS

Care of a cast may not be delegated to assistive personnel (AP). Depending on the state's nurse practice act and the organization's policies and procedures, care of a cast may be delegated to licensed practical/vocational nurses (LPN/LVNs). The decision to delegate must be based on careful analysis of the patient's needs and circumstances as well as the qualifications of the person to whom the task is being delegated. Refer to the Delegation Guidelines in Appendix A.

(continued on page 612)

Skill 9-16 ▶ Caring for a Patient With a Cast *(continued)*

EQUIPMENT
- Disposable cleansing wipes or washcloth, towel, skin cleanser, and basin of warm water
- Waterproof pads
- Tape
- Pillows
- PPE, as indicated

ASSESSMENT

Review the patient's health record and prescribed interventions to determine the need for cast care and care of the affected area. Perform a pain assessment and administer the prescribed medication in sufficient time to allow for the full effect of the analgesic before starting care. Assess the neurovascular status of the affected extremity, including distal pulses, color, temperature, presence of edema, capillary refill to fingers or toes, and sensation and motion. Assess the skin distal to the cast. Note any indications of infection, including any foul odor from the cast, pain, fever, edema, and extreme warmth over an area of the cast. Assess for complications of immobility, including alterations in skin integrity, reduced joint movement, decreased peristalsis, constipation, alterations in respiratory function, and signs of **thrombophlebitis**. Inspect the condition of the cast. Be alert for cracks, dents, or the presence of drainage from the cast. Assess the patient's knowledge of cast care.

ACTUAL OR POTENTIAL HEALTH PROBLEMS AND NEEDS

Many actual or potential health problems or issues may require the use of this skill as part of related interventions. An appropriate health problem or issue may include:
- Altered skin integrity risk
- Risk for impaired peripheral neurovascular function
- ADL deficit

OUTCOME IDENTIFICATION AND PLANNING

The expected outcomes to achieve when caring for a patient with a cast are that the cast remains intact, and the patient does not experience neurovascular compromise. Other outcomes include that the patient is free from infection, the patient experiences only mild pain and slight edema or soreness, the patient experiences only slight limitations of range-of-joint motion, the skin around the cast edges remains intact, the patient participates in activities of daily living (ADLs), and the patient verbalizes an understanding of and demonstrates appropriate cast-care techniques.

IMPLEMENTATION

ACTION	RATIONALE
1. Review the health record and the care plan to determine the need for cast care and care for the affected body part.	Reviewing the health record and care plan validates the correct patient and correct procedure.
2. Perform hand hygiene. Put on PPE, as indicated.	Hand hygiene and PPE prevent the spread of microorganisms. PPE is required based on transmission precautions.
3. Identify the patient. Explain the procedure to the patient.	Patient identification validates the correct patient and correct procedure. Discussion and explanation help allay anxiety and prepare the patient for what to expect.
4. Close the curtains around the bed and close the door to the room, if possible. Place the bed at an appropriate and comfortable working height (VHACEOSH, 2016).	Closing the door or curtains provides for privacy. Proper bed height helps reduce back strain while you are performing the procedure.
5. If a plaster cast was applied, handle the casted extremity or body area with the palms of your hands for the first 24 to 36 hours, until the cast is fully dry.	Proper handling of a plaster cast prevents dents in the cast, which may create pressure areas on the inside of the cast.
6. If the cast is on an extremity, **elevate the affected area at heart level as prescribed, making sure pressure is evenly distributed under the cast. Maintain the normal curvatures and angles of the cast.**	Elevation promotes venous return and reduces swelling. Maintaining curvatures and angles maintains proper joint alignment. Evenly distributed pressure prevents molding and denting of the cast and development of pressure areas.

ACTION

7. **Do not rest cast on pillows while drying.** Keep cast (plaster) uncovered until fully dry.

8. Assess the condition of the cast. Be alert for cracks, dents, or the presence of drainage from the cast. Perform skin assessment, particularly around edges of the cast, and neurovascular assessment according to facility policy, as often as every 1 to 2 hours. **Assess for pain, edema, inability to move body parts distal to the cast, pallor, pulses, and abnormal sensations. If the cast is on an extremity, compare it with the noncasted extremity (Figure 1).**

9. If breakthrough bleeding or drainage is noted on the cast, mark the area on the cast, according to facility policy (Figure 2). Indicate the date and time next to the area. Follow prescribed interventions or facility policy regarding the amount of drainage that needs to be reported to the health care team.

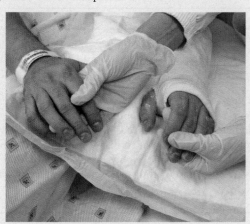

FIGURE 1. Assessing skin and neurovascular function, comparing with noncasted extremity.

10. Assess for signs of infection. Monitor the patient's temperature. Assess for a foul odor from the cast, increased pain, or extreme warmth over an area of the cast.

11. Reposition the patient every 2 hours. Provide back and skin care frequently. Encourage range-of-motion exercise for unaffected joints. Encourage the patient to cough and breathe deeply.

12. Instruct the patient to report pain, odor, drainage, changes in sensation, abnormal sensation, or the inability to move fingers or toes of the affected extremity.

13. Place the bed in the lowest position, with the side rails up. Make sure the call bell and other essential items are within easy reach.

14. Remove PPE, if used. Perform hand hygiene.

RATIONALE

Resting the cast on a pillow can increase the risk of thermal injury to the extremity as a result of the exothermic reactions during maturing and hardening of the cast materials (Sabeh et al., 2020). Keeping the cast uncovered allows heat and moisture to dissipate and air to circulate to speed drying.

Assessment helps detect abnormal neurovascular function or infection and allows for prompt intervention. Assessing the neurovascular status determines the circulation and oxygenation of tissues. Pressure within a cast may increase with edema and lead to compartment syndrome.

Marking the area provides a baseline for monitoring the amount of bleeding or drainage.

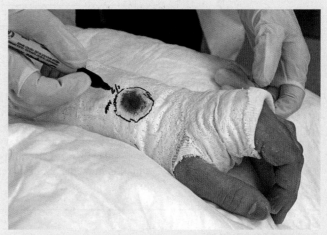

FIGURE 2. Marking any breakthrough bleeding on cast, indicating date and time.

Infection deters healing. Assessment allows for early detection and prompt intervention.

Repositioning promotes even drying of the cast and reduces the risk for the development of pressure areas under the cast. Frequent skin and back care prevents patient discomfort and skin breakdown. ROM exercises maintain joint function of unaffected areas. Coughing and deep breathing reduce the risk for respiratory complications associated with immobility.

Pressure within a cast may increase with edema and lead to compartment syndrome. The patient's understanding of signs and symptoms allows for early detection and prompt intervention.

Having the bed at the proper height and leaving the call bell and other items within reach ensures patient safety.

Proper removal of PPE reduces the risk for infection transmission and contamination of other items. Hand hygiene prevents the spread of microorganisms.

(*continued on page 614*)

Skill 9-16 ▶ Caring for a Patient With a Cast *(continued)*

EVALUATION

The expected outcomes have been met when the patient has exhibited a cast that is intact without evidence of neurovascular compromise to the affected body part, the patient has remained free from infection, the patient has verbalized only mild pain and slight edema or soreness, the patient has maintained range-of-joint motion, the patient has demonstrated intact skin at cast edges, the patient is able to perform ADLs, and the patient has verbalized an understanding of and demonstrated appropriate cast-care techniques.

DOCUMENTATION

Guidelines

Document all assessments and care provided. Document the patient's response to the cast, repositioning, and any teaching.

Sample Documentation

> 9/1/25 0845 Fiberglass cast in place on right lower extremity from just below knee to toes. Patient repositioned from right side to back. Cast clean and dry; edges padded. No signs of irritation noted. Patient able to move toes freely. Skin tone on right toes somewhat paler tone compared with left toes; toes warm and dry. Capillary refill less than 2 seconds. Patient denies any numbness, tingling, or pain. Right lower extremity elevated on two pillows. Patient verbalized an understanding of the need to report any complaints of pain, pressure, numbness, tingling, or decreased ability to move toes.
> —*P. Collins, RN*

DEVELOPING CLINICAL REASONING AND CLINICAL JUDGMENT

UNEXPECTED SITUATIONS AND ASSOCIATED INTERVENTIONS

- *Patient, who has a cast on his hand and forearm, has been experiencing pain relief in the extremity with ice application and oral analgesics. He now reports pain unrelieved by the analgesic and a feeling of tightness in his arm. In addition, his fingers are cool, with sluggish capillary refill:* Compartment syndrome may be developing. Adjust the arm so that it is no higher than heart level. This enhances arterial perfusion and controls edema. Notify the health care team of the situation immediately. Prepare for bivalving of the cast (cutting of the cast in half longitudinally) to relieve pressure.

SPECIAL CONSIDERATIONS

General Considerations

- Explain that itching under the cast is normal, but the patient should not stick objects down or in the cast to scratch. Scratching the skin inside the cast could cause an injury or infection (MFMER, 2020; Sebeh et al., 2020). As suggested by the Mayo Clinic, to relieve itchy skin under a cast, turn a hair dryer on a **cool setting** and aim it under the cast (MFMER, 2020).
- Ice can be used to reduce swelling and edema. Loosely wrap an ice pack covered in a thin towel around the cast at the level of the injury. Wrapping the ice pack in a towel keeps the cast dry. Applying the ice over a larger surface area around the cast is more effective at reducing edema (MFMER, 2020).
- Begin patient teaching immediately after the cast is applied and continue until the patient or a significant other can provide care.
- If a cast is applied after surgery or trauma, monitor vital signs (the most accurate way to assess for bleeding).
- Synthetic casts are lightweight, easy to clean, and somewhat water resistant. A fiberglass cast with a waterproof liner may be immersed in water without affecting the cast integrity (MFMER, 2020).

Infant and Child Considerations

- Do not allow the child to put anything inside the cast. Avoid placing powder, lotion, or deodorant on or near the cast (MFMER, 2020).
- Remove toys, hazardous floor rugs, pets, or other items that might cause the child to stumble.
- Keep in mind that synthetic casts come in different colors and with designs, such as cartoons and stripes. These features may make the experience more pleasant for a child.

- Cover cast with two layers of plastic sealed with duct tape for bathing and do not submerge or hold under running water (AAOS, 2020; MFMER, 2020).
- Instruct the parents/guardians/caregivers of an infant/child with a cast not to alter standard car seats to accommodate a cast. Specially designed car seats and restraints are available for travel in a car (UNC Tar Heel Trauma, 2018).
- Instruct the parents/guardians/caregivers of an infant/child with a cast to immediately report the following symptoms to their health care provider (MFMER, 2020). If your child:
  - Feels increasing pain and tightness in the injured limb
  - Feels numbness or tingling in the injured hand or foot
  - Feels burning or stinging under the cast
  - Develops excessive swelling below the cast
  - Can't move the toes or fingers of the injured limb, or the toes or fingers turn blue or cold
  - Tells you the cast feels too tight or too loose
  - Develops red or raw skin around the cast
  - Develops a crack, soft spots or a foul odor in the cast, or gets the cast soaking wet

Older Adult Considerations

- Older adults may experience changes in circulation related to their age. They may have slow or poor capillary refill related to peripheral vascular disease. Obtain baseline information for comparison after the cast is applied. Use more than one neurovascular assessment to assess circulation. Compare extremities or sides of the body for symmetry.

Community-Based Care Considerations

- Instruct patients to rest the extremity, apply ice to the extremity, and elevate the extremity for the first 24 to 72 hours to prevent pain and swelling after the application of the cast (AAOS, 2020; MFMER, 2020).
- To control itching after the cast is dry, use a hair dryer on **cool setting** to blow cool air into the cast (Hinkle et al., 2022; MFMER, 2020). Instruct patients to never insert an object into the cast and report a wet cast to their health care provider (Hinkle & Cheever, 2018).
- Instruct patients to immediately to report the following symptoms to their health care provider (AAOS, 2020; Hinkle et al., 2022):
  - Increased pain and/or the feeling that the cast is too tight, which may indicate excessive swelling
  - Numbness and tingling in the hand or foot, which may be caused by too much pressure on the nerves
  - Burning and stinging, which may be caused by too much pressure on the skin
  - Excessive swelling below the cast, indicating compromised circulation
  - Loss of active movement of toes or fingers, indicating neurovascular compromise

Skill 9-17 ▶ Applying Skin Traction and Caring for a Patient in Skin Traction

Traction is the application of a pulling force to a part of the body to promote and maintain alignment to an injured part of the body (Flynn, 2018, as cited in Hinkle et al., 2022, p. 1173). Skin traction is applied directly to the skin, exerting force over a large area of skin/soft tissue to transmit indirect pull/traction on the bone (Choudhry et al., 2020). The force may be applied using adhesive or nonadhesive traction tape or a boot, belt, or halter. It is used to stabilize a fracture leg, decrease muscle spasms and pain, and immobilize an area before surgery (Hinkle et al., 2022). Traction is primarily used as short-term intervention until other interventions, such as external or internal fixation, are possible (Hinkle et al., 2022). The use of skin traction has decreased, and its use is controversial, with conflicting evidence related to benefit and appropriateness of use (Biz et al., 2019; Brox et al., 2015; Choudhry et al., 2020; Etxebarría-Foronda & Caeiro-Rey, 2018). However, skin traction may still be prescribed for some patients and therefore nurses must be familiar with basic principles and guidelines for implementation.

Traction must be applied in the correct direction and magnitude to obtain the therapeutic effects desired. The affected body part is immobilized by pulling with equal force on each end of the injured area, mixing traction and countertraction. Weights provide the pulling force or traction.

(continued on page 616)

Skill 9-17 ▶ Applying Skin Traction and Caring for a Patient in Skin Traction *(continued)*

The use of additional weights or positioning of the patient's body weight against the traction pull provides the countertraction. See Box 9-2 Principles of Effective Traction.

Types of skin traction for adults include Buck's extension traction (lower leg), and the pelvic belt (Hinkle et al., 2022). Nursing care for skin traction includes setting the traction up, applying the traction, monitoring the application and patient response, and preventing complications from the therapy and immobility.

Box 9-2 | Principles of Effective Traction

- Countertraction must be applied for effective traction.
- Traction must be continuous to be effective.
- Skeletal traction is never interrupted.
- Weights are not removed unless intermittent traction is prescribed.
- Patient must maintain good body alignment in the center of the bed.
- Ropes must be unobstructed.
- Weights must hang free.

Source: Adapted from Hinkle, J. L., Cheever, K. H., & Overbaugh, K. J. (2022). *Brunner & Suddarth's textbook of medical-surgical nursing* (15th ed.). Wolters Kluwer.

DELEGATION CONSIDERATIONS	The application of, and care for a patient with, skin traction may not be delegated to assistive personnel (AP). Depending on the state's nurse practice act and the organization's policies and procedures, this care may be delegated to licensed practical/vocational nurses (LPN/LVNs). The decision to delegate must be based on careful analysis of the patient's needs and circumstances as well as the qualifications of the person to whom the task is being delegated. Refer to the Delegation Guidelines in Appendix A.
EQUIPMENT	• Bed with traction frame and trapeze • Weights • Velcro straps or other straps • Rope and pulleys • Boot with footplate • Graduated compression stocking, as appropriate • Nonsterile gloves and/or other PPE, as indicated • Skin-cleansing supplies
ASSESSMENT	Assess the patient's health record and the prescribed interventions to determine the type of traction, traction weight, and line of pull. Assess the traction equipment to ensure proper function, including inspecting the ropes for fraying and proper positioning. Assess the patient's body alignment. Perform skin and neurovascular assessments. Assess for complications of immobility, including alterations in respiratory function, skin integrity, urinary and bowel elimination, and muscle weakness, contractures, thrombophlebitis, pulmonary embolism, and fatigue.
ACTUAL OR POTENTIAL HEALTH PROBLEMS AND NEEDS	Many actual or potential health problems or issues may require the use of this skill as part of related interventions. An appropriate health problem or issue may include: • Acute pain • Risk for impaired peripheral neurovascular function • ADL deficit
OUTCOME IDENTIFICATION AND PLANNING	The expected outcomes to achieve when applying and caring for a patient in skin traction are that the traction is maintained with the appropriate counterbalance, and the patient maintains proper body alignment. Other outcomes that may be appropriate include that the patient reports an increased level of comfort, and the patient is free from injury.

IMPLEMENTATION

ACTION	RATIONALE
1. Review the health record and the plan of care to determine the type of traction being used and care for the affected body part.	Reviewing the health record and care plan validates the correct patient and correct procedure.

ACTION

2. Perform hand hygiene. Put on PPE, as indicated.

3. Identify the patient. Explain the procedure to the patient, emphasizing the importance of maintaining counterbalance, alignment, and position.

4. Perform a pain assessment and assess for muscle spasm. Administer prescribed medications in sufficient time to allow for the full effect of the analgesic and/or muscle relaxant.

5. Close the curtains around the bed and close the door to the room, if possible. Place the bed at an appropriate and comfortable working height (VHACEOSH, 2016).

Applying Skin Traction

6. Ensure the traction apparatus is attached securely to the bed. Assess the traction setup.

7. Check that the ropes move freely through the pulleys. Check that all knots are tight and are positioned away from the pulleys. Pulleys should be free from the linens.

8. Place the patient in a supine position with the foot of the bed elevated slightly. The patient's head should be near the head of the bed and in alignment.

9. Assess the skin of the affected extremity for abrasions and circulatory status. Cleanse the affected area. Place the compression stocking on the affected limb, as appropriate.

10. Place the traction boot over the patient's leg (Figure 1). Be sure the patient's heel is in the heel of the boot. Secure the boot with the straps.

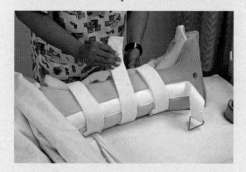

FIGURE 1. Applying traction boot with a compression stocking in place on leg.

11. Attach the traction cord to the boot footplate. Pass the rope over the pulley fastened at the end of the bed. Attach the weight to the hook on the rope, usually 5 to 8 lb for an adult (Figure 2). Gently let go of the weight. **The weight should hang freely, not touching the bed or the floor.**

RATIONALE

Hand hygiene and PPE prevent the spread of microorganisms. PPE is required based on transmission precautions.

Patient identification validates the correct patient and correct procedure. Discussion and explanation help allay anxiety and prepare the patient for what to expect.

Assessing pain and administering analgesics promote patient comfort.

Closing the door or curtains provides for privacy. Proper bed height prevents back and muscle strain.

Assessment of traction setup and weights promotes safety.

Checking ropes and pulleys ensures that weight is being applied correctly, promoting accurate counterbalance and traction function.

Proper patient positioning maintains proper counterbalance and promotes safety.

The skin and circulation should not be compromised to avoid negative consequences related to use of skin traction (Hinkle et al., 2022). Skin care aids in preventing skin breakdown. Use of graduated compression stockings prevents edema and neurovascular complications.

The boot provides a means for attaching traction; proper application ensures proper pull.

Weight attachment applies the pull for the traction. Gently releasing the weight prevents a quick pull on the extremity and possible injury and pain. Properly hanging weights and correct patient positioning ensure accurate counterbalance and traction function.

(continued on page 618)

Skill 9-17 ▶ Applying Skin Traction and Caring for a Patient in Skin Traction *(continued)*

ACTION

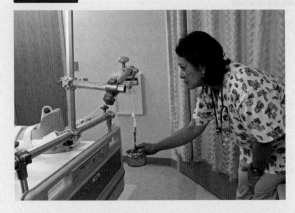

FIGURE 2. Applying weight for skin traction.

12. **Check the patient's alignment with the traction in place.**

13. **Check the boot for placement and alignment. Make sure the line of pull is parallel to the bed and not angled downward.**

14. Place the bed in the lowest position that still allows the weight to hang freely. Make sure the call bell and other essential items are within easy reach.

15. Remove PPE, if used. Perform hand hygiene.

Caring for a Patient With Skin Traction

16. Perform a skin-traction assessment per facility policy. This assessment includes checking the traction equipment, examining the affected body part, maintaining proper body alignment, and performing skin and neurovascular assessments.

17. Remove the straps every 4 hours per the prescribed interventions or facility policy. Check bony prominences for skin breakdown, abrasions, and pressure areas. Remove the boot, per prescribed interventions or facility policy, every 8 hours. Put on gloves and wash, rinse, and thoroughly dry the skin.

18. Assess the extremity distal to the traction for edema, and assess peripheral pulses (Figure 3). Assess the temperature, color, and capillary refill (Figure 4), and compare with the unaffected limb (Hinkle et al., 2022). Check for pain, inability to move body parts distal to the traction, pallor, and abnormal sensations. Assess for indicators of deep vein thrombosis, including calf tenderness and swelling.

19. Replace the traction; remove gloves and dispose of them appropriately. Perform hand hygiene.

20. Check the boot for placement and alignment. **Make sure the line of pull is parallel to the bed and not angled downward.**

RATIONALE

Proper alignment is necessary for proper counterbalance and ensures patient safety.

Misalignment causes ineffective traction and may interfere with healing. A properly positioned boot prevents pressure on the heel.

Proper bed positioning ensures effective application of traction without patient injury. Having the call bell and other items in easy reach contributes to patient safety.

Proper removal of PPE decreases the risk for infection transmission and contamination of other items. Hand hygiene prevents the spread of microorganisms.

Assessment provides information to determine proper application and alignment, thereby reducing the risk for injury. Misalignment causes ineffective traction and may interfere with healing.

Removing the straps provides assessment information for early detection and prompt intervention of potential complications should they arise. Washing the area enhances circulation to skin; thorough drying prevents skin breakdown. Using gloves prevents transfer of microorganisms.

Doing so helps detect signs of abnormal neurovascular function and allows for prompt intervention. Assessing neurovascular status determines the circulation and oxygenation of tissues. Pressure within the traction boot may increase with edema.

Replacing traction is necessary to provide immobilization and facilitate healing. Proper disposal of gloves prevents the transmission of microorganisms. Hand hygiene prevents the spread of microorganisms.

Misalignment causes ineffective traction and may interfere with healing. A properly positioned boot prevents pressure on the heel.

ACTION

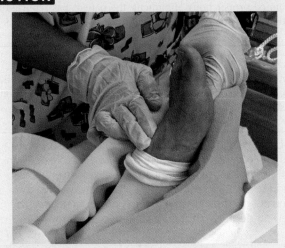

FIGURE 3. Assessing distal pulses.

21. **Ensure the patient is positioned in the center of the bed, with the affected leg aligned with the trunk of the patient's body. Check overall alignment of the patient's body.**

22. Examine the weights and pulley system. **Weights should hang freely, off the floor and bed. Knots should be secure. Ropes should move freely through the pulleys. The pulleys should not be constrained by knots (Figure 5).**

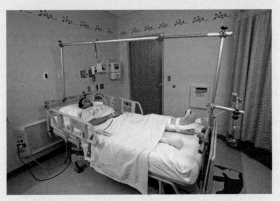

FIGURE 5. Skin traction in place.

23. Keep the bedsheets wrinkle free.

24. Perform range-of-motion (ROM) exercises on all unaffected joint areas, unless contraindicated. Encourage the patient to cough and deep breathe every 2 hours.

25. Raise the side rails. Place the bed in the lowest position that still allows the weight to hang freely. Make sure the call bell and other essential items are within easy reach.

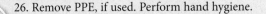

26. Remove PPE, if used. Perform hand hygiene.

RATIONALE

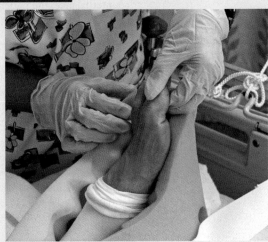

FIGURE 4. Assessing capillary refill.

Misalignment interferes with the effectiveness of traction and may lead to complications.

Checking the weights and pulley system ensures proper application and reduces the risk for patient injury from traction application.

Wrinkles may create areas of increased pressure and contribute to alterations in skin integrity and patient discomfort.

ROM exercises maintain joint function. Coughing and deep breathing help to reduce the risk for respiratory complications related to immobility.

Raising the side rails promotes patient safety. Proper bed positioning ensures effective application of traction without patient injury. Having the call bell and other items in easy reach contributes to patient safety.

Proper removal of PPE decreases the risk for infection transmission and contamination of other items. Hand hygiene prevents the spread of microorganisms.

(continued on page 620)

Skill 9-17 ▶ Applying Skin Traction and Caring for a Patient in Skin Traction *(continued)*

EVALUATION

The expected outcomes have been met when traction has been maintained with the appropriate counterbalance, the patient has maintained proper body alignment, the patient has reported an increased level of comfort, and the patient has remained free from injury.

DOCUMENTATION

Guidelines

Document the time, date, type, amount of weight used, and the site where the traction was applied. Include the skin assessment and care provided before application. Document the patient's response to the traction and the neurovascular status of the extremity.

Sample Documentation

6/3/25 1500 Patient complaining of pain in left hip due to fracture, rating it 7/10. Administered oxycodone (2 tablets). Pain rated 3/10, 30 minutes later. Buck's extension traction with 5 lb of weight applied to left extremity. Skin intact. Pedal pulses present and equal, feet pale pink, warm, and dry, with brisk capillary refill bilaterally. Patient able to wiggle toes freely. Denies numbness or tingling. Patient lying flat in bed with head of bed elevated approximately 15 degrees. Surgery planned for tomorrow.
                                                                        —L. James, RN

DEVELOPING CLINICAL REASONING AND CLINICAL JUDGMENT

UNEXPECTED SITUATIONS AND ASSOCIATED INTERVENTIONS

- *Patient in Buck's traction reports pain in the heel of the affected leg:* Remove traction and perform skin and neurovascular assessments. Reapply the traction and reassess the neurovascular status in 15 to 20 minutes. Communicate with the health care team regarding the findings.

SPECIAL CONSIDERATIONS

General Considerations

- Unless contraindicated, encourage the patient to do active flexion–extension ankle exercise and calf-pumping exercises at regular intervals to decrease venous stasis.
- Be alert for pressure on peripheral nerves with skin traction. Take care with Buck's traction to avoid pressure on the peroneal nerve at the point where it passes around the neck of the fibula just below the knee (Hinkle et al., 2022).
- Assess patients who are in traction for extended periods for the development of helplessness, isolation, confinement, and loss of control. Diversional activities, therapeutic communication, and frequent visits by staff and significant others are an important part of care.

Older Adult Considerations

- Be extra vigilant with older adults in skin traction. Older adults are susceptible to alterations in skin integrity due to a decreased amount of subcutaneous fat and thinner, drier, more fragile skin, as well as constipation due to being confined to bed.

Skill 9-18 ▶ Caring for a Patient in Skeletal Traction

Traction is the application of a pulling force to a part of the body to promote and maintain alignment to an injured part of the body (Hinkle et al., 2022). Skeletal traction provides pull to a body part by attaching weight directly to the bone through pins, screws, wires, or tongs inserted into the bone (Choudhry et al., 2020). It is used to immobilize a body part for prolonged periods. This method of traction is used to treat fractures of the femur, tibia, and cervical spine.

Traction must be applied in the correct direction and magnitude to obtain the therapeutic effects desired. The affected body part is immobilized by pulling with equal force on each end of the injured area, mixing traction and countertraction. Weights provide the pulling force or traction. The use of additional weights or positioning of the patient's body weight against the traction pull provides the countertraction. See Box 9-2 Principles of Effective Traction in Skill 9-17.

Nursing responsibilities related to skeletal traction include maintaining the traction, maintaining body alignment, monitoring neurovascular status, promoting exercise, preventing complications from the therapy and immobility, and preventing infection by providing pin-site care. A growing evidence base supports effective management of pin sites but with no clear consensus (Cam & Korkmaz, 2014; Ktistakis et al., 2015; Lagerquist et al., 2012; Lethaby et al., 2013). There remains considerable diversity of practice in caring for pin sites (Abbariao, 2018; Kazmers et al., 2016; Lethaby et al., 2013: Walker et al., 2018). Pin-site care varies based on prescribed interventions and facility policy. Dressings may be applied for the first 48 to 72 hours, and then sites may be left open to air (Abbariao, 2018). Pin-site care may be performed frequently in the first 48 to 72 hours after application, when drainage may be heavy; other evidence suggests pin care should begin after the first 48 to 72 hours (Abbariao, 2018). Pin-site care may be done daily or weekly or not at all (Georgiades, 2018; Lagerquist et al., 2012; Timms & Pugh, 2012). Pin-site care is completed using aseptic technique in the immediate postoperative period. Refer to specific patient prescribed interventions and facility guidelines.

DELEGATION CONSIDERATIONS

The care of a patient with skeletal traction may not be delegated to assistive personnel (AP). Depending on the state's nurse practice act and the organization's policies and procedures, care for these patients may be delegated to licensed practical/vocational nurses (LPN/LVNs). The decision to delegate must be based on careful analysis of the patient's needs and circumstances as well as the qualifications of the person to whom the task is being delegated. Refer to the Delegation Guidelines in Appendix A.

EQUIPMENT

- Sterile applicators
- Cleansing agent for pin care, sterile normal saline for initial cleaning, but may be an antimicrobial such as chlorhexidine or povidone-iodine (Hickey & Strayer, 2020; Sáenz-Jalón et al., 2020; Walker et al., 2018), per prescribed intervention or facility policy
- Sterile container
- Antimicrobial ointment, per prescribed intervention or facility policy

- Sterile gauze or dressing, per prescribed intervention or facility policy
- Analgesic, as prescribed
- Sterile or nonsterile gloves for performing pin care, depending on prescribed intervention or facility policy
- Additional PPE, as indicated

ASSESSMENT

Review the patient's health record and care plan to determine the type of traction, traction weight, and line of pull. Assess the traction equipment to ensure proper function, including inspecting the ropes for fraying and proper positioning. Assess the patient's body alignment. Assess the patient's pain and need for analgesia before providing care. Perform skin and neurovascular assessments. Inspect the pin insertion sites for inflammation and infection, including swelling, cloudy or offensive drainage, pain, or redness. Assess for complications of immobility, including alterations in respiratory function, constipation, alterations in skin integrity, alterations in urinary elimination, and muscle weakness, contractures, thrombophlebitis, pulmonary embolism, and fatigue.

ACTUAL OR POTENTIAL HEALTH PROBLEMS AND NEEDS

Many actual or potential health problems or issues may require the use of this skill as part of related interventions. An appropriate health problem or issue may include:
- ADL deficit
- Infection risk
- Disturbed body image

OUTCOME IDENTIFICATION AND PLANNING

The expected outcomes to achieve when applying and caring for a patient in skeletal traction are that the traction is maintained appropriately, and the patient maintains proper body alignment. Other outcomes that may be appropriate include that the patient reports an increased level of comfort, and the patient is free from infection and injury.

(continued on page 622)

Skill 9-18 ▸ Caring for a Patient in Skeletal Traction *(continued)*

IMPLEMENTATION

ACTION	RATIONALE
1. Review the health record and the care plan to determine the type of traction being used and the prescribed care.	Reviewing the health record and care plan validates the correct patient and correct procedure.
2. Perform hand hygiene. Put on PPE, as indicated.	Hand hygiene and PPE prevent the spread of microorganisms. PPE is required based on transmission precautions.
3. Identify the patient. Explain the procedure to the patient, emphasizing the importance of maintaining counterbalance, alignment, and position.	Patient identification validates the correct patient and correct procedure. Discussion and explanation help allay anxiety and prepare the patient for what to expect.
4. Perform a pain assessment and assess for muscle spasm. Administer prescribed medications in sufficient time to allow for the full effect of the analgesic and/or muscle relaxant.	Assessing for pain and administering analgesics promote patient comfort.
5. Close the curtains around the bed and close the door to the room, if possible. Place the bed at an appropriate and comfortable working height (VHACEOSH, 2016).	Closing the door or curtains provides for privacy. Proper bed height prevents back and muscle strain.
6. Ensure the traction apparatus is attached securely to the bed. Assess the traction setup, including application of the prescribed amount of weight. **Be sure that the weights hang freely, not touching the bed or the floor (Figure 1).**	Proper traction application reduces the risk of injury by promoting accurate counterbalance and traction function.

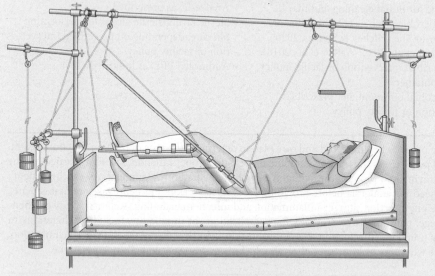

FIGURE 1. Skeletal traction in place, weights hanging freely. (*Source:* From Farrell, M. [2017]. *Smeltzer & Bare's Textbook of Medical-Surgical Nursing* [4th Australia/New Zealand edition]; Lippincott Williams & Wilkins Pty Ltd.)

ACTION	RATIONALE
7. **Check that the ropes move freely through the pulleys. Check that all knots are tight and are positioned away from the pulleys. Pulleys should be free from the linens.**	Free ropes and pulleys ensure accurate counterbalance and traction function.
8. Check the alignment of the patient's body, as prescribed.	Proper alignment maintains an effective line of pull and prevents injury.
9. Perform a skin assessment. Pay attention to pressure points, including the ischial tuberosity, popliteal space, Achilles tendon, sacrum, and heel.	Skin assessment provides early intervention for skin irritation, impaired tissue perfusion, and other complications.

ACTION

10. Perform a neurovascular assessment. Assess the extremity distal to the traction for edema and peripheral pulses. Assess the temperature and color and compare with the unaffected limb. Check for pain, inability to move body parts distal to the traction, pallor, and abnormal sensations. Assess for indicators of deep vein thrombosis, including calf tenderness, and swelling.

11. Assess the site at and around the pins for redness, edema, and odor. Assess for skin tenting, prolonged or purulent drainage, elevated body temperature, elevated pin-site temperature, and bowing or bending of the pins.

12. Provide pin-site care, based on prescribed interventions and/or facility policy and procedure.

    a. Using sterile technique, open the applicator package and pour the cleansing agent into the sterile container.

    b. Put on the sterile gloves.

    c. Place the applicators into the solution.

    d. **Clean the pin site, starting at the insertion area and working outward, away from the pin site (Figure 2).**

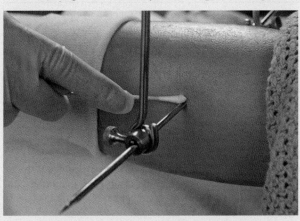

FIGURE 2. Cleaning around pin sites with normal saline on an applicator.

    e. **Use each applicator once. Use a new applicator for each pin site.** Depending on prescribed intervention and facility policy, gently remove crusts or scabs appearing at the pin site if they can be removed easily; leave in place if there is difficulty during removal.

13. Depending on prescribed interventions and facility policy, apply the antimicrobial ointment to pin sites and apply a dressing. Remove gloves and dispose of them appropriately. Perform hand hygiene.

RATIONALE

Neurovascular assessment aids in early identification and allows for prompt intervention should compromised circulation and oxygenation of tissues develop.

Pin sites provide a possible entry for microorganisms. Skin inspection allows for early detection and prompt intervention should complications develop.

Performing pin-site care may help to reduce the risk of pin site infection and associated complications (Abbariao, 2018; Sáenz-Jalón et al., 2020; Kazmers et al., 2016; Lethaby et al., 2013).

Using sterile technique in the initial 2 to 3 days may reduce the risk for transmission of microorganisms (Hickey & Strayer, 2020; Kazmers et al., 2016).

Gloves prevent contact with blood and/or body fluids.

Cleaning from the center outward ensures movement from the least to most contaminated area.

Using an applicator once reduces the risk of transmission of microorganisms. Removal of crusts is controversial; some evidence suggests removal of crusts prevents excessive pressure at site and allows for drainage and prevents infection (Abbariao, 2018; Cam & Korkmaz, 2014; Walker et al., 2018). Other evidence suggests crusts should be left in place to act as a biologic barrier to prevent introduction of microorganisms and decrease the risk of pint site infection (Abbariao, 2018; Georgiades, 2018; Walker et al., 2018).

Antimicrobial ointment may help reduce the risk of infection (Hickey & Strayer, 2020; Kazmers et al., 2016; Lethaby et al., 2013). A dressing may aid in protecting the pin sites from contamination and in containing any drainage. Disposing of gloves reduces the risk of microorganism transmission. Hand hygiene prevents the spread of microorganisms.

(continued on page 624)

Skill 9-18 ▶ Caring for a Patient in Skeletal Traction *(continued)*

ACTION	**RATIONALE**
14. Perform range-of-motion (ROM) and active exercises on all noninvolved joints, unless contraindicated. Encourage the patient to cough and deep breathe every 2 hours.	ROM and active exercises promote joint, help maintain muscle strength and tone, and promote circulation (Hinkle et al., 2022). Coughing and deep breathing reduce the risk of respiratory complications related to immobility.
15. Place the bed in the lowest position that still allows the weight to hang freely. Make sure the call bell and other essential items are within easy reach.	Proper bed positioning ensures effective application of traction without patient injury. Having the call bell and other items in easy reach contributes to patient safety.
16. Remove PPE, if used. Perform hand hygiene.	Proper removal of PPE reduces the risk for infection transmission and contamination of other items. Hand hygiene prevents the spread of microorganisms.

EVALUATION

The expected outcomes have been met when the traction was maintained appropriately, the patient has maintained proper body alignment, the patient has reported an increased level of comfort, and the patient is free from infection and injury.

DOCUMENTATION

Guidelines

Document the time, date, type of traction, and the amount of weight used. Include skin and pin-site assessments, and pin-site care. Document the patient's response to the traction and the neurovascular status of the extremity.

Sample Documentation

> 6/5/25 1020 Pin-site care performed. Pin sites cleaned with normal saline and open to the air. Sites slightly red with serosanguineous crusting noted. Neurovascular status intact. Balanced suspension skeletal traction maintained as prescribed.
>
> —M. Leroux, RN

DEVELOPING CLINICAL REASONING AND CLINICAL JUDGMENT

UNEXPECTED SITUATIONS AND ASSOCIATED INTERVENTIONS

- *While performing a pin-site assessment for your patient with skeletal traction, you note that several of the pins move and slide in the pin tract:* Assess the patient for other symptoms, including signs of infection at the pin sites, pain, and fever. Assess for neurovascular changes. Communicate with the health care team regarding the findings.

SPECIAL CONSIDERATIONS

- Normal changes at the pin site related to the inflammatory response after insertion include redness, warmth, and serosanguineous drainage and usually subside 72 hours after insertion (Hinkle et al., 2022). If a pin site becomes unusually painful or tender, or if you notice any fluid discharge after the initial insertion period, it may be a signal that the pin has loosened or become infected. Other signs of infection may include the presence of purulent drainage, tenting of the skin at pin site, odor and fever (Hinkle et al., 2022). Communicate these symptoms to the health care team.
- Assess the patient for chronic conditions, such as diabetes mellitus, peripheral vascular disease, and chronic obstructive pulmonary disease, which can increase a patient's risk for complications when skeletal traction is in use.
- Never remove the weights from skeletal traction unless a life-threatening situation occurs. Removal of the weights interferes with therapy and can result in injury to the patient.
- Jarring movements can disrupt traction. Use smooth, coordinated effort whenever you must reposition the patient.
- Inspect the pin sites for inflammation and evidence of infection at least every 8 hours. Prevention of osteomyelitis is of utmost importance (Abbariao, 2018; Kazmers et al., 2016).

EVIDENCE FOR PRACTICE ▶

EXTERNAL FIXATOR PIN-SITE CARE

Different methods of cleansing external fixator percutaneous pin sites have been suggested to prevent pin-site infections, with no clear consensus on a cleansing regimen or other aspects of pin-site care (Kazmers et al., 2016; Lathaby et al., 2013). Chlorhexidine-alcohol solution and povidone-iodine solution are commonly used to provide pin-site care. Is there a significant difference between the number and severity of infections in fixators among those who are cared for using one or the other of these solutions?

Related Evidence

Sáenz-Jalón, M., Sarabia-Cobo, C. M., Bartolome, E. R., Fernández, M. S., Vélez, B., Escudero, M., Miguel, M. E., Artabe, P., Cabañas, I., Fernández, A., Garcés, C., & Couceiro, J. (2020). A randomized clinical trial on the use of antiseptic solutions for the pin-site care of external fixators: Chlorhexidine-alcohol versus povidone-iodine. *Journal of Trauma Nursing, 27*(3), 146–150. https://doi.org/10.1097/JTN.0000000000000503

This randomized clinical trial investigated the superiority of chlorhexidine-alcohol solution versus povidone-iodine solution for external fixator pin-site care in pin-site infection. The study took place in one hospital in Spain with 128 patients who underwent placement of an external fixator. Participants were randomly assigned to receive pin-site care using either a 2% chlorhexidine-alcohol solution or a 10% povidone-iodine solution. The average number of pins per patient was 4.3 with a total 568 of pins initially available for analysis. Ultimately, 489 pins were analyzed for the development of a pin-site infection, with 79 pins not analyzed for various reasons, including improper collection of the sample and inappropriate condition of the sample upon arrival to the laboratory. The majority of patients (82%) remained free of pin-site infection. Results indicated no significant differences of rate of infection between groups. Statistically significant differences were found regarding time and infection variables. The longer the person had the fixator, the higher the risk of infection (*P* = .002). The researchers concluded both chlorhexidine-alcohol and povidone-iodine solutions are equally effective for preventing infection in external fixator pin sites. The researchers suggested other factors should also be taken into consideration when developing pin-site care guidelines, including cost and simplicity of use to optimal care.

Relevance for Nursing Practice

The results of this study suggest that implementing pin-site care with either antimicrobial solution is effective in preventing pin-site infections and that other factors should also be considered to ensure consistent implementation of pin-site care. Nurses should consider adoption of evidence-based pin-site care guidelines to support quality patient care and improve patient outcomes.

EVIDENCE FOR PRACTICE ▶

EXTERNAL FIXATOR PIN-SITE CARE

The goal of pin-site care is to reduce the risk for or, when possible, prevent pin-site infection. Removal of crusts from pin sites is controversial; some evidence suggests removal of crusts prevents excessive pressure at site and allows for drainage and prevents infection (Abbariao, 2018; Cam & Korkmaz, 2014; Walker et al., 2018). Other evidence suggest crusts should be left in place to act as a biologic barrier to prevent introduction of microorganisms and decrease the risk of pin-site infection (Abbariao, 2018; Georgiades, 2018; Walker et al., 2018).

Related Evidence

Georgiades, D. S. (2018). A systematic integrative review of pin site crusts. *Orthopaedic Nursing, 37*(1), 36–42. https://doi.org/10.1097/NOR.0000000000000416

Refer to details in Skill 9-19, Evidence for Practice.

Skill 9-19 ▶ Caring for a Patient With an External Fixation Device

External fixation devices are used to manage fractures with soft tissue damage and complicated fractures, correct defects, treat nonunion, and lengthen limbs (Hinkle et al., 2022). External fixators consist of one of a variety of frames to hold pins that are drilled into or through bones. External fixators provide stable support for severely crushed or splintered fractures and access to, and treatment for, soft tissue injuries. The use of these devices allows treatment of the fracture and damaged soft tissues while promoting patient comfort, early mobility, and active exercise of adjacent uninvolved joints. Complications related to disuse and immobility are minimized. Nursing responsibilities include reassuring the patient, maintaining the device, monitoring neurovascular status, promoting exercise, preventing complications from the therapy, preventing infection by providing pin-site care, and providing teaching to ensure compliance and self-care.

A growing evidence base supports effective management of pin sites, but with no clear consensus (Cam & Korkmaz, 2014; Ktistakis et al., 2015; Lagerquist et al., 2012; Lethaby et al., 2013). There remains considerable diversity of practice in caring for pin sites (Abbariao, 2018; Kazmers et al., 2016; Lethaby et al., 2013: Walker et al., 2018). Pin-site care varies based on prescribed interventions and facility policy. Dressings may be applied for the first 48 to 72 hours, and then sites may be left open to air (Abbariao, 2018). Pin-site care may be performed frequently in the first 48 to 72 hours after application, when drainage may be heavy; other evidence suggests pin care should begin after the first 48 to 72 hours (Abbariao, 2018). Pin-site care may be done daily or weekly or not at all (Georgiades, 2018; Lagerquist et al., 2012; Timms & Pugh, 2012). Pin-site care is completed using aseptic technique in the immediate postoperative period. Refer to specific patient prescribed interventions and facility guidelines.

Nurses play a major role in preparing the patient psychologically for the application of an external fixator. The devices appear clumsy and large. In addition, the nurse needs to clarify misconceptions regarding pain and discomfort associated with the device.

DELEGATION CONSIDERATIONS

The care of a patient with an external fixator device may not be delegated to assistive personnel (AP). Depending on the state's nurse practice act and the organization's policies and procedures, care for these patients may be delegated to licensed practical/vocational nurses (LPN/LVNs). The decision to delegate must be based on careful analysis of the patient's needs and circumstances as well as the qualifications of the person to whom the task is being delegated. Refer to the Delegation Guidelines in Appendix A.

EQUIPMENT

Equipment varies with the type of fixator and the type and location of the fracture, but may include:
- Sterile applicators
- Cleansing agent for pin care, sterile normal saline for initial cleaning, but may be an antimicrobial such as chlorhexidine or povidone-iodine (Hickey & Strayer, 2020; Sáenz-Jalón et al., 2020; Walker et al., 2018, per prescribed intervention or facility policy)
- Ice bag
- Antimicrobial ointment, per prescribed intervention or facility policy
- Sterile gauze or dressing, per prescribed intervention or facility policy
- Analgesic, as prescribed
- Sterile or nonsterile gloves for performing pin care, depending on prescribed intervention or facility policy
- Additional PPE, as indicated

ASSESSMENT

Review the patient's health record and care plan to determine the type of device being used and prescribed care. Assess the patient's pain and need for analgesia before providing care. Assess the external fixator to ensure proper function and position. Perform skin and neurovascular assessments. Inspect the pin-insertion sites for signs of inflammation and infection, including swelling, cloudy or offensive drainage, pain, or redness. Assess the patient's knowledge regarding the device and self-care activities and responsibilities.

ACTUAL OR POTENTIAL HEALTH PROBLEMS AND NEEDS	Many actual or potential health problems or issues may require the use of this skill as part of related interventions. An appropriate health problem or issue may include: • Infection risk • Knowledge deficiency • Disturbed body image
OUTCOME IDENTIFICATION AND PLANNING	The expected outcome to achieve when caring for a patient with an external fixator device is that the patient shows no evidence of complication, such as infection, contractures, venous stasis, thrombus formation, or skin breakdown. Additional outcomes that may be appropriate include that the patient shows signs of healing, the patient reports an increased level of comfort, and the patient is free from injury.

IMPLEMENTATION

ACTION	RATIONALE
1. Review the health record and the care plan to determine the type of device being used and prescribed care.	Reviewing the health record and care plan validates the correct patient and correct procedure.
2. Perform hand hygiene. Put on PPE, as indicated.	Hand hygiene and PPE prevent the spread of microorganisms. PPE is required based on transmission precautions.
3. Identify the patient. Explain the procedure to the patient. Assure the patient that there will be little pain after the fixation device is in place. Reinforce that the patient will be able to adjust to the device and will be able to move about with the device, allowing them to resume normal activities more quickly.	Patient identification validates the correct patient and correct procedure. Discussion and explanation allay anxiety and prepare the patient psychologically for the application of the device.
4. **After the fixation device is in place (Figure 1), apply ice to the surgical site, as prescribed or per facility policy. Elevate the affected body part, if appropriate.**	Ice and elevation help reduce swelling, relieve pain, and reduce bleeding.

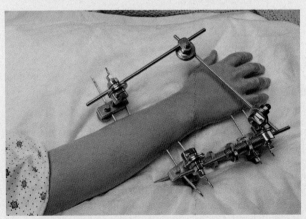

FIGURE 1. External fixation device in place.

5. Perform a pain assessment and assess for muscle spasm. Administer prescribed medications in sufficient time to allow for the full effect of the analgesic and/or muscle relaxant.	Pain assessment and analgesic administration help promote patient comfort.
6. Administer analgesics, as prescribed, before exercising or mobilizing the affected body part.	Administration of analgesics promotes patient comfort and facilitates movement.

(continued on page 628)

Skill 9-19 ▶ Caring for a Patient With an External Fixation Device *(continued)*

ACTION	**RATIONALE**
7. Perform neurovascular assessments, per facility policy or prescribed interventions, usually every 2 to 4 hours for 24 hours, then every 4 to 8 hours. Assess the affected body part for color, motion, sensation, edema, capillary refill, and pulses. If appropriate, compare with the unaffected side. Assess for pain not relieved by analgesics, and for burning, tingling, and numbness.	Assessment promotes early detection and prompt intervention for abnormal neurovascular function, nerve damage, or circulatory impairment. Assessment of neurovascular status determines the circulation and oxygenation of tissues.
8. Close the curtains around the bed and close the door to the room, if possible. Place the bed at an appropriate and comfortable working height (VHACEOSH, 2016).	Closing the door or curtains provides for privacy. Proper bed height prevents back and muscle strain.
9. Assess the pin site for redness, edema, tenting of the skin, prolonged or purulent drainage, and bowing, bending, or loosening of the pins. Monitor body temperature.	Assessing pin sites aids in early detection of infection and stress on the skin and allows for appropriate intervention.
10. Provide pin-site care, based on prescribed interventions and/or facility policy and procedure.	Performing pin-site care may help to reduce the risk of pin-site infection and associated complications (Abbariao, 2018; Sáenz-Jalón et al., 2020; Kazmers et al., 2016; Lethaby et al., 2013).
a. Using sterile technique, open the applicator package and pour the cleansing agent into the sterile container.	Using sterile technique in the initial 2 to 3 days may reduce the risk for transmission of microorganisms (Hickey & Strayer, 2020; Kazmers et al., 2016).
b. Put on the sterile gloves.	Gloves prevent contact with blood and/or body fluids.
c. Place the applicators into the solution.	
d. **Clean the pin site starting at the insertion area and working outward, away from the pin site (Figure 2).**	Cleaning from the center outward promotes movement from the least to most contaminated area.

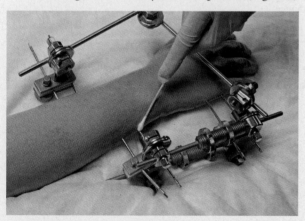

FIGURE 2. Cleaning around pin sites with normal saline on an applicator.

e. **Use each applicator once. Use a new applicator for each pin site.** Depending on prescribed intervention and facility policy, gently remove crusts or scabs appearing at the pin site if they can be removed easily; leave in place if there is difficulty during removal.	Using an applicator once reduces the risk of transmission of microorganisms. Removal of crusts is controversial; some evidence suggests removal of crusts prevents excessive pressure at site and allows for drainage and prevents infection (Abbariao, 2018; Cam & Korkmaz, 2014; Walker et al., 2018). Other evidence suggests crusts should be left in place to act as a biologic barrier to prevent introduction of microorganisms and decrease the risk of pint site infection (Abbariao, 2018; Georgiades, 2018; Walker et al., 2018).
11. Depending on prescribed interventions and facility policy, apply the antimicrobial ointment to pin sites and apply a dressing. Remove gloves and dispose of them appropriately. Perform hand hygiene.	Antimicrobial ointment may help reduce the risk of infection (Hickey & Strayer, 2020; Kazmers et al., 2016; Lethaby et al., 2013). A dressing may aid in protecting the pin sites from contamination and in containing any drainage. Disposing of gloves reduces the risk of microorganism transmission. Hand hygiene prevents the spread of microorganisms.

ACTION

12. Perform range-of-motion (ROM) and active exercises on all noninvolved joint areas, unless contraindicated. Encourage the patient to cough and deep breathe every 2 hours.

13. Place the bed in the lowest position. Make sure the call bell and other essential items are within easy reach.

 14. Remove PPE, if used. Perform hand hygiene.

RATIONALE

ROM and active exercises promote joint, help maintain muscle strength and tone, and promote circulation (Hinkle et al., 2022). Coughing and deep breathing reduce the risk of respiratory complications related to immobility.

Proper bed positioning ensures effective application of traction without patient injury. Leaving the call bell and other items within reach ensures patient safety.

Proper removal of PPE reduces the risk for infection transmission and contamination of other items. Hand hygiene prevents the spread of microorganisms.

EVALUATION

The expected outcomes have been met when the patient has exhibited an external fixation device in place with pin sites that are clean, dry, and intact, without evidence of infection; the patient has remained free of complications, such as contractures, venous stasis, thrombus formation, or skin breakdown; the patient has reported an increased level of comfort; the patient has remained free of injury, and the patient has demonstrated knowledge of pin-site care.

DOCUMENTATION

Guidelines

Document the time, date, and type of device in place. Include the skin assessment, pin-site assessment, and pin-site care. Document the patient's response to the device and the neurovascular status of the affected area.

Sample Documentation

7/6/25 1020 External fixator in place on left forearm. Pin-site care performed. Pin sites cleaned with normal saline and open to the air. Sites slightly red with serosanguineous crusting noted. Neurovascular status intact. Instruction given regarding ROM exercises to left fingers and elbow; patient verbalizes an understanding and is able to demonstrate.
—B. Clapp, RN

DEVELOPING CLINICAL REASONING AND CLINICAL JUDGMENT

SPECIAL CONSIDERATIONS

- Normal changes at the pin site related to the inflammatory response after insertion include redness, warmth, and serosanguineous drainage, and usually subside 72 hours after insertion (Hinkle et al., 2022). If a pin site becomes unusually painful or tender, or if you notice any fluid discharge after the initial insertion period, it may be a signal that the pin has loosened or become infected. Other signs of infection may include the presence of purulent drainage, tenting of the skin at pin site, odor, and fever (Hinkle et al., 2022). Communicate these symptoms to the health care team.
- Teach the patient and significant others how to provide pin-site care and how to recognize the signs of pin-site infection. External fixator devices are in place for prolonged periods. Clean technique can be used at home instead of sterile technique.
- Teach the patient and significant others to identify early signs of infection, signs of a loose pin, and how to contact the orthopedic team, if necessary.
- Reinforce the importance of keeping the affected body part elevated when sitting or lying down to prevent edema.
- Do not adjust the clamps on the external fixator frame. It is the physician's or advanced practice professional's responsibility to adjust the clamps.

(continued on page 630)

Skill 9-19 ▶ Caring for a Patient With an External Fixation Device *(continued)*

- Fractures often require additional treatment and stabilization with a cast or molded splint after the fixator device is removed.
- Patients may be encouraged to shower after removing the pin site dressing and allow water to rinse the frame and use an antibacterial liquid soap to wash the affected limb, followed by the prescribed pin site care (Kazmers et al., 2016; Walker et al., 2018).

EVIDENCE FOR PRACTICE ▶

EXTERNAL FIXATOR PIN SITES—CLINICAL EVIDENCE REVIEW

The goal of pin-site care is to reduce the risk for or, when possible, prevent pin-site infection. Removal of crusts from pin sites is controversial; some evidence suggests removal of crusts prevents excessive pressure at site and allows for drainage and prevents infection (Abbariao, 2018; Cam & Korkmaz, 2014; Walker et al., 2018). Other evidence suggests crusts should be left in place to act as a biologic barrier to prevent introduction of microorganisms and decrease the risk of pin-site infection (Abbariao, 2018; Georgiades, 2018; Walker et al., 2018).

Related Evidence

Georgiades, D. S. (2018). A systematic integrative review of pin site crusts. *Orthopaedic Nursing*, *37*(1), 36–42. https://doi.org/10.1097/NOR.0000000000000416

The aim of this systematic review was to explore the effectiveness of pin-site crusts as a biologic dressing versus the removal of pin-site crusts in pin-site care and prevention of pin-site infection. A systematic search was conducted using CINAHL, Cochrane Library, and ProQuest, resulting in 29 initial studies. Five studies that met the inclusion criteria were appraised using the Mixed Method Appraisal Tool. Findings of a narrative synthesis revealed that pin-site crusts have similar properties to that of a dressing, as the crusts are able to act as a barrier between the insertion site of the pin and the external environment, which can reduce infection. The authors concluded pin-site crusts could reduce risk of pin-site infection and could be maintained in place.

Relevance for Nursing Practice

The results of this study suggest that pin-site crusts could be left in place as a biologic dressing, decreasing patients' risk of pin-site infection and improving patient outcomes. Nurses should consider adoption of evidence-based pin-site care guidelines to support quality patient care and improve patient outcomes.

Refer to details in Skill 9-19, Evidence for Practice.

EVIDENCE FOR PRACTICE ▶

EXTERNAL FIXATOR PIN-SITE CARE

Different methods of cleansing external fixator percutaneous pin sites have been suggested to prevent pin-site infections, with no clear consensus on a cleansing regimen or other aspects of pin-site care (Kazmers et al., 2016; Lathaby et al., 2013). Chlorhexidine-alcohol solution and povidone-iodine solution are commonly used to provide pin-site care. Is there a significant difference between the number and severity of infections in fixators among those who are cared for using one or the other of these solutions?

Related Evidence

Sáenz-Jalón, M., Sarabia-Cobo, C. M., Bartolome, E. R., Fernández, M. S., Vélez, B., Escudero, M., Miguel, M. E., Artabe, P., Cabañas, I., Fernández, A., Garcés, C., & Couceiro, J. (2020). A randomized clinical trial on the use of antiseptic solutions for the pin-site care of external fixators: Chlorhexidine-alcohol versus povidone-iodine. *Journal of Trauma Nursing*, *27*(3), 146–150. https://doi.org/10.1097/JTN.0000000000000503

Refer to details in Skill 9-18, Evidence for Practice.

Enhance Your Understanding

Focusing on Patient Care: Developing Clinical Reasoning and Clinical Judgment

Consider the case scenarios at the beginning of the chapter as you answer the following questions to enhance your understanding and apply what you have learned.

QUESTIONS

1. You are preparing to discharge Bobby Rowden from the emergency room. Discuss the teaching you should include for Bobby and his parents related to his injury and his plaster cast.

2. A pneumatic compression device has been prescribed as part of the interventions for Esther Levitz. You bring the pump and sleeves into the room, and she asks, "What is that? It looks like a torture machine!" How will you respond?

3. You are caring for Manuel Esposito the evening before his surgery. Your assessment of his affected extremity reveals skin that is warm to the touch, rapid capillary refill, and positive sensation and movement. What other assessments should you perform as part of your care for Mr. Esposito?

You can find suggested answers after the Bibliography at the end of this chapter.

Integrated Case Study Connection

The case studies in the back of the book focus on integrating concepts. Refer to the following case studies to enhance your understanding of the concepts and skills in this chapter.

- Basic Case Studies: Abigail Cantonelli, page 1193.
- Intermediate Case Studies: Jason Brown, page 1215; Kent Clark, page 1217.

Bibliography

Abbariao, M. (2018). Can pin-site infection be prevented? *KaiTiak Nursing New Zealand, 24*(9), 27–29.

Adamczyk, M. A. (2018). Reducing intensive care unit staff musculoskeletal injuries with implementation of a safe patient handling and mobility program. *Critical Care Nursing Quarterly, 41*(3), 264–271.

American Academy of Orthopaedic Surgeons (AAOS). (2015, February). *How to use crutches, canes, and walkers.* https://orthoinfo.aaos.org/en/recovery/how-to-use-crutches-canes-and-walkers/

American Academy of Orthopaedic Surgeons (AAOS). (2020, March). *OrthoInfo. Care of casts and splints.* https://orthoinfo.aaos.org/en/recovery/care-of-casts-and-splints

American Association of Critical-Care Nurses (AACN). (2016, October 1). *Practice alert. Preventing venous thromboembolism in adults.* https://www.aacn.org/clinical-resources/practice-alerts/venous-thromboembolism-prevention

American Geriatrics Society, Health in Aging Foundation. (2019, June). *Tip sheet: Choosing the right cane or walker.* https://www.healthinaging.org/tools-and-tips/tip-sheet-choosing-right-cane-or-walker

Arnold, M., Needham, D. M., & Nydahl, P. (2018). International round table discussion: Early Mobility. *International Journal of Safe Patient Handling & Mobility (SPHM), 8*(1), 57–64.

Arnold, M. (2019). Functional assessments for safe patient mobilization across the continuum of care. *International Journal of Safe Patient Handling & Mobility (SPHM), 9*(3), 111–121.

Baptiste-McKinney, A., & Halvorson, B. (2018). The use of friction-reducing devices in a safe patient handling & mobility program. *International Journal of Safe Patient Handling & Mobility (SPHM), 8*(3), 132–141.

Biz, C., Fantoni, I., Crepaldi, N., Zonta, F., Buffon, L., Corradin, M., Lissandron, A., & Ruggieri, P. (2019). Clinical practice and nursing management of preoperative skin or skeletal traction for hip fractures in elderly patients: A cross-sectinal three-institution study. *International Journal of Orthopaedic and Trauma Nursing, 32,* 32–40. https://doi.org/10.1016/j.ijotn.2018.10.002

Boynton, T., Kumpar, D., & VanGilder, C. (2020). The Bedside Mobility Assessment Tool 2.0. *American Nurse Journal, 15*(7), 18–22.

Bram, J. T., Gambone, A. J., DeFrancesco, C. J., Striano, B. M., & Ganley, T. J. (2019). Use of continuous passive motion reduces rates of arthrofibrosis after anterior cruciate ligament reconstruction in a pediatric population. *Orthopedics, 42*(1), e81–e85. https://doi.org/10.3928/01477447-20181120-04

Brox, W. T., Roberts, K. C., Taksali, S., Wright, D. G., Wixted, J. J., Tubb, C. C., Patt, J. C., Templeton, K. J., Dickman, E., Adler, R. A., Macauley, W. B., Jackman, J. M., Annaswamy, T., Adelman, A. M., Hawthorne, C. G., Olson, S. A., Mendelson, D. A., LeBoff, M. S., Camacho, P. A., ... Sevarino, K. (2015). The American Academy of Orthopaedic Surgeons evidence-based guideline on management of hip fractures in the elderly. *Journal of Bone and Joint Surgery American, 97*(14), 1196–1199. https://doi.org/10.2106/JBJS.O.00229

Burns, S. M., & Delgado, S. A. (2019). *AACN Essentials of critical care nursing* (4th ed.). McGraw-Hill Education.

Cam, R., & Korkmaz, F. D. (2014). The effect of long-term care and follow-up on complications in patients with external fixators. *International Journal of Nursing Practice, 20*(1), 89–96. https://doi.org/10.1111/ijn.12126

Canterbury District Health Board. (2018). *Thrombo-embolus deterrent (TED) stockings. Patient information.* Department of General Surgery. https://www.cdhb.health.nz/Patients-Visitors/patient-information-pamphlets/Documents/Thrombo-Embolus%20Deterrent-Stockings-2582.pdf

Chen, M. C., Lin, C. C., Ko, J. Y., & Kuo, F. C. (2020). The effects of immediate programmed cryotherapy and continuous passive motion in patients after computer-assisted total knee arthroplasty: A prospective, randomized controlled trial. *Journal of Orthopaedic Surgery and Research, 15*(1), 379. https://doi.org/10.1186/s13018-020-01924-y

Cho, S. H., Lee, J. H., & Jang, S. H. (2015). Efficacy of pulmonary rehabilitation using cervical range of motion exercise in stroke patients with tracheostomy tubes. *Journal of Physical Therapy Science, 27*(5), 1329–1331. https://doi.org/10.1589/jpts.27.1329

Choudhry, B., Leung, B., Filips, E., & Dhaliwal, K. (2020, August 25). Keeping the traction on in orthopaedics. *Cureus, 12*(8), e10034. https://doi.org/10.7759/cureus.10034

Cleveland Clinic. (2019). *How to use crutches.* https://my.clevelandclinic.org/health/articles/15543-how-to-use-crutches

Eliopoulos, C. (2018). *Gerontological nursing* (9th ed.). Wolters Kluwer.

Enos, L. (2018). The role of ceiling lifts in a safe patient handling and mobility program. *International Journal of Safe Patient Handling and Movement, 8*(1), 25–45.

Enos, L. (2019). A comprehensive review of patient slings. *International Journal of Safe Patient Handling and Movement, 9*(1), 15–36.

Etxebarría-Foronda, I., & Caeiro-Rey, J. R. (2018). The usefulness of preoperative traction in hip fracture. *Journal of Osteoporosis & Mineral Metabolism, 10*(2), 98–102. https://doi.org/10.4321/S1889-836X2018000200007

Fragala, G., Boynton, T., Conti, M. T., Cyr, L., Enos, L., Kelly, D., McGann, N., Mullen, K., Salsbury, S., & Vollman, K. (2016). Patient-handling injuries: Risk factors and risk-reduction strategies. *American Nurse Today, 11*(5), 40–44.

Francis, R. (2020). What's new in SPHM. ANA's revised safe patient handling and mobility standards are coming soon. *American Nurse Journal, 15*(5), 66–70.

Francis, R., & Dawson, J. M. (2016). Special report: Preventing patient-handling injuries in nurses. *American Nurse Today, 11*(5), 37–38.

Georgiades, D. S. (2018). A systematic integrative review of pin site crusts. *Orthopaedic Nursing, 37*(1), 36–42. https://doi.org/10.1097/NOR.0000000000000416

Gillespie, T., & Lane, S. (2018). Moving the bariatric patient. *Critical Care Nursing Quarterly, 41*(3), 297–301. https://doi.org/10.1097/CNQ.0000000000000209

Hickey, J. V., & Strayer, A. L. (2020). *The clinical practice of neurological and neurosurgical nursing* (8th ed.). Wolters Kluwer.

Hinkle, J. L., Cheever, K. H., & Overbaugh, K. J. (2022). *Brunner & Suddarths's textbook of medical-surgical nursing* (15th ed.). Wolters Kluwer.

Jarvis, C., & Echkardt, A. (2020). *Physical examination & health assessment* (8th ed.). Elsevier.

Jensen, S. (2019). *Nursing health assessment: A best practice approach* (3rd ed.). Wolters Kluwer.

Jootun, D., & Pryde, A. (2013). Moving and handling of patients with dementia. *Journal of Nursing Education and Practice, 3*(2), 126–131. https://doi.org/https://doi.org/10.5430/jnep.v3n2p126

Kazmers, N. H., Fragomen, A. T., & Rozbrunch, S. R. (2016). Prevention of pin site infection in external fixation: A review of the literature. *Strategies in Trauma and Limb Reconstruction, 11*(2), 75–85. https://doi.org/10.1007/s11751-016-0256-4

Ktistakis, I., Guerado, E., & Giannoudis, P. V. (2015). Pin-site care: Can we reduce the incidence of infections? *Injury, 46*(Suppl 3), S35–S39. https://doi.org/10.1016/S0020-1383(15)30009-7

Kyle, T., & Carman, S. (2021). *Essentials of pediatric nursing* (4th ed.). Wolters Kluwer.

Lagerquist, D., Dabrowski, M., Dock, C., Fox, A., Daymond, M., Sandau, K. E., & Halm, M. (2012). Care of external fixator pin sites. *American Journal of Critical Care, 21*(4), 288–292. https://doi.org/10.4037/ajcc2012600

Lethaby, A., Temple, J., & Santy-Tomlinson, J. (2013). Pin site care for preventing infections associated with external bone fixators and pins. *The Cochrane Database of Systematic Reviews, 3*(12), CD004551. https://doi.org/10.1002/14651858.CD004551.pub3

Liu, B., Moore, J. E., Almaawiy, U., Chan, W. H., Khan, S., Ewusie, J., Hamid, J. S., Straus, S. E., & MOVE ON Collaboration. (2018). Outcomes of Mobilisation of Vulnerable Alders in Ontario (MOVE ON): A multisite interrupted time series evaluation of an implementation intervention to increase patient mobilisation. *Age and Ageing, 47*(1), 112–119. https://doi.org/10.1093/ageing/afx128

Mayo Foundation for Medical Education and Research (MFMER). (2019a, August 21). *Healthy lifestyle. Walker tips.* https://www.mayoclinic.org/healthy-lifestyle/healthy-aging/multimedia/walker/sls-20076469

Mayo Foundation for Medical Education and Research (MFMER). (2019b, August 21). *Healthy lifestyle. Cane tips.* https://www.mayoclinic.org/healthy-lifestyle/healthy-aging/multimedia/canes/sls-20077060

Mayo Foundation for Medical Education and Research (MFMER). (2020, April 21). *Cast care: Do's and don'ts.* https://www.mayoclinic.org/healthy-lifestyle/childrens-health/in-depth/cast-care/art-20047159

Mokhtari, R., Adib-Hajbaghery, M., & Rezaei, M. (2020). The effects of cast-related training for nurses on the quality of cast care: A quasi-experimental study. *International Journal of Orthopaedic and Trauma Nursing, 38*, 100768. https://doi.org/10.1016/j.ijotn.2020.100768

Monaghan, H. M. (2018). The role of mobile floor-based lifts in a safe patient handling and mobility program. *International Journal of Safe Patient Handling & Mobility (SPHM), 8*(2), 91–99.

Morton, P. G., & Fontaine, D. K. (2018). *Critical care nursing: A holistic approach* (11th ed.). Wolters Kluwer.

Muir, M., & Archer-Heese, G. (2009). Essentials of a bariatric patient handling program. *The Online Journal of Issues in Nursing, 14*(1), Manuscript 5. https://doi.org/10.3912/OJIN.Vol14No1Man05

Muñoz-Figueroa, G. P., & Ojo, O. (2015). Venous thromboembolism: Use of graduated compression stockings. *British Journal of Nursing, 24*(13), 680, 682–685. https://doi.org/10.12968/bjon.2015.24.13.680

Nack, B., Combs, J., & Herron-Foster, B. J. (2019). An interdisciplinary approach: Answering the how, when, and where of early mobility technology. *International Journal of Safe Patient Handling & Mobility (SPHM), 9*(2), 57–67.

National Institute for Health and Care Excellence (NICE) (UK). (2019). *Venous thromboembolism in over 16s: Reducing the risk of hospital-acquired deep vein thrombosis or pulmonary embolism.* NICE Guideline. https://www.nice.org.uk/guidance/ng89

National Institute for Occupational Safety and Health (NIOSH). (2013, August 2). *Safe patient handling and movement (SPHM).* Centers for Disease Control and Prevention. https://www.cdc.gov/niosh/topics/safepatient/default.html

Occupational Safety & Health Administration (OSHA) and Joint Commission. (2017). OSHA & worker safety. Handling with care. Practicing safe patient handling. Environment of Care News. https://www.jcrinc.com/-/media/jcr/jcr-documents/about-jcr/osha-alliance/pages_from_ecn_20_2017_08-2.pdf?db=web&hash=E471E08D9AC494C0D2C740FD4103DACD

Peterson, M. J., Kahn, J. A., Kerrigan, M. V., Gutmann, J. M., & Harrow, J. J. (2015). Pressure ulcer risk of patient handling sling use. *Journal of Rehabilitation Research & Development, 52*(3), 291–300. https://doi.org/10.1682/JRRD.2014.06.0140

Rabe, E., Partsch, H., Morrison, N., Meissner, M. H., Mosti, G., Lattimer, C. R., Carpentier, P. H., Gaillard, S., Jünger, M., Urbanek, T., Hafner, J., Patel, M., Wu, S., Caprini, J., Lurie, F., & Hirsch, T. (2020). Risks and contraindications of medical compression treatment– A critical reappraisal. An international consensus statement. *Phlebology, 35*(7), 447–460. https://doi.org/10.1177/0268355520909066

Rex, C. (2018). Continuous passive motion therapy after total knee arthroplasty. *Nursing, 48*(5), 55–57.

Sabeh, K., Aiyer, A., Summers, S., & Hennrikus, W. (2020). Cast application techniques for common pediatric injuries: A review. *Current Orthopaedic Practice, 31*(3), 277–287. https://doi.org/10.1097/BCO.0000000000000859

Sachdeva, A., Dalton, M., & Lees, T. (2018). Graduated compression stockings for prevention of deep vein thrombosis. *Cochrane Database of Systematic Reviews, 11*(11), CD001484. https://doi.org/10.1002/14651858.CD001484.pub4

Sáenz-Jalón, M., Sarabia-Cobo, C. M., Bartolome, E. R., Fernández, M. S., Vélez, B., Escudero, M., Miguel, M. E., Artabe, P., Cabañas, I., Fernández, A., Garcés, C., & Couceiro, J. (2020). A randomized clinical trial on the use of antiseptic solutions for the pin-site care of external fixators: Chlorhexidine-alcohol versus povidone-iodine. *Journal of Trauma Nursing, 27*(3), 146–150. https://doi.org/10.1097/JTN.0000000000000503

Silbert-Flagg, J., & Pillitteri, A. (2018). *Maternal and child health nursing* (8th ed.). Wolters Kluwer.

Smith, S. R., Gibbs, R. L., Rosen, B. S., & Lee, J. T. (2015). The critical lift zone: Recognizing the need for safe patient handling equipment across the broader spectrum of patient weights. *International Journal of Safe Patient Handling & Mobility, 5*(3), 108–116.

Spruce, L. (2020). Safe patient handling and movement. *AORN Journal, 112*(1), 63–71. http://doi.org/10.1002/aorn.13094

Tasheva, P., Vollenweider, P., Kraege, V., Roulet, G., Lamy, O., Marques-Vidal, P., & Méan, M. (2020).

Association between physical activity levels in the hospital setting and hospital-acquired functional decline in elderly patients. *JAMA Network Open, 3*(1), e1920185. https://doi.org/10.1001/jamanetworkopen.2019.20185

Taylor, C., Lynn, P., & Bartlett, J. (2023). *Fundamentals of nursing: The art and science of person-centered care* (10th ed.). Wolters Kluwer.

Timms, A., & Pugh, H. (2012). Pin site care: Guidance and key recommendations. *Nursing Standard, 27*(1), 50–55; quiz 56. https://doi.org/10.7748/ns2012.09.27.1.50.c9271

Toughy, T. A., & Jett, K. (2018). *Ebersol and Hess' gerontological nursing & healthy aging* (5th ed.). Elsevier.

UNC Tar Heel Trauma. (2018). Special needs are seats and adaptive restraints. University of North Carolina Health Care. https://tarheeltrauma.org/child-injury-prevention/special-needs-seats/

U. S. Department of Veteran Affairs. (2016, December 21). Public health. Safe patient handling and mobility (SPHM). https://www.publichealth.va.gov/employeehealth/patient-handling/index.asp

U.S. National Library of Medicine, MedlinePlus. (2020, November 23). *How to make a sling.* https://medlineplus.gov/ency/article/000017.htm

VA Mobile Health. (n.d.). *Safe patient handling.* (Version 1.3.3). [Mobile app]. U. S. Department of Veteran Affairs. https://mobile.va.gov/app/safe-patient-handling

VHA Center for Engineering & Occupational Safety and Health (CEOSH). (2015). *Bariatric safe patient handling and mobility guidebook: A resource guide for care of persons of size.* https://www.asphp.org/wp-content/uploads/2011/05/Baraiatrice-SPHM-guidebook-care-of-Person-of-Size.pdf

VHA Center for Engineering & Occupational Safety and Health (CEOSH). (2016). *Safe patient handling and mobility guidebook.* http://www.tnpatientsafety.com/pubfiles/Initiatives/workplace-violence/sphm-pdf.pdf

Walker, J. A., Scammell, B. E., & Bayston, R. (2018). A web-based survey to identify current practice in skeletal pin site management. *International Wound Journal, 15*(2), 250–257. https://doi.org/10.1111/iwj.12858

Warees, W. M., Clayton, L. & Slane, M. (2020, August 28). Crutches. StatPearls. National Center for Biotechnology Information. https://www.ncbi.nlm.nih.gov/books/NBK539724/

Weber, J. R., & Kelley, J. H. (2018). *Health assessment in nursing* (6th ed.). Wolters Kluwer.

Wilson, K., Devito, D., Zavotsky, K. E., Rusay, M., Allen, M., & Huang, S. (2018). Keep it moving and remember to P.A.C. (pharmacology, ambulation, and compression) for venous thromboembolism prevention. *Orthopaedic Nursing, 37*(6), 339–345. https://doi.org/10.1097/NOR.0000000000000497

Wintersgill, W. (2019). Gait belts 101: A tool for patient and nurse safety. *American Nurse Today, 14*(5), 31–34.

Wirries, N., Ezechieli, M., Stimpel, K., & Skutek, M. (2020). Impact of continuous passive motion on rehabilitation following total knee arthroplasty. *Physiotherapy Research International, 25*(4), e1869. https://doi.org/10.1002/pri.1869

Yang, X., Li, G. H., Wang, H. J., & Wang, C. Y. (2019). Continuous passive motion after total knee arthroplasty: A systematic review and meta-analysis of associated effects on clinical outcomes. *Archives of Physical Medicine & Rehabilitation, 100*(9), 1763–1778. https://doi.org/10.1016/j.apmr.2019.02.001

SUGGESTED ANSWERS FOR FOCUSING ON PATIENT CARE: DEVELOPING CLINICAL REASONING AND CLINICAL JUDGMENT

1. Teaching that should be included for Bobby and his parents related to his injury and his plaster cast includes the following: keeping the extremity elevated to reduce edema; handling the cast with the palm of the hands for the first 24 to 36 hours; keeping the cast uncovered until fully dry; reporting pain, odor, drainage, changes in sensation, abnormal sensation, or the inability to move his fingers; and avoiding putting anything in the cast.

2. Reassure the patient, Esther Levitz, that the device will not hurt. Explain how the pneumatic compression device works and the rationale for its use. In addition, describe potential adverse symptoms, such as pain or discomfort in the legs and changes in sensation that the patient should report while the pneumatic compression device is in use.

3. Additional assessments that should be performed as part of Mr. Esposito's care include the following: assessing the traction equipment to ensure proper function, including inspecting the ropes for fraying and proper positioning; assessing the patient's body alignment; performing skin and neurovascular assessments; assessing pin sites; performing a pain assessment; assessing for complications of immobility, including alterations in respiratory function, skin integrity, urinary and bowel elimination, and muscle weakness, contractures, thrombophlebitis, pulmonary embolism, and fatigue.

10

Comfort and Pain Management

Focusing on Patient Care

This chapter will help you develop some of the skills related to comfort and pain management that may be necessary to care for the following patients:

Mildred Simpson, is a 75-year-old woman recovering from a total hip replacement.

Joseph Watkins, age 45, comes to the emergency department because of acute pain in his lower back that started when he was moving furniture.

Jerome Batiste, age 60, has been diagnosed with bone cancer and is being discharged with an order for patient-controlled analgesia (PCA) at home.

Refer to Focusing on Patient Care: Developing Clinical Reasoning and Clinical Judgment at the end of the chapter to apply what you learn.

Learning Outcomes

After completing the chapter, you will be able to accomplish the following:

1. Promote patient comfort.
2. Give a back massage.
3. Apply and care for a patient using a transcutaneous electrical nerve stimulation (TENS) unit.
4. Care for a patient receiving PCA.
5. Care for a patient receiving epidural analgesia.
6. Care for a patient receiving continuous wound perfusion pain management.

Nursing Concepts

- Assessment
- Clinical decision making/clinical judgment
- Comfort
- Safety
- Teaching and learning/patient education

Comfort is an important need and ensuring a patient's comfort is a major nursing responsibility. Providing comfort can be as simple as straightening the patient's bed linens, offering to hold the patient's hand, or assisting with hygiene needs. Often, providing comfort includes providing pain relief. The classic definition of pain that is probably of greatest benefit to nurses and patients is that offered by McCaffery (1968): "Pain is whatever the experiencing person says it is, existing whenever the experiencing person says it does" (p. 95). This definition rests on the belief that the only one who can be a real authority on whether, and how, a person is experiencing pain is that person; pain is the individual experience and description of a sensation or feeling (Sonneborn & Williams, 2020). The International Association for the Study of Pain (IASP) further defines pain as "an unpleasant sensory and emotional experience associated with, or resembling that associated with, actual or potential tissue damage" (IASP, 2020, para. 3). Additional key factors that define pain include (IASP, 2020):

- Pain is always a personal experience, influenced by biological, psychological, and social factors.
- Individuals learn the concept of pain through life experiences.
- A person's report of an experience as pain should be respected.
- Pain may have adverse effects on function and social and psychological well-being.
- Verbal description is only one of several behaviors to express pain; inability to communicate does not negate the possibility that a person experiences pain.

Differences in individual pain perception and response to pain, as well as the multiple and diverse causes of pain, require the use of accurate knowledge and appropriate interventions to promote comfort and relieve pain. The most important of these are the nurse's belief that the patient's pain is real, a willingness to become involved in the patient's pain experience, and competence in collaborating to develop effective pain management regimens. It is important for nurses to understand the pathophysiology of pain and of the crucial role pain assessment plays in pain management (IASP, 2020; Sonneborn & Williams, 2020).

Assessment of pain is an integral part of providing nursing care, including individualized pain assessment, treatment, and management. Fundamentals Review 10-1 outlines factors to include in a pain assessment. Because pain is subjective, self-report is generally considered the most reliable way to assess pain and the nurse should use this method whenever possible; however as noted above, a verbal description is only one of several behaviors to express pain (IASP, 2020; Sonneborn & Williams, 2020). Pasero and McCaffery (2011) identified, additional methods to assess a person's pain that are still relevant today and include the following: identification of pathologic conditions or procedures that may be causing pain; take into account the report of a family member/caregiver, another person close to the patient, or caregiver who is familiar with the patient; the nonverbal behaviors that may indicate the presence of pain (restlessness, grimacing, crying, clenching fists, protecting the painful area); and physiologic measures (increased blood pressure and pulse), although most research verifies that **reliance on vital signs to indicate the presence of pain should be minimized** (Herr et al., 2019). The absence of an increase in vital signs does not mean that pain is not present. Infants, young children, patients who are nonverbal or have difficulty communicating verbally, and cognitively impaired adults, such as those with dementia, are at high risk for underassessment and undertreatment/overtreatment of pain (Herr et al., 2019).

Use of a pain guide and a pain scale should be part of the initial and continued assessment of pain and evaluation of pain control measures. Choosing an appropriate tool for patient assessment is necessary to obtain an accurate assessment and valid pain ratings. Fundamentals Review 10-2 is one example of a pain assessment tool. Pain assessment guides and pain scales eliminate guesswork and biases when dealing with the patient's pain; help the nurse appreciate what the person is experiencing; analyze findings that will help prepare an appropriate nursing response to the patient's pain; and facilitate improved outcomes (Taylor et al., 2023). Alternative approaches to pain assessment for special populations ensure that unacceptable levels of pain are addressed and treated. For example, a nurse caring for a patient in an intensive care unit would use a valid and reliable pain assessment tool that considers the unresponsive and/or noncommunicative nature of the patient. Fundamentals Review 10-3 provides a listing of pain assessment scales that can be used in adults and children who can self-report, as well as scales that can be used to assess pain in adults and children who cannot self-report discomfort and pain. Fundamentals Review 10-4 is an example of a scale that can be used to assess discomfort and pain in patients who are unable to self-report. A comprehensive pain assessment must also include discussion of the patient's expectations for pain relief. The patient and health care team need to set mutually agreed upon goals that are acceptable and satisfactory, and that facilitate recovery. For example, it may not be possible to have a pain rating of zero after a surgical procedure when the movement required to prevent complications naturally causes some pain or discomfort. Having this conversation and setting a realistic, mutually agreed upon goal facilitates the patient's recognition and report of pain that is unacceptable. Setting pain management goals also provides the nurse the opportunity to establish rapport, discuss individualized pain management interventions, and evaluate the plan with the patient and caregivers (Taylor et al., 2023).

This chapter covers skills to assist the nurse in providing for patient comfort, including pain relief. Refer to *Fundamentals of Nursing* (Taylor et al., 2023) textbook for further, in-depth discussions of the physiology, assessment, and treatment of pain.

Fundamentals Review 10-1

GENERAL GUIDELINES FOR PAIN ASSESSMENT

Factors to Assess	Questions and Approaches
Characteristics of the pain	
Location	*Where is your pain? Is it external or internal? Generalized, localized, radiation?*
	Asking the patient with **acute pain** to point to the painful area with one finger may help to localize the pain. Patients with chronic pain may have difficulty trying to localize their pain.
Duration/ Chronology	*Onset of the pain? Pain episode last? How often does a pain episode occur? How does the pain develop and progress? Has the pain changed since it first began? If so, how?*
Intensity/Severity	Ask the patient to indicate the severity of pain currently experienced using a scale. One example of a scale appears below.
	Note that it is important to give patients *zero/no pain* as an option.
	0 1 2 3 4 5 6 7 8 9 10
	No pain Mild Moderate Severe Pain as bad as it can be
	It is also helpful to ask how much pain the patient has (on the same scale) when the pain is at its least and at its worst:
	Least_____ Worst_____
Quality and character	*What words would you use to describe your pain?*
Aggravating or causal factors	*What makes the pain occur or increase in intensity? What makes it worse?*
Alleviating or relieving factors	*What makes the pain go away or lessen? What makes it better? What methods of relief have you tried in the past? How long were they used? How effective were they?*
	Pharmacologic and **nonpharmacologic** methods of relief currently in effect for hospitalized patients should be apparent from the chart. It is important to verify the use of current prescriptions and their effectiveness with the patient. Outpatients may need to be asked to record a medication profile, a thorough and accurate account of all medications they are taking.
Contributing or related factors	*Are there any other factors that seem to relate consistently to your pain? Any other symptoms that occur just before the pain begins?*
Physiologic responses Vital signs (blood pressure, pulse, respirations)[a] Skin color Perspiration	Signs of sympathetic stimulation can occur with acute pain but need not be present to verify the presence of pain. Signs of parasympathetic stimulation (decreased blood pressure and pulse, rapid and regular respirations, pupil constriction, nausea and vomiting, and warm, dry skin) may occur, especially with prolonged, severe pain, visceral, or deep pain.

Fundamentals Review 10-1   continued

GENERAL GUIDELINES FOR PAIN ASSESSMENT

Factors to Assess	Questions and Approaches
Pupil size	
Nausea	
Muscle tension	Observe. Ask the patient whether they are aware of any tight, tense muscles.
Anxiety	Are signs of anxiety evident? May include decreased attention span or ability to follow directions, frequent asking of questions, shifting topics of conversation, avoiding discussion of feelings, acting out, somatizing.
Behavioral responses	
Posture, gross motor activities	Does patient rub or support a particular area? Make frequent position changes? Walk, pace, kneel, or assume a rolled-up position? Does patient rest a particular body part? Protect an area from stimulation? Lie quietly? In acute pain, postural and gross motor activities are often altered; in **chronic pain**, the only signs of change may be postures characteristic of withdrawal.
Facial features	Does the patient have a pinched look? Are there facial grimaces? Knotted brow? Overall taut, anxious appearance? A look of fatigue is more characteristic of chronic pain.
Verbal expressions	Does the patient sigh, moan, scream, cry, or repetitively use the same words?
Affective responses	
Anxiety	*Do you feel anxious? Are you afraid? If so, how bad are these feelings?*
Depression	*Do you feel depressed, down, or low? If so, how bad are these feelings? Are your feelings about yourself mostly good or bad? Do you have feelings of failure? Do you see yourself or your illness as a burden to those you care about?*
Interactions with others	How does the patient act when they are in pain in the presence of others? How does the patient respond to others when they are not in pain? How do significant others and caregivers respond to the patient when the patient is in pain? When the patient is not in pain?
Degree to which pain interferes with patient's life (use past performance as baseline)	*Does the pain interfere with sleep? If so, to what extent? Is fatigue a major factor in the pain experience? Is the conduct of intimate or peer relationships affected by the pain? Is work function affected? Participation in recreational–diversional activities?* An activity diary is often helpful—sometimes crucial. One to several weeks of hourly activity recorded by the patient may be necessary. Pain level, food intake, and sleep–rest periods are noted along with activities performed. Separate diaries for inpatient and outpatient episodes may be necessary because hospitalization markedly affects the nature and type of activities performed.
Perception of pain and meaning to patient	*Are you worried about your illness? Do you see any connection between your pain and the nature or course of illness? If so, how do you see them as related? Do you find any meaning in your pain? If so, is this beneficial or detrimental to you? Are you struggling to find some meaning for your pain?*
Adaptive mechanisms used to cope with pain	*What do you usually do to relieve stress? How well do these things work? What techniques do you use at home to help cope with the pain? How well have they worked? Do you use these in the hospital? If not, why not?*
Outcomes	*Pain management goals? What would you like to be doing right now, this week, this month, if the pain were better controlled? How much would the pain have to decrease (on the 0 to 10 or other scale) for you to begin to accomplish these goals? What is your pain goal (on the 0 to 10 or other scale)?* Keep in mind that a response of "NO pain" may not be an option for some patients. Helping a patient to identify a realistic goal promotes effective pain management.
Factors that may affect expression of pain	Patterned attitudes related to cultural, ethnic and/or social group; family, sex, biological sex, gender and age variables; spirituality; religious beliefs and spirituality; environment and support people; anxiety and other stressors; past pain experience

[a]Increases in vital signs may occur briefly in acute pain and may be absent in chronic pain (Pasero & McCaffery, 2011). **Reliance on vital signs to indicate the presence of pain should be minimized** (Herr et al., 2019). The absence of an increase in vital signs does not mean that pain is not present (Pasero & McCaffery, 2011).

Source: Adapted from Taylor, C., Lynn, P., & Bartlett, J. (2023). *Fundamentals of nursing: The art and science of person-centered care* (10th ed.). Wolters Kluwer.

Fundamentals Review 10-2

PAIN ASSESSMENT TOOL

Prescott, Martin	**Gender:** Male	**Diagnosis:** Diverticular disease	**Adm Provider:**
MRN: 22432	**DOB:** 8/29/1971	**Isolation Precaution:** Standard	**Facility:** General Mass
Allergies: None	**Age:** 46 Years	**Adv Directive:** Full Code	**Room:** 2
	Height: 67 in		**Adm On:** 2/21/2018 15:49 [0 day(s)]
	Weight: 175 lb		

Patient Info   Assessment   ADLs   Notes   Nursing Dx   Orders   MAR   I/O   Vital Signs   Diagnostics   OT   Flowsheet

HEENT   Neuro   Cardio   Respiratory   GI   GU   Musculoskeletal   Mental Health   Pain Scale   Integumentary   Vascular Access

Add New Site

Documented By: [▼]

Documented At: [0] days [0] hours [0] minutes [after admission   ▼]

Pain Location: [   ]

Onset: [0] days [0] hours [0] minutes [after admission   ▼]

Pain Duration: [   ]

Pain Frequency: [▼]

Type Of Pain: [▼]

Pain Goal: [▼]

[Pain Goal Comments

]

Aggravating Factors:
☐ Movement
☐ Coughing
☐ Breathing
☐ Eating

[Aggravating Factors Comments

]

Alleviating Factors:
☐ Rest
☐ Compression
☐ Medication
☐ Ice
☐ Immobility

[Alleviating Factors Comments

]

Pain Scale Used: [   ]

Pain Rating: [▼]

Pain Characteristics:
☐ Aching
☐ Throbbing
☐ Dull
☐ Stabbing
☐ Burning
☐ Piercing
☐ Sore
☐ Crushing
☐ Radiating

Notes:
[

]

Fundamentals Review 10-3

PAIN ASSESSMENT SCALES

Resource	Website	Indications
COMFORT Scale	https://www.verywell.com/pain-scales-assessment-tools-4020329	Infants, children, adults who are unable to use Numerical Rating Pain Scale or Wong-Baker Faces Pain Rating Scale
CRIES Pain Scale	https://www.verywell.com/pain-scales-assessment-tools-4020329	Neonates (0 to 6 months)
FLACC Scale	https://www.verywell.com/pain-scales-assessment-tools-4020329	Infants and children (2 months to 7 years) who are unable to validate the presence of or quantify the severity of pain
FPS-R (Faces Pain Scale, Revised)	https://www.iasp-pain.org/Education/Content.aspx?ItemNumber=1519&navItemNumber=577	Young children in parallel with numerical self-rating scales (0 to 10). Patients choose the depiction of a facial expression that best corresponds with their pain
PAINAD Scale	https://hign.org/sites/default/files/2020-06/Try_This_Dementia_2.pdf	Patients whose dementia is so advanced that they cannot verbally communicate
Payen Behavioral Pain Scale	https://www.mdcalc.com/behavioral-pain-scale-bps-pain-assessment-intubated-patients	Can be used with intubated, critically ill patients; measures bodily indicators of pain and tolerance of intubation
Wong-Baker Faces Pain Rating Scale	https://www.verywell.com/pain-scales-assessment-tools-4020329	Adults and children (>3 years) in all patient care settings
0–10 Numerical Rating Pain Scale	https://www.verywell.com/pain-scales-assessment-tools-4020329	Adults and children (>9 years) in all patient care settings who are able to use numbers to rate the intensity of their pain

Fundamentals Review 10-4

FLACC BEHAVIORAL SCALE

This display presents two ways of demonstrating the FLACC Behavioral Scale.

Categories	Scoring		
	0	**1**	**2**
Face	No particular expression or smile	Occasional grimace or frown, withdrawn, disinterested	Frequent to constant frown, clenched jaw, quivering chin
Legs	Normal position or relaxed	Uneasy, restless, tense	Kicking, or legs drawn up
Activity	Lying quietly, normal position, moves easily	Squirming, shifting back and forth, tense	Arched, rigid, or jerking
Cry	No cry (awake or asleep)	Moans or whimpers, occasional complaint	Crying steadily, screams or sobs, frequent complaints
Consolability	Content, relaxed	Reassured by occasional touching, hugging, or being talked to, distractible	Difficult to console or comfort

Each of the five categories (**F**) Face; (**L**) Legs; (**A**) Activity; (**C**) Cry; (**C**) Consolability is scored from 0 to 2, which results in a total score between 0 and 10.

Patients who are awake: Observe for at least 1 to 2 minutes. Observe legs and body uncovered. Reposition the patient or observe activity; assess body for tenseness and tone. Initiate consoling interventions, if needed.

Patients who are asleep: Observe for at least 2 minutes or longer. Observe body and legs uncovered. If possible, reposition the patient. Touch the body and assess for tenseness and tone.

Face

Score 0 points if patient has a relaxed face, eye contact, and interest in surroundings.

Score 1 point if patient has a worried look to face, with eyebrows lowered, eyes partially closed, cheeks raised, mouth pursed.

Score 2 points if patient has deep furrows in forehead, with closed eyes, open mouth, and deep lines around the nose/lips.

Legs

Score 0 points if patient has usual tone and motion to limbs (legs and arms).

Score 1 point if patient has increased tone; rigidity; tense, intermittent flexion/extension of limbs.

Score 2 points if patient has hypertonicity, legs pulled tight, exaggerated flexion/extension of limbs, tremors.

Activity

Score 0 points if patient moves easily and freely, with normal activity/restrictions.

Score 1 point if patient shifts positions, is hesitant to move or is guarding, has tense torso, pressure on body part.

Score 2 points if patient is in fixed position, rocking, has side-to-side head movements, is rubbing body part.

Cry

Score 0 points if patient has no cry/moan (awake or asleep).

Score 1 point if patient has occasional moans, cries, whimpers, sighs.

Score 2 points if patient has frequent/continuous moans, cries, grunts.

Consolability

Score 0 points if patient is calm and does not require consoling.

Score 1 point if patient responds to comfort by touch or talk in 30 seconds to a minute.

Score 2 points if patient requires constant consoling or is unable to be consoled after an extended time.

Whenever feasible, behavioral measurement of pain should be used in conjunction with self-report. When self-report is not possible, interpretation of pain behaviors and decision making regarding treatment of pain requires careful consideration of the context in which pain behaviors were observed.

Each category is scored on the 0 to 2 scale, which results in a total score of 0 to 10.

Assessment of Behavioral Scale

0 = Relaxed and comfortable

1–3 = Mild discomfort

4–6 = Moderate pain

7–10 = Severe discomfort/pain

Source: Printed with permission. © 2002, *The Regents of the University of Michigan.* All rights reserved.

Skill 10-1 ▶ Promoting Patient Comfort

The nurse can promote increased comfort and relieve patient discomfort and pain through various interventions and therapies. Interventions can include comfort measures, emotional support, nonpharmacologic interventions, and the administration of analgesics and/or other medications to remove or alter the intensity of painful stimuli. Nonpharmacologic methods of comfort and pain management can diminish the emotional components of pain, strengthen coping abilities, give patients a sense of control, contribute to pain relief, decrease fatigue, and promote sleep (Bauldoff et al., 2020; Georga et al., 2019; Kiley et al., 2018; Labus et al., 2019). The Joint Commission (2018) supports the use of nonpharmacologic and nonopioid interventions for pain management, identifying that the use of nonopioid treatment options may be helpful in eliminating or reducing the need for/use of opioid analgesics. Refer as well to the Evidence for Practice display at the end of this skill.

The following skill identifies potential interventions to address discomfort and pain. The interventions are listed sequentially for teaching purposes; the order is not sequential and should be adjusted based on patient assessment and nursing judgment. Not every intervention discussed will be appropriate for every patient. Additional interventions for discomfort and pain are discussed in other chapters. Refer to Chapter 5 for nursing skills related to administering medications for pain relief. The application of heat or cold therapy is discussed in Chapter 8. Chapter 9 provides details related to patient positioning to promote patient comfort.

DELEGATION CONSIDERATIONS	The assessment of a patient's pain is not delegated to assistive personnel (AP). Depending on the state's nurse practice act and the organization's policies and procedures, some or all of the parts of assessment of a patient's pain may be delegated to licensed practical/vocational nurses (LPN/LVNs). The use of nonpharmacologic interventions related to patient comfort may be delegated to AP as well as to LPN/LVNs. The decision to delegate must be based on careful analysis of the patient's needs and circumstances as well as the qualifications of the person to whom the task is being delegated. Refer to the Delegation Guidelines in Appendix A.
EQUIPMENT	• Pain assessment tool and pain scale • Oral hygiene supplies • Nonsterile gloves, if necessary • Additional PPE, as indicated • Additional supplies, depending on specific intervention utilized
ASSESSMENT	Review the patient's health record and plan of care for information about the patient's status and contraindications to any of the potential interventions. Inquire about any allergies. Assess the patient's level of discomfort. Assess the patient's pain using an appropriate assessment tool and pain scale. Assess the characteristics of any pain and for other symptoms that often occur with the pain, such as headache or restlessness. Ask the patient what interventions have and have not been successful in the past to promote comfort and relieve pain. Assess the patient's vital signs. Check the patient's medication administration record for the time an analgesic was last administered. Assess cultural beliefs and influences related to the pain experience. Assess the patient's response to a particular intervention to evaluate effectiveness and presence of adverse effects. Refer to assessment details included in Fundamentals Review 10-1, 10-2, 10-3, and 10-4.
ACTUAL OR POTENTIAL HEALTH PROBLEMS AND NEEDS	Many actual or potential health problems or issues may require the use of this skill as part of related interventions. An appropriate health problem or issue may include: • Acute pain • Chronic pain • Discomfort
OUTCOME IDENTIFICATION AND PLANNING	The expected outcome to achieve is that the patient experiences relief from discomfort and/or pain without adverse effect. Other outcomes that may be appropriate include that the patient experiences decreased anxiety and improved relaxation; is able to participate in activities of daily living (ADLs); and verbalizes an understanding of, and satisfaction with, the comfort and pain management plan.

(continued on page 642)

Skill 10-1 ▶ Promoting Patient Comfort *(continued)*

IMPLEMENTATION

ACTION	RATIONALE
1. Perform hand hygiene and put on PPE, if indicated.	Hand hygiene and PPE prevent the spread of microorganisms. PPE is required based on transmission precautions.
2. Identify the patient.	Identifying the patient ensures the right patient receives the intervention and helps prevent errors.
3. Discuss pain with the patient, acknowledging that the patient's pain exists. Discuss the patient's expectations for comfort and pain relief. Explain how interventions to address discomfort, pain management therapies, and pain medications work together to alleviate discomfort and provide pain relief. Encourage the patient to collaborate in the plan of care to address discomfort and for pain relief.	These measures promote a collaborative relationship in which the patient is treated with respect. Pain discussion and patient involvement strengthen the nurse–patient relationship and promote pain relief (Taylor et al., 2023). Explanation encourages patient understanding and engagement and reduces apprehension.
4. Assess the patient's level of comfort and pain using an appropriate assessment tool and measurement scale (see Fundamentals Review 10-1 through 10-4).	Accurate assessment is necessary to guide treatment/relief interventions and evaluate the effectiveness of pain control measures.
5. Provide pharmacologic interventions, if indicated and prescribed.	Analgesics and **adjuvant** drugs reduce perception of pain and alter responses to discomfort.
6. Adjust the patient's environment to promote comfort.	The environment can improve or detract from the patient's sense of well-being and can be a source of stimulation that aggravates pain and reduces comfort.
a. Adjust and maintain the room temperature per the patient's preference.	A too-warm or too-cool environment can be a source of stimulation that aggravates pain and reduces comfort.
b. Reduce harsh lighting but provide adequate lighting per the patient's preference.	Harsh lighting can be a source of stimulation that aggravates pain and reduces comfort.
c. Reduce harsh and unnecessary noise. Avoid having conversations immediately outside the patient's room.	Noise, including talking, can be a source of stimuli that aggravates pain and reduces comfort.
d. Close the room door and/or curtain whenever possible.	Closing the door or curtain provides privacy and reduces noise and other extraneous stimuli that may aggravate pain and reduce comfort (Aparício & Panin, 2020; Goeren et al., 2018.)
e. Provide good ventilation in the patient's room. Reduce unpleasant odors by promptly emptying bedpans, urinals, and emesis basins after use. Remove trash and laundry promptly.	Odors can be a source of stimuli that aggravate pain and reduce comfort.
7. Prevent unnecessary interruptions and coordinate patient activities to group activities together. Allow for and plan rest periods without disturbance.	Frequent interruptions and disturbances for assessment or treatment can be a source of stimuli that aggravate pain and reduce comfort. Fatigue reduces tolerance for pain and can increase the pain experience.
8. Assist the patient to change position frequently. Assist the patient to a comfortable position, maintaining good alignment and supporting extremities, as needed. Raise the head of the bed, as appropriate (see Chapter 9 for more information on positioning).	Positioning in proper alignment with supports ensures that the patient will be able to maintain the desired position and reduces pressure.
9. Provide oral hygiene as often as necessary (every 1 or 2 hours if necessary) to keep the mouth and mucous membranes clean and moist. This is especially important for patients who cannot drink or are not permitted fluids by mouth (see Chapter 7 for additional information about oral care).	Moisture helps maintain the integrity of mucous membranes. Dry mucous membranes can be a source of stimuli that aggravate pain and reduce comfort.

ACTION	RATIONALE
10. Ensure the availability of appropriate fluids for drinking, unless contraindicated. Make sure the patient's water pitcher or a water bottle is filled and within reach. Have other fluids of the patient's choice available.	Thirst and dry mucous membranes can be sources of stimuli that reduce comfort and aggravate pain.
11. Remove physical situations that might cause discomfort.	
a. Change soiled and/or wet dressings; replace soiled and/or wet bed linens.	Moisture can cause discomfort and irritation to skin.
b. Smooth wrinkles in bed linens.	Wrinkled bed linens apply pressure to skin and can cause discomfort and irritation to skin.
c. Ensure patient is not lying or sitting on tubes, tubing, wires, or other equipment.	Tubing and equipment apply pressure to skin and can cause discomfort and irritation to skin.
12. Assist the patient, as necessary, with ambulation, and active or passive range-of-motion exercises, as appropriate (see Chapter 9 for more information about activity).	Activity prevents stiffness and loss of mobility, which can reduce comfort and aggravate pain.
13. Assess the patient's spiritual needs related to the pain experience. Ask the patient if they would like a spiritual counselor to visit.	Some people's spiritual beliefs facilitate positive coping with the effects of illness, including pain (Minton et al., 2018; Taylor et al., 2023).
14. Consider the use of distraction. Distraction requires the patient to focus on something other than the discomfort and pain.	Focused attention on pain may increase the perception of pain. Preoccupation with other things has been observed to decrease the experience of discomfort and pain. Distraction requires the patient to focus attention on something other than the pain. It is not entirely clear whether distraction raises the threshold of pain or increases **pain tolerance** (Taylor et al., 2023).
a. Have the patient recall a pleasant experience or focus attention on an enjoyable experience.	
b. Offer age or developmentally appropriate games, toys, books, audiobooks, access to television, and/or videos, or other items of interest to the patient.	
c. Encourage the patient to hold or stroke a loved person, pet, or toy.	
d. Offer access to music the patient prefers. Turn on the music when pain begins, or before anticipated painful stimuli. The patient can close their eyes and concentrate on listening. Raising or lowering the volume as pain increases or decreases can be helpful.	
15. Consider the use of guided imagery.	Guided imagery incorporates mental images to enhance an overall sense of well-being and to promote relaxation, helping the patient to gradually become less aware of the discomfort or pain (Krau, 2020; Taylor et al., 2023). Positive emotions evoked by the image help reduce the pain experience and improve patient comfort (Krau, 2020).
a. Help the patient to identify a scene or experience that the patient describes as happy, pleasant, or peaceful.	
b. Encourage the patient to begin with several minutes of focused breathing, relaxation, or meditation (refer to specific information in Steps 16 and 17).	
c. Help the patient concentrate on the peaceful, pleasant image.	
d. If indicated, read a description of the identified scene or experience, using a soothing, soft voice.	
e. Encourage the patient to concentrate on the details of the image, such as its sight, sounds, smells, tastes, and touch.	

(continued on page 644)

Skill 10-1 ▶ Promoting Patient Comfort *(continued)*

ACTION	RATIONALE

ACTION

16. Consider the use of relaxation activities, such as deep breathing.

   a. Have the patient sit or recline comfortably and place their hands on their stomach. Ask them to close their eyes.

   b. Ask the patient to mentally count to maintain a comfortable rate and rhythm. Have the patient inhale slowly and deeply while letting the abdomen expand as much as possible. Have the patient hold their breath for a few seconds.

   c. Tell the patient to exhale slowly through the mouth, blowing through puckered lips. Have the patient continue to count to maintain comfortable rate and rhythm, concentrating on the rise and fall of the abdomen.

   d. When the patient's abdomen feels empty, have the patient begin again with a deep inhalation.

   e. Encourage patient to practice at least twice a day, for 10 minutes, and then use the technique, as needed, to assist with pain management.

17. Consider the use of relaxation activities, such as progressive muscle relaxation.

   a. Assist the patient to a comfortable position.

   b. Direct the patient to focus on a particular muscle group. Start with the muscles of the jaw, then repeat with the muscles of the neck, shoulder, upper and lower arm, hand, abdomen, buttocks, thigh, lower leg, and foot.

   c. Ask the patient to tighten the muscle group and note the sensation that the tightened muscles produce. After 5 to 7 seconds, tell the patient to relax the muscles all at once and concentrate on the sensation of the relaxed state, noting the difference in feeling in the muscles when contracted and relaxed.

   d. Have the patient continue to tighten-hold-relax each muscle group until the entire body has been covered.

   e. Encourage the patient to practice at least twice a day, for 10 minutes, and then use the technique, as needed, to assist with pain management.

18. Consider the use of cutaneous stimulation, such as the intermittent application of heat or cold, or both (see Chapter 8 for additional information on heat and cold therapy).

RATIONALE

Relaxation techniques reduce skeletal muscle tension and lessen anxiety, both of which can reduce comfort and aggravate pain. Relaxation can also be a distraction, providing help in reducing the pain experience (Helming et al., 2021; Taylor et al., 2023; Ward, 2016).

Relaxation techniques reduce skeletal muscle tension and lessen anxiety, both of which can reduce comfort and aggravate pain. Relaxation can also be a distraction, providing help in reducing the pain experience (Hasanpour-Dehkordi et al., 2019; Taylor et al., 2023; Ward, 2016).

Heat helps relieve pain by stimulating specific nerve fibers, closing the gate that allows the transmission of pain stimuli to centers in the brain. Heat accelerates the inflammatory response to promote healing and reduces muscle tension to promote relaxation and help to relieve muscle spasms and joint stiffness. Cold reduces blood flow to tissues and decreases the local release of pain-producing substances, such as histamine, serotonin, and bradykinin, and reduces the formation of edema and inflammation.

Cold reduces muscle spasm, alters tissue sensitivity (producing numbness), and promotes comfort by slowing the transmission of pain stimuli (Taylor et al., 2023).

ACTION	RATIONALE
19. Consider the use of cutaneous stimulation, such as massage (see Skill 10-2).	Cutaneous stimulation techniques stimulate the skin's surface, closing the gating mechanism in the spinal cord, decreasing the number of pain impulses that reach the brain for perception. Massage has been suggested as having positive effects on patient outcomes, including promotion of sleep, fatigue (Ahmadidarrehsima et al., 2018), and reduction of anxiety (Ayik & Özden, 2018; Hsu et al., 2019; Jagan et al., 2019; Kudo & Sasaki, 2020).
20. Discuss consideration of consultation with a nurse trained in healing touch (HT)/therapeutic touch (TT) with the patient.	HT and TT are complementary health approaches that have proved valuable as an adjunct to traditional health interventions (Taylor et al., 2023). Studies have indicated that HT and TT are effective in reducing pain and anxiety and promoting patient comfort and health (Bagci & Yucel, 2020; Davis et al., 2020; Weaver, 2017). TT has been suggested as a means to address comfort during end-of-life care (Tabatabaee et al., 2016).
21. Discuss the potential for use of cutaneous stimulation, such as transcutaneous electrical nerve stimulation (TENS) or electrical muscle stimulation (EMS, ESTIM, E-Stim) with the patient and the health care team (see Skill 10-3).	Cutaneous stimulation techniques stimulate the skin's surface, closing the gating mechanism in the spinal cord, decreasing the number of pain impulses that reach the brain for perception.
22. Discuss the potential for use of other complementary health approaches (CHA) and integrative health care IH) interventions, such as aromatherapy, humor, mindfulness, acupuncture and dry needling, hypnosis, biofeedback, or animal-assisted activities (AAA) and animal-assisted intervention (AAI), with the patient and the health care team.	CHA and IH can be practiced in all health care settings a part of a holistic pain management strategy (Ayik & Özden, 2018; Jaruzel et al., 2019; Sandvik et al., 2020; Taylor et al., 2023).
23. Remove equipment and return patient to a position of comfort. Remove gloves, if used. Perform hand hygiene. Raise the side rail and lower the bed.	Equipment removal and repositioning promote patient comfort. Removing gloves properly and hand hygiene reduce the risk for infection transmission and contamination of other items. Lowering the bed promotes patient safety.
24. Remove additional PPE, if used. Perform hand hygiene.	Proper removal of PPE reduces the risk for infection transmission and contamination of other items. Hand hygiene prevents transmission of microorganisms.
25. Evaluate the patient's response to interventions. Reassess level of discomfort or pain using original assessment tools. Reassess and alter care plan, as appropriate.	Evaluation allows for individualization of plan of care and promotes optimal patient comfort.

EVALUATION

The expected outcomes have been met when the patient experiences relief from discomfort and/or pain without adverse effect; experiences decreased anxiety and improved relaxation; is able to participate in activities of daily living (ADLs); and verbalizes an understanding of, and satisfaction with, the comfort and pain management plan.

DOCUMENTATION

Guidelines

Document pain assessment and other significant assessments. Document comfort and pain relief therapies used and patient responses. Record CHA and IH interventions to consider, if appropriate. Document reassessment of comfort and pain after interventions, at an appropriate interval, based on specific interventions used.

(continued on page 646)

Skill 10-1 ▶ Promoting Patient Comfort *(continued)*

Sample Documentation

> <u>5/12/25</u> 2030 Patient reports increased pain in lower extremities, rating the pain at 5/10, and described it as burning and constant, consistent with previous pain. Medicated with oxycodone 5 mg PO, as ordered for breakthrough pain. Patient using relaxation and deep-breathing techniques, as well as listening to music. Reviewed instructions for use of relaxation and deep breathing; patient verbalized understanding.
> —*R. Curry, RN*
>
> <u>5/12/25</u> 2145 Patient reports pain reduced to 2/10. OOB to solarium with family.
> —*R. Curry, RN*

DEVELOPING CLINICAL REASONING AND CLINICAL JUDGMENT

UNEXPECTED SITUATIONS AND ASSOCIATED INTERVENTIONS

- *Patient reports or assessment reveals, ineffective/or lack of pain relief:* Reassess pain and evaluate response to implemented therapies. Implement additional or alternate interventions until desired level of comfort is achieved.
- *Intervention increases patient discomfort or pain:* Immediately stop intervention. Document intervention used and the effect. Communicate changes in the patient's condition to the health care team, as appropriate. Revise plan of care, noting adverse effect of intervention, so other caregivers avoid using same intervention.

SPECIAL CONSIDERATIONS

General Considerations

- The use of complementary, integrative, and adjunct therapies is often a "try-and-see" process. Many interventions can be tried to achieve the best combination for a particular patient. People respond to pain differently; what works for one person may not help another.

Infant and Child Considerations

- Assessment, measurement, and treatment of discomfort and pain in infants and children frequently involve the use of more than one technique. Pain scales have been developed for various pediatric populations (Wrona & Czarnecki, 2021). Communication and collaboration with parents, guardians, caregivers, or other people important to the patient is vital for accurate pediatric pain assessment and management (Kyle & Carman, 2021; Taylor et al., 2023).
- Nonpharmacologic therapies can be very beneficial in decreasing acute and chronic pain, as well as pain related to procedures in infants and children (Kyle & Carman, 2021) and should be tailored to the developmental level of the child and their individual needs (Wrona & Czarnecki, 2021).
- Age-appropriate nonpharmacological pain management interventions include:
  - Infants: breastfeeding, oral sucrose, non-nutritive sucking, swaddling (Ceylan & Bolışık, 2018) and rocking the infant back and forth (swaying) (Wrona & Czarnecki, 2021)
  - Toddlers: bubbles, toys, books, secure hugging by a parent (comfort hold) (Wrona & Czarnecki, 2021)
  - School-age children: secure hugging by a parent during procedures (comfort hold), video games, toys, books, bubbles (Wrona & Czarnecki, 2021)

Older Adult Considerations

- In addition to medical problems, poor positioning or posture, inactivity, emotional issues, and adverse drug reactions could be at the root of new or worsened pain. Improving these underlying factors is the first step in pain management (Eliopoulos, 2018, p. 170).
- Pain negatively impacts on the emotional well-being, functional ability, sleep, coping, and resources of older adults. Although pain is not a normal part of aging, pain occurs secondary to many chronic illnesses that are present in older adults (Taylor et al., 2023).
- Assessment of pain in the older adult can be problematic. Vision or hearing impairments may influence the assessment format. Multiple-drug regimens that are common in older people can also affect reliable reporting of pain. Many older adults view pain as a forecast of serious illness or death, thus are reluctant to admit its occurrence or report it. Boredom, loneliness, and depression may affect an older adult's perception and report of pain (Taylor et al., 2023).

EVIDENCE FOR PRACTICE ▶

NONPHARMACOLOGICAL THERAPIES AND PATIENT COMFORT

Complementary health approaches are increasingly being integrated into patient care plans related to the management of pain. Nurses can implement nonpharmacologic therapies in all health care settings as part of a holistic pain management strategy (Taylor et al., 2023).

Related Evidence

Kovach, C. R., Putz, M., Guslek, B., & McInnes, R. (2019). Do warmed blankets change pain, agitation, mood or analgesic use among nursing home residents? *Pain Management Nursing*, *20*(6), 526–531. https://doi.org/10.1016/j.pmn.2019.07.002

The purpose of this quality improvement project was to describe the use of warmed blankets in a nursing home setting and examine if the use was associated with changes in pain, agitation, mood, or analgesic use. The project was conducted at one urban, 160-bed, skilled long-term care facility in Wisconsin. Residents of the facility who were not using a transdermal drug or who did not have an acute injury, acute inflammatory process, multiple sclerosis, open skin wound, or any other condition that might be worsened by superficial heat were eligible to receive a warming blanket ($n = 141$). Warmed blankets were unfolded and placed over residents with pain, agitation, or thermal discomfort. Short-term changes in pain and agitation from baseline (prior to application of the blanket) to 30 minutes after application of the blanket and to the next shift after application were examined using the Revised FACES Pain Scale for participants who could self-report, the PAINAD for those who could not self-report, and the Brief Agitation Rating Scale. Comparisons were made from 1 month before to 1 month after warmed blanket use between those receiving the warmed blanket and a randomly selected group who did not receive a warmed blanket. Long-term outcomes measured included the number of pain complaints, pain severity, prn analgesic use, agitation, and mood. There were statistically significant decreases in both pain level and agitation among baseline, 20 minutes after application, and the subsequent shift assessments ($P < .001$). There were also long-term changes in the number of pain complaints ($P < .040$), severity of pain complaints ($P < .009$), and as-needed analgesic use ($P < .011$). There were no statistically significant differences between the treated group and comparison group on any long-term measures. The authors concluded that warmed blankets have potential for reducing pain, short-term agitation, and discomfort in residents of long-term care facilities and should be considered to increase resident comfort.

Relevance to Nursing Practice

Nurses should collaborate with the health care team to integrate nonpharmacological therapies to address patient comfort and pain management. Nurses should consider individual patient preferences when planning interventions for the management of pain and consider complementary health approaches to provide holistic care to their patients.

Skill 10-2 ▶ Giving a Back Massage

Massage has many benefits, including general relaxation; improved circulation; decreased symptom distress and anxiety; improved sleep quality; and provision of a means of communicating with the patient through the use of touch (Ahmadidarrehsima et al., 2018; Ayik & Özden, 2018; Hsu et al., 2020; Jagan et al., 2020; Kudo & Sasaki, 2020; Taylor et al., 2023; Westman & Blaisdell, 2016). A back massage can be incorporated into the patient's bath, as part of care before bedtime, or at any time to promote increased patient comfort.

An effective back massage should take 4 to 6 minutes to complete. A lotion is usually applied; warm it before applying to the back. Be aware of the patient's health issues when considering giving a back massage. A back massage may not be appropriate for patients with burns or healing wounds, deep vein thrombosis, fractures, severe osteoporosis, or severe thrombocytopenia (MFMER, 2021). Position the patient on their abdomen or, if this is contraindicated, on their side for a back massage.

(*continued on page 648*)

Skill 10-2 ▶ Giving a Back Massage *(continued)*

DELEGATION CONSIDERATIONS	Providing a back massage may be delegated to assistive personnel (AP) as well as to licensed practical/vocational nurses (LPN/LVNs). The decision to delegate must be based on careful analysis of the patient's needs and circumstances as well as the qualifications of the person to whom the task is being delegated. Refer to the Delegation Guidelines in Appendix A.

EQUIPMENT	<ul><li>Pain assessment tool and pain scale</li><li>Lotion or oil, to which the patient has no allergy or aversion (Westman & Blaisdell, 2016)</li></ul> <ul><li>Bath blanket</li><li>Towel</li><li>Nonsterile gloves, if indicated</li><li>Additional PPE, as indicated</li></ul>

ASSESSMENT	Review the patient's health record and plan of care for information about the patient's status and contraindications to back massage. Ask the patient about any conditions that might require modifications or that might contraindicate a massage. Inquire about any allergies, such as to lotions or scents. Ask if the patient has any preferences for lotion or has their own lotion. Assess the patient's pain using an appropriate assessment tool and pain scale. Assess the characteristics of any pain and for other symptoms that often occur with the pain, such as headache or restlessness. Ask the patient what interventions have and have not been successful in the past to promote comfort and relieve pain. Assess the patient's vital signs. Check the patient's medication administration record for the time an analgesic was last administered. Assess cultural beliefs and influences related to the pain experience. Assess the patient's response to a particular intervention to evaluate effectiveness and presence of adverse effects. If appropriate, administer an analgesic early enough prior to the massage so that it has time to take effect. Refer to assessment details included in Fundamentals Review 10-1, 10-2, 10-3, and 10-4.

ACTUAL OR POTENTIAL HEALTH PROBLEMS AND NEEDS	Many actual or potential health problems or issues may require the use of this skill as part of related interventions. An appropriate health problem or issue may include:<ul><li>Discomfort</li><li>Acute anxiety</li><li>Impaired sleep</li></ul>

OUTCOME IDENTIFICATION AND PLANNING	The expected outcomes to achieve are that the patient reports increased comfort and/or decreased pain, and that the patient is relaxed. Other outcomes that may be appropriate include that the patient experiences decreased anxiety and improved relaxation, and the patient verbalizes an understanding of the use of back massage.

IMPLEMENTATION

ACTION	**RATIONALE**
1. Perform hand hygiene and put on PPE, if indicated.	Hand hygiene and PPE prevent the spread of microorganisms. PPE is required based on transmission precautions.
2. Identify the patient.	Identifying the patient ensures the right patient receives the intervention and helps prevent errors.
3. Offer a back massage to the patient and explain the procedure.	Explanation encourages patient understanding and engagement and reduces apprehension.
4. Put on gloves, if indicated.	Gloves are not usually necessary. Gloves prevent contact with blood and body fluid.
5. Close the room door and/or the curtain around the bed. Turn down the lights, if possible, and adjust the room temperature for patient comfort (Westman & Blaisdell, 2016).	Closing the door or curtain provides privacy, promotes relaxation, and reduces noise and stimuli that may aggravate pain and reduce comfort (Aparício & Panin, 2020; Goeren et al., 2018). Lowering the lights, reducing noise, and adjusting the temperature of the room create a calming environment (Westman & Blaisdell, 2016).

ACTION

6. Assess the patient's pain using an appropriate assessment tool and measurement scale (see Fundamentals Review 10-1 through 10-4). Ask the patient if they have any aversion to touch (Westman & Blaisdell, 2016).

7. Raise the bed to a comfortable working position (VHA Center for Engineering & Occupational Safety and Health [CEOSH], 2016), and lower the side rail.

8. Assist the patient to a comfortable position, preferably the prone or side-lying position. Remove the covers and move the patient's gown just enough to expose the patient's back from the shoulders to sacral area. Drape the patient, as needed, with the bath blanket.

9. Warm the lubricant or lotion in the palm of your hand, or place the container in small basin of warm water. During the massage, observe the patient's skin for reddened areas or injury. **Avoid areas of injury, such as wounds, burns, and pressure ulcers and areas with rashes, tubes, and IV access/lines** (Westman & Blaisdell, 2016). See Chapter 8 for detailed information regarding skin assessment.

10. Using light, gliding strokes (*effleurage*), apply lotion to patient's shoulders, back, and sacral area (Figure 1).

11. Place your hands beside each other at the base of the patient's spine and stroke upward to the shoulders and back downward to the buttocks in slow, continuous strokes (Figure 2). Continue for several minutes.

RATIONALE

Accurate assessment is necessary to guide treatment and pain relief interventions and to evaluate the effectiveness of pain control measures. Patients with posttraumatic stress disorder or previous negative experience with massage may not want to receive massage (Westman & Blaisdell, 2016).

Having the bed at the proper height prevents back and muscle strain.

This position exposes an adequate area for massage. Draping the patient provides privacy and warmth.

Cold lotion causes chilling and discomfort. Massage of these areas could result in further injury and is contraindicated (Westman & Blaisdell, 2016).

Effleurage relaxes the patient and lessens tension.

Continuous contact is soothing and stimulates circulation and muscle relaxation.

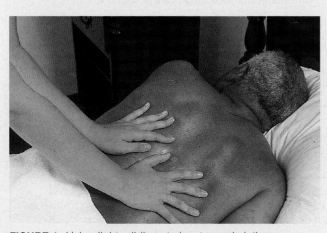

FIGURE 1. Using light, gliding strokes to apply lotion.

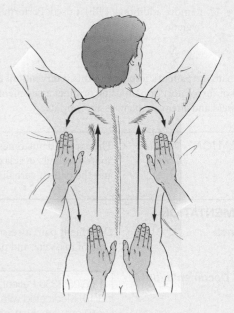

FIGURE 2. Stroking upward to shoulders and back downward to the buttocks.

12. Massage the patient's shoulders, entire back, areas over iliac crests, and sacrum with circular, stroking motions, keeping hands in contact with the patient's skin. Continue for several minutes, applying additional lotion, as necessary.

A firm stroke with continuous contact promotes relaxation.

(*continued on page 650*)

Skill 10-2 ▶ Giving a Back Massage *(continued)*

ACTION

13. Knead the patient's back by gently alternating grasping and compression motions (*pétrissage*) (Figure 3).

14. Complete the massage with additional long, stroking movements that eventually become lighter in pressure (Figure 4).

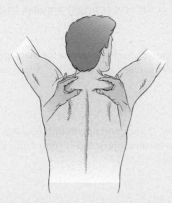

FIGURE 3. Kneading the patient's back.

15. If excess lotion remains, use the towel to pat the patient dry.

16. Remove gloves, if worn, and perform hand hygiene. Reposition patient's gown and covers. Raise side rail and lower bed. Assist patient to a position of comfort.

17. Remove additional PPE, if used. Perform hand hygiene.

18. Evaluate the patient's response to this intervention. Reassess level of discomfort or pain using original assessment tools. Reassess and alter care plan, as appropriate.

RATIONALE

Kneading increases blood circulation.

Long, stroking motions are soothing and promote relaxation; continued stroking with gradual lightening of pressure helps extend the feeling of relaxation.

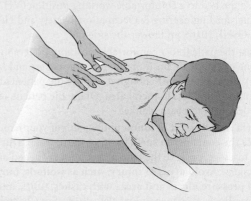

FIGURE 4. Using long strokes with lessening pressure.

Drying provides comfort and reduces the feeling of moisture on the back.

Removal of gloves and hand hygiene prevent transmission of microorganisms. Repositioning bedclothes, linens, and the patient helps to promote patient comfort and safety.

Proper removal of PPE reduces the risk for infection transmission and contamination of other items. Hand hygiene prevents transmission of microorganisms.

Reassessment allows for individualization of the patient's plan of care and promotes optimal patient comfort.

EVALUATION

The expected outcomes have been met when the patient reports increased comfort, decreased pain, and/or feelings of relaxation; the patient experiences decreased anxiety and improved relaxation; and the patient verbalizes an understanding of the use of back massage.

DOCUMENTATION

Guidelines

Document pain assessment and other significant assessments. Document massage use, length of time of massage, and patient response.

Sample Documentation

12/6/25 2330 Patient reports inability to sleep and increased pain at surgical site, rated 3/10. Medicated with acetaminophen 650 mg, as prescribed. Back massage administered ×10 minutes. Skin intact without redness. Patient reports increased comfort and relaxation; "I feel like I can sleep now."

—B. Black, RN

12/6/25 2400 Patient reports pain level 0/10.

—B. Black, RN

DEVELOPING CLINICAL REASONING AND CLINICAL JUDGMENT

UNEXPECTED SITUATIONS AND ASSOCIATED INTERVENTIONS

- Patient cannot lie prone, so you are giving them a back massage while they are lying on their side. However, as you begin to massage the back, the patient cannot maintain the side-lying position: If possible, have the patient hold on to the side rail on the side to which they are facing. If this is not possible or the patient cannot assist, use pillows and bath blankets to prevent the patient from rolling. If necessary, enlist the help of another person to maintain the patient's position. If possible, experiment with other positions based on the patient's condition and comfort, such as leaning forward against a pillow on the bedside table while sitting in a chair.
- While massaging the patient's back, you notice a 5-cm reddened area on the patient's sacrum: Note this observation in the patient's health record and communicate it to the health care team. Do not massage the area. When the back massage is completed, position the patient off the sacral area, using supports to maintain the patient's position, and institute a turning schedule.

SPECIAL CONSIDERATIONS

General Considerations

- Before giving a back massage, assess the patient's body structure and skin condition, and tailor the duration and intensity of the massage accordingly. If you are giving a back massage at bedtime, have the patient ready for bed beforehand so the massage can help them fall asleep.
- Massage only the hands, feet, or scalp of patients with sepsis, fever over 100°F, sickle cell or HIV crisis, thrombocytopenia, or meningitis (Westman & Blaisdell, 2016).
- Check in frequently with the patient during the massage, asking how the massage feels and adjust the pressure and technique based on the patient's preferences (Westman & Blaisdell, 2016).

Infant and Child Considerations

- Hold infants and small children in a comfortable, well-supported position, such as against the chest or across the lap.
- Oil or lotion should be odorless and edible in case the infant or child gets some in their mouth (MFMER, 2020).

Older Adult Considerations

- Be gentle with massage. The skin on older adults is often fragile and dry.
- Reduce pressure, provide short massage sessions, and consider alternative positions, such as supine or seated positions for massage with older adults (Durand, 2020).

EVIDENCE FOR PRACTICE ▶

MASSAGE AND ANXIETY AND SLEEP

Patient comfort is attained through management of many factors. Pharmacologic interventions alone may not address all of the factors involved in the patient's experiences with discomfort and pain. Can alternative approaches to managing patient discomfort help improve patient experiences and outcomes?

Related Research

Ayik, C., & Özden, D. (2018). The effects of preoperative aromatherapy massage on anxiety and sleep quality of colorectal surgery patients: A randomized controlled study. *Complementary Therapies in Medicine, 36,* 93–99. https://doi.org/10.1016/j.ctim.2017.12.002

The aim of this study was to examine the effects of aromatherapy massage on anxiety and sleep quality in patients undergoing colorectal surgery in the preoperative period. Eighty patients undergoing colorectal surgery were randomly assigned to experimental and control groups. Participants in the experimental group ($n = 40$) received aromatherapy back massage using 5% lavender oil for 10 minutes the night before surgery and the morning of surgery. The control group ($n = 40$) received standard nursing care. The preoperative anxiety level and sleep quality of the participants was measured in the afternoon on the day prior to surgery and again in the morning of surgery. Participants in the experimental group received the two massages

(continued on page 652)

Skill 10-2 ▶ Giving a Back Massage   *(continued)*

after baseline measurement and prior to the second measurement. There was no baseline difference between the groups. A statistically significant difference was found between the experimental and control group in terms of the anxiety and sleep quality mean scores recorded on the morning of surgery. It was determined that the anxiety and sleep quality mean score of the experimental group after aromatherapy massage on the morning of surgery decreased when compared to that of the evening before surgery. The researchers concluded that aromatherapy massage with lavender oil increased the sleep quality and reduced the level of anxiety in patients with colorectal surgery in the preoperative period.

The authors suggested the use of lavender oil massage may be recommended to reduce anxiety and increase sleep quality and patient satisfaction in the preoperative period.

Relevance to Nursing Practice

Massage is an economical intervention that is easily incorporated into nursing practice. Evidence suggests that massage can be an important part of decreasing discomfort and increasing patient's well-being. Nurses should consider making time to incorporate this intervention into their practice.

Skill 10-3 ▶ Applying and Caring for a Patient Using a Transcutaneous Electrical Nerve Stimulation Unit

Transcutaneous electrical nerve stimulation (TENS) is a noninvasive technique for providing pain relief that involves the use of low-voltage electrical stimulation. This electrical stimulation is thought stimulate nerve cells that block the transmission of painful impulses and/or stimulation raises the level of endorphins that block the perception of pain (Cleveland Clinic, 2020; NHS, 2021). The TENS unit consists of a battery-powered portable unit, lead wires, and cutaneous electrode pads that are applied to or around the painful area (Figure 1). TENS therapy is used to treat acute and chronic pain related to multiple health problems, including osteoarthritis-related problems, fibromyalgia-related problems, bursitis, low back pain, and tendonitis (Cleveland Clinic, 2020).

TENS should not be applied to wounds due to osteomyelitis; areas recently treated with radiation; on the head; near reproductive organs or genitals; or in persons who have trouble communicating or who have mental impairment (Cleveland Clinic, 2020). Never place electrodes over the carotid sinus nerves; laryngeal or pharyngeal muscles (the front or sides of the neck); the eyes or temples; chest and upper back at the same time; irritated, infected, or broken skin; numb areas or areas of the body that lack or have reduced sensation; or varicose veins (NHS, 2021).

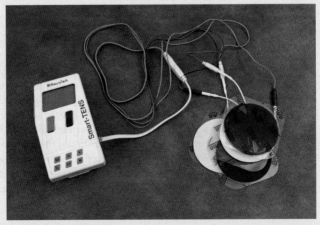

FIGURE 1. TENS unit.

TENS therapy prescribed by a health care provider. The TENS unit can be applied intermittently throughout the day or worn for extended periods. There are many different manufacturers of TENS units. **Nurses need to be familiar with the particular unit in use by their patient and to refer to the specific manufacturer's recommendations for use.**

DELEGATION CONSIDERATIONS

The application and monitoring of use of a TENS unit is not delegated to assistive personnel (AP). Depending on the state's nurse practice act and the organization's policies and procedures, the application and monitoring of use of a TENS unit may be delegated to licensed practical/vocational nurses (LPN/LVNs). The decision to delegate must be based on careful analysis of the patient's needs and circumstances as well as the qualifications of the person to whom the task is being delegated. Refer to the Delegation Guidelines in Appendix A.

EQUIPMENT

- TENS unit
- Self-adhering electrodes
- Pain assessment tool and pain scale
- Disposable cleansing washcloths or skin cleanser, water, towel, and washcloth
- PPE, as indicated

ASSESSMENT

Review the patient's health record and plan of care for specific instructions related to TENS therapy, including the prescribed intervention and conditions indicating the need for therapy. Review the patient's health record for conditions that might contraindicate therapy or require modifications of therapy, such as the presence of an implantable device, (cardioverter/defibrillator, neurostimulator, bone growth stimulator, and indwelling blood pressure monitor); diagnosis of cancer; pregnancy; epilepsy; deep vein thrombosis or thrombophlebitis; bleeding disorder; heart disease, heart failure, or arrhythmias (Cleveland Clinic, 2020). Determine the location of electrode placement in consultation with the prescribing health care provider and based on the patient's report of pain. Assess the patient's understanding of TENS therapy and the rationale for its use.

Inspect the skin of the area designated for electrode placement for irritation, redness, or breakdown. Assess the patient's pain and level of discomfort using an appropriate assessment tool. Assess the characteristics of any pain. Assess for other symptoms that often occur with the pain, such as headache or restlessness. Ask the patient what interventions have and have not been successful in the past to promote comfort and relieve pain. Assess the patient's vital signs. Check the patient's medication administration record for the time an analgesic was last administered. Assess the patient's response to a particular intervention to evaluate effectiveness and presence of any adverse effect. Refer to assessment details included in Fundamentals Review 10-1, 10-2, 10-3, and 10-4.

Check the unit to ensure proper functioning and review the manufacturer's instructions for use.

ACTUAL OR POTENTIAL HEALTH PROBLEMS AND NEEDS

Many actual or potential health problems or issues may require the use of this skill as part of related interventions. An appropriate health problem or issue may include:
- Acute pain
- Chronic pain
- Knowledge deficiency

OUTCOME IDENTIFICATION AND PLANNING

The expected outcome to achieve is that the patient verbalizes decreased discomfort and pain without experiencing any injury or skin irritation or alteration in skin integrity. Other appropriate outcomes may include the patient verbalizing an understanding of the therapy, use of the device, and the reason for its use.

IMPLEMENTATION

ACTION	**RATIONALE**
1. Perform hand hygiene and put on PPE, if indicated.	Hand hygiene and PPE prevent the spread of microorganisms. PPE is required based on transmission precautions.

(continued on page 654)

Skill 10-3 ▶ **Applying and Caring for a Patient Using a Transcutaneous Electrical Nerve Stimulation Unit** *(continued)*

ACTION	**RATIONALE**
2. Identify the patient.	Identifying the patient ensures that the right patient receives the intervention and helps prevent errors.
3. Show the patient the TENS device, and explain its function and the reason for its use.	Explanation encourages patient understanding and engagement and reduces apprehension.
4. Assess the patient's pain using an appropriate assessment tool and measurement scale (see Fundamentals Review 10-1 through 10-4).	Accurate assessment is necessary to guide treatment and relief interventions and evaluate the effectiveness of pain control measures.
5. Inspect the area where the electrodes are to be placed. Clean the patient's skin using the disposable cleansing wipe or skin cleanser and water. Dry the area thoroughly.	Inspection ensures that the electrodes will be applied to intact skin. Cleaning and drying help ensure that the electrodes will adhere.
6. Remove the adhesive backing from the self-adhering electrodes and apply them to the specified location (Figure 2).	Application to the proper location enhances the success of the therapy. Gel is necessary to promote conduction of the electrical current.
7. **Check the placement of the electrodes; leave at least a 2-inch (5-cm) space between them.**	Proper spacing is necessary to reduce the risk of burns due to the proximity of the electrodes.
8. **Check the controls on the TENS unit to make sure that they are off.** Connect the wires to the electrodes (if not already attached) and plug them into the unit.	Having controls off prevents flow of electricity. This connection completes the electrical circuit necessary to stimulate the nerve fibers.
9. Turn on the unit and adjust the intensity setting to the lowest intensity (Figure 3) and determine if the patient can feel a tingling, burning, or buzzing sensation. Then adjust the intensity to the prescribed amount or the setting most comfortable for the patient. Secure the unit to the patient.	Using the lowest setting at first introduces the patient to the sensations. Adjusting the intensity is necessary to provide the proper amount of stimulation.

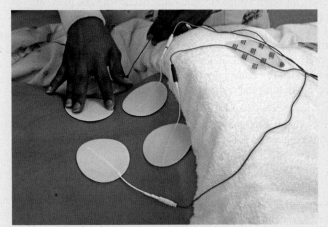
FIGURE 2. Applying TENS electrodes.

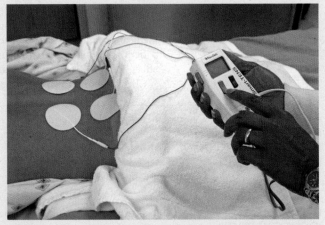
FIGURE 3. Turning on TENS unit.

10. Set the pulse width (duration of each pulsation) as indicated or recommended.	The pulse width determines the depth and width of the stimulation.
11. Assess the patient's pain level during therapy.	Pain assessment helps evaluate the effectiveness of therapy.
a. If intermittent use is ordered, turn the unit off after the specified duration of treatment and remove the electrodes. Clean the patient's skin at the electrode sites.	TENS therapy can be ordered for intermittent or continuous use. Skin care reduces the risk for irritation and breakdown.

ACTION

b. If continuous therapy is ordered, periodically remove the electrodes from the skin (after turning off the unit) to inspect the area and clean the skin, according to facility policy. Reapply the electrodes and continue therapy. Change the electrodes according to the manufacturer's directions.

12. When therapy is discontinued, turn off the unit and remove the electrodes. Clean the patient's skin. Clean the unit and replace the batteries.

 13. Remove PPE, if used. Perform hand hygiene.

RATIONALE

Periodic removal of electrodes allows for skin assessment. Skin care reduces the risk for irritation and breakdown. Reapplication ensures continued therapy.

Turning off the unit and removing electrodes when therapy is discontinued reduces the risk of injury to the patient. Skin care reduces the risk for irritation and breakdown. Cleaning the unit and replacing the batteries ensures that the unit is ready for future use.

Proper removal of PPE reduces the risk for infection transmission and contamination of other items. Hand hygiene prevents transmission of microorganisms.

EVALUATION

The expected outcomes have been met when the patient verbalizes decreased discomfort and pain without injury or skin irritation or alteration in skin integrity, and the patient verbalizes an understanding of the therapy, use of the device, and the reason for its use.

DOCUMENTATION

Guidelines

Document the date and time of application; patient's initial pain assessment; skin assessment; electrode placement location; intensity and pulse width; duration of therapy; pain assessments during therapy and patient's response; and time of removal or discontinuation of therapy.

Sample Documentation

> 5/28/25 1105 Patient reports severe lower back pain, rating it as 9/10 on pain scale. Identified lower sacral area as site of pain. TENS therapy ordered for 30 to 45 minutes. Electrodes applied to right and left sides of sacral area. Intensity initially set at 80 pulses/sec with pulse width of 80 microseconds. Pain rating at 7/10 after 15 minutes of therapy. Intensity increased to 100 pulses/sec, with a pulse width increased to 100 microseconds. Pain rating at 5/10 after 15 minutes at increased settings. Therapy continued for an additional 15 minutes and discontinued. Patient rated pain at 3/10 at end of session. Skin on lower sacral area clean, dry, and intact without evidence of irritation or breakdown. Patient instructed to report increasing pain.
>
> —K. Lewin, RN

DEVELOPING CLINICAL REASONING AND CLINICAL JUDGMENT

UNEXPECTED SITUATIONS AND ASSOCIATED INTERVENTIONS

- *While receiving TENS therapy, the patient reports pain and intolerable paresthesia:* Check the settings, connections, and placement of the electrodes. Adjust the settings and reposition the electrodes, as necessary.
- *During a TENS therapy session, the patient reports muscle twitching:* Assess the patient and check the intensity setting. Readjust the intensity to a lower setting because the patient is most likely experiencing overstimulation.
- *While assessing the skin where the electrodes are placed for a patient receiving continuous TENS therapy, you notice some irritation and redness:* Clean and dry the area thoroughly. Reposition the electrodes in the same area, avoiding the irritated and reddened area.

(continued on page 656)

Skill 10-3 ▶ Applying and Caring for a Patient Using a Transcutaneous Electrical Nerve Stimulation Unit *(continued)*

SPECIAL CONSIDERATIONS

- Never place electrodes over the carotid sinus nerves; laryngeal or pharyngeal muscles (the front or sides of the neck); the eyes or temples; chest and upper back at the same time; irritated, infected, or broken skin; numb areas; or varicose veins (NHS Choices, 2021).
- Whenever electrodes are being repositioned or removed, first turn off the unit.

Community-Based Care Considerations

- Patient and/or family/caregiver teaching is essential and should include an explanation of the manufacturer's directions, instructions on where to place the electrodes, and the importance of placing the electrodes on clean, unbroken skin (Bauldoff et al., 2020). The patient/family/caregiver should assess the skin daily at the electrode locations for signs of irritation (Bauldoff et al., 2020).

EVIDENCE FOR PRACTICE ▶

TENS AND POSTOPERATIVE PAIN

Patient comfort is attained through management of many factors. Achieving pain relief and/or pain control is a large contributor to achieving patient comfort. Pharmacologic interventions alone may not address all of the factors involved in the pain experience. Do alternative approaches to managing pain that supplement medication administration help achieve effective pain management?

Related Evidence

Zhou, J., Dan, Y., Yixian, Y., Lyu, M., Zhong, J., Wang, Z., Zhu, Y., & Liu, L. (2020). Efficacy of transcutaneous electronic nerve stimulation in postoperative analgesia after pulmonary surgery: A systematic review and meta-analysis. *American Journal of Physical Medicine & Rehabilitation*, 99(3), 241–249. https://doi.org/10.1097/PHM.0000000000001312

The aim of this study was to identify the analgesic efficacy and safety of transcutaneous electronic nerve stimulation (TENS) in postoperative pain after pulmonary surgery. Four data bases (PubMed, Embase, Web of Science, and CENTRAL) were systematically searched from their inception to June 2019. The continuous variables were pooled as the weighted mean difference with correlated 95% confidence interval. Subgroup analyses, sensitivity analyses, and quality assessment were completed. Ten studies were included; pooled results indicated that TENS conferred lower pain intensity score when compared with the placebo group on the first through the fifth postoperative days; postoperative day 1 ($P = .004$), postoperative day 2 ($P = .002$), postoperative day 3 ($P = .03$), postoperative day 4 ($P < .001$), and postoperative day 5 ($P < .001$). There were no significant findings related to sensitivity analyses. The researchers concluded TENS might be an effective supplementary analgesic regimen in multimodal analgesia to decrease pain intensity after pulmonary surgery.

Relevance to Nursing Practice

Nurses have an important role in providing interventions to assist patients in controlling pain and educating patients about analgesic interventions. Nurses should consider the appropriateness of inclusion of nonpharmacologic interventions, such as TENS, in collaboration with health care providers and patients when planning care for patients experiencing or likely to experience pain. Nurses have a responsibility to be informed and knowledgeable regarding all methods of analgesia and work to provide a plan of care that addresses individual patient needs.

Skill 10-4 ▶ Caring for a Patient Receiving Patient-Controlled Analgesia

Patient-controlled analgesia (PCA) allows patients to self-administer small doses of analgesic within a prescribed time interval, controlling the administration of their own medication within predetermined safety limits (Bauldoff et al., 2020). This approach can be used with oral analgesic agents as well as with infusions of opioid analgesic agents by intravenous, subcutaneous, sublingual, **epidural**, and **perineural routes** (Golembiewski et al., 2016; Katz et al., 2017). PCA provides effective individualized analgesia and comfort. This drug delivery system can be used to manage acute and chronic pain in a health care facility or the home, in a wide range of clinical situations (Nijland et al., 2019).

The PCA system used to deliver an intravenous opioid analgesic permits the patient to self-administer medication (bolus doses) with episodes of increased pain or painful activities. A timing device electronically controls the PCA pump. The PCA system consists of a computerized, portable infusion pump containing a reservoir or chamber for a syringe or other reservoir that is prefilled with the prescribed medication, usually an opioid, or dilute anesthetic solution in the case of epidural administration (D'Arcy, 2013; Hinkle et al., 2022). When pain occurs, the patient pushes a button that activates the PCA device to deliver a small, preset bolus dose of the analgesic. A dose interval that is programmed into the PCA unit prevents reactivation of the pump and administration of another dose during that period of time (bolus; commonly 6 to 8 minutes). The pump mechanism can also be programmed to deliver only a specified amount of analgesic within a given time interval (basal rate; most commonly every hour or, occasionally, every 4 hours). These safeguards limit the risk for overmedication and allow the patient to evaluate the effect of the previous dose. PCA pumps also have a locked safety system that prohibits tampering with the device (Karch, 2020; Pasero & McCaffery, 2011).

The proper selection of patients for PCA is vital for a safe, positive experience (Grissinger, 2019). Suitable candidates for this type of delivery system include people who are alert and capable of controlling the unit. The Institute for Safe Medication Practices (ISMP, 2016) identifies people for whom this type of pain relief is not recommended, including confused older adults, infants and very young children, cognitively impaired patients, patients with conditions for which oversedation poses a significant health risk (e.g., asthma and sleep apnea), and patients who are taking other medications that potentiate opioids. PCA has proven safe for use in developmentally normal children as young as 4 to 6 years of age (DiGiusto et al., 2014; Pasero & McCaffery, 2011). All patients should be assessed for level of risk of opioid-induced advancing sedation and respiratory depression; the plan of care and monitoring strategies should be driven by reassessment according to level of risk (Jungquist et al., 2020).

Nursing responsibilities for patients receiving medications via a PCA system include collaboration with the health care team and the patient to ensure appropriate patient selection criteria, patient/family/caregiver teaching, knowledge of the appropriate drugs used with PCA, initial device setup, monitoring the device to ensure proper functioning, and frequent assessment of the patient's response, including pain and discomfort control, respiratory status and sedation screening, and presence of adverse effects (Gorski et al., 2021). Box 10-1 (on page 658) outlines guidelines for safe and effective use of PCA. Additional information related to epidural infusions is discussed in Skill 10-5.

DELEGATION CONSIDERATIONS

The care related to PCA is not delegated to assistive personnel (AP). Depending on the state's nurse practice act and the organization's policies and procedures, specific aspects of the care related to PCA, such as monitoring the infusion and assessment of patient response, may be delegated to licensed practical/vocational nurses (LPN/LVNs). The decision to delegate must be based on careful analysis of the patient's needs and circumstances as well as the qualifications of the person to whom the task is being delegated. Refer to the Delegation Guidelines in Appendix A.

EQUIPMENT

- PCA system, including programmable smart infusion pump device with dose error-reductions systems
- Syringe (or appropriate reservoir for device) filled with prescribed medication
- PCA system tubing
- Antimicrobial swabs
- Appropriate label for syringe and tubing, based on facility policy and procedure
- Second clinician to verify medication and programmed pump information, according to facility policy

(continued on page 658)

Skill 10-4 ▶ Caring for a Patient Receiving Patient-Controlled Analgesia *(continued)*

- Pain assessment tool and pain scale
- Electronic medication administration record (eMAR) or medication administration record (MAR)
- Gloves
- Additional PPE, as indicated

Box 10-1 | Guidelines for Safe and Effective Use of Patient-Controlled Analgesia

Safe patient-controlled analgesia (PCA) use requires proper patient selection, education, assessment, and monitoring (ISMP, 2016). Use the following tips as guidelines to ensure optimal patient comfort and safety when caring for patients receiving PCA.

- Be aware of patient groups who generally are not good candidates for PCA, including infants and very young children, patients with cognitive impairment, patients with conditions for which oversedation poses a significant health risk (e.g., asthma and sleep apnea), and patients who are taking other medications that potentiate opioids.
- All patients should be assessed for level of risk of opioid-induced advancing sedation and respiratory depression; the plan of care and monitoring strategies should be driven by reassessment according to level of risk.
- Caution is required when PCA is used in older adults; patients who are obese or have asthma, sleep apnea or other respiratory disease; patients taking other drugs that potentiate opioids, such as muscle relaxants, antiemetics, and sleeping medications; and patients who are morbidly obese.
- Use standard medical order sets and prefilled syringes with standard drug concentrations.

- Check PCA orders/prescriptions ensuring that they include the medication, the initial loading dose, demand (bolus) dose, lockout interval, and an hourly maximum administration rate. Some prescriptions include a continuous infusion rate.
- Be familiar with the particular PCA infusion device in use at a facility. Use programmable smart infusion pump technology with dose error-reductions systems (ISMP, 2020).
- Ensure that PCA pumps are programmed correctly. Check pump settings at least once every 4 hours. Two nurses should verify PCA programming when initiating infusion or making a change in infusion settings.
- Place warning signs on all PCA pumps that say "For patient use only."
- Assess pain level, alertness, sedation, pulse oximetry, capnography, and vital signs, including respiratory rate and quality, at least every 4 hours or more often as needed, such as during the first 24 hours of treatment and at night, when nocturnal hypoxia may develop.
- Teach patients and family members/caregivers about the danger of PCA use by anyone other than the patient.

Source: Adapted from Casey, G. (2015). Capnography: Monitoring CO2. *Nursing New Zealand, 21*(9), 20–24; Cooney, M. F., Czarnecki, M., Dunwoody, C., Eksterowicz, N., Merkel, S., Oakes, L., & Wuhrman, E. (2013). American Society for Pain Management nursing position statement with clinical practice guidelines: Authorized agent controlled analgesia. *Pain Management Nursing, 14*(3), 176–181; Gorski, L. A., Hadaweay, L., Hagle, M. E., Broadhurst, D., Clare, S., Kleidon, T., Meyer, B. M., Nickel, B., Rowley, S., Sharpe, E., & Alexander, M. (2021). Infusion therapy standards of practice. Infusion Nurses Society (INS). *Journal of Infusion Nursing, 44*(1S), S1–S231. https://www.ins1.org/publications/infusion-therapy-standards-of-practice/; Institute for Safe Medication Practices (ISMP). (2016). *Acute Care ISMP Medication Safety Alert!® Worth repeating…Recent PCA by proxy event suggests reassessment of practices that may have fallen by the wayside.* https://www.ismp.org/Newsletters/acutecare/showarticle.aspx?id=1149; Institute for Safe Medication Practices (ISMP). (2003; updated 2017). *Acute Care ISMP Medication Safety Alert!® Part II: How to prevent errors. Safety issues with patient-controlled analgesia.* http://www.ismp.org/newsletters/acutecare/articles/20030724.asp; Institute for Safe Medication Practices (ISMP). (2013). *Acute Care ISMP Medication Safety Alert!® Fatal PCA adverse events continue to happen…Better patient monitoring is essential to prevent harm.* https://www.ismp.org/newsletters/acutecare/showarticle.aspx?id=50; and Jungquist, C. R., Quinlan-Cowell, A., Vallerand, A., Carlisle, H. L., Cooney, M., Dempsey, S. J., Dunwoody, D., Maly, A., Meloche, K., Mehyers, A., Sawyer, J., Singh, N., Sullivan, D., Watson, C., & Polomano, R. C. (2020). American Society for Pain Management nursing guidelines on monitoring for opioid-induced advancing sedation and respiratory depression: Revisions. *Pain Management Nursing, 21*(1), 7–25. https://doi.org/10.1016/j.pmn.2019.06.007; and Lisi, D. M. (2013). Patient-controlled analgesia and the older patient. *US Pharmacist, 38*(3), HS2–HS6. https://www.uspharmacist.com/article/patient-controlled-analgesia-and-the-older-patient

ASSESSMENT

Review the patient's health record and plan of care for specific instructions related to PCA therapy, including the prescribed intervention and conditions indicating the need for therapy. Check the health record for the prescribed drug, initial loading dose, dose for self-administration, and lockout interval. Check to ensure proper functioning of the unit. Assess the patient's level of consciousness and understanding of PCA therapy and the rationale for its use. Inquire about any allergies.

Review the patient's history for conditions that might contraindicate therapy, such as respiratory limitations, history of substance abuse, or psychiatric disorder. Review the patient's health record and assess for factors contributing to an increased risk for adverse effects, such as the use of a continuous basal infusion, the patient's age (older age, infant [prematurity, developmental delay, underweight, age <1 year]), morbid obesity, upper abdominal or thoracic surgery, known or suspected sleep disorder breathing problems, preexisting pulmonary and/or cardiac disease, renal insufficiency, impaired liver function, history of smoking, concurrent use of sedating medications (Gorski et al., 2021; Jungquist et al., 2020). Determine the prescribed route for administration. Inspect the site to be used for the infusion for signs of infiltration or infection. If the route is via an IV infusion, ensure that the access is patent, and the current solution is compatible with the drug ordered.

Assess the patient's level of consciousness and vital signs. Assess the patient's pain and level of discomfort using an appropriate assessment tool and pain scale (refer to Fundamentals Review 10-1 through 10-4). Assess the characteristics of any pain, and for other symptoms that often occur with the pain, such as headache or restlessness. Ask the patient what interventions have and have not been successful in the past to promote comfort and relieve pain.

Assess the patient's vital signs. Assess the patient's respiratory status, including rate, depth, and rhythm; oxygen saturation level using pulse oximetry; and level of carbon dioxide concentration using capnography. Assess the patient's sedation score (Table 10-1). Determine the patient's response to the intervention to evaluate effectiveness and for the presence of adverse effects.

Table 10-1 Pasero Opioid-Induced Sedation Scale (POSS)

PATIENT ASSESSMENT CHARACTERISTICS	SEDATION SCORE	ACTION
Sleeping, easy to arouse	S	No action necessary
Awake and alert	1	No action needed
Occasionally drowsy, but easily aroused	2	No action needed
Frequently drowsy, arousable, drifts off during conversation	3	Requires action; decrease dose
Somnolent, minimal or no response to stimuli	4	Unacceptable, stop opioid, consider administering naloxone

Source: Used with permission. © 1994, Pasero C. Used with permission. As cited in Pasero, C., McCaffery, M. (2011). *Pain assessment and pharmacologic management* (p. 510). Mosby/Elsevier.

ACTUAL OR POTENTIAL HEALTH PROBLEMS AND NEEDS	Many actual or potential health problems or issues may require the use of this skill as part of related interventions. An appropriate health problem or issue may include: • Acute pain • Risk for medication side effect • Knowledge deficiency
OUTCOME IDENTIFICATION AND PLANNING	The expected outcome to achieve is that the patient reports increased comfort and/or decreased pain without adverse effects, oversedation, or respiratory depression. Other appropriate outcomes may include that the patient verbalizes an understanding of the reason of use of the therapy, the patient verbalizes and demonstrates an understanding of the use of the therapy, and the patient's family/caregiver verbalizes an understanding that the PCA is to be used only by the patient.

IMPLEMENTATION

ACTION

1. Gather equipment. Check the medication prescribed against the original order in the health record, depending on facility policy and the medication order system in place. Clarify any inconsistencies. Check the patient's health record for allergies.

RATIONALE

The prescription is the legal record of prescribed medication interventions. This comparison helps to identify errors that may have occurred when orders were transcribed. Computer provider order-entry (CPOE) systems allow prescribers to send electronic medication prescriptions directly to the pharmacy located in a health care facility and to outpatient pharmacies.

(continued on page 660)

Skill 10-4 ▶ Caring for a Patient Receiving Patient-Controlled Analgesia *(continued)*

ACTION	RATIONALE
2. Know the actions, special nursing considerations, safe dose ranges, purpose of administration, and adverse effects of the medications to be administered. Consider the appropriateness of the medication for this patient.	This knowledge aids the nurse in evaluating the therapeutic effect of the medication in relation to the patient's health status and can also be used to educate the patient about the medication.
3. Prepare the medication syringe or other reservoir for administration, based on facility policy (see Chapter 5 for additional information).	Proper preparation and administration procedures prevent errors.
4. Perform hand hygiene and put on PPE, if indicated.	Hand hygiene and PPE prevent the spread of microorganisms. PPE is required based on transmission precautions.
5. Identify the patient.	Identifying the patient ensures that the right patient receives the intervention and helps prevent errors.
6. Show the patient/family/caregiver the device, and explain its function and the reason for use. Explain the purpose and action of the medication to the patient.	Explanation encourages patient understanding and engagement and reduces apprehension.
7. Plug the PCA device into the electrical outlet, if necessary. Check status of battery power, if appropriate.	The PCA device requires a power source (electricity or battery) to run. Most units will alarm to acknowledge a low battery state.
8. Close the door to the room or pull the bedside curtain. **Identify the patient. Compare the information with the eMAR/MAR. The patient should be identified using at least two of the following methods** (The Joint Commission, 2021). Refer to Chapter 5 for additional information related to medication administration.	Closing the door or pulling the curtain provides for patient privacy. Identifying the patient ensures the right patient receives the medications and helps prevent errors. The patient's room number or physical location is not used as an identifier (The Joint Commission, 2021). Replace the identification band if it is missing or inaccurate in any way.
9. Complete necessary assessments before administering medication. Assess the IV site for presence of inflammation or infiltration or other signs of complications. Check allergy bracelet or ask patient about allergies. Assess the patient's pain using an appropriate assessment tool and measurement scale (see Fundamentals Review 10-1 through 10-4).	Assessment is a prerequisite to medication administration. IV medication must be given directly into a vein for safe administration. Accurate assessment is necessary to guide treatment and relief interventions and to evaluate the effectiveness of pain control measures.
10. **Check the label on the prefilled drug syringe or reservoir with the medication record and patient identification, verifying the drug, concentration, dose, and rate of infusion (Figure 1). Obtain verification of information from a second clinician, according to facility policy.** Scan the bar code on the package, if required.	This action verifies that the correct drug and dosage will be administered to the correct patient. An independent double check by two clinicians is recommended prior to initiation of the PCA and when the syringe, solution container, drug, or rate is changed (Gorski et al., 2021). Confirmation of information by a second clinician helps prevent errors.

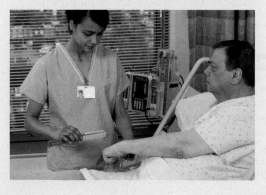

FIGURE 1. Checking label on prefilled drug syringe with patient identification.

ACTION

11. Scan the patient's barcode on the identification band, if required (The Joint Commission, 2021). **Based on facility policy, the third check of the medication label may occur at this point. If so, read the label and recheck the label with the eMAR/MAR before administering the medications to the patient.**

12. Connect tubing to prefilled syringe or other reservoir and place into the PCA device (Figure 2). **Prime the tubing.** Attach label to tubing, based on facility policy.

13. Set the PCA device to administer the loading dose, if ordered, and then program the device based on the prescribed intervention, **verifying the drug, concentration, dose, and rate of infusion, dose interval, and lockout interval (Figure 3). Obtain verification of information from a second clinician, according to facility policy.**

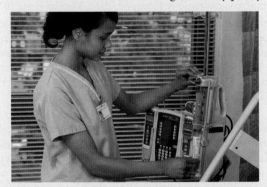

FIGURE 2. Placing syringe/reservoir into PCA device.

14. Put on gloves. Depending on facility policy, remove the passive disinfection cap from the connection port on the IV infusion tubing or other access site, based on route of administration. Alternatively, use an antimicrobial swab to clean the connection port. Connect the PCA tubing to the patient's IV infusion line or appropriate access site, based on the specific site used. Secure the site per facility policy and procedure. Remove gloves. Perform hand hygiene. Initiate the therapy by activating the appropriate button on the pump. Lock the PCA device, per facility policy.

15. Ensure the patient control (dosing button) is within the patient's reach. Attach the warning sign to the PCA control cord and/or PCA infusion device, per facility policy. Reinforce the steps for use with the patient and the need to press the button each time they need relief from pain (Figure 4).

RATIONALE

Scanning of the patient's barcode on identification band provides an additional check to ensure that the medication is given to the right patient. Many facilities require the *third* check to occur at the bedside, after identifying the patient and before administration. If facility policy directs the *third* check at this time, this *third* check ensures accuracy and helps prevent errors.

Doing so prepares the device to deliver the drug. Priming the tubing purges air from the tubing and reduces the risk for air embolism. Labeling tubing allows for identification of purpose of infusion, reducing confusion in the presence of multiple infusions.

These actions ensure that the appropriate drug dosage will be administered. An independent double check by two clinicians is recommended prior to initiation of the PCA and when the syringe, solution container, drug, or rate is changed (Gorski et al., 2021). Confirmation of information by a second clinician helps prevent errors.

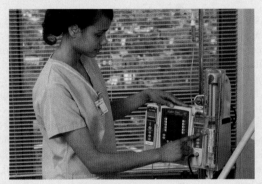

FIGURE 3. Programming PCA device.

Gloves prevent contact with blood and body fluids. Passive disinfection caps contain an antiseptic-impregnated sponge that dispenses the antiseptic over the connector's top and threads and provides continuous disinfection of the needleless connection versus intermittent disinfection when using antimicrobial wipes (Barton, 2019; Casey et al., 2018). Venous access device entry points, end-caps, and needleless connectors must be vigorously scrubbed and disinfected prior to each access to reduce the risk for introduction of microorganisms and prevent venous access device-related infection (Flynn et al., 2019; Gorski et al., 2021). Friction is needed to physically remove microorganisms from the top, sides, and threads of the needleless connector or end cap. Allow the antiseptic to dry completely (5 to 20 seconds) to ensure complete effectiveness (INS, 2021; Slater et al., 2018). Removal of gloves and hand hygiene prevent transmission of microorganisms. Connection and initiation are necessary to allow drug delivery to the patient. Locking the device prevents tampering with the settings.

The patient control (dosing button) must be within reach to enable patient use. Warning sign/label provides warning/reinforcement for the patient, family members/caregivers, and staff that the button is to be pressed only by the patient to reduce the risk for adverse effect (ISMP, 2016). Reinforcement of instructions promotes correct use of the device.

(*continued on page 662*)

Skill 10-4 ▶ Caring for a Patient Receiving Patient-Controlled Analgesia *(continued)*

ACTION

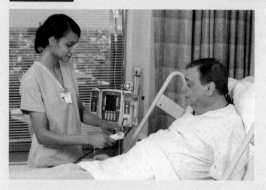

FIGURE 4. Reinforcing the need to press button to administer pain medication.

RATIONALE

16. Initiate continuous capnography and/or pulse oximetry, based on facility policy.

Continuous capnography and/or pulse oximetry has been suggested for use in all patients receiving PCA opioids for early detection of opioid-induced respiratory depression; continuous capnography should be used in all patients receiving supplemental oxygen (Fazio & Firestone, 2020; Khanna et al., 2020).

17. Assess the patient's response to the medication: Assess the patient's pain at least every 4 hours or more often, as needed, based on patient's individual risk factors. Monitor vital signs, especially respiratory status, including respiratory rate, depth, and quality and oxygen saturation every 2 to 4 hours or more often, as needed, based on patient's individual risk factors and situation.

The plan of care and monitoring strategies should be driven by reassessment according to level of risk (Jungquist et al., 2020). Continued assessment at frequent intervals helps evaluate the effectiveness of the drug and reduce the risk for complications (Fazio & Firestone, 2020; Gorski et al., 2021; Jungquist et al., 2017a, 2017b).

18. Assess the patient's response to the medication: Assess the patient's sedation score (see Table 10-1) and end-tidal carbon dioxide level (capnography) at least every 4 hours or more often, as needed, based on patient's individual risk factors.

The plan of care and monitoring strategies should be driven by reassessment according to level of risk (Jungquist et al., 2020). Sedation occurs before clinically significant respiratory depression (Hall & Stanley, 2019). Respiratory depression can occur with the use of opioid analgesics (Fazio & Firestone, 2020; Hall & Stanley, 2019). Capnography provides an earlier warning of respiratory depression as compared to continuous oximetry (Casey, 2015; Gorski et al., 2021; Jungquist et al., 2017a, 2017b).

19. Assess the infusion site periodically, according to facility policy and nursing judgment. Assess the patient's use of the medication, noting number of attempts and number of doses delivered. Replace the drug syringe when it is empty.

Continued assessment of the infusion site is necessary for early detection of problems (Gorski et al., 2021). Continued assessment of the patient's use of medication and effect is necessary to ensure adequate pain control without adverse effect. Replacing the syringe ensures continued drug delivery.

20. Make sure the patient control (dosing button) is within the patient's reach.

Easy access to the control is essential for the patients to use the device.

21. Remove gloves and additional PPE, if used. Perform hand hygiene.

Proper removal of PPE reduces the risk for infection transmission and contamination of other items. Hand hygiene prevents transmission of microorganisms.

EVALUATION

The expected outcomes have been met when the patient reports increased comfort and/or decreased pain without adverse effects, oversedation, and respiratory depression; the patient displays an understanding of use of the therapy and the reason for its use; and the patient's family/caregiver verbalizes an understanding that the PCA is to be used only by the patient.

DOCUMENTATION

Guidelines

Document the date and time PCA therapy was initiated, initial assessments, drug and loading dose administered, if appropriate, and individual dosing and time interval. Document patient teaching and patient's response. Document continued pain, sedation level, vital signs and assessments, and patient's response to therapy.

Sample Documentation

6/1/25 0645 Patient returned from surgery with PCA therapy with morphine sulfate 1 mg/mL in place via IV infusion. Device programmed to deliver 0.1 mg at 10-minute lockout intervals. Patient reports moderate to severe abdominal pain, rating pain as 6 to 8/10 on a pain-rating scale. Patient instructed to press PCA button for pain relief. Vital signs within acceptable parameters. Respiratory rate 16 breaths/min, regular rhythm and depth. Oxygen saturation 96%; partial pressure end-tidal CO_2 (PetCO$_2$) 36%. IV of 1,000 mL D5LR infusing at 100 mL/min; IV site clean and dry without evidence of infiltration or infection.

—P. Joyner, RN

6/1/25 0715 Patient rates pain at 4/10. Respirations 16 breaths/min, regular rhythm and depth. Encouraged patient to take deep breaths and cough. Lying on right side with the support of two pillows and head of bed elevated 30 degrees.

—P. Joyner, RN

DEVELOPING CLINICAL REASONING AND CLINICAL JUDGMENT

UNEXPECTED SITUATIONS AND ASSOCIATED INTERVENTIONS

- *While receiving PCA therapy, the patient's respiratory rate drops to 10 breaths/min, with a sedation score of 3 via sedation scale (Pasero Opioid-Induced Sedation Scale [POSS]):* Stop the PCA infusion if basal infusion is present. Notify the health care team. Discontinue the basal infusion; if no basal infusion is being used, then reduce the medication dosage. Increase the frequency of sedation and respiratory rate monitoring to every 15 minutes. Arouse the patient every 15 minutes and encourage deep breathing (Jungquist et al., 2017a; Pasero & McCaffery, 2011).
- *While receiving PCA therapy, the patient is somnolent, with a sedation score of 4 via sedation scale (POSS):* Stop the medication infusion immediately. Stimulate the patient; raise the head of bed to seated position (if not contraindicated) and talk to patient (Jungquist et al., 2017a). Call the rapid response team (RRT) (Jungquist et al., 2017a). Notify the health care team. Administer oxygen and an opioid antagonist, such as naloxone, based on facility policy (ISMP, 2017). The dose of naloxone is titrated to effect—reversing the oversedation and respiratory depression, not reversing analgesia (Morton & Fontaine, 2018).
- *The patient's IV infusion line becomes infiltrated:* Stop the PCA infusion and IV infusion. Remove the IV catheter and restart the IV line in another site. Once the site is established, resume the IV and PCA infusion. Provide site care to the infiltration site based on facility policy.
- *The patient's subcutaneous infusion site becomes infiltrated:* Stop the PCA infusion. Remove the administration device. Obtain new administration equipment and restart the infusion at another site. Once the site is established, resume the PCA infusion. Provide site care to the infiltration site based on facility policy.

SPECIAL CONSIDERATIONS

General Considerations

- A wide variety of PCA devices are available on the market. Check the manufacturer's instructions and facility policies before using any one device.
- Provide individualized patient and caregiver education appropriate to the duration of therapy and care setting, treatment options, the purpose of PCA therapy, frequency of monitoring, expected outcomes, precautions, potential side effects, symptoms to report, and how dose will be adjusted (Gorski et al., 2021).

(continued on page 664)

Skill 10-4 ▶ Caring for a Patient Receiving Patient-Controlled Analgesia *(continued)*

- All patients should be assessed for level of risk of opioid-induced advancing sedation and respiratory depression; the plan of care and monitoring strategies should be driven by reassessment according to level of risk (Jungquist et al., 2020).
- Continuous capnography and/or pulse oximetry has been suggested for use in all patients receiving PCA opioids for early detection of opioid-induced respiratory depression; continuous capnography should be used in all patients receiving supplemental oxygen (Fazio & Firestone, 2020; Khanna et al., 2020).
- Adults and children who are cognitively and physically able to use the PCA equipment and are able to understand that pressing a button can result in pain relief are appropriate candidates for PCA therapy (DiGiusto et al., 2014; Gorski et al., 2021; Pasero & McCaffery, 2011).
- Opioid analgesia via a continuous subcutaneous infusion is a safe, effective alternative when IV access is not available and oral analgesia is no longer possible. Candidates for subcutaneous infusion of analgesia are often patients requiring hospice and palliative care (Thomas & Barclay, 2015). Equipment consists of a small-gauge needle inserted subcutaneously, and an infusion pump and administration set that is clearly labeled *subcutaneous infusion*. This setup delivers the opioid in a small amount of fluid (Taylor et al., 2023). Nurses can initiate subcutaneous infusion therapy once competence has been validated. Assessment includes monitoring of vital signs, pain level, and the insertion site for leakage, bleeding, or other complications (Gorski et al., 2021).
- PCA by proxy refers to activation of the PCA dosing button by anyone other than the patient (Grissinger, 2019). PCA by proxy is not recommended (Grissinger, 2019; ISMP, 2016). PCA by proxy can cause serious analgesic overdoses resulting in oversedation, respiratory depression, and death (Grissinger, 2019; ISMP, 2016). Institutions must verify that they have protocols in place to protect against unauthorized PCA delivery and it is recommended that clear warning labels stating, "WARNING: BUTTON TO BE PRESSED ONLY BY THE PATIENT" be attached to PCA pumps and tubing (Grissinger, 2019; ISMP, 2016).
- Some facilities and health care agencies have developed clinical practice guidelines for authorized agent–controlled analgesia (AACA) for patients who are unable to independently utilize PCA (Cooney et al., 2013). In these cases, one family member or nurse is designated as the primary pain manager and *only* that person can press the PCA button for the patient (Benjenk et al., 2020). The patient and the caregiver must be assessed for appropriateness of use of AACA (Gorski et al., 2021). In the case of family members, the primary pain manager must be chosen

Box 10-2 | Guidelines for Safe Implementation of Authorized Agent–Controlled Analgesia

Authorized agent–controlled analgesia (AACA) can be implemented to provide prompt, safe, and effective pain relief for the patient who, because of cognitive or physical limitations, is unable to self-administer analgesics using an analgesic pump (Benjenk et al., 2020; Cooney et al., 2013; Gorski et al., 2021). Use the following tips as guidelines to ensure optimal patient comfort and safety when caring for patients receiving AACA.

- Limit the number of authorized agents to one at a given time; alternative authorized agents may be designated to provide respite and/or coverage.
- Use standard AACA medical order sets.
- Provide patient and family/caregiver education regarding the principles of AACA, requirements of an authorized agent, specific policies and procedures related to AACA, and the negative consequences of unauthorized activation of the analgesic infusion pump dosing button.

- Document the identity of the authorized agent(s) and caregiver-authorized agent, as well as education provided and feedback.
- Ensure that authorized agents only activate the dosing button if the patient is awake and/or the patient's words or behavior indicate that the patient is in pain or pain is anticipated. Authorized agents should verbalize an understanding of how to recognize pain, sedation, and respiratory depression.

Source: Adapted with permission from Cooney, M. F., Czarnecki, M., Dunwoody, C., Eksterowicz, N., Merkel, S., Oakes, L., & Wuhrman, E. (2013). American Society for Pain Management nursing position statement with clinical practice guidelines: Authorized agent controlled analgesia. *Pain Management Nursing, 14*(3), 176–181. https://doi.org/10.1016/j.pmn.2013.07.003

carefully and taught to assess for pain and the adverse effect of the medication (Gorski et al., 2021). In addition, nursing staff must be vigilant in assessing the patient's need for and response to the medication, following the same assessment guidelines previously discussed. It is very important to follow facility guidelines to ensure safe administration (Benjenk et al., 2020; Cooney et al., 2013; D'Arcy, 2013). Box 10-2 outlines guidelines for safe implementation of AACA.

- If using a device that provides continuous and bolus doses, the cumulative doses per hour should not exceed the total hourly dose prescribed by the health care provider.
- Encourage the patient to practice coughing and deep breathing to promote ventilation and prevent pooling of secretions.
- An opioid antagonist, such as naloxone, must be readily available in case the patient develops respiratory complications related to drug therapy. The dose of naloxone is titrated to effect—reversing the oversedation and respiratory depression, not reversing analgesia (Morton & Fontaine, 2018). If naloxone is administered, continue to closely assess the patient for oversedation and respiratory depression, as the half-life of naloxone (1.5 to 2 hours) is shorter than most opioids (Morton & Fontaine, 2018).

Infant and Child Considerations

- PCA can be an effective method of pain control for a child. When determining the appropriateness of this therapy for a child, consider the child's chronologic age and developmental level, ability to understand (cognitive level), and motor skills (Pasero & McCaffery, 2011). It is essential to assess each child individually and consider their developmental level and psychosocial factors in determining appropriate PCA use. The child must have the necessary intellect, manual dexterity, and strength to operate the device (Kyle & Carman, 2021).

Community-Based Care Considerations

- Be sure that the patient understands how to use the PCA device properly. Teach the patient how the device works, when to contact the health care provider, and signs and symptoms of adverse reactions and of drug tolerance.
- Provide individualized patient and caregiver education appropriate to the duration of therapy and care setting, treatment options, the purpose of PCA therapy, frequency of monitoring, expected outcomes, precautions, potential side effects, symptoms to report, and how dose will be adjusted (Gorski et al., 2021).
- Advise the patient, particularly those with preexisting cardiac disease and older adults, to change positions gradually to prevent orthostatic hypotension and syncope, which can result from use of an opioid analgesic (Chen & Ashburn, 2015).
- Ensure that a reliable adult is available who can provide backup assistance should the patient have difficulty.
- Collaborate to obtain a referral to a community-based health care provider team to continue teaching and provide assessment of the therapy.

EVIDENCE FOR PRACTICE ▶

AUTHORIZED AGENT–CONTROLLED ANALGESIA

Patient-controlled analgesia is commonly used for pain management. However, many patients are unable to use patient-controlled analgesia due to physical or cognitive limitations (Benjenk et al., 2020). Is authorized agent–controlled analgesia, in which a nurse or designated care giver activates the analgesia device, an effective option for management of pain in these patients?

Related Evidence
Benjenk, I., Messing, J., Lenihan, M. J., Hernandez, M., Amdur, R., Sirajuddin, S., Davison, D., Schroeder, M. E., & Sarani, B. (2020). Authorized agent-controlled analgesia for pain management in critically ill adult patients. *Critical Care Nurse, 40*(3), 31–36. https://doi.org/10.4037/ccn2020323

The aim of this retrospective pilot study was to evaluate the efficacy of authorized agent–controlled analgesia in critically ill adult patients. Authorized agent–controlled analgesia (AACA) was initiated as a pain management intervention for 46 patients in a medical-surgical adult intensive care unit. Pain was measured using the Critical-Care Pain Observation Tool for

(continued on page 666)

Skill 10-4 ▶ Caring for a Patient Receiving Patient-Controlled Analgesia *(continued)*

the 24 hours before and after initiation of AACA, administered by nurses only. The mean pain score from before to after initiation decreased 69% ($P < .001$). When the results were controlled for time, sedative administration, and opioid medication administration, the effect of AACA initiation on pain scores remained significant ($P < .001$). The researchers concluded the use of AACA is associated with a reduction in pain in critically ill patients and suggested AACA as an effective means of providing analgesia in this patient population.

Relevance to Nursing Practice

Nurses have an important role in providing interventions to assist patients in controlling pain and improving comfort. Nurses have a responsibility to be informed and knowledgeable regarding all methods of analgesia and work to provide a plan of care that addresses individual patient needs.

EVIDENCE FOR PRACTICE ▶

ASSESSMENT OF OPIOID-INDUCED SEDATION

Opioids are used as part of the plan of care for pain management for patients in a variety of circumstances. There is a need to balance the achievement of adequate pain control while avoiding adverse effects, such as opioid-induced sedation and respiratory depression. Nurses must carefully monitor for oversedation and respiratory depression (Taylor et al., 2023). Assessment should include use of a sedation scale. There are several tools available to support these assessments. What is the evidence supporting use of these tools?

Related Evidence

Hall, K. R., & Stanley, A. Y. (2019). Literature review: Assessment of opioid-related sedation and the Pasero Opioid Sedation Scale. *Journal of PeriAnesthesia Nursing, 34*(1), 132–142. https://doi.org/10.1016/j.jopan.2017.12.009

The purpose of this literature review was to examine sedation scales and monitoring practices, specifically evaluating utilization of the Pasero Opioid Sedation Scale (POSS) in the clinical setting. Publications from January 2009 to June 2016 were searched using PubMed, the Cumulative Index to Nursing and Allied Health Literature, and Google Scholar Databases. Search terms included monitor, monitoring, opioid-induced, Pasero Opioid Sedation Scale, respiratory depression, and sedation. MeSH terms used were monitoring, physiologic; analgesics, opioid; respiratory insufficiency/complications/nursing, and prevention and control. The initial literature search identified 14 articles for review and analysis. Six articles were selected for review based on titles and abstracts: three descriptive survey-based design, two quasi-experimental design, and one evidence-based practice project. Of the six, two articles evaluated the safety and efficacy of the POSS in a clinical environment; one evidence-based practice project standardized the way nurses assess for and monitor opioid-induced sedation in general care areas; one investigated the validity and reliability of three sedation scales, including the POSS; and two studies evaluated monitoring practices related to sedation and respiratory depression. The researchers concluded there was a need for further research, as there was limited publication regarding implementation of a POSS in the PACU and other clinical settings. The authors also concluded additional research or evidence-based practice projects should be conducted to evaluate the tool's application to the general population, improved outcomes, and financial impact. The researchers suggested that, overall, the literature supports the goal of the POSS, citing the potential for fewer opioid-related adverse events and increased confidence among nursing staff.

Relevance to Nursing Practice

Nurses have an important role in monitoring for adverse effects related to health care interventions. Use of appropriate assessment tools can support critical assessments by nurses to support clinical reasoning and clinical judgment, contributing to delivery of safe, effective nursing care.

Skill 10-5 ▶ Caring for a Patient Receiving Epidural Analgesia

Epidural analgesia can be used to provide pain relief during the immediate postoperative period (particularly after thoracic, abdominal, orthopedic, and vascular surgery), procedural pain, trauma pain, and for chronic pain situations (Schrieber, 2015). Epidural pain management is also being used with infants and children (Gai et al., 2020; Kyle & Carman, 2021). Spinal analgesia using opioids has a longer duration than other routes and significantly less opioid is needed to achieve affective pain relief (Morton & Fontaine, 2018). Absolute contraindications include an allergic response to analgesics being used, coagulation disorders, anticoagulants, and localized infection or sepsis; relative contraindications include hypotension or compromised cardiovascular system, increased intracranial pressure, spinal abnormalities, and certain neurological conditions (Taylor et al., 2023). The anesthesiologist or radiologist usually inserts the catheter in the mid-lumbar region into the epidural space that exists between the walls of the vertebral canal and the dura mater or outermost connective tissue membrane surrounding the spinal cord. For temporary therapy, the catheter exits directly over the spine, and the tubing is positioned over the patient's shoulder with the end of the catheter taped to the chest. For long-term therapy, the catheter may be tunneled subcutaneously and made to exit on the side of the body or on the abdomen (Figure 1).

The epidural analgesia can be administered using medications such as preservative-free fentanyl, hydromorphone, or morphine, combined with a local anesthetic (bupivacaine, levobupivacaine or ropivacaine) as a bolus dose (either one time or intermittently), via a continuous infusion pump, or by a patient-controlled epidural analgesia (PCEA) pump (Morton & Fontaine, 2018; Polomano et al., 2017; Schrieber, 2015; Wong & Lim, 2018). Epidural catheters used for the management of acute pain are typically removed within 5 days after surgery, when oral medication can be substituted for pain relief (Gai et al., 2020; Galligan, 2020). Additional information specific to PCA administration is discussed in Skill 10-4.

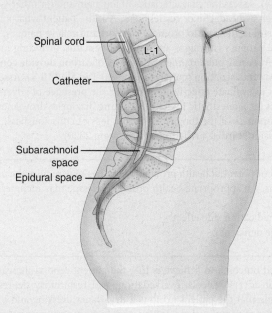

FIGURE 1. Placement of an epidural catheter for long-term use.

DELEGATION CONSIDERATIONS

The care related to epidural analgesia is not delegated to assistive personnel (AP). Depending on the state's nurse practice act and the organization's policies and procedures, specific aspects of the care related to epidural analgesia, such as monitoring the infusion and assessment of patient response, may be delegated to licensed practical/vocational nurses (LPN/LVNs). The decision to delegate must be based on careful analysis of the patient's needs and circumstances as well as the qualifications of the person to whom the task is being delegated. Refer to the Delegation Guidelines in Appendix A.

(continued on page 668)

Skill 10-5 ▶ Caring for a Patient Receiving Epidural Analgesia   *(continued)*

EQUIPMENT

- Infusion device
- Epidural infusion tubing
- Prescribed epidural analgesic solutions
- Electronic medication administration record (eMAR) or medication administration record (MAR)
- Pain assessment tool and/or measurement scale
- Transparent dressing or gauze pads
- Labels for epidural infusion line
- Tape
- Emergency drugs and equipment, such as naloxone, oxygen, endotracheal intubation set, handheld resuscitation bag, per facility policy
- Gloves
- Additional PPE, as indicated
- Additional PCA equipment, based on prescribed administration; refer to Skill 10-4

ASSESSMENT

Review the patient's health record and plan of care for specific instructions related to epidural analgesia therapy, including the prescribed intervention and conditions indicating the need for therapy. Check the health record for the prescribed drug; if epidural PCA, check the initial loading dose, dose for self-administration, and lockout interval. Review the patient's history for conditions that might contraindicate therapy, such as an allergic response to analgesics being used, coagulation disorders, anticoagulants, and localized infection or sepsis; relative contraindications include hypotension or compromised cardiovascular system, increased intracranial pressure, spinal abnormalities, and certain neurological conditions (Schrieber, 2015; Taylor et al., 2023). Check to ensure proper functioning of the infusion device. Assess the patient's understanding of epidural analgesia therapy and the rationale for its use.

Assess the patient's level of consciousness and vital signs. Assess the patient's level of discomfort and pain using an appropriate assessment tool and pain scale (refer to Fundamentals Review 10-1 through 10-4). Assess the characteristics of any pain and for other symptoms that often occur with the pain, such as headache or restlessness. Ask the patient what interventions have and have not been successful in the past to promote comfort and relieve pain.

Assess the patient's vital signs and respiratory status, including rate, depth, and rhythm, oxygen saturation level using pulse oximetry and level of carbon dioxide concentration using capnography. Assess the patient's sedation score (see Table 10-1 in Skill 10-4). Assess the patient's response to the intervention to evaluate effectiveness and for the presence of adverse effects. Assess for signs and symptoms of local anesthetic toxicity, including dizziness, drowsiness, tinnitus, circumoral numbness and numbness of the tongue, agitation, loss of consciousness, seizure, bradycardia/tachycardia, hypotension, cardiac arrhythmias (Galligan, 2020).

ACTUAL OR POTENTIAL HEALTH PROBLEMS AND NEEDS

Many actual or potential health problems or issues may require the use of this skill as part of related interventions. An appropriate health problem or issue may include:

- Acute pain
- Risk for medication side effect
- Knowledge deficiency

OUTCOME IDENTIFICATION AND PLANNING

The expected outcome to achieve is that the patient reports increased comfort and/or decreased pain without adverse effects, oversedation, and respiratory depression. Other appropriate outcomes include that the patient exhibits a dry, intact dressing and a catheter exit site free of signs and symptoms of complications, injury, or infection, and the patient displays an understanding of use of the therapy and the reason for its use.

IMPLEMENTATION

ACTION	RATIONALE
1. Gather equipment. Check the medication prescribed against the original order in the health care record, depending on facility policy and the medication order system in place. Clarify any inconsistencies. Check the patient's health record for allergies.	The prescription is the legal record of prescribed medication interventions. This comparison helps to identify errors that may have occurred when orders were transcribed. Computer provider order-entry (CPOE) systems allow prescribers to send electronic medication prescriptions directly to the pharmacy located in a health care facility and to outpatient pharmacies.

ACTION	**RATIONALE**
2. Know the actions, special nursing considerations, safe dose ranges, purpose of administration, and adverse effects of the medications to be administered. Consider the appropriateness of the medication for this patient.	This knowledge aids the nurse in evaluating the therapeutic effect of the medication in relation to the patient's disorder and can also be used to educate the patient about the medication.
3. Prepare the medication syringe or other reservoir for administration, based on facility policy (see Chapter 5 for additional information).	Proper preparation and administration prevent errors.
4. Perform hand hygiene and put on PPE, if indicated.	Hand hygiene and PPE prevent the spread of microorganisms. PPE is required based on transmission precautions.
5. Identify the patient.	Identifying the patient ensures that the right patient receives the intervention and helps prevent errors.
6. Show the patient the device, and explain the function of the device and the reason for its use. Explain the purpose and action of the medication to the patient.	Explanation encourages patient understanding and engagement and reduces apprehension.
7. Close the door to the room or pull the bedside curtain. **Identify the patient. Compare the information with the eMAR/MAR. The patient should be identified using at least two of the following methods** (The Joint Commission, 2021). Refer to Chapter 5 for additional information related to medication administration.	Closing the door or curtain provides for patient privacy. Identifying the patient ensures the right patient receives the medications and helps prevent errors. The patient's room number or physical location is not used as an identifier (The Joint Commission, 2021). Replace the identification band if it is missing or inaccurate in any way.
8. Complete necessary assessments before administering the medication. Check allergy bracelet or ask the patient about allergies. Assess the patient's pain using an appropriate assessment tool and measurement scale (see Fundamentals Review 10-1 through 10-4).	Assessment is a prerequisite to administration of medications. Accurate assessment is necessary to guide treatment and relief interventions and to evaluate the effectiveness of pain control measures.
9. **Have an ampule of 0.4-mg naloxone and a syringe at the bedside, according to facility policy.**	Naloxone reverses the respiratory depressant effect of opioids.
10. **Check the label on the prefilled drug syringe or reservoir with the medication record and patient identification, verifying the drug, concentration, dose, and rate of infusion. Obtain verification of information from a second clinician, according to facility policy.** Scan the bar code on the package, if required.	This action verifies that the correct drug and dosage will be administered to the correct patient. An independent double check by two clinicians is recommended prior to initiation of the PCA and when the syringe, solution container, drug, or rate is changed (Gorski et al., 2021). Confirmation of information by a second clinician helps prevent errors.
11. Scan the patient's barcode on the identification band, if required (The Joint Commission, 2021). **Based on facility policy, the third check of the medication label may occur at this point. If so, read the label and recheck the label with the eMAR/MAR before administering the medications to the patient.**	Scanning of the patient's barcode on identification band provides an additional check to ensure that the medication is given to the right patient. Many facilities require the *third* check to occur at the bedside, after identifying the patient and before administration. If facility policy directs the *third* check at this time, this *third* check ensures accuracy and helps prevent errors.
12. After the catheter has been inserted and the infusion initiated by the anesthesiologist or radiologist, **verify the drug, concentration, dose, and rate of infusion; if epidural PCA is in use, verify the dose interval, and lockout interval. Obtain verification of information from a second clinician, according to facility policy.**	These actions ensure that the appropriate drug dosage will be administered. An independent double check by two clinicians is recommended prior to initiation of the PCA and when the syringe, solution container, drug, or rate is changed (Gorski et al., 2021). Confirmation of information by a second clinician helps prevent errors.

(continued on page 670)

Skill 10-5 ▶ Caring for a Patient Receiving Epidural Analgesia *(continued)*

ACTION	RATIONALE

ACTION

13. Tape all connection sites. **Label the bag, tubing, and pump apparatus "For Epidural Infusion Only." Do not administer any other opioid or adjuvant drugs without the approval of the clinician responsible for the prescribed epidural analgesia.**

14. Put on gloves. Assess the catheter exit site and apply a transparent dressing over the catheter insertion site, if not already in place (Figure 2). Secure the catheter and tubing, based on facility policy. Remove gloves and additional PPE, if used. Perform hand hygiene.

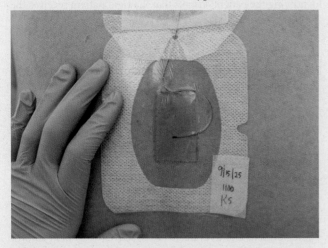

15. Refer to Skill 10-4 for additional considerations if the epidural analgesia is being administered as PCA.

16. Initiate continuous capnography and/or pulse oximetry, based on facility policy.

17. Monitor the infusion rate according to facility policy. Assess the patient's response to the medication: Assess the patient's pain at least every 4 hours or more often, as needed, based on patient's individual risk factors. Monitor vital signs, especially respiratory status, including respiratory rate, depth, and quality and oxygen saturation every 2 to 4 hours or more often, as needed, based on patient's individual risk factors and situation.

18. Assess the patient's response to the medication: Assess the patient's sedation score (see Table 10-1 in Skill 10-4) and end-tidal carbon dioxide level (capnography) at least every 4 hours or more often, as needed, based on patient's individual risk factors.

RATIONALE

Taping prevents accidental dislodgement. Labeling prevents inadvertent administration of other IV medications through this setup (Morton & Fontaine, 2018). Additional opioid or adjuvant medication may potentiate the action of the epidural analgesic, increasing the risk for respiratory depression (Kyle & Carman, 2021).

The transparent dressing protects the site while still allowing assessment. Securing of catheter and tubing prevents accidental displacement and removal. Proper removal of PPE reduces the risk for infection transmission and contamination of other items. Hand hygiene reduces transmission of microorganisms.

FIGURE 2. Assessing the epidural catheter exit site.

Patient-controlled analgesia (PCA) requires additional patient education and nursing intervention to provide safe nursing care and promote optimal patient outcomes. Refer to Skill 10-4.

Continuous capnography and/or pulse oximetry has been suggested for use in all patients receiving PCA opioids for early detection of opioid-induced respiratory depression; continuous capnography should be used in all patients receiving supplemental oxygen (Fazio & Firestone, 2020; Khanna et al., 2020).

Monitoring the infusion rate prevents incorrect administration of the medication. The plan of care and monitoring strategies should be driven by reassessment according to level of risk (Jungquist et al., 2020). Continued assessment at frequent intervals helps evaluate the effectiveness of the drug and reduce the risk for complications (Fazio & Firestone, 2020; Gorski et al., 2021; Jungquist et al., 2017a, 2017b).

The plan of care and monitoring strategies should be driven by reassessment according to level of risk (Jungquist et al., 2020). Sedation occurs before clinically significant respiratory depression (Hall & Stanley, 2019). Respiratory depression can occur with the use of opioid analgesics (Fazio & Firestone, 2020; Hall & Stanley, 2019). Capnography provides an earlier warning of respiratory depression as compared to continuous oximetry (Casey, 2015; Gorski et al., 2021; Jungquist et al., 2017a, 2017b).

ACTION	**RATIONALE**
	Opioids can depress the respiratory center in the medulla. A change in the level of consciousness is usually the first sign of altered respiratory function.
19. Keep the head of bed elevated 30 degrees unless contraindicated.	Elevation of the patient's head minimizes upward migration of the opioid in the spinal cord, thus decreasing the risk for respiratory depression.
20. Monitor the patient's blood pressure and pulse.	Hypotension can result from the use of epidural analgesia (NHS, Hull University Teaching Hospitals, 2018).
21. Monitor urinary output and assess for bladder distention.	Epidural analgesia can cause urinary retention (NHS, Hull University Teaching Hospitals, 2018).
22. Assess motor strength and sensation every 4 hours or as specified by facility policy.	The catheter may migrate into the intrathecal space and allow opioids to block the transmission of nerve impulses completely through the spinal cord to the brain.
23. Monitor for adverse effects (pruritus, nausea, decreased gastric motility, headache, constipation, and vomiting) (Gai et al., 2020; Galligan, 2020; Kyle & Carman, 2021; UHN, 2017). Monitor for signs and symptoms of local anesthetic toxicity, including dizziness, drowsiness, tinnitus, circumoral numbness and numbness of the tongue, agitation, loss of consciousness, seizure, bradycardia/tachycardia, hypotension, cardiac arrhythmias (Galligan, 2020).	Opioids may spread into the trigeminal nerve, causing itching, or resulting in nausea and vomiting owing to slowed gastrointestinal function or stimulation of a chemoreceptor trigger zone in the brain (Galligan, 2020). Medications are available to treat these adverse effects. Neonates; infants; older adults; and patients with chronic renal, cardiac, or liver disease are at increased risk of local anesthetic toxicity (El-Boghdadly et al., 2018).
24. Assess for signs of infection, hematoma, or abscess at the insertion site.	Inflammation or local infection or hematoma can develop at the catheter insertion site (Taylor et al., 2023).
25. Assess the catheter-site dressing for drainage, based on facility policy. Notify the anesthesia provider or pain management team immediately of any abnormalities. Change the dressing over the catheter exit site per facility policy using aseptic technique. Change the infusion tubing as specified by facility policy.	The catheter-site dressing should remain clean, dry, and intact. Abnormalities in the dressing may indicate leakage of cerebrospinal fluid or catheter dislodgement. Dressing and tubing changes using aseptic technique reduce the risk for infection.
26. If using epidural PCA, make sure the patient control (dosing button) is within the patient's reach.	Easy access to the control is essential for the patients to use the device.
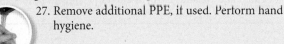 27. Remove additional PPE, if used. Perform hand hygiene.	Proper removal of PPE reduces the risk for infection transmission and contamination of other items. Hand hygiene prevents transmission of microorganisms.

EVALUATION

The expected outcomes have been met when the patient verbalizes pain relief and/or increased comfort; the patient exhibits a dry, intact dressing and a catheter exit site free of signs and symptoms of complications, injury, or infection; and the patient verbalizes an understanding of the use of the therapy and the reason for its use.

DOCUMENTATION

Guidelines Document the date and time the epidural therapy was initiated, catheter patency; the condition of the insertion site and dressing; sedation score, oxygen saturation, vital signs, and other assessment information; the infusion rate and solution; any tubing change; any other analgesics administered; and the patient's response to the therapy. Document patient teaching and patient's response.

(continued on page 672)

Skill 10-5 ▶ Caring for a Patient Receiving Epidural Analgesia *(continued)*

Sample Documentation

> 6/3/25 0935 Continuous morphine infusion via epidural catheter in place; see medication administration record. Exit site clean and slightly moist. Transparent dressing in place. Patient rates pain 2/10. Temperature 98.2°F; pulse, 76 beats/min; respirations 16 breaths/min and effortless; blood pressure, 110/70 mm Hg. Pulse oximetry 96% on oxygen via nasal cannula at 2 L/min; partial pressure end-tidal CO_2 ($PetCO_2$) 38%. Patient alert and quickly responds to verbal stimuli. Sedation score of 1. Bladder nonpalpable; urine output of 100 mL over the last 2 hours. Denies nausea, vomiting, or itching. Able to detect sensation of cold in lower extremities bilaterally. Able to wiggle toes and flex and dorsiflex feet bilaterally. Lower extremity muscle strength equal and moderately strong bilaterally.
>
> —T. James, RN

DEVELOPING CLINICAL REASONING AND CLINICAL JUDGMENT

UNEXPECTED SITUATIONS AND ASSOCIATED INTERVENTIONS

- *While receiving epidural analgesia, the patient's sedation score drops below 3 (Pasero Opioid-Induced Sedation Scale [POSS]) and/or has a respiratory rate of <10 breaths or has shallow respirations:* Immediately notify the anesthesiologist/health care team. Stop the epidural infusion, if indicated, according to facility procedure. Encourage the patient to take deep, slow breaths, if possible. Prepare to administer oxygen and an opioid antagonist, such as naloxone, via a peripheral IV site.
- *Patient demonstrates weakness and loss of sensation in the lower extremities while receiving epidural analgesia:* Reassess the patient's lower extremities for motor and sensory function. If positive for sensorimotor loss, notify the health care team and expect to decrease or stop the epidural infusion and possible removal of the catheter.
- *While receiving epidural analgesia, the patient suddenly develops a severe headache. Inspection of the catheter site reveals clear drainage on the dressing:* Stop the epidural infusion and notify the health care team immediately. The catheter may have migrated and entered the dura.
- *Patient demonstrates signs/symptoms of local anesthetic toxicity:* Immediately stop the epidural infusion; assess the patient's airway, breathing, and circulation and address any abnormal findings; support the patient with high-glow oxygen therapy; and notify the health care team (Galligan, 2020). Anticipate administration of lipid emulsion to act as an antidote to the local anesthetic (The Association of Anaesthetists of Great Britain and Ireland, 2010, as cited in Galligan, 2020, p. 82).

SPECIAL CONSIDERATIONS

General Considerations

- Epidural infusion administration sets have no injection ports to prevent accidental infusion of other drugs via the infusion (Morton & Fontaine, 2018).
- Clearly label the medication infusion bag, tubing, and pump apparatus "For Epidural Infusion Only" to prevent accidental infusion of other drugs with preservatives that could cause neural damage, resulting in paralysis or death (Morton & Fontaine, 2018, p. 144).
- Notify the anesthesiologist or pain management team immediately if the patient exhibits any of the following: respiratory rate below 10 breaths/min, continued report of unmanaged pain, leakage at the insertion site, fever, inability to void, paresthesia, itching, or headache or any other questionable assessment findings (Schreiber, 2015).
- Do not administer other sedatives or analgesics, unless ordered by the anesthesiologist or pain management team, to avoid oversedation.
- Always ensure that the patient receiving epidural analgesia has a peripheral IV line in place, either as a continuous IV infusion or as an intermittent infusion device, to allow immediate administration of emergency drugs, if warranted.
- An opioid antagonist, such as naloxone, must be readily available in case the patient develops respiratory complications related to drug therapy. The dose of naloxone is titrated to effect—reversing the oversedation and respiratory depression, not reversing analgesia (Morton & Fontaine, 2018). If naloxone is administered, continue to closely assess the patient for

oversedation and respiratory depression, as the half-life of naloxone (1.5 to 2 hours) is shorter than most opioids (Morton & Fontaine, 2018).
- Keep in mind that drugs given via the epidural route diffuse slowly and can cause adverse reactions, including excessive sedation, for up to 12 hours after the infusion has been discontinued.
- PCEA catheter removal generally occurs within 5 days after insertion; if the epidural catheter has been tunneled under the skin after insertion, it can remain in place for up to 10 days (Galligan, 2020). Typically, an anesthesiologist orders analgesics and removes the catheter. However, facility policy may allow a specially trained nurse to remove the catheter. Once the epidural catheter has been removed, continue sensory and motor assessments for 24 hours or longer, depending on facility policy (Galligan, 2020).
- Be aware that no resistance should be felt during the removal of an epidural catheter. Assess the catheter to confirm the catheter tip is intact. Assess the exit site for bleeding and infection (Schreiber, 2015).
- Before removal of the epidural catheter, it is important to consider the patient's current level of pain management and ensure that appropriate alternative analgesia has been planned to maintain adequate pain management (Galligan, 2020).

Infant and Child Considerations
- When epidural analgesia is administered, additional opioid analgesics are not administered in order to prevent complications such as respiratory depression, pruritus, nausea, vomiting, and urinary retention (Kyle & Carman, 2021, p. 410).

Community-Based Care Considerations
- If the patient is discharged from a care setting to a community-based setting (e.g., home) soon after removal of the epidural catheter, provide patient/family/caregiver education regarding ongoing after care and safety advice related to potential late side effects, as sensory and motor effects are possible for 24 hours or longer after catheter removal (Galligan, 2020; Macintyre & Schug, 2015, as cited in Galligan, 2020, p. 81).

Skill 10-6 ▶ Caring for a Patient Receiving Continuous Wound Perfusion Pain Management

Continuous wound perfusion or infiltration management systems are one strategy to be considered as a component of multimodal analgesia (Cinar et al., 2021; Mijovski et al., 2020; Polomano et al., 2017). **Continuous wound perfusion pain management systems** deliver a continuous infusion of local analgesia to intraarticular and wound sites (Polomano et al., 2017). These systems are used as an adjuvant in the management of postoperative pain in a wide range of surgical procedures (Cinar et al., 2021; Porter et al., 2021; Singh et al., 2017). The system consists of a balloon-type pump filled with local anesthetic and a catheter placed near an incision, in a nerve close to a surgical site, or in a wound bed (Figure 1). The catheter is placed during surgery and is not sutured into place; the site dressing holds it in place. The catheter delivers a consistent flow rate and uniform distribution to the surgical site. Continuous wound perfusion may also be delivered via patient-controlled analgesia systems (Mijovski et al., 2020).

Continuous wound perfusion catheters decrease postoperative pain and opioid use and side effects and have been associated with decreased postoperative nausea and vomiting as well as increased and earlier patient mobility (Cinar et al. 2021; Li et al., 2020; Mijovksi et al., 2020; Porter et al., 2021; Singh et al., 2017). The following skill outlines general guidelines for the care of a patient with a continuous wound perfusion pain management system with a balloon-type pump. There are many different systems and applications of this intervention. **Nurses need to be familiar with the particular device and system in use by their patient and to refer to the specific manufacturer's recommendations and facility policies for use.**

(continued on page 674)

Skill 10-6 ▶ Caring for a Patient Receiving Continuous Wound Perfusion Pain Management *(continued)*

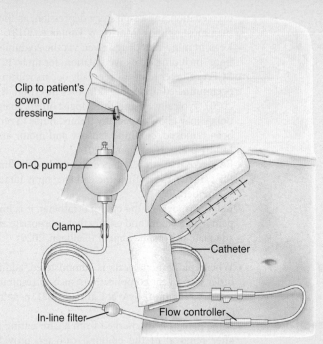

Clip to patient's gown or dressing

On-Q pump

Clamp

In-line filter

Catheter

Flow controller

FIGURE 1. Wound perfusion pain management system consists of a balloon (pump), filter, and catheter that deliver a specific amount of prescribed local anesthetic at the rate determined by the prescribing health care provider. (*Source:* Redrawn from I-Flow Corporation, a Kimberly-Clark Health Care Company, with permission.)

DELEGATION CONSIDERATIONS	Care related to continuous wound perfusion pain management systems is not delegated to assistive personnel (AP). Depending on the state's nurse practice act and the organization's policies and procedures, specific aspects of the care related to continuous wound perfusion pain management systems, such as monitoring the infusion and assessment of patient response, may be delegated to licensed practical/vocational nurses (LPN/LVNs). The decision to delegate must be based on careful analysis of the patient's needs and circumstances as well as the qualifications of the person to whom the task is being delegated. Refer to the Delegation Guidelines in Appendix A.
EQUIPMENT	• Electronic medication administration record (eMAR) or medication administration record (MAR) • Pain assessment tool and pain scale • Gauze and tape, or other dressing, based on facility policy • Gloves • Additional PPE, as indicated
ASSESSMENT	Review the patient's health record and plan of care for specific instructions related to continuous wound perfusion analgesia therapy, including the prescribed intervention and conditions indicating the need for therapy. Review the patient's history for allergy to the prescribed medication. Assess the patient's understanding of a continuous wound perfusion pain management system and the rationale for its use. Assess the patient's level of discomfort and pain using an appropriate assessment tool and pain scale (refer to Fundamentals Review 10-1 through 10-4). Assess the characteristics of any pain. Assess for other symptoms that often occur with the pain, such as headache or restlessness. Assess the surgical site (see Chapter 8). Ask the patient what interventions have and have not been successful in the past to promote comfort and relieve pain. Assess for signs of adverse effect that require immediate action: increase in pain; fever, chills, sweats; bowel or bladder changes; difficulty breathing; redness, warmth, discharge, or excessive bleeding from the catheter site; pain, swelling, or a large bruise around the catheter site; dizziness or

lightheadedness; blurred vision; ringing or buzzing in the ears; metal taste in the mouth; numbness and/or tingling around the mouth, fingers or toes; or drowsiness or confusion (Avanos Medical, 2018d).

Assess the catheter insertion–site dressing (see Chapter 8). Assess the patient's vital signs and respiratory status, including rate, depth, and rhythm, and oxygen saturation level using pulse oximetry. Assess the patient's response to the intervention to evaluate its effectiveness and for the presence of adverse effects.

ACTUAL OR POTENTIAL HEALTH PROBLEMS AND NEEDS	Many actual or potential health problems or issues may require the use of this skill as part of related interventions. An appropriate health problem or issue may include: • Acute pain • Knowledge deficiency • Infection risk
OUTCOME IDENTIFICATION AND PLANNING	The expected outcome to achieve is that the patient reports increased comfort and/or decreased pain without adverse effects. Other appropriate outcomes may include that the patient exhibits a dry, intact dressing with the continuous wound perfusion system catheter in place; the patient remains free from infection; and the patient demonstrates an understanding of the functioning of the wound perfusion system and the reason for its use.

IMPLEMENTATION

ACTION

1. Check the medication prescribed against the original health care provider's order, depending on facility policy and the medication order system in place. Clarify any inconsistencies. Check the patient's health record for allergies.

2. Know the actions, special nursing considerations, safe dose ranges, purpose of administration, and adverse effects of the medications to be administered. Consider the appropriateness of the medication for this patient.

3. Perform hand hygiene and put on PPE, if indicated.

4. Identify the patient.

5. Close the door to the room or pull the bedside curtain.

6. Assess the patient's pain using an appropriate assessment tool and measurement scale (see Fundamentals Review 10-1 through 10-4). Administer postoperative analgesic, if necessary, as ordered.

7. Check the medication label attached to the pain management system balloon. Compare it with the health care provider's order and eMAR or MAR, per facility policy. Assess patient for signs of adverse reaction. Refer to discussion in the previous Assessment section. Assess the patient's vital signs.

RATIONALE

The prescription is the legal record of prescribed medication interventions. This comparison helps to identify errors that may have occurred when orders were transcribed. Computer provider order-entry (CPOE) systems allow prescribers to send electronic medication prescriptions directly to the pharmacy located in a health care facility and to outpatient pharmacies.

This knowledge aids the nurse in evaluating the therapeutic effect of the medication in relation to the patient's disorder and can also be used to educate the patient about the medication.

Hand hygiene and PPE prevent the spread of microorganisms. PPE is required based on transmission precautions.

Identifying the patient ensures that the right patient receives the intervention and helps prevent errors.

Closing the door or curtain provides for patient privacy.

Continuous wound perfusion pain management is an adjuvant therapy; patients may require postoperative pain medication, with reduced frequency. Accurate assessment is necessary to guide treatment and relief interventions and to evaluate the effectiveness of pain control measures.

Checking the medication label with the order and MAR ensures correct therapy for the patient. These symptoms may indicate local anesthetic toxicity (Avanos Medical, 2018d). Changes in vital signs may indicate adverse effect.

(*continued on page 676*)

Skill 10-6 ▶ Caring for a Patient Receiving Continuous Wound Perfusion Pain Management *(continued)*

ACTION

8. Put on gloves. Assess the wound perfusion system. Inspect tubing for kinks; check that the white tubing clamps are open (see Figure 1). Check filter in tubing, which should be unrestricted and free from tape (see Figure 1).

9. Check the flow controller to ensure it is in contact with the patient's skin. Tape in place, as necessary (see Figure 1).

10. Check the insertion-site dressing. Ensure that it is intact. Assess for leakage and dislodgement. Assess for redness, warmth, swelling, pain at site, and drainage.

11. Review the device with the patient. Review the function of the device and reason for its use. Reinforce the purpose and action of the medication to the patient. If the device is used in the community setting or the patient will be discharged with the device in place, provide patient teaching regarding use. Refer to the discussion in the Community-Based Care Considerations section at the end of the Skill.

To Remove the Catheter

12. Check to ensure that infusion is complete. Infusion is complete when the delivery time has passed, and the balloon is no longer inflated.

13. Perform hand hygiene. Identify the patient. Put on gloves. Remove the catheter-site dressing. Loosen adhesive skin closure strips at the catheter site.

14. Grasp the catheter close to the patient's skin at the insertion site. Gently pull catheter to remove. Catheter should be easy to remove and not painful. Do not tug or quickly pull on the catheter during removal. Check the distal end of the catheter for the black marking.

15. Cover the puncture site with a dry dressing, according to facility policy.

16. Dispose of the balloon, tubing, and catheter, according to facility policy.

17. Remove gloves and additional PPE, if used. Perform hand hygiene.

RATIONALE

Gloves prevent contact with blood and body fluids. Tubing must be unclamped and free of kinks and/or crimping to maintain consistent flow of analgesic. Tape over filter interferes with properly functioning system.

Checking the flow restrictor for adequate contact ensures accurate flow rate.

Transparent dressing holds the catheter in place. Dressing must stay in place to prevent accidental dislodgement or removal. These symptoms may indicate infection.

Explanation encourages patient understanding and engagement and reduces apprehension.

Depending on the size and volume of the balloon, the infusion typically lasts 2 to 5 days. Infusion time should be recorded in the operative note or postoperative instructions. The balloon will no longer appear full, the outside bag will be flat, and a hard tube can be felt in the middle of the balloon (Avanos Medical, 2015).

Hand hygiene and use of gloves reduce the risk of infection transmission. Identifying the patient ensures that the right patient receives the intervention and helps prevent errors. Loosening of materials allows the catheter to be free of constraints.

Gentle removal prevents patient discomfort and accidental breakage of the catheter (Avanos Medical, 2018e). Checking for the black mark at the distal end ensures the entire catheter was removed (Avanos Medical, 2018e).

Covering the wound prevents contamination.

Proper disposal reduces the risk for infection transmission and contamination of other items.

Proper removal of PPE reduces the risk for infection transmission and contamination of other items. Hand hygiene prevents transmission of microorganisms.

EVALUATION

The expected outcomes have been met when the patient reports increased comfort and/or decreased pain without adverse effects; the patient exhibits a dry, intact dressing with the continuous wound perfusion system catheter in place; the patient remains free from infection; and the patient demonstrates an understanding of the functioning of the wound perfusion system and the reason for its use.

DOCUMENTATION

Guidelines

Document system patency, the condition of the insertion site, system, and dressing, vital signs and assessment information, analgesics administered, and the patient's response to the therapy.

Sample Documentation

> 6/3/25 0935 Continuous wound perfusion pain management system in place. Exit site clean and dry. Transparent dressing in place. Temperature 98.7°F; pulse, 82 beats/min; respirations, 14 breaths/min and effortless; blood pressure, 112/74 mm Hg. Pulse oximetry 96% on room air. Patient alert and quickly responds to verbal stimuli. Denies nausea, vomiting, vision changes, paresthesias, dizziness, or ringing in ears. Patient rates pain in RLE 3/10. Ibuprofen 800 mg po given as ordered.
>
> *—T. James, RN*
>
> 6/3/20 51035 Patient reports pain in RLE 1/10. OOB to ambulate length of hall with wife.
> *—T. James, RN*

DEVELOPING CLINICAL REASONING AND CLINICAL JUDGMENT

UNEXPECTED SITUATIONS AND ASSOCIATED INTERVENTIONS

- *Patient reports and/or your assessment identifies the following symptoms:* increase in pain; fever, chills, sweats; bowel or bladder changes; difficulty breathing; redness, warmth, discharge, or excessive bleeding from the catheter site; pain, swelling, or a large bruise around the catheter site; dizziness or lightheadedness; blurred vision; ringing or buzzing in the ears; metal taste in the mouth; numbness and/or tingling around the mouth, fingers or toes; or drowsiness or confusion (Avanos Medical, 2018d). Close the clamp on the system tubing to stop the infusion. Report the symptoms to the health care team immediately. The presence of any of these symptoms may indicate local anesthetic toxicity (Avanos Medical, 2018d).
- *Catheter and tubing are accidentally pulled out:* Check the distal end of the catheter for the black marking to ensure the entire catheter was removed. Assess the insertion site. Cover the site with a dry, sterile dressing. Notify the health care team. Assess the patient's level of pain and administer analgesic, as ordered.
- *Resistance is encountered and/or the catheter stretches during its removal:* Stop. Do not continue to try to remove the catheter. Wait 30 to 60 minutes and attempt to remove the catheter again. The patient's body movements may relieve constriction on the catheter to allow easier removal. If catheter is still difficult to remove, contact the patient's health care provider. Do not forcefully remove the catheter. Do not continue to apply tension if the catheter begins to stretch (Avanos Medical, 2018e).

SPECIAL CONSIDERATIONS

General Considerations

- During the infusion, the pump will gradually lose its shape and flatten. Be aware that a change in the appearance and size of the pump may not be evident for more than 24 hours after surgery, owing to the slow flow rate of the device (Avanos Medical, 2018b).
- Do not expect to observe a fluid level line in the balloon and fluid moving through the system tubing (Avanos Medical, 2015).
- Over time, expect to see the outside bag on the balloon becoming looser, with creases beginning to form in the bag. As the medication is delivered, the pump will gradually become smaller (Avanos Medical, 2015).
- Do not tape or cover the filter (Avanos Medical, 2015).
- Ensure the tubing clamp remains open and avoid kinks in the pump tubing (Avanos Medical, 2015).
- Do not forcefully remove the catheter (Avanos Medical, 2018e).
- Do not reuse or refill balloon. System is intended for one-time use.
- Protect the balloon and catheter site from water. Do not submerge the pump in water (Avanos Medical, 2015).
- Clip the balloon to the patient's clothing to prevent the application of tension on the system and site.
- Avoid placing cold therapy in the area of the flow controller (see Figure 1). Contact with cold therapy will decrease flow rate (Avanos Medical, 2015).

(continued on page 678)

Skill 10-6 ▶ Caring for a Patient Receiving Continuous Wound Perfusion Pain Management *(continued)*

Community-Based Care Considerations

- Instruct patients to immediately close the clamp on the pump tubing and call their health care provider or 911 if they experience any of the following symptoms (Avanos Medical, 2018b): increased pain; fever, chills, sweats; bowel or bladder changes; difficulty breathing; redness, warmth, discharge, or excessive bleeding from the catheter site; pain, swelling, or large bruise around the catheter site; dizziness or lightheadedness, blurred vision, ringing in the ears; numbness and/or tingling around the mouth, fingers or toes; metal taste in the mouth; or drowsiness or confusion.
- Patients may experience numbness at and around the surgical site and should take care to avoid injury at the site (Avanos Medical, 2018e).
- Patients may be instructed to remove the ON-Q* catheter at home. Provide written details and explanation. Instruct the patient to contact their health care provider for any issues with removal or if they do not see the black marking on the catheter upon removal (Avanos Medical, 2018e).

Enhance Your Understanding

Focusing on Patient Care: Developing Clinical Reasoning and Clinical Judgment

Consider the case scenarios at the beginning of the chapter as you answer the following questions to enhance your understanding and apply what you have learned.

QUESTIONS

1. Since their surgery, Mildred Simpson has been spending most of the time in bed. A special pillow is placed between their legs to keep their hips in abduction. The nurse offers to give Mrs. Simpson a back massage. What areas would be most important for the nurse to address when performing this skill?

2. The health care provider decides to admit Joseph Watkins to the hospital for evaluation of his back pain. Intermittent TENS therapy is ordered and is to be started in the emergency department. How would the nurse initiate this therapy?

3. Jerome Batiste and their wife are concerned about using the PCA device at home. What information would the nurse provide to help alleviate their concerns?

You can find suggested answers after the Bibliography at the end of this chapter.

Integrated Case Study Connection

The case studies in the back of the book focus on integrating concepts. Refer to the following case studies to enhance your understanding of the concepts and skills in this chapter.

Bibliography

Ahmadidarrehsima, S., Mohammadpourhodki, R., Ebrahimi, H., Keramati, M., & Dianatinasab, M. (2018). Effect of foot reflexology and slow stroke back massage on the severity of fatigue in patients undergoing hemodialysis: A semi-experimental study. *Journal of Complementary and Integrative Medicine, 15*(4). https://doi.org/10.1515/jcim-2017-0183

American Massage Therapy Association. (2011). *Massage and the aging body*. https://www.amtamassage.org/articles/3/MTJ/detail/2315

Aparício, C., & Panin, F. (2020). Interventions to improve inpatients' sleep quality in intensive care units and acute wards: A literature review. *British Journal of Nursing, 29*(13), 770–776. https://doi.org/10.12968/bjon.2020.29.13.770

Avanos Medical. (2018a). *ON-Q* pain relief system. How it works*. [Video]. https://myon-q.com/

Avanos Medical. (2018b). *ON-Q* pain relief system. My ON-Q* pump*. https://myon-q.com/on-q-pump/

Avanos Medical. (2018c). *ON-Q* pain relief system. Why ON-Q* for post-op pain relief?* https://myon-q.com/why-on-q/

Avanos Medical. (2018d). *ON-Q* pain relief system. Effective pain relief. Getting patients back to normal faster*. https://avanospainmanagement.com/solutions/acute-pain/on-q-pain-relief-system/

Avanos Medical. (2018e). *ON-Q* catheter removal*. http://1797f0cd94.nxcli.net/wp-content/uploads/2019/09/ap_patient-brochure_catheterremoval-mk-00456-rev1_90d.pdf

Avanos Medical. (2018f, May). *ON-Q* pain relief system. Pain relief that's better for everybody*. [Brochure]. http://1797f0cd94.nxcli.net/wp-content/uploads/2019/09/ap_patient-brochure_general-mk-00453-rev-1_90d.pdf

Avanos Medical. Halyard Health, Inc. (2015). *ON-Q* pain relief system. Patient guidelines*. http://1797f0cd94.nxcli.net/wp-content/uploads/2019/09/on-q-patient-guidelines-15-h1-832-0-00.pdf

Ayik, C., & Özden, D. (2018). The effects of preoperative aromatherapy massage on anxiety and sleep quality of colorectal surgery patients: A randomized controlled study. *Complementary Therapies in Medicine, 36*, 93–99. https://doi.org/10.1016/j.ctim.2017.12.002

Bagci, H., & Yucel, S.C. (2020). A systematic review of the studies about Therapeutic Touch after the year of 2000. *International Journal of Caring Sciences, 13*(1), 231.

Barton, A. (2019). The case for using a disinfecting cap for needlefree connectors. *British Journal of Nursing, 28*(14), S22–S27. https://doi.org/10.12968/bjon.2019.28.14.S??

Bauldoff, G., Gubrud, P., & Carno, M. A. (2020). *LeMone and Burke's medical-surgical nursing: Clinical reasoning in patient care* (7th ed.). Pearson.

Benjenk, I., Messing, J., Lenihan, M. J., Hernandez, M., Amdur, R., Sirajuddin, S., Davison, D., Schroeder, M. E., & Sarani, B. (2020). Authorized agent-controlled analgesia for pain management in critically ill adult patients. *Critical Care Nurse, 40*(3), 31–36. https://doi.org/10.4037/ccn2020323

Blackburn, L., Abel, S., Green, L., Johnson, K., & Panda, S. (2019). The use of comfort kits to optimize adult cancer pain management. *Pain Management Nursing, 20*(1), 25–31. https://doi.org/10.1016/j.pmn.2018.01.004

Booker, S. Q., & Haedtke, C. (2016). Assessing pain in verbal older adults. *Nursing, 46*(2), 65–68.

Bosch-Alcaraz, A., Falcó-Pegueroles, A., & Jordan, I. (2018). A literature review of comfort in the paediatric critical care patient. *Journal of Clinical Nursing, 27*(13–14), 2546–2557. https://doi.org/10.1111/jocn.14345

Casey, A. L., Karpanen, T. J., Nightingale, P., & Elliot, T. S. J. (2018). An in vitro comparison of standard cleaning to a continuous passive disinfection cap for the decontamination of needle-free connectors. *Antimicrobial Resistance & Infection Control, 7*, 50. https://doi.org/10.1186/s13756-018-0342-0

Casey, G. (2015). Capnography: Monitoring CO2. *Nursing New Zealand, 21*(9), 20–24.

Ceylan, S. S., & Bolışık, B. (2018). Effects of swaddled and sponge bathing methods on signs of stress and pain in premature newborns: Implications for evidence-based practice. *Worldviews on Evidence-Based Nursing, 15*(4), 296–303. https://doi.org/10.1111/wvn.12299

Chen, A., & Ashburn, M. A. (2015). Cardiac effects of opioid therapy. *Pain Medicine, 16*(S1), S27–S31. https://doi.org/10.1111/pme.12915

Cinar, H. U., Celik, H. K., & Celik, B. (2021). The efficacy of the ON-Q elastomeric pump system in post-thoracotomy acute pain control. *Nigerian Journal of Clinical Practice, 24*(5), 651–659. https://doi.org/10.4103/njcp.njcp_203_20

Cleveland Clinic. (2020, January 15). *Transcutaneous electrical nerve stimulation (TENS)*. https://my.clevelandclinic.org/health/treatments/15840-transcutaneous-electrical-nerve-stimulation-tens

Cooney, M. F., Czarnecki, M., Dunwoody, C., Eksterowicz, N., Merkel, S., Oakes, L., & Wuhrman, E. (2013). American Society for Pain Management nursing position statement with clinical practice guidelines: Authorized agent controlled analgesia. *Pain Management Nursing, 14*(3), 176–181. https://doi.org/10.1016/j.pmn.2013.07.003

D'Arcy, Y. (2013). PCA by proxy: Taking the patient out of patient-controlled analgesia: This controversial practice can be done safely in carefully controlled circumstances. *Dimensions of Critical Care Nursing, 32*(4), 200–203. https://doi.org/10.1097/DCC.0b013e31829d3bff

Davis, T. M., Friesen, M. A., Lindgren, V., Golino, A., Jackson, R., Mangione, L., Swengros, D., & Anderson, J. G. (2020). The effect of Healing Touch on critical care patients' vital signs. A pilot study. *Holistic Nursing Practice, 34*(4), 244–251. https://doi.org/10.1097/HNP.0000000000000394

DiGiusto, M., Bhalla, T., Martin, D., Foerschler, D., Jones, M. J., & Tobias, J. (2014). Patient-controlled analgesia in the pediatric population: Morphine versus hydromorphone. *Journal of Pain Research, 7*, 471–475. https://doi.org/10.2147/JPR.S64497

Durand, M. (2020, August 1). *Massage therapy for seniors*. American Massage Therapy Association. https://www.amtamassage.org/publications/massage-therapy-journal/massage-for-elderly/

El-Boghdadly, K., Pawa, A., & Chin, K. J. (2018). Local anesthetic systemic toxicity: Current perspectives. *Local Regional Anesthesia, 11*, 35–44. https://doi.org/10.2147/LRA.S154512

Eliopoulos, C. (2018). *Gerontological nursing* (9th ed.). Wolters Kluwer Health.

Fazio, S., & Firestone, R. (2020, May). *Fatal patient-controlled analgesia (PCA) opioid-induced respiratory depression*. Patient Safety Network. https://psnet.ahrq.gov/web-mm/fatal-patient-controlled-analgesia-pca-opioid-induced-respiratory-depression

Flaherty, E., & Horgas, A. L. (2020). *ConsultGeri. Try this: Series. Pain assessment for older adults*. Hartford Institute for Geriatric Nursing. https://hign.org/consultgeri/try-this-series/pain-assessment-older-adults

Flynn, J.M., Larsen, E.N., Keogh, S., Ullman, A.J., & Rickard, C.M. (2019). Methods for microbial needle-less connector decontamination: A systematic review and meta-analysis. *American Journal of Infection Control, 47*(8), 956–965. https://doi.org/10.1016/j.ajic.2019.01.002

Gai, N., Naser, B., Hanley, J., Peliowski, A., Hayes, J., & Aoyama, K. (2020). A practical guide to acute pain management in children. *Journal of Anesthesia, 34*(3), 421–433. https://doi.org/10.1007/s00540-020-02767-x

Galligan M. (2020). Care and management of patients receiving epidural analgesia. *Nursing Standard, 35*(12), 77–82. https://doi.org/10.7748/ns.2020.e11573

Georga, G., Chrousos, G., Artemiadis, A., Panagiotis, P. P., Bakakos, P., & Darviri, C. (2019). The effect of stress management incorporating progressive muscle relaxation and biofeedback-assisted relaxation breathing on patients with asthma: A randomised controlled trial. *Advances in Integrative Medicine, 6*(2), 73–77. https://doi.org/10.1016/j.aimed.2018.09.001

Goeren, D., John, S., Meskill, K., Iacono, L., Wahl, S., & Scanlon, K. (2018). Quiet Time: A noise reduction initiative in a neurosurgical intensive care unit. *Critical Care Nursing, 38*(4), 38–45. https://doi.org/10.4037/ccn2018219

Golembiewski, J., Dasta, J., & Palmer, P. P. (2016). Evolution of patient-controlled analgesia: From intravenous to sublingual treatment. *Hospital Pharmacy, 51*(3), 214–229. https://doi.org/10.1310/hpj5103-214

Gorski, L. A., Hadaway, L., Hagle, M. E., Broadhurst, D., Clare, S., Kleidon, T., Meyer, B. M., Nickel, B., Rowley, S., Sharpe, E., & Alexander, M. (2021). Infusion therapy standards of practice. Infusion Nurses Society (INS). *Journal of Infusion Nursing, 44*(1S), S1-S231. https://www.ins1.org/publications/infusion-therapy-standards-of-practice/

Grissinger, M. (2019). Worth repeating: PCA by proxy event suggests reassessment of practices that may have fallen by the wayside. *Pharmacy & Therapeutics, 44*(10), 580–581.

Hall, K. R., & Stanley, A. Y. (2019). Literature review: Assessment of opioid-related sedation and the Pasero Opioid Sedation Scale. *Journal of PeriAnesthesia Nursing, 34*(1), 132–142. https://doi.org/10.1016/j.jopan.2017.12.009

Hasanpour-Dehkordi, A., Solati, K., Tali, S. S., & Dayani, M. A. (2019). Effect of progressive muscle relaxation with analgesic on anxiety status and pain in surgical patients. *British Journal of Nursing, 28*(3), 174–178. https://doi.org/10.12968/bjon.2019.28.3.174

Helming, M. A. B., Shields, D. A., Avino, K. M., & Rosa, W. E. (Eds.). (2021). *Dossey & Keegan's holistic nursing: A handbook for practice* (8th ed.). Jones & Bartlett Learning.

Herr, K., Coyne, P. J., Ely, E., Gélinas, C., & Manworren, R. C. B. (2019). ASPMN 2019 position statement: Pain assessment in the patient unable to self-report. *Pain Management Nursing, 20*(5), 402–403. https://doi.org/10.1016/j.pmn.2019.07.007

Hess, D. R., MacIntyre, N. R., Galvin, W. F., & Mishoe, S. C. (2021). *Respiratory care: Principles and practice* (4th ed.). Jones & Bartlett Learning.

Hinkle, J. L., Cheever, K. H., & Overbaugh, K. J. (2022). *Brunner & Suddarth's textbook of medical-surgical nursing* (15th ed.). Wolters Kluwer.

Hogan-Quigley, B., Palm, M. L., & Bickley, L. (2017). *Bates' nursing guide to physical examination and history taking* (2nd ed.). Wolters Kluwer.

Horgas, A. L. (2020). *ConsultGeri. Try this: Series. Assessing pain in older adults with dementia*. Hartford Institute for Geriatric Nursing. https://hign.org/consultgeri/try-this-series/assessing-pain-older-adults-dementia

Hsu, W. C., Guo, S. E., & Chang, C. H. (2019). Back massage intervention for improving health and sleep quality among intensive care unit patients. *Nursing in Critical Care, 21*(5), 313–319. https://doi.org/10.1111/nicc.12428

Institute for Safe Medication Practices (ISMP). (2013). *Acute Care ISMP Medication Safety Alert!® Fatal PCA adverse events continue to happen…Better patient monitoring is essential to prevent harm*. https://www.ismp.org/resources/fatal-pca-adverse-events-continue-happen-better-patient-monitoring-essential-prevent-harm?id=50

Institute for Safe Medication Practices (ISMP). (2016, September 22). *Acute Care ISMP Medication Safety Alert!® Worth repeating…Recent PCA by proxy event suggests reassessment of practices that may have fallen by the wayside*. https://www.ismp.org/resources/worth-repeating-recent-pca-proxy-event-suggests-reassessment-practices-may-have-fallen?id=1149

Institute for Safe Medication Practices (ISMP). (2017). *Acute Care ISMP Medication Safety Alert!® Part II: How to prevent errors. Safety issues with patient-controlled analgesia*. https://www.ismp.org/resources/safety-issues-pca-part-ii-how-prevent-errors

Institute for Safe Medication Practices (ISMP). (2020). *ISMP targeted medication safety best practices for hospitals*. https://www.ismp.org/guidelines/best-practices-hospitals

Institute of Medicine (IOM). (2011). *Relieving pain in America: A blueprint for transforming prevention, care, education, and research*. The National Academies Press. https://www.nap.edu/catalog/13172/relieving-pain-in-america-a-blueprint-for-transforming-prevention-care

International Association for the Study of Pain (IASP). (2020, July 16). *IASP announces revised definition of pain*. https://www.iasp-pain.org/PublicationsNews/NewsDetail.aspx?ItemNumber=10475

International Council of Nurses (ICN). (2019). *Nursing diagnosis and outcome statements*. https://www.icn.ch/sites/default/files/inline-files/ICNP2019-DC.pdf

Jagan, S., Park, T., & Papathanassoglou, E. (2019). Effects of massage on outcomes of adult intensive care unit patients: A systematic review. *Nursing in Critical Care, 24*(6), 414–429. https://doi.org/10.1111/nicc.12417

Jaruzel, C. B., Gregoski, M., Mueller, M., Faircloth, A., & Kelechi, T. (2019). Aromatherapy for preoperative anxiety: A pilot study. *Journal of PeriAnesthesia Nursing, 34*(2), 259–264. https://doi.org/10.1016/j.jopan.2018.05.007

Jarvis, C., & Echkardt, A. (2020). *Physical examination & health assessment* (8th ed.). Elsevier.

Jensen, S. (2019). *Nursing health assessment: A best practice approach* (3rd ed.). Wolters Kluwer.

The Joint Commission. (2018, August). *Quick safety. Non-pharmacologic and non-opioid solutions for pain management*. Issue 44. https://www.jointcommission.org/-/media/tjc/documents/resources/pain-management/qs_nonopioid_pain_mgmt_8_15_18_finall.pdf

The Joint Commission. (2021). *Hospital: 2021 National Patient Safety Goals*. https://www.jointcommission.org/standards/national-patient-safety-goals/hospital-national-patient-safety-goals/

Jungquist, C. R., Quinlan-Cowell, A., Vallerand, A., Carlisle, H. L., Cooney, M., Dempsey, S. J., Dunwoody, D., Maly, A., Meloche, K., Mehyers, A., Sawyer, J., Singh, N., Sullivan, D., Watson, C., & Polomano, R. C. (2020). American Society for Pain Management nursing guidelines on monitoring for opioid-induced advancing sedation and respiratory depression: Revisions. *Pain Management Nursing, 21*(1), 7–25. https://doi.org/10.1016/j.pmn.2019.06.007

Jungquist, C. R., Smith, K., Nicely, K. L. W., & Polomano, R. C. (2017a). Monitoring hospitalized adult patients for opioid-induced sedation and respiratory depression. *The American Journal of Nursing, 117*(3 Suppl 1), S27–S35. https://doi.org/10.1097/01.NAJ.0000513528.79557.33

Jungquist, C. R., Vallerand, A. H., Sicoutris, C., Kwon, K. N., & Polomano, R. C. (2017b). Assessing and managing acute pain: A call to action. *The American Journal of Nursing, 117*(3 Suppl 1), S4–S11. https://doi.org/10.1097/01.NAJ.0000513526.33816.0e

Karch, A. M. (2020). *Focus on nursing pharmacology* (8th ed.). Wolters Kluwer.

Katz, P., Takyar, S., Palmer, P., & Liedgens, H. (2017). Sublingual, transdermal and intravenous patient-controlled analgesia for acute post-operative pain: Systematic literature review and mixed treatment comparison. *Current Medical Research and Opinion, 33*(5), 899–910. https://doi.org/10.1080/03007995.2017.1294559

Khanna, A. K., Bergese, S. D., Jungquist, C. R., Morimatsu, H., Uezono, S., Lee, S., Ti, L. K., Urman, R. D., McIntyre, R. Jr., Tornero, C., Dahan, A., Saager, L. Weingarten, T. N., Wittmann, M., Auckley, D., Brazzi, L., Le Guen, M., Soto, R., Schramm, F...Overdyk, F. J. (2020). Prediction of opioid-induced respiratory depression on inpatient wards using continuous capnography and oximetry: An international prospective, observational trial. *Anesthesia & Analgesia, 131*(4), 1012–1024. https://doi.org/10.1213/ANE.0000000000004788

Kiley, K. A., Sehgal, A. R., Neth, S., Dolata, J., Pike, E., Spilsbury, J. C., & Albert, J. M. (2018). The effectiveness of guided imagery in treating compassion fatigue and anxiety of mental health workers. *Social Work Research, 42*(1), 33–43. https://doi.org/10.1093/swr/svx026

Kovach, C. R., Putz, M., Guslek, B., & McInnes, R. (2019). Do warmed blankets change pain, agitation, mood or analgesic use among nursing home residents? *Pain Management Nursing, 20*(6), 526–531. https://doi.org/10.1016/j.pmn.2019.07.002

Krau, S. D. (2020). The multiple uses of guided imagery. *Nursing Clinics of North America, 55*(4), 467–474. https://doi.org/10.1016/j.cnur.2020.06.013

Kudo, Y., & Sasaki, M. (2020). Effect of a hand massage with a warm hand bath on sleep and relaxation in elderly women with disturbance of sleep: A crossover trial. *Japan Journal of Nursing Science, 17*(3), e12327. https://doi.org/10.1111/jjns.12327

Kyle, T., & Carman, S. (2021). *Essentials of pediatric nursing* (4th ed.). Wolters Kluwer Health.

Labus, N., Wilson, C., & Arena, S. (2019). Mind-body therapies as a therapeutic intervention for pain management. *Home Healthcare Now, 37*(5), 293–294. https://doi.org/10.1097/NHH.0000000000000809

Li, K., Ji, C., Luo, D., Feng, H., Yang, K., & Xu, H. (2020). Wound infiltration with ropivacaine as an adjuvant to patient controlled analgesia for transforaminal lumbar interbody fusion: A retrospective study. *BMC Anesthesiology, 20*, 288. https://doi.org/10.1186/s12871-020-01205-5

Lisi, D. M. (2013). Patient-controlled analgesia and the older patient. *US Pharmacist, 38*(3), HS2–HS6. https://www.uspharmacist.com/article/patient-controlled-analgesia-and-the-older-patient

Mayo Foundation for Medical Education and Research (MFMER). (2020, April 8). *Infant massage: Understand this soothing therapy*. https://www.mayoclinic.org/healthy-lifestyle/infant-and-toddler-health/in-depth/infant-massage/art-20047151

Mayo Foundation for Medical Education and Research (MFMER). (2021, January 12). *Massage: Get in touch with its many benefits*. https://www.mayoclinic.org/healthy-lifestyle/stress-management/in-depth/massage/art-20045743

McCaffery, M. (1968). Nursing practice theories related to cognition, bodily pain, and man-environment interactions. UCLA Students' Store.

Merkel, S., Voepel-Lewis, T., & Malviya, S. (2002). Pain assessment in infants and young children: The FLACC Scale. *The American Journal of Nursing, 102*(10), 55–58.

Mijovski, G., Podbregar, M., Kšela, J., Jenko, M., & Šošarič, M. (2020). Effectiveness of wound infusion of 0.2% ropivacaine by patient control analgesia pump after minithoracotomy aortic valve replacement: A randomized, double-blind, placebo-controlled trial. *BMC Anesthesiology, 20*(1), 172. https://doi.org/10.1186/s12871-020-01093-9

Minton, M. E., Isaacson, M. J., Varilek, B.M., Stadick, J. L., & O'Connell-Persuad, S. (2018). A willingness to go there: Nurses and spiritual care. *Journal of Clinical Nursing, 27*(1–2), 173–181. https://doi.org/10.1111/jocn.13867

Morton, P. G., & Fontaine, D. K. (2018). *Critical care nursing: A holistic approach* (11th ed.). Wolters Kluwer.

Muirhead, R., & Kynoch, K. Safety and effectiveness of parent/nurse controlled analgesia on patient outcomes in the neonatal intensive care unit: A systematic review protocol. *JBI Database Systematic Reviews and Implementation Reports, 16*(10), 1959–1964. https://doi.org/10.11124/JBISRIR-2017-003711

National Health Service (NHS) (UK). (2021, August 10). *TENS (transcutaneous electrical nerve stimulation)*. https://www.nhs.uk/conditions/transcutaneous-electrical-nerve-stimulation-tens/

National Health Service (NHS) (UK). Hull University Teaching Hospitals. (2018, October 8). *Patient controlled epidural analgesia*. https://www.hey.nhs.uk/patient-leaflet/patient-controlled-epidural-analgesia/

Nijland, L., Schmidt, P., Frosch, M., Wager, J., Hübner-Möhler, B., Drake, R., & Zernikow, B. (2019). Subcutaneous or intravenous opioid administration by patient-controlled analgesia in cancer pain: A systematic literature review. *Supportive Care in Cancer, 27*(1), 33–42. https://doi.org/10.1007/s00520-018-4368-x

Norris, T. L. (2019). *Porth's essentials of pathophysiology* (5th ed.). Wolters Kluwer.

Pasero, C., & McCaffery, M. (2011). *Pain assessment and pharmacologic management*. Elsevier.

Polomano, R. C., Fillman, M., Giordano, N. A., Vallerand, A. H., Nicely, K. L. W., & Jungquist, C. R. (2017). Multimodal analgesia for acute postoperative and trauma-related pain. *The American Journal of Nursing, 117*(3 Suppl 1), S12–S26. https://doi.org/10.1097/01.NAJ.0000513527.71934.73

Porter, A. C., Behrendt, N. J., Zaretsky, M. V., Liechty, K. W., Wood, C., Chow, F., & Galan, H. L. (2021). Continuous local bupivacaine wound infusion reduces oral opioid use for acute postoperative pain control following myelomeningocele repair. *American Journal of Obstetrics & Gynecology, 3*(2), 100296. https://doi.org/10.1016/j.ajogmf.2020.100296

Problem-based care plans. (2020). In *Lippincott Advisor*. Wolters Kluwer. https://advisor.lww.com/lna/home.do permission statement

Salicath, J. H., Yeoh, E. C., & Bennett, M. H. (2018, August 30). Epidural analgesia versus patient-controlled intravenous analgesia for pain following intra-abdominal surgery in adults. *Cochrane Database of Systematic Reviews, 8*(8), CD010434. https://doi.org/10.1002/14651858.CD010434.pub2

Sandvik, R. K., Olsen, B. F., Rygh, L. J., & Moi, A. L. (2020). Pain relief from nonpharmacological interventions in the intensive care unit: A scoping review. *Journal of Clinical Nursing, 29*(9–10), 1488–1498. https://doi.org/10.1111/jocn.15194

Schreiber, M. L. (2015). Nursing care considerations: The epidural catheter. *Medsurg Nursing, 24*(4), 273–276.

Silbert-Flagg, J., & Pillitteri, A. (2018). *Maternal and child health nursing* (8th ed.). Wolters Kluwer.

Singh, A., Jindal, P., Khurana, G., & Kumar, R. (2017). Post-operative effectiveness of continuous wound infiltration, continuous epidural infusion and intravenous patient-controlled analgesia on post-operative pain management in patients undergoing spinal surgery. *Indian Journal of Anaesthesia, 61*(7), 562–569. https://doi.org/10.4103/ija.IJA_684_16

Slater, K., Fullerton, F., Cooke, M., Snell, S., & Rickard, C.M. (2018). Needleless connector drying time-how long does it take? *American Journal of Infection Control, 46*(9), 1080–1081. http://doi.org/10.1016/j.ajic.2018.05.007

Sonneborn, O., & Williams, A. (2020). How does the 2020 revised definition of pain impact nursing practice? *Journal of Perioperative Nursing, 33*(4), e25–e28. https://doi.org/10.26550/2209-1092.1104

Tabatabaee, A., Tafreshi, M. Z., Rassouli, M., Aledavood, S. A, AlaviMajd, H., & Farahmand, S. K. (2016). Effect of therapeutic touch in patients with cancer: A literature review. *Medical Archives, 70*(2), 142–147. DOI: 10.5455/medarh.2016.70.142-147

Taylor, C., Lynn, P., & Bartlett, J. (2023). *Fundamentals of nursing: The art and science of person-centered care* (10th ed.). Wolters Kluwer.

Thomas, T., & Barclay, S. (2015). Continuous subcutaneous infusion in palliative care: A review of current practice. *International Journal of Palliative Nursing, 21*(2), 60, 62–64. https://doi.org/10.1268/ijpn.2015.21.2.60

University Health Network (UHN). (2017, March). Managing your pain with patient controlled analgesia (PCA). Anesthesiology and pain management. https://www.uhn.ca/PatientsFamilies/Health_Information/Health_Topics/Documents/Managing_Your_Pain_with_PCA.pdf

VHA Center for Engineering & Occupational Safety and Health (CEOSH). (2016). *Safe patient handling and mobility guidebook*. http://www.tnpatientsafety.com/pubfiles/Initiatives/workplace-violence/sphm-pdf.pdf

Ward, C. W. (2016). Non-pharmacologic methods of postoperative pain management. *Medsurg Nursing, 25*(1), 9–10.

Weaver, M. (2017). Healing Touch: Positively sharing energy in a pediatric hospital. *Journal of Pain and Symptom Management, 54*(2), 259–261. https://doi.org/10.1016/j.jpainsymman.2016.12.340

Webb, R. J., & Shelton, C. P. (2015). The benefits of authorized agent controlled analgesia (AACA) to control pain and other symptoms at the end of life. *Journal of Pain and Symptom Management, 50*(3), 371–374. https://doi.org/10.1016/j.jpainsymman.2015.03.015

Westman, K. F., & Blaisdell, C. (2016). Many benefits, little risk: The use of massage in nursing practice. *The American Journal of Nursing, 116*(1), 34–39; quiz 40-41. https://doi.org/10.1097/01.NAJ.0000476164.97929.f2

Wong, J., & Lim, S. S. T. (2018). Epidural analgesia in a paediatric teaching hospital: Trends, developments, and a brief review of literature. *Proceedings of Singapore Healthcare, 27*(1), 49–54. https://doi.org/10.1177/2010105817733997

Wrona, S., & Czarnecki, M. L. (2021). Pediatric pain management. An individualized, multimodal, and interprofessional approach is key for success. *American Nurse Journal, 16*(3), 6–11.

Zhou, J., Dan, Y., Yixian, Y., Lyu, M., Zhong, J., Wang, Z., Zhu, Y., & Liu, L. (2020). Efficacy of transcutaneous electronic nerve stimulation in postoperative analgesia after pulmonary surgery: A systematic review and meta-analysis. *American Journal of Physical Medicine & Rehabilitation, 99*(3), 241–249. https://doi.org/10.1097/PHM.0000000000001312

SUGGESTED ANSWERS FOR FOCUSING ON PATIENT CARE: DEVELOPING CLINICAL REASONING AND CLINICAL JUDGMENT

1. Review the patient's health record and care plan for information about the patient's status and contraindications to back massage, and review the prescribed intervention for the patient's activity level. Because of the surgery, it will probably be difficult for Mrs. Simpson to lie in a prone position; assess their ability to turn to their side for the massage. It will be necessary to maintain the position of the abductor pillow, to prevent adduction of her hip. Assess the patient's level of pain. Check the patient's medication administration record for the time an analgesic was last administered. If appropriate, administer an analgesic sufficiently early so it has time to take effect before beginning the massage. Assess for the need to obtain assistance of another caregiver to assist the patient to their side and maintain that position for the massage. Include an assessment of the patient's skin integrity, because of the increased risk for impaired skin integrity.

2. Review the patient's health record and care plan for specific instructions related to TENS therapy, including the order and conditions indicating the need for therapy, and prescribed settings. Review the patient's history for conditions that might contraindicate therapy, such as pacemaker insertion, cardiac monitoring, or electrocardiography. Determine the location of electrode placement in consultation with the ordering health care provider and based on the patient's report of pain. Assess the patient's understanding of TENS therapy and the rationale for its use. Explain the rationale for the use of TENS therapy and patient instructions.

   Before initiating therapy, inspect the skin of the area designated for electrode placement for irritation, redness, or breakdown. Assess the patient's pain and level of discomfort using an appropriate assessment tool. Check the unit to ensure proper functioning and review the manufacturer's instructions for use.

3. Provide teaching for Mr. Batiste and their wife concerning the rationale for the use of a PCA and how a PCA works. Show the equipment as part of the explanation and provide a written copy of the information. Include information regarding safety mechanisms built into the device, as well as guidelines for adverse effects. Instruct the patient and their wife regarding symptoms that should be reported to the health care provider. They should be aware that community-based care provider/nurse will be consulted to continue support at home. The patient and/or their wife should be able to verbalize and demonstrate an understanding of information.

11

Nutrition

Focusing on Patient Care

This chapter will help you develop some of the skills related to nutrition needed to care for the following patients:

Paula Williams, age 78, who is recovering from a cerebrovascular accident (CVA), or stroke. The nurse needs to help her with breakfast.

Jack Mason, a 62-year-old man, has severe dysphagia related to progressive muscle weakness. He is NPO and receiving enteral nutrition through a nasogastric tube. He and his wife are considering the placement of a gastrostomy tube for long-term nutrition.

Cole Brenau, age 12, has cystic fibrosis and needs to increase his caloric intake through gastrostomy tube feedings at nighttime.

Refer to Focusing on Patient Care: Developing Clinical Reasoning and Clinical Judgment at the end of the chapter to apply what you learn.

Learning Outcomes

After completing the chapter, you will be able to accomplish the following:

1. Assist a patient with eating.
2. Confirm placement of a nasogastric feeding tube.
3. Administer a tube feeding.
4. Care for a gastrostomy tube.

Nursing Concepts

- Assessment
- Clinical Decision Making/Clinical Judgment
- Nutrition
- Safety

Good **nutrition** is vital for life and health. Important **nutrients**, found in food, are needed for the body to function. A varied diet is necessary to provide all of the essential nutrients that a person needs. Poor nutrition can seriously decrease a person's level of wellness. An adequate diet provides a balanced intake of all essential nutrients in appropriate amounts. Details related to appropriate dietary intake can be found in the *Dietary Guidelines for Americans 2020–2025* at https://www.dietaryguidelines.gov/resources/2020-2025-dietary-guidelines-online-materials. Refer to information found in *Fundamentals of Nursing*, 10th edition, or a nutrition text for details related to sources, functions, and significance of carbohydrates, protein, and fat. Nurses incorporate nutrition into all aspects of thoughtful person-centered nursing care and are involved in all aspects of nutritional care.

Because of the significant influence that adequate nutrition plays in restoring and maintaining health and disease prevention, the nurse integrates nutritional assessment into the care of the patient (Fundamentals Review 11-1). Factors that may affect nutritional status are discussed in Fundamentals Review 11-2.

This chapter addresses skills necessary to care for patients with nutritional needs, including assisting a patient with eating, confirming the placement of a feeding tube, administering a tube feeding, and caring for a gastrostomy feeding tube. Nasogastric tubes are also used to decompress or to drain unwanted fluid and air from the stomach, monitor bleeding in the gastrointestinal (GI) tract, to remove undesirable substances (lavage), or to help treat an intestinal obstruction. Insertion and removal of nasogastric tubes for feeding and any of these other purposes is accomplished using essentially the same procedure and is discussed in Chapter 13.

Fundamentals Review 11-1

CLINICAL OBSERVATIONS FOR NUTRITIONAL ASSESSMENT

Body Area	Signs of Good Nutritional Status	Signs of Poor Nutritional Status
General appearance	Alert, responsive	Listless, apathetic, and cachexic
General vitality	Endurance, energetic, sleeps well, vigorous	Easily fatigued, no energy, falls asleep easily, looks tired, apathetic
Weight	Normal for height, age, body build	Overweight or underweight
Hair	Shiny, lustrous, firm, not easily plucked, healthy scalp	Dull and dry, brittle, loss of color, easily plucked, thin and sparse
Face	Uniform skin color; healthy appearance, not swollen	Dark skin over cheeks and under eyes, flaky skin, facial edema (moon face), pale skin color
Eyes	Bright, clear, moist; no sores at corners of eyelids; membranes moist and healthy pink color; no prominent blood vessels	Pale eye membranes, dry eyes (xerophthalmia), increased vascularity, dull or scarred cornea
Lips	Good pink color, smooth, moist, not chapped or swollen	Swollen and puffy (cheilosis); angular lesion at corners of mouth or fissures or scars (stomatitis)
Tongue	Deep red, surface papillae present	Smooth appearance, beefy red or magenta colored, swollen, hypertrophy or atrophy
Teeth	Straight, no crowding, no cavities, no pain, bright, no discoloration, well-shaped jaw	Cavities, mottled appearance, malpositioned, missing teeth
Gums	Firm, good pink color, no swelling or bleeding	Spongy, bleed easily, marginal redness, recessed, swollen, and inflamed
Glands	No enlargement of the thyroid, face not swollen	Enlargement of the thyroid (goiter), enlargement of the parotid (swollen cheeks)

(continued)

Fundamentals Review 11-1 continued

CLINICAL OBSERVATIONS FOR NUTRITIONAL ASSESSMENT

Body Area	Signs of Good Nutritional Status	Signs of Poor Nutritional Status
Skin	Smooth, good color, slightly moist; no signs of rashes, swelling, or color irregularities	Rough, dry, flaky, swollen, pale, pigmented, lack of fat under the skin, fat deposits around the joints, bruises, petechiae
Nails	Firm, pink	Spoon shaped (koilonychia), brittle, pale, ridged
Skeleton	Good posture, no malformations	Poor posture, beading of the ribs, bowed legs or knock-knees, prominent scapulas, chest deformity at diaphragm
Muscles	Well developed, firm, good tone, some fat under the skin	Flaccid, poor tone, wasted, underdeveloped, difficulty walking
Extremities	No tenderness	Weak and tender, presence of edema
Abdomen	Flat	Swollen
Nervous system	Normal reflexes, psychological stability	Decrease in or loss of ankle and knee reflexes, psychomotor changes, mental confusion, depression, sensory loss, motor weakness, loss of sense of position, loss of vibration, burning and tingling of the hands and feet (paresthesia)
Cardiovascular system	Normal heart rate and rhythm, no murmurs, normal blood pressure for age	Cardiac enlargement, tachycardia, elevated blood pressure
GI system	No palpable organs or masses (liver edge may be palpable in children)	Hepatosplenomegaly, enlarged liver or spleen

Source: Adapted from Dudek, S. G. (2022). *Nutrition essentials for nursing practice* (9th ed.). Wolters Kluwer; Jarvis, C., & Echkardt, A. (2020). *Physical examination & health assessment* (8th ed.). Elsevier.

Fundamentals Review 11-2

FACTORS THAT MAY AFFECT NUTRITIONAL STATUS

- Social determinants of health
- Socioeconomic status
- Illiteracy
- Language barriers
- Lack of caregiver or social support
- Knowledge of nutrition
- Access to reliable, healthy food options
- Psychosocial factors (meaning of food)
- Medical conditions that involve malabsorption, such as Crohn disease or cystic fibrosis
- Age
- Medical conditions that may affect desire to eat, such as chemotherapy treatment or pregnancy accompanied by morning sickness

- Conditions that involve physical limitations, weakness, and/or fatigue
- Dysphagia
- Culture
- Medications
- Alcohol abuse
- Religion
- Megadoses of nutrient substances
- Alterations in mental status

Skill 11-1 ▶ Assisting a Patient With Eating

A variety of oral diets are available in health care settings and may be prescribed for use at home. A diet is prescribed based on the individual person's condition. Table 11-1 outlines several commonly prescribed modified consistency diets and therapeutic diets. Many patients can independently meet their nutritional needs by feeding themselves. Other patients, especially the very young and some older adult patients, such as people with arthritis of the hands, may have difficulty opening juice containers, for example. Patients with paralysis of the upper extremities or advanced dementia may be unable to feed themselves. The nurse should ensure patients receive the assistance they need to maintain sufficient oral intake to meet their nutritional needs, either by assisting the patients as needed, or delegating as appropriate.

The skill of assisting a patient with eating is frequently delegated to assistive personnel (AP). However, the nurse remains responsible for the initial and ongoing assessment of the patient for potential complications related to feeding. Before this skill can be delegated, it is paramount for the nurse to make sure that the AP has been educated to observe for any swallowing difficulties and has knowledge of **aspiration** precautions. Box 11-1 (on page 686) outlines special considerations and interventions for assisting patients with dementia or other alterations in cognition with eating. Box 11-2 (on page 686) discusses special considerations and interventions for assisting patients with **dysphagia** with eating.

Table 11-1 Modified Consistency and Selected Therapeutic Diets

DIET AND DESCRIPTION	INDICATIONS
Modified Consistency Diets	
Clear-Liquid Diet: Composed only of clear fluids or foods that become fluid at body temperature. Requires minimal digestion and leaves minimal residue. Includes clear broth, coffee, tea, clear fruit juices (apple, cranberry, grape), gelatin, popsicles, commercially prepared clear liquid supplements.	Preparation for bowel surgery and lower endoscopy; acute gastrointestinal disorders; initial postoperative diet
Puréed Diet: Also known as a blenderized liquid diet because the diet is made up of liquids and foods blenderized to liquid form. All foods are allowed.	After oral or facial surgery; chewing and swallowing difficulties
Mechanically Altered Diet: Regular diet with modifications for texture. Excludes most raw fruits and vegetables and foods with seeds, nuts, and dried fruits. Foods are chopped, ground, mashed or soft.	Chewing and swallowing difficulties; after surgery to the head, neck, or mouth
Selected Therapeutic Diets	
Consistent-Carbohydrate Diet: Total daily carbohydrate content is consistent; emphasizes general nutritional balance. **Calories** based on attaining and maintaining healthy weight. High-fiber and heart-healthy fats encouraged; sodium and saturated fats are limited.	Type 1 and type 2 diabetes, gestational diabetes, impaired glucose tolerance
Fat-Restricted Diet: Low-fat diets are intended to lower the patient's total intake of fat.	Chronic cholecystitis (inflammation of the gallbladder) to decrease gallbladder stimulation; cardiovascular disease, to help prevent atherosclerosis
High-Fiber Diet: Emphasis on increased intake of foods high in fiber.	Prevent or treat constipation; irritable bowel syndrome; diverticulosis
Low-Fiber Diet: Fiber limited to <10 g/day.	Before surgery; ulcerative colitis; diverticulitis; Crohn disease
Sodium-Restricted Diet: Sodium limit may be set at 500–3,000 mg/day	Hypertension; heart failure; acute and chronic renal disease, liver disease
Renal Diet: Reduce workload on kidneys to delay or prevent further damage; control accumulation of uremic toxins. Protein restriction 0.6–1 g/kg/day; sodium restriction 1,000–3,000 mg/day; potassium and fluid restrictions dependent on patient situation	Nephrotic syndrome; chronic kidney disease; diabetic kidney disease

(continued on page 686)

Skill 11-1 ▶ Assisting a Patient With Eating *(continued)*

Box 11-1 — Special Considerations and Interventions for Assisting Patients With Dementia or Other Alterations in Cognition With Eating

- Change the environment in which meals occur.
- Assess the area where meals are served. Create a home-like environment by preparing food close to the place where it will be served to stimulate senses.
- Observe as many former rituals as possible, such as handwashing and saying a blessing.
- Avoid clutter and distractions.
- Maintain a pleasant, well-lighted room. Play calming music.
- Keep food as close to its original form as possible; try "finger foods" that are easy to pick up.
- Serve meals in the same place at the same time and in the company of others.
- Provide longer and continuous facilitation at mealtimes.
- Check food temperatures to prevent accidental mouth burns.
- Assist as needed. Be alert for cues from the patient. Turning away may signal that the patient has had enough to eat or that the patient needs to slow down. Leaning

forward with an open mouth usually means the patient is ready for more food.
- Stroking the underside of the chin may help promote swallowing.
- Provide one or two food items at a time. Offer small, frequent eating opportunities. A whole tray of food may be overwhelming.
- Ensure that the patient's glasses and hearing aid are working properly.
- Demonstrate what you want the patient to do. State the goal clearly, and then mimic the action with exaggerated motions.
- Provide foods and between-meal snacks that are easy to consume using the hands.
- Use adaptive feeding equipment, as needed, such as weighted utensils, large-handled cups, and larger or smaller silverware than standard.
- Promote family/caregiver involvement to encourage eating.

Source: Adapted from Alzheimer's Association. Alzheimer's and Dementia Caregiver Center. (n.d.). *Food and eating.* Retrieved September 26, 2020, from https://www.alz.org/help-support/caregiving/daily-care/food-eating; Dudek, S. (2022). *Nutrition essentials for nursing practice* (9th ed.). Wolters Kluwer; Liu, W., Williams, K., Batchelor-Murphy, M., Perkhounkova, Y., & Hein, M. (2019). Eating performance in relation to intake of solid and liquid food in nursing home residents with dementia: A secondary behavioral analysis of mealtime videos. *International Journal of Nursing Studies, 96,* 18–26. https://doi.org/10.1016/j.ijnurstu.2018.12.010; and Mendes, A. (2018). Optimising nutritional intake in people with dementia on hospital wards. *British Journal of Nursing, 27*(20), 1206. https://doi.org/10.12968/bjon.2018.27.20.1206.

Box 11-2 — Special Considerations and Interventions for Assisting Patients With Dysphagia With Eating

- Provide at least a 30-minute rest period prior to mealtime. A rested person will likely have less difficulty swallowing.
- Sit the patient upright, preferably in a chair. If bed rest is mandatory, elevate the head of the bed to a 90-degree angle. Maintain upright position for 30 minutes after the meal.
- Provide mouth care immediately before meals to enhance the sense of taste.
- Avoid rushed or forced feeding. Adjust the rate of feeding and size of bites to the patient's tolerance. Allow patient to control the eating process if possible.
- Collaborate to obtain a speech therapy consult for swallowing evaluation.
- Initiate a nutrition consult for appropriate diet modification such as chopping, mincing, or pureeing of foods and liquid consistency (thin, nectar-thick, honeylike, spoon-thick).

- Keep in mind that some patients may find thickened liquids unpalatable and thus drink insufficient fluids.
- Reduce or eliminate distractions at mealtime so that the patient can focus attention on swallowing; discourage chatting during the meal.
- Alternate solids and liquids.
- Assess for signs of aspiration during eating: sudden appearance of severe coughing; choking; cyanosis; voice change, hoarseness, and/or gurgling after swallowing; frequent throat clearing after meals; or regurgitation through the nose or mouth.
- Inspect oral cavity for retained food.
- Avoid or minimize the use of sedatives and hypnotics since these agents may impair the cough reflex and swallowing.

Source: Adapted from Dudek, S. (2022). *Nutrition essentials for nursing practice* (9th ed.). Wolters Kluwer; Holdoway, A., & Smith, A. (2020). Meeting nutritional need and managing patients with dysphagia. *Journal of Community Nursing, 34*(2), 52–59; Metheny, N. (n.d.). *Issue #20. General assessment series. Preventing aspiration in older adults with dysphagia.* Retrieved September 26, 2020, from https://hign.org/consultgeri/try-this-series/preventing-aspiration-older-adults-dysphagia; and Nazarko, L. (2020). Dysphagia: A guide for nurses in general practice. *Practice Nursing, 31*(4), 162–168. https://doi.org/10.12968/pnur.2020.31.4.162

DELEGATION CONSIDERATIONS

Assisting patients to eat may be delegated to assistive personnel (AP) as well as to licensed practical/vocational nurses (LPN/LVNs). See previous discussion. The decision to delegate must be based on careful analysis of the patient's needs and circumstances as well as the qualifications of the person to whom the task is being delegated. Refer to the Delegation Guidelines in Appendix A.

EQUIPMENT	
	• Prepared food, based on prescribed diet • Wet wipes for hand hygiene, or access to hand gel/skin cleanser and water • Mouth care materials • Patient's dentures, eyeglasses, hearing aid, if needed • Special adaptive utensils, as needed • Napkins, protective covering, or towel • PPE, as indicated

ASSESSMENT

Before assisting the patient, confirm the type of diet that has been ordered for the patient. Also, it is important to assess for any food allergies and religious or cultural preferences. Check to make sure the patient does not have any scheduled laboratory or diagnostic studies that may impact whether they are able to eat a meal. Before beginning the feeding, assess for any barriers to eating, such as swallowing difficulties or weakness and/or fatigue. Assess the patient's abdomen. Inspect the abdomen for distention and firmness; auscultate for bowel sounds or peristalsis and palpate the abdomen for distention and tenderness. If the abdomen is distended, consider measuring the abdominal girth at the umbilicus to establish a baseline.

ACTUAL OR POTENTIAL HEALTH PROBLEMS AND NEEDS

Many actual or potential health problems or issues may require the use of this skill as part of related interventions. An appropriate health problem or issue may include:
• Impaired Self Feeding
• Aspiration risk
• Impaired Swallowing

OUTCOME IDENTIFICATION AND PLANNING

The expected outcome to achieve when assisting a patient with feeding is that the patient consumes a variety of food consistent with the prescribed diet and individual circumstances to attain and maintain ideal body weight. Other outcomes include that the patient does not aspirate during or after the meal, and the patient expresses contentment related to eating, as appropriate.

IMPLEMENTATION

ACTION	RATIONALE
1. Check the prescribed interventions for the type of diet prescribed for the patient.	This ensures the correct diet for the patient.
2. Perform hand hygiene and put on PPE, if indicated.	Hand hygiene and PPE prevent the spread of microorganisms. PPE is required based on transmission precautions.
3. Identify the patient.	Identifying the patient ensures the right patient receives the intervention and helps prevent errors.
4. Discuss the procedure with the patient and assess the patient's ability to assist in the bathing process.	Discussion and explanation promotes reassurance and facilitates patient engagement.
5. **Assess level of consciousness and for physical limitations and decreased hearing or visual acuity. If the patient uses a hearing aid or wears glasses or dentures, provide, as needed. Ask if the patient has any cultural or religious preferences and food likes and dislikes, if possible.**	Alertness is necessary for the patient to swallow and consume food. Using a hearing aid, glasses, and dentures for chewing facilitates the intake of food. Patient preferences should be considered in food selection as much as possible to increase the intake of food and maximize the benefit of the meal.
6. Pull the patient's bedside curtain. Assess the abdomen. Ask the patient if they have any nausea. Ask the patient if they have any difficulty swallowing. Assess the patient for nausea or pain and administer an antiemetic or analgesic, as needed.	This provides for privacy. A functioning GI tract is essential for digestion. The presence of pain or nausea will diminish appetite. If the patient is medicated, wait for the appropriate time for absorption of the medication before beginning the feeding.
7. Offer to assist the patient with any elimination needs.	This promotes comfort and may avoid interruptions for toileting during meals.

(continued on page 688)

Skill 11-1 ▶ Assisting a Patient With Eating *(continued)*

ACTION	RATIONALE

8. Provide hand hygiene and mouth care, as needed.

This may improve appetite and promote comfort.

 9. Remove any bedpans or undesirable equipment and odors, if possible, from the vicinity where the meal will be eaten. Perform hand hygiene.

Unpleasant odors and equipment may decrease the patient's appetite. Hand hygiene prevents the spread of microorganisms.

10. Open the patient's bedside curtain. Assist to, or position the patient in, a high-Fowler or sitting position in the bed or chair. Position the bed in the low position if the patient remains in bed.

Proper positioning improves swallowing ability and reduces the risk of aspiration.

11. Place a napkin or a towel over the patient if desired and as necessary.

This prevents soiling of the patient's gown.

12. Check the food tray to make sure that it is the correct tray before serving. Place the tray on the overbed table so the patient can see the food, if able. Ensure that hot foods are hot and cold foods are cold. Use caution with hot beverages, allowing sufficient time for cooling, if needed. Ask the patient for their preference related to what foods are desired first. Cut food into small pieces, as needed. Observe swallowing ability throughout the meal.

This ensures that the correct tray is given to the patient. Encouraging the patient choice promotes patient dignity and respect. Close observation is necessary to assess for signs of aspiration or difficulty with meal.

13. If possible, sit facing the patient at their eye level while eating is taking place (Figure 1). If the patient is able, encourage them to hold finger foods and feed themselves as much as possible. Converse with patient during the meal and make eye contact, as appropriate. **If, however, the patient has dysphagia, limit questioning or conversation that would require patient response during eating.** Play relaxation music if the patient desires..

Sitting at the patient's eye level and making eye contact create a more relaxed, person-centered atmosphere. In general, optimal mealtime involves social interaction and conversation. Talking during eating is contraindicated for patients with dysphagia because of increased risk for aspiration.

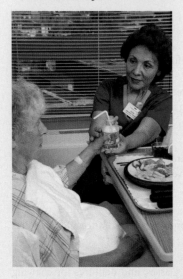

FIGURE 1. Sitting facing the patient at the patient's eye level and encouraging patient to feed themselves.

14. Allow enough time for the patient to chew and swallow the food adequately. The patient may need to rest for short periods during eating.

Eating requires energy, and many medical conditions can weaken patients. Rest can restore energy for eating.

15. When the meal is completed or the patient is unable to eat any more, remove the tray from the room. **Note the amount and types of food consumed. Note the volume of liquid consumed.**

Nutrition plays an important role in healing and overall health. If the patient is not eating enough to meet nutritional requirements, alternative methods need to be considered. Noting the amount and type of food and volume of liquids consumed allows for accurate documentation of intake.

ACTION

16. Reposition the overbed table; remove the protective covering; offer hand hygiene, as needed; and offer toileting. Assist the patient to a position of comfort and relaxation.

17. Remove PPE, if used. Perform hand hygiene.

RATIONALE

This promotes the comfort of the patient, meets possible elimination needs, and facilitates digestion.

Proper removal of PPE reduces the risk for infection transmission and contamination of other items. Hand hygiene prevents the spread of microorganisms.

EVALUATION

The expected outcomes have been met when the patient has consumed an adequate amount of nutrients consistent with the prescribed diet and individual circumstances to attain and maintain ideal body weight. In addition, the patient did not aspirate during or after the meal, and the patient has expressed contentment related to eating.

DOCUMENTATION

Guidelines

Document the assessment of the abdomen. Note that the head of the bed was elevated to at least 30 to 45 degrees. Note any swallowing difficulties and the patient's response to the meal. Document the percentage of the intake from the meal. If the patient had a poor intake, document the need for further consultation with the health care team and dietitian, as needed. Record any pertinent teaching that was conducted. Record liquids consumed on intake and output record, as appropriate.

Sample Documentation

12/23/25 0730 Patient's abdomen soft, nondistended, positive bowel sounds. HOB elevated to 45 degrees. Gag reflex intact. Awake. Fed full liquid tray; consumed about 50%; ate most of the oatmeal, 120 mL of cranberry juice. Some conversation during the meal. Patient remains with HOB elevated, watching TV. Call bell in reach.
—S. Essner, RN

DEVELOPING CLINICAL REASONING AND CLINICAL JUDGMENT

UNEXPECTED SITUATIONS AND ASSOCIATED INTERVENTIONS

- *Patient states that they do not want to eat anything on the tray:* Explore with the patient the reason why they do not want to eat anything on the tray. Assess for psychological factors that impact nutrition. Malnutrition is sometimes found with depression in the older adult population. Mutually develop a plan to address the lack of nutritional intake and consult the dietitian, as needed.
- *Patient states that they feel nauseated and cannot eat:* Remove the tray from the patient's room. Explore with the patient the desirability of eating small amounts of foods or liquids, such as crackers or ginger ale, if the patient's diet permits. Administer antiemetic as prescribed and encourage patient to retry small amounts of food after medication has had time to take effect.

SPECIAL CONSIDERATIONS

- Patients with arthritis of the hands may benefit from use of special utensils with modified handles that facilitate an easier grip. Contact an occupational therapist for guidance on adaptive equipment.
- A visually impaired patient may benefit from use of special plate guards, utensils, double handles, and compartmentalized plates. These patients may be guided to feed themselves through use of a "clock" pattern. For example, the chicken is placed at 6 o'clock; the vegetables at 3 o'clock.
- Refer to Box 11-1 for interventions and considerations related to assisting patients with alterations in cognition.
- For the patient with dysphagia, suggest small bites of food such as puddings, ground meat, or cooked vegetables. Advise the patient not to talk while swallowing and to swallow twice after each bite. Refer to Box 11-2 for additional considerations for this patient population.

(continued on page 690)

Skill 11-1 ▶ Assisting a Patient With Eating *(continued)*

EVIDENCE FOR PRACTICE ▶

NUTRITION SUPPORT STRATEGIES AND DEMENTIA

People living with dementia often lose some or all of the ability to feed themselves, which often is a source of significant challenges for caregivers. What are effective nutrition support strategies that have potential to be of assistance to these caregivers?

Related Research

Liu, W., Williams, K., Batchelor-Murphy, M., Perkhounkova, Y., & Hein, M. (2019). Eating performance in relation to intake of solid and liquid food in nursing home residents with dementia: A secondary behavioral analysis of mealtime videos. *International Journal of Nursing Studies*, *96*, 18–26. https://doi.org/10.1016/j.ijnurstu.2018.12.010.

This study examined the association between intake and characteristics of eating performance cycles among nursing home residents with dementia. An eating performance cycle was defined for this study as the process of getting food from the plate or container, transporting it into the mouth, and chewing and swallowing it. A secondary analysis of mealtime video clips from a nursing home communication training study was conducted. The 111 video clips involved 25 residents and 29 staff in 9 nursing homes. The Cue Utilization and Engagement in Dementia Mealtime video-coding scheme was used to code the characteristics of eating performance cycles, including eating technique (resident completed, staff facilitated), type of food (solid, liquid), duration of each eating performance cycle, and intake outcome (intake, no intake). The Generalized Linear Mixed Model was used to examine the interaction effects of eating technique by type of food, eating technique by duration, and type of food by duration on intake outcome. A total of 1,122 eating performance cycles were coded from the video clips. The majority of the cycles (85.7%) resulted in intake of liquid or solid food, with the rest (14.3%) resulting in no intake. As the duration of the eating performance cycle increased, staff-facilitated cycles resulted in greater odds of intake than resident-completed cycles (odds ratio [OR] = 17.80 vs. 2.73); and cycles involving liquid food resulted in greater odds of intake than cycles involving solid food (OR = 15.42 vs. 3.15). The odds of intake were greater for resident-completed cycles than for staff-facilitated cycles regardless of the type of food being involved in the cycle (OR = 3.60 for liquid food, OR = 10.69 for solid food). The researchers concluded that interventions to improve oral intake should support resident independence in eating performance. In addition, liquid food should be provided when residents struggle with solid food and staff should provide longer and continuous facilitation at mealtimes. The researchers suggested that innovative mealtime assistance and staff training are important interventions to promote eating performance and intake.

Relevance for Nursing Practice

People with dementia are at risk for reduced nutritional intake with the potential for weight loss and malnutrition. This study suggests that health care professionals should consider interventions to support optimal nutritional intake for individuals with dementia. Nurses are involved in all aspects of nutritional care and have a responsibility to assist patients and their care givers in attaining and maintaining adequate nutritional intake. Nurses must utilize appropriate interventions to provide appropriate education and support to achieve this outcome.

Skill 11-2 ▶ Confirming Placement of a Nasogastric Tube

Verify correct placement of the nasogastric tube after the initial insertion, before beginning a feeding or instilling medications or liquids, and at regular intervals during continuous feedings (Metheny et al., 2019). This decreases the risk that the tip of the tube is situated in the stomach or intestine, preventing inadvertent administration of substances into the wrong place. A misplaced feeding tube in the lungs or pulmonary tissue places the patient at risk for aspiration, pneumonia, and even death (Lamont et al., 2011, as cited in Anderson, 2018a). Radiographic examination, measurement of tube length and measurement of tube marking, measurement of aspirate pH, and monitoring of carbon dioxide have been suggested to confirm feeding tube placement (Anderson, 2018a; Irving et al., 2018; Metheny et al., 2019). The use of two or more of these techniques in conjunction with each other increases the likelihood of correct tube placement (AACN, 2020; Anderson, 2019; Anderson, 2018a; Dias et al., 2019; Rahimi et al., 2015). An old technique of auscultation of air injected into a feeding tube has been proved unreliable and is not suggested for use (AACN, 2020; Anderson, 2018a; Boeykens et al., 2014; Boullata et al., 2017; Irving et al., 2018; Metheny et al., 2019). Recommendations for use of visual inspection of gastric aspirate are conflicting; this method should be used cautiously if part of policy and procedure guidelines and with consideration to the potential for inaccuracy (AACN, 2020; Dias et al., 2019; Mak & Tam, 2020; Metheny et al., 2019). When bedside methods to check placement suggest the tube has been displaced, a radiograph should be requested to determine the tube's location (AACN, 2020).

Allow a 1-hour interval after the patient has received medication or completed an intermittent feeding before testing pH of gastric fluid. Feedings should never be interrupted solely for the purpose of pH testing; however, if a feeding is interrupted as part of preparation for a test or procedure, testing of the pH may be desired. Fasting gastric pH is usually 5 or less, even in patients receiving gastric-acid inhibitors (AACN, 2020). The pH of feeding tube aspirates is likely to approach fasting levels if nutritional feedings have been off for at least 1 hour (AACN, 2020; Irving et al., 2018). When continuous feedings are in use, pH may become less helpful, because the nutritional formula may buffer the pH of GI secretions (Judd, 2020).

Use of pH test strips calibrated in units of 0.5 and approved for use with human secretions should be used to ensure accuracy in testing gastric pH (Anderson, 2018a; Metheny et al., 2019). There is considerable variation in the evidence guidelines related to the pH values to distinguish between gastric and respiratory aspirates (Metheny et al., 2019). The lower the pH, obviously, the stronger the evidence for placement in the stomach and not the respiratory tract (Metheny et al., 2019). Suggested limits for a safe range to identify gastric secretions vary and include a pH of ≤ 4.0, ≤ 5.0, or ≤ 5.5; suggested limit for respiratory secretions is a pH of ≥ 6.0 (AACN, 2020; Dias et al., 2019; Metheny et al., 2019). Nurses should be certain to follow facility policy, procedure, and practice guidelines. If placement is in doubt, a radiograph should be obtained to verify tube placement (AACN, 2020; Boullata et al., 2017).

DELEGATION CONSIDERATIONS	The confirmation of placement of a nasogastric tube is not delegated to assistive personnel (AP). Depending on the state's nurse practice act and the organization's policies and procedures, confirmation of placement of a nasogastric tube may be delegated to licensed practical/vocational nurses (LPN/LVNs). The decision to delegate must be based on careful analysis of the patient's needs and circumstances as well as the qualifications of the person to whom the task is being delegated. Refer to the Delegation Guidelines in Appendix A.
EQUIPMENT	• Normal saline solution or sterile water, for irrigation, depending on facility policy • Tongue blade • Irrigation set, including a large syringe (20 to 50 mL) • Bath towel or disposable pad • Nonsterile, disposable gloves • Additional PPE, as indicated • Tape measure, or other measuring device • pH test strip (calibrated in units of 0.5 and approved for use with human secretions) • Stethoscope
ASSESSMENT	Assess for signs of respiratory distress; coughing, choking, dyspnea may occur when a tube is inadvertently positioned in the airway (AACN, 2020). Inspect the abdomen for distention and firmness; auscultate for bowel sounds or peristalsis and palpate the abdomen for distention and tenderness. If the abdomen is distended, consider measuring the abdominal girth at the umbilicus to establish a baseline. Assess the time when the patient last received medication or tube feeding.

(continued on page 692)

Skill 11-2 ▶ Confirming Placement of a Nasogastric Tube *(continued)*

ACTUAL OR POTENTIAL HEALTH PROBLEMS AND NEEDS

Many actual or potential health problems or issues may require the use of this skill as part of related interventions. An appropriate health problem or issue may include:
- Risk for Impaired Nutritional Status
- Injury risk
- Aspiration risk

OUTCOME IDENTIFICATION AND PLANNING

The expected outcomes to achieve when confirming placement of an NG tube are that the tube is located in the patient's stomach without any complications, and the patient does not exhibit signs and symptoms of aspiration.

IMPLEMENTATION

ACTION	RATIONALE
1. Gather equipment.	Assembling equipment provides for an organized approach to the task.
2. Perform hand hygiene and put on PPE, if indicated.	Hand hygiene and PPE prevent the spread of microorganisms. PPE is required based on transmission precautions.
3. Identify the patient.	Identifying the patient ensures the right patient receives the intervention and helps prevent errors.
4. Explain the procedure to the patient, including the rationale for confirming tube placement. Answer any questions as needed.	Explanation facilitates patient engagement.
5. Assemble equipment on the overbed table or other surface within reach.	Arranging items nearby is convenient, saves time, and avoids unnecessary stretching and twisting of muscles on the part of the nurse.
6. Close the patient's bedside curtain or door. Raise the bed to a comfortable working height (VHACEOSH, 2016). Perform respiratory and abdominal assessments as described above. Drape the chest/work area with a bath towel or disposable pad.	Closing curtains or the door provides for patient privacy. Having the bed at the proper height prevents back and muscle strain. Assessment is vital to detect changes in the patient's condition before initiating the intervention. The protective drape prevents accidental soiling of bed linens and patient clothing with stomach contents.
7. Confirm placement of the nasogastric tube in the patient's stomach using at least two methods. The first method utilized should be measurement of the exposed length of tube.	With the exception of radiographic examination, which is usually done immediately after insertion to verify initial tube placement, the use of two or more of these techniques in conjunction with each other increases the likelihood of correct tube placement (AACN, 2020; Anderson, 2019; Anderson, 2018a; Dias et al., 2019; Rahimi et al., 2015). Any change in the length of the exposed tube may indicate dislodgement (AACN, 2020; Boullata et al., 2017). If a significant change in the external length is observed, use other bedside tests to help determine if the tube has become dislocated (Boullata et al., 2017).
8. Put on gloves. Verify the position of the marking on the tube at the nostril. Measure length of the exposed tube and compare with the documented length (Figure 1).	Gloves prevent contact with blood and body fluids and transfer of microorganisms. The tube should be marked with an indelible marker at the nostril or the centimeter marking on the tube noted at the time it was placed (AACN, 2020; Irving et al., 2018; Judd, 2020). This marking should be assessed at regular intervals and each time the tube is used (AACN, 2020). Tube length should be checked and compared with this initial measurement, in conjunction with pH measurement and visual assessment of aspirate. Any change in the length of the exposed tube may indicate dislodgement (AACN, 2020; Boullata et al., 2017).

ACTION

9. Verify how much time has elapsed since the patient has received medication or completed an intermittent feeding. Attach a syringe to the end of the tube and aspirate a small amount (5 to 10 mL) of gastric secretions (Figure 2). If unable to obtain a specimen, reposition the patient and flush the tube with an air bolus, then apply negative pressure to the plunger (AACN, 2020). It may be necessary to retry several times. Slowly apply negative pressure to withdraw fluid.

RATIONALE

The pH of feeding tube aspirates is likely to approach fasting levels if nutritional feedings have been off for at least 1 hour (AACN, 2020; Irving et al., 2018). However, when continuous feedings are in use, pH may become less helpful, because the nutritional formula may buffer the pH of GI secretions (Judd, 2020). The tube is in the stomach if its contents can be aspirated: the pH of the aspirate can then be tested to determine gastric placement. Difficulty in aspiration may be due to a blocked tube or the tip of the tube not being positioned in fluid. Injecting an air bolus will help remove the blockage, and repositioning the patient will help place the tip of the tube in the fluid. This action may be necessary several times in order to obtain aspirate.

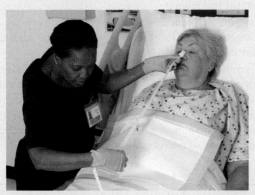

FIGURE 1. Measuring the length of the exposed nasogastric tube.

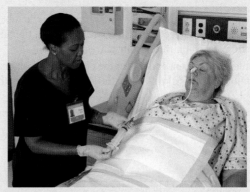

FIGURE 2. Aspirating gastric contents.

10. Measure the pH of aspirated fluid using pH test strips calibrated in units of 0.5 and approved for use with human secretions (Figure 3). Place a drop of gastric secretions onto the pH test strip or place a small amount of secretions in a plastic cup and dip the pH test strip into it. Within 30 seconds, compare the color on the test strip with the chart supplied by the manufacturer.

The pH of gastric contents is acidic (<5.5). Suggested limits for a safe range are (AACN, 2020; Anderson, 2018a; Dias et al., 2019; Metheny et al., 2019):

- Stomach: ≤4.0, ≤5.0, or ≤5.5 (depending on evidence source)
- Intestines: ≥7.0
- Respiratory tract: ≥6.0

This method will not effectively differentiate between intestinal fluid and pleural fluid.

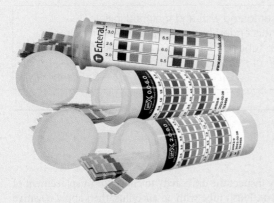

FIGURE 3. pH test strips to measure pH of aspirated fluid.

(continued on page 694)

Skill 11-2 ▶ Confirming Placement of a Nasogastric Tube *(continued)*

ACTION	**RATIONALE**
11. Use capnography if available. Refer to the *General Considerations* below.	A carbon dioxide detector is helpful in detecting when a feeding tube is in the tracheobronchial tree but is not sufficiently sensitive and specific to preclude the need for a confirming radiograph before initial use of a feeding tube (AACN, 2020).
12. If it is not possible to aspirate contents, assessments to check placement are inconclusive, the exposed tube length has changed, or there are any other indications that the tube may not be in place, check placement by radiograph (x-ray) of the placement of the tube based on facility policy.	X-ray is considered the most reliable method for identifying the position of the NG tube (AACN, 2020; Boullata et al., 2017).
13. Flush the tube with 30 to 50 mL of water for irrigation. Disconnect the syringe from the tubing and cap the end of the tubing.	Flushing the tube prevents occlusion (Bischoff et al., 2020; Boullata et al., 2017; Drummond Hayes, 2018). Capping the tube deters the entry of microorganisms and prevents leakage onto the bed linens.
14. Clamp the tube and remove the syringe. Cap the tube, reattach it to the feeding delivery set, or attach the tube to suction, based on the circumstances.	Capping or reattachment to the feeding delivery set or reattachment to suction allows for appropriate treatment for individual patients.
15. Remove equipment and return the patient to a position of comfort. Remove gloves. Raise the side rail and lower the bed.	This promotes patient comfort and safety. Removing gloves properly reduces the risk for infection transmission and contamination of other items.
16. Remove additional PPE, if used. Perform hand hygiene.	Proper removal of PPE reduces the risk for infection transmission and contamination of other items. Hand hygiene prevents transmission of microorganisms.

EVALUATION

The expected outcomes have been met when the tube has been determined to be located in the patient's stomach without complications, and the patient has not exhibited signs and symptoms of aspiration.

DOCUMENTATION

Guidelines

Document the type of nasogastric tube that is present. Record the criteria that were used to confirm tube placement. Document respiratory and abdominal assessment findings. Include subjective data, such as any reports from the patient of abdominal pain or nausea or any other patient response.

Sample Documentation

> 10/29/25 1015 Position of NG tube was compared with and matched initial measurement on insertion. Abdomen nondistended and soft; patient denies pain or nausea. Scant residual aspirated; pH 3.9. Tube flushed with 60 mL water with ease. Patient instructed to call for nurse for pain or nausea or other concerns.
> —S. Essner, RN

DEVELOPING CLINICAL REASONING AND CLINICAL JUDGMENT

UNEXPECTED SITUATIONS AND ASSOCIATED INTERVENTIONS

• *No gastric contents can be aspirated*: Visually inspect the oral cavity to check for misplacement of tube/coiling in mouth. Reposition the patient. Flush tube with an air bolus, then apply negative pressure to the plunger. Repeat as needed. Refer to Step 9 above.

**SPECIAL
CONSIDERATIONS**
General Considerations

- Check tube placement before administering any fluids, medications, or feeding, using multiple techniques: x-ray, external length, external verification marking, pH testing, and carbon dioxide monitoring (if available). Consistent inability to withdraw fluid from tube may indicate displacement of the tube from the stomach into the esophagus (AACN, 2020).
- Signs of respiratory distress may be absent in patients with an impaired level of consciousness when nasogastric tubes are inadvertently positioned in the airway (AACN, 2020).
- Sterile water should be used for tube flushes in immunocompromised or critically ill patients (Allen, 2015; Boullata et al., 2017).
- Gastric pH ≥6 is of no benefit in predicting tube location in the GI tract or in ruling out tracheopulmonary placement (Boullata et al., 2017).
- Monitoring for carbon dioxide to determine NG tube position and/or dislodgement has been investigated (Hess et al., 2021). This involves the use of colorimetric end-tidal CO_2 detector to detect the presence of carbon dioxide, which would indicate tube positioning in the patient's airway (Hess et al., 2021). Monitoring for carbon dioxide may be helpful to detect placement of a feeding tube in the tracheobronchial tree (AACN, 2020; Boullata et al., 2017; Hess et al., 2021). However, this technique may be unreliable, as it cannot differentiate placement in the mouth and carbon dioxide may not be detected when the tube is in the patient's airway if the ports in the tube are occluded (Gilber & Burns, 2010, as cited in AACN, 2020).

**EVIDENCE
FOR PRACTICE ▶**

VERIFICATION OF FEEDING TUBE PLACEMENT
American Association of Critical Care Nurses (AACN). (2020, January 29). *AACN practice alert. Initial and ongoing verification of feeding tube placement in adults.* https://www.aacn.org/
  Practice alerts are directives from AACN that are supported by authoritative evidence to ensure excellence in practice and a safe and humane work environment. These directives provide guidance and standardize practice as well as identify/inform about new advances and trends. The AACN has provided directives addressing best practice for verification of feeding tube placement in adults. Expected practice includes radiographic confirmation of correct tube placement of all blindly inserted small-bore or large-bore tubes prior to initial use for feedings or medication administration, tubes inserted with assistance from an electromagnetic tube placement device, and gastric decompression tubes that are later used for other purposes. The tube's exit site from the nose or mouth should be marked and length documented immediately after radiographic confirmation of correct tube placement. The mark should be observed routinely, and the external tube measured to assess for a change in length of the external portion of the tube. Bedside techniques to assess tube location should be used at regular intervals and at 4-hour intervals after feedings are started (AACN, 2020) to determine if the tube has remained in its intended position.

Skill 11-3 ▶ Administering a Tube Feeding (Open System)

Skill Variation: *Administering a Tube Feeding Using a Prefilled Tube-Feeding Set (Closed System)*

Depending on the patient's physical, health, and nutritional requirements and status, feeding through the NG tube or other GI tube might be ordered. The steps for administering feedings are similar regardless of the tube used. Feeding can be provided by bolus, intermittent continuous or continuous infusion (Anderson, 2018b; Bischoff et al., 2020). Bolus formula administration involves administering a 200 to 400 mL volume over a 15- to 60-minute period, depending on patient tolerance, using a 50-mL syringe (no feeding pump) (Bischoff et al., 2020). The total feed volume is divided into four to six feedings throughout the day (Bischoff et al., 2020). Intermittent

(continued on page 696)

Skill 11-3 ▶ Administering a Tube Feeding (Open System) *(continued)*

continuous feeding is the administration of nutritional formula and fluids by giving a volume of formula over a period of time at regular intervals using a feeding pump (Anderson, 2018b; Bischoff et al., 2020). Continuous feeding is the administration of a small volume of formula over a longer period of time, for as much as 12, 18, or 24 hours. Use of a feeding pump delivers nutritional formula and fluid at a set rate over a specified period of time (Anderson, 2018b). Volume-based feeding protocols are another approach to deliver enteral nutrition. Refer to the discussion in the *Special Considerations* below. Box 11-3 provides criteria to evaluate enteral feeding tolerance.

The procedure below describes using open systems and a feeding pump; the skill variation at the end of the skill describes using a closed system.

Box 11-3 ▏ Monitoring for Tolerance of Enteral Nutrition

Patient tolerance of the volume and type of formula must be monitored daily (Boullata et al., 2017; McClave, Taylor, et al., 2016). Criteria to consider when evaluating patient feeding tolerance include:

- Absence of nausea, vomiting
- Absence of diarrhea and constipation
- Absence of abdominal pain and feelings of fullness
- Absence of distention
- Achievement of target goal nutrition administration
- Presence of bowel sounds within normal limits

*Gastric residual volume (GRV) is not a suitable parameter to determine feeding intolerance and has been shown to be a poor marker of true gastric volume, gastric emptying, risk of aspiration, pneumonia, and poor outcomes (Hartwell et al., 2018; McClave, DiBaise, et al., 2016; McClave, Taylor, et al., 2016; Pars & Çavuşoğlu, 2019). Some evidence for practice suggests measurement of GRV may only be necessary during initiation and advancement of enteral nutrition (EN) (Roveron et al., 2018; Singer et al., 2019). If GRV checks are part of facility policy and procedure, automatic cessation of EN should be avoided for GRVs <500 mL in the absence of other signs of intolerance (Boullata et al., 2017; McClave, Taylor, et al., 2016; Roveron et al., 2018). Evaluate the significance of a single high gastric residual volume in relation to other indicators of GI intolerance, including abdominal distention, abdominal discomfort, nausea, and vomiting (AACN, 2018).

DELEGATION CONSIDERATIONS

The administration of a tube feeding is not usually delegated to assistive personnel (AP) in the acute care setting. The administration of a tube feeding in some settings may be delegated to assistive personnel (AP) who have received appropriate training, after assessment of tube placement and patency by the registered nurse. Depending on the state's nurse practice act and the organization's policies and procedures, the administration of a tube feeding may be delegated to licensed practical/vocational nurses (LPN/LVNs). The decision to delegate must be based on careful analysis of the patient's needs and circumstances as well as the qualifications of the person to whom the task is being delegated. Refer to the Delegation Guidelines in Appendix A.

EQUIPMENT

- Prescribed tube-feeding formula at room temperature
- Feeding bag or prefilled tube-feeding set
- Stethoscope
- Nonsterile gloves
- Additional PPE, as indicated
- Alcohol preps
- Disposable pad or towel
- Large syringe (20 to 50 mL)

- Enteral feeding pump (if ordered)
- Rubber band
- Clamp (Hoffman or butterfly)
- IV pole
- Water for irrigation and hydration, as needed
- pH test strip (calibrated in units of 0.5 and approved for use with human secretions)
- Tape measure, or other measuring device

ASSESSMENT

Assess for signs of respiratory distress; coughing, choking, dyspnea may occur when a tube is inadvertently positioned in the airway (AACN, 2020). Assess the abdomen by inspecting for presence of distention, auscultate for bowel sounds, and palpate the abdomen for firmness or tenderness. If the abdomen is distended, consider measuring the abdominal girth at the umbilicus. If the patient reports any tenderness or nausea, exhibits any rigidity or firmness of the abdomen, and if bowel sounds are absent, confer with health care provider before administering the tube feeding. Assess for patient and/or family/caregiver understanding, if appropriate, for the rationale for the tube feeding and address any questions or concerns expressed by the patient and family members/caregivers.

ACTUAL OR POTENTIAL HEALTH PROBLEMS AND NEEDS	Many actual or potential health problems or issues may require the use of this skill as part of related interventions. An appropriate health problem or issue may include: • Aspiration risk • Knowledge deficiency • Effective Response to Enteral Nutrition
OUTCOME IDENTIFICATION AND PLANNING	The expected outcome to achieve when administering an enteral feeding is that the patient achieves target goal nutrition administration without nausea, vomiting, gastric distention, diarrhea, constipation, or pain. Additional expected outcomes may include that the patient does not exhibit signs and symptoms of aspiration, the patient demonstrates an increase in weight, and the patient verbalizes knowledge related to tube feeding.

IMPLEMENTATION

ACTION

1. Gather equipment. Check amount, concentration, type, and frequency of tube feeding in the patient's health record. Check the formula expiration date.

2. Perform hand hygiene and put on PPE, if indicated.

3. Identify the patient.

4. Explain the procedure to the patient. Answer any questions, as needed.

5. Assemble equipment on the overbed table or other surface within reach.

6. Close the patient's bedside curtain or door. Raise the bed to a comfortable working position, usually elbow height of the caregiver (VHACEOSH, 2016). Perform respiratory and abdominal assessments as described above.

7. **Position the patient as upright as possible with the head of the bed elevated at least 30 to 45 degrees or as near-normal position for eating as possible.** Patient should remain in this position during feeding and for 1 hour afterward. **Patients for whom the semi-recumbent position is contraindicated or who cannot tolerate a semi-Fowler position should be placed in a reverse- or anti-Trendelenburg position** (Boullata et al., 2017; Roveron et al., 2018).

8. Put on gloves. Confirm placement of the nasogastric tube in the patient's stomach using at least two methods (refer to Skill 11-2).

9. If assessments to check placement are inconclusive, the exposed tube length has changed, or there are any other indications that the tube may not be in place, check placement by radiograph (x-ray) of placement of tube, based on facility policy.

RATIONALE

This provides for an organized approach to the task. Checking ensures that correct feeding will be administered. Outdated formula may be contaminated.

Hand hygiene and PPE prevent the spread of microorganisms. PPE is required based on transmission precautions.

Identifying the patient ensures the right patient receives the intervention and helps prevent errors.

Explanation facilitates patient engagement.

Organization facilitates performance of the task.

Closing curtains or the door provides for patient privacy. Having the bed at the proper height prevents back and muscle strain. Assessment is vital to detect changes in the patient's condition before initiating the intervention.

These positions minimize possibility of reflux, aspiration, and pneumonia (McClave, Taylor, et al., 2016; Roveron et al., 2018).

Gloves prevent contact with blood and body fluids. With the exception of radiographic examination, which is usually done immediately after insertion to verify initial tube placement, the use of two or more of these techniques in conjunction with each other increases the likelihood of correct tube placement (AACN, 2020; Anderson, 2019; Anderson, 2018a; Dias et al., 2019; Rahimi et al., 2015).

Radiographic confirmation is considered the most reliable method for identifying the position of the NG tube (AACN, 2020; Boullata et al., 2017).

(continued on page 698)

Skill 11-3 ▶ Administering a Tube Feeding (Open System) *(continued)*

ACTION

10. If gastric residual volume (GRV) checks are part of facility policy and procedure, check GRV: After multiple steps have been taken to ensure that the feeding tube is located in the stomach or small intestine, aspirate all gastric contents with the syringe and measure to check for gastric residual—the amount of feeding remaining in the stomach. Return the residual based on facility policy. Proceed with feeding if the amount of residual does not exceed facility policy or the limit indicated in the health record. Refer to additional information in the *Special Considerations* below.

11. Flush tube with 30 to 50 mL of water for irrigation. Disconnect syringe from tubing and cap end of tubing while preparing the formula feeding equipment. Remove gloves. Perform hand hygiene.

12. Put on gloves before preparing, assembling, and handling any part of the feeding system.

13. Administer feeding.

When Using a Feeding Bag Administration System and Gravity (Bolus; Open System)

a. Label the bag and/or tubing with date and time. Hang the bag on the IV pole and adjust to about 12 inches above the stomach. Clamp tubing.

b. Check the expiration date of the formula. Cleanse top of feeding container with a disinfectant before opening it (Figure 1). Pour formula into the feeding bag and allow solution to run through tubing. Close the clamp.

c. Attach feeding administration set to the feeding tube (Figure 2), open clamp, and regulate drip according to the prescribed rate or allow feeding to run in over 30 minutes.

RATIONALE

GRV has been used to monitor for tolerance of enteral nutrition; however, there is little support for this intervention as routine measurement for most patients, and it is not considered best practice and should not be used as part of routine care to monitor enteral nutrition (McClave, Taylor, et al., 2016; Ozen et al., 2018; Parker et al., 2019; Pars & Çavuşoğlu, 2019; Rysavy et al., 2020). GRV is not a suitable parameter to determine feeding intolerance (McClave, Taylor, et al., 2016; Pars & Çavuşoğlu, 2019). GRV has been shown to be a poor marker of true gastric volume; gastric emptying; and risk of aspiration, pneumonia, and poor outcomes (Hartwell et al., 2018; McClave, DiBaise, et al., 2016). The use of GRVs as a monitor for tolerance increases the risk of tube clogging and decreases attainment of nutritional goals as a result of disruption of delivery of enteral nutrition (McClave, DiBaise, et al., 2016).

Flushing the tube prevents occlusion (Bischoff et al., 2020; Boullata et al., 2017; Drummond Hayes, 2018). Capping the tube deters the entry of microorganisms and prevents leakage onto the bed linens. Hand hygiene prevents transmission of microorganisms.

Gloves prevent contact with blood and body fluids and deter transmission of contaminants to feeding equipment and/or formula.

Labeling date and time of first use allows for disposal of bag and tubing within 24 hours, to deter growth of microorganisms. Proper feeding bag height reduces risk of formula being introduced too quickly.

Cleansing the container top with alcohol minimizes risk for contaminants entering feeding bag. Formula displaces air in the tubing.

Introducing formula at an appropriate rate allows the stomach to accommodate to the feeding and decreases GI distress.

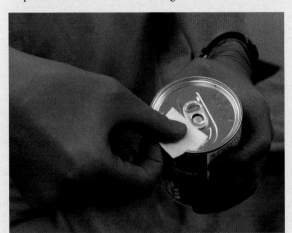

FIGURE 1. Cleaning top of feeding container with alcohol before opening it.

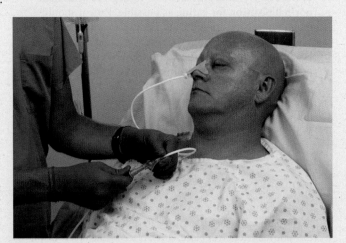

FIGURE 2. Attaching feeding administration set to NG tube.

ACTION

d. **Add 30 to 60 mL (1 to 2 oz) of water for irrigation to feeding bag when feeding is almost completed** (Figure 3) and allow it to run through the tube.

e. Clamp the tubing immediately after water has been instilled. Disconnect the feeding administration set from the feeding tube. Clamp the tube and cover the end with cap (Figure 4).

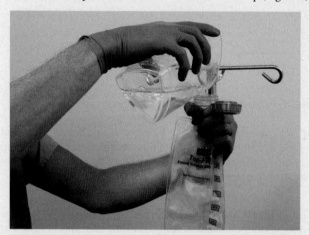

FIGURE 3. Pouring water into feeding bag.

When Using a Large Syringe (Bolus; Open System)

a. Remove the plunger from the 30- or 60-mL syringe (Figure 5).

b. Attach the syringe to the feeding tube and pour a pre-measured amount of tube-feeding formula into the syringe (Figure 6). Open the clamp on the feeding tube and allow the formula to enter the tube. Regulate the rate, fast or slow, by the height of the syringe. **Do not push the formula with the syringe plunger.**

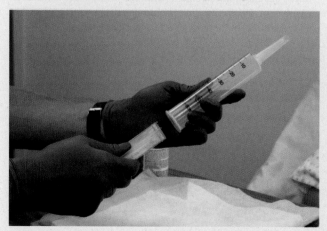

FIGURE 5. Removing plunger from a 60-mL syringe.

RATIONALE

Water rinses the feeding from the tube and helps to keep it patent as well as provides hydration for the patient. Feeding tubes should be flushed with at least 30 mL of water before starting and after completion of bolus feedings and every 4 to 8 hours during continuous feeding (Bischoff et al., 2020; Boullata et al., 2017; Roveron et al., 2018), based on the patient's fluid needs and restrictions (Boullata et al., 2017).

Clamping the tube prevents air from entering the stomach. Capping the tube deters entry of microorganisms and covering end of tube protects patient and linens from fluid leakage from tube.

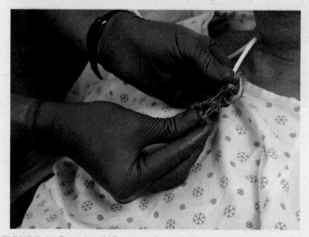

FIGURE 4. Capping NG tube after it is clamped.

Introducing the formula at a slow, regular rate allows the stomach to accommodate to the feeding and decreases GI distress. The higher the syringe is held, the faster the formula flows.

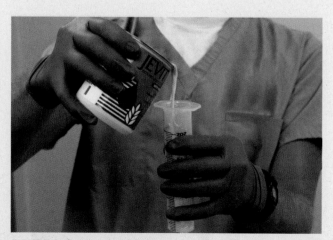

FIGURE 6. Pouring formula into syringe.

(continued on page 700)

Skill 11-3 ▶ Administering a Tube Feeding (Open System) *(continued)*

ACTION	RATIONALE

ACTION

c. When feeding is almost completed, **add 30 to 60 mL (1 to 2 oz) of water for irrigation to the syringe** (Figure 7) and allow it to run through the tube.

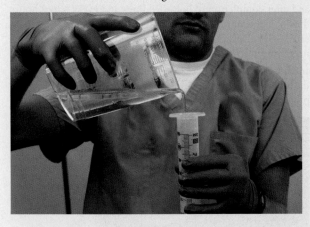

RATIONALE

Water rinses the feeding from the tube and helps to keep it patent as well as provides hydration for the patient. Feeding tubes should be flushed with at least 30 mL of water before starting and after completion of bolus feedings (Bischoff et al., 2020; Boullata et al., 2017; Roveron et al., 2018), based on the patient's fluid needs and restrictions (Boullata et al., 2017).

FIGURE 7. Pouring water into almost-empty syringe.

d. When the syringe has emptied, hold it high, clamp the tube, and disconnect it from the tube. Cover the end of the tube with the cap.

By holding syringe high, the formula will not backflow out of tube and onto patient. Clamping the tube prevents air from entering the stomach. Capping end of tube deters entry of microorganisms and prevents fluid leakage from tube.

When Using an Enteral Feeding Pump (Open System)

a. Close the flow-regulator clamp on tubing and fill the feeding bag with prescribed formula, as described in Steps 13a and 13b. Place a label on the bag with patient's name, date, and time the feeding was hung.

Closing the clamp prevents the formula from moving through the tubing until the nurse is ready. Labeling date and time of first use allows for disposal of the bag and tubing within 24 hours, to deter growth of microorganisms.

b. Hang the feeding container on the IV pole. Open the clamp on tubing and allow the solution to flow through the tubing.

This primes the tubing, removing air in the tubing and preventing air from being forced into the stomach or intestines.

c. Connect the administration setup to the feeding pump, following the manufacturer's directions. Set the prescribed rate (Figure 8).

Feeding pumps vary. Some of the newer pumps have built-in safeguards that protect the patient from complications. Safety features include cassettes that prevent free flow of formula, automatic tube flush, safety tips that prevent accidental attachment to an IV setup, and various audible and visible alarms. The rate of infusion begins at the recommended rate, based on guidelines from the dietician or nutrition nurse specialist, and the rate is advanced in increments until the desired rate is achieved (Anderson, 2018b); feeding should be advanced to goal within 48 to 72 hours of initiation (McClave, DiBaise, et al., 2016).

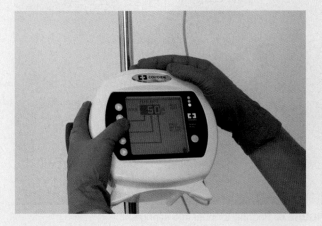

FIGURE 8. Setting infusion rate on pump.

ACTION

d. **Flush the tube with at least 30 mL of water at least every 4 to 8 hours during continuous feeding. Verify placement (refer to Skill 11-2) before administering flush.**

14. Remove equipment and return the patient to a position of comfort. Remove gloves. Perform hand hygiene. Raise the side rail and lower the bed.

15. Put on gloves. Wash and clean equipment or replace according to facility policy. Remove gloves. Perform hand hygiene.

16. Monitor patient tolerance of enteral nutrition. Observe the patient's response during and after tube feeding and signs of tolerance at least daily. Refer to Box 11-3 for criteria to evaluate tolerance of enteral feeding.

17. **Have the patient remain in an upright position for at least 1 hour after feeding.** Refer to Step 7.

18. **Remove additional PPE, if used. Perform hand hygiene.**

RATIONALE

Feeding tubes should be flushed with at least 30 mL of water before starting and after completion of bolus feedings; every 4 to 8 hours during continuous feeding (Bischoff et al., 2020; Boullata et al., 2017; Roveron et al., 2018); and before and after medication administration (Drummond Hayes, 2018) to prevent blockage, based on the patient's fluid needs and restrictions (Boullata et al., 2017).

This promotes patient comfort and safety. Removing gloves properly reduces the risk for infection transmission and contamination of other items. Hand hygiene prevents transmission of microorganisms.

Gloves prevent contamination and deter spread of microorganisms. Reusable systems are cleansed with soap and water with each use and replaced every 24 hours. Refer to facility policy and manufacturer's guidelines for specifics on equipment care.

Patient tolerance of the volume and type of formula must be monitored daily (Boullata et al., 2017; McClave, Taylor, et al., 2016).

This minimizes possibility of reflux, aspiration, and pneumonia and should be implemented unless contraindicated (McClave, Taylor, et al., 2016; Roveron et al., 2018).

Proper removal of PPE reduces the risk for infection transmission and contamination of other items. Hand hygiene prevents transmission of microorganisms.

EVALUATION

The expected outcomes have been met when the patient has achieved target goal nutrition administration without nausea, vomiting, gastric distention, diarrhea, constipation, or pain; the patient did not exhibit signs and symptoms of aspiration; the patient has demonstrated an increase in weight; and the patient has verbalized knowledge related to tube feeding.

DOCUMENTATION

Guidelines

Document the type of NG tube or gastrostomy/jejunostomy tube that is present. Record the criteria that were used to confirm tube placement before feeding was initiated and during administration, as indicated. Record respiratory and abdominal assessments. If GRVs are part of facility policy and procedure, record the amount of gastric residual volume that was obtained. Document the position of the patient, the type of feeding, and the method and the amount of feeding. Include any relevant patient teaching. Document results of evaluation of tolerance of enteral feeding.

Sample Documentation

10/29/25 1815 Position of NG tube was compared with initial measurement on insertion; no change in measurement. No signs of respiratory distress. Abdomen nondistended and soft; patient denies pain or nausea. HOB raised to 45 degrees. Gastric aspirate pH 3.9. 150 mL of Jevity 1.2 Cal administered over 30 minutes. Tube flushed with 60-mL water with ease. Patient instructed to call for nurse for pain or nausea or other concerns related to feeding.

—S. Essner, RN

(continued on page 702)

Skill 11-3 ▶ Administering a Tube Feeding (Open System) *(continued)*

DEVELOPING CLINICAL REASONING AND CLINICAL JUDGMENT

UNEXPECTED SITUATIONS AND ASSOCIATED INTERVENTIONS

- *Nasogastric tube is identified not to be in stomach or intestine:* Tube must be in the stomach before feeding. If the tube is in misplaced, the patient is at increased risk for aspiration. Anticipate replacement of feeding tube. Refer to Skill 13-8.
- *Patient reports nausea after tube feeding:* Ensure that the head of the bed remains elevated and that suction equipment is at the bedside. Assess for other signs and symptoms of changes in tolerance to enteral feeding. Check the medication record to see if any antiemetics have been ordered for the patient. Consider collaborating with the health care team to review administration rate, volume, and type of nutritional formula. Monitor for pattern of nausea related to enteral feeding.
- *When attempting to aspirate contents, the nurse notes that tube is clogged:* Feeding tubes are prone to blockage, due to protein-rich formula solutions, the viscosity of the feeding formulas and relatively small diameter of the feeding tube lumens, the use of the tubes for medication administration, and inadequate water flushes (Bischoff et al., 2020; Drummond Hayes, 2018). Try to remove the clog: use air bolus or attach a 30- or 60-mL piston syringe to the feeding tube and pull back the plunger to help dislodge the clog. Fill the syringe with warm water and attempt to flush. If met with resistance, use gentle back and forth motion of the plunger to help loosen the clog. If necessary, clamp the tube to allow the warm water to penetrate the clog for up to 20 minutes and then attempt to flush (Boullata et al., 2017). The tube may have to be replaced. To prevent clogs, ensure that adequate flushing is completed after each feeding and before and after medication administration (Bischoff et al., 2020; Drummond Hayes, 2018).

SPECIAL CONSIDERATIONS

- There is no benefit from stopping feedings during short periods of lowering of the head of the bed (such as turning the patient) (Boullata et al., 2017). If a prolonged procedure will require lowering of the head of the bed, feedings should be stopped during this period; feedings should be promptly restarted when the procedure is ended or as feasible.
- If GRV checks are part of facility policy and procedure, automatic cessation of enteral nutrition should be avoided for GRVs < 500 mL in the absence of other signs of intolerance (Boullata et al., 2017; McClave, Taylor, et al., 2016; Roveron et al., 2018).
- Volume-based feeding protocols in which 24-hour or daily volumes are targeted instead of hourly rates have been shown to increase volume of nutrition delivered (Heyland et al., 2013, as cited in McClave, Taylor, et al., 2016). This type of method empowers nurses to increase feeding rates to make up for volume lost for scheduled and unscheduled interruptions or while enteral nutrition is held and increase attainment of nutritional goals, supporting optimal nutritional intake (Kinikin et al., 2020; McClave, Taylor, et al., 2016).
- Feedings into the intestine are always continuous and include initiation at a lower rate with a gradual increase in the rate until the target rate identified to meet nutritional goals is met (Bischoff et al., 2020).
- A combination of methods, such as overnight continuous feeding and bolus feeding during the day, may be used for some patients to best meet their needs and allow for autonomy and lifestyle preferences (Bischoff et al., 2020). For other patients, cyclic feeding, administering continuous feeding for a portion of the 24-hour period, may be implemented. The usual routine is to feed the patient for 12 to 16 hours, most often overnight. Cyclic feeding allows the patient to attempt eating regular meals during the day, if this is possible, making ambulation and activity easier.
- Tolerance to gastric feeding can be improved through use of a prokinetic agent, continuous infusion, and elevation of the head of the bed (McClave, DiBaise, et al., 2016).
- Sterile water should be used for tube flushes in immunocompromised or critically ill patients (Allen, 2015; Boullata et al., 2017).
- If GRV checks are part of facility policy and procedure, evaluate the significance of a single high gastric residual volume in relation to other indicators of GI intolerance, including abdominal distention, abdominal discomfort, nausea, and vomiting (AACN, 2018).
- Immediately refrigerate formulas reconstituted in advance. Discard unused reconstituted and refrigerated formulas within 24 hours of preparation (Boullata et al., 2017).

- Discard unused reconstituted formulas exposed to room temperature after 4 hours (Boullata et al., 2017).
- Some feeding equipment allows for the addition of water for flushes to a second feeding container, which enters the system through a second set of tubing. The feeding pump will automatically administer the preset volume of flush at the preset frequency.

Skill Variation ▶ Administering a Tube Feeding Using a Prefilled Tube-Feeding Set (Closed System)

Prefilled tube-feeding sets, which are considered closed systems, are frequently used to provide patient nourishment. Closed systems contain sterile feeding solutions in ready-to-hang containers (Figure A). This method reduces the opportunity for bacterial contamination of the feeding formula. In general, these prefilled feedings are administered via an enteral pump.

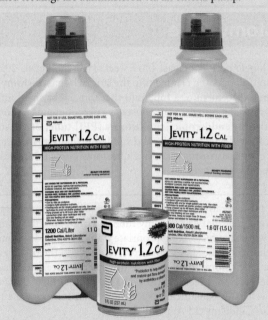

FIGURE A. Prefilled tube feedings in plastic containers and ready-to-use feeding in a can. (*Source:* Reprinted with permission from Abbott Nutrition, a division of Abbott Laboratories.)

1. Check amount, concentration, type, and frequency of tube feeding in the patient's health record.
2. Gather all equipment, checking the feeding solution and container for correct solution and expiration date. Label formula container with patient's name, type of solution, and prescribed rate. Label administration tubing/set with date and time.
3. Perform hand hygiene. Put on PPE, as indicated.

4. Identify the patient and explain the procedure.

5. Put on gloves.
6. Verify feeding tube placement of the feeding tube; refer to Skill 11-2.
7. If GRVs are part of facility policy and procedure, check and record the amount of gastric residual volume. Return residual to the stomach, as indicated by facility policy.
8. Flush the tube with 30 mL of water.
9. Put on nonsterile gloves; remove the screw-on cap and attach the administration setup with the drip chamber and tubing.
10. Hang the feeding container on the IV pole and connect it to the feeding pump, allowing solution to flow through the tubing, following the manufacturer's directions.
11. Attach the feeding setup to the patient's feeding tube.
12. Open the clamp of the patient's feeding tube.
13. Turn on the pump.
14. Set the pump at the prescribed rate of flow and remove gloves. Perform hand hygiene.

15. Observe the patient's response during the tube feeding.
16. Continue to assess the patient for signs and symptoms of GI distress, such as nausea, abdominal distention, or absence of bowel sounds.
17. Have the patient remain in the upright position throughout the feeding and for at least 1 hour after feeding.
18. After the prescribed amount of feeding has been administrated (or according to facility policy), turn off the pump, put on nonsterile gloves, clamp the feeding tube, and disconnect it from the feeding set tube, capping the end of the feeding set.
19. Flush the feeding tube with 30 to 60 mL of water.
20. Clamp the feeding tube. Cover the end of the tube with the cap.
21. Continue as directed in Skill 11-3, Steps 14–18.

(*continued on page 704*)

Skill 11-3 ▶ Administering a Tube Feeding (Open System) *(continued)*

EVIDENCE FOR PRACTICE ▶

ASPEN SAFE PRACTICES FOR ENTERAL NUTRITION THERAPY
Boullata, J. I., Carrera, A. L., Harvey, L., Escuro, A. A., Hudson, L., Mays, A., Wessel, J. J., Bajpai, S., Beebe, M. L., Kinn, T. J., Klang, M. G., Lord, L., Martin, K., Pompeii-Wolfe, C., Sullivan, J., Wood, A., Malone, A., Guenter, P., & ASPEN Safe Practices for Enteral Nutrition Therapy, American Society for Parenteral and Enteral Nutrition. (2017). ASPEN safe practices for enteral nutrition therapy. *Journal of Parenteral and Enteral Nutrition, 41*(1), 15–103. https://doi.org/10.1177/0148607116673053.

    The American Society for Parenteral and Enteral Nutrition (ASPEN) *Safe Practices for Enteral Nutrition Therapy* guideline provides recommendations based on the available evidence and expert consensus for safe practices for patients receiving enteral nutrition.

    Refer to details in Skill 11-2, Evidence for Practice.

Skill 11-4 ▶ Caring for a Gastrostomy Tube

When enteral feeding is required for a longer period (at least 4 to 6 weeks) (Bischoff et al., 2020), an enterostomal tube may be placed through an opening created into the stomach (**gastrostomy tube**) or into the jejunum (**jejunostomy tube**). Placement of a tube into the stomach or small intestine can be accomplished by a surgeon or gastroenterologist via endoscopy (**percutaneous endoscopic gastrostomy [PEG] tube** and **percutaneous endoscopic jejunostomy [PEJ] tube**) or via surgery (open or laparoscopically). Providing care at the insertion site and validating tube patency are nursing responsibilities. Site care is the same for a gastrostomy and a jejunostomy. Box 11-3 in Skill 11-3 provides criteria to evaluate enteral feeding tolerance.

DELEGATION CONSIDERATIONS

The care of a gastrostomy tube, in the postoperative period, is not delegated to assistive personnel (AP) in the acute care setting. The care of a healed gastrostomy tube site in some settings may be delegated to assistive personnel (AP) who have received appropriate training, after assessment of the tube by the registered nurse. Depending on the state's nurse practice act and the organization's policies and procedures, the care of a gastrostomy tube may be delegated to licensed practical/vocational nurses (LPN/LVNs). The decision to delegate must be based on careful analysis of the patient's needs and circumstances as well as the qualifications of the person to whom the task is being delegated. Refer to the Delegation Guidelines in Appendix A.

EQUIPMENT

- Nonsterile gloves
- Additional PPE, as indicated
- Washcloth, towel, and skin cleanser or cotton-tipped applicators and sterile saline solution (depending on patient circumstances)
- Gauze (if needed)

ASSESSMENT

Assess the gastrostomy or jejunostomy tube site, noting any drainage, pressure injury, erythema, inflammation, erosion, or hypergranulation tissue. Assess for pain. Assess the tube position and the position of the external fixation device. Refer to details in the Implementation section of this Skill. Check to ensure that the tube is securely stabilized and has not become dislodged. Assess the tension of the tube. If the tension is too great, the internal anchoring device may erode into the gastric wall (Roveron et al, 2018). Excessive traction may also contribute to enlargement of the stoma and development of leakage around the tube (Roveron et al., 2018).

ACTUAL OR POTENTIAL HEALTH PROBLEMS AND NEEDS	Many actual or potential health problems or issues may require the use of this skill as part of related interventions. An appropriate health problem or issue may include: • Knowledge deficiency • Altered skin integrity • Infection risk
OUTCOME IDENTIFICATION AND PLANNING	The expected outcomes to achieve when caring for a gastrostomy tube are that the patient does not exhibit signs and symptoms of drainage, pressure injury, erythema, inflammation, erosion, or hypergranulation tissue at the tube insertion site, and the tube remains in place. In addition, the patient verbalizes little discomfort related to tube placement and verbalizes an understanding of the care needed for the gastrostomy tube, as appropriate.

IMPLEMENTATION

ACTION	**RATIONALE**
1. Gather equipment. Verify the prescribed interventions or facility policy and procedure regarding site care.	Assembling equipment provides for an organized approach to the task. Verification ensures the patient receives the correct intervention.
2. Perform hand hygiene and put on PPE, if indicated.	Hand hygiene and PPE prevent the spread of microorganisms. PPE is required based on transmission precautions.
3. Identify the patient.	Identifying the patient ensures the right patient receives the intervention and helps prevent errors.
4. Explain the procedure to the patient. Answer any questions, as needed.	Explanation facilitates patient engagement.
5. Assess for presence of pain at the tube-insertion site. If pain is present, offer the patient analgesic medication per the prescribed interventions and wait for the medication to take effect before beginning insertion-site care.	Feeding tubes can be uncomfortable, especially in the first few days after insertion. Analgesic medication may permit the patient to tolerate the insertion site care more easily. After the first few days, pain at the site should diminish (Roveron et al., 2018).
6. Pull the patient's bedside curtain. Assemble equipment on the bedside table, within reach. Raise the bed to a comfortable working position (VHACEOSH, 2016).	This provides for privacy. Assembling equipment provides for organized approach to the task. An appropriate working height facilitates comfort and proper body mechanics for the nurse.
7. Put on gloves. Assess the gastrostomy site, as described above.	Gloves prevent contact with blood and body fluids. Assessment is vital to detect changes in the patient's condition before initiating the intervention.
8. Measure the length of the exposed tube, comparing it with the initial measurement after insertion. Alternatively, examine the mark on the tube at the skin; the mark should be at skin level at the insertion site.	Tube length should be checked and compared with the initial measurement or marking daily (Roveron et al., 2018). A change in the length of the exposed tube may indicate displacement.
9. Beginning 24 hours after placement of the tube and for the first week, cleanse the stoma and peristomal skin with sterile saline to remove any discharge or material around the tube (Bischoff et al., 2020; Roveron et al., 2018) (Figure 1). Pat the skin around the insertion site dry. If necessary, cover the stoma with sterile gauze to absorb exudate or other fluids (Roveron et al., 2018).	Cleaning the new site with sterile saline solution prevents the introduction of microorganisms into the wound (Roveron et al., 2018). Crust and drainage can harbor bacteria and lead to skin breakdown. Drying the skin thoroughly prevents skin breakdown. Gauze absorbs drainage.

(continued on page 706)

Skill 11-4 ▶ Caring for a Gastrostomy Tube *(continued)*

ACTION	RATIONALE
10. After the first week to 10 days, wet a washcloth and apply a small amount of skin cleanser onto the washcloth. Gently cleanse around the insertion, removing any crust or drainage (Bischoff et al., 2020; Roveron et al., 2018) (Figure 2).	Crust and drainage can harbor bacteria and lead to skin breakdown. Removing the cleanser helps to prevent skin irritation. If able, the patient may shower and cleanse the site with soap and water. Drying the skin thoroughly prevents skin breakdown. Placing the dressing above the external fixation device avoids excessive tension (Roveron et al., 2018). Gauze absorbs drainage.
Rinse the site, removing all cleanser. Pat the skin around the insertion site dry. If necessary, based on facility policy and patient situation, place a gauze dressing above the external fixation device. Alternatively, if the exterior fixation device is 5 mm above the skin, the dressing may be placed under the exterior fixation device, if the dressing is not too thick (Roveron et al., 2018).	

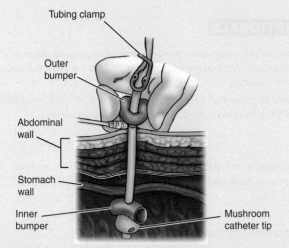

FIGURE 1. Wiping gastric tube site with cotton-tipped applicator and sterile saline.

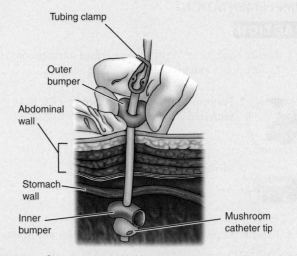

FIGURE 2. Cleaning site with skin cleanser, water, and washcloth.

ACTION	RATIONALE
11. After the first 24 hours, gently rotate the position of the gastrostomy tube 360 degrees. **Rotation of the tube should be done at least once a week and no more than once a day** (Roveron et al., 2018).	Rotation of the tube prevents adherence to the tract and adhesion (Roveron et al., 2018).
12. After the first 7 to 10 days, loosen the exterior fixation device and gently push the tube into the stomach 2 to 3 cm, then gently pull it back until it reaches the area of minimal resistance (the gastric wall). **Push/pull of the tube should be done at least once a week and no more than once a day** (Bischoff et al., 2020; Roveron et al., 2018). Assess that the guard or external bumper is not digging into the surrounding skin. The external fixation device should be 0.5 to 1 cm above the skin (Bischoff et al., 2020; Roveron et al., 2018). **Avoid placing any tension on the tube.**	The gastrocutaneous tract heals in 7 to 10 days (Roveron et al., 2018). This maneuver reduces the risk for buried bumper syndrome (Bischoff et al., 2020; Roveron et al., 2018). Proper placement prevents/avoids excessive tube movement and enlargement of the stoma (Roveron et al., 2018). The external fixation device should be 0.5 to 1 cm above the skin to avoid excessive tension between the interior and exterior fixation devices and to reduce the risk of ischemia, necrosis, infection, and buried bumper syndrome (Bischoff et al., 2020; Roveron et al., 2018). Excessive distance between the external fixation device and the skin could lead to fixation of the gastric wall to the abdominal wall and formation of a gastrocutaneous fistula (Roveron et al., 2018). Excessive traction may contribute to enlargement of the stoma and the development of leakage around the tube (Roveron et al., 2018).
13. For most patients, the site can be left open to air unless there is drainage. Avoid the use of creams or powders around the stoma (Roveron et al., 2018).	Dressing is not necessary in the absence of drainage (Bischoff et al., 2020; Roveron et al., 2018). Avoiding use of creams or powders around the stoma prevents growth of pathogens (Roveron et al., 2018).

ACTION

14. If the tube is not in use, check that the cap is securely in place.

15. Secure the gastrostomy tube to the patient's abdomen in a way that stabilizes the tube and avoids excessive traction (Boullata et al., 2017; Pars & Çavuşoğlu, 2019; Roveron et al., 2018). Assess the integrity of the tape or device used to secure the tube to the stomach.

16. Remove gloves. Perform hand hygiene. Lower the bed and assist the patient to a position of comfort, as needed.

17. Remove additional PPE, if used. Perform hand hygiene.

RATIONALE

The cap should remain closed when the tube is not in use to deter entry of microorganisms and prevent leakage from the tube.

Excessive friction may result in development of peristomal hypergranulation tissue (Bischoff et al., 2020; Roveron et al., 2018). Excessive traction may contribute to enlargement of the stoma and the development of leakage around the tube (Roveron et al., 2018).

Removing gloves reduces the risk for infection transmission and contamination of other items. Hand hygiene prevents transmission of microorganisms. Lowering the bed and assisting the patient ensure patient safety and comfort.

Proper removal of PPE reduces the risk for infection transmission and contamination of other items. Hand hygiene prevents transmission of microorganisms.

EVALUATION

The expected outcomes have been met when the patient has not exhibited signs and symptoms of drainage, pressure injury, erythema, inflammation, erosion, or hypergranulation tissue at the tube-insertion site, and the patient has verbalized little discomfort related to tube placement as well as an understanding of the care needed for the gastrostomy tube, as appropriate.

DOCUMENTATION

Guidelines

Document the site care that was provided, including the substance used to cleanse the tube site. Record the assessment of the site, including the surrounding skin and measurement of length of external tube and comparison to length on insertion. Note the presence of any drainage, recording the amount and color, and pressure injury, erythema, inflammation, erosion, or hypergranulation tissue. Note the rotation and/or push/pull of the tube. Note the external fixator position. Comment on the patient's response to the care, if the patient experienced any pain, and if an analgesic was administered. Record any patient instruction that was provided.

Sample Documentation

10/10/25 1145 Gastrostomy tube site cleansed with skin cleanser and water. No change in measurement of tube length from initial measurement. Tube rotated without difficulty. Site is of consistent tone with surrounding skin, without any signs of skin breakdown. Small amount of clear crust noted on tube. Patient tolerated site care without incident. Wife at bedside, actively participating in tube care.
—S. Essner, RN

DEVELOPING CLINICAL REASONING AND CLINICAL JUDGMENT

UNEXPECTED SITUATIONS AND ASSOCIATED INTERVENTIONS

- *Gastrostomy tube is leaking large amount of drainage:* Check tension of tube. If there is a large amount of slack between the internal guard and the external bumper, drainage can leak out of site. Apply gentle pressure to the tube while pressing the external bumper closer to the skin (0.5 to 1 cm from skin) (Bischoff et al., 2020; Roveron et al., 2018). If the tube has an internal balloon holding it in place (similar to a urinary catheter balloon), check to make sure that the balloon is inflated properly.
- *Skin irritation is noted around insertion site:* Investigate the cause of the irritation. Address the cause of the leakage; apply skin barrier or zinc oxide–based skin protectant (Bischoff et al., 2020). If the skin is erythematous and appears to be broken down, gastric fluids may be leaking from the site. Gastric fluids have a low pH and are very acidic. Address the leakage. If the skin has a patchy, red rash, the cause could be candidiasis (yeast). Consult with the health care team regarding the use of an antifungal powder. Ensure that the site is kept dry.

(continued on page 708)

Skill 11-4 ▶ Caring for a Gastrostomy Tube *(continued)*

- *Site appears erythematous and patient reports pain at site:* Consult with the health care team; the patient could be developing an infection at the site.
- *Patient reports severe pain that does not respond to routine analgesics; when the tube is used for feeding/hydration; or when site care is provided during the first 72 hours after placement of the tube:* Discontinue any type of administration through the tube and notify the health care team (Roveron et al., 2018).

SPECIAL CONSIDERATIONS

General Considerations

- Feeding tubes should be flushed with at least 30 mL of water before starting and after completion of bolus feedings, every 4 to 8 hours during continuous feeding, and before and after medication administration (Bischoff et al., 2020; Boullata et al., 2017; Pars & Çavuşoğlu, 2019; Roveron et al., 2018), based on the patient's fluid needs and restrictions (Boullata et al., 2017).
- Avoid occlusive dressings at gastrostomy site; occlusive dressings promote a moist wound environment and can lead to skin maceration (Bischoff et al., 2020).
- Glycerin hydrogel or glycogel dressings may be used as an alternative to gauze dressings (Bischoff et al., 2020). Use of this type of dressing removes the need for daily dressing changes (Bischoff et al., 2020).
- Do not place a dressing between the skin and external fixation device unless drainage is present. Change the dressing immediately when soiled, to prevent skin complications.
- If the length of the exposed tube has changed or marking on tube is not visible, do not use the tube. Consult with the health care team regarding the finding.
- If the patient experiences pain during nutritional infusion, prolonged pain after the procedure, passage of nutritional formula or medications through the stoma, or bleeding from the site, stop the enteral nutrition feeding immediately and consult with the health care team (Roveron et al., 2018, p. 331).

Community-Based Care Considerations

- Advise patients and caregivers to stop the enteral nutrition feeding immediately and contact their health care provider if the patient experiences pain during nutritional infusion, prolonged pain after the procedure, passage of nutritional formula or medications through the stoma, or bleeding from the site (Roveron et al., 2018, p. 331).
- For patients with a well-healed exit site, showering, bathing, and swimming (it is advisable to cover the site with a waterproof dressing when swimming in public pools) is possible after a few weeks (Bischoff et al., 2020).
- All information related to home enteral nutrition should be provided to patients and family members/caregivers verbally and in writing and/or pictures (Bischoff et al., 2020).

EVIDENCE FOR PRACTICE ▶

CLINICAL PRACTICE GUIDELINES FOR NURSING MANAGEMENT OF PERCUTANEOUS ENDOSCOPIC GASTROSTOMY AND JEJUNOSTOMY TUBES

The Italian Association of Stoma care Nurses and the Italian Association of Gastroenterology Nurses and Associates *Clinical Practice Guidelines for Nursing Management of Percutaneous Endoscopic Gastrostomy and Jejunostomy Tubes (PEG/PEJ) in Adult Patients* guidelines provide recommendations for nursing management of percutaneous endoscopic gastrostomy or jejunostomy (PEG/PEJ) tubes based on the available evidence and expert consensus. These guidelines provide best practices related to preparation for PEG/PEJ procedures and perioperative monitoring, monitoring during the initial 72 hours after tube placement, management of the stoma and tube, administering nutrition and medications, preventing reflux or aspiration of gastric contents, nursing management of common complications, education for patients and caregivers, and tube replacement and methods to assess tube position.

EVIDENCE FOR PRACTICE ▶

ASPEN SAFE PRACTICES FOR ENTERAL NUTRITION THERAPY

Boullata, J. I., Carrera, A. L., Harvey, L., Escuro, A. A., Hudson, L., Mays, A., Wessel, J. J., Bajpai, S., Beebe, M. L., Kinn, T. J., Klang, M. G., Lord, L., Martin, K., Pompeii-Wolfe, C., Sullivan, J., Wood, A., Malone, A., Guenter, P., & ASPEN Safe Practices for Enteral Nutrition Therapy, American Society for Parenteral and Enteral Nutrition. (2017). ASPEN safe practices for enteral nutrition therapy. *Journal of Parenteral and Enteral Nutrition, 41*(1), 15–103. https://doi.org/10.1177/0148607116673053

Refer to details in Skill 11-3, Evidence for Practice.

Enhance Your Understanding

Focusing on Patient Care: Developing Clinical Reasoning and Clinical Judgment

Consider the case scenarios at the beginning of the chapter as you answer the following questions to enhance your understanding and apply what you have learned.

QUESTIONS

1. Ms. Williams tells the nurse that she hates hospital food and is too tired to eat. How can the nurse help Ms. Williams maintain her nutritional intake while recovering from her stroke?

2. Mr. Mason confides he is having "a lot of pain" in his throat and his nose feels "really sore." What assessments and nursing interventions should be a part of Mr. Mason's nursing care while he has the nasogastric tube?

3. The nurse is responsible for providing information to Cole and his family/caregivers regarding home management of his gastrostomy tube and tube feedings. What information will the nurse include in the patient teaching?

You can find suggested answers after the Bibliography at the end of this chapter.

Integrated Case Study Connection

The case studies in the back of the book focus on integrating concepts. Refer to the following case studies to enhance your understanding of the concepts and skills in this chapter.

- Basic Case Studies: Claudia Tran, page 1201.

Bibliography

Allen, S. M. (2015). As a flushing agent for enteral nutrition, does sterile water compared to tap water affect the associated risk of infection in critically ill patients? *Alabama Nurse, 42*(1), 5–6.

Alzheimer's Association. Alzheimer's and Dementia Caregiver Center. (2020). *Food and eating.* Retrieved September 26, 2020, from https://www.alz.org/help-support/caregiving/daily-care/food-eating

American Association of Critical Care Nurses (AACN). (2018, May 17). *AACN practice alert. Prevention of aspiration in adults.* https://www.aacn.org/clinical-resources/practice-alerts/prevention-of-aspiration

American Association of Critical Care Nurses (AACN). (2020, January 29). *AACN practice alert. Initial and ongoing verification of feeding tube placement in adults.* https://www.aacn.org/

Anderson, L. (2018a). Fine-bore nasogastric tube feeding: Reducing the risks. *British Journal of Nursing, 27*(12), 674–675.

Anderson, L. (2018b). Delivering artificial nutrition and hydration safely by feeding pumps. *British Journal of Nursing, 27*(18), 1032–1033.

Anderson, L. (2019). Enteral feeding tubes: An overview of nursing care. *British Journal of Nursing, 28*(12), 748–754. https://doi.org/10.12968/bjon.2019.28.12.748

Batchelor-Murphy, M., & Amella, E. J. (2020). *Eating and feeding issues in older adults with dementia. Part II: Interventions.* Retrieved September 27, 2020, from https://hign.org/consultgeri/try-this-series/eating-and-feeding-issues-older-adults-dementia-part-ii-interventions

Bischoff, S. C., Austin, P., Boeykens, K., Chourdakis, M., Cuerda, C., Jonkers-Schuitema, C., Lichota, M., Nyulasi, I., Schneider, S. M., Stanga, Z., & Pironi, L. (2020). ESPEN guideline on home enteral nutrition. *Clinical Nutrition, 39*(1), 5–22. https://doi.org/10.1016/j.clnu.2019.04.022

Boeykens, K., Steeman, E., & Dyusburgh, I. (2014). Reliability of pH measurement and the auscultatory method to confirm the position of a nasogastric tube. *International Journal of Nursing Studies, 51*(11), 1427–1433. https://doi.org/10.1016/j.ijnurstu.2014.03.004

Boullata, J. I., Carrera, A. L., Harvey, L., Escuro, A. A., Hudson, L., Mays, A., Wessel, J. J., Bajpai, S., Beebe, M. L., Kinn, T. J., Klang, M. G., Lord, L., Martin, K., Pompeii-Wolfe, C., Sullivan, J., Wood, A., Malone, A., & Guenter, P., & ASPEN Safe Practices for Enteral Nutrition Therapy, American Society for Parenteral and Enteral Nutrition. (2017). ASPEN safe practices for enteral nutrition therapy. *Journal of Parenteral and Enteral Nutrition, 41*(1), 15–103. https://doi.org/10.1177/0148607116673053

Dias, F. S. B., Almeida, B. P., Alvares, B. R., Jales, R. M., Caldas, J. P. S., & Carmona, E. V. (2019). Use of pH reagent strips to verify gastric tube placement in newborns. *Revista Latino-Americana de Enfermagem*, 27, e3227. https://doi.org/10.1590/1518-8345.3150.3227

Drummond Hayes, K., & Drummond Hayes, D. (2018). Best practices for unclogging feeding tubes in adults. *Nursing*, 48(6), 66. https://doi.org/10.1097/01.NURSE.0000532744.80506.5e

Dudek, S. (2022). *Nutrition essentials for nursing practice* (9th ed.). Wolters Kluwer.

Dunlap, J. J., & Patterson, S. (2019). Focus on clinical assessment. Assessing dysphagia. *Gastroenterology Nursing*, 42(3), 302–305. https://doi.org/10.1097/SGA.0000000000000472

Eliopoulos, C. (2018). *Gerontological nursing* (9th ed.). Wolters Kluwer.

Fetherstonhaugh, D., Haesler, E., & Bauer, M. (2019). Promoting mealtime function in people with dementia: A systematic review of studies undertaken in residential aged care. *International Journal of Nursing Studies*, 96, 99–118. https://doi.org/10.1016/j.ijnurstu.2019.04.005

Fischbach, F. T., & Fischbach, M. A. (2018). *A manual of laboratory and diagnostic tests* (10th ed.). Wolters Kluwer.

Hartwell, J. L., Cotton, A., & Rozycki, G. (2018). Optimizing nutrition for the surgical patient: An evidenced based update to dispel five common myths in surgical nutrition care. *The American Surgeon*, 84(6), 831–835. https://doi.org/10.1177/000313481808400627

Healthy People 2030. (n.d.). *Social determinants of health*. Office of Disease Prevention and Health Promotion. https://health.gov/healthypeople/objectives-and-data/social-determinants-health

Hess, D. R., MacIntyre, N. R., Galvin, W. F., & Mishoe, S. C. (2021). *Respiratory care. Principles and practice* (4th ed.). Jones & Bartlett Learning.

Hinkle, J. L., Cheever, K. H., & Overbaugh, K. J. (2022). *Brunner & Suddarths's textbook of medical-surgical nursing* (15th ed.). Wolters Kluwer.

Holdoway, A., & Smith, A. (2020). Meeting nutritional need and managing patients with dysphagia. *Journal of Community Nursing*, 34(2), 52–59.

International Council of Nurses (ICN). (2019). *Nursing diagnosis and outcome statements*. https://www.icn.ch/sites/default/files/inline-files/ICNP2019-DC.pdf

Irving, S. Y., Rempel, G., Lyman, B., Sevilla, W. M. A., Northington, L., Guenter, P., & The American Society for Parenteral and Enteral Nutrition. (2018). Pediatric nasogastric tube placement and verification: Best practice recommendations from the NOVEL Project. *Nutrition in Clinical Practice*, 33(6), 921–927. https://doi.org/10.1002/ncp.10189

Jarvis, C., & Eckhardt, A. (2020). *Physical examination & health assessment* (8th ed.). Elsevier.

Jennings Dunlap, J., & Patterson, S. (2019). Focus on clinical assessment. Assessing dysphagia. *Gastroenterology Nursing*, 42(3), 302–305. https://doi.org/10.1097/SGA.0000000000000472

Jensen, S. (2019). *Nursing health assessment. A best practice approach* (3rd ed.). Wolters Kluwer.

Jordan, E. A., & Moore, S. C. (2020). Enteral nutrition in critically ill adults: Literature review of protocols. *Nursing in Critical Care*, 25(1), 24–30. https://doi.org/10.1111/nicc.12475

Judd, M. (2020). Confirming nasogastric tube placement in adults. *Nursing*, 50(4), 43–46. https://doi.org/10.1097/01.NURSE.0000654032.78679.f1

Kinikin, J., Phuillipp, R., & Altamirano, C. (2020). Using volume-based tube feeding to increase nutrient delivery in patients on a rehabilitation unit. *Rehabilitation Nursing*, 45(4), 186–194. doi: 10.1097/rnj. 0000000000000211

Kyle, T., & Carman, S. (2021). *Essentials of pediatric nursing* (4th ed.). Wolters Kluwer.

Liu, W., Williams, K., Batchelor-Murphy, M., Perkhounkova, Y., & Hein, M. (2019). Eating performance in relation to intake of solid and liquid food in nursing home residents with dementia: A secondary behavioral analysis of mealtime videos. *International Journal of Nursing Studies*, 96, 18–26. https://doi.org/10.1016/j.ijnurstu.2018.12.010

Lyman, B., Peyton, C., & Healey, F. (2018). Reducing nasogastric tube misplacement through evidence-based practice. *American Nurse Today*, 13(11), 6–11.

Mak, M. Y., & Tam, G. (2020). Ultrasonography for nasogastric tube placement verification: An additional reference. *British Journal of Community Nursing*, 25(7), 328–344. DOI: 10.12968/bjcn.2020.25.7.328

McClave, S. A., DiBaise, J. K., Mullin, G., & Martindale, R. G. (2016). ACG clinical guideline: Nutrition therapy in the adult hospitalized patient. *The American Journal of Gastroenterology*, 111(3), 315–334. https://doi.org/10.1038/ajg.2016.28

McClave, S. A., Taylor, B. E., Martindale, R. G., Warren, M. M., Johnson, D. R., Braunschweig, C., McCarthy, M. S., Davanos, E., Rice, T. W., Cresci, G. A., Gervasio, J. M., Sacks, G. S., Roberts, P. R., Compher, C., & American Society for Parenteral and Enteral Nutrition and Society of Critical Care Medicine. (2016). Guidelines for the provision and assessment of nutrition support therapy in the adult critically ill patient. *Journal of Parenteral and Enteral Nutrition*, 40(2), 159–211. https://doi.org/10.1177/0148607115621863

Metheny, N. (n.d.). *Preventing aspiration in older adults with dysphagia*. Retrieved December 15, 2021, from https://hign.org/consultgeri/try-this-series/preventing-aspiration-older-adults-dysphagia

Metheny, N. A., Krieger, M. M., Healey, F., & Meert, K. L. (2019). A review of guidelines to distinguish between gastric and pulmonary placement of nasogastric tubes. *Heart & Lung*, 48(3), 226–235. https://doi.org/10.1016/j.hrtlng.2019.01.003

Morton, P.G., & Fontaine, D. K. (2018). *Critical care nursing. A holistic approach* (11th ed.). Wolters Kluwer.

Nazarko, L. (2020). Dysphagia: A guide for nurses in general practice. *Practice Nursing*, 31(4), 162–168. https://doi.org/10.12968/pnur.2020.31.4.162

Norris, T. L. (2019). *Porth's essentials of pathophysiology* (5th ed.). Wolters Kluwer.

Ozen, N., Blot, S., Ozen, V., Donmez, A. A., Gurun, P., Cinar, F. I., & Labeau, S. (2018). Gastric residual volume measurement in the intensive care unit: An international survey reporting nursing practice. *Nursing in Critical Care*, 23(5), 263–269. doi: 10.1111/nicc.12378

Palese, A., Bressan, V., Kasa, T., Meri, M., Hayter, M., & Watson, R. (2018). Interventions maintaining eating independence in nursing home residents: A multicentre qualitative study. *BMC Geriatrics*, 18(1), 292. https://doi.org/10.1186/s12877-018-0985-y

Parker, L. A., Weaver, M., Murgas Torrazza, R. J., Shuster, J., LI, N., Krueger, C., & Neu, J. (2019). Effect of gastric residual evaluation on enteral intake in extremely preterm infants. *JAMA Pediatrics*, 173(6), 534–543. https://doi.org/10.1001/jamapediatrics.2019.0800

Parker, L. A., Withers, J. H., & Talaga, E. (2018). Comparison of neonatal nursing practices for determining feeding tube insertion length and verifying gastric placement with current best evidence. *Advances in Neonatal Care*, 18(4), 307–317. https://doi.org/10.1097/ANC.0000000000000526

Pars, H., & Çavuşoğlu, H. (2019). A literature review of percutaneous endoscopic gastrostomy. Dealing with complications. *Gastroenterology Nursing*, 42(4), 351–359. https://doi.org/10.1097/SGA.0000000000000320359

Problem-based care plans. (2020). In *Lippincott advisor*. Wolters Kluwer. https://advisor.lww.com/lna/home.do

Rahimi, M., Farhadi, K., Ashtarian, H., & Changaei, F. (2015). Confirming nasogastric tube position: Methods and restrictions. A narrative review. *Journal of Nursing and Midwifery Sciences*, 2(1), 55–62. https://doi.org/10.4103/2345-5756.231420

Roveron, G., Antonini, M., Barbierato, M., Calandrino, V., Canese, G., Chiurazzi, L. F., Coniglio, G., Gentini, G., Marchetti, M., Minucci, A., Nembrini, L., Neri, V., Trovato, P., & Ferrara, F. (2018). Clinical practice guidelines for the nursing management of percutaneous endoscopic gastrostomy and jejunostomy (PEG/PEJ) in adult patients. *Journal of Wound, Ostomy, and Continence Nursing*, 45(4), 326–334. https://doi.org/10.1097/WON.0000000000000442

Rysavy, M. A., Watkins, P. L., Colaizy, T. T., & Das, A. (2020). Is routine evaluation of gastric residuals for premature infants safe or effective? *Journal of Perinatology*, 40(3), 540–543. https://doi.org/10.1038/s41372-019-0582-8

Semerdzhieva, E., & Reid, B. (2019). Getting the fundamentals right: Assisting patients with eating and drinking. *Nursing & Residential Care*, 21(10), 562–565.

Shellnutt, C. (2019). The evidence on feeding initiation after percutaneous endoscopic gastrostomy tube placement. *Gastroenterology Nursing*, 42(5), 420–427. https://doi.org/10.1097/SGA.0000000000000393

Silbert-Flagg, J., & Pillitteri, A. (2018). *Maternal and child health nursing* (8th ed.). Wolters Kluwer.

Singer, P., Blaser, A. R., Berger, M. M., Alhazzani, W., Calder, P. C., Casaer, M. P., Hiesmayr, M., Mayer, K., Montejo, J. C., Pichard, C., Preiser, J. C., van Zanten, A. R. H., Oczkowski, S., Szczeklik, W., & Bischoff, S. C. (2019). ESPEN guideline on clinical nutrition in the intensive care unit. *Clinical Nutrition*, 38(1), 48–79. https://doi.org/10.1016/j.clnu.2018.08.037

Taylor, C., Lynn, P., & Bartlett, J. (2023). *Fundamentals of nursing: The art and science of person-centered care* (10th ed.). Wolters Kluwer.

Toughy, T. A., & Jett, K. (2018). *Ebersol and Hess' gerontological nursing & healthy aging* (5th ed.). Elsevier.

VHA Center for Engineering & Occupational Safety and Health (CEOSH). (2016). Safe patient handling and mobility guidebook. http://www.tnpatientsafety.com/pubfiles/Initiatives/workplace-violence/sphm-pdf.pdf

Weber, J. R., & Kelley, J. H. (2018). *Health assessment in nursing* (6th ed.). Wolters Kluwer.

Wilson, J., Tingle, A., Bak, A., Greene, C., Tsiami, A., & Loveday, H. (2020). Improving fluid consumption of older people in care homes: An exploration of the factors contributing to under-hydration. *Nursing and Residential Care*, 22(3), 139–146.

SUGGESTED ANSWERS FOR FOCUSING ON PATIENT CARE: DEVELOPING CLINICAL REASONING AND CLINICAL JUDGMENT

1. Explore the patient's usual food preferences and habits. Choose foods that the patient prefers from facility menus. In addition, encourage Ms. Williams' family/caregivers to bring favorite foods from home. Food choices should focus on foods that are easy to eat and nutrient dense. Provide rest periods before mealtimes, so she is not overly tired. Assist the patient to a comfortable position for meals, help her with hand hygiene, and ensure she has clean dentures in place, and her glasses, as appropriate. Encourage her family/caregivers to visit during mealtimes, to provide as normal a social environment as possible. Cut food and open packages as necessary, to limit the amount of exertion by the patient. Suggest she eat small portions, keeping some food items to snack on as the day progresses. Frequent small servings are not as tiring. Allow enough time for the patient to chew and swallow the food adequately. The patient may need to rest for short periods during eating. If Ms. Williams is agreeable, feed her a portion of the meal, to avoid overtiring.

2. Assess the patient's level of comfort every 4 hours and PRN. Offer analgesic as prescribed. Offer oral hygiene at least every 4 hours or more often. Discuss the potential for topical analgesic, such as analgesic throat spray, with the health care team. Reassess pain after interventions. Assess the patient's oral and nasal mucous membranes, as well as nasal skin, at least every shift. Ensure the device anchoring the tube is not pulled taut, creating pressure on the nose. Resecure the NG tube with new commercially prepared device or tape every 24 hours; clean skin thoroughly and apply skin barrier. Resecure in a slightly different position to prevent excessive pressure in one area of nostril.

3. Patients who are caring for a gastrostomy tube at home should understand the care of the tube, tube site, nutritional feeding routine, and potential adverse effects, with the accompanying actions. Provide Cole and his family/caregivers with the date his tube was placed, the procedure used to place the tube, the tube size, how the tube is anchored, and the calibration measurement at skin level or the length of the external tube. Discuss, provide written information, and obtain a return demonstration for the care of the tube and tube site, as well as the feeding procedure. Teaching should include the formula type, frequency, rate of infusion, checking tube placement, and checking gastric residual, based on prescribed therapeutic regimen. Review infection control measures, such as handwashing before starting, refrigerating formula between use, disposing of unused formula after 24 hours, and measuring out only 4 hours of formula at a time. The length of the tube or calibration mark at the skin should be checked prior to each feeding or use of the tube. Cole should be in a sitting position for the feeding and for 1 hour afterward. Skin care for tube site includes washing the area with the cleansing agent identified by the health care team, rinsing, and patting dry. Cole should assess the site daily for swelling, redness, and drainage. Cole and his family/caregivers should verbalize an understanding of these instructions, as well as a knowledge of signs and symptoms that should be communicated to the health care team. These include the presence of nausea or vomiting, pain, and fever. Cole and his family/caregivers should also understand proper procedure if the gastrostomy tube should come out or become dislodged.

12

Urinary Elimination

Focusing on Patient Care

This chapter will help you develop some of the skills related to urinary elimination that may be necessary to care for the following patients:

Ralph Bellows, age 73, has been admitted with a stroke. Due to incontinence and skin breakdown, Ralph's nurse has decided to include the application of an external urinary sheath (condom catheter) in their plan of care.

Grace Halligan, age 24, is pregnant and has been placed on bed rest. They need to void but cannot get out of bed.

Mike Wimmer, age 36, receives peritoneal dialysis. Mike has noticed that the insertion site around the catheter is becoming tender and reddened.

Refer to Focusing on Patient Care: Developing Clinical Reasoning and Clinical Judgment at the end of the chapter to apply what you learn.

Learning Outcomes

After completing the chapter, you will be able to accomplish the following:

1. Assist with the use of a bedpan.
2. Assist with use of a urinal.
3. Assist with use of a bedside commode.
4. Assess bladder volume using an ultrasound bladder scanner.
5. Apply an external urinary sheath (external urine collection device male genitalia).
6. Apply an external urine collection system (female genitalia).
7. Catheterize the urinary bladder of a patient with female genitalia.
8. Catheterize the urinary bladder of a patient with male genitalia.
9. Remove an indwelling urinary catheter.
10. Administer continuous closed bladder irrigation.
11. Empty and change a stoma appliance on a urinary diversion.
12. Care for a suprapubic urinary catheter.
13. Care for a peritoneal dialysis catheter.
14. Care for hemodialysis access.

Nursing Concepts

- Assessment
- Clinical Decision Making/Clinical Judgment
- Elimination
- Functional Ability
- Infection
- Safety

Urine is excreted from the kidneys via the ureters to the bladder, where it is stored and eliminated via the urethra. Elimination from the urinary tract helps to rid the body of waste products and materials that exceed bodily needs. Numerous factors affect the amount and quality of urine produced by the body and the manner in which it is excreted. Some patients experience urinary elimination problems affecting fluid and electrolyte balance, hydration, skin integrity, comfort, and self-concept. Many health problems, medications, and health care interventions can affect urinary elimination. Nurses play an important role in preventing and managing urinary elimination problems.

This chapter covers skills that the nurse may use to promote urinary elimination. An assessment of the urinary system is required as part of providing interventions outlined in many of these skills. Refer to Fundamentals Review 12-1 for a review of the male and female genitourinary tracts. Fundamentals Review 12-2 summarizes factors that may affect urinary elimination.

Fundamentals Review 12-1

ANATOMY OF THE GENITOURINARY TRACT

- The main components of the urinary tract are the kidneys, ureters, bladder, and urethra.

- The average female urethra is 1.6 inches (4 cm) long; the average male urethra is 8 inches (20 cm) long (Norris, 2020).

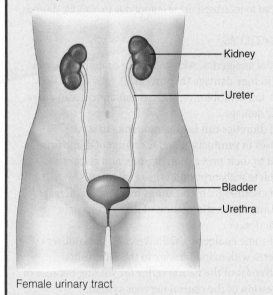

Female urinary tract

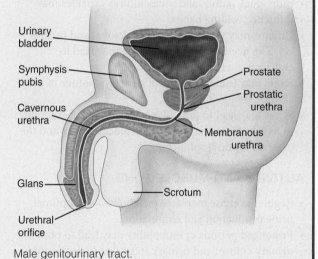

Male genitourinary tract.

Fundamentals Review 12-2

FACTORS AFFECTING URINARY ELIMINATION

Numerous factors affect the amount and quality of urine produced by the body and the manner in which it is excreted.

EFFECTS OF AGING

- Diminished ability of kidneys to concentrate urine may result in nocturia.
- Hypertrophy of the bladder muscle and thickening of the bladder decreases the ability of the bladder

to expand and reduces storage capacity, resulting in increased frequency of urination.
- Decreased bladder contractility leading to urine retention and stasis with an increased risk of urinary tract infection (UTI).
- Neuromuscular problems, degenerative joint problems, alterations in thought processes, and weakness may interfere with voluntary control of urination and the ability to reach a toilet in time.

(continued)

Fundamentals Review 12-2   continued

FACTORS AFFECTING URINARY ELIMINATION

FOOD AND FLUID INTAKE

- Dehydration leads to increased fluid reabsorption by the kidneys, leading to decreased and concentrated urine production.
- Fluid overload leads to excretion of a large quantity of dilute urine.
- Consumption of alcoholic beverages leads to increased urine production due to their inhibition of antidiuretic hormone release.
- Ingestion of foods high in water content may increase urine production.
- Ingestion of foods and beverages high in sodium content leads to decreased urine formation due to sodium and water reabsorption and retention.
- Ingestion of certain foods (e.g., asparagus, onions, beets) may lead to alterations in the odor or color of urine.

PSYCHOLOGICAL VARIABLES

- Individual, family, and sociocultural variables may influence voiding habits.
- Patients may view voiding as a personal and private act. The need to ask for assistance may lead to embarrassment and/or anxiety.
- Stress may lead to voiding of smaller amounts of urine at more frequent intervals.
- Stress may lead to difficulty emptying the bladder due to its effects on relaxation of perineal muscles and the external urethral sphincter.

ACTIVITY AND MUSCLE TONE

- Regular exercise increases metabolism and optimal urine production and elimination.
- Prolonged periods of immobility may lead to poor urinary control and urinary stasis due to decreased bladder and sphincter tone.
- Use of indwelling urinary catheters leads to loss of bladder tone because the bladder muscle is not being stretched by filling with urine.
- Childbearing, muscle atrophy related to menopausal hormonal changes, and trauma-related muscle damage lead to decreased muscle tone.

PATHOLOGIC CONDITIONS

- Congenital urinary tract abnormalities, polycystic kidney disease, urinary tract infection, urinary calculi (kidney stones), hypertension, diabetes mellitus, gout, and certain connective tissue disorders lead to altered quantity and quality of urine.
- Diseases that reduce physical activity or lead to generalized weakness (e.g., arthritis, Parkinson disease, degenerative joint disease) interfere with toileting.
- Cognitive deficits and psychiatric conditions may interfere with ability or desire to control urination voluntarily.
- Fever and diaphoresis (profuse perspiration) lead to conservation of body fluids.
- Other pathologic conditions, such as congestive heart failure, may lead to fluid retention and decreased urine output.
- High blood–glucose levels, such as with diabetes mellitus, may lead to increased urine output due to osmotic diuresis.

MEDICATIONS

- Abuse of analgesics, such as aspirin or ibuprofen, can cause kidney damage (nephrotoxic).
- Use of some antibiotics, such as gentamicin, can cause kidney damage.
- Use of diuretics can lead to moderate to severe increases in production and excretion of dilute urine, related to their prevention of water and certain electrolyte reabsorption in the renal tubules.
- Use of cholinergic medications may lead to increased urination due to stimulation of detrusor muscle contraction.
- Use of some analgesics, sedatives, and tranquilizers interferes with urination due to the diminished effectiveness of the neural reflex for voiding because of suppression of the central nervous system.
- Use of certain drugs causes changes to the color of urine. Anticoagulants may cause hematuria (blood in the urine) or a pink or red color. Diuretics can lighten the color of urine to pale yellow. Phenazopyridine can cause orange or orange-red urine. Amitriptyline and B-complex vitamins can cause green or blue-green urine. Levodopa (L-dopa) and injectable iron compounds can cause brown or black urine.

Skill 12-1 ► Assisting With the Use of a Bedpan

Skill Variation: *Assisting With the Use of a Bedpan When the Patient Has Limited Movement*

Patients who cannot get out of bed because of physical limitations or prescribed interventions need to use a bedpan or urinal for voiding. Patients with male genitalia usually prefer to use the urinal for voiding (see Skill 12-2) and the bedpan for defecation; patients with female genitalia usually prefer to use the bedpan for both. Many patients find it difficult and embarrassing to use the bedpan. When a patient uses a bedpan, promote comfort and normalcy, and respect the patient's privacy as much as possible. Be sure to maintain a professional manner. In addition, provide skin care, perineal hygiene, and hand hygiene after bedpan use.

Regular bedpans have a rounded, smooth upper end and a tapered, open lower end. The upper end fits under the patient's buttocks toward the sacrum, with the open end toward the foot of the bed (Figure 1A). A special bedpan called a *fracture bedpan* is frequently used for patients with fractures of the femur or lower spine. Smaller and flatter than the ordinary bedpan, this type of bedpan is helpful for patients who cannot easily raise themselves onto the regular bedpan (see Figure 1B). The fracture pan has a shallow, narrow upper end with a flat wide rim, and a deeper, open lower end. The upper end fits under the patient's buttocks toward the sacrum, with the deeper, open lower end toward the foot of the bed.

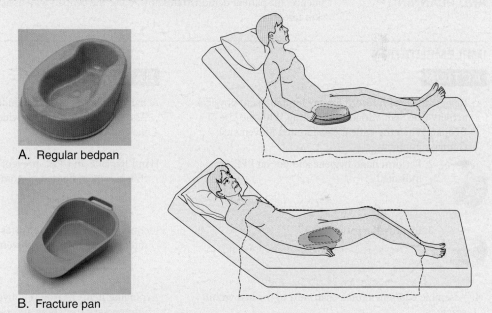

A. Regular bedpan

B. Fracture pan

FIGURE 1. A. Regular (standard) bedpan. Position a standard bedpan like a regular toilet seat—the buttocks are placed on the wide, rounded shelf, with the open end pointed toward the foot of the bed. **B.** Fracture pan. Position a fracture pan with the thin edge toward the head of the bed.

DELEGATION CONSIDERATIONS

Assisting a patient with the use of a bedpan may be delegated to assistive personnel (AP) as well as to licensed practical/vocational nurses (LPN/LVNs). The decision to delegate must be based on careful analysis of the patient's needs and circumstances as well as the qualifications of the person to whom the task is being delegated. Refer to the Delegation Guidelines in Appendix A.

EQUIPMENT

- Bedpan (regular or fracture)
- Toilet tissue
- Disposable clean gloves
- Additional PPE, as indicated
- Cover for bedpan or urinal (disposable waterproof pad or cover)
- Disposable washcloths and skin cleanser
- Moist towelettes, skin cleanser and water, or hand sanitizer

(continued on page 716)

Skill 12-1 ▶ Assisting With the Use of a Bedpan *(continued)*

ASSESSMENT	Assess the patient's usual elimination habits. Determine why the patient needs to use a bedpan (e.g., prescribed bed rest or immobilization). Also assess the patient's degree of limitation and ability to help with activity. Assess for health problems, such as hip surgery or spinal injury, which would contraindicate certain actions by the patient. Check for the presence of drains, dressings, intravenous fluid infusion sites/equipment, traction, or any other devices that could interfere with the patient's ability to help with the procedure or that could become dislodged. Assess the characteristics of the urine and the patient's skin.
ACTUAL OR POTENTIAL HEALTH PROBLEMS AND NEEDS	Many actual or potential health problems or issues may require the use of this skill as part of related interventions. An appropriate health problem or issue may include: • Functional urinary incontinence • Toileting ADL deficit • Deconditioning
OUTCOME IDENTIFICATION AND PLANNING	The expected outcome to achieve when offering a bedpan is that the patient is able to void (or defecate) with assistance. Other appropriate outcomes may include that the patient maintains continence, the patient demonstrates how to use the bedpan with assistance, and the patient maintains skin integrity.

IMPLEMENTATION

ACTION	**RATIONALE**
1. Review the health record for any limitations in physical activity (see Skill Variation: Assisting With the Use of a Bedpan When the Patient Has Limited Movement). Gather equipment.	Activity limitations may contraindicate certain actions by the patient. Assembling equipment provides for an organized approach to the task.
2. Perform hand hygiene and put on PPE, if indicated.	Hand hygiene and PPE prevent the spread of microorganisms. PPE is required based on transmission precautions.
3. Identify the patient.	Identifying the patient ensures the right patient receives the intervention and helps prevent errors.
4. Assemble equipment on a chair next to the bed within reach.	Arranging items nearby is convenient, saves time, and prevents unnecessary stretching and twisting of muscles on the part of the nurse.
5. Close the curtains around the bed and close the door to the room, if possible. Discuss the procedure with the patient and assess the patient's ability to assist with the procedure as well as personal hygiene preferences.	This ensures the patient's privacy. Discussion promotes reassurance and provides knowledge about the procedure. Dialogue encourages patient participation and allows for individualized nursing care.
6. Unless contraindicated, apply powder to the rim of the bedpan. Place the bedpan and cover on a chair next to the bed. Put on gloves.	Powder helps keep the bedpan from sticking to the patient's skin and makes it easier to remove. Powder is not applied if the patient has respiratory problems, is allergic to powder, or if a urine specimen is needed (could contaminate the specimen). The bedpan on the chair allows for easy access. Gloves prevent contact with blood and body fluids.
7. Adjust the bed to a comfortable working height (VHACEOSH, 2016). Place the patient in a supine position, with the head of the bed elevated about 30 degrees, unless contraindicated.	Having the bed at the proper height prevents back and muscle strain. The supine position is necessary for correct placement of the patient on the bedpan.

ACTION

8. Fold the top linen back just enough to allow placement of the bedpan. If there is no waterproof pad on the bed and time allows, consider placing a waterproof pad under the patient's buttocks before placing the bedpan (Figure 2).

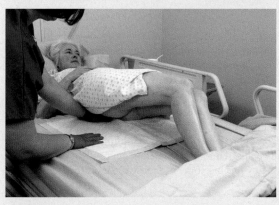

9. Ask the patient to bend their knees. Have the patient lift their hips upward. Assist the patient, if necessary, by placing your hand that is closest to the patient palm up, under the lower back, and assist with lifting. Slip the bedpan into place with the other hand (Figure 3).

10. **Ensure that the bedpan is in proper position and the patient's buttocks are resting on the rounded shelf of the regular bedpan or the shallow rim of the fracture bedpan.** Remove gloves. Perform hand hygiene.

11. Raise the head of the bed as near to sitting position as tolerated, unless contraindicated. Cover the patient with bed linens.

12. **Place the call bell and toilet tissue within easy reach. Place the bed in the lowest position.** Leave the patient if it is safe to do so. Use side rails appropriately (Figure 4).

RATIONALE

Folding back the linen in this manner minimizes unnecessary exposure, while still allowing the nurse to place the bedpan. The waterproof pad will protect the bed should there be a spill.

FIGURE 2. Placing waterproof pad under patient's buttocks. (*Note: Covers should be folded back just enough to work, not expose patient unnecessarily. Covers in this series of photos have been pulled back to show action.*)

The nurse uses less energy when the patient can assist by placing some of their weight on the heels.

Having the bedpan in the proper position prevents spills onto the bed, ensures patient comfort, and prevents injury to the skin from a misplaced bedpan. Proper removal of gloves prevents transmission of microorganisms. Hand hygiene deters the spread of microorganisms.

This position makes it easier for the patient to void or defecate, avoids strain on the patient's back, and allows gravity to aid in elimination. Covering promotes warmth and privacy.

Falls can be prevented if the patient does not have to reach for items they need. Placing the bed in the lowest position promotes patient safety. Leaving the patient alone, if possible, promotes self-esteem and shows respect for privacy. Side rails assist the patient in repositioning.

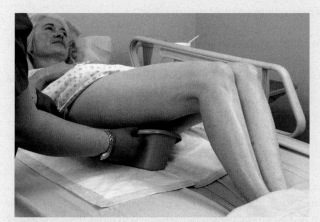

FIGURE 3. Assisting patient to raise hips upward and positioning the bedpan. (*Note: Covers should be folded back just enough to work, not expose patient unnecessarily. Covers in this series of photos have been pulled back to show action.*)

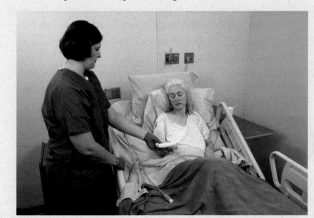

FIGURE 4. Placing call bell within patient's reach and handing patient toilet tissue.

(*continued on page 718*)

Skill 12-1 ▶ Assisting With the Use of a Bedpan *(continued)*

ACTION	RATIONALE
13. Remove additional PPE, if used. Perform hand hygiene.	Proper removal of PPE prevents transmission of microorganisms. Hand hygiene deters the spread of microorganisms.

Removing the Bedpan

ACTION	RATIONALE
14. Perform hand hygiene and put on gloves and additional PPE, as indicated. Adjust the bed to a comfortable working height (VHACEOSH, 2016). Have a receptacle, such as a plastic trash bag, handy for discarding tissue.	Hand hygiene deters the spread of microorganisms. Gloves prevent exposure to blood and body fluids. Having the bed at the proper height prevents back and muscle strain. Proper disposal of soiled tissue prevents transmission of microorganisms.
15. Lower the head of the bed, if necessary, to about 30 degrees. Place a waterproof pad on a bedside chair or the floor; have a second waterproof pad accessible. Remove the bedpan in the same manner in which it was offered, being careful to hold it steady. Ask the patient to bend their knees and lift the buttocks up from the bedpan. Assist the patient, if necessary, by placing your hand that is closest to the patient palm up, under the lower back, and assist with lifting.	Lowering the head of the bed facilitates repositioning by the patient. Preparing a place to place the bedpan provides for an organized approach to the task. Holding the bedpan steady prevents spills. The nurse uses less energy when the patient can assist by placing some of their weight on the heels.
16. Place the bedpan on the bedside chair and cover it with the waterproof pad.	Covering the bedpan helps to prevent the spread of microorganisms.
17. If the patient needs assistance with hygiene, wrap tissue around your hand several times, and wipe the patient clean, using one stroke from the pubic area toward the anal area. Discard the tissue. Use a warm, moist disposable washcloth and skin cleanser to clean the perineal area. Assist the patient to turn on their side away from you and spread the buttocks to clean the anal area.	Cleaning the area from the front to back minimizes fecal contamination of the vagina and urinary meatus. Cleaning the patient after they have used the bedpan prevents offensive odors and skin irritation.
18. Do not place toilet tissue in the bedpan if a specimen is required, or if output is being recorded. Place toilet tissue in an appropriate receptacle.	Mixing toilet tissue with a specimen makes laboratory examination more difficult and interferes with accurate output measurement.
19. Make sure the linens under the patient are dry. Replace or remove the pad under the patient, as necessary. Remove your gloves and perform hand hygiene. Assist the patient to a comfortable position and ensure that the patient is covered.	Positioning helps to promote patient comfort. Removing contaminated gloves prevents the spread of microorganisms.
20. Raise the side rail. Lower the bed height and adjust the head of the bed to a comfortable position. Reattach the call bell.	These actions promote patient safety.
21. Offer the patient supplies to wash and dry their hands, assisting as necessary.	Washing hands after using the urinal helps prevent the spread of microorganisms.
22. Put on gloves. Empty and clean the bedpan, measuring urine in a graduated container, as necessary. Discard the trash receptacle with used toilet paper per facility policy.	Gloves prevent exposure to blood and body fluids. Cleaning reusable equipment helps prevent the spread of microorganisms.
23. Remove additional PPE, if used. Perform hand hygiene.	Proper removal of PPE reduces the risk for infection transmission and contamination of other items. Hand hygiene prevents the spread of microorganisms.

EVALUATION The expected outcome has been met when the patient was able to void or defecate using the bedpan. Other outcomes have been met when the patient has remained dry, has not experienced episodes of incontinence, has demonstrated measures to assist with using the bedpan, and has not experienced alterations in skin integrity.

DOCUMENTATION

Guidelines

Document the patient's tolerance of the activity. Record the amount of urine voided on the intake and output record, if appropriate. Document any other assessments, such as unusual urine characteristics or alterations in the patient's skin.

Sample Documentation

> <u>12/06/25</u> 0730 Patient placed on fracture bedpan with a two-person assist. Voided 400-mL dark yellow urine; strong odor noted. Perineal skin intact, without redness or irritation. Specimen sent for urinalysis as prescribed.
>
> —*S. Barnes, RN*

DEVELOPING CLINICAL REASONING AND CLINICAL JUDGMENT

SPECIAL CONSIDERATIONS

- A fracture bedpan is usually more comfortable for the patient, but it does not hold as large a volume as the regular bedpan (see Figure 1).
- Very thin and older adult patients often find it easier and more comfortable to use the fracture bedpan.
- The bedpan should not be left in place for extended periods because this can result in excessive pressure and irritation to the patient's skin.

Skill Variation ▶ Assisting With the Use of a Bedpan When the Patient Has Limited Movement

Patients who are unable to lift themselves onto the bedpan or who have activity limitations that prohibit the required actions can be assisted onto the bedpan in an alternative manner using these actions:

1. Review the patient's health record for any limitations in physical activity. Gather equipment.

  2. Put on PPE, as indicated, and perform hand hygiene. Check the patient's identification band.

3. Place the bedpan and cover on the chair next to the bed. Close the curtains around the bed and close the door to the room, if possible.
4. Discuss the procedure with the patient and assess the patient's ability to assist with the procedure as well as personal hygiene preferences.
5. Unless contraindicated, apply powder to the rim of the bedpan.
6. Adjust the bed to a comfortable working height (VHACEOSH, 2016). Place the patient in a supine position, with the head of the bed elevated about 30 degrees, unless contraindicated. Put on gloves.
7. Fold the top linen just enough to turn the patient, while minimizing exposure. If no waterproof pad is on the bed and time allows, consider placing a waterproof pad under the patient's buttocks before placing the bedpan.
8. Assist the patient to roll to their opposite side or turn the patient into a side-lying position.

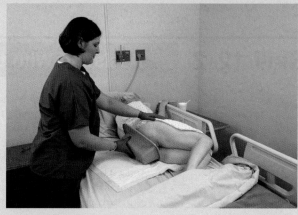

FIGURE A. Rolling patient on side to place bedpan. (*Note: Covers should be folded back just enough to work, not expose patient unnecessarily. Covers in photo pulled back to show action for photo.*)

9. Hold the bedpan firmly against the patient's buttocks, with the upper end of the bedpan under the patient's buttocks toward the sacrum, and down into the mattress (Figure A).
10. Keep one hand against the bedpan. Apply gentle pressure to ensure the bedpan remains in place as you assist the patient to roll back onto the bedpan.

 11. Ensure that the bedpan is in the proper position and the patient's buttocks are resting on rounded shelf of the regular bedpan or the shallow rim of the fracture bedpan. Remove gloves, and PPE, if used. Perform hand hygiene.

(continued)

Skill 12-1 ▶ Assisting With the Use of a Bedpan *(continued)*

Skill Variation ▶ Assisting With the Use of a Bedpan When the Patient Has Limited Movement *(continued)*

12. Raise the head of the bed as near to sitting position as tolerated, unless contraindicated. Cover the patient with bed linens.

13. Place the call bell and toilet tissue within easy reach. Place the bed in the lowest position. Leave the patient if it is safe to do so. Use side rails appropriately.

 14. Remove PPE, if used. Perform hand hygiene.

To Remove the Bedpan

 15. Perform hand hygiene and put on gloves, and additional PPE, as indicated. Raise the bed to a comfortable working height. Have a receptacle handy for discarding tissue.

16. Lower the head of the bed. Grasp the closest side of the bedpan. Apply gentle pressure to hold the bedpan flat and steady. Assist the patient to roll to their opposite side or turn the patient into a side-lying position with the assistance of a second caregiver. Remove the bedpan and set it on the chair. Cover the bedpan.

 17. If the patient needs assistance with hygiene, wrap tissue around your hand several times, and wipe the patient clean, using one stroke from the pubic area toward the anal area. Discard the tissue. Use a warm, moist disposable washcloth and skin cleanser to clean the perineal area. Place the patient on their side and spread the buttocks to clean the anal area. Remove gloves and perform hand hygiene.

18. Return the patient to a comfortable position. Make sure the linens under the patient are dry and that the patient is covered.

19. Offer the patient supplies to wash and dry their hands, assisting as necessary.

20. Raise the side rail. Lower the bed height and adjust the head of the bed to a comfortable position. Reattach the call bell.

 21. Put on gloves. Empty and clean the bedpan, measuring urine in a graduated container, as necessary. Remove gloves and additional PPE, if used. Perform hand hygiene.

Skill 12-2 ▶ Assisting With the Use of a Urinal

Patients who have a penis and cannot get out of bed because of physical limitations or prescribed interventions usually prefer to use the urinal (Figure 1) for voiding as a matter of convenience. Alternatively, use of a urinal in the standing position facilitates emptying of the bladder. Patients who are unable to stand alone may benefit from assistance when voiding into a urinal. If the patient is unable to stand, the urinal may be used in bed. Patients may also use a urinal in the bathroom to facilitate measurement of urinary output. Many patients find it embarrassing to use the urinal. Promote comfort and normalcy as much as possible, while respecting the patient's privacy. Provide skin care, perineal hygiene, and hand hygiene after urinal use and maintain a professional manner.

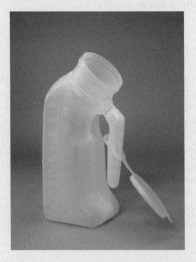

FIGURE 1. Urinal.

DELEGATION CONSIDERATIONS	Assisting a patient with the use of a urinal may be delegated to assistive personnel (AP) as well as to licensed practical/vocational nurses (LPN/LVNs). The decision to delegate must be based on careful analysis of the patient's needs and circumstances as well as the qualifications of the person to whom the task is being delegated. Refer to the Delegation Guidelines in Appendix A.
EQUIPMENT	• Urinal with end cover (usually attached) • Toilet tissue • Clean gloves • Additional PPE, as indicated • Disposable washcloths and skin cleanser • Moist towelettes, skin cleanser and water, or hand sanitizer
ASSESSMENT	Assess the patient's usual elimination habits. Determine why the patient needs to use a urinal (e.g., a prescribed intervention for strict bed rest or immobilization). Also assess the patient's degree of limitation and ability to help with activity. Assess for health problems, such as hip surgery or spinal injury, which would contraindicate certain actions by the patient. Check for the presence of drains, dressings, intravenous fluid infusion sites/equipment, traction, or any other devices that could interfere with the patient's ability to help with the procedure or that could become dislodged. Assess the characteristics of the urine and the patient's skin.
ACTUAL OR POTENTIAL HEALTH PROBLEMS AND NEEDS	Many actual or potential health problems or issues may require the use of this skill as part of related interventions. An appropriate health problem or issue may include: • Functional urinary incontinence • Toileting ADL deficit • Activity intolerance
OUTCOME IDENTIFICATION AND PLANNING	The expected outcome to achieve when offering a urinal is that the patient is able to void with assistance. Other appropriate outcomes may include that the patient maintains continence, the patient demonstrates how to use the urinal, and the patient maintains skin integrity.

IMPLEMENTATION

ACTION	**RATIONALE**
1. Review the patient's health record for any limitations in physical activity. Gather equipment.	Activity limitations may contraindicate certain actions by the patient. Assembling equipment provides for an organized approach to the task.
2. Perform hand hygiene and put on PPE, if indicated.	Hand hygiene and PPE prevent the spread of microorganisms. PPE is required based on transmission precautions.
3. Identify the patient.	Identifying the patient ensures the right patient receives the intervention and helps prevent errors.
4. Assemble equipment on a chair next to the bed within reach.	Arranging items nearby is convenient, saves time, and prevents unnecessary stretching and twisting of muscles on the part of the nurse.
5. Close the curtains around the bed and close the door to the room, if possible. Discuss the procedure with the patient and assess the patient's ability to assist with the procedure as well as personal hygiene preferences.	This ensures the patient's privacy. Discussion promotes reassurance and provides knowledge about the procedure. Dialogue encourages patient participation and allows for individualized nursing care.
6. Put on gloves.	Gloves prevent exposure to blood and body fluids.

(continued on page 722)

Skill 12-2 ▶ Assisting With the Use of a Urinal *(continued)*

ACTION	**RATIONALE**
7. Assist the patient to an appropriate position, as necessary: standing at the bedside, lying on one side or back, sitting in bed with the head elevated, or sitting on the side of the bed.	These positions facilitate voiding and emptying of the bladder.
8. If the patient remains in the bed, fold the linens just enough to allow for proper placement of the urinal.	Folding back the linen in this manner minimizes unnecessary exposure, while still allowing the nurse to place the urinal.
9. If the patient is not standing, have them spread their legs slightly. **Hold the urinal close to the penis and position the penis completely within the urinal (Figure 2). Keep the bottom of the urinal lower than the penis.** If necessary, assist the patient to hold the urinal in place.	Slight spreading of the legs allows for proper positioning of the urinal. Placing the penis completely within the urinal and keeping the bottom lower than the penis avoids urine spills.

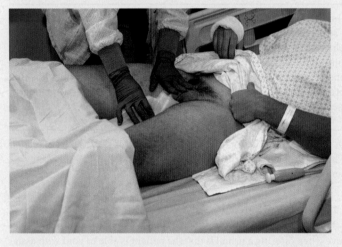

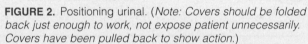

FIGURE 2. Positioning urinal. (*Note: Covers should be folded back just enough to work, not expose patient unnecessarily. Covers have been pulled back to show action.*)

10. Remove gloves. Perform hand hygiene. Cover the patient with the bed linens.	Proper removal of gloves reduces transmission of microorganisms. Hand hygiene deters the spread of microorganisms. Covering promotes warmth and privacy.
11. Place the call bell and toilet tissue within easy reach. Have a receptacle, such as a plastic trash bag, handy for discarding tissue. Ensure the bed is in the lowest position. Leave the patient if it is safe to do so. Use side rails appropriately.	Falls can be prevented if the patient does not have to reach for items they need. Placing the bed in the lowest position promotes patient safety. Leaving the patient alone, if possible, promotes self-esteem and shows respect for privacy. Side rails assist the patient in repositioning.
12. Remove additional PPE, if used. Perform hand hygiene.	Proper removal of PPE reduces transmission of microorganisms. Hand hygiene deters the spread of microorganisms.

Removing the Urinal

13. Perform hand hygiene. Put on gloves and additional PPE, as indicated.	Hand hygiene and PPE prevent the spread of microorganisms. Gloves prevent exposure to blood and body fluids. PPE is required based on transmission precautions.
14. Pull back the patient's bed linens just enough to remove the urinal. Remove the urinal. Cover the open end of the urinal. Place it on the bedside chair. If the patient needs assistance with hygiene, wrap tissue around your hand several times, and wipe the patient dry. Discard the tissue in the receptacle. Use a warm, moist disposable washcloth and skin cleanser to clean the perineal area, as necessary, and as per patient request.	Covering the end of the urinal helps to prevent the spread of microorganisms. Cleaning the patient after they have used the urinal prevents offensive odors and skin irritation.

ACTION	**RATIONALE**

15. Return the patient to a comfortable position. Make sure the linens under the patient are dry. Remove gloves and perform hand hygiene.

Proper positioning promotes patient comfort. Removing contaminated gloves and hand hygiene prevent the spread of microorganisms.

16. Ensure the patient is covered, and the call bell is in reach.

This promotes patient comfort and safety.

17. Offer the patient supplies to wash and dry their hands, assisting as necessary.

Washing hands after using the urinal helps prevent the spread of microorganisms.

18. Put on gloves. Empty and clean the urinal, measuring urine in a graduated container, as necessary. Discard the trash receptacle with used toilet paper per facility policy.

Measurement of urine volume is required for accurate intake and output records.

19. Remove gloves and additional PPE, if used, and perform hand hygiene.

Gloves prevent exposure to blood and body fluids. Proper removal of PPE reduces the risk for infection transmission and contamination of other items. Hand hygiene prevents the spread of microorganisms.

EVALUATION

The expected outcome has been met when the patient voided using the urinal. Other outcomes have been met when the patient has remained dry, has not experienced episodes of incontinence, has demonstrated measures to assist with using the urinal, and has not experienced impaired skin integrity.

DOCUMENTATION

Guidelines

Document the patient's tolerance of the activity. Record the amount of urine voided on the intake and output record, if appropriate. Document any other assessments, such as unusual urine characteristics or alterations in the patient's skin.

Sample Documentation

> 12/06/25 0730 Patient using urinal at bedside to void. Voided 600-mL yellow urine. Perineal skin intact, without redness or irritation. Reinforced need for continued use of urinal for recording accurate output. Patient verbalized an understanding of instructions.
>
> —S. Barnes, RN

DEVELOPING CLINICAL REASONING AND CLINICAL JUDGMENT

SPECIAL CONSIDERATIONS

- The urinal should not be left in place for extended periods because pressure and irritation to the patient's skin can result. If the patient is unable to use alone or with assistance, consider other interventions, such as assisting the patient to use a bedside commode or applying an external urine collection device (see Skills 12-3 and 12-5).
- It may be necessary to assist patients who have difficulty holding the urinal in place, such as those with limited upper extremity movement or alteration in mentation, to prevent spillage of urine.
- The urinal may also be used standing or sitting at the bedside or in the patient's bathroom, if patient is able to do so.

Skill 12-3 ▶ Assisting With the Use of a Bedside Commode

Patients who experience difficulty getting to the bathroom may benefit from the use of a bedside commode. Bedside commodes are portable toilet substitutes that can be used for voiding and defecation (Figure 1). A bedside commode can be placed close to the bed for easy use. Many have armrests attached to the legs that may interfere with ease of transfer. The legs usually have some type of end cap on the bottom to reduce movement, but care must be taken to prevent the commode from moving during transfer, resulting in patient injury or falls.

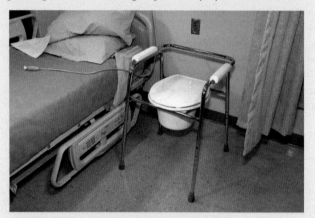

FIGURE 1. Bedside commode.

DELEGATION CONSIDERATIONS	Assisting a patient with the use of a commode may be delegated to assistive personnel (AP) as well as to licensed practical/vocational nurses (LPN/LVNs). The decision to delegate must be based on careful analysis of the patient's needs and circumstances as well as the qualifications of the person to whom the task is being delegated. Refer to the Delegation Guidelines in Appendix A.
EQUIPMENT	• Commode with cover (usually attached) • Toilet tissue • Nonsterile gloves • Additional PPE, as indicated • Disposable washcloths and skin cleanser • Moist towelettes, skin cleanser and water, or hand sanitizer
ASSESSMENT	Assess the patient's usual elimination habits. Determine why the patient needs to use a commode, such as weakness or unsteady gait. Assess the patient's degree of limitation and ability to help with the activity. Check for the presence of drains, dressings, intravenous fluid infusion sites/equipment, or other devices that could interfere with the patient's ability to help with the procedure or that could become dislodged. Assess the characteristics of the urine and the patient's skin.
ACTUAL OR POTENTIAL HEALTH PROBLEMS AND NEEDS	Many actual or potential health problems or issues may require the use of this skill as part of related interventions. An appropriate health problem or issue may include: • Fall risk • Functional urinary incontinence • Toileting ADL deficit
OUTCOME IDENTIFICATION AND PLANNING	The expected outcome to achieve when assisting with the use of a commode is that the patient is able to void or defecate with assistance. Other appropriate outcomes may include that the patient maintains continence, demonstrates how to use the commode, maintains skin integrity, and remains free from injury.

IMPLEMENTATION

ACTION	RATIONALE

1. Review the patient's health record for any limitations in physical activity. Gather equipment.

Physical limitations may require adaptations in performing the skill. Assembling equipment provides for an organized approach to the task.

2. Obtain assistance for a patient transfer from another staff member and/or appropriate transfer equipment, as indicated (refer to Chapter 9).

Assistance from another person or use of appropriate transfer equipment may be required to transfer the patient safely to the commode.

3. Perform hand hygiene and put on PPE, if indicated.

Hand hygiene and PPE prevent the spread of microorganisms. PPE is required based on transmission precautions.

4. Identify the patient.

Identifying the patient ensures the right patient receives the intervention and helps prevent errors.

5. Close the curtains around the bed and close the door to the room, if possible. Discuss the procedure with the patient and assess the patient's ability to assist with the procedure as well as personal hygiene preferences.

This ensures the patient's privacy. Discussion promotes reassurance and provides knowledge about the procedure. Dialogue encourages patient participation and allows for individualized nursing care.

6. Place the commode close to, and parallel with, the bed. Raise or remove the seat cover (refer to Figure 1).

This allows for easy access.

7. Encourage the patient to make use of the stand-assist device, as necessary. Cue the patient to stand. Assist the patient to pivot and turn to the commode. **While bracing one commode leg with your foot, ask the patient to place their hands one at a time on the armrests. Assist the patient to lower themself slowly onto the commode seat.**

Use of a stand-assist device decreases the risk of injury to the nurse and to the patient. Standing and then pivoting ensures safe patient transfer. Bracing the commode leg with a foot prevents the commode from shifting while the patient is sitting down. The patient uses their own arm for support and stability.

8. Cover the patient with a blanket. Place call bell and toilet tissue within easy reach. Leave the patient if it is safe to do so. Remove PPE, if used, and perform hand hygiene.

Covering the patient promotes warmth. Falls can be prevented if the patient does not have to reach for items they need. Leaving the patient alone, if possible, promotes self-esteem and shows respect for privacy. Proper removal of PPE reduces the risk for infection transmission and contamination of other items. Hand hygiene prevents the spread of microorganisms.

Assisting Patient off the Commode

9. Perform hand hygiene. Put on gloves and additional PPE, as indicated.

Hand hygiene deters the spread of microorganisms. Gloves prevent exposure to blood and body fluids.

10. Assist the patient to a standing position. If the patient needs assistance with hygiene, wrap toilet tissue around your hand several times, and wipe the patient clean, using one stroke from the pubic area toward the anal area. Discard the tissue in an appropriate receptacle, according to facility policy, and continue with additional tissue until the patient is dry. Discard the tissue in the receptacle. Use a warm, moist disposable washcloth and skin cleanser to clean the perineal area, as necessary, and as per patient request.

Cleaning the area from front to back minimizes fecal contamination of the vagina and urinary meatus. Cleaning the patient after they have used the commode prevents offensive odors and irritation to the skin.

11. Do not place toilet tissue in the commode if a specimen is required, or if output is being recorded. Replace or lower the seat cover.

Mixing toilet tissue with a specimen makes laboratory examination more difficult and interferes with accurate output measurement. Covering the commode helps to prevent the spread of microorganisms.

(continued on page 726)

Skill 12-3 ▶ Assisting With the Use of a Bedside Commode *(continued)*

ACTION	RATIONALE
12. Remove your gloves. Perform hand hygiene. Return the patient to the bed or chair. If the patient returns to the bed, raise the side rails, as appropriate. Ensure that the patient is covered, and the call bell is readily within reach.	Removing contaminated gloves prevents the spread of microorganisms. Hand hygiene prevents the spread of microorganisms. Returning the patient to the bed or chair promotes patient comfort. Side rails assist with patient movement in the bed. Having the call bell readily available promotes patient safety.
13. Offer the patient supplies to wash and dry their hands, assisting as necessary.	Washing hands after using the commode helps prevent the spread of microorganisms.
14. Put on clean gloves. Empty and clean the commode, measuring urine in a graduated container, as necessary.	Gloves prevent exposure to blood and body fluids. Accurate measurement of urine is necessary for accurate intake and output records.
15. Remove gloves and additional PPE, if used. Perform hand hygiene.	Proper removal of PPE reduces the risk for infection transmission and contamination of other items. Hand hygiene prevents the spread of microorganisms.

EVALUATION

The expected outcome has been met when the patient successfully used the bedside commode. Other outcomes have been met when the patient has remained dry, has not experienced episodes of incontinence, has demonstrated measures to assist with using the commode, and has not experienced impaired skin integrity or falls.

DOCUMENTATION

Guidelines

Document the patient's tolerance of the activity, including their ability to use the commode. Record the amount of urine voided and/or stool passed on the intake and output record, if appropriate. Document any other assessments, such as unusual urine or stool characteristics or alterations in the patient's skin.

Sample Documentation

> 07/06/25 0730 Patient using commode at bedside to void with assistance of one for transfer. Voided 325-mL yellow urine. Perineal skin intact and slightly red. Perineal hygiene provided, and skin protectant applied. Reinforced need for continued use of commode related to patient's unsteady gait. Patient verbalized an understanding of instructions and states they will call for assistance when getting up to use commode.
> —S. Barnes, RN

DEVELOPING CLINICAL REASONING AND CLINICAL JUDGMENT

SPECIAL CONSIDERATIONS

- The commode can be left within the patient's reach, to be used without assistance, if appropriate and safe to do so, based on patient's activity limitations and mobility. Adjust the room door or curtain to provide privacy for the patient in the event the commode is used.

Skill 12-4 ▶ Assessing Bladder Volume Using an Ultrasound Bladder Scanner

A portable bladder ultrasound scanner is an accurate, reliable, and noninvasive device used to assess bladder volume. Bladder scanners do not pose a risk for the development of a urinary tract infection, unlike intermittent catheterization, which may also be used to determine bladder volume. A bladder scanner may be used when there is urinary frequency, absent or decreased urine output, bladder distention, or inability to void, and when establishing intermittent catheterization schedules (AHRQ, 2020). Protocols can be established to guide the decision to catheterize a patient. Some scanners offer the ability to print the scan results for documentation purposes.

Scanning may be done with the patient siting or supine, but the most accurate measurements are obtained when the patient is supine (AHRQ, 2020). Ensure the biologic sex setting on the device is set correctly on the device. If a patient with female genitalia has had a hysterectomy, the male button is pushed (AHRQ, 2020). A postvoid residual (PVR) volume less than 50 mL indicates adequate bladder emptying. A PVR of greater than 300 to 500 mL is recommended as the guideline for intermittent catheterization; a PVR of 100 mL or more may indicate the bladder is not emptying completely (NIDDK, 2014).

This skill provides general directions to use a bladder scanner; always refer to facility policies and the manufacturer's directions for device in use.

DELEGATION CONSIDERATIONS

The assessment of bladder volume using an ultrasound bladder scanner is not delegated to assistive personnel (AP). Depending on the state's nurse practice act and the organization's policies and procedures, this procedure may be delegated to licensed practical/vocational nurses (LPN/LVNs). The decision to delegate must be based on careful analysis of the patient's needs and circumstances as well as the qualifications of the person to whom the task is being delegated. Refer to the Delegation Guidelines in Appendix A.

EQUIPMENT

- Bladder scanner
- Ultrasound gel or bladder scan gel pad
- Alcohol wipe or other sanitizer recommended by the scanner manufacturer and/or facility policy
- Clean gloves
- Additional PPE, as indicated
- Paper towel or washcloth

ASSESSMENT

Assess the patient for the need to check bladder volume, including signs of urinary retention, measurement of PVR volume, verification that the bladder is empty, identification of obstruction in an indwelling catheter, and evaluation of bladder distention to determine if catheterization is necessary. Verify as a prescribed intervention, if required by facility. Many facilities' policies identify the use of a bladder scanner as a nursing judgment.

ACTUAL OR POTENTIAL HEALTH PROBLEMS AND NEEDS

Many actual or potential health problems or issues may require the use of this skill as part of related interventions. An appropriate health problem or issue may include:
- Urinary retention
- Urinary frequency
- Impaired urination

OUTCOME IDENTIFICATION AND PLANNING

The expected outcome to achieve when using a bladder scanner is that the volume of urine in the bladder will be accurately measured.

(continued on page 728)

Skill 12-4 ▸ Assessing Bladder Volume Using an Ultrasound Bladder Scanner *(continued)*

IMPLEMENTATION

ACTION	**RATIONALE**
1. Review the patient's health record for any limitations in physical activity. Gather equipment.	Physical limitations may require adaptations in performing the skill. Assembling equipment provides for an organized approach to the task.
2. Perform hand hygiene and put on PPE, if indicated.	Hand hygiene and PPE prevent the spread of microorganisms. PPE is required based on transmission precautions.
3. Identify the patient.	Identifying the patient ensures the right patient receives the intervention and helps prevent errors.
4. Close the curtains around the bed and close the door to the room, if possible. Discuss the procedure with the patient and assess the patient's ability to assist with the procedure as well as personal hygiene preferences.	This ensures the patient's privacy. Discussion promotes reassurance and provides knowledge about the procedure. Dialogue encourages patient participation and allows for individualized nursing care.
5. Adjust the bed to a comfortable working height (VHACEOSH, 2016). Place the patient in a supine position. Drape the patient. Stand on the patient's right side if you are right-handed or on the patient's left side if you are left-handed.	Having the bed at the proper height prevents back and muscle strain. Proper positioning allows accurate assessment of bladder volume. Keeping the patient covered as much as possible promotes patient comfort and privacy. Positioning allows for ease of use of your dominant hand for the procedure.
6. Put on gloves.	Gloves prevent contact with blood and body fluids.
7. Press the ON button. Wait until the device warms up. Press the SCAN button to turn on the scanning screen.	Many devices require a few minutes to prepare the internal programs.
8. Press the appropriate biologic sex button. The icon for male or female will appear on the screen (Figure 1).	The device must be programmed for the biologic sex of the patient by pushing the correct button on it. If a patient with female genitalia has had a hysterectomy, the male button is pushed (AHRQ, 2020).
9. Clean the scanner head with the appropriate cleaner (Figure 2).	Cleaning the scanner head deters transmission of microorganisms.

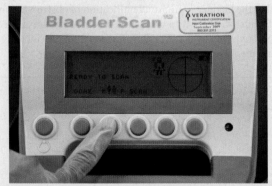

FIGURE 1. Identifying icon for patient's biologic sex. (*Source:* Used with permission from Shutterstock. *Photo by B. Proud.*)

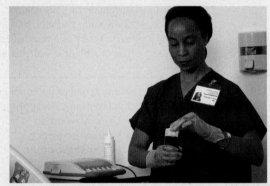

FIGURE 2. Cleaning scanner head. (*Source:* Used with permission from Shutterstock. *Photo by B. Proud.*)

10. Gently palpate the patient's **symphysis pubis** (anterior midline junction of pubic bones). Place a generous amount of ultrasound gel (Figure 3A) or gel pad (Figure 3B) midline on the patient's abdomen, about 1 to 1.5 inches above the symphysis pubis. Alternatively, depending on facility policy, apply ultrasound gel to the scanner head (AHRQ, 2020).	Palpation identifies the proper location and allows for correct placement of the scanner head over the patient's bladder.

ACTION

RATIONALE

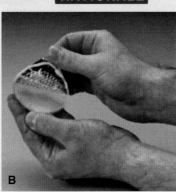

FIGURE 3. **A.** Placing ultrasound gel about 1 to 1.5 inches above symphysis pubis. **B.** Gel pad. (*Source:* Used with permission from Shutterstock. *Photo by B. Proud.*)

11. Place the scanner head on the gel or gel pad, **with the directional icon on the scanner head toward the patient's head. Aim the scanner head toward the bladder (point the scanner head slightly downward toward the coccyx)** (Figure 4A). Press and release the scan button (Figure 4B).

Proper placement allows for accurate reading of urine in the bladder (AHRQ, 2020; Widdall, 2015).

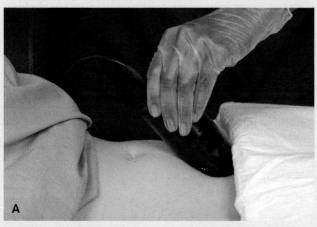

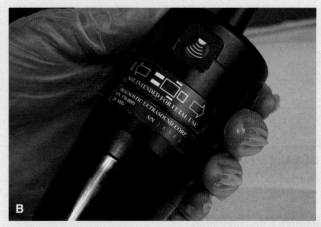

FIGURE 4. **A.** Positioning scanner head with directional icon toward patient's head and aiming the scanner head toward the bladder. **B.** Scan button. (*Source:* Used with permission from Shutterstock. *Photos by B. Proud.*)

12. Observe the image on the scanner screen, which includes the volume measured and an aiming display with crosshairs. **If the crosshairs are not centered on the bladder image, adjust the scanner head and rescan until the bladder image is centered on the crosshairs** (Figure 5).

This action allows for accurate reading of urine in the bladder.

13. Once the image is centered, press and hold the DONE button until it beeps. Read the volume measurement on the screen. Print the results, if required, by pressing PRINT.

This action provides for accurate documentation of reading.

14. Use a washcloth or paper towel to remove the remaining gel from the patient's skin. Alternatively, gently remove the gel pad from the patient's skin. Return the patient to a comfortable position. Remove your gloves and perform hand hygiene. Ensure that the patient is covered.

Removal of the gel promotes patient comfort. Removing contaminated gloves prevents the spread of microorganisms. Hand hygiene prevents the spread of microorganisms.

15. Lower the bed height and adjust the head of the bed to a comfortable position. Reattach the call bell, if necessary.

These actions promote patient safety.

(*continued on page 730*)

| Skill 12-4 | Assessing Bladder Volume Using an Ultrasound Bladder Scanner *(continued)* |

ACTION

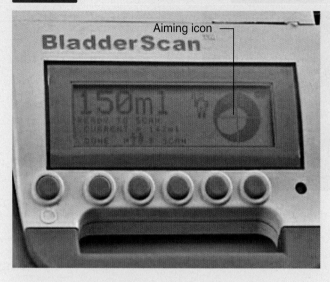

Aiming icon

FIGURE 5. Centering image on crossbars.

16. Put on gloves. Clean the scanner head according to the manufacturer's instructions and/or facility policy.

17. Remove gloves and any additional PPE, if used. Perform hand hygiene.

RATIONALE

Cleaning equipment prevents transmission of microorganisms.

Proper removal of PPE reduces the risk for infection transmission and contamination of other items. Hand hygiene prevents the spread of microorganisms.

EVALUATION

The expected outcome has been met when the volume of urine in the bladder is accurately measured.

DOCUMENTATION

Guidelines

Document the assessment data that led to the use of the bladder scanner, relevant symptoms, the urine volume measured, and the patient's response.

Sample Documentation

> <u>7/06/25</u> 1130 Patient has not voided 8 hours after catheter removal. Patient denies feelings of discomfort, pressure, and pain. Bladder not palpable. Bladder scanned for 120 mL of urine. Patient encouraged to increase oral fluid intake to eight 6-oz glasses today. Dr. Liu notified of assessment. Prescribed rescan in 4 hours if patient does not void.
>
> —B. Clapp, RN

DEVELOPING CLINICAL REASONING AND CLINICAL JUDGMENT

UNEXPECTED SITUATIONS AND ASSOCIATED INTERVENTIONS

- *You press the wrong icon for the patient's biologic sex when initiating the scanner:* Turn scanner off and back on. Reenter information using the correct biologic sex button.
- *You have reason to believe the bladder is full, based on assessment data, but the scanner reveals little to no urine in the bladder:* Ensure proper positioning of the scanner head. Place a generous amount of ultrasound gel or gel pad midline on the patient's abdomen, about 1 to 1.5 inches above the symphysis pubis. Place the scanner head on the gel or gel pad, with the directional icon on the scanner head toward the patient's head. Aim the scanner head toward the bladder (point the scanner head slightly downward toward the coccyx). Ensure that the bladder image is centered on the crossbars.

SPECIAL CONSIDERATIONS

- Ensure use of an adequate amount of ultrasound gel. Do not use lubricant (Widdall, 2015).
- Bladder volume measurements may be inaccurate in the presence of intraabdominal fluid, such as ascites (Schallom et al., 2020).
- If the patient is very thin or obese, use more ultrasound gel (AHRQ, 2020).
- If the patient has a large amount of lower abdominal hair, apply the gel directly to the skin (AHRQ, 2020).
- Ask or assist patients who are overweight or have larger abdominal tissue to hold their abdomen up and away from area to be scanned to reduce risk for interference, resulting in inaccurate measurement (Widdall, 2015).
- The use of bladder scanning can be used to reduce catheterization rates and associated complications (Institute for Healthcare Improvement [IHI], 2011).
- Bladder scanning in combination with intermittent catheterization may be beneficial in the management of postoperative urinary retention to avoid placement of an indwelling catheter (IHI, 2011).

Skill 12-5 ▶ Applying an External Urinary Sheath

When voluntary control of urination is difficult or not possible for patients with a penis, an alternative to an indwelling catheter is the condom-type **urinary sheath**, one type of external urine collection device for use on the penis (Newman, 2020b; Panchisin, 2016; Smart, 2014). This soft, pliable sheath made of silicone or latex material is applied externally to the penis and directs urine away from the body. Most devices are self-adhesive. The external urinary catheter is connected to drainage tubing and a collection bag and can be used with a leg bag.

Nursing care of a patient with a urinary sheath includes vigilant skin care to prevent excoriation. This includes removing the urinary sheath daily, washing the penis with skin cleanser and water and drying carefully, and inspecting the skin for irritation. In hot, humid weather, more frequent changing may be required. Always follow the manufacturer's instructions for applying the external urinary sheath because there are several variations. In all cases, take care to fasten the urinary sheath securely enough to prevent leakage, yet not so tightly as to constrict the blood vessels in the area. When using sheath-type devices, the tip of the tubing should be kept 1 to 2 inches (2.5 to 5 cm) beyond the tip of the penis to prevent irritation to the sensitive glans area.

Maintaining free urinary drainage is another nursing priority. Institute measures to prevent the tubing from becoming kinked and urine from backing up in the tubing. Urine can lead to excoriation of the glans, so position the tubing that collects the urine from the external urinary sheath so that it draws urine away from the penis.

Always use a measuring or sizing guide supplied by the manufacturer to ensure the correct size of sheath is applied. Apply skin barriers, such as Cavilon™ or Skin-Prep™, to the penis to protect penile skin from irritation and changes in integrity.

DELEGATION CONSIDERATIONS

The application of an external urinary sheath may be delegated to assistive personnel (AP) as well as to licensed practical/vocational nurses (LPN/LVNs). The decision to delegate must be based on careful analysis of the patient's needs and circumstances as well as the qualifications of the person to whom the task is being delegated. Refer to the Delegation Guidelines in Appendix A.

EQUIPMENT

- External urinary sheath (condom catheter) in appropriate size
- Skin protectant, such as Cavilon™ or Skin-Prep™
- Velcro leg strap, catheter-securing device, or tape
- Bath blanket
- Reusable leg bag with tubing or urinary drainage setup

(continued on page 732)

Skill 12-5 ▶ Applying an External Urinary Sheath *(continued)*

- Premoistened disposable washcloths or
  - Basin with warm water
  - Skin cleanser, towel, washcloth
- Disposable gloves
- Additional PPE, as indicated
- Washcloth and towel
- Scissors

ASSESSMENT	Assess the patient's knowledge of the need for use of the urinary sheath. Ask the patient about any allergies, especially to latex or tape. Assess the size of the patient's penis to ensure that the appropriate-sized external urinary sheath is used; size is determined by penile diameter at the base of the penile shaft (Newman, 2020a). Inspect the penile skin and the skin in the groin and scrotal area, noting any areas of redness, irritation, or breakdown.
ACTUAL OR POTENTIAL HEALTH PROBLEMS AND NEEDS	Many actual or potential health problems or issues may require the use of this skill as part of related interventions. An appropriate health problem or issue may include: • Toileting ADL deficit • Functional urinary incontinence • Altered skin integrity risk
OUTCOME IDENTIFICATION AND PLANNING	The expected outcome to achieve when applying an external urinary sheath is that the patient's urine is diverted into the urine collection device, and the patient's skin remains clean, dry, intact, and without evidence of irritation or breakdown.

IMPLEMENTATION

ACTION	**RATIONALE**
1. Gather equipment.	Assembling equipment provides for an organized approach to the task.
2. Perform hand hygiene and put on PPE, if indicated.	Hand hygiene and PPE prevent the spread of microorganisms. PPE is required based on transmission precautions.
3. Identify the patient.	Identifying the patient ensures the right patient receives the intervention and helps prevent errors.
4. Close the curtains around the bed and close the door to the room, if possible. Discuss the procedure with the patient. Ask the patient if they have any allergies, especially to latex.	This ensures the patient's privacy. Discussion promotes reassurance and provides knowledge about the procedure. Dialogue encourages patient participation and allows for individualized nursing care. Some external urinary sheaths are made of latex.
5. Assemble equipment on the overbed table or other surface within reach.	Arranging items nearby is convenient, saves time, and prevents unnecessary stretching and twisting of muscles on the part of the nurse.
6. Adjust the bed to a comfortable working height (VHACEOSH, 2016). Stand on the patient's right side if you are right-handed, or on patient's left side if you are left-handed.	Having the bed at the proper height prevents back and muscle strain. Positioning on one side allows for ease of use of your dominant hand for device application.
7. Prepare the urinary drainage setup or reusable leg bag for attachment to the external urinary sheath.	This provides for an organized approach to the task.
8. Position the patient on their back with the thighs slightly apart. Drape the patient so that only the area around the penis is exposed. Slide the waterproof pad under the patient.	Positioning allows access to the site. Draping prevents unnecessary exposure and promotes warmth. The waterproof pad will protect bed linens from moisture.

ACTION	**RATIONALE**

9. Put on gloves. Trim the pubic hair at the base of the penis.

Gloves prevent contact with blood and body fluids. Trimming the pubic hair prevents pulling of hair by adhesive; do not shave hair to avoid irritation associated with shaving (Newman, 2020a).

10. Clean the genital area with a washcloth, skin cleanser, and warm water. If the patient is uncircumcised, retract the foreskin and clean the glans of the penis. Replace the foreskin. Clean the tip of the penis first, moving the washcloth in a circular motion from the meatus outward. Wash the shaft of the penis using downward strokes toward the pubic area. Rinse and dry. Remove gloves. Perform hand hygiene.

Washing removes urine, secretions, and microorganisms. The penis must be clean and dry to minimize skin irritation. If the foreskin is left retracted, it may cause venous congestion in the glans of the penis, leading to edema. Hand hygiene prevents the spread of microorganisms.

11. Put on gloves. Apply skin protectant to the penis and allow it to dry.

Gloves prevent contact with blood and body fluids. Skin protectant minimizes the risk of skin irritation from adhesive and moisture and increases the adhesive's ability to adhere to skin.

12. Roll the external urinary sheath outward onto itself. Grasp the penis firmly with your nondominant hand. Apply the external urinary sheath by rolling it onto the penis with your dominant hand (Figure 1). **Leave 1 to 2 inches (2.5 to 5 cm) of space between the tip of the penis and the end of the external urinary sheath.**

Rolling the external urinary sheath outward allows for easier application. The space prevents irritation to the tip of the penis and allows free drainage of urine.

13. Apply pressure to the sheath at the base of the penis for 10 to 15 seconds.

Application of pressure ensures good adherence of the adhesive to the skin.

14. Connect the external urinary sheath to the drainage setup (Figure 2). Avoid kinking or twisting drainage tubing.

The collection device keeps the patient dry. Kinked tubing encourages backflow of urine.

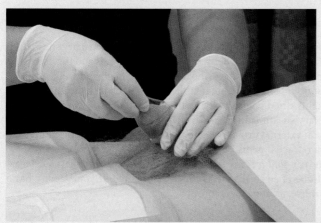

FIGURE 1. Unrolling sheath onto penis.

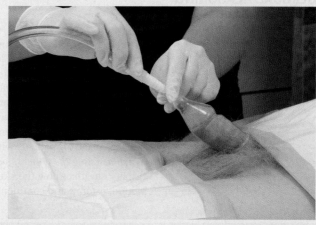

FIGURE 2. Connecting external urinary sheath to drainage setup.

15. Remove gloves. Perform hand hygiene. Secure the drainage tubing to the patient's inner thigh with the Velcro leg strap, catheter securement device, or tape. Leave some slack in the tubing for leg movement.

Proper attachment prevents tension on the sheath and potential inadvertent removal. Hand hygiene prevents the spread of microorganisms.

16. Assist the patient to a comfortable position. Cover the patient with bed linens. Place the bed in the lowest position.

Positioning and covering provide warmth and promote comfort. The bed in the lowest position promotes patient safety.

17. Secure the drainage bag below the level of the bladder. Check that the drainage tubing is not kinked and that movement of the side rails does not interfere with the drainage bag.

This facilitates drainage of urine and prevents the backflow of urine.

(continued on page 734)

Skill 12-5 ▶ Applying an External Urinary Sheath *(continued)*

ACTION

18. Remove equipment. Remove additional PPE, if used. Perform hand hygiene.

RATIONALE

Proper disposal of equipment prevents transmission of microorganisms. Proper removal of PPE reduces the risk for infection transmission and contamination of other items. Hand hygiene prevents the spread of microorganisms.

EVALUATION

The expected outcome has been met when the patient's urine has been diverted into the urine collection device, and the patient's skin has remained clean, dry, intact, and without evidence of irritation or breakdown.

DOCUMENTATION

Guidelines

Document the assessment data supporting the decision to use an external urinary sheath, the application of the external urinary sheath, and the condition of the patient's skin. Record urine output on the intake and output record.

Sample Documentation

7/12/25 1910 Patient incontinent of urine; states: "It just comes too fast. I can't get to the bathroom in time." Perineal skin slightly reddened. Discussed rationale for use of external urinary sheath. Patient and wife agreeable to trying external urinary sheath. Medium-sized external urinary sheath applied; urine draining into collection bag without leakage. Leg bag in place for daytime use. Patient verbalized understanding of need to call for assistance to empty drainage bag.

—*B. Clapp, RN*

DEVELOPING CLINICAL REASONING AND CLINICAL JUDGMENT

UNEXPECTED SITUATIONS AND ASSOCIATED INTERVENTIONS

- *External urinary sheath leaks with every voiding:* Check the size of the external urinary sheath. If it is too big or too small, it may leak. Check the space between the tip of the penis and the end of the external urinary sheath. If this space is too small, the urine has no place to go and will leak out.
- *External urinary sheath will not stay on patient:* Ensure that the external urinary sheath is correct size, and that the penis is thoroughly dried before applying the external urinary sheath. Remind the patient that the external urinary sheath is in place, so that they do not tug at the tubing. If the patient has a retracted penis, an external urinary sheath may not be the best choice; there are pouches made for patients with a retracted penis.
- *When assessing the patient's penis, you find a break in skin integrity:* Do not reapply the external urinary sheath. Allow the skin to be open to the air as much as possible. If your facility has a wound, ostomy, and continence nurse, arrange for a consult.

EVIDENCE FOR PRACTICE ▶

PREVENTION OF CATHETER-ASSOCIATED INFECTIONS

Centers for Disease Control and Prevention (CDC). (2015, October). *Healthcare-associated infections (HAIs). Catheter-associated urinary tract infections (CAUTI).* https://www.cdc.gov/hai/ca_uti/uti.html

This site provides resources for health care providers and patients, including the CDC guidelines for prevention of catheter-associated infections. These guidelines recommend considering the use of alternatives to indwelling urethral catheterization in selected patients, when appropriate, such as the use of external urinary sheaths in cooperative patients with male genitalia without urinary retention or bladder outlet obstruction.

Skill 12-6 ▶ Applying an External Urine Collection Device (Female Genitalia)

When voluntary control of urination is difficult or not possible for patients with female genitalia, an alternative to an indwelling catheter is a female external urine collection device (Beeson & Davis, 2018; Dublynn & Episcopia, 2019; Gentile et al., 2020; Newman, 2020a). Use of this device minimizes the risk for skin injury associated with incontinence and infection associated with an indwelling urinary catheter (Beeson & Davis, 2018; Dublynn & Episcopia, 2019; Gentile et al., 2020). The device consists of a "wick" that conforms to the perineal area between the labia against the urethra (Figure 1), collection tubing, and a collection canister (Figure 2). It is connected to low continuous suction providing a sump mechanism to collect and measure urine output. The device also delivers continuous air flow to promote a microclimate environment to the perineum (Beeson & Davis, 2018). Use of these devices reduces the use of indwelling catheters and decreases CAUTI events (Dublynn & Episcopia, 2019; Gentile et al., 2020).

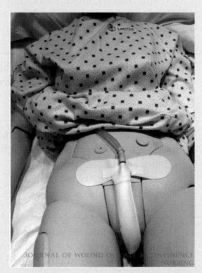

FIGURE 1. External urine collection device in place, secured to the suprapubic region. (*Source:* The PureWick™ System includes the PureWick™ Female External Catheter [wick] and the PureWick™ Urine Collection System. Courtesy and © Becton, Dickinson and Company. Reprinted with permission.)

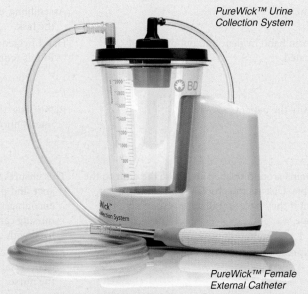

PureWick™ Urine Collection System

PureWick™ Female External Catheter

FIGURE 2. External urine collection system (female genitalia). (*Source:* Beeson, T., & Davis, C. [2018, March/April]. Urinary management with an external female collection device. *Journal of Wound Ostomy & Continence Nursing, 45*[2],187–189.)

(continued on page 736)

Skill 12-6 ▶ Applying an External Urine Collection Device (Female Genitalia) *(continued)*

DELEGATION CONSIDERATIONS	The application of an external urine collection device may be delegated to assistive personnel (AP) as well as to licensed practical/vocational nurses (LPN/LVNs). The decision to delegate must be based on careful analysis of the patient's needs and circumstances as well as the qualifications of the person to whom the task is being delegated. Refer to the Delegation Guidelines in Appendix A.

EQUIPMENT	• External urine collection system (base, collection canister, collector tubing)
	• Female external catheter (wick)
	• Bath blanket
	• Premoistened disposable washcloths or
	  • Basin with warm water
	  • Skin cleanser, towel, washcloth
	• Disposable gloves
	• Additional PPE, as indicated

ASSESSMENT	Assess the patient's knowledge of the need for use of the external urine collection device. Ask the patient about any allergies, especially to adhesive or tape. Inspect the labial and perineal skin, noting any areas of redness, irritation, or breakdown.
ACTUAL OR POTENTIAL HEALTH PROBLEMS AND NEEDS	Many actual or potential health problems or issues may require the use of this skill as part of related interventions. An appropriate health problem or issue may include: • Toileting ADL deficit • Functional urinary incontinence • Altered skin integrity risk
OUTCOME IDENTIFICATION AND PLANNING	The expected outcome to achieve when applying an external urine collection device is that the patient's urine is diverted into the urine collection device, and the patient's skin remains clean, dry, intact, and without evidence of irritation or breakdown.

IMPLEMENTATION

ACTION	RATIONALE
1. Gather equipment.	Assembling equipment provides for an organized approach to the task.
2. Perform hand hygiene and put on PPE, if indicated.	Hand hygiene and PPE prevent the spread of microorganisms. PPE is required based on transmission precautions.
3. Identify the patient.	Identifying the patient ensures the right patient receives the intervention and helps prevent errors.
4. Close the curtains around the bed and close the door to the room, if possible. Discuss the procedure with the patient. Ask the patient if they have any allergies, especially to adhesive or tape.	This ensures the patient's privacy. Discussion promotes reassurance and provides knowledge about the procedure. Dialogue encourages patient participation and allows for individualized nursing care. Some external urine collection devices are stabilized with an adhesive securement device.
5. Assemble equipment on the overbed table or other surface within reach.	Arranging items nearby is convenient, saves time, and prevents unnecessary stretching and twisting of muscles on the part of the nurse.
6. Adjust the bed to a comfortable working height (VHACEOSH, 2016). Stand on the patient's right side if you are right-handed, or on patient's left side if you are left-handed.	Having the bed at the proper height prevents back and muscle strain. Positioning on one side allows for ease of use of your dominant hand for device application.

ACTION	RATIONALE
7. Prepare the urine collection system; attach the collection tubing to the canister. Set the canister in the base. Turn the system on.	This provides for an organized approach to the task.
8. Put on gloves. Position the patient in the dorsal recumbent position with their knees flexed, feet about 2 ft apart, with their legs abducted. Drape the patient with the bath blanket so that only the perineal area is exposed. Slide the waterproof pad under the patient.	Gloves prevent contact with blood and body fluids. Positioning allows access to the site. Draping prevents unnecessary exposure and promotes warmth. The waterproof pad will protect bed linens from moisture.
9. Clean the perineal area with a washcloth, skin cleanser, and warm water. Rinse and dry. Assess the perineal skin. Remove gloves. Perform hand hygiene.	Washing removes urine, secretions, and microorganisms. The perineal skin must be clean and dry to minimize skin irritation. Hand hygiene prevents the spread of microorganisms.
10. Put on gloves. Remove the external catheter (wick) from the packaging and connect to the collection tubing.	Gloves prevent contact with blood and body fluids.
11. Gently separate the patient's labia and tuck the soft gauze side of the external catheter (wick) between the separated gluteus and labia. The external catheter (wick) should be fitted snugly against the body and urethral opening. The top of the gauze on the catheter/wick should be aligned with the pubic bone (refer to Figure 1).	Proper placement is essential for collection of urine. Urine is diverted away from the skin using suction and pulled into the collection tubing.
12. The collection tubing should rest on the patient's stomach. Depending on the particular external collection device in use, remove the paper backing from the securement adhesive, and attach to the patient's suprapubic skin (refer to Figure 1).	The collection tubing carries urine to the collection canister. The adhesive securement device helps prevent dislodgment.
13. Remove gloves. Perform hand hygiene. Assist the patient to place their legs back together and then to a comfortable position. Cover the patient with bed linens. Place the bed in the lowest position.	Positioning and covering provide warmth and promote comfort. The bed in the lowest position promotes patient safety.
14. Remove additional PPE, if used. Perform hand hygiene.	Proper removal of PPE reduces the risk for infection transmission and contamination of other items. Hand hygiene prevents the spread of microorganisms.
15. Discard and replace the external catheter (wick) at least once every 8 to 12 hours or when soiled (Becton, Dickinson and Company, 2020).	This maintains patency of the system and reduces risk of skin irritation.

EVALUATION The expected outcomes have been met when the patient's urine has been diverted into the urine collection device, and the patient's skin has remained clean, dry, intact, and without evidence of irritation or breakdown.

DOCUMENTATION Document the assessment data supporting the decision to use an external urine collection device, the application of the external urine collection device, and the condition of the patient's skin. Record urine output on the intake and output record.

Sample Documentation

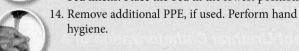

6/12/25 1410 Patient incontinent of urine several times, patient denies awareness of need to void "until it's too late." Discussed rationale for use of external urine collection device. Patient agreeable to trying external urine collection device. Patient verbalized understanding of need to call for assistance to remove device prior to getting out of bed.

(continued on page 738)

Skill 12-6 ▶ Applying an External Urine Collection Device (Female Genitalia) *(continued)*

DEVELOPING CLINICAL REASONING AND CLINICAL JUDGMENT

SPECIAL CONSIDERATIONS

General Considerations

- Replace the external catheter (wick) immediately if soiled with blood or feces (Becton, Dickinson and Company, 2020).
- The external catheter should not be used for patients who are experiencing skin irritation or altered skin integrity in device contact areas (Becton, Dickinson and Company, 2020).
- Excessive movement or the side-lying position may dislodge the external catheter (wick) (CDC, 2019); frequent patient assessment may be necessary to confirm maintenance of correct placement. Provide the patient with education regarding possible consequences of excessive movement.

EVIDENCE FOR PRACTICE ▶

PREVENTION OF CATHETER-ASSOCIATED INFECTIONS

Centers for Disease Control and Prevention. (2019, November 21). *CDC/STRIVE infection control training. Targeted prevention strategies. Catheter-associated urinary tract infection (CAUTI)—WB4222. CAUTI 103: Alternatives to the indwelling urinary catheter.* https://www.cdc.gov/infectioncontrol/training/strive.html#anchor_CAUTI

This site provides competency-based training modules for health care providers and patients, addressing targeted prevention strategies for catheter-associated urinary tract infection prevention. This module addresses alternatives to indwelling urinary catheters, including external urinary catheters/devices.

Skill 12-7 ▶ Catheterizing the Urinary Bladder of a Patient With Female Genitalia

Skill Variation: *Intermittent Urethral Catheterization of a Patient With Female Genitalia*

Urinary catheterization is the introduction of a catheter (tube) through the urethra into the bladder for the purpose of withdrawing urine. Catheter-associated urinary tract infections (CAUTIs) remain one of the most common causes of health care–associated infections in the United States (Knill et al., 2018). The best way to prevent a CAUTI is to use urinary catheters only when absolutely necessary (ANA, n.d.; Panchisin, 2016). The CDC provides parameters to guide the decision to insert an indwelling urinary catheter (Gould et al., 2019). When use of a urinary catheter is deemed necessary, it should be performed using strict aseptic technique, left in place only as long as needed, and removed as soon as possible (ANA, 2014; Gould et al., 2019; Gyesi-Appiah et al., 2020; SUNA, 2015).

If a catheter is to remain in place for continuous drainage, an **indwelling urethral catheter** is used. Indwelling catheters are also called *retention* or *Foley catheters*. The indwelling urethral catheter is designed so that it does not slip out of the bladder. A balloon is inflated to ensure that the catheter remains in the bladder once it is inserted (Figure 1A).

Intermittent urethral catheters (straight catheters) are used to drain the bladder for shorter periods (Figure 1B). Intermittent catheterization should be considered as an alternative to short- or long-term indwelling urethral catheterization to reduce CAUTIs (Gould et al., 2019). Intermittent catheterization is the preferred bladder management method for patients with urinary retention and bladder-emptying dysfunctions and following surgical interventions (Beauchemin et al., 2018; Gould et al., 2019). Certain advantages to intermittent catheterization, including the lower risks of

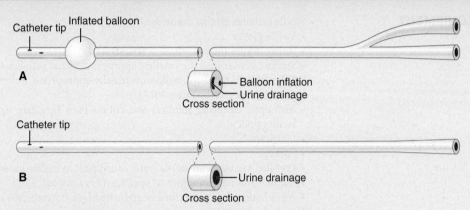

FIGURE 1. A. Indwelling urethral catheter. **B.** Intermittent urethral catheter.

CAUTI and complications, may make it a more desirable and safer option than indwelling catheterization (Panchisin, 2016; Wilson, 2015).

Some facilities have adopted a two-person urinary catheter insertion protocol, in which one nurse catheterizes the patient and one observes to ensure that the nurse inserting the catheter follows sterile technique and performs the procedure correctly (Belizario, 2015; Rhone et al., 2017). Implementation of the two-person urinary catheter insertion protocol has been shown to decrease CAUTI (Belizario, 2015; Fletcher-Gutowski & Cecil, 2019; Rhone et al., 2017).

The following procedure reviews insertion of an indwelling catheter. The procedure for an intermittent catheter follows as a Skill Variation. Guidelines for caring for a patient with an indwelling catheter are summarized in Box 12-1.

Box 12-1 Guidelines for Care of the Patient With an Indwelling Catheter

- Use an indwelling catheter only when necessary. In addition, consider evidence-based practice guidelines and facility policy to ensure the catheter is removed at the earliest time possible, to limit use to the shortest duration possible (ANA, 2014; Gould et al., 2019; SUNA, 2015).
- Wash hands before and after caring for the patient.
- Use the smallest appropriate-sized catheter that will allow effective drainage (ANA, 2014; SUNA, 2015; Yates, 2017a).
- Use sterile technique when inserting a catheter.
- Secure the catheter properly to the patient's thigh or abdomen after insertion (ANA, 2014; Holroyd, 2019; SUNA, 2015; Yates, 2016).
- Keep the drainage bag below the level of the patient's bladder to maintain drainage of urine and prevent the backflow of urine into the patient's bladder (ANA, 2014; Gould et al., 2019).
- Keep the drainage bag and tubing off the ground (ANA, 2014; Gould et al., 2019).
- Maintain a closed system (Gould et al., 2019).

- If necessary, obtain urine samples using aseptic technique via the sampling port on a closed system (Gould et al., 2019).
- Keep the catheter free from obstruction to maintain free flow to the urine.
- Avoid irrigation, unless needed, to relieve or prevent obstruction (Gould et al., 2019; SUNA, 2015).
- Ensure that the patient maintains adequate fluid intake (Hill & Mitchell, 2018).
- Empty the drainage bag regularly; prevent contact of the drainage spout with nonsterile collection/measuring container (Gould et al., 2019).
- Provide daily routine personal hygiene as outlined in Chapter 7; clean the perineal area thoroughly, especially around the meatus, daily and after each bowel movement. Rinse the area well. Cleanse the catheter by cleaning gently from the meatus outward. Do not use powders and lotions after cleaning. Do not use antibiotic or other antimicrobial cleaners or betadine at the urethral meatus (Gould et al., 2019; Herter & Kazer, 2010).

DELEGATION CONSIDERATIONS

The catheterization of the urinary bladder is not delegated to assistive personnel (AP). Depending on the state's nurse practice act and the organization's policies and procedures, catheterization of the urinary bladder may be delegated to licensed practical/vocational nurses (LPN/LVNs). The decision to delegate must be based on careful analysis of the patient's needs and circumstances as well as the qualifications of the person to whom the task is being delegated. Refer to the Delegation Guidelines in Appendix A.

(continued on page 740)

Skill 12-7 ▶ Catheterizing the Urinary Bladder of a Patient With Female Genitalia *(continued)*

EQUIPMENT

- Sterile catheter kit that contains:
  - Sterile gloves
  - Sterile drapes (one of which is **fenestrated**)
  - Sterile catheter (use the smallest appropriate-sized catheter that will allow effective drainage; a 14F with a 5- to 10-mL balloon is usually appropriate, unless another size is prescribed [ANA, 2014; SUNA 2021b; Yates, 2017a])
  - Antiseptic cleansing solution and cotton balls or gauze squares; antiseptic swabs (based on facility policy)
  - Lubricant
  - Forceps
  - Prefilled syringe with sterile water (sufficient to inflate indwelling catheter balloon)
  - Sterile specimen container (if specimen is required)
  - Anesthetic gel, as prescribed or indicated (see Assessments below)
- Flashlight or lamp
- Waterproof, disposable pad
- Sterile, disposable urine collection bag and drainage tubing (may be connected to catheter in catheter kit)
- Catheter-securing device
- Disposable gloves
- Additional PPE, as indicated
- Washcloth, skin cleanser, and warm water to perform perineal hygiene before and after catheterization

ASSESSMENT

Assess the patient's usual elimination habits. Assess the patient's degree of limitations and ability to help with activity. Assess for health problems, such as hip surgery or spinal injury, which would contraindicate certain actions by the patient. Assess for the presence of any other conditions that may interfere with passage of the catheter or contraindicate insertion of the catheter, such as urethral strictures or bladder cancer. Check for the presence of drains, dressings, intravenous fluid infusion sites/equipment, traction, or any other devices that could interfere with the patient's ability to help with the procedure or that could become dislodged. Assess bladder fullness before performing the procedure, either by palpation or with a handheld bladder ultrasound device. Question the patient about any allergies, especially to latex or iodine. Ask the patient if they have ever been catheterized. If they had an indwelling catheter previously, ask why and for how long it was used. The patient may have urethral strictures, which may make catheter insertion more difficult. Assess for the need to use anesthetic gel; the use of anesthetic gel is usually not necessary for patients with female anatomy but should be considered if it is the patient's first catheterization or if a difficulty catheterization is anticipated (SUNA, 2021a). Assess the characteristics of the urine and the patient's skin.

ACTUAL OR POTENTIAL HEALTH PROBLEMS AND NEEDS

Many actual or potential health problems or issues may require the use of this skill as part of related interventions. An appropriate health problem or issue may include:
- Urinary retention
- Infection risk
- Total urinary incontinence

OUTCOME IDENTIFICATION AND PLANNING

The expected outcomes to achieve when catheterizing the urinary bladder is that the catheter is successfully inserted without adverse effect, the patient's urinary elimination is maintained, and the patient's bladder is not distended. Other appropriate outcomes may include that the patient's skin remains clean, dry, intact, and without evidence of irritation or breakdown, and the patient verbalizes an understanding of the purpose for and care of the catheter, as appropriate.

IMPLEMENTATION

ACTION	RATIONALE

1. Review the patient's health record for any limitations in physical activity. Confirm the prescribed intervention for indwelling catheter insertion.

Physical limitations may require adaptations in performing the skill. Verifying the prescribed intervention ensures that the correct intervention is administered to the right patient.

2. Gather equipment. Obtain assistance from another staff member, if necessary or based on facility policy.

Assembling equipment provides for an organized approach to the task. Assistance from another person may be required to perform the intervention safely.

3. Perform hand hygiene and put on PPE, if indicated.

Hand hygiene and PPE prevent the spread of microorganisms. PPE is required based on transmission precautions.

4. Identify the patient.

Identifying the patient ensures the right patient receives the intervention and helps prevent errors.

5. Close the curtains around the bed and close the door to the room, if possible. Discuss the procedure with the patient and assess the patient's ability to assist with the procedure. Ask the patient if they have any allergies, especially to latex or iodine.

This ensures the patient's privacy. Discussion promotes reassurance and provides knowledge about the procedure. Dialogue encourages patient participation and allows for individualized nursing care. Some catheters and gloves in kits are made of latex. Some antiseptic solutions contain iodine.

6. Provide good lighting. Artificial light is recommended (use of a flashlight requires an assistant to hold and position it). Place a trash receptacle within easy reach.

Good lighting is necessary to see the meatus clearly. A readily available trash receptacle allows for prompt disposal of used supplies and reduces the risk of contaminating the sterile field.

7. Assemble equipment on the overbed table or other surface within reach.

Arranging items nearby is convenient, saves time, and prevents unnecessary stretching and twisting of muscles on the part of the nurse.

8. Adjust the bed to a comfortable working height (VHACEOSH, 2016). Stand on the patient's right side if you are right-handed or on the patient's left side if you are left-handed.

Having the bed at the proper height prevents back and muscle strain. Positioning allows for ease of use of your dominant hand for catheter insertion.

9. Assist the patient to a dorsal recumbent position with their knees flexed, feet about 2 ft apart, and legs abducted. Drape the patient (Figure 2). Alternatively, the Sims', or lateral, position can be used. Place the patient's buttocks near the edge of the bed with their shoulders at the opposite edge and their knees drawn toward the chest (Figure 3). Allow the patient to lie on either side, depending on which position is easiest for the nurse and best for the patient's comfort. Slide a waterproof pad under the patient.

Proper positioning allows adequate visualization of the urinary meatus. Patients with female genitalia should lie with their knees bent and legs spread apart (SUNA, 2021a; Yates, 2017b). Embarrassment, chilliness, and tension can interfere with catheter insertion; draping the patient will promote comfort and relaxation. The Sims' position may allow better visualization and be more comfortable for the patient, especially if hip and knee movements are difficult. The smaller area of exposure is also less stressful for the patient. The waterproof pad will protect bed linens from moisture.

10. Put on clean gloves. Clean the perineal area with a washcloth, skin cleanser, and warm water, using a different corner of the washcloth with each stroke. Wipe from above the orifice downward toward the sacrum (front to back). Rinse and dry. Remove gloves. Perform hand hygiene again.

Gloves reduce the risk of exposure to blood and body fluids. Cleaning reduces microorganisms near the urethral meatus and provides an opportunity to visualize the perineum and landmarks before the procedure. Hand hygiene reduces the spread of microorganisms.

11. Prepare the urine drainage setup if a separate urine collection system is to be used. Secure it to the bed frame, according to the manufacturer's directions.

This facilitates connection of the catheter to the drainage system and provides for easy access.

(continued on page 742)

Skill 12-7 ▶ Catheterizing the Urinary Bladder of a Patient With Female Genitalia *(continued)*

ACTION

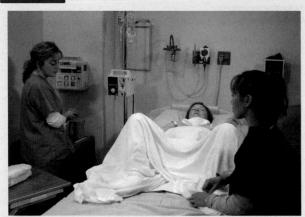

FIGURE 2. Patient in dorsal recumbent position and draped properly.

12. Open the sterile catheterization tray on a clean overbed table using sterile technique.

13. Put on sterile gloves. Grasp the upper corners of the drape and unfold the drape without touching nonsterile areas. Fold back a corner on each side to make a cuff over your gloved hands. Ask the patient to lift their buttocks and slide the sterile drape under them with your gloves protected by the cuff.

14. Based on facility policy, position the fenestrated sterile drape. Place a fenestrated sterile drape over the perineal area, exposing the labia (Figure 4). (*Note:* The fenestrated drape is not shown in the remaining illustrations in order to provide a clear view of the procedure.)

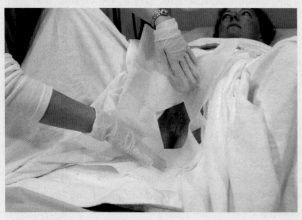

15. Place the sterile tray on the drape between the patient's thighs. If the patient is in the side-lying position, place the sterile tray near the patient's legs close to the sterile drape.

16. Open all the supplies. Remove the cap from the prefilled sterile saline syringe and attach it to the balloon inflation port on the catheter. Open the package of antiseptic swabs. Alternatively, fluff cotton balls in a tray before pouring antiseptic solution over them. Open the specimen container if a specimen is to be obtained. If using anesthetic gel, remove the cap from the prefilled syringe. Open and squirt lubricant in the tray.

RATIONALE

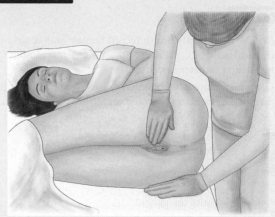

FIGURE 3. Demonstration of side-lying position.

Placement of equipment near the worksite increases efficiency. Sterile technique protects the patient and prevents transmission of microorganisms.

The drape provides a sterile field close to the meatus. Covering the gloved hands will help keep the gloves sterile while placing the drape.

The drape expands the sterile field and protects against contamination. Use of a fenestrated drape may limit visualization and is considered optional by some health care providers and/or facility policies.

FIGURE 4. Patient with fenestrated drape in place over perineum.

The sterile setup should be arranged so that the nurse's back is not turned to it, nor should it be out of the nurse's range of vision. This provides easy access to supplies.

It is necessary to open all supplies and prepare for the procedure while both hands are sterile.

ACTION

17. Remove the cover from the catheter and lubricate 1 to 2 inches of the catheter tip (SUNA, 2021b).

18. With the thumb and one finger of your nondominant hand, spread the labia and identify the meatus (Figure 5). **Be prepared to maintain separation of the labia with one hand until the catheter is inserted and urine is flowing well and continuously.** If the patient is in the side-lying position, lift the upper buttock and labia to expose the urinary meatus (Figure 6).

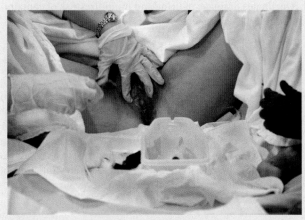

FIGURE 5. Using dominant hand to separate and hold labia open.

19. Use your dominant hand to pick up an antiseptic swab, or use forceps to pick up a cotton ball. **Clean one labial fold, top to bottom (from above the meatus down toward the rectum), then discard the swab/cotton ball (Figure 7). Using a new swab/cotton ball for each stroke, continue to clean the other labial fold, then use a third to clean directly over the meatus.** Discard each swab/cotton ball after one use.

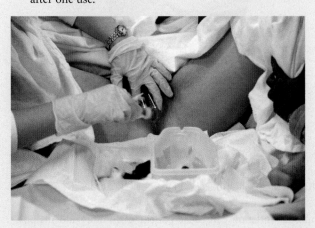

RATIONALE

Lubrication facilitates catheter insertion and reduces tissue trauma (SUNA, 2021a).

Smoothing the area immediately surrounding the meatus helps to make it visible. Allowing the labia to drop back into position may contaminate the area around the meatus as well as the catheter. The nondominant hand is now contaminated.

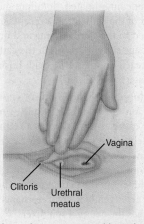

FIGURE 6. Exposing urinary meatus with patient in side-lying position.

Moving from an area where there is likely to be less contamination to an area where there is more contamination helps prevent the spread of microorganisms. Cleaning the meatus last helps reduce the possibility of introducing microorganisms into the bladder.

FIGURE 7. Wiping perineum with cotton ball held by forceps. Wipe in one direction—from top to bottom.

(*continued on page 744*)

Skill 12-7 ▶ Catheterizing the Urinary Bladder of a Patient With Female Genitalia *(continued)*

ACTION	RATIONALE

ACTION

20. If using anesthetic gel, with your noncontaminated, dominant hand, pick up the anesthetic syringe. Gently place nozzle of gel near the urethral orifice and apply some gel (SUNA, 2021b). Gently place nozzle at the meatus and slowly squeeze at least 5 mL of gel into the urethra (SUNA, 2021b). Allow the gel to dwell for approximately 3 to 5 minutes before starting the catheter insertion (SUNA, 2021b). Additional lubrication with a water-based lubricant may not be needed.

21. With your noncontaminated, dominant hand, place the drainage end of the catheter in a receptacle. If the catheter is pre-attached to the sterile tubing and drainage container (closed drainage system), position the catheter and setup within easy reach on the sterile field. Ensure that the clamp on the drainage bag is closed.

22. **Using your dominant hand, hold the catheter 2 to 3 inches from the tip and insert slowly into the urethra (Figure 8). Advance the catheter until there is a return of urine (approximately 2 to 3 inches [4.8 to 7.2 cm]). Once urine drains, advance the catheter another 2 to 3 inches (4.8 to 7.2 cm). Do not force the catheter through the urethra into the bladder.** Ask the patient to breathe deeply, and rotate the catheter gently if slight resistance is met as the catheter reaches the external sphincter.

23. Hold the catheter securely at the meatus with your nondominant hand. Use your dominant hand to inflate the catheter balloon (Figure 9). Inject the entire volume of sterile water supplied in a prefilled syringe. Remove the syringe from the port.

RATIONALE

The use of anesthetic gel is usually not necessary for patients with female anatomy but should be considered if it is the patient's first catheterization or if a difficulty catheterization is anticipated (SUNA, 2021a).

This facilitates drainage of urine and minimizes risk of contaminating sterile equipment.

The female urethra is about 1.5 to 2.5 inches (3.6 to 6.0 cm) long. Applying force on the catheter is likely to injure mucous membranes. The sphincter relaxes and the catheter can enter the bladder easily when the patient relaxes. Advancing an indwelling catheter an additional 2 to 3 inches (4.8 to 7.2 cm) ensures placement in the bladder and facilitates inflation of the balloon without damaging the urethra.

Bladder or sphincter contraction could push the catheter out. The balloon anchors the catheter in place in the bladder. The manufacturer provides the appropriate amount of sterile water for the size of the catheter in the kit; as a result, use the entire syringe provided in the kit. Removal of the syringe from the injection port prevents the sterile water from pushing back into the syringe and resulting balloon deflation.

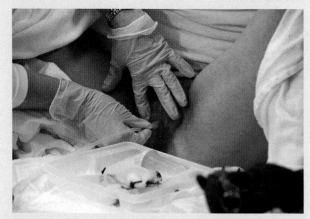

FIGURE 8. Inserting catheter with dominant hand while nondominant hand holds labia apart.

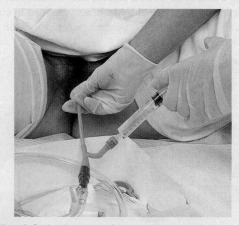

FIGURE 9. Inflating balloon of indwelling catheter.

24. Pull gently on the catheter after the balloon is inflated to feel resistance.

Improper inflation can cause patient discomfort and malpositioning of the catheter.

25. Attach the catheter to the drainage system if not already pre-attached (Figure 10).

The closed drainage system minimizes the risk for microorganisms being introduced into the bladder (Gould et al., 2019).

ACTION

26. Remove equipment and dispose of it according to facility policy. Discard the syringe in a sharps container. Wash and dry the perineal area, as needed.

 27. Remove gloves. Perform hand hygiene. **Secure the catheter tubing to the patient's inner thigh with a catheter-securing device (Figure 11).** Leave some slack in the catheter for leg movement.

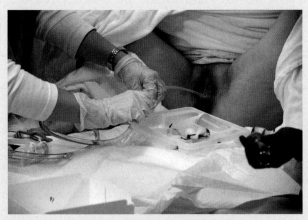

FIGURE 10. Attaching catheter to drainage bag.

28. Assist the patient to a comfortable position. Cover the patient with bed linens. Place the bed in the lowest position.

29. Secure the drainage bag below the level of the bladder. Check that the drainage tubing is not kinked and that movement of side rails does not interfere with the catheter or drainage bag.

30. Put on gloves. Obtain a urine specimen immediately, if needed, from the drainage bag. Label the specimen. Send the urine specimen to the laboratory promptly or refrigerate it.

 31. Remove gloves and additional PPE, if used. Perform hand hygiene.

RATIONALE

Proper disposal prevents the spread of microorganisms. Placing the syringe in a sharps container prevents reuse. Cleaning promotes comfort and appropriate personal hygiene.

Proper securement prevents tension on the catheter; reduces risk for catheter displacement, expulsion, migration, and trauma; and increases patient comfort (Holroyd, 2019). Hand hygiene prevents the spread of microorganisms. Whether to secure the drainage tubing over or under the leg depends on gravity flow, the patient's mobility, and the patient's comfort.

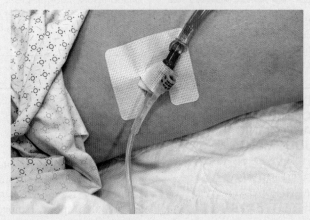

FIGURE 11. Catheter secured to leg.

Positioning and covering provides warmth and promotes comfort.

This facilitates drainage of urine and prevents the backflow of urine (ANA, 2014; Gould et al., 2019).

The catheter system is sterile. Obtaining a specimen immediately allows access to the sterile system. Keeping the urine at room temperature may cause microorganisms, if present, to grow and distort laboratory findings.

Proper removal of PPE reduces the risk for infection transmission and contamination of other items. Hand hygiene prevents the spread of microorganisms.

EVALUATION

The expected outcomes have been met when the catheter has been inserted without adverse effect, the patient's urinary elimination has been maintained, and the patient's bladder has not distended. Other outcomes have been met when the patient's skin has remained clean, dry, intact, and without evidence of irritation or breakdown, and the patient has verbalized an understanding of the purpose for and care of the catheter, as appropriate.

(continued on page 746)

Skill 12-7 ▶ Catheterizing the Urinary Bladder of a Patient With Female Genitalia *(continued)*

DOCUMENTATION

Guidelines

Document the type and size of catheter and balloon inserted, as well as the amount of fluid used to inflate the balloon. Document the patient's tolerance of the activity. Record the amount of urine obtained through the catheter and any specimen obtained. Document any other assessments, such as unusual urine characteristics or alterations in the patient's skin. Record urine amount on intake and output record, if appropriate.

Sample Documentation

Lippincott
DocuCare

Practice documenting
catheterization of the
female urinary bladder in
Lippincott DocuCare.

7/14/25 0915 Patient's primary care provider notified of palpable bladder (3 cm below umbilicus) and the patient's inability to void; 750 mL of urine noted with bladder scan. A 14F Foley catheter inserted without difficulty; 10 mL of sterile water injected into balloon port; 700-mL clear yellow urine returned. Patient states, "Oh, I feel much better now." Bladder is no longer palpable. Patient tolerated procedure without adverse event.

—B. Clapp, RN

DEVELOPING CLINICAL REASONING AND CLINICAL JUDGMENT

UNEXPECTED SITUATIONS AND ASSOCIATED INTERVENTIONS

- *No urine flow is obtained, and you note that the catheter is in the vaginal orifice:* Leave the catheter in place as a marker. Obtain new sterile gloves and catheter kit. Start the procedure over and attempt to place the new catheter directly above the misplaced catheter. Once the new catheter is correctly in place, remove the catheter in the vaginal orifice. Because of the risk of cross-infection, never remove a catheter from the vagina and insert it into the urethra.
- *Patient moves legs during procedure:* If no supplies have been contaminated, ask the patient to hold still and continue with the procedure. If supplies have been contaminated, stop the procedure and start over. If necessary, get an assistant to remind the patient to hold still.
- *Urine flow is initially well established, and urine is clear, but after several hours flow dwindles:* Check the tubing for kinking. If patient has changed position, the tubing and drainage bag may need to be moved to facilitate drainage of urine.
- *Urine leaks out of the meatus around the catheter:* Do not increase the size of the indwelling catheter. Make sure the smallest-sized catheter with a 10-mL balloon is used. Large catheters cause bladder and urethral irritation and trauma. Large balloon-fill volumes occupy more space inside the bladder and put added weight on the base of the bladder. Irritation of the bladder wall and detrusor muscle can cause leakage. If leakage persists, consider an evaluation for urinary tract infection. Ensure that the correct amount of solution was used to inflate the balloon. Underfilling the balloon can cause the catheter to dislodge into the urethra, causing urethral spasm, pain, and discomfort. If you suspect underfill, do not attempt to push the catheter farther into the bladder. Remove the catheter and replace with a new catheter. Assess the patient for constipation. A bowel full of stool can cause pressure on the catheter lumen and prevent the drainage of urine. Implement interventions to prevent/treat constipation.

SPECIAL CONSIDERATIONS

General Considerations

- Some facilities have adopted a two-person urinary catheter insertion protocol, in which one nurse catheterizes the patient and one observes to ensure that the nurse inserting the catheter follows sterile technique and performs the procedure correctly (Belizario, 2015; Rhone et al., 2017). Implementation of the two-person urinary catheter insertion protocol has been shown to decrease CAUTI (Belizario, 2015; Fletcher-Gutowski & Cecil, 2019; Rhone et al., 2017).
- The use of anesthetic gel is usually not necessary for patients with female anatomy but should be considered if it is the patient's first catheterization or if a difficulty catheterization is anticipated (SUNA, 2021a).

- Check for patient allergy before use of anesthetic gel. Anesthetic gel instilled into the patient's urethra should be administered at 3 to 5 minutes before catheterization to ensure sufficient anesthetic effect (SUNA, 2021b).
- Be familiar with facility policy and/or primary health care provider guidelines for the maximum amount of urine to remove from the bladder at the time of insertion.
- If the patient is unable to lift their buttocks or maintain the required position for the procedure, the assistance of another staff member may be necessary to place the drape under the patient and to help the patient maintain the required position.
- Supplies can be opened and prepared on the overbed table, moving the tray onto the bed just before cleansing the patient.
- If there is not an immediate flow of urine after the catheter has been inserted, several measures may prove helpful:
  - Have the patient take a deep breath, which helps to relax the perineal and abdominal muscles.
  - Rotate the catheter slightly, because a drainage hole may be resting against the bladder wall.
  - Raise the head of the patient's bed to increase pressure in the bladder area.
  - Assess the patient's intake to ensure adequate fluid intake for urine production.
  - Assess the catheter and drainage tubing for kinks and occlusion.
- If the catheter cannot be advanced, have the patient take several deep breaths. Rotate the catheter half a turn and try to advance it. If you are still unable to advance, remove the catheter. Notify the health care team.
- Some catheter kits do not contain the catheter. This allows you to select a catheter and balloon size separately.
- Maintain a constant downward flow of urine. Check tubing frequently to ensure kinks and dependent loops (low points) are not present in the tubing (ANA, 2014; Gould et al., 2019; Wuthier et al., 2016). Check to see that the patient is not lying on the drainage tubing and compressing it.
- Keep the catheter drainage bag below the level of the bladder at all times (ANA, 2014; Gould et al., 2019).
- Keep the drainage bag off the floor at all times to reduce the risk of infection (ANA, 2014; Gould et al., 2019). The floor is grossly contaminated.

Infant and Child Considerations

- Size 6F to 8F is used for infants and young children (Kyle & Carman, 2021). Size 8F to 12F catheters are commonly used for older children (Kyle & Carman, 2021).
- Distraction, such as blowing bubbles, deep breathing, or singing a song, can help the child relax.
- Consider use of lidocaine jelly to anesthetize and lubricate the area before insertion of the catheter, decreasing the child's discomfort and anxiety. Refer to facility policy regarding prescribing requirements and use.

Community-Based Care Considerations

- Intermittent catheterization, performed by the patient or a caregiver in the home, may be necessary for patients with spinal cord injuries or other neurologic conditions. Although the risk for UTI is always present, practice guidelines support the use of clean, rather than sterile, technique in the home environment (Bardsley, 2015a; Beauchemin et al., 2018; Gould et al., 2019; Wilson, 2015a). The procedure for self-intermittent catheterization is essentially the same as that used by the nurse to catheterize a patient, using clean, nonsterile technique (Collins, 2019; Leach, 2018). Box 12-2 outlines important information related to patient intermittent self-catheterization (ISC).
- Single-use catheters and no-touch catheters are options for use for ISC in the home setting (Beauchemin et al., 2018). The past practice of catheter reuse in community settings, instructing patients to wash and reuse the same catheter for multiple catheterizations, is not recommended; no evidence-based guidelines on cleaning or disposing of a reused catheter are available (Beauchemin et al., 2018; Newman, 2019b).

(continued on page 748)

Skill 12-7 ▶ Catheterizing the Urinary Bladder of a Patient With Female Genitalia *(continued)*

Box 12-2 | Patient Intermittent Self-Catheterization

- Explain the reason for self-catheterization and corresponding health issues related to the need for catheterization.
- Explain the benefits of self-catheterization, including reducing high postvoid residual volumes, reduced risk of urinary tract infection compared to an indwelling urinary catheterization, and improved quality of life.
- Explain potential complications, such as bleeding and the risk of urinary tract infections, and what to do if they occur.
- Ensure privacy and dignity.
- Include discussion regarding the frequency of intermittent catheterization and how to incorporate it into the patient's usual daily routine.
- Explain the anatomy of the urinary tract, hygiene, and preparation of the catheter.
- Demonstrate how to open, hold, and use the catheter.

- Explain catheterization process; demonstrate process; observe return demonstration by patient.
- Explore process to obtain supplies and assist with an informed choice of a catheter that suits the patient and their lifestyle.
- Provide information in an appropriate format (such as written materials or video, in appropriate language) to reinforce instruction.
- Allow the patient adequate time to ask questions.
- Provide information about how to recognize a urinary tract infection and other signs/symptoms to report to the health care team.
- Explain that aids are available to help meet the challenges of intermittent self-catheterization for patients with poor eyesight, reduced mobility, and/or reduced manual dexterity.

Source: Adapted from Balhi, S., & Mrabet, M. K. (2020). Teaching patients clean intermittent self-catheterisation: Key points. *British Journal of Community Nursing, 25*(12), 586–593; Bardsley, A. (2015b). Assessing and teaching female intermittent self-catheterization. *British Journal of Community Nursing, 20* (7), 344–346; Collins, L. (2019). Intermittent self-catheterisation: Good patient education and support are key. *British Journal of Nursing, 28*(15), 964–966; Davis, C., & Rantell, A. (2018). Selecting an intermittent self-catheter: Key considerations. *British Journal of Nursing, 27*(15), S11–S16; Hillery, S. (2020). Intermittent self-catheterisation: A person-centred approach. *British Journal of Nursing, 29*(15), 858–860; Leach, D. (2018). Teaching patients a clean intermittent self-catheterisation technique. *British Journal of Nursing, 27*(6), 296–298; Logan, K. (2020). An exploration of men's experiences of learning intermittent self-catheterisation with a silicone catheter. *British Journal of Nursing, 29*(2), 84–90; Mangnall, J. (2015). Managing and teaching intermittent catheterisation. *British Journal of Community Nursing, 20* (2), 82–88; and Wilson, M. (2015a). Clean intermittent self-catheterisation: Working with patients. *British Journal of Nursing, 24*(2), 76–85.

Skill Variation ▶ Intermittent Urethral Catheterization of a Patient With Female Genitalia

1. Check the health record for the prescribed intervention of intermittent urethral catheterization. Review the patient's health record for any limitations in physical activity. Gather equipment. Obtain assistance from another staff member, if necessary.

2. Perform hand hygiene. Put on PPE, as indicated.

3. Identify the patient. Discuss the procedure with the patient and assess the patient's ability to assist with the procedure. Ask the patient if they have any allergies, especially to latex or iodine.

4. Close the curtains around the bed and close the door to the room, if possible.
5. Provide good lighting. Artificial light is recommended (use of a flashlight requires an assistant to hold and position it). Place a trash receptacle within easy reach.
6. Assemble equipment on the overbed table or other surface within reach.
7. Raise the bed to a comfortable working height. Stand on the patient's right side if you are right-handed, or the patient's left side if you are left-handed.

8. Put on gloves. Assist the patient to the dorsal recumbent position with their knees flexed, feet about 2 ft apart, and legs abducted. Drape the patient. Alternatively, use the Sims', or lateral, position. Place the patient's buttocks near the edge of the bed with their shoulders at the opposite edge and their knees drawn toward her chest. Slide a waterproof drape under the patient.

9. Clean the perineal area with a washcloth, skin cleanser, and warm water, using a different corner of the washcloth with each stroke. Wipe from above the orifice downward toward the sacrum (front to back). Rinse and dry. Remove gloves. Perform hand hygiene.

10. Open the sterile catheterization tray on a clean overbed table using sterile technique.
11. Put on sterile gloves. Grasp the upper corners of the drape and unfold the drape without touching nonsterile areas. Fold back a corner on each side to make a cuff over your gloved hands. Ask the patient to lift their buttocks and slide the sterile drape under them with your gloves protected by the cuff.
12. Place a fenestrated sterile drape over the perineal area, exposing the labia, if appropriate.

13. Place the sterile tray on the drape between the patient's thighs.
14. Open all the supplies. Open the package of antiseptic swabs. Alternatively, fluff cotton balls in a tray before pouring antiseptic solution over them. Open the specimen container if a specimen is to be obtained.
15. Lubricate 1 to 2 inches of the catheter tip.
16. With the thumb and one finger of your nondominant hand, spread the labia and identify the meatus. If the patient is in the side-lying position, lift the upper buttock and labia to expose the urinary meatus. **Be prepared to maintain separation of the labia with one hand until the catheter is inserted and urine is flowing well and continuously.**
17. Use your dominant hand to pick up an antiseptic swab/cotton ball. **Clean one labial fold, top to bottom (from above the meatus down toward the rectum), then discard the swab/cotton ball. Using a new swab/cotton ball for each stroke, continue to clean the other labial fold, then directly over the meatus.**
18. With your noncontaminated dominant hand, pick up the lubricant syringe. Gently insert the tip of the syringe with lubricant into the urethra and instill the 5 to 10 mL of lubricant.
19. With your noncontaminated, dominant hand, place the drainage end of the catheter in a receptacle. If a specimen is required, place the end into the specimen container in the receptacle.
20. **Using your dominant hand, hold the catheter 2 to 3 inches from the tip and insert slowly into the urethra. Advance the catheter until there is a return of urine (approximately 2 to 3 inches [4.8 to 7.2 cm]). Do not force the catheter through the urethra into the bladder.** Ask the patient to breathe deeply, and rotate the catheter gently if slight resistance is met as the catheter reaches the external sphincter.

21. Hold the catheter securely at the meatus with the nondominant hand while the bladder empties. If a specimen is being collected, remove the drainage end of the tubing from the specimen container after the required amount is obtained, and allow urine to flow into the receptacle. Set the specimen container aside and place the lid on the container.
22. Allow the bladder to empty. Withdraw the catheter slowly and smoothly after urine has stopped flowing. Remove equipment and dispose of it according to facility policy. Discard the syringe in a sharps container to prevent reuse. Wash and dry the perineal area, as needed.
23. Remove gloves. Perform hand hygiene. Assist the patient to a comfortable position. Cover the patient with bed linens. Place the bed in the lowest position.
24. Put on gloves. Secure the container lid and label the specimen. Send the urine specimen to the laboratory promptly or refrigerate it.
25. Remove gloves and additional PPE, if used. Perform hand hygiene.

Note: Intermittent catheterization in the home is performed using clean technique (Collins, 2019; Leach, 2018). Single-use catheters and no-touch catheters are options for use for intermittent self-catheterization (ISC) in the home setting (Beauchemin et al., 2018). The past practice of catheter reuse in community settings, instructing patients to wash and reuse the same catheter for multiple catheterizations, is not recommended; no evidence-based guidelines on cleaning or disposing of a reused catheter are available (Beauchemin et al., 2018; Newman, 2019b).

Box 12-2 outlines information related to patient ISC.

EVIDENCE FOR PRACTICE ▶

PREVENTION OF CATHETER-ASSOCIATED INFECTIONS
Gould, C. V., Umscheid, C. A., Agarwal, R. K., Kuntz, G., Pegues, D. A., & the Healthcare Infection Control Practices Advisory Committee (HICPAC). (2019 [update]). *Guideline for prevention of catheter-associated urinary tract infections 2009. Centers for Disease Control and Prevention, 31*(4). https://www.cdc.gov/infectioncontrol/pdf/guidelines/cauti-guidelines-H.pdf

These guidelines provide evidence-based recommendations to guide care for patients requiring catheterization of the urinary bladder to prevent CAUTI.

(continued on page 750)

| Skill 12-7 ▶ | Catheterizing the Urinary Bladder of a Patient With Female Genitalia *(continued)* |

EVIDENCE FOR PRACTICE ▶

ANTIMICROBIALS FOR MEATAL CLEANING

Guidelines for catheter insertion and control of CAUTIs in hospitalized patients include the recommended practice of cleaning of the urethral meatus prior to catheterization to reduce the risk of introducing bacteria during catheter insertion (Mitchell & Hill, 2018). Is the use of an antimicrobial for meatal cleaning effective?

Related Research

Fasugba, O., Cheng, A. S., Gregory, V., Graves, N., Koerner, J., Collignon, P., Gardner, A., & Mitchell, B. G. (2019). Chlorhexidine for meatal cleaning in reducing catheter-associated urinary tract infections: A multicentre stepped-wedge randomised controlled trial. *Lancet Infectious Diseases, 19*(6), 611–619. https://doi.org/10.1016/S1473-3099(18)30736-9

The purpose of this randomized-controlled trial was to evaluate the efficacy of using chlorhexidine compared with normal saline for meatal cleaning before catheter insertion in reducing the incidence of catheter-associated asymptomatic bacteriuria and urinary tract infection. Participants included patients requiring a urinary catheter at three public and private hospitals in Australia with an intensive care unit and more than 30,000 admissions per year. Hospitals were randomly assigned to an intervention crossover date using a computer-generated randomization system every 8 weeks. During the first 8 weeks of the study, no hospitals were exposed to the intervention (control phase), after which each hospital sequentially crossed over from the control to the intervention every 8 weeks. The intervention consisted of the use of 0.1% chlorhexidine solution for meatal cleaning before urinary catheterization; 0.9% normal saline was used for meatal cleaning before urinary catheterization during the control phase. The total number of participants in all three hospitals was 1,642, with 697 (42%), in the control phase and 945 (58%) in the intervention period. The number of cases of catheter-associated asymptomatic bacteriuria and urinary tract infection were assessed within 7 days of catheter insertion. In the control period, there were 13 catheter-associated urinary tract infections and 29 catheter-associated asymptomatic bacteriuria events. During the intervention period, there were 4 catheter-associated urinary tract infections and 16 catheter-associated asymptomatic bacteriuria cases. The intervention was associated with a 74% reduction in the incidence of catheter-associated asymptomatic bacteriuria ($p = .026$) and a 94% decrease in the incidence of catheter-associated urinary tract infection ($p = .00080$). The researchers concluded the use of chlorhexidine solution for meatal cleaning before urinary catheter insertion is associated with improved patient outcomes related to decreased incidence of catheter-associated asymptomatic bacteriuria and urinary tract infection and has the potential to improve patient safety.

Relevance to Nursing Practice

Nurses are an integral part of the committees involved in the development of policy and procedures for health care organizations. Nurses have a responsibility to use interventions to improve patient outcomes, in this case, in reducing the risk for CAUTI in patients with indwelling urinary catheters. Integration of the best evidence is an integral part of providing evidence-based practice, and nurses should consider this and other evidence to ensure the best patient outcomes related to use of indwelling urinary catheters.

Refer to Skill 12-8 for additional evidence related to urinary catheterization.

Skill 12-8 ▶ Catheterizing the Urinary Bladder of a Patient With Male Genitalia

Skill Variation: *Intermittent Urethral Catheterization of a Patient With Male Genitalia*

Urinary catheterization is the introduction of a catheter (tube) through the urethra into the bladder for the purpose of withdrawing urine. Catheter-associated urinary tract infections (CAUTIs) remain one of the most common causes of health care–associated infections in the United States (Knill et al., 2018). The best way to prevent a CAUTI is to use urinary catheters only when absolutely necessary (ANA, n.d.; Panchisin, 2016). The CDC provides parameters to guide the decision to insert an indwelling urinary catheter (Gould et al., 2019). When the use of a urinary catheter is deemed necessary, it should be performed using strict aseptic technique, left in place only as long as needed, and removed as soon as possible (ANA, 2014; Gould et al., 2019; Gyesi-Appiah et al., 2020; SUNA, 2015).

If a catheter is to remain in place for continuous drainage, an indwelling urethral catheter is used. Indwelling catheters are also called *retention* or *Foley catheters.* The indwelling urethral catheter is designed so that it does not slip out of the bladder. A balloon is inflated to ensure that the catheter remains in the bladder once it is inserted (see Figure 1A, Skill 12-7).

Intermittent urethral catheters, or straight catheters, are used to drain the bladder for shorter periods (see Figure 1B, Skill 12-7). Intermittent catheterization should be considered as an alternative to short- or long-term indwelling urethral catheterization to reduce CAUTIs (Gould et al., 2019). Intermittent catheterization is the preferred bladder management method for patients with urinary retention and bladder-emptying dysfunctions and following surgical interventions (Beauchemin et al., 2018; Gould et al., 2019). Certain advantages to intermittent catheterization, including the lower risks of CAUTI and complications, may make it a more desirable and safer option than indwelling catheterization (Panchisin, 2016; Wilson, 2015).

Some facilities have adopted a two-person urinary catheter insertion protocol, in which one nurse catheterizes the patient and one observes to ensure that the nurse inserting the catheter follows sterile technique and performs the procedure correctly (Belizario, 2015; Rhone et al., 2017). Implementation of the two-person urinary catheter insertion protocol has been shown to decrease CAUTI (Belizario, 2015; Fletcher-Gutowski & Cecil, 2019; Rhone et al., 2017).

The following procedure reviews insertion of an indwelling catheter into the urinary bladder of a patient with male genitalia. The procedure for intermittent catheterization of a urinary bladder of a patient with male genitalia follows as a Skill Variation. Guidelines for caring for a patient with an indwelling catheter are summarized in Box 12-1, located within Skill 12-7.

DELEGATION CONSIDERATIONS

The catheterization of the urinary bladder is not delegated to assistive personnel (AP). Depending on the state's nurse practice act and the organization's policies and procedures, catheterization of the urinary bladder may be delegated to licensed practical/vocational nurses (LPN/LVNs). The decision to delegate must be based on careful analysis of the patient's needs and circumstances as well as the qualifications of the person to whom the task is being delegated. Refer to the Delegation Guidelines in Appendix A.

EQUIPMENT

- Sterile catheter kit that contains:
  - Sterile gloves
  - Sterile drapes (one of which is fenestrated)
  - Sterile catheter (use the smallest appropriate-size catheter, usually a 14F catheter with a 5- to 10-mL balloon [ANA, 2014; SUNA, 2021d; Yates, 2017a])
  - Antiseptic cleansing solution and cotton balls or gauze squares; antiseptic swabs
  - Lubricant
  - Forceps
  - Prefilled syringe with sterile water (sufficient to inflate indwelling catheter balloon)
  - Sterile basin (usually base of kit serves as this)
  - Sterile specimen container (if specimen is required)
  - Anesthetic gel, as prescribed or indicated (see Assessments below)
- Flashlight or lamp
- Waterproof, disposable pad

(continued on page 752)

Skill 12-8 ▶ Catheterizing the Urinary Bladder of a Patient With Male Genitalia *(continued)*

- Sterile, disposable urine collection bag and drainage tubing (may be connected to catheter in catheter kit)
- Catheter-securing device
- Disposable gloves
- Additional PPE, as indicated
- Washcloth, skin cleanser, and warm water to perform perineal hygiene before and after catheterization

ASSESSMENT

Assess the patient's usual elimination habits. Assess the patient's degree of limitations and ability to help with activity. Assess for health problems, such as hip surgery or spinal injury, which would contraindicate certain actions by the patient. Assess for the presence of any other conditions that may interfere with passage of the catheter or contraindicate insertion of the catheter, such as urethral strictures or bladder cancer. Check for the presence of drains, dressings, intravenous fluid infusion sites/equipment, traction, or any other devices that could interfere with the patient's ability to help with the procedure or that could become dislodged. Assess bladder fullness before performing the procedure, either by palpation or with a handheld bladder ultrasound device. Question the patient about any allergies, especially to latex or iodine. Ask the patient if they have ever been catheterized. If they had an indwelling catheter previously, ask why and for how long it was used. The patient may have urethral strictures, which may make catheter insertion more difficult. If the patient is age 50 years or older, ask if they have had any prostate problems. Prostate enlargement typically is noted to begin around age 50 years. Assess for the need to use anesthetic gel; the use of anesthetic gel inserted in the urethra prior to catheterization is an option in for patients with male anatomy and should be considered if it is the patient's first catheterization or if a difficulty catheterization is suspected (SUNA, 2021d). Assess the characteristics of the urine and the patient's skin.

ACTUAL OR POTENTIAL HEALTH PROBLEMS AND NEEDS

Many actual or potential health problems or issues may require the use of this skill as part of related interventions. An appropriate health problem or issue may include:
- Urinary retention
- Infection risk
- Total urinary incontinence

OUTCOME IDENTIFICATION AND PLANNING

The expected outcomes to achieve when catheterizing the urinary bladder is that the catheter is successfully inserted without adverse effect, the patient's urinary elimination is maintained, and the patient's bladder is not distended. Other appropriate outcomes may include that the patient's skin remains clean, dry, intact, and without evidence of irritation or breakdown, and the patient verbalizes an understanding of the purpose for and care of the catheter, as appropriate.

IMPLEMENTATION

ACTION	RATIONALE
1. Review the patient's health record for any limitations in physical activity. Confirm the prescribed intervention for indwelling catheter insertion.	Physical limitations may require adaptations in performing the skill. Verifying the prescribed intervention ensures that the correct intervention is administered to the right patient.
2. Gather equipment. Obtain assistance from another staff member, if necessary.	Assembling equipment provides for an organized approach to the task. Assistance from another person may be required to perform the intervention safely.
3. Perform hand hygiene and put on PPE, if indicated.	Hand hygiene and PPE prevent the spread of microorganisms. PPE is required based on transmission precautions.
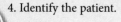 4. Identify the patient.	Identifying the patient ensures the right patient receives the intervention and helps prevent errors.

ACTION

5. Close the curtains around the bed and close the door to the room, if possible. Discuss the procedure with the patient and assess the patient's ability to assist with the procedure. Ask the patient if they have any allergies, especially to latex or iodine.

6. Provide good lighting. Artificial light is recommended (use of a flashlight requires an assistant to hold and position it). Place a trash receptacle within easy reach.

7. Assemble equipment on the overbed table or other surface within reach.

8. Adjust the bed to a comfortable working height (VHACEOSH, 2016). Stand on the patient's right side if you are right-handed, or the patient's left side if you are left-handed.

9. Position the patient on their back with their thighs slightly apart. Drape the patient so that only the area around the penis is exposed. Slide a waterproof pad under the patient.

10. Put on gloves. Clean the genital area with a washcloth, skin cleanser, and warm water. Clean the tip of the penis first, moving the washcloth in a circular motion from the meatus outward. Wash the shaft of the penis using downward strokes toward the pubic area. Rinse and dry. Remove gloves. Perform hand hygiene.

11. Prepare the urine drainage setup if a separate urine collection system is to be used. Secure it to the bed frame according to the manufacturer's directions.

12. Open the sterile catheterization tray on a clean overbed table or other flat surface, using sterile technique.

13. Put on sterile gloves. Open the sterile drape and place it on the patient's thighs. Place the fenestrated drape with the opening over the penis (Figure 1).

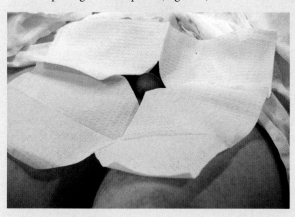

FIGURE 1. Patient lying supine with fenestrated drape +over penis.

14. Place the catheter setup on or next to the patient's legs on the sterile drape.

RATIONALE

This ensures the patient's privacy. Discussion promotes reassurance and provides knowledge about the procedure. Dialogue encourages patient participation and allows for individualized nursing care. Some catheters and gloves in kits are made of latex. Some antiseptic solutions contain iodine.

Good lighting is necessary to see the meatus clearly. A readily available trash receptacle allows for prompt disposal of used supplies and reduces the risk of contaminating the sterile field.

Arranging items nearby is convenient, saves time, and prevents unnecessary stretching and twisting of muscles on the part of the nurse.

Having the bed at the proper height prevents back and muscle strain. Positioning allows for ease of use of your dominant hand for catheter insertion.

Proper positioning allows adequate visualization of the urinary meatus. This prevents unnecessary exposure and promotes warmth. The waterproof pad will protect bed linens from moisture.

Gloves reduce the risk of exposure to blood and body fluids. Cleaning the penis reduces microorganisms near the urethral meatus. Hand hygiene reduces the spread of microorganisms.

This facilitates connection of the catheter to the drainage system and provides for easy access.

Placement of equipment near the worksite increases efficiency. Sterile technique protects the patient and prevents the spread of microorganisms.

The drape provides a sterile field close to the meatus.

The sterile setup should be arranged so that the nurse's back is not turned to it, nor should it be out of the nurse's range of vision. This provides easy access to supplies.

(continued on page 754)

Skill 12-8 ▶ Catheterizing the Urinary Bladder of a Patient With Male Genitalia *(continued)*

ACTION

15. Open all the supplies. Remove the cap from the prefilled sterile saline syringe and attach it to the balloon inflation port on the catheter. Open the package of antiseptic swabs. Alternatively, fluff cotton balls in a tray before pouring antiseptic solution over them. Open the specimen container if a specimen is to be obtained. If using anesthetic gel, remove the cap from the prefilled syringe. Open and squirt lubricant in the tray.

16. Remove the cover from the catheter and lubricate 5 to 7 inches of the catheter tip (SUNA, 2021d).

17. Lift the penis with your nondominant hand. Retract the foreskin in an uncircumcised patient. **Be prepared to keep your hand in this position until the catheter is inserted and urine is flowing well and continuously.** Use your dominant hand to pick up an antiseptic swab, or use forceps to pick up a cotton ball. **Using a circular motion, clean the penis, moving from the meatus down the glans of the penis (Figure 2). Repeat this cleansing motion two more times, using a new swab/cotton ball each time. Discard each swab/cotton ball after one use.**

18. Hold the penis with slight upward tension and perpendicular to the patient's body at a 90-degree angle to the patient's thighs (SUNA, 2021d). If using anesthetic gel, use your noncontaminated dominant hand to pick up the anesthetic syringe. Gently insert the tip of the syringe with anesthetic into the meatus and inject approximately 5 to 10 mL into the urethra (SUNA, 2021d) (Figure 3). Allow the gel to dwell for approximately 3 to 5 minutes before starting the catheter insertion (SUNA, 2021d).

RATIONALE

It is necessary to open all supplies and prepare for the procedure while both hands are sterile. The use of anesthetic gel inserted in the urethra prior to catheterization is an option in for patients with male anatomy and should be considered if it is the patient's first catheterization or if a difficulty catheterization is suspected (SUNA, 2021d).

Lubrication facilitates catheter insertion, reduces urethral trauma, and reduces discomfort during insertion (SUNA, 2021d).

The hand touching the penis becomes contaminated. Cleansing the area around the meatus and under the foreskin in the uncircumcised patient helps prevent infection. Moving from the meatus toward the base of the penis prevents bringing microorganisms to the meatus.

This position extends the urethra and straightens the curvature of the penis (SUNA, 2021d). The use of anesthetic gel inserted in the urethra prior to catheterization is an option in for patients with male anatomy and should be considered if it is the patient's first catheterization or if a difficulty catheterization is suspected (SUNA, 2021d).

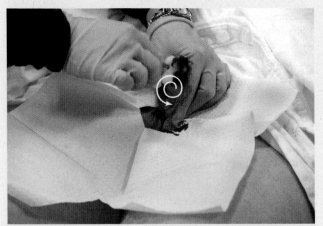

FIGURE 2. Lifting penis with gloved nondominant hand and cleaning meatus with cotton ball held with forceps in gloved dominant hand.

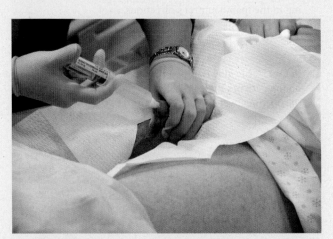

FIGURE 3. Inserting syringe into urethra and instilling lubricant.

19. With your noncontaminated, dominant hand, place the drainage end of the catheter in a receptacle. If the catheter is pre-attached to the sterile tubing and drainage container (closed drainage system), position the catheter and setup within easy reach on the sterile field. Ensure that the clamp on the drainage bag is closed.

This facilitates drainage of urine and minimizes risk of contaminating sterile equipment.

ACTION

20. Use your noncontaminated, dominant hand to pick up the catheter and hold it 3 to 4 inches from the tip. Ask the patient to bear down as if voiding. **Insert the catheter tip into the meatus (Figure 4). Ask the patient to take deep breaths. Advance the catheter about 7 to 10 inches into the urethra; urine should begin to flow through the tubing. Once urine flow is established, insert the catheter 2 more inches further, to the bifurcation or "Y" juncture of the ports (SUNA, 2021d). Do not use force to introduce the catheter.** If the catheter resists entry, ask the patient to breathe deeply and rotate the catheter slightly.

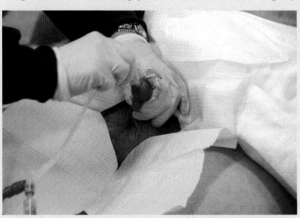

RATIONALE

Bearing down eases the passage of the catheter through the urethra. The male urethra is about 20 cm long. Having the patient take deep breaths or twisting the catheter slightly may ease the catheter past resistance at the sphincters. Insert indwelling catheters in patients with male genitalia to the catheter bifurcation (the "Y" level created by the balloon filling and urinary drainage ports) to assure the balloon is within the bladder and to avoid inadvertent inflation of the balloon in the urethra (ANA, 2014; SUNA, 2021d).

FIGURE 4. Inserting catheter using dominant hand.

21. Hold the catheter securely at the meatus with your nondominant hand. Use your dominant hand to inflate the catheter balloon. Inject the entire volume of sterile water supplied in the prefilled syringe. Once the balloon is inflated, the catheter may be gently pulled back into place. **Replace the foreskin, if present, over the catheter.** Lower the penis.

Bladder or sphincter contraction could push the catheter out. The balloon anchors the catheter in place in the bladder. The manufacturer provides the appropriate amount of solution for the size of the catheter in the kit; as a result, use the entire syringe provided in the kit.

22. Pull gently on the catheter after the balloon is inflated to feel resistance.

Improper inflation can cause patient discomfort and malpositioning of the catheter.

23. Attach the catheter to the drainage system, if necessary.

The closed drainage system minimizes the risk for microorganisms being introduced into the bladder (Gould et al., 2019).

24. Remove equipment and dispose of it according to facility policy. Discard the syringe in a sharps container. Wash and dry the perineal area, as needed.

Proper disposal prevents the spread of microorganisms. Placing the syringe in a sharps container prevents reuse. Cleaning promotes comfort and appropriate personal hygiene.

25. Remove gloves. Perform hand hygiene. **Secure the catheter tubing to the patient's inner thigh or lower abdomen (with the penis directed toward the patient's chest) with a catheter-securing device.** Leave some slack in the catheter for leg movement.

Proper securement prevents tension on the catheter; reduces risk for catheter displacement, expulsion, migration, and trauma; and increases patient comfort (Holroyd, 2019). Hand hygiene prevents the spread of microorganisms. Whether to take the drainage tubing over or under the leg depends on gravity flow, the patient's mobility, and the comfort of the patient.

26. Assist the patient to a comfortable position. Cover the patient with bed linens. Place the bed in the lowest position.

Positioning and covering provides warmth and promotes comfort.

27. Secure the drainage bag below the level of the bladder. Check that the drainage tubing is not kinked and that movement of the side rails does not interfere with the catheter or drainage bag.

This facilitates drainage of urine and prevents the backflow of urine (ANA, 2014; Gould et al., 2019).

(continued on page 756)

Skill 12-8 ▶ Catheterizing the Urinary Bladder of a Patient With Male Genitalia *(continued)*

ACTION	**RATIONALE**
28. Put on gloves. Obtain a urine specimen immediately, if needed, from the drainage bag. Label the specimen. Send the urine specimen to the laboratory promptly or refrigerate it.	The catheter system is sterile. Obtaining a specimen immediately allows access to the sterile system. Keeping the urine at room temperature may cause microorganisms, if present, to grow and distort laboratory findings.
29. Remove gloves and additional PPE, if used. Perform hand hygiene.	Proper removal of PPE reduces the risk for infection transmission and contamination of other items. Hand hygiene prevents the spread of microorganisms.

EVALUATION

The expected outcomes have been met when the catheter has been inserted without adverse effect, the patient's urinary elimination has been maintained, and the patient's bladder has not distended. Other outcomes have been met when the patient's skin has remained clean, dry, intact, and without evidence of irritation or breakdown, and the patient has verbalized an understanding of the purpose for and care of the catheter, as appropriate.

DOCUMENTATION

Guidelines

Document the type and size of catheter and balloon inserted as well as the amount of fluid used to inflate the balloon. Document the patient's tolerance of the activity. Record the amount of urine obtained through the catheter and any specimen obtained. Document any other assessments, such as unusual urine characteristics or alterations in the patient's skin. Record the urine amount on the intake and output record, if appropriate.

Sample Documentation

Lippincott DocuCare

Practice documenting catheterization of the male urinary bladder in *Lippincott DocuCare*.

> 7/14/25 1830 Patient unable to void for 8 hours and reports, "I feel like I have to go to the bathroom." Bladder scanned for 540-mL urine. Primary care provider notified; 10-mL prescribed 2% lidocaine jelly instilled before catheterization; 14F Foley catheter inserted without difficulty; 10 mL of sterile water injected into 5-mL balloon port; 525-mL clear yellow urine returned. Patient reports decreased bladder pressure. Patient tolerated procedure without adverse event.
>
> —B. Clapp, RN

DEVELOPING CLINICAL REASONING AND CLINICAL JUDGMENT

UNEXPECTED SITUATIONS AND ASSOCIATED INTERVENTIONS

- *You cannot insert the catheter past 3 to 4 inches; rotating the catheter and having the patient breathe deeply are of no help:* If still unable to place the catheter, notify the health care team. Repeated catheter placement attempts can traumatize the urethra. Anticipate the possible insertion of a coudé catheter by a urologist or advanced practice professional.
- *Patient is obese or has a retracted penis:* Have an assistant available to place their fingers on either side of the pubic area and press backward to bring the penis out of the pubic cavity. Hold the patient's penis up and forward. The catheter still needs to be inserted to the bifurcation; the length of the urethra has not changed.
- *Urine leaks out of meatus around the catheter:* Do not increase the size of the indwelling catheter. Make sure the smallest-sized catheter with a 10-mL balloon is used. Large catheters cause bladder and urethral irritation and trauma. Large balloon-fill volumes occupy more space inside the bladder and put added weight on the base of the bladder. Irritation of the bladder wall and detrusor muscle can cause leakage. If leakage persists, consider an evaluation for urinary tract infection. Ensure that the correct amount of solution was used to inflate the balloon. Underfilling the balloon can cause the catheter to dislodge into the urethra, causing urethral spasm, pain, and discomfort. If you suspect underfill, do not attempt to push the catheter farther into the bladder.

Remove the catheter and replace with a new catheter. Assess the patient for constipation. A bowel full of stool can cause pressure on the catheter lumen and prevent the drainage of urine. Implement interventions to prevent/treat constipation.

- *Urine flow is initially well established, and urine is clear, but after several hours urine flow dwindles:* Check the tubing for kinking. If the patient has changed position, the tubing and drainage bag may need to be moved to facilitate drainage of urine.

SPECIAL CONSIDERATIONS

General Considerations

- Some facilities have adopted a two-person urinary catheter insertion protocol, in which one nurse catheterizes the patient and one observes to ensure that the nurse inserting the catheter follows sterile technique and performs the procedure correctly (Belizario, 2015; Rhone et al., 2017). Implementation of the two-person urinary catheter insertion protocol has been shown to decrease CAUTI (Belizario, 2015; Fletcher-Gutowski & Cecil, 2019; Rhone et al., 2017).
- Assess for the need to use anesthetic gel; the use of anesthetic gel inserted in the urethra prior to catheterization is an option in for patients with male anatomy and should be considered if it is the patient's first catheterization or if a difficulty catheterization is suspected (SUNA, 2021d).
- Check for patient allergy before use of anesthetic gel. Anesthetic gel instilled into the patient's urethra should be administered at least 5 minutes before catheterization to ensure sufficient anesthetic effect (Yates, 2017b).
- Be familiar with facility policy and/or primary health care provider guidelines for the maximum amount of urine to remove from the bladder at the time of insertion.
- Supplies can be opened and prepared on the overbed table, moving the tray onto the bed just before cleansing the patient.
- If there is not an immediate flow of urine after the catheter has been inserted, several measures may prove helpful:
  - Have the patient take a deep breath, which helps to relax the perineal and abdominal muscles.
  - Rotate the catheter slightly because a drainage hole may be resting against the bladder wall.
  - Raise the head of the patient's bed to increase pressure in the bladder area.
  - Assess the patient's intake to ensure adequate fluid intake for urine production.
  - Assess the catheter and drainage tubing for kinks and occlusion.
  - Urethral strictures, false passages, prostatic enlargement, and postsurgical bladder-neck contractures can make urethral catheterization difficult and may require the services of a urologist. If there is any question as to the location of the catheter, do not inflate the balloon. Remove the catheter and notify the health care team (SUNA, 2021c).
- If the catheter cannot be advanced, having the patient take several deep breaths may be helpful. Rotate the catheter half a turn, and try to advance it. If you are still unable to advance it, remove the catheter. Notify the health care team.
- Some catheter kits do not contain the catheter. This allows you to select a catheter and balloon size separately.
- Maintain a constant downward flow of urine. Check tubing frequently to ensure kinks and dependent loops (low points) are not present in the tubing (ANA, 2014; Gould et al., 2019; Wuthier et al., 2016). Check to see that the patient is not lying on the drainage tubing and compressing it.
- Keep the catheter drainage bag below the level of the bladder at all times (ANA, 2014; Gould et al., 2019).
- Keep the drainage bag off the floor at all times to reduce the risk of infection (ANA, 2014; Gould et al., 2019). The floor is grossly contaminated.

Infant and Child Considerations

- Size 6F to 8F is used for infants and young children (Kyle & Carman, 2021). Size 8F to 12F catheters are commonly used for older children (Kyle & Carman, 2021).
- Distraction, such as blowing bubbles, deep breathing, or singing a song, can help the child relax.
- Consider the use of lidocaine jelly to anesthetize and lubricate the area before insertion of the catheter, decreasing the child's discomfort and anxiety. Refer to facility policy regarding prescribing requirements and use.

(continued on page 758)

Skill 12-8 ▶ Catheterizing the Urinary Bladder of a Patient With Male Genitalia *(continued)*

Older Adult Considerations

- If resistance is met while inserting a catheter, and rotating does not help, it is important to never force the catheter. The resistance may be caused by enlargement of the prostate gland, which is commonly seen in men over age 50 years. A special crook-tipped catheter called a coudé catheter, inserted by the urologist or advanced practice professional, may be required to maneuver past the prostate gland.

Community-Based Care Considerations

- Intermittent catheterization, performed by the patient or a caregiver in the home, may be necessary for patients with spinal cord injuries or other neurologic conditions. Although the risk for UTI is always present, and practice guidelines support the use of clean, rather than sterile, technique in the home environment (Bardsley, 2015a; Beauchemin et al., 2018; Gould et al., 2019; Wilson, 2015a). The procedure for self-intermittent catheterization is essentially the same as that used by the nurse to catheterize a patient, using clean, nonsterile technique (Collins, 2019; Leach, 2018). Box 12-2 (page 748) outlines important information related to patient intermittent self-catheterization (ISC).
- Single-use catheters and no-touch catheters are options for use for ISC in the home setting (Beauchemin et al., 2018). The past practice of catheter reuse in community settings, instructing patients to wash and reuse the same catheter for multiple catheterizations, is not recommended; no evidence-based guidelines on cleaning or disposing of a reused catheter are available (Beauchemin et al., 2018; Newman, 2019b).

Skill Variation ▶ Intermittent Urethral Catheterization of a Patient With Male Genitalia

1. Check the health record for the prescribed intervention of intermittent urethral catheterization. Review the patient's health record for any limitations in physical activity. Gather supplies. Obtain assistance from another staff member, if necessary.

2. Perform hand hygiene. Put on PPE, as indicated.

3. Identify the patient. Discuss the procedure with the patient and assess the patient's ability to assist with the procedure. Ask the patient if they have any allergies, especially to latex or iodine.

4. Close the curtains around the bed and close the door to the room, if possible.

5. Provide good lighting. Artificial light is recommended (use of a flashlight requires an assistant to hold and position it). Place a trash receptacle within easy reach.

6. Assemble equipment on the overbed table or other surface within reach.

7. Raise the bed to a comfortable working height. Stand on the patient's right side if you are right-handed, or the patient's left side if you are left-handed.

8. Position the patient on their back with their thighs slightly apart. Drape the patient so that only the area around the penis is exposed. Slide a waterproof pad under the patient.

9. Put on gloves. Clean the genital area with a washcloth, skin cleanser, and warm water. Clean the tip of the penis first, moving the washcloth in a circular motion from the meatus outward. Wash the shaft of the penis using downward strokes toward the pubic area. Rinse and dry. Remove gloves. Perform hand hygiene.

10. Open the sterile catheterization tray on a clean overbed table using sterile technique.

11. Put on sterile gloves. Open the sterile drape and place it on the patient's thighs. Place the fenestrated drape with the opening over the penis.

12. Place the catheter setup on or next to the patient's legs on the sterile drape.

13. Open all the supplies. Open the package of antiseptic swabs. Alternatively, fluff cotton balls in a tray before pouring antiseptic solution over them. Open the specimen container if a specimen is to be obtained. If using anesthetic gel, remove the cap from the prefilled syringe. Open and squirt lubricant in the tray.

14. Remove the cover from the catheter and lubricate 5 to 7 inches of the catheter tip.

15. Lift the penis with your nondominant hand. Retract the foreskin in an uncircumcised patient. **Be prepared to keep your hand in this position until the catheter is inserted and urine is flowing well and continuously.**

16. Use your dominant hand to pick up an antiseptic swab/cotton ball. **Using a circular motion, clean the penis, moving from the meatus down the glans of the penis. Repeat this cleansing motion two more times, using a swab/cotton ball each time. Discard each swab/cotton ball after one use.**

17. Hold the penis with slight upward tension and perpendicular to the patient's body at a 90-degree angle to the patient's thighs (SUNA, 2021d). If using anesthetic gel, use your noncontaminated dominant hand to pick up the anesthetic syringe. Gently insert the tip of the syringe with anesthetic into the meatus and inject approximately 5 to 10 mL into the urethra (SUNA, 2021d). Allow the gel to dwell for approximately 3 to 5 minutes before starting the catheter insertion (SUNA, 2021d).

18. With your noncontaminated, dominant hand, place the drainage end of the catheter in a receptacle. If a specimen is required, place the end into the specimen container in the receptacle.

19. **Use your dominant hand to pick up the catheter and hold it 3 or 4 inches from the tip. Ask the patient to bear down as if voiding. Insert the catheter tip into the meatus. Ask the patient to take deep breaths as you advance the catheter 7 to 10 inches or until urine flows. Do not force the catheter through the urethra into the bladder.** Ask the patient to breathe deeply, and rotate the catheter gently if slight resistance is met as the catheter reaches the external sphincter.

20. Hold the catheter securely at the meatus with your non-dominant hand while the bladder empties. If a specimen is being collected, remove the drainage end of the tubing from the specimen container after the required amount is obtained and allow urine to flow into the receptacle. Set the specimen container aside and place the lid on the container.

21. Allow the bladder to empty. Withdraw the catheter slowly and smoothly after urine has stopped flowing. Remove equipment and dispose of it according to facility policy. Discard the syringe in a sharps container to prevent reuse. Wash and dry the genital area, as needed. Replace the foreskin in the forward position, if necessary.

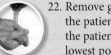

22. Remove gloves. Perform hand hygiene. Assist the patient to a comfortable position. Cover the patient with bed linens. Place the bed in the lowest position.

23. Put on clean gloves. Secure the container lid and label the specimen. Send the urine specimen to the laboratory promptly or refrigerate it.

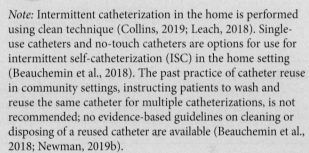

24. Remove gloves and additional PPE, if used. Perform hand hygiene.

Note: Intermittent catheterization in the home is performed using clean technique (Collins, 2019; Leach, 2018). Single-use catheters and no-touch catheters are options for use for intermittent self-catheterization (ISC) in the home setting (Beauchemin et al., 2018). The past practice of catheter reuse in community settings, instructing patients to wash and reuse the same catheter for multiple catheterizations, is not recommended; no evidence-based guidelines on cleaning or disposing of a reused catheter are available (Beauchemin et al., 2018; Newman, 2019b).

Box 12-2 (page 748) outlines information related to patient ISC.

EVIDENCE FOR PRACTICE ▶	**PREVENTION OF CATHETER-ASSOCIATED INFECTIONS**

PREVENTION OF CATHETER-ASSOCIATED INFECTIONS

Gould, C. V., Umscheid, C. A., Agarwal, R. K., Kuntz, G., Pegues, D. A., & the Healthcare Infection Control Practices Advisory Committee (HICPAC). (2019 [update]). *Guideline for prevention of catheter-associated urinary tract infections 2009. Centers for Disease Control and Prevention, 31*(4). https://www.cdc.gov/infectioncontrol/guidelines/cauti/index.html

These guidelines provide evidence-based recommendations to guide care for patients requiring catheterization of the urinary bladder to prevent CAUTI.

Refer to Skill 12-7 for additional evidence related to urinary catheterization.

Skill 12-9 ▶ Removing an Indwelling Urinary Catheter

Removal of an indwelling catheter is performed using clean technique. Take care to prevent trauma to the urethra during the procedure. Completely deflate the catheter balloon before catheter removal to avoid irritation and damage to the urethra and meatus. The patient may experience burning or irritation the first few times they void after removal, due to urethral irritation. If the catheter was in place for more than a few days, decreased bladder muscle tone and swelling of the urethra may cause the patient to experience difficulty voiding or an inability to void. Monitor the patient for urinary retention. It is important to encourage adequate oral fluid intake to promote adequate urinary output. Check facility policy regarding the length of time the patient is allowed to accomplish successful voiding after catheter removal.

DELEGATION CONSIDERATIONS

Removal of an indwelling catheter is not delegated to assistive personnel (AP). Depending on the state's nurse practice act and the organization's policies and procedures, removal of an indwelling catheter may be delegated to licensed practical/vocational nurses (LPN/LVNs). The decision to delegate must be based on careful analysis of the patient's needs and circumstances as well as the qualifications of the person to whom the task is being delegated. Refer to the Delegation Guidelines in Appendix A.

EQUIPMENT

- Syringe sufficiently large to accommodate the volume of solution used to inflate the balloon (volume used to inflate the catheter balloon should be recorded in the health record; balloon size/inflation volume is printed on the balloon inflation valve on the catheter at the bifurcation)
- Waterproof, disposable pad
- Disposable gloves
- Additional PPE, as indicated
- Washcloth, skin cleanser, and warm water to perform perineal hygiene after catheter removal

ASSESSMENT

Check the policies and procedures for the facility related to continued use of indwelling urinary catheters; check the health record for a prescribed intervention to remove the catheter. Assess for discharge or encrustation around the urethral meatus. Assess urine output, including color and current amount in the drainage bag.

ACTUAL OR POTENTIAL HEALTH PROBLEMS AND NEEDS

Many actual or potential health problems or issues may require the use of this skill as part of related interventions. An appropriate health problem or issue may include:
- Urinary tract infection
- Infection risk

OUTCOME IDENTIFICATION AND PLANNING

The expected outcome to achieve when removing an indwelling catheter is that the catheter will be removed without difficulty and with minimal patient discomfort. Other appropriate outcomes include that the patient voids without discomfort after catheter removal; the patient voids a minimum of 250 mL of urine within 6 to 8 hours of catheter removal; the patient's skin remains clean, dry, intact, and without evidence of irritation or breakdown; and the patient verbalizes an understanding of the need to maintain adequate fluid intake, as appropriate.

IMPLEMENTATION

ACTION	RATIONALE
1. Confirm the prescribed intervention for catheter removal in the health record. Gather equipment.	Verifying the prescribed intervention ensures that the correct intervention is administered to the right patient. Assembling equipment provides for an organized approach to the task.
2. Perform hand hygiene and put on PPE, if indicated.	Hand hygiene and PPE prevent the spread of microorganisms. PPE is required based on transmission precautions.

ACTION	**RATIONALE**

3. Identify the patient.

Identifying the patient ensures the right patient receives the intervention and helps prevent errors.

4. Close the curtains around the bed and close the door to the room, if possible. Discuss the procedure with the patient and assess the patient's ability to assist with the procedure.

This ensures the patient's privacy. Discussion promotes reassurance and provides knowledge about the procedure. Dialogue encourages patient participation and allows for individualized nursing care.

5. Adjust the bed to a comfortable working height (VHACEOSH, 2016). Stand on the patient's right side if you are right-handed, or on the patient's left side if you are left-handed.

Having the bed at the proper height prevents back and muscle strain. Positioning allows for ease of use of your dominant hand for catheter removal.

6. Position the patient as for catheter insertion. Drape the patient so that only the area around the catheter is exposed. Slide a waterproof pad between the legs of a patient with female genitalia or over the patient's thighs for patients with male genitalia.

Positioning allows access to the site. Draping prevents unnecessary exposure and promotes warmth. The waterproof pad will protect bed linens from moisture and serve as a receptacle for the used catheter after removal.

7. Remove the device used to secure the catheter to the patient's thigh or abdomen.

This action permits removal of catheter.

8. Insert the syringe into the balloon inflation port. Allow the pressure within the balloon to force the syringe plunger back and fill the syringe with water (Yates, 2017c) (Figure 1). **Do not cut the inflation port** (Yates, 2017c). **Check that the volume of fluid in the syringe is equal to the volume inserted.**

Removal of sterile water deflates the balloon to allow for catheter removal. All the sterile water must be removed to prevent injury to the patient. Aspiration by pulling on the syringe plunger may result in collapse of the inflation lumen; contribute to the formation of creases, ridges, or cuffing at the balloon area; and increase the catheter balloon diameter size on deflation, resulting in difficult removal and urethral trauma. *Note:* Silicon catheters may not give back the same volume, as fluid can be lost from the balloon by osmosis (Yates, 2017c).

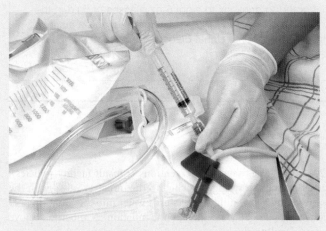

FIGURE 1. Removing fluid from balloon.

9. Caution patients with male genitalia that there may be potential discomfort as the deflated balloon passes through the prostatic urethra (Yates, 2017c). Caution patients with female genitalia that they may experience a stinging sensation and discomfort (Yates, 2017c). Ask the patient to take several slow, deep breaths. **Slowly and gently remove the catheter.** Place it on the waterproof pad and wrap it in the pad.

Slow, deep breathing helps to relax the sphincter muscles. Slow, gentle removal prevents trauma to the urethra. Using a waterproof pad prevents contact with the catheter and urine.

10. Wash and dry the perineal area, as needed.

Cleaning promotes comfort and appropriate personal hygiene.

11. Remove gloves. Perform hand hygiene. Assist the patient to a comfortable position. Cover the patient with bed linens. Place the bed in the lowest position.

These actions provide warmth and promote comfort and safety.

(continued on page 762)

Skill 12-9 ▶ Removing an Indwelling Urinary Catheter *(continued)*

ACTION

12. Put on gloves. Remove equipment and dispose of it according to facility policy. Note characteristics and amount of urine in the drainage bag.

13. Remove gloves and additional PPE, if used. Perform hand hygiene.

RATIONALE

Proper disposal prevents the spread of microorganisms. Observing the characteristics ensures accurate documentation.

Proper removal of PPE reduces the risk for infection transmission and contamination of other items. Hand hygiene prevents the spread of microorganisms.

EVALUATION

The expected outcomes have been met when the catheter has been removed without difficulty and with minimal patient discomfort; the patient has voided without discomfort after catheter removal and a minimum of 250 mL of urine within 6 to 8 hours of catheter removal; the patient's skin has remained clean, dry, intact, and without evidence of irritation or breakdown; and the patient has verbalized an understanding of the need to maintain adequate fluid intake, as appropriate.

DOCUMENTATION

Guidelines

Document the type and size of catheter removed and the amount of fluid removed from the balloon. Also document the patient's tolerance of the procedure. Record the amount of urine in the drainage bag. Note the time the patient is due to void. Document any other assessments, such as unusual urine characteristics or alterations in the patient's skin. Also record urine amount on intake and output record, if appropriate.

Sample Documentation

7/14/25 0800 Removed 15-mL fluid from catheter balloon; 14F Foley removed without difficulty; 500 mL of clear yellow urine noted in drainage bag at time of removal. Patient due to void by 1600. Patient instructed to drink six to eight 6-oz glasses of fluid in the course of the day, and that it may take some time for the passage of urine on his own; patient verbalized understanding of instructions. Urinal placed at bedside, with patient demonstrating appropriate use.

—B. Clapp, RN

DEVELOPING CLINICAL REASONING AND CLINICAL JUDGMENT

UNEXPECTED SITUATIONS AND ASSOCIATED INTERVENTIONS

- *Balloon will not deflate:* Yates (2017c) suggests several interventions (consult facility policies), including trying a different syringe; leaving the syringe attached to the inflation valve, with the plunger removed, for 20 minutes; inserting a few milliliters of sterile water into the inflation port to help clear any blockage; and attaching a 25-gauge needle into the inflation chamber just above the cuff and drawing back, to bypass a faulty valve.
- *Resistance is felt while attempting to pull out catheter:* Stop pulling the catheter. Reattach the syringe to the balloon inflation port and aspirate to make sure all the sterile water has been removed. Reattempt catheter removal. If resistance is still present, stop the removal and notify the health care team.

SPECIAL CONSIDERATIONS

- Have alternate toileting measures available, as necessary, based on patient assessment. A bedside commode, urinal, or bedpan may be necessary if the patient is unable to get to the bathroom promptly.
- Refer to facility policy and the manufacturer's recommendation regarding balloon deflation. Aspiration by pulling on the syringe plunger may result in collapse of the inflation lumen; contribute to the formation of creases, ridges, or cuffing at the balloon area; and increase the catheter balloon diameter size on deflation, resulting in difficult removal and urethral trauma.
- WOCN has developed a consensus-based algorithm for patient assessment and selection and use of bladder management strategies after indwelling catheter removal. Visit the WOCN website at https://www.wocn.org/learning-center/clinical-tools/ to access the interactive Interventions Post Catheter Removal (iPCaRe) tool (WOCN, n.d.).

PREVENTION OF CATHETER-ASSOCIATED INFECTIONS
Practice Guideline
Gould, C. V., Umscheid, C. A., Agarwal, R. K., Kuntz, G., Pegues, D. A., & the Healthcare Infection Control Practices Advisory Committee (HICPAC). (2019 [update]). *Guideline for prevention of catheter-associated urinary tract infections 2009. Centers for Disease Control and Prevention*, 31(4). https://www.cdc.gov/infectioncontrol/pdf/guidelines/cauti-guidelines-H.pdf
These guidelines provide evidence-based recommendations to guide care for patients requiring catheterization of the urinary bladder to prevent CAUTI.

Skill 12-10 ▶ Administering a Continuous Closed Bladder or Catheter Irrigation

Routine intermittent irrigation of long-term catheters is not recommended (Gould et al., 2019). Unless obstruction is anticipated, as might occur with bleeding after prostatic or bladder surgery, bladder irrigation is not recommended and should be avoided (Gould et al., 2019; SUNA, 2015). In these situations, sediment or debris, as well as blood clots, might block the catheter, preventing the flow of urine out of the catheter. Irrigations might also be used to instill medications that will act directly on the bladder wall.

Irrigating a catheter through a closed system is preferred to opening the catheter because opening the catheter could lead to contamination and infection (Gould et al., 2019). Closed-system irrigation via a triple-lumen catheter (Figure 1) is suggested to prevent obstruction and maintain a closed system (Figure 2 on page 764) and is recommended to prevent the introduction of pathogens into the bladder (Gould et al., 2019).

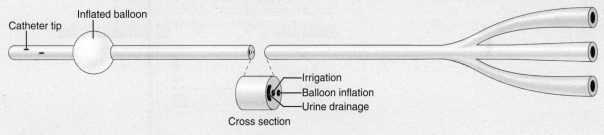

FIGURE 1. A triple-lumen catheter.

DELEGATION CONSIDERATIONS

The administration of continuous closed bladder irrigation is not delegated to assistive personnel (AP). Depending on the state's nurse practice act and the organization's policies and procedures, administration of continuous closed bladder irrigation may be delegated to licensed practical/vocational nurses (LPN/LVNs). The decision to delegate must be based on careful analysis of the patient's needs and circumstances as well as the qualifications of the person to whom the task is being delegated. Refer to the Delegation Guidelines in Appendix A.

EQUIPMENT

- Sterile irrigating solution (at room temperature or warmed to body temperature)
- Sterile tubing with drip chamber and clamp for connection to irrigating solution
- IV pole
- IV pump (if bladder is being irrigated with a solution containing medication)
- Three-way indwelling catheter in place in patient's bladder
- Indwelling catheter drainage setup (tubing and collection bag)
- Alcohol or other disinfectant swab
- Bath blanket
- Disposable gloves
- Additional PPE, as indicated

(continued on page 764)

Skill 12-10 ► Administering a Continuous Closed Bladder or Catheter Irrigation *(continued)*

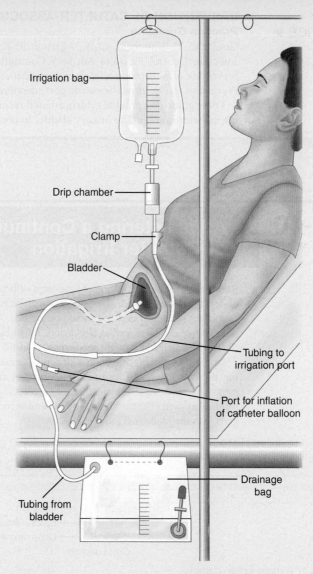

FIGURE 2. A continuous bladder irrigation (CBI) setup.

Labels in figure:
- Irrigation bag
- Drip chamber
- Clamp
- Bladder
- Tubing to irrigation port
- Port for inflation of catheter balloon
- Drainage bag
- Tubing from bladder

ASSESSMENT	Verify the prescribed intervention in the health record for continuous bladder irrigation, including type and amount of irrigant or irrigation parameters. Assess the catheter to ensure that it has an irrigation port (if the patient has an indwelling catheter already in place) (three-way indwelling catheter). Assess the characteristics of urine present in the tubing and drainage bag. Review the patient's health record for, and ask the patient about, any allergies to medications. Before performing the procedure, assess the bladder for fullness either by palpation or with a handheld bladder ultrasound device. Assess for signs of adverse effects, which may include pain, bladder spasm, bladder distention /fullness, or lack of drainage from the catheter.
ACTUAL OR POTENTIAL HEALTH PROBLEMS AND NEEDS	Many actual or potential health problems or issues may require the use of this skill as part of related interventions. An appropriate health problem or issue may include: • Impaired urination • Infection risk

OUTCOME IDENTIFICATION AND PLANNING

The expected outcomes to achieve are that the irrigation is administered without adverse effect, and the patient exhibits free-flowing urine through the catheter. Initially, clots or debris may be noted. These should decrease over time, with the patient ultimately exhibiting urine that is free of clots or debris. Other outcomes may include that the continuous bladder irrigation continues without adverse effect, drainage is greater than the hourly amount of irrigation solution being placed in the bladder, and the patient exhibits no signs and symptoms of infection.

IMPLEMENTATION

ACTION	RATIONALE
1. Confirm the prescribed intervention for continuous catheter irrigation in the health record, including infusion parameters. If irrigation is to be implemented via gravity infusion, calculate the drip rate. Often, titration to keep the urine clear of blood or clots is prescribed.	Verifying the prescribed intervention ensures that the correct intervention is administered to the right patient. The solution must be administered via gravity at the appropriate rate as prescribed.
2. Gather equipment.	Assembling equipment provides for an organized approach to the task.
3. Perform hand hygiene and put on PPE, if indicated.	Hand hygiene and PPE prevent the spread of microorganisms. PPE is required based on transmission precautions.
4. Identify the patient.	Identifying the patient ensures the right patient receives the intervention and helps prevent errors.
5. Close the curtains around the bed and close the door to the room, if possible. Discuss the procedure with the patient.	This ensures the patient's privacy. Discussion promotes reassurance and provides knowledge about the procedure. Dialogue encourages patient participation and allows for individualized nursing care.
6. Assemble equipment on the overbed table or other surface within reach.	Arranging items nearby is convenient, saves time, and prevents unnecessary stretching and twisting of muscles on the part of the nurse.
7. Adjust the bed to a comfortable working height (VHACEOSH, 2016).	Having the bed at the proper height prevents back and muscle strain.
8. Empty the catheter drainage bag and measure the amount of urine, noting the amount and characteristics of the urine.	Emptying the drainage bag allows for accurate assessment of drainage after the irrigation solution is instilled. Assessment of urine provides a baseline for future comparison.
9. Assist the patient to a comfortable position and expose the irrigation port on the catheter setup. Place a waterproof pad under the catheter and irrigation port.	This provides adequate visualization. The waterproof pad protects the patient and bed from leakage.
10. Prepare the sterile irrigation bag for use as directed by the manufacturer. Clearly label the solution as "Bladder Irrigant." Include the date and time on the label. Hang the bag on the IV pole 2.5 to 3 ft above the level of the patient's bladder. Close the tubing clamp and insert the sterile tubing with drip chamber to the container using aseptic technique (Figure 3). Release the clamp and remove the protective cover on the end of the tubing without contaminating it. Allow the solution to flush the tubing and remove air (Figure 4). Clamp the tubing and replace the end cover.	Proper labeling provides accurate information for caregivers. Sterile solution not used within 24 hours of opening should be discarded. Aseptic technique prevents contamination of solution irrigation system. Priming the tubing before attaching irrigation clears air from the tubing that might cause bladder distention.

(continued on page 766)

Skill 12-10 ▶ Administering a Continuous Closed Bladder or Catheter Irrigation *(continued)*

ACTION	RATIONALE

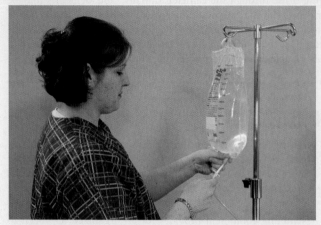

FIGURE 3. Inserting tubing into solution bag.

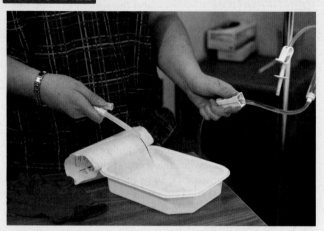

FIGURE 4. Removing air from irrigation tubing.

11. Put on gloves. **Cleanse the irrigation port on the catheter with an alcohol swab. Using aseptic technique, attach the irrigation tubing to the irrigation port of the three-way indwelling catheter (Figure 5).**

Aseptic technique prevents the spread of microorganisms into the bladder.

12. Check the drainage tubing to make sure the clamp, if present, is open.

An open clamp prevents accumulation of solution in the bladder.

13. **Release the clamp on the irrigation tubing and regulate the flow at the determined drip rate, according to the prescribed rate (Figure 6).** If the bladder irrigation is to be done with a medicated solution, use an electronic infusion device to regulate the flow.

This allows for continual gentle irrigation without causing discomfort to the patient. An electronic infusion device regulates the flow of the medication.

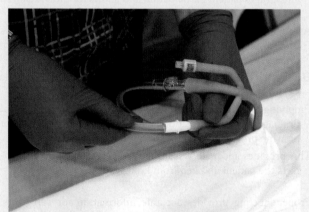

FIGURE 5. Attaching irrigation tubing to irrigation port on catheter.

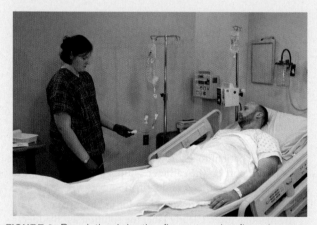

FIGURE 6. Regulating irrigation flow rate using flow clamp.

14. Remove gloves. Perform hand hygiene. Assist the patient to a comfortable position. Cover the patient with bed linens. Place the bed in the lowest position.

Positioning and covering provide warmth and promote comfort and safety. Hand hygiene prevents the spread of microorganisms.

15. Assess the patient's response to the procedure and the quality and amount of drainage.

Assessment is necessary to determine the effectiveness of the intervention and to detect adverse effects.

16. Remove equipment. Remove additional PPE, if used. Perform hand hygiene.

Proper disposal of equipment prevents transmission of microorganisms. Proper removal of PPE reduces the risk for infection transmission and contamination of other items. Hand hygiene prevents the spread of microorganisms.

ACTION

17. As the irrigation fluid container nears empty, clamp the administration tubing. Do not allow the drip chamber to empty. Disconnect the empty bag and attach a new full irrigation solution bag.

18. Put on gloves to empty the drainage collection bag as each new container is hung. Record initiation of the new container and volume of drainage.

RATIONALE

This eliminates the need to separate the tubing from the catheter and clear air from the tubing. Opening the drainage system provides access for microorganisms.

Gloves protect against exposure to blood, body fluids, and microorganisms. Accurate recording of the volume of the irrigation solution infused and catheter drainage allows for accurate calculation of urinary output.

EVALUATION

The expected outcomes have been met when the irrigation has been administered without adverse effect, the patient has exhibited free-flowing urine through the catheter, the continuous bladder irrigation has continued without adverse effect, drainage from the catheter has been greater than the hourly amount of irrigation solution being placed in the bladder, and the patient has exhibited no signs and symptoms of infection.

DOCUMENTATION

Guidelines

Document the baseline assessment of the patient. Document the amount and type of irrigation solution used and the patient's tolerance of the procedure. Record the urine amount emptied from the drainage bag before the procedure and the amount of irrigant used on the intake and output record. Record the amount of urine and irrigant emptied from the drainage bag. **Subtract the amount of irrigant instilled from the total volume of drainage to obtain the volume of urine output.**

Sample Documentation

12/14/25 1330 Foley catheter replaced with three-way Foley catheter. Bladder nonpalpable. Continuous bladder irrigation with normal saline initiated at 100 mL/hr. Patient tolerated procedure without adverse effect. Drainage from bladder slightly cloudy, light cherry colored. No evidence of clots.

—B. Clapp, RN

DEVELOPING CLINICAL REASONING AND CLINICAL JUDGMENT

UNEXPECTED SITUATIONS AND ASSOCIATED INTERVENTIONS

- *Continuous bladder irrigation begins, and hourly drainage is less than amount of irrigation being given:* Palpate for bladder distention. If the patient is lying supine, rolling them onto their side may help increase the amount of drainage. Check to make sure that the tubing is not kinked. If return flow remains decreased, notify the health care team.
- *Bladder irrigation is not flowing at prescribed rate, even with clamp wide open:* Check the tubing for kinks or pressure points. Raise the bag slightly and then check the flow of the irrigation solution. Frequently check the flow rate of the irrigation solution.

SPECIAL CONSIDERATIONS

- Patients with long-term indwelling urinary catheters and their health care providers should monitor the "life" of the patient's catheter to anticipate and preempt blockage from encrustation, crystalline formation, sediment, and debris, often related to formation of biofilms to avoid the need for irrigation (Dean & Ostaszkiewicz, 2019; Pelling et al., 2019).

(*continued on page 768*)

Skill 12-10 ▶ Administering a Continuous Closed Bladder or Catheter Irrigation *(continued)*

Skill 12-11 ▶ Emptying and Changing a Stoma Appliance on a Urinary Diversion

Skill Variation: *Applying a Two-Piece Stoma Appliance on a Urinary Diversion*

Urinary diversions may be used as part of the treatment for patients with obstructions or tumors in the urinary tract, a neurogenic bladder, radiation cystitis, or congenital anomalies of the lower urinary tract. An **ileal conduit** (also known as a urostomy) is the most common type of incontinent cutaneous urinary diversion (Berti-Hearn & Elliott, 2019; Goldberg et al., 2018). An ileal conduit involves a surgical resection of the small intestine, with transplantation of the ureters to the isolated segment of small bowel. This separated section of the small intestine is then brought to the abdominal wall, where urine is excreted through a **stoma**, a surgically created opening on the body surface. Such diversions are usually permanent, and the patient wears an external appliance to collect the urine because urine elimination from the stoma cannot be controlled voluntarily. Appliances are available in a one-piece (barrier backing already attached to the pouch) or two-piece (separate pouch that fastens to the barrier backing) system and choice of use is based on the physical needs and personal preferences of the patient (Goldberg et al., 2018). The appliance is usually changed every 3 to 7 days, although it could be changed more often (American Cancer Society, 2019; Berti-Hearn & Elliott, 2019; O'Flynn, 2018; Stelton, 2019). Proper application minimizes the risk for skin breakdown around the stoma. This skill addresses changing a one-piece appliance. A one-piece appliance consists of a pouch with an integral adhesive section that adheres to the patient's skin. The adhesive flange is generally made from hydrocolloid. The accompanying Skill Variation addresses changing a two-piece appliance.

The appliance is usually changed after a time of low fluid intake, such as in the early morning. Urine production is less at this time, making changing the appliance easier. Proper application minimizes the risk for skin breakdown around the stoma. Box 12-3 summarizes guidelines for care of the patient with a urinary diversion.

DELEGATION CONSIDERATIONS

The emptying of a stoma appliance on a urinary diversion may be delegated to assistive personnel (AP) as well as to licensed practical/vocational nurses (LPN/LVNs). The changing of a stoma appliance on a urinary diversion may be delegated to LPN/LVNs. The decision to delegate must be based on careful analysis of the patient's needs and circumstances as well as the qualifications of the person to whom the task is being delegated. Refer to the Delegation Guidelines in Appendix A.

Box 12-3	Guidelines for Care of the Patient With a Urinary Diversion

- Keep the patient as free of odors as possible. If the patient has an external appliance, empty the appliance frequently.
- Inspect the patient's stoma regularly. It should ideally protrude about 1 to 3 cm above skin level and be dark pink to red in color and moist (Berti-Hearn & Elliott, 2019; Stelton, 2019). A pale stoma may indicate anemia, and a dark or purple-blue stoma may reflect compromised circulation or ischemia. Bleeding around the stoma and its stem should be minimal. The edges of the stoma should appear secure to the surrounding skin (Stelton, 2019). The pulling away of the stoma from the peristomal skin is called mucocutaneous separation or stoma dehiscence (Stelton, 2019) and occurs more often in patients who are at risk for impaired healing, including patients with diabetes, poor nutritional status or who received high-dose steroid therapy or chemotherapy before surgery (Butler, 2009). Notify the health care team promptly if bleeding persists or is excessive, if color changes occur in the stoma, or if it appears the stoma is separating from the peristomal skin (Stelton, 2019).
- Note the size of the stoma, which usually stabilizes within 6 to 8 weeks (Stelton, 2019). Most stomas protrude 0.5 to 1 inch from the abdominal surface and may initially appear swollen and edematous. After 6 weeks, the edema usually subsides. If an abdominal dressing is in place at the incision site after surgery, check it frequently for drainage and bleeding.
- Keep the skin around the stoma site (peristomal area) clean and dry. If care is not taken to protect the skin around the stoma, irritation or infection may occur. Assess the peristomal (around the stoma) skin; peristomal skin should be intact and appear consistent with that of the rest of the abdomen, without pain or discomfort (Burch, 2018). In patients with light skin tones, the peristomal

skin should not be reddened; in patients with darker skin tones, the skin should not have darker discolorations (Stelton, 2019). A leaking or ill-fitted stoma appliance will cause moisture-associated skin damage (Berti-Hearn & Elliott, 2019) (refer to the discussion earlier in the chapter). Candida or yeast infections can also occur around the stoma if the area is not kept dry.
- Measure the patient's fluid intake and output. Careful monitoring of the patient's urinary output is necessary to monitor fluid balance.
- Monitor the return of intestinal function and peristalsis. Initially after surgery, peristalsis is inhibited. Remember, the patient had a bowel resection as part of the urinary diversion procedure.
- Monitor for mucus in the urine from an ileal conduit, which is a normal finding (Berti-Hearn & Elliott, 2019). The isolated segment of small intestine continues to produce mucus as part of its normal functioning.
- Explain each aspect of care to the patient and explain what their role will be when they begin self-care. Patient teaching is one of the most important aspects of ostomy care and should include family members/caregivers, when appropriate. Teaching can begin before surgery so that the patient has adequate time to absorb the information.
- Encourage the patient to participate in care and to look at the stoma. Patients normally experience emotional depression during the early postoperative period. Help the patient to cope by listening, explaining, and being available and supportive. A visit from a representative of the local ostomy support group may be helpful. Patients usually begin to accept their altered body image when they are willing to look at the stoma, make neutral or positive statements concerning the ostomy, and express interest in learning self-care.

EQUIPMENT

- Premoistened disposable washcloths or
  - Basin with warm water
  - Skin cleanser, towel, washcloth
- Silicone-based adhesive remover
- Gauze squares
- Skin protectant, such as Skin-Prep™
- Ostomy appliance
- Stoma-measuring guide
- Graduated container
- Ostomy belt (optional)
- Disposable gloves
- Additional PPE, as indicated
- Waterproof, disposable pad
- Small plastic trash bag

ASSESSMENT

Assess the current urinary diversion appliance, observing product style, condition of appliance, and stoma (if bag is clear). Note the length of time the appliance has been in place. Determine the patient's knowledge of urinary diversion care, including their level of self-care and ability to manipulate the equipment. After the appliance is removed, assess the stoma and the skin surrounding the urinary diversion. The stoma should ideally protrude about 1 to 3 cm above skin level and be dark pink to red in color and moist (Berti-Hearn & Elliott, 2019; Stelton, 2019). The peristomal skin should look like the skin on the rest of the abdomen (Stelton, 2019). Assess the condition of any abdominal scars or incisional areas, if surgery to create the urinary diversion was recent.

(continued on page 770)

Skill 12-11 ▶ Emptying and Changing a Stoma Appliance on a Urinary Diversion *(continued)*

ACTUAL OR POTENTIAL HEALTH PROBLEMS AND NEEDS	Many actual or potential health problems or issues may require the use of this skill as part of related interventions. An appropriate health problem or issue may include: • Altered body image perception • Altered skin integrity risk • Knowledge deficiency
OUTCOME IDENTIFICATION AND PLANNING	The expected outcome to achieve when changing a patient's urinary stoma appliance is that the stoma appliance is applied correctly to the skin to allow urine to drain freely and without leakage. Other outcomes may include that the patient exhibits a moist red stoma with intact skin surrounding the stoma, the patient demonstrates knowledge of how to apply the appliance, and the patient verbalizes positive self-image.

IMPLEMENTATION

ACTION	RATIONALE
1. Gather equipment.	Assembling equipment provides for an organized approach to the task.
2. Perform hand hygiene and put on PPE, if indicated.	Hand hygiene and PPE prevent the spread of microorganisms. PPE is required based on transmission precautions.
3. Identify the patient.	Identifying the patient ensures the right patient receives the intervention and helps prevent errors.
4. Close the curtains around the bed and close the door to the room, if possible. Explain to the patient what you are going to do and why. Encourage the patient to observe or participate, if possible and as appropriate.	This ensures the patient's privacy. Explanation relieves anxiety and facilitates engagement. Having the patient observe or assist encourages self-acceptance and helps the patient develop self-care skills.
5. Assemble equipment on the overbed table or other surface within reach.	Arranging items nearby is convenient, saves time, and prevents unnecessary stretching and twisting of muscles on the part of the nurse.
6. Assist the patient to a comfortable sitting or lying position in bed or a standing or sitting position in the bathroom. If the patient is in bed, adjust the bed to a comfortable working height (VHACEOSH, 2016). Place a waterproof pad under the patient at the stoma site.	Either position should allow the patient to view the procedure in preparation for learning to perform it independently. Lying flat or sitting upright facilitates smooth application of the appliance. Having the bed at the proper height prevents back and muscle strain. A waterproof pad protects linens and the patient from moisture.

Emptying the Appliance

ACTION	RATIONALE
7. Put on gloves. Hold the end of the appliance over a bedpan, toilet, or measuring device. Remove the end cap from the spout. Open the spout and empty the contents into the bedpan, toilet, or measuring device (Figure 1).	Gloves protect the nurse from exposure to blood and body fluids. Emptying the pouch before handling it reduces the likelihood of spilling the excretions.
8. Close the spout. Wipe the spout with toilet tissue. Replace the cap.	Drying the spout removes any urine.
9. Remove equipment. Remove gloves. Perform hand hygiene. Assist the patient to a comfortable position.	Proper removal of PPE prevents the transmission of microorganisms. Positioning ensures patient comfort. Hand hygiene prevents the spread of microorganisms.
10. If the appliance is not to be changed, place the bed in the lowest position. Remove additional PPE, if used. Perform hand hygiene.	Lowering the bed promotes patient safety. Proper removal of PPE reduces the risk for infection transmission and contamination of other items. Hand hygiene prevents the spread of microorganisms.

ACTION

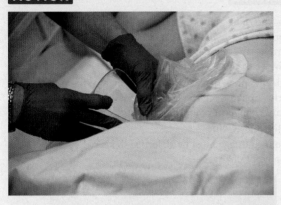

FIGURE 1. Emptying urine into graduated container.

RATIONALE

Changing the Appliance

11. Place a disposable waterproof pad on the overbed table or other work area. Open the premoistened disposable washcloths or set up the washbasin with warm water and the rest of the supplies. Place a trash bag within reach.

12. Put on gloves. Place a waterproof pad under the patient at the stoma site. Empty the appliance, if necessary, as described in Steps 6 to 8.

13. Put on gloves. Use two hands to gently remove the appliance faceplate, starting at the top and keeping the abdominal skin taut (Figure 2). Remove the appliance faceplate from the skin by pushing the skin from the appliance rather than pulling the appliance from the skin (Figure 3). Apply a silicone-based adhesive remover by spraying or wiping with the remover wipe, as indicated.

The pad protects the surface. Organization facilitates performance of the procedure.

The waterproof pad protects linens and the patient from moisture. Emptying the contents before removal prevents accidental spillage of fecal material.

Gloves prevent contact with blood and body fluids. The seal between the surface of the faceplate and the skin must be broken before the faceplate can be removed. Harsh handling of the appliance can damage the skin and impair the development of a secure seal in the future. Silicone-based adhesive remover loosens the adhesive bond to make removal easier and less likely to damage the skin and is particularly beneficial for patients with fragile skin and those at increased risk for medical adhesive–related skin injury/stripping (Collier, 2019; LeBlanc et al., 2019; Swift et al., 2020).

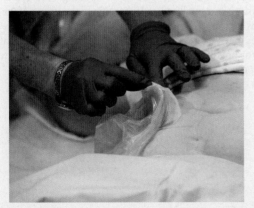

FIGURE 2. Gently removing appliance faceplate from skin.

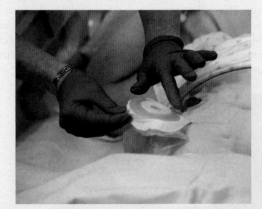

FIGURE 3. Pushing skin from appliance rather than pulling appliance from skin.

14. Place the appliance in the trash bag, if disposable. If reusable, set it aside to wash in lukewarm soap and water and allow it to air dry after the new appliance is in place.

Thorough cleaning and airing of the appliance reduces odor and deterioration of the appliance. For aesthetic and infection control purposes, used appliances should be discarded appropriately.

(continued on page 772)

Skill 12-11 ▶ Emptying and Changing a Stoma Appliance on a Urinary Diversion *(continued)*

ACTION	**RATIONALE**
15. Clean the skin around the stoma with mild skin cleanser and water or a cleansing agent and a washcloth (Figure 4). Remove all old adhesive from the skin; additional adhesive remover may be used. Do not apply lotion to the peristomal area.	Cleaning the skin removes excretions and old adhesive and skin protectant. Excretions or a buildup of other substances can irritate and damage the skin. Lotion will prevent a tight adhesive seal.
16. Gently pat the area dry. **Make sure the skin around the stoma is thoroughly dry.** Assess the stoma and the condition of the surrounding skin.	Careful drying prevents trauma to the skin and stoma. An intact, properly applied urinary collection device protects skin integrity. Any change in color and size of the stoma may indicate circulatory problems.
17. Place one or two gauze squares over the stoma opening (Figure 5).	Continuous drainage must be absorbed to keep the skin dry during appliance change.

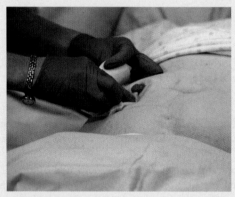

FIGURE 4. Cleaning stoma with cleansing agent and washcloth.

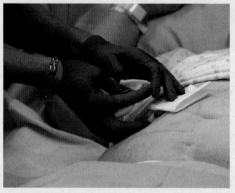

FIGURE 5. Placing one or two gauze squares over stoma opening.

18. Apply skin protectant/barrier film to a 2-inches (5-cm) radius around the stoma, and allow it to dry completely, which takes about 30 seconds.	The skin needs protection from the potentially excoriating effect of the appliance adhesive (WOCN, 2018). The skin must be perfectly dry before the appliance is placed to get good adherence and to prevent leaks.
19. Lift the gauze squares for a moment and measure the stoma opening, using the measurement guide. Replace the gauze. Trace the same-size opening on the back center of the appliance. Cut the opening 1/8 inch (2 to 3 mm) larger than the stoma size (Hill, 2020) (Figure 6). Use a finger to gently smooth the wafer edges after cutting. Check that the spout is closed, and the end cap is in place.	The appliance should fit snugly around the stoma, with only 1/8 inch of skin visible around the opening. A faceplate opening that is too small can cause trauma to the stoma. If the opening is too large, exposed skin will be irritated by urine. Wafer edges may be uneven after cutting and could cause irritation to and/or pressure on the stoma. A closed spout and secured end cap prevent urine from leaking from the appliance.

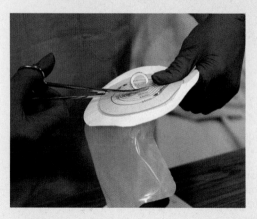

FIGURE 6. Cutting the faceplate opening 1/8 inch larger than stoma size.

ACTION

20. Remove the paper backing from the appliance faceplate. Quickly remove the gauze squares and discard appropriately; ease the appliance over the stoma. Gently press them onto the skin while smoothing over the surface (Figure 7). Apply gentle, even pressure to the appliance for approximately 30 seconds (Burch, 2019a; Hill, 2020).

RATIONALE

The appliance is effective only if it is properly positioned and adhered securely. Pressure on the faceplate allows the faceplate to mold to the patient's skin and improves the seal.

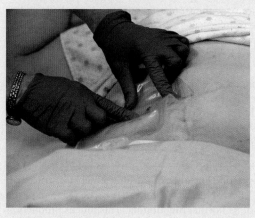

FIGURE 7. Applying faceplate over stoma.

21. Secure the optional belt to the appliance and around the patient.

An elasticized belt helps support the appliance for some people.

22. Remove gloves. Perform hand hygiene. Assist the patient to a comfortable position. Cover the patient with bed linens. Place the bed in the lowest position.

Removing gloves reduces risk of transmission of microorganisms. Hand hygiene prevents the spread of microorganisms. Positioning and covering provide warmth and promote comfort. The bed in the lowest position promotes patient safety.

23. Put on gloves. Remove or discard any remaining equipment and assess the patient's response to the procedure.

The patient's response may indicate acceptance of the ostomy as well as the need for health teaching.

24. Remove gloves and additional PPE, if used. Perform hand hygiene.

Proper removal of PPE reduces the risk for infection transmission and contamination of other items. Hand hygiene prevents the spread of microorganisms.

EVALUATION

The expected outcomes have been met when the ileal conduit appliance has been emptied and/or changed without trauma to the stoma or peristomal skin or leaking; urine has drained freely into the appliance; the skin surrounding the stoma has remained clean, dry, and intact; and the patient has showed an interest in learning to perform the pouch change and has verbalized positive self-image.

DOCUMENTATION

Guidelines

Document the procedure, including the appearance of the stoma, condition of the peristomal skin, characteristics of the urine, the patient's response to the procedure, and pertinent patient teaching.

Sample Documentation

7/23/25 1245 Ileal conduit appliance changed. Mr. Jones present. Mrs. Jones asking questions about care for ileal conduit, states, "I don't know if I'll ever be able to care for this thing at home." Tearful at times. Patient encouraged to express feelings. Patient agreed to talk with wound, ostomy, and continence nurse about concerns. Mr. Jones very supportive, also asking appropriate questions. Patient states they would like to watch change one more time before they attempt to do it. Stoma is moist and red, peristomal skin intact, draining yellow urine with small amount of mucus.

—B. Clapp, RN

(*continued on page 774*)

Skill 12-11 ▶ Emptying and Changing a Stoma Appliance on a Urinary Diversion *(continued)*

DEVELOPING CLINICAL REASONING AND CLINICAL JUDGMENT

UNEXPECTED SITUATIONS AND ASSOCIATED INTERVENTIONS

- *You remove appliance and find an area of skin excoriated:* Make sure that the appliance is not cut too large. Skin that is exposed inside of the ostomy appliance will become excoriated. Assess for the presence of a fungal skin infection. Consult with the wound, ostomy, and continence nurse to identify appropriate treatment. Cleanse the skin thoroughly and pat dry. Apply products made for excoriated skin before placing the appliance over the stoma. Frequently check the faceplate to ensure that a seal has formed and that there is no leakage. Document the assessment findings and related interventions in the patient's record.
- *Faceplate is leaking after applying a new appliance:* Remove the appliance, clean the skin, and start over.
- *You are ready to place the faceplate and notice that the opening is cut too large:* Discard the appliance and begin over. A faceplate that is cut too large may lead to excoriation of the skin and leakage.
- *Stoma is dark brown or black:* The stoma should appear pink to red, shiny, and moist. Alterations may indicate compromised circulation. If the stoma is dark brown or black, suspect ischemia and necrosis. Notify the health care team immediately.

SPECIAL CONSIDERATIONS

- Patients with urinary diversions created using a portion of the gastrointestinal (GI) tract will experience the presence of mucus in the urine (Berti-Hearn & Elliott, 2019). The segment of the GI tract continues to produce mucus, as part of its normal functioning. This mucus production does not decrease over time but is usually not a problem for patients with an ileal conduit (Berti-Hearn & Elliott, 2019).
- Key components in postoperative education before the patient is discharged from the hospital include assessment and care of the stoma and peristomal skin, pouch emptying, changing the appliance, drainage collectors, common complications, clothing, fluid guidelines, medications, and obtaining supplies (Goldberg et al., 2018).

Skill Variation ▶ Applying a Two-Piece Stoma Appliance on a Urinary Diversion

A two-piece colostomy appliance is composed of a pouch and a separate adhesive faceplate that attach together (Figure A). The faceplate is left in place for a period of time, depending on the type being used and specific patient circumstances, but usually every 3 to 7 days (American Cancer Society, 2019; Berti-Hearn & Elliott, 2019; O'Flynn, 2018; Stelton, 2019). The pouch/bag may be replaced as needed during this time.

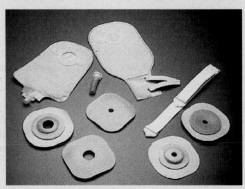

FIGURE A. Two-piece appliances.

1. Gather necessary equipment.

2. Perform hand hygiene and put on PPE, if indicated.

3. Identify the patient.

4. Close the curtains around the bed and close the door to room, if possible. Explain to the patient what you are going to do and why. Encourage the patient to observe or participate, if possible and as appropriate.
5. Assemble equipment on the overbed table or other surface within reach.
6. Assist the patient to a comfortable sitting or lying position in bed or a standing or sitting position in the bathroom.
7. Place a disposable pad on the work surface. Open the premoistened disposable washcloths or set up the washbasin with warm water and the rest of the supplies. Place a trash bag within reach.

8. Put on gloves. Place a waterproof pad under the patient at the stoma site. Empty the appliance as described previously in Skill 12-11.

9. Use two hands to gently remove the pouch faceplate from the skin by pushing the skin from the appliance rather than pulling the appliance from the skin. Start at the top of the appliance, while keeping the abdominal skin taut. Apply a silicone-based adhesive remover by spraying or wiping with the remover wipe, as indicated.

10. Place the appliance in the trash bag, if disposable. If reusable, set it aside to wash in lukewarm soap and water and allow it to air dry after the new appliance is in place.

11. Clean the skin around the stoma with a mild skin cleanser and water or a cleansing agent and a washcloth. Remove all old adhesive from skin; additional adhesive remover may be used. Do not apply lotion to the peristomal area.

12. Gently pat the area dry. Make sure the skin around the stoma is thoroughly dry. Assess the stoma and the condition of the surrounding skin. Place one or two gauze squares over the stoma opening.

13. Apply skin protectant/barrier film to a 2-inches (5-cm) radius around the stoma, and allow it to dry completely, which takes about 30 seconds.

14. Lift the gauze squares for a moment and measure the stoma opening, using the measurement guide. Replace the gauze. Trace the same-size opening on the back center of the appliance faceplate. Cut the opening 1/8 inch (2 to 3 mm) larger than the stoma size (Hill, 2020).

15. Remove the backing from the faceplate. Quickly remove the gauze squares and ease the faceplate over the stoma. Gently press them onto the skin while smoothing over the surface (Figure B). Apply gentle, even pressure to the appliance for approximately 30 seconds (Burch, 2019a; Hill, 2020).

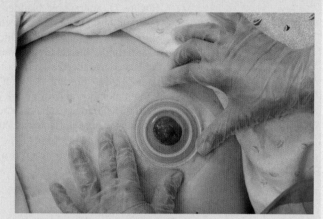

FIGURE B. Gently pressing faceplate to skin.

16. Apply the appliance pouch to the faceplate following the manufacturer's directions. Check that the spout is closed, and the end cap is in place. If using a "click" system, lay the ring on the pouch over the ring on the faceplate. Ask the patient to tighten their stomach muscles, if possible. Beginning at one edge of the ring, push the pouch ring onto the faceplate ring. A "click" should be heard when the pouch is secured onto the faceplate.

17. Remove gloves. Perform hand hygiene. Assist the patient to a comfortable position. Cover the patient with bed linens. Place the bed in the lowest position.

18. Put on gloves. Remove or discard equipment and assess the patient's response to the procedure.

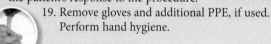

19. Remove gloves and additional PPE, if used. Perform hand hygiene.

EVIDENCE FOR PRACTICE ▶

EVIDENCE-BASED PRACTICE GUIDELINE
Providing Care for Patients With Ostomies

Goldberg, M., Colwell, J., Burns, S., Carmel, J., Fellows, J., Hendren, S., Livingston, V., Nottingham, C. U., Pittman, J., Rafferty, J., Salvadalena, G., Steinberg, G., & Wound, Ostomy and Continence Nurses Society. Guideline Development Task Force. (2018). WOCN Society Clinical Guideline. Management of the adult patient with a fecal or urinary ostomy—An executive summary. *Journal of Wound, Ostomy and Continence Nursing, 45*(1), 50–58. https://doi.org/10.1097/WON.0000000000000396

These guidelines provide evidence-based recommendations to guide care for patients with ostomies, prevent or decrease complications, and improve patient outcomes.

Skill 12-12 ▶ Caring for a Suprapubic Urinary Catheter

A **suprapubic urinary catheter** is an indwelling catheter used for long-term continuous urinary drainage. This type of catheter is surgically inserted through a small incision above the pubic area (Figure 1). Suprapubic bladder drainage diverts urine from the urethra when injury, stricture, prostatic obstruction, or gynecologic or abdominal surgery has compromised the flow of urine through the urethra (Hill & Mitchell, 2018). A suprapubic catheter may be preferred over indwelling urethral catheters for long-term urinary drainage (Gibson et al., 2019). Suprapubic catheters are associated with decreased risk of contamination with organisms from fecal material, elimination of damage to the urethra; does not interfere with sexual activity; increased comfort for patients with limited mobility; and lower risk of CAUTIs (Buehrle et al., 2020; Gibson et al., 2019; Hooton et al., 2010). The drainage tube may be secured with sutures and should be secured with a catheter fixation device or tape (Holroyd, 2019). Care of the patient with a suprapubic catheter includes skin care around the insertion site; care of the drainage tubing and drainage bag is the same as for an indwelling catheter (refer to Box 12-1 on page 739).

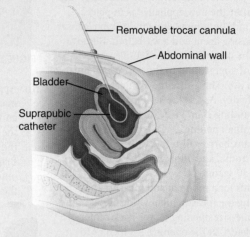

Removable trocar cannula
Abdominal wall
Bladder
Suprapubic catheter

FIGURE 1. A suprapubic catheter positioned in bladder.

DELEGATION CONSIDERATIONS	The care of a suprapubic urinary catheter, in the postoperative period, is not delegated to assistive personnel (AP) in the acute care setting. The care of a healed suprapubic catheter site in some settings may be delegated to assistive personnel (AP) who have received appropriate training, after assessment of the catheter by the registered nurse. Depending on the state's nurse practice act and the organization's policies and procedures, the care of a suprapubic urinary catheter may be delegated to licensed practical/vocational nurses (LPN/LVNs). The decision to delegate must be based on careful analysis of the patient's needs and circumstances as well as the qualifications of the person to whom the task is being delegated. Refer to the Delegation Guidelines in Appendix A.

EQUIPMENT	• Premoistened disposable washcloths or
	  • Basin with warm water
	  • Skin cleanser, towel, washcloth
	• Disposable gloves
	• Additional PPE, as indicated
	• Velcro tube holder or tape to secure tube
	• Drainage sponge (if necessary)
	• Plastic trash bag
	• Sterile cotton-tipped applicators and sterile saline solution (if the patient has a new suprapubic catheter)

ASSESSMENT	Assess the suprapubic catheter and bag, observing the condition of the catheter and the drainage bag connected to the catheter, and the product style. If a dressing is in place at the insertion site, assess the dressing for drainage. Inspect the site around the suprapubic catheter, looking for drainage, erythema, or excoriation. Assess the method used to secure the catheter in place. If sutures are present, assess for intactness. Also, assess the characteristics of the urine in the drainage bag. Assess the patient's knowledge of caring for a suprapubic catheter.

ACTUAL OR POTENTIAL HEALTH PROBLEMS AND NEEDS	Many actual or potential health problems or issues may require the use of this skill as part of related interventions. An appropriate health problem or issue may include: • Impaired urination • Infection risk • Knowledge deficiency

OUTCOME IDENTIFICATION AND PLANNING	The expected outcomes to be achieved when caring for a suprapubic catheter are that the catheter site and the patient's skin remains clean, dry, intact, and without evidence of irritation or break-down, and that the patient verbalizes an understanding of the purpose for, and care of, the catheter, as appropriate. Other appropriate outcomes include that the patient's urinary elimination is maintained, and the patient's bladder is not distended.

IMPLEMENTATION

ACTION	RATIONALE
1. Gather equipment.	Assembling equipment provides for an organized approach to task.
2. Perform hand hygiene and put on PPE, if indicated.	Hand hygiene and PPE prevent the spread of microorganisms. PPE is required based on transmission precautions.
3. Identify the patient.	Identifying the patient ensures the right patient receives the intervention and helps prevent errors.
4. Close the curtains around the bed and close the door to the room, if possible. Explain to the patient what you are going to do and why. Encourage the patient to observe or participate, if possible.	This ensures the patient's privacy. Explanation relieves anxiety and facilitates engagement. Having the patient observe or assist encourages self-acceptance.
5. Assemble equipment on the overbed table or other surface within reach.	Arranging items nearby is convenient, saves time, and prevents unnecessary stretching and twisting of muscles on the part of the nurse.
6. Adjust the bed to a comfortable working height (VHACEOSH, 2016). Assist the patient to a supine position. Place a waterproof pad under the patient at the tube exit site.	Having the bed at the proper height prevents back and muscle strain. The supine position is usually the best way to gain access to the suprapubic urinary catheter. A waterproof pad protects linens and patient from moisture.
7. Put on gloves. Gently remove the old dressing, if one is in place. Place dressing in the trash bag. Remove gloves. Perform hand hygiene.	Gloves prevent contact with blood and body fluids. Proper disposal of contaminated dressing and hand hygiene deter the spread of microorganisms.
8. Assess the exit site and surrounding skin.	Any changes in assessment could indicate potential infection.
9. Put on gloves. Remove one disposable washcloth from the package or wet a washcloth with warm water and apply skin cleanser. **Gently cleanse around the suprapubic exit site (Figure 2).** Remove any encrustations. Alternatively, if this is a new suprapubic catheter, use sterile cotton-tipped applicators and sterile saline to clean the site until the incision has healed. Moisten the applicators with the saline. **Clean in a circular motion from the insertion site outward (Figure 3).**	Gloves prevent contact with blood and body fluids. Using a gentle skin cleanser helps to protect the skin. The exit site is the most common area of skin irritation with a suprapubic catheter. If encrustations are left on the skin, they provide a medium for bacteria and an area of skin irritation.
10. Rinse the area of all cleanser. Pat dry.	The skin needs to be kept dry to prevent any irritation.

(continued on page 778)

Skill 12-12 ▶ Caring for a Suprapubic Urinary Catheter *(continued)*

ACTION

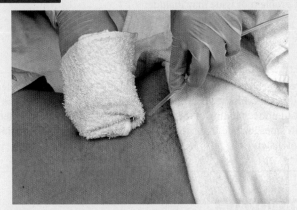

FIGURE 2. Cleaning area around catheter site with skin cleanser and water.

11. If the exit site has been draining, place a small drain sponge around the catheter to absorb any drainage (Figure 4). Be prepared to change this sponge throughout the day, depending on the amount of drainage. Do not cut a 4 × 4 gauze to make a drain sponge.

12. Remove gloves. Perform hand hygiene. Form a loop in the tubing and anchor it on the patient's abdomen with a catheter fixation device or tape (Holroyd, 2019) (Figure 5).

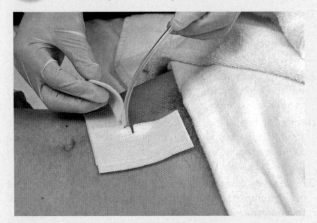

FIGURE 4. Applying small drain sponge around catheter.

13. Assist the patient to a comfortable position. Cover the patient with bed linens. Place the bed in the lowest position.

14. Put on gloves. Remove or discard equipment and assess the patient's response to the procedure.

15. Remove gloves and additional PPE, if used. Perform hand hygiene.

RATIONALE

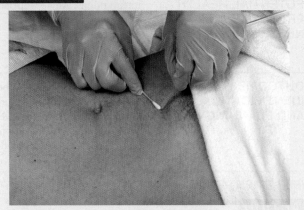

FIGURE 3. Using a sterile cotton-tipped applicator for cleaning.

A small amount of drainage from the exit site is normal. The sponge needs to be changed when it becomes soiled to prevent skin irritation and breakdown. The fibers from a cut 4 × 4 gauze may enter the exit site and cause irritation or infection.

Proper removal of gloves and hand hygiene deter the spread of microorganisms. Anchoring the catheter and tubing absorbs any tugging, preventing tension on, and irritation to, the skin or bladder (Queensland Spinal Cord Injuries Service, 2019).

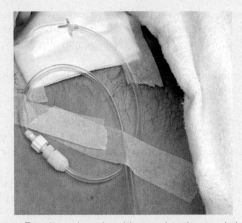

FIGURE 5. Forming a loop in tubing and taping to abdomen.

Positioning and covering provide warmth and promote comfort. The bed in the lowest position promotes patient safety.

Gloves prevent contact with blood and body fluids. The patient's response may indicate acceptance of the catheter or the need for health teaching.

Proper removal of PPE reduces the risk for infection transmission and contamination of other items. Hand hygiene prevents the spread of microorganisms.

EVALUATION

The expected outcomes have been met when the patient's skin has remained clean, dry, intact, and without evidence of irritation or breakdown; the patient has verbalized an understanding of the purpose for, and care of, the catheter, as appropriate; the patient's urinary elimination has been maintained; and the patient's bladder has not distended.

DOCUMENTATION

Guidelines

Document the appearance of the catheter exit site and surrounding skin, urine amount and characteristics, and the patient's reaction to the procedure.

Sample Documentation

> 7/12/25 1845 Suprapubic catheter care performed. Patient assisted in care. Skin is slightly erythematous on right side where catheter was taped. Catheter taped to left side. Small amount of yellow, clear drainage noted on drain sponge. Patient would like to try to go without drain sponge at this time. Instructions given to call nurse if amount of drainage increases. Moderate amount of clear yellow urine continues to drain from catheter into collection bag.
>
> —B. Clapp, RN

DEVELOPING CLINICAL REASONING AND CLINICAL JUDGMENT

UNEXPECTED SITUATIONS AND ASSOCIATED INTERVENTIONS

- *When cleaning the site, the catheter becomes dislodged and pulls out:* Notify the health care team. It takes approximately 4 weeks for the suprapubic tract to become established, the time at which it can be safely changed (SUNA, 2016). The site of insertion can close fairly quickly prior to the establishment of the tract, so prompt attention is needed (Mount Sinai, 2019; Queensland Spinal Cord Injuries Service, 2019). If this is a well-healed site, the health care provider or advanced practice nurse can replace a new catheter easily. If this is a new suprapubic tube, the primary care provider may want to assess for any trauma to the bladder wall.
- *Exit site is extremely excoriated:* Consult the wound, ostomy, and incontinence nurse for evaluation. A skin protectant or barrier may need to be applied as well as more frequent cleansing of the area and changing of the drain sponge (if applied).

SPECIAL CONSIDERATIONS

- Depending on the patient's situation, they may have both a suprapubic and indwelling urethral catheter. Urine will drain from both catheters; usually, drainage from the suprapubic catheter is the larger volume.
- If the suprapubic catheter is not draining into the bag but, instead, has a valve at the end of the catheter, open the valve at least every 6 hours (or more frequently depending on the prescribed intervention in the health record or institutional policy) to drain the urine from the bladder.
- Powder, creams, or sprays should not be used at the insertion site (Mount Sinai, 2019; Queensland Spinal Cord Injuries Service, 2019).
- Encourage patients to drink adequate fluids to keep the urine clear and free flowing (Mount Sinai, 2019; Queensland Spinal Cord Injuries Service, 2019).
- Keep the drainage bag below the insertion site level to prevent backflow of urine into the bladder (Mount Sinai, 2019; Queensland Spinal Cord Injuries Service, 2019).

Skill 12-13 ▶ Caring for a Peritoneal Dialysis Catheter

Peritoneal dialysis is a method of removing fluid and wastes from the body of a patient with kidney failure, using blood vessels in the abdominal lining (peritoneum) to fill in for the kidneys, with the help of a special fluid (dialysate) washed in and out of the peritoneal space. A catheter (a thin, soft silicone rubber tube) inserted through the abdominal wall into the peritoneal cavity allows dialysate to be infused and then drained from the body (Figure 1). The exit site should be protected and kept clean and dry to allow for healing, which may take up to 6 weeks (Bridger, 2019). Daily exit-site dressing changes are not started for 2 weeks, with dressings only reinforced if needed to minimize catheter manipulation (George, 2019a). Once the exit site has healed, routine exit-site care is provided daily (George, 2019a). The catheter insertion site is a site for potential infection, possibly leading to catheter tunnel infection and **peritonitis**; therefore, meticulous care is needed. The incidence of exit-site infections can be reduced through a cleansing regimen by the patient or caregiver. Until the site is healed care is performed using aseptic technique, to reduce the risk for a health care–acquired infection. Once healed, clean technique can be used by the patient and caregivers.

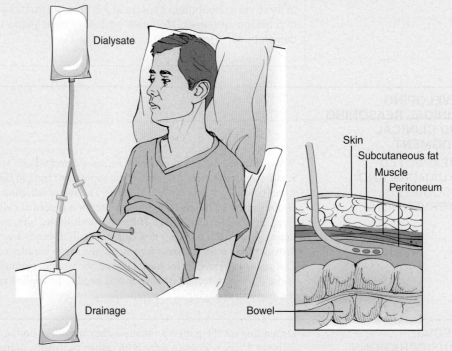

FIGURE 1. Position of catheter in peritoneal space. Patient is set up for peritoneal dialysis.

DELEGATION CONSIDERATIONS

The care of a peritoneal dialysis catheter is not delegated to assistive personnel (AP). Depending on the state's nurse practice act and the organization's policies and procedures, care of a peritoneal dialysis catheter may be delegated to licensed practical/vocational nurses (LPN/LVNs). The decision to delegate must be based on careful analysis of the patient's needs and circumstances as well as the qualifications of the person to whom the task is being delegated. Refer to the Delegation Guidelines in Appendix A.

EQUIPMENT

- Face masks (2)
- Sterile gloves
- Nonsterile gloves
- Additional PPE, as indicated
- Antimicrobial cleansing agent, per facility policy
- Sterile gauze squares (4)
- Sterile basin
- Sterile drain sponge
- Transparent, occlusive site dressing
- Topical antimicrobial, such as mupirocin or gentamicin, depending on prescribed interventions and facility policy
- Sterile applicator
- Plastic trash bag
- Bath blanket

ASSESSMENT	Inspect the peritoneal dialysis catheter exit site for any erythema, drainage, bleeding, tenderness, swelling, skin irritation or breakdown, or leakage. These signs could indicate exit-site or tunnel infection. Assess the abdomen for tenderness, pain, and guarding. Assess the patient for nausea, vomiting, and fever, which could indicate peritonitis. Assess the patient's knowledge about measures used to care for the exit site.
ACTUAL OR POTENTIAL HEALTH PROBLEMS AND NEEDS	Many actual or potential health problems or issues may require the use of this skill as part of related interventions. An appropriate health problem or issue may include: • Altered skin integrity risk • Knowledge deficiency • Infection risk
OUTCOME IDENTIFICATION AND PLANNING	The expected outcomes to achieve when performing care for a peritoneal dialysis catheter are that the peritoneal dialysis catheter dressing change is completed using aseptic technique without trauma to the site or patient; the site is clean, dry, intact, and without evidence of inflammation or infection; and the patient participates in self-care, as appropriate.

IMPLEMENTATION

ACTION

RATIONALE

1. Review the patient's health record for prescribed interventions related to catheter site care. Gather equipment.

This ensures appropriate interventions for the patient. Assembling equipment provides for an organized approach to the task.

 2. Perform hand hygiene and put on PPE, if indicated.

Hand hygiene and PPE prevent the spread of microorganisms. PPE is required based on transmission precautions.

 3. Identify the patient.

Identifying the patient ensures the right patient receives the intervention and helps prevent errors.

4. Close the curtains around the bed and close the door to the room, if possible. Explain to the patient what you are going to do and why. Encourage the patient to observe or participate, if possible.

This ensures the patient's privacy. Discussion promotes engagement and helps to minimize anxiety. Having the patient observe or assist encourages self-acceptance.

5. Assemble equipment on the overbed table or other surface within reach.

Arranging items nearby is convenient, saves time, and prevents unnecessary stretching and twisting of muscles on the part of the nurse.

6. Adjust the bed to a comfortable working height (VHACEOSH, 2016). Assist the patient to a supine position. Expose the abdomen, draping the patient's chest with the bath blanket, exposing only the catheter site.

Having the bed at the proper height prevents back and muscle strain. The supine position is usually the best way to gain access to the peritoneal dialysis catheter. Use of a bath blanket provides patient warmth and prevents unnecessary exposure.

7. Put on nonsterile gloves. Put on one of the facemasks; have the patient put on the other mask.

Gloves protect the nurse from contact with blood and bodily fluids. Use of facemasks deters the spread of microorganisms.

8. Gently remove old dressing, noting odor, amount, and color of drainage; leakage; and condition of the skin around the catheter. Discard the dressing in an appropriate container.

Drainage, leakage, and skin condition can indicate problems with the catheter, such as infection.

(continued on page 782)

Skill 12-13 ▶ Caring for a Peritoneal Dialysis Catheter *(continued)*

ACTION	RATIONALE
9. Remove gloves and discard. Perform hand hygiene. Set up a sterile field. Open the packages. Using aseptic technique, place two sterile gauze squares in the basin with an antimicrobial agent. Leave two sterile gauze squares opened on the sterile field. Alternatively (based on facility's policy), place sterile antimicrobial swabs on the sterile field. Place the sterile applicator on the field. Squeeze a small amount of the topical antimicrobial on one of the gauze squares on the sterile field.	Hand hygiene prevents the spread of microorganisms. Until the catheter site has healed, aseptic technique is necessary for site care to prevent infection.
10. Put on sterile gloves. Pick up the dialysis catheter with your nondominant hand. **With the antimicrobial- or sterile normal saline-soaked gauze/swab, cleanse the skin around the exit site using a circular motion, starting at the exit site and then slowly going outward 2 inches** (Bridger, 2019). Scabs or crusts should never be removed forcibly to avoid creating open areas susceptible to infection (George, 2019a).	Aseptic technique is necessary to prevent infection. The antimicrobial agent cleanses the skin and removes any drainage or crust from the wound, reducing the risk for infection.
11. **Continue to hold the catheter with your nondominant hand.** After the skin has dried, clean the catheter with an antimicrobial-soaked gauze, beginning at the exit site, going around the catheter, and then moving up to end of the catheter. Gently remove crusted secretions on the tube, if necessary.	Movement of the catheter should be minimal in the immediate postoperative period (Bridger, 2019). Antimicrobial agents cleanse the catheter and remove any drainage or crust from the tube, reducing the risk for infection.
12. Using the sterile applicator, apply the prescribed topical antimicrobial to the catheter exit site.	Application of topical antimicrobial at the catheter exit site prevents exit-site infection and peritonitis (Bridger, 2019; George, 2019b; National Kidney Foundation, 2019; Szeto et al., 2017).
13. Place a sterile drain sponge around the exit site. Then place a 4 × 4 gauze over the exit site. Cover it with a dressing. Remove gloves and then masks. Perform hand hygiene.	The drain sponge and 4 × 4 gauze are used to absorb any drainage from the exit site. Occlusion of the site with a dressing deters site contamination. Once the site is covered, masks and gloves are no longer necessary. Hand hygiene prevents the spread of microorganisms.
14. Label the dressing with the date, time of change, and your initials.	Other personnel working with the catheter will know information related to site care.
15. Coil the exposed length of tubing and anchor the catheter to the patient's abdomen with tape or a commercial device (Bridger, 2019; George, 2019b).	Anchoring the catheter absorbs any tugging, preventing tension on, and irritation to, the skin or abdomen.
16. Assist the patient to a comfortable position. Cover the patient with bed linens. Place the bed in the lowest position.	Positioning and covering provide warmth and promote comfort. A bed in the low position promotes patient safety.
17. Put on gloves. Remove or discard equipment and assess the patient's response to the procedure.	These actions deter the spread of microorganisms. The patient's response may indicate acceptance of the catheter or the need for health teaching.
18. Remove gloves and additional PPE, if used. Perform hand hygiene.	Proper removal of PPE reduces the risk for infection transmission and contamination of other items. Hand hygiene prevents the spread of microorganisms.

EVALUATION The expected outcomes have been met when the peritoneal dialysis catheter dressing change has been completed using aseptic technique without trauma to the site or to the patient; the site has remained clean, dry, intact, and without evidence of redness, irritation, or excoriation; the patient's fluid balance has been maintained; and the patient has verbalized appropriate measures to care for the site.

DOCUMENTATION

Guidelines

Document the dressing change, including the condition of the skin surrounding the exit site, drainage, or odor; the patient's reaction to the procedure; and any patient teaching provided.

Sample Documentation

> <u>8/22/25</u> 1530 Peritoneal dialysis catheter dressing changed; skin surrounding catheter slightly erythematous but remains intact. Small amount of clear drainage, approximately the size of a dime without odor, noted on drain sponge. Patient asking appropriate questions regarding dressing change. Verbalized an understanding of explanations.
>
> —B. Clapp, RN

DEVELOPING CLINICAL REASONING AND CLINICAL JUDGMENT

UNEXPECTED SITUATIONS AND ASSOCIATED INTERVENTIONS

- *Patient reports pain when you palpate the abdomen; purulent or cloudy drainage is present, site is red or swollen, or foul odor is noted when old dressing is removed:* Notify the health care team immediately (George, 2019b). Any of these signs could indicate a site infection or peritonitis.
- *You note that the old dressing is saturated with clear fluid:* Replace the dressing to prevent skin breakdown. Notify the health care team. A frequent complication is leakage from the exit site. Frequently check the dressing, especially after the patient has had solution placed in the abdominal cavity.

SPECIAL CONSIDERATIONS

General Considerations

- Instruct patients to avoid showering for 2 to 3 weeks, until the site has healed; site care should be performed after every shower (Bridger, 2019; George, 2019b; National Kidney Foundation, 2019).
- Remind patients performing their own site care of the importance of good handwashing before self-care (George, 2019a; National Kidney Foundation, 2019; NIDDK, 2018a).
- Discourage patients from wearing tight clothes and belts around the exit site.

Community-Based Care Considerations

- Once the catheter site is healed, clean technique can be used by the patient and caregivers.
- Teach patients the signs of exit-site infection and encourage them to contact their health care team for prompt intervention.

Skill 12-14 ▶ Caring for a Hemodialysis Access (Arteriovenous Fistula or Graft)

Hemodialysis, a mechanical way of filtering waste products and excess electrolytes from the blood, requires access to the patient's vascular system to remove and return blood from the patient's body. This vascular access, an arteriovenous (AV) fistula or AV graft, allows for access to the bloodstream. A temporary or permanent double-lumen central venous catheter can also be used to provide vascular access for hemodialysis (ANNA, 2018). If a catheter is used (Figure 1 on page 784), the site is cared for in the same manner as a central venous access device (see Skill 16-7). An **arteriovenous fistula** is a surgically created passage that connects an artery and vein (Figure 2 on page 784). An **arteriovenous graft** is a surgically created connection between an artery and vein using a synthetic material (Figure 3 on page 784). Accessing a hemodialysis arteriovenous graft or fistula is done only by specially trained health care team members.

(continued on page 784)

Skill 12-14 ▶ Caring for a Hemodialysis Access (Arteriovenous Fistula or Graft) *(continued)*

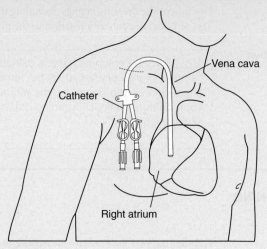

FIGURE 1. Central catheter for hemodialysis.

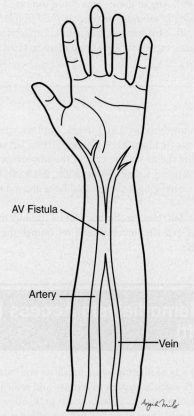

FIGURE 2. Arteriovenous fistula for hemodialysis.

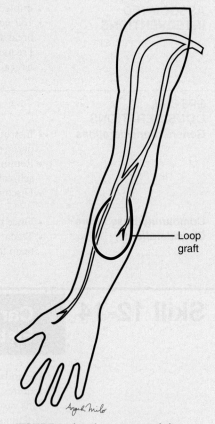

FIGURE 3. Arteriovenous graft for hemodialysis.

DELEGATION CONSIDERATIONS

The assessment of, and care for, a hemodialysis access is not delegated to assistive personnel (AP). Depending on the state's nurse practice act and the organization's policies and procedures, these procedures may be delegated to licensed practical/vocational nurses (LPN/LVNs). The decision to delegate must be based on careful analysis of the patient's needs and circumstances as well as the qualifications of the person to whom the task is being delegated. Refer to the Delegation Guidelines in Appendix A.

EQUIPMENT

- Stethoscope
- PPE, as indicated

ASSESSMENT

Ask the patient how much they know about caring for the site. Ask the patient to describe important observations to be made. Note the location of the access site. Assess the site for signs of infection, including inflammation, edema, and drainage, and for healing of the incision. Assess for patency by assessing for presence of bruit and thrill (refer to the explanation in Step 4).

ACTUAL OR POTENTIAL HEALTH PROBLEMS AND NEEDS

Many actual or potential health problems or issues may require the use of this skill as part of related interventions. An appropriate health problem or issue may include:
- Altered skin integrity risk
- Knowledge deficiency
- Infection risk

OUTCOME IDENTIFICATION AND PLANNING

The expected outcomes to achieve when caring for a hemodialysis catheter are that the graft or fistula remains patent, the patient verbalizes appropriate care measures and observations to be made, and the patient demonstrates appropriate care measures.

IMPLEMENTATION

ACTION

RATIONALE

1. Perform hand hygiene and put on PPE, if indicated.

Hand hygiene and PPE prevent the spread of microorganisms. PPE is required based on transmission precautions.

2. Identify the patient.

Identifying the patient ensures the right patient receives the intervention and helps prevent errors.

3. Close the curtains around the bed and close the door to the room, if possible. Explain to the patient what you are going to do and why.

This ensures the patient's privacy. Explanation relieves anxiety and facilitates engagement.

4. Question the patient about the presence of muscle weakness and cramping; changes in temperature; and sensations, such as numbness, tingling, pain, burning, itchiness; and pain.

This aids in determining the patency of the hemodialysis access as well as the presence of complications.

5. Inspect the area over the access site for continuity of skin color. Inspect for any redness, warmth, tenderness, edema, rash, blemishes, bleeding, tremors, and twitches. Inspect the muscle strength and the patient's ability to perform range of motion in the extremity/body part with the hemodialysis access.

Inspection aids in determining the patency of the hemodialysis access as well as the status of the patient's circulatory, neurologic, and muscular function and presence of infection. Compare with the opposite body area/part.

6. Put on gloves if the site is not completely healed. Palpate over the access site, feeling for a **thrill** or pulse/vibration (Morton & Fontaine, 2018) (Figure 4). Palpate pulses above and below the site. Palpate the continuity of the skin temperature along and around the extremity. Check capillary refill in fingers or toes of the extremity with the fistula or graft.

Gloves prevent contact with blood and body fluids. Palpation aids in determining the patency of the hemodialysis access as well as the status of the patient's circulatory, neurologic, and muscular function and presence of infection. Compare with the opposite body area/part.

7. Remove gloves and perform hand hygiene. Auscultate over the access site with the bell of the stethoscope, listening for a **bruit** or swishing/blowing (Morton & Fontaine, 2018).

Proper removal of gloves and hand hygiene prevents the spread of microorganisms. Palpation aids in determining the patency of the hemodialysis access.

(continued on page 786)

Skill 12-14 ▶ Caring for a Hemodialysis Access (Arteriovenous Fistula or Graft) *(continued)*

ACTION	RATIONALE

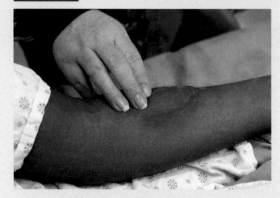

FIGURE 4. Palpating access site for thrill.

8. Ensure that a sign is placed over the head of the bed informing the health care team which arm is affected. **Do not measure blood pressure, perform a venipuncture, or start an IV on the access arm** (National Kidney Foundation, 2017).

The affected arm should not be used for any other procedures, such as obtaining blood pressure, which could lead to clotting of the graft or fistula. Venipuncture or IV access could lead to an infection of the affected arm and could cause the loss of the graft or fistula.

9. Instruct the patient not to sleep with the arm with the access site under the head or body (National Kidney Foundation, 2017).

This could lead to clotting of the fistula or graft.

10. Instruct the patient not to lift heavy objects with, or put pressure on, the arm with the access site. Advise the patient not to carry heavy bags (including purses) on the shoulder of that arm (National Kidney Foundation, 2017).

This could lead to clotting of the fistula or graft.

11. Remove PPE, if used. Perform hand hygiene.

Proper removal of PPE reduces the risk for infection transmission and contamination of other items. Hand hygiene prevents the spread of microorganisms.

EVALUATION

The expected outcomes have been met when the access site has an audible bruit and a palpable thrill, the site has remained intact without signs of adverse complications or pain, and the patient has verbalized appropriate information about caring for the access site and observations to be made.

DOCUMENTATION

Guidelines

Document assessment findings, including the presence or absence of a bruit and thrill. Document any patient education and patient response.

Sample Documentation

5/10/25 0830 Arteriovenous fistula patent in left upper arm. Area without redness, pain, or edema; skin at site similar to surrounding skin tone. Patient denies pain and tenderness. Positive bruit and thrill noted. Patient verbalized understanding the importance of avoiding venipuncture in left arm.

—B. Clapp, RN

DEVELOPING CLINICAL REASONING AND CLINICAL JUDGMENT

UNEXPECTED SITUATIONS AND ASSOCIATED INTERVENTIONS

- *Thrill is diminished or not palpable and/or bruit is diminished or not audible:* Notify the health care team. The thrill and bruit are caused by arterial blood flowing into the vein. If these signs are not present, the access may be clotting off.
- *Site is warm to touch, erythematous, or painful or has a skin blemish:* Notify the health care team. These signs can indicate a site infection.

SPECIAL CONSIDERATIONS

- Teach patients the importance of not wearing tight clothes or jewelry on the access arm and avoiding carrying or doing anything that would put pressure on the access (National Kidney Foundation, 2017).
- Patients should be aware that they should not allow anyone to use a blood pressure cuff on the access arm or let anyone draw blood from the access arm (NIDDK, 2018b).
- Teach patients to check the pulse (thrill) in the access every day (Latif, 2018).
- Teach patients to be aware of signs of possible complications and to call their health care provider right away if they notice any of these problems (Latif, 2018):
  - Bleeding from the vascular access site
  - Signs of infection (redness, swelling, soreness, pain, warmth, pus around site)
  - Fever ≥100.3°F
  - Pulse (thrill) in the access slowing down or not present
  - Access arm swelling
  - Hand on the access arm getting cold, numb, or weak

EVIDENCE FOR PRACTICE ▶

HEMODIALYSIS AND PATIENT FATIGUE

Patients receiving chronic hemodialysis experience troubling symptoms that cause distress and anxiety, and adversely affect their quality of life. Fatigue is common and can be debilitating. How can nurses assist patients in dealing with this issue?

Related Research

Karadag, E., & Baglama, S. S. (2019). The effect of aromatherapy on fatigue and anxiety in patients undergoing hemodialysis treatment. A randomized controlled study. *Holistic Nursing Practice, 33*(4), 222–229. https://doi.org/10.1097/HNP.0000000000000334

The aim of this randomized-controlled study was to examine the effect of the application of lavender oil on fatigue and anxiety levels in patients undergoing hemodialysis treatment. A power analysis determined that 60 participants were needed. The participants were randomly assigned to the intervention ($n = 30$) and control groups ($n = 30$). Patients in both groups completed the Fatigue Severity Scale (FSS) and Beck Anxiety Inventory (BAI) on the initial day of the study. Patients in the intervention group inhaled 2% lavender oil for 20 minutes before hemodialysis during weekly (2 to 3 days/week) hemodialysis sessions for 30 days. Patients in the control group underwent routine care during hemodialysis without the application of lavender oil for 30 days. The FSS and BAI were completed by participants in both groups at the end of day 30. There was no significant difference ($p = .208$) between pretest–posttest scores of FSS in the control group, with a significant increase in anxiety levels at the end of the 30 days ($p = .001$). In the intervention group, a statistically significant difference was identified between pretest and posttest scores of the FSS ($p = .001$) and the BAI ($p = .001$). Comparison of the FSS and BAI scores of the patients in the control and intervention groups before and after the intervention revealed a statistically significant difference in favor of the intervention group ($p < .05$). The researchers concluded that lavender aromatherapy decreased fatigue and anxiety levels in patients undergoing hemodialysis. The researchers suggested lavender aromatherapy should be considered as an effective nursing intervention to reduce the fatigue and anxiety of patients undergoing hemodialysis treatment.

Relevance to Nursing Practice

This information can be valuable to nurses caring for these patients and may be useful in planning evidence-based nursing interventions to support patients with fatigue and anxiety. The information can also be used to plan and implement appropriate patient education related to the fatigue and anxiety associated with hemodialysis; devising ways to manage symptoms is important to improve quality of life.

Enhance Your Understanding

Focusing on Patient Care: Developing Clinical Reasoning and Clinical Judgment

Consider the case scenarios at the beginning of the chapter as you answer the following questions to enhance your understanding and apply what you have learned.

QUESTIONS

1. When checking Ralph Bellow's external urinary sheath, you notice that, although the sheath is still in place, Mr. Bellow's bed is soaked with urine and there is very little urine in the catheter tubing. What should you do?

2. Grace Halligan is asking to go to the bathroom; they say, "I don't think I can go on a bedpan." You recheck the prescribed interventions and notice that Ms. Halligan is on strict bed rest. How can you help alleviate her concerns about using a bedpan?

3. Mike Wimmer notices that his peritoneal dialysis catheter insertion site is reddened and tender. He phones to ask what should be done. What should you tell Mike?

You can find suggested answers after the Bibliography at the end of this chapter.

Integrated Case Study Connection

The case studies in the back of the book focus on integrating concepts. Refer to the following case studies to enhance your understanding of the concepts and skills in this chapter.

- Basic Case Studies: Tiffany Jones, page 1195.
- Intermediate Case Studies: Lucille Howard, page 1219.
- Advanced Case Studies: Robert Espinoza, page 1230.

Bibliography

Agency for Healthcare Research and Quality (AHRQ). (2020, October). *Toolkit for reducing catheter-associated urinary tract infections in hospital units: Implementation guide.* Appendix C. Sample bladder scan policy. https://www.ahrq.gov/hai/cauti-tools/impl-guide/implementation-guide-appendix-c.html

American Association of Critical-Care Nurses (AACN). (2016, August 1). *Prevention of CAUTI in adults.* https://www.aacn.org/clinical-resources/practice-alerts/prevention-of-cauti-in-adults

American Cancer Society. (2019, October 16). *Caring for a urostomy.* https://www.cancer.org/treatment/treatments-and-side-effects/treatment-types/surgery/ostomies/urostomy/management.html

American Nephrology Nurses Association (ANNA). (2018). *Vascular access fact sheet.* https://www.annanurse.org/download/reference/practice/vascularAccessFactSheet.pdf

American Nephrology Nurses Association (ANNA). (2019). *Peritoneal dialysis fact sheet.* https://www.annanurse.org/download/reference/practice/pdFactSheet.pdf

American Nurses Association (ANA). (n.d.). *ANA CAUTI Prevention Tool.* Retrieved December 16, 2020, from https://www.nursingworld.org/practice-policy/work-environment/health-safety/infection-prevention/ana-cauti-prevention-tool/

American Nurses Association (ANA). (2014). *Streamlined evidence-based RN tool: Catheter associated urinary tract infection (CAUTI) prevention.* https://www.nursingworld.org/~4aede8/globalassets/practiceandpolicy/innovation-evidence/clinical-practice-material/cauti-prevention-tool/anacautipreventiontool-final-19dec2014.pdf

Balhi, S., & Mrabet, M. K. (2020). Teaching patients clean intermittent self-catheterisation: Key points. *British Journal of Community Nursing, 25*(12), 586–593.

Bardsley, A. (2015a). Safe and effective catheterization for patients in the community. *British Journal of Community Nursing, 20*(4), 166–172. https://doi.org/10.12968/bjcn.2015.20.4.166

Bardsley, A. (2015b). Assessing and teaching female intermittent self-catheterization. *British Journal of Community Nursing, 20*(7), 344–346. https://doi.org/10.12968/bjcn.2015.20.7.344

Bauldoff, G., Gubrud, P., & Carno, M. A. (2020). *LeMone and Burke's Medical-surgical nursing: Clinical reasoning in patient care* (7th ed.). Pearson.

Beauchemin, L., Newman, D. K., Le Danseur, M., Jackson, A., & Ritmiller, M. (2018). Best practices for clean intermittent catheterization. *Nursing, 48*(9), 49–54. https://doi.org/10.1097/01.NURSE.0000544216.23783.bc

Becton Dickinson and Company (BD). (2020). *BD PureWick™ Urine Collection System. How it works.* https://www.purewickathome.com/purewick-how-it-works/

Beeson, T., & Davis, C. (2018). Urinary management with an external female collection device. *Journal of Wound, Ostomy and Continence Nursing, 45*(2), 187–189. https://doi.org/10.1097/WON.0000000000000417

Belizario, S. M. (2015). Preventing urinary tract infections with a two-person catheter insertion procedure. *Nursing, 45*(3), 67–69. https://doi.org/10.1097/01.NURSE.0000460736.74021.69

Berti-Hearn, L., & Elliott, B. (2019). Urostomy care. A guide for home care clinicians. *Home Healthcare Now, 37*(5), 248–255.

Bridger, S. (2019). Peritoneal dialysis access management: More than skin deep. *The Canadian Association of Nephrology Nurses and Technologists Journal, 29*(4), 11–19.

Buehrle, D. J., Clancy, C. J., & Decker, B. K. (2020). Suprapubic catheter placement improves antimicrobial stewardship among Veterans Affairs nursing care facility residents. *American Journal of Infection Control, 48*(10), 1264–1266. DOI: 10.1016/j.ajic.2020.01.005

Burch, J. (2018). Stoma-related complications and treatments. *Nursing & Residential Care, 20*(9), 430–433. https://doi.org/10.12968/nrec.2018.20.9.430

Burch, J. (2019a). Supporting residents to care for a stoma independently. *Nursing and Residential Care, 21*(5), 276–280. https://doi.org/10.12968/nrec.2019.21.5.276

Burch, J. (2019b). Peristomal skin care considerations for community nurses. *British Journal of Community Nursing, 24*(9), 414–418. https://doi.org/10.12968/bjcn.2019.24.9.414

Butler, D. L. (2009). Early postoperative complications following ostomy surgery. *Journal of Wound, Ostomy and Continence Nursing, 36*(5), 513–519.

Centers for Disease Control and Prevention (CDC). (2015, October). *Healthcare-associated infections (HAIs). Catheter-associated urinary tract infections (CAUTI).* https://www.cdc.gov/hai/ca_uti/uti.html

Centers for Disease Control and Prevention (CDC). (2019, November 21). *CDC/STRIVE infection control training. Targeted prevention strategies. Catheter-associated urinary tract infection (CAUTI)—WB4222. CAUTI 103: Alternatives to the indwelling urinary catheter.* https://www.cdc.gov/infectioncontrol/training/strive.html#anchor_CAUTI

Collier, M. (2019). Minimising pain and medical adhesive related skin injuries in vulnerable patients. *British Journal of Nursing, 28*(15), S26–S32. doi: 10.12968/bjon.2019.28.15.S26

Collins, L. (2019). Intermittent self-catheterisation: Good patient education and support are key. *British Journal of Nursing, 28*(15), 964–966. https://doi.org/10.12968/bjon.2019.28.15.964

Dean, J., & Ostaszkiewicz, J. (2019). Current evidence about catheter maintenance solutions for management of catheter blockage in long-term urinary catheterisation. *Australian and New Zealand Continence Journal, 25*(3), 74–80.

Dublynn, T., & Episcopia, B. (2019). Female external catheter use: A new bundle element to reduce CAUTI [Poster Presentation]. APIC 46th Annual Educational Conference & International Meeting. In: *American Journal of Infection Control, 47*(Supplement), S39–S40. https://doi.org/10.1016/j.ajic.2019.04.093

Eliopoulos, C. (2018). *Gerontological nursing* (9th ed.). Wolters Kluwer Health.

Engberg, S., Clapper, J., McNichol, L., Thompson, D., Welch, V. W., & Gray, M. (2020). Current evidence related to intermittent catheterization. *Journal of Wound, Ostomy and Continence Nursing, 47*(2), 140–165. https://doi.org/10.1097/WON.0000000000000625

Fasugba, O., Cheng, A. S., Gregory, V., Graves, N., Koerner, J., Collignon, P., Gardner, A., & Mitchell, B. G. (2019). Chlorhexidine for meatal cleaning in reducing catheter-associated urinary tract infections: A multicentre stepped-wedge randomised controlled trial. *Lancet Infectious Diseases, 19*(6), 611–619. https://doi.org/10.1016/S1473-3099(18)30736-9

Fischbach, F. T., & Fischbach, M. A. (2018). *A manual of laboratory and diagnostic tests* (10th ed.). Wolters Kluwer.

Fletcher-Gutowski, S., & Cecil, J. (2019). Is 2-person urinary catheter insertion effective in reducing CAUTI? *American Journal of Infection Control, 47*(12), 1508–1509. https://doi.org/10.1016/j.ajic.2019.05.014

Gattinger, H., Werner, B., & Saxer, S. (2013). Patient experience with bedpans in acute care: A cross-sectional study. *Journal of Clinical Nursing, 22*(15–16), 2216–2224. https://doi.org/10.1111/jocn.12203

Gentile, P., Jacob, J., & Ashraf, S. (2020). Implementation of a female external urinary catheter reduces indwelling urinary catheter use and catheter-associated urinary tract infections [Poster presentation]. Sixth Decennial International Conference on Healthcare-Associated Infections, Atlanta, GA. In: *Infection Control & Hospital Epidemiology, 41*(S1), S482–S483. https://doi.org/10.1017/ice.2020.1158

George, C. (2019a). Caring for patients receiving peritoneal dialysis: Part I. *MedSurg Nursing, 28*(4), 227–233.

George, C. (2019b). Caring for patients receiving peritoneal dialysis: Part II. *MedSurg Nursing, 28*(5), 287–292.

Gibson, K. E., Neill, S., Tuma, E., Meddings, J., & Mody, L. (2019). Indwelling urethral versus suprapubic catheters in nursing home residents: Determining the safest option for long-term use. *Journal of Hospital Infection, 102*(), 219–225. https://doi.org/10.1016/j.jhin.2018.07.027

Gill, B. C., Firoozi, F., & Rackley, R. R. (2018, June 20). *Injectable bulking agents for incontinence*. Medscape. https://emedicine.medscape.com/article/447068-overview

Goldberg, M., Colwell, J., Burns, S., Carmel, J., Fellows, J., Hendren, S., Livingston, V., Nottingham, C. U., Pittman, J., Rafferty, J., Salvadalena, G., Steinberg, G., & Wound, Ostomy and Continence Nurses Society. Guideline Development Task Force. (2018). WOCN Society Clinical Guideline. Management of the adult patient with a fecal or urinary ostomy—An executive summary. *Journal of Wound, Ostomy and Continence Nursing, 45*(1), 50–58. https://doi.org/10.1097/WON.0000000000000396

Gould, C. V., Umscheid, C. A., Agarwal, R. K., Kuntz, G., Pegues, D. A., & the Healthcare Infection Control Practices Advisory Committee (HICPAC). (2019 [update]). Guideline for prevention of catheter-associated urinary tract infections 2009. *Centers for Disease Control and Prevention, 31*(4). https://www.cdc.gov/infectioncontrol/pdf/guidelines/cauti-guidelines-H.pdf

Gray, M., Skinner, C., & Kaler, W. (2016). External collection devices as an alternative to the indwelling urinary catheter. Evidence-based review and expert clinical panel deliberations. *Journal of Wound Ostomy and Continence Nursing, 43*(3), 301–307. https://doi.org/10.1097/WON.0000000000000220

Gyesi-Appiah, E., Brown, J., & Clifton, A. (2020). Short-term urinary catheters and their risks: An integrated review. *British Journal of Community Nursing, 25*(11), 538–544. doi: 10.12968/bjcn.2020.25.11.538

Herter, R., & Kazer, M. W. (2010). Best practices in urinary catheter care. *Home Healthcare Nurse, 28*(6), 342–349. https://doi.org/10.1097/NHH.0b013e3181df5d79

Hill, B. (2020). Stoma care: Procedures, appliances, and nursing considerations. *British Journal of Nursing, 29*(22) (Stoma Care Supplement), S14–S19. https://doi.org/10.12968/bjon.2020.29.22.s14

Hill, B., & Mitchell, M. (2018). Urinary catheters. Part 1. *British Journal of Nursing, 27*(21), 1234–1236. https://doi.org/10.12968/bjon.2018.27.21.1234

Hill, B., & Mitchell, A. (2020). Catheter application in the care home. *Nursing and Residential Care, 22*(4), 1–8. https://doi.org/10.12968/nrec.2020.22.4.9

Holroyd, S. (2019). The importance of indwelling urinary catheter securement. *British Journal of Nursing, 28*(15), 976–977. https://doi.org/10.12968/bjon.2019.28.15.976

Hooton, T. M., Bradley, S. F., Cardenas, D. D., Colgan, R., Geerlings, S. E., Rice, J. C., Saint, S., Schaeffer, A. J., Tambayh, P. A., Tenke, P., Nicolle, L. E., & Infectious Diseases Society of America. (2010). Diagnosis, prevention, and treatment of catheter-associated urinary tract infection in adults: 2009 international clinical practice guidelines from the Infectious Diseases Society of America. *Clinical Infectious Diseases, 50*(5), 625–663. https://doi.org/10.1086/650482

Institute for Healthcare Improvement (IHI). (2011). *How-to guide: Prevent catheter-associated urinary tract infection.* http://www.ihi.org/resources/Pages/Tools/HowtoGuidePreventCatheterAssociatedUrinaryTractInfection.aspx

Jarvis, C., & Echkardt, A. (2020). *Physical examination & health assessment* (8th ed.). Elsevier.

Jensen, S. (2019). *Nursing health assessment. A best practice approach* (3rd ed.). Wolters Kluwer.

Kaiser Permanente. (2020a, July 17). *Learning about how to use a bedpan.* https://healthy.kaiserpermanente.org/health-wellness/health-encyclopedia/he.learning-about-how-to-use-a-bedpan.abs2394

Kaiser Permanente. (2020b, July 17). *Learning about how to use a urinal.* https://healthy.kaiserpermanente.org/health-wellness/health-encyclopedia/he.learning-about-how-to-use-a-urinal.abs2410

Kaiser Permanente. (2020c, July 17). *Caregiving: Using a bedpan or urinal.* https://healthy.kaiserpermanente.org/health-wellness/health-encyclopedia/he.caregiving-using-a-bedpan-or-urinal.abq1767

Kaiser Permanente. (2020d, July 17). *Caregiving: Using a bedside commode (toilet).* https://healthy.kaiserpermanente.org/health-wellness/health-encyclopedia/he.caregiving-using-a-bedside-commode-toilet.abq1769

Kaiser Permanente. (2020e, July 17). Learning about using a bedside commode. https://healthy.kaiserpermanente.org/health-wellness/health-encyclopedia/he.learning-about-using-a-bedside-commode.abs2388

Karadag, E., & Baglama, S. S. (2019). The effect of aromatherapy on fatigue and anxiety in patients undergoing hemodialysis treatment. A randomized controlled study. *Holistic Nursing Practice, 33*(4), 222–229. https://doi.org/10.1097/HNP.0000000000000334

Kyle, T., & Carman, S. (2021). *Essentials of pediatric nursing* (4th ed.). Wolters Kluwer.

Knill, L., Maduro, R., & Payne, J. E. (2018). Targeting zero CAUTIs. *American Nurse Today, 13*(11), 54–57.

Latif, W. (2018). Taking care of your vascular access for hemodialysis. *MedlinePlus.* https://medlineplus.gov/ency/patientinstructions/000591.htm

Leach, D. (2018). Teaching patients a clean intermittent self-catheterisation technique. *British Journal of Nursing, 27*(6), 296–298. https://doi.org/10.12968/bjon.2018.27.6.296

LeBlanc, K., Whiteley, I., McNichol, L., Salfadalena, G., & Gray, M. (2019). Peristomal medical adhesive-related skin injury. Results of an international consensus meeting. *Journal of Wound, Ostomy and Continence Nursing, 46*(2), 125–136. DOI: 10.1097/WON.0000000000000513

Mangnall, J. (2015). Managing and teaching intermittent catheterisation. *British Journal of Community Nursing, 20*(2), 82–88.

Mayo Foundation for Medical Education and Research (MFMER). (2019a, July 23). *Tests and procedures. Hemodialysis.* https://www.mayoclinic.org/tests-procedures/hemodialysis/about/pac-20384824

Mayo Foundation for Medical Education and Research (MFMER). (2019b, April 24). *Tests and procedures. Peritoneal dialysis.* https://www.mayoclinic.org/tests-procedures/peritoneal-dialysis/about/pac-20384725

Mitchell, M., & Hill, B. (2018). Urinary catheters: Part 2. Catheterisation in males and females. *British Journal of Nursing, 27*(22), 1306–1310. https://doi.org/10.12968/bjon.2018.27.22.1306

Morton, P. G., & Fontaine, D. K. (2018). *Critical care nursing. A holistic approach* (11th ed.). Wolters Kluwer.

Mount Sinai. (2019, January 31). *Suprapubic catheter care.* https://www.mountsinai.org/health-library/selfcare-instructions/suprapubic-catheter-care

National Institute of Diabetes and Digestive and Kidney Diseases (NIDDK). (2014, February). *Urodynamic testing.* https://www.niddk.nih.gov/health-information/diagnostic-tests/urodynamic-testing

National Institute of Diabetes and Digestive and Kidney Diseases (NIDDK). (2018a, January). *Peritoneal dialysis.* https://www.niddk.nih.gov/health-information/kidney-disease/kidney-failure/peritoneal-dialysis

National Institute of Diabetes and Digestive and Kidney Diseases (NIDDK). (2018b, January). *Hemodialysis.* https://www.niddk.nih.gov/health-information/kidney-disease/kidney-failure/hemodialysis

National Kidney Foundation (NKF). (2017, February 3). *Hemodialysis access.* https://www.kidney.org/atoz/content/hemoaccess#:~:text=A%20hemodialysis%20access%2C%20or%20vascular,placed%20by%20a%20minor%20surgery

National Kidney Foundation (NKF). (2019, February 28). *Taking care of your peritoneal dialysis (PD) catheter.* https://www.kidney.org/atoz/content/taking-care-your-peritoneal-dialysis-pd-catheter

National Kidney Foundation (NKF). (2020, July 2). *Peritoneal dialysis. What you need to know.* https://www.kidney.org/atoz/content/peritoneal

Newman, D. K. (2013). *Designs—Indwelling urinary catheters.* UroToday. https://www.urotoday.com/urinary-catheters-home/indwelling-catheters/description/designs.html

Newman, D. K. (2019a). Evidence-based practice guideline. Prompted voiding for individuals with urinary incontinence. *Journal of Gerontological Nursing, 45*(2), 14–26. https://doi.org/10.3928/00989134-20190111-03

Newman, D. K. (2019b, November 28). *Urinary catheters. Intermittent catheters. Description.* UroToday. https://www.urotoday.com/urinary-catheters-home/intermittent-catheters/description/definition-intermittent-catheters.html

Newman, D. K. (2020a). *Bladder health. Types and materials—external urine collection devices.* UroToday. https://www.urotoday.com/library-resources/bladder-health/120651-types-and-materials-external-urine-collection-devices.html

Newman, D. K. (2020b, April 10). *Introduction: External urinary catheters.* UroToday. https://www.urotoday.com/library-resources/bladder-health/120599-introduction-external-urinary-catheters.html

Newman, D. K. (2021). Intermittent self-catheterization patient education checklist. *Urologic Nursing, 41*(2), 97–109. https://doi.org/10.7257/1053-816X.2021.41.2.97

Norris, T. L. (2020). *Porth's essentials of pathophysiology* (5th ed.). Wolters Kluwer.

O'Flynn, S. K. (2018). Care of the stoma: Complications and treatments. *British Journal of Community Nursing, 23*(8), 382–387. doi: 10.12968/bjcn.2018.23.8.382

Palmer, S. J. (2020). Overview of stoma care for community nurses. *British Journal of Community Nursing, 25*(7), 340–344. https://doi.org/10.12968/bjcn.2020.25.7.340

Panchisin, T. L. (2016). Improving outcomes with the ANA CAUTI Prevention Tool. *Nursing, 46*(3), 55–59. https://doi.org/10.1097/01.NURSE.0000480603.14769.d6

Pelling, H., Nzakizwanayo, J., Milo, S., Denham, E. L., MacFarlane, W. M., Bock, L. J., Sutton, J. M., Jones, B. V. (2019). Bacterial biofilm formation on indwelling urethral catheters. *Letters in Applied Microbiology, 68*(4), 277–293. https://doi.org/10.1111/lam.13144

Queensland Spinal Cord Injuries Service. (2019, August). *Fact sheet. Caring for and changing our supra-pubic catheter (SPC).* Queensland Government, Australia. https://www.health.qld.gov.au/__data/assets/pdf_file/0024/422619/spc-care.pdf

Rhone, C., Breiter, Y., Benson, L., Petri, H., Thompson, P., & Murphy, C. (2017). The impact of two-person indwelling urinary catheter insertion in the emergency department using technical and socio-adaptive interventions. *Journal of Clinical Outcomes Management, 24*(10), 451–456.

Schallom, M., Prentice, D., Sona, C., Vyers, K., Arroyo, C., Wessman, B., & Ablordeppey, E. (2020). Accuracy of measuring bladder volumes with ultrasound and bladder scanning. *American Journal of Critical Care, 29*(6), 458–467. https://doi.org/10.4037/ajcc2020741

Shah, S. M. (2019, January 31). *Suprapubic catheter care.* MedlinePlus. https://medlineplus.gov/ency/patientinstructions/000145.htm

Silbert-Flagg, J., & Pillitteri, A. (2018). *Maternal and child health nursing* (8th ed.). Wolters Kluwer.

Smart, C. (2014). Male urinary incontinence and the urinary sheath. *British Journal of Nursing, 23*(9), S20–S25.

Society of Urologic Nurses and Associates (SUNA). (2015). Clinical practice guidelines. *Care of the patient with an indwelling catheter.* [Brochure]. Author.

Society of Urologic Nurses and Associates (SUNA). (2016). Clinical practice guidelines. *Suprapubic catheter replacement.* [Brochure]. Author.

Society of Urologic Nurses and Associates (SUNA). (2021a). Clinical practice procedure. Urinary catheterization of the adult female. *Urologic Nursing, 41*(2), 65–69. https://www.suna.org/resource/urinary-catheter-care

Society of Urologic Nurses and Associates (SUNA). (2021b). Clinical practice procedure. Insertion of an indwelling urethral catheter in the adult female. *Urologic Nursing, 41*(2), 76–109. https://www.suna.org/download/catheterInsertionFemaleCCP.pdf

Society of Urologic Nurses and Associates (SUNA). (2021c). Clinical practice procedure. Urinary catheterization of the adult male. *Urologic Nursing, 41*(2), 70–75. https://www.suna.org/download/catheterizationMaleCCP.pdf

Society of Urologic Nurses and Associates (SUNA). (2021d). Clinical practice procedure. Insertion of an indwelling urethral catheter in the adult male. *Urologic Nursing, 41*(2), 86–109.

Stelton, S. (2019). Stoma and peristomal skin care: A clinical review. *American Journal of Nursing, 119*(6), 38–45.

Strouse, A. C. (2015). Appraising the literature on bathing practices and catheter-associated urinary tract infection prevention. *Urologic Nursing, 35*(1), 11–17. https://doi.org/10.7257/1053-816X.2015.35.1.11

Swift, T., Westgate, G., Van Onselen, J., & Lee, S. (2020). Developments in silicone technology for use in stoma care. *British Journal of Nursing, 29*(6), S6–S15. https://doi.org/10.12968/bjon.2020.29.6.S6

Szeto, C. C., Li, P. K. T., Johnson, D. W., Bernardini, J., Dong, J., Figueiredo, A. E., Ito, Y., Kazancioglu, R., Moraes, T., Van Esch, S., & Brown, E. A. (2017). ISPD catheter-related infection recommendations: 2017

update. *Peritoneal Dialysis International Journal, 37*(2), 141–154. https://doi.org/10.3747/pdi.2016.00120

Taylor, C., Lynn, P., & Bartlett, J. (2023). *Fundamentals of nursing: The art and science of person-centered care* (10th ed.). Wolters Kluwer.

Tielemans, C., & Voegeli, D. (2019). Silicone-based adhesive removers for preventing peristomal skin complications caused by mechanical trauma. *Gastrointestinal Nursing, 17*(Suppl 9), S22–S28. https://doi.org/10.12968/gasn.2019.17.Sup9.S22

Trossle, C., Malmberg, L., Nikoleris, G., Diegel, O., Nordqvist, P., Hajdu, T., Kjellson, F., & Malmqvist, U. (2020). Evaluation of a novel medical device to facilitate gel instillation during change of long-term indwelling urinary catheters-A randomized controlled pilot study. *Urologic Nursing, 40*(3), 121–128. https://doi.org/10.7257/1053-816X.2020.40.3.121

United Ostomy Associations of America, Inc. (2017). *Urostomy guide.* https://www.ostomy.org/wp-content/uploads/2018/03/UrostomyGuide.pdf

VHA Center for Engineering & Occupational Safety and Health (CEOSH). (2016). *Safe patient handling and mobility guidebook.* http://www.tnpatientsafety.com/pubfiles/Initiatives/workplace-violence/sphm-pdf.pdf

Widdall, D. A. (2015). Considerations for determining a bladder scan protocol. *Journal of the Australasian Rehabilitation Nurses' Association, 18*(3), 22–27.

Wilson, M. (2015). Clean intermittent self-catheterisation: Working with patients. *British Journal of Nursing, 24*(2), 76–85. https://doi.org/10.12968/bjon.2015.24.2.76

Wolters Kluwer. (2022). Problem-based care plans. In *Lippincott Advisor.* Wolters Kluwer.

Wound, Ostomy and Continence Nurses Society (WOCN). (2018). *Basic ostomy skin care: A guide for*

patients and health care providers. https://www.ostomy.org/wp-content/uploads/2018/11/wocn_basic_ostomy_skin_care_2018.pdf

Wound, Ostomy and Continence Nurses Society (WOCN). (n.d.). Clinical tools. Interventions post catheter removal. Retrieved January 23, 2021, from https://www.wocn.org/learning-center/clinical-tools/

Wuthier, P., Sublett, K., & Riehl, L. (2016). Urinary catheter dependent loops as a potential contributing cause of bacteriuria: An observational study. *Urologic Nursing, 36*(1), 7–16. https://doi.org/10.7257/1053-816X.2016.36.1.7

Yates, A. (2016). Indwelling urinary catheterisation: What is best practice? *British Journal of Nursing, 25*(9), S4–S13.

Yates, A. (2017a). Urinary catheters 1: Male catheterisation. *Nursing Times, 113*(1), 32–34. https://www.nursingtimes.net/clinical-archive/continence/urinary-catheters-1-male-catheterisation-2-05-12-2016/

Yates, A. (2017b). Urinary catheters 2: Inserting a catheter into a female patient. *Nursing Times, 113*(2), 50–52. https://www.nursingtimes.net/clinical-archive/continence/urinary-catheters-2-inserting-a-catheter-into-a-female-patient-16-01-2017/

Yates, A. (2017c). Urinary catheters 6: Removing an indwelling urinary catheter. *Nursing Times, 113*(6), 33–35. https://www.nursingtimes.net/clinical-archive/continence/urinary-catheters-6-removing-an-indwelling-urinary-catheter-15-05-2017/

Yates, A. (2018). Catheter securing and fixation devices: Their role in preventing complications. *British Journal of Nursing, 27*(6), 290–294. https://doi.org/10.12968/bjon.2018.27.6.290

SUGGESTED ANSWERS FOR FOCUSING ON PATIENT CARE: DEVELOPING CLINICAL REASONING AND CLINICAL JUDGMENT

1. Assess the patency of the external urinary sheath. Lack of adhesion of the sheath on the penis or resistance to gravity flow of urine would allow urine to leak around the sheath. You should assess for the presence of these conditions, as well as the condition of the patient's skin. Take care to fasten the external urinary sheath securely enough to prevent leakage, yet not so tightly as to constrict the blood vessels in the area. In addition, the tip of the tubing should be kept 1 to 2 inches (2.5 to 5 cm) beyond the tip of the penis to prevent irritation to the sensitive glans area. Maintaining free urinary drainage is another nursing priority. Institute measures to prevent the tubing from becoming kinked and urine from backing up in the tubing. Urine can lead to excoriation of the glans, as well as separation of the sheath from the skin, so position the tubing that collects the urine from the external urinary sheath so that it draws urine away from the penis.

Always use a measuring or sizing guide supplied by the manufacturer to ensure the correct size of sheath is applied. Skin barriers, such as 3M or Skin-Prep, can be applied to the penis to protect penile skin from irritation and changes in integrity. In addition, nursing care of a patient with an external urinary sheath includes vigilant skin care to prevent excoriation. This includes removing the external urinary sheath daily, washing the penis with skin cleanser and water and drying carefully, and inspecting the skin for irritation. In hot and humid weather, more frequent changing may be required. Always follow the manufacturer's instructions for applying the external urinary sheath because there are several variations.

2. Discuss and confirm the continued need for bedrest with the health care team, if appropriate. Begin by assessing what the patient understands about the reason they are required to use the bedpan for elimination. Based on this information, reinforce the rationale for the use of the bedpan. Promote comfort and normalcy as much as possible, while respecting the patient's privacy. Determine if a regular bedpan or a fracture pan would be most appropriate for Ms. Halligan. Also be sure to provide skin care and perineal hygiene after bedpan use and maintain a professional manner.

3. Obtain additional assessment data regarding the catheter site. Assessment data should include the presence of erythema, drainage, bleeding, tenderness, swelling, skin irritation or breakdown, or leakage. These signs could indicate exit-site or tunnel infection. In addition, inquire about any tenderness, pain, and guarding of the abdomen, as well as nausea, vomiting, and fever, which could indicate peritonitis. Assess the patient's knowledge about measures to care for the exit site. Remind Mr. Wimmer that exit-site and catheter care includes avoiding baths and public pools; the importance of good handwashing before self-care; and that he should be maintaining a dressing over the site.

Because he is experiencing site redness and tenderness, which could indicate an infection, instruct Mr. Wimmer to contact his health care provider for an appointment to have his catheter and exit site evaluated.

Bowel Elimination

Focusing on Patient Care

This chapter will help you develop some of the skills related to bowel elimination necessary to care for the following patients:

Hugh Levens, age 64, has been placed on a bowel program after a fall left them paralyzed from the waist down.

Isaac Greenberg, age 9, has been having blood in their stools. They are scheduled for a colonoscopy as an outpatient. Isaac and their mother need teaching about the preparation for the procedure, which includes a small-volume cleansing enema.

Maria Blakely, age 26, has recently received an ileostomy. Maria is having problems with the appliance and is concerned about skin irritation.

Refer to Focusing on Patient Care: Developing Clinical Reasoning and Clinical Judgment at the end of the chapter to apply what you learn.

Learning Outcomes

After completing the chapter, you will be able to accomplish the following:

1. Administer a large-volume cleansing enema.
2. Administer a small-volume cleansing enema.
3. Administer a retention enema.
4. Remove stool digitally.
5. Apply a fecal incontinence collection device.
6. Empty and change an ostomy appliance.
7. Irrigate a colostomy.
8. Insert a nasogastric tube.
9. Irrigate a nasogastric tube connected to suction.
10. Remove a nasogastric tube.

Nursing Concepts

- Assessment
- Clinical Decision Making/Clinical Judgment
- Elimination
- Functional Ability
- Safety

Elimination of the waste products of digestion is a natural process critical for human functioning. Patients differ widely in their expectations about bowel elimination, their usual pattern of **defecation**, and the ease with which they speak about bowel elimination or bowel problems. Although most people have experienced minor acute bouts of **diarrhea** or **constipation**, some patients experience severe or chronic bowel elimination problems affecting their fluid and electrolyte balance, hydration, nutritional status, skin integrity, comfort, and self-concept. Moreover, many illnesses, diagnostic tests, medications, and surgical treatments can affect bowel elimination. Nurses play an integral role in preventing and managing bowel elimination problems.

This chapter covers skills the nurse may use to promote bowel elimination. Understanding the anatomy of the gastrointestinal (GI) system is integral to performing the skills in this chapter (Fundamentals Review 13-1). An abdominal assessment is required as part of providing the interventions outlined in many of these skills. Refer to Skill 3-7 in Chapter 3. Fundamentals Review 13-2 summarizes factors that may affect bowel elimination. Fundamentals Review 18-2 in Chapter 18 reviews the characteristics of stool.

Fundamentals Review 13-1

ANATOMY OF THE GASTROINTESTINAL TRACT

- The GI tract begins with the mouth and continues to the esophagus, the stomach, the small intestine, and the large intestine. It ends at the anus.
- From the mouth to the anus, the GI tract is approximately 9 m (30 ft) long.
- The small intestine consists of the duodenum, jejunum, and ileum.

- The large intestine consists of the cecum, colon (ascending, transverse, descending, and sigmoid), and rectum.
- Accessory organs of the GI tract include the teeth, salivary glands, gallbladder, liver, and pancreas.

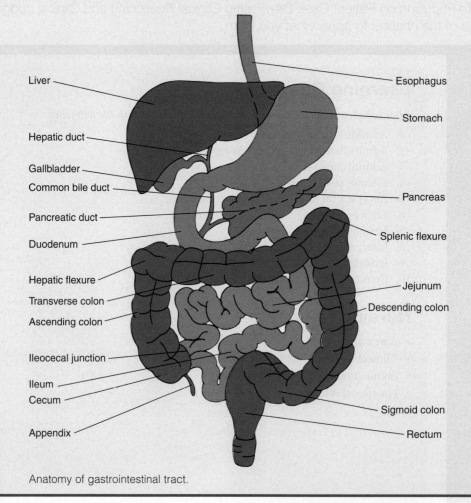

Anatomy of gastrointestinal tract.

Fundamentals Review 13-2

FACTORS THAT AFFECT BOWEL ELIMINATION

- Mobility: Regular exercise improves GI motility and muscle tone, whereas inactivity decreases both. Adequate tone in the abdominal muscles, the diaphragm, and the perineal muscles is essential for ease of defecation.
- Food and Fluids: Foods high in fiber help keep stool moving through the intestines. Adequate fluid intake keeps stools from becoming dry and hard. Adequate fluid also helps fiber to keep stool soft and bulky and prevents dehydration from being a contributing factor to constipation.
- Medications: Some antibiotics and laxatives may cause stool to become loose and more frequent. Diuretics may lead to dry, hard, and less frequent stools. Opioids decrease GI motility, leading to constipation.
- Intestinal diversions: Ileostomies normally have liquid, foul-smelling stool. Sigmoid colostomies normally have pasty, formed stool.

Skill 13-1 ▶ Administering a Large-Volume Cleansing Enema

Cleansing (evacuant) **enemas** are given to remove feces from the colon. Some of the reasons for administering a cleansing enema include relieving constipation or **fecal impaction**, evacuating the bowel before surgery to prevent involuntary escape of fecal material during surgical procedures, and promoting visualization of the intestinal tract by radiographic or endoscopic examination. Cleansing enemas are classified as either large or small volume. This skill addresses administering a large-volume enema. (Small-volume enemas are addressed in Skill 13-2.)

Large-volume enemas are known as hypotonic or isotonic, depending on the solution used. Hypotonic (tap water) and isotonic (normal saline solution) enemas are large-volume enemas that result in rapid colonic emptying. However, using large volumes of solution (adults: 500 to 1,000 mL; infants: less than 250 mL [Kyle & Carman, 2021]) may be dangerous for patients with weakened intestinal walls, such as those with bowel inflammation or bowel infection. The enema solution should be at or just above body temperature and warmed, if necessary, by placing the container with the enema solution in a container of warm water (Dougherty & Lister, 2015, as cited in Mitchell, 2019b, p. 155). See Table 13-1 (on page 794) for a list of commonly used enema solutions.

DELEGATION CONSIDERATIONS

The administration of some types of enemas may be delegated to assistive personnel (AP) who have received appropriate training. The administration of a large-volume cleansing enema may be delegated to licensed practical/vocational nurses (LPN/LVNs). The decision to delegate must be based on careful analysis of the patient's needs and circumstances as well as the qualifications of the person to whom the task is being delegated. Refer to the Delegation Guidelines in Appendix A.

EQUIPMENT

- Enema solution as prescribed at or just above body temperature (Dougherty & Lister, 2015, as cited in Mitchell, 2019b, p. 155) in the prescribed amount (amount will vary depending on the type of solution, patient's age, and patient's ability to retain the solution; average cleansing enema for an adult may range from 500 to 1,000 mL)
- Disposable enema set, which includes a solution container and tubing
- Water-soluble lubricant
- IV pole
- Necessary additives, as prescribed
- Waterproof pad
- Bath thermometer (if available)
- Bath blanket
- Bedpan or commode and toilet tissue
- Disposable gloves
- Additional PPE, as indicated
- Paper towel
- Washcloth, skin cleanser, and towel

(continued on page 794)

Skill 13-1 ▶ Administering a Large-Volume Cleansing Enema *(continued)*

Table 13-1 Commonly Used Enema Solutions

SOLUTION	AMOUNT	ACTION	TIME TO TAKE EFFECT	ADVERSE EFFECTS
Tap water (hypotonic)	500–1,000 mL	Distends intestine, increases peristalsis, softens stool	15 minutes	Can lead to fluid and electrolyte imbalance, water intoxication. Should not be used in children
Normal saline (isotonic)	500–1,000 mL	Distends intestine, increases peristalsis, softens stool	15 minutes	
Soap	500–1,000 mL (concentrate at 3–5 mL/1,000 mL)	Distends intestine, irritates intestinal mucosa, which stimulates peristalsis, softens stool	10–15 minutes	Must only use Castile soap; other soaps will cause significant rectal mucosa irritation or damage
Phosphate (hypertonic)	70–130 mL	Draws fluids out of the interstitial space into the colon, leading to distention which stimulates peristalsis. Commonly used, commercially prepared (Fleet Enema)	5–10 minutes	Avoid in patients who are dehydrated or where phosphate retention could be a concern. Can be irritating to rectum
Oil (mineral, olive, or cottonseed oil)	150–200 mL	Lubricates stool and intestinal mucosa. Often used as a retention enema. If able, patient may need to hold solution for 30–60 minutes	30 minutes	

ASSESSMENT

Ask the patient when they had their last bowel movement. Assess the patient's abdomen, including auscultating for bowel sounds and palpating for tenderness and/or firmness. Because the goal of a cleansing enema is to increase peristalsis, which should increase bowel sounds, assess the abdomen before and after the enema. Assess the rectal area for any **fissures, hemorrhoids,** sores, or rectal tears. If any of these are present, take added care while inserting the tube. Assess the results of the patient's laboratory work, specifically the platelet count and white blood cell (WBC) count. Rectal agents should be avoided in patients at risk of thrombocytopenia, leukopenia, and/or mucositis and manipulation of the rectum and anus, including administration of enemas, should be avoided in immunocompromised patients and/or patients at risk for myelosuppression and mucositis (NCI, 2020). Enemas are also contraindicated for patients with bowel obstruction or paralytic ileus (Mitchell, 2019b) and in situations in which administration could cause circulatory overload, mucosal damage, necrosis, perforation, or hemorrhage or following any GI or gynecologic surgery in which sutures may be ruptured (Dougherty & Lister, 2015, as cited in Mitchell, 2019b, p. 154). Assess for dizziness, lightheadedness, diaphoresis, and clammy skin. The enema may stimulate a **vagal response or stimulus,** which increases parasympathetic stimulation, causing a decrease in heart rate.

ACTUAL OR POTENTIAL HEALTH PROBLEMS AND NEEDS

Many actual or potential health problems or issues may require the use of this skill as part of related interventions. An appropriate health problem or issue may include:

- Acute pain
- Constipation
- Constipation risk

OUTCOME IDENTIFICATION AND PLANNING

The expected outcome to achieve when administering a cleansing enema is that the patient expels feces. Other appropriate outcomes may include that the patient verbalizes decreased discomfort, abdominal distention is absent, and the patient remains free of any evidence of trauma to the rectal mucosa or other adverse effects.

IMPLEMENTATION

ACTION	RATIONALE
1. Review the patient's health record for any limitations in physical activity. Verify the prescribed intervention for the enema. Gather equipment.	Physical limitations may require adaptations in performing the skill. Verifying the prescribed intervention ensures that the correct intervention is administered to the right patient. Assembling equipment provides for an organized approach to the task.
2. Perform hand hygiene and put on PPE, if indicated.	Hand hygiene and PPE prevent the spread of microorganisms. PPE is required based on transmission precautions.
3. Identify the patient.	Identifying the patient ensures the right patient receives the intervention and helps prevent errors.
4. Explain the procedure to the patient and provide the rationale as to why the enema is needed. Discuss the associated discomforts that may be experienced and possible interventions that may allay this discomfort. Answer any questions, as needed.	Explanation facilitates patient engagement and reduces anxiety.
5. Assemble equipment on the overbed table or other surface within reach.	Arranging items nearby is convenient, saves time, and avoids unnecessary stretching and twisting of muscles on the part of the nurse.
6. Close the curtains around the bed and close the door to the room, if possible. Discuss where the patient will defecate. Have a bedpan, commode, or nearby bathroom ready for use.	This ensures the patient's privacy. Explanation relieves anxiety and facilitates patient engagement. The patient is better able to relax and participate if they are familiar with the procedure and know everything is in readiness when the urge to defecate is felt. Defecation usually occurs within 5 to 15 minutes.
7. Warm the enema solution to at or just above body temperature by placing the container with the enema solution in the amount prescribed in a container of warm water, and check the temperature with a thermometer, if available. If a thermometer is not available, warm and test on your inner wrist. If tap water is used, adjust the temperature as it flows from the faucet.	Enema solution should be at or just above body temperature and warmed, if necessary, by placing the container with the enema solution in a container of warm water (Dougherty & Lister, 2015, as cited in Mitchell, 2019b, p. 155). Warming the solution prevents chilling the patient, adding to the discomfort of the procedure. A cold solution could cause cramping; a too-warm solution could cause trauma to intestinal mucosa.
8. Add the enema solution to the enema set solution container. Release the clamp and allow fluid to progress through the tube before reclamping.	This causes any air to be expelled from the tubing. Although allowing air to enter the intestine is not harmful, it may further distend the intestine.
9. Adjust the bed to a comfortable working height (VHACEOSH, 2016). Position the patient on their left side (Sims position), with the upper thigh pulled toward the abdomen, if possible, or the knee–chest position, as dictated by patient comfort and condition. Fold the top linen back just enough to allow access to the patient's rectal area. Drape the patient with the bath blanket, as necessary, to maintain privacy and warmth. Place a waterproof pad under the patient's hip.	Having the bed at the proper height prevents back and muscle strain. The Sims or knee–chest position facilitates flow of solution via gravity into the rectum and colon, optimizing solution retention. Folding back the linen in this manner minimizes unnecessary exposure and promotes the patient's comfort and warmth. The waterproof pad will protect the bed.
10. Put on gloves.	Gloves prevent contact with contaminants and body fluids.

(continued on page 796)

Skill 13-1 ▶ Administering a Large-Volume Cleansing Enema *(continued)*

ACTION

11. Elevate the solution so that it is no higher than 18 inches (45 cm) above the level of the anus (Figure 1). Plan to give the solution slowly over a period of 5 to 10 minutes. Hang the container on an IV pole or hold it at the proper height.

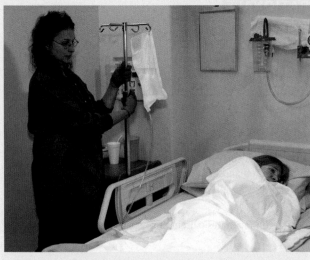

12. Generously lubricate the end of the rectal tube 2 to 3 inches (5 to 7 cm). A disposable enema set may have a prelubricated rectal tube.

13. Lift a buttock to expose the anus. Ask the patient to take several deep breaths. Slowly and gently insert the enema tube 4 to 5 inches (10 to 12.5 cm) for an adult. Direct it at an angle pointing toward the umbilicus, not the bladder (Figure 2).

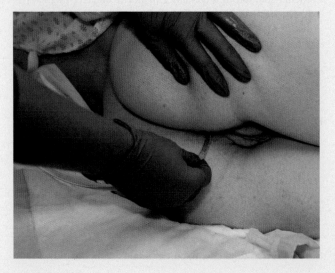

RATIONALE

Gravity forces the solution to enter the intestine. The amount of pressure determines the rate of flow and pressure exerted on the intestinal wall. Giving the solution too quickly causes rapid distention and pressure, poor defecation, or damage to the mucous membrane.

FIGURE 1. Adjusting height of solution container.

Lubrication facilitates passage of the rectal tube through the anal sphincter and prevents injury to the mucosa.

Good visualization of the anus helps prevent injury to tissues. Deep breathing helps relax the anal sphincters. The anal canal is about 1 to 2 inches (2.5 to 5 cm) long. Insertion 4 to 5 inches (10 to 12.5 cm) ensures the tube is inserted past the external and internal anal sphincters (Dougherty & Lister, 2015, as cited in Mitchell, 2019b, p. 155); further insertion may damage the intestinal mucous membrane. The suggested angle follows the normal intestinal contour and thus will help to prevent perforation of the bowel. Slow insertion of the tube minimizes spasms of the intestinal wall and sphincters.

FIGURE 2. Inserting enema tip into anus, directing tip toward umbilicus.

ACTION

14. If resistance is met while inserting the tube, permit a small amount of solution to enter, withdraw the tube slightly, and then continue to insert it. **Do not force entry of the tube.** Ask the patient to take several deep breaths.

15. Introduce the solution slowly over a period of 5 to 10 minutes. Hold the tubing all the time that solution is being instilled. Assess for dizziness, lightheadedness, nausea, diaphoresis, and clammy skin during administration. **If the patient experiences any of these symptoms, stop the procedure immediately, monitor the patient's heart rate and blood pressure, and notify the health care team.**

16. Clamp the tubing or lower the container if the patient has the urge to defecate or cramping occurs (Figure 3). Instruct the patient to take small, fast breaths or to pant.

17. After the solution has been given, clamp the tubing (Figure 4) and remove the tube. Have a paper towel ready to receive the tube as it is withdrawn.

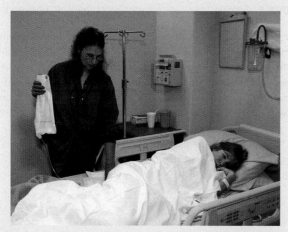

FIGURE 3. Holding bag lower to slow flow of enema solution.

18. Return the patient to a comfortable position. Encourage the patient to hold the solution until the urge to defecate is strong, usually in about 10 to 15 minutes. Make sure the linens under the patient are dry. Remove your gloves and ensure that the patient is covered. Perform hand hygiene.

19. Raise the side rail. Lower the bed height and adjust the head of the bed to a comfortable position.

20. Remove additional PPE, if used. Perform hand hygiene.

RATIONALE

Resistance may be due to spasms of the intestine or failure of the internal sphincter to open. The solution may help to reduce spasms and relax the sphincter, thus making continued insertion of the tube safe. Forcing a tube may injure the intestinal mucosa wall. Taking deep breaths helps relax the anal sphincter.

Introducing the solution slowly helps prevent rapid distention of the intestine and a desire to defecate. Assessment allows for detection of a vagal response. The enema may stimulate a vagal response, which increases parasympathetic stimulation, causing a decrease in heart rate.

These techniques help relax muscles and prevent premature expulsion of the solution.

Wrapping the tube in a paper towel prevents dripping of the solution.

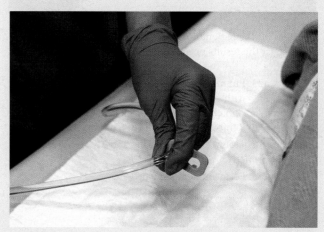

FIGURE 4. Clamping tubing before removing.

This amount of time usually allows muscle contractions to become sufficient to produce good results. Dry linens promote patient comfort. Removing contaminated gloves and performing hand hygiene prevent the spread of microorganisms.

Positioning promotes comfort and safety.

Proper removal of PPE reduces the risk for infection transmission and contamination of other items. Hand hygiene prevents the spread of microorganisms.

(continued on page 798)

Skill 13-1 ▶ Administering a Large-Volume Cleansing Enema *(continued)*

ACTION	RATIONALE
21. When the patient has a strong urge to defecate, place them in a sitting position on a bedpan or assist them to a commode or a nearby bathroom. Offer toilet tissues, if not in the patient's reach (Figure 5). Stay with the patient or have the call bell readily accessible.	The sitting position is most natural and facilitates defecation. Fall prevention is a high priority due to the urgency of reaching the commode.

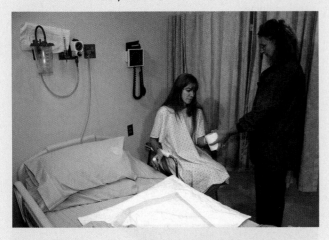

FIGURE 5. Offering toilet tissue to patient on bedside commode.

ACTION	RATIONALE
22. Remind the patient not to flush the commode before you inspect the results of the enema.	The results need to be observed and recorded. Additional enemas may be necessary if the health care provider has prescribed enemas "until clear." Refer to "Special Considerations" below.
23. Put on gloves and assist the patient, if necessary, with cleaning the anal area. Offer washcloths, skin cleanser, and water for handwashing. Remove gloves. Perform hand hygiene.	Cleaning the anal area and proper hygiene deter the spread of microorganisms. Gloves prevent contact with contaminants and body fluids. Hand hygiene deters the spread of microorganisms.
24. Leave the patient clean and comfortable. Care for equipment properly.	Bacteria that grow in the intestine can be spread to others if equipment is not properly cleaned.
25. Perform hand hygiene.	Hand hygiene deters the spread of microorganisms.

EVALUATION   The expected outcomes have been met when the patient has expelled feces, the patient has verbalized decreased discomfort, abdominal distention has not occurred, and the patient has remained free of any evidence of trauma to the rectal mucosa or other adverse effect.

DOCUMENTATION

Guidelines   Document the amount and type of enema solution used; amount, consistency, and color of stool; pain assessment rating; assessment of the perineal area for any irritation, tears, or bleeding; and the patient's reaction to the procedure.

Sample Documentation

> 7/22/25 1310 800-mL tap water enema given via rectum. Large amount of soft, brown stool returned. No irritation, tears, or bleeding noted in perineal area. Patient reported "stomach cramping," which was relieved when enema was released. Rates pain as 0 after evacuation of enema.
>
> —*K. Sanders, RN*

DEVELOPING CLINICAL REASONING AND CLINICAL JUDGMENT

UNEXPECTED SITUATIONS AND ASSOCIATED INTERVENTIONS

- *Solution does not flow into rectum:* Reposition the rectal tube. If solution will still not flow, remove the tube, and check for any fecal contents clogging the tube.
- *Patient cannot retain enema solution for adequate amount of time:* The patient may need to be placed on a bedpan in the supine position while receiving the enema. The head of the bed may be elevated 30 degrees for the patient's comfort.
- *Patient cannot tolerate large amount of enema solution:* Amount and length of administration may have to be modified if the patient begins to report pain.
- *Patient reports severe cramping with introduction of enema solution:* Lower the solution container and check the temperature and flow rate. If the solution is too cold or the flow rate too fast, severe cramping may occur.

SPECIAL CONSIDERATIONS

General Considerations

- Rectal agents should be avoided in patients at risk of thrombocytopenia, leukopenia, and/or mucositis, and manipulation of the rectum and anus, including administration of enemas, should be avoided in immunocompromised patients and/or patients at risk for myelosuppression and mucositis (NCI, 2020). These actions can lead to development of anal fissures or abscesses, which are portals for infection (NCI, 2020).
- If the patient experiences fullness or pain, or if fluid escapes around the tube, stop administration. Wait 30 seconds to a minute and then restart the flow at a slower rate. If symptoms persist, stop administration, and contact the health care team.
- If the order states the enema is to be given "until clear," check with the health care team before administering more than three enemas. Severe fluid and electrolyte imbalances may occur if the patient receives more than three cleansing enemas. Results are considered clear whenever there are no more pieces of stool in the enema return. The solution may be colored but still considered a clear return.

Infant and Child Considerations

- When administering an enema to a child, use isotonic solutions. Plain water is not used because it is hypotonic and can cause rapid fluid shift and fluid overload (Silbert-Flagg & Pillitteri, 2018).
- Appropriate fluid volume for an enema (Silbert-Flagg & Pillitteri, 2018):
  - Infant: 250 mL or less
  - Toddler or preschooler: 250 to 350 mL
  - School-aged child: 300 to 500 mL
  - Adolescent: 500 mL
- Position the infant or toddler on their abdomen with knees bent. Position the child or adolescent on their left side with the right leg flexed toward the chest (Cincinnati Children's, 2018).
- Insert the tubing into the rectum 2 to 3 inches (5 to 7.5 cm) for children (ages 2 to 10 years); 1 to 1.5 inches (2.5 to 4 cm) for infants (Cincinnati Children's, 2018).

Older Adult Considerations

- If the older adult cannot retain the enema solution, administer the enema with the patient on the bedpan in the supine position. For comfort, elevate the head of the bed 30 degrees, if necessary, and use pillows appropriately.

EVIDENCE FOR PRACTICE ▶

MILK AND MOLASSES ENEMAS

Constipation is a common condition (Wangui-Verry et al., 2019). Enemas may be used as part of interventions to relieve constipation. There are several types of enema solutions; milk and molasses enemas has traditionally been used by nurses and other health care providers for severe constipation that has not resolved with standard interventions. However, there has been little research examining the safety and efficacy of this type of enema (Wangui-Verry et al., 2019).

(continued on page 800)

Skill 13-1 ▸ Administering a Large-Volume Cleansing Enema *(continued)*

Related Research

Wangui-Verry, J., Farrington, M., Matthews, G., & Tucker, S. J. (2019). CE: Original Research: Are milk and molasses enemas safe for hospitalized adults? A retrospective electronic health record review. *American Journal of Nursing, 119*(9), 24–28. https://doi.org/10.1097/01. NAJ.0000580148.43193.76

The purpose of this study was to evaluate the safety of milk and molasses enemas for hospitalized adults with constipation that persisted after use of standard treatment interventions. Data were obtained retrospectively from the electronic health records (EHRs) of patients at an academic medical center over a period of 4 years. The final sample ($n = 196$) was chosen by random selection from the EHRs of 615 adult patients who had received a milk and molasses enema during this time frame. Data collected included patient demographics and presenting medical characteristics as well as three safety outcomes associated with milk and molasses enemas. Safety outcomes of interest included bloating, flatus, and bleeding; serious complications including allergic reactions, bacteremia, bowel perforation, electrolyte abnormalities, abdominal compartment syndrome, cardiac arrhythmia, dehydration, death, and sodium and potassium changes. Findings indicated no milk and molasses enema–associated allergic reactions, bacteremia, bowel perforation, electrolyte abnormalities, abdominal compartment syndrome, cardiac arrhythmia, dehydration, or death. Sodium and potassium levels remained within normal limits during hospitalization, with no significant changes noted before or after milk and molasses enema administration. The authors concluded that the use of milk and molasses enemas for relief of constipation did not result in safety concerns in hospitalized adults. The authors suggested the findings indicated that this treatment is safe, and further study examining its efficacy in adults was warranted.

Relevance to Nursing Practice

There are still many health care practices that are based on tradition. Nurses are in an excellent position to consider existing evidence and to investigate practices for which there is little to no evidence related to use. The use of milk and molasses enemas to relieve constipation has been an intervention grounded in tradition but appears to have support for use as a treatment option for adults when other treatments have been ineffective.

Skill 13-2 ▸ Administering a Small-Volume Cleansing Enema

Cleansing (evacuant) enemas are given to remove feces from the colon. Some of the reasons for administering a cleansing enema include relieving constipation or fecal impaction, evacuating the bowel before surgery to prevent involuntary escape of fecal material during surgical procedures, and promoting visualization of the intestinal tract by radiographic or endoscopic examination. Cleansing enemas are classified as either large or small volume. This skill addresses administering a small-volume enema. (Large-volume enemas are addressed in Skill 13-1.)

Small-volume enemas (adult: 118 to 197 mL) are also known as hypertonic (phosphate and sodium citrate) enemas. These hypertonic solutions work by drawing water into the colon, which stimulates the defecation reflex. They may be contraindicated in patients for whom sodium and/or water retention is a problem (NICE, 2017, as cited in Mitchell, 2019b, p. 154). Phosphate enemas should not be used in older adults (Toughy & Jett, 2018). Hypertonic solution enemas are also contraindicated for patients with renal impairment or reduced renal clearance because such patients have compromised ability to excrete phosphate adequately, with resulting hyperphosphatemia (Dougherty & Lister, 2015, as cited in Mitchell, 2019b, p. 154).

DELEGATION CONSIDERATIONS

The administration of some types of enemas may be delegated to assistive personnel (AP) who have received appropriate training. The administration of a small-volume cleansing enema may be delegated to licensed practical/vocational nurses (LPN/LVNs). The decision to delegate must be based on careful analysis of the patient's needs and circumstances as well as the qualifications of the person to whom the task is being delegated. Refer to the Delegation Guidelines in Appendix A.

EQUIPMENT

- Commercially prepared enema with rectal tip
- Water-soluble lubricant
- Waterproof pad
- Bath blanket
- Bedpan or commode and toilet tissue
- Disposable gloves
- Additional PPE, as indicated
- Paper towel
- Washcloth, skin cleanser, and towel

ASSESSMENT

Ask the patient when they had their last bowel movement. Assess the patient's abdomen, including auscultating for bowel sounds and palpating the abdomen. Because the goal of a cleansing enema is to increase peristalsis, which should increase bowel sounds, assess the abdomen before and after the enema. Inspect the rectal area for any fissures, hemorrhoids, sores, or rectal tears. If any of these are noted, take added care while administering the enema. Check the results of the patient's laboratory work, specifically the platelet count and white blood cell (WBC) count. Rectal agents should be avoided in patients at risk of thrombocytopenia, leukopenia, and/or mucositis, and manipulation of the rectum and anus, including administration of enemas, should be avoided in immunocompromised patients and/or patients at risk for myelosuppression and mucositis (NCI, 2020). Enemas are also contraindicated for patients with bowel obstruction or paralytic ileus (Mitchell, 2019b) and in situations in which administration could cause circulatory overload, mucosal damage, necrosis, perforation or hemorrhage or following any GI or gynecologic surgery in which sutures may be ruptured (Doughery & Lister, 2015, as cited in Mitchell, 2019b, p. 154). Assess for dizziness, lightheadedness, diaphoresis, and clammy skin. The enema may stimulate a vagal response or stimulus, which increases parasympathetic stimulation, causing a decrease in heart rate.

ACTUAL OR POTENTIAL HEALTH PROBLEMS AND NEEDS

Many actual or potential health problems or issues may require the use of this skill as part of related interventions. An appropriate health problem or issue may include:
- Acute pain
- Constipation
- Constipation risk

OUTCOME IDENTIFICATION AND PLANNING

The expected outcomes to achieve when administering a cleansing enema are that the patient expels feces and reports a decrease in pain and discomfort. In addition, the patient remains free of any evidence of trauma to the rectal mucosa.

IMPLEMENTATION

ACTION	RATIONALE
1. Review the patient's health record for any limitations in physical activity. Verify the prescribed intervention for the enema. Gather equipment.	Physical limitations may require adaptations in performing the skill. Verifying the prescribed intervention ensures that the correct intervention is administered to the right patient. Assembling equipment provides for an organized approach to the task.
2. Perform hand hygiene and put on PPE, if indicated.	Hand hygiene and PPE prevent the spread of microorganisms. PPE is required based on transmission precautions.

(continued on page 802)

Skill 13-2 ▶ Administering a Small-Volume Cleansing Enema *(continued)*

ACTION	RATIONALE

3. Identify the patient.

Identifying the patient ensures the right patient receives the intervention and helps prevent errors.

4. Explain the procedure to the patient and provide the rationale for why the tube is needed. Discuss the associated discomforts that may be experienced and possible interventions that may allay this discomfort. Answer any questions, as needed.

Explanation facilitates patient engagement and reduces anxiety.

5. Assemble equipment on the overbed table or other surface within reach.

Arranging items nearby is convenient, saves time, and avoids unnecessary stretching and twisting of muscles on the part of the nurse.

6. Close the curtains around the bed and close the door to the room, if possible. Discuss where the patient will defecate. Have a bedpan, commode, or nearby bathroom ready for use.

This ensures the patient's privacy. Explanation relieves anxiety and facilitates patient engagement. The patient is better able to relax and participate if they are familiar with the procedure and know everything is in readiness when the urge to defecate is felt. Defecation usually occurs within 5 to 15 minutes.

7. Warm the enema solution to at or just above body temperature by placing the container with the enema solution in the amount prescribed in a container of warm water, and check the temperature with a thermometer, if available. If a thermometer is not available, warm and test on your inner wrist.

The enema solution should be at or just above body temperature and warmed, if necessary, by placing the container with the enema solution in a container of warm water (Dougherty & Lister, 2015, as cited in Mitchell, 2019b, p. 155). Warming the solution prevents chilling the patient, adding to the discomfort of the procedure. A cold solution could cause cramping; a too-warm solution could cause trauma to intestinal mucosa.

8. Adjust the bed to a comfortable working height (VHACEOSH, 2016). Position the patient on their left side (Sims position), with the upper thigh pulled toward the abdomen, if possible, or the knee–chest position, as dictated by patient comfort and condition. Fold the top linen back just enough to allow access to the patient's rectal area. Drape the patient with the bath blanket, as necessary, to maintain privacy and provide warmth. Place a waterproof pad under the patient's hip.

Having the bed at the proper height prevents back and muscle strain. The Sims or knee–chest position facilitates flow of solution via gravity into the rectum and colon, optimizing retention of solution. Folding back the linen in this manner minimizes unnecessary exposure and promotes the patient's comfort and warmth. The waterproof pad will protect the bed.

9. Put on gloves.

Gloves prevent contact with contaminants and body fluids.

10. Remove the cap (Figure 1) and generously lubricate the end of the rectal tube 2 to 3 inches (5 to 7 cm). Purge the air from the enema nozzle, based on the manufacturer's guidance (Mitchell, 2019b).

Lubrication facilitates passage of the rectal tube through the anal sphincter and prevents injury to the mucosa. Introduction of air into the colon causes distention of the walls and unnecessary discomfort for the patient (Mitchell, 2019b).

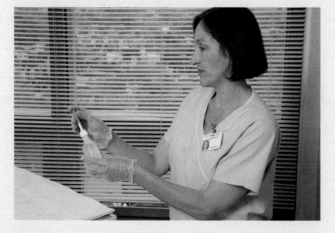

FIGURE 1. Removing cap from prepackaged enema solution container.

ACTION

11. Lift a buttock to expose the anus. Ask the patient to take several deep breaths. Slowly and gently insert the enema rectal tube 4 to 5 inches (10 to 12.5 cm) for an adult. Direct it at an angle pointing toward the umbilicus, not bladder (Figure 2). **Do not force entry of the tube.**

12. Compress the container with your hands (Figure 3). Roll the end of the enema container up on itself, from the bottom, toward the rectal tip. Administer all the solution in the container. Assess for dizziness, lightheadedness, nausea, diaphoresis, and clammy skin during administration. **If the patient experiences any of these symptoms, stop the procedure immediately, monitor the patient's heart rate and blood pressure, and notify the health care team.**

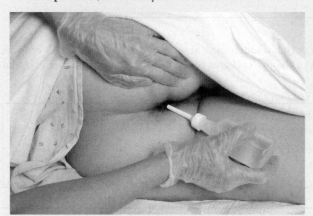

FIGURE 2. Inserting tube into rectum, directing toward umbilicus.

13. After the solution has been given, remove the tube, **keeping the container compressed.** Have a paper towel ready to receive the tube as it is withdrawn.

14. Return the patient to a comfortable position. Encourage the patient to hold the solution until the urge to defecate is strong, usually in about 10 to 15 minutes. Make sure the linens under the patient are dry. Remove gloves and ensure that the patient is covered. Perform hand hygiene.

15. Raise the side rail. Lower the bed height and adjust the head of the bed to a comfortable position.

16. Remove additional PPE, if used. Perform hand hygiene.

17. When the patient has a strong urge to defecate, place them in a sitting position on a bedpan or assist them to a commode or the bathroom. Stay with the patient or have the call bell readily accessible.

RATIONALE

Good visualization of the anus helps prevent injury to tissues. Deep breathing helps relax the anal sphincters. The anal canal is about 1 to 2 inches (2.5 to 5 cm) long. Insertion 4 to 5 inches (10 to 12.5 cm) ensures the tube is inserted past the external and internal anal sphincters (Dougherty & Lister, 2015, as cited in Mitchell, 2019b, p. 155); further insertion may damage the intestinal mucous membrane. The suggested angle follows the normal intestinal contour, helping prevent perforation of the bowel. Slow insertion of the tube minimizes spasms of the intestinal wall and sphincters. Forcing a tube may injure the intestinal mucosa wall.

Rolling the container aids administration of all its contents. Assessment allows for detection of a vagal response. The enema may stimulate a vagal response, which increases parasympathetic stimulation, causing a decrease in heart rate.

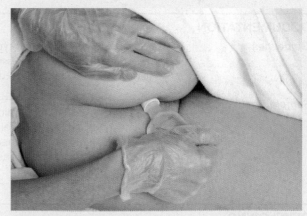

FIGURE 3. Compressing container.

If the container is released, a vacuum will form, allowing some of the enema solution to reenter the container.

This amount of time usually allows muscle contractions to become sufficient to produce good results. Dry linens promote patient comfort. Removing contaminated gloves and performing hand hygiene prevents the spread of microorganisms.

Positioning promotes patient safety.

Proper removal of PPE reduces the risk for infection transmission and contamination of other items. Hand hygiene prevents the spread of microorganisms.

The sitting position is most natural and facilitates defecation. Fall prevention is a high priority due to the urgency of reaching the commode.

(continued on page 804)

Skill 13-2 ▶ Administering a Small-Volume Cleansing Enema *(continued)*

ACTION	**RATIONALE**
18. Remind the patient not to flush the toilet or empty the commode before you inspect the results of the enema.	The results need to be observed and recorded. Additional enemas may be necessary if the health care provider has prescribed enemas "until clear." Refer to "Special Considerations" on the following page.
19. Put on gloves and assist the patient, if necessary, with cleaning of the anal area. Offer washcloths, skin cleanser, and water for handwashing. Remove gloves. Perform hand hygiene.	Cleaning the anal area and proper hygiene deter the spread of microorganisms. Hand hygiene prevents the spread of microorganisms.
20. Leave the patient clean and comfortable. Care for equipment properly.	Bacteria that grow in the intestine can be spread to others if equipment is not properly cleaned.
21. Perform hand hygiene.	Hand hygiene deters the spread of microorganisms.

EVALUATION

The expected outcomes have been met when the patient has expelled feces, the patient has verbalized decreased discomfort, abdominal distention has not occurred, and the patient has remained free of any evidence of trauma to the rectal mucosa or other adverse effect.

DOCUMENTATION

Guidelines

Document the amount and type of enema solution used; amount, consistency, and color of stool; pain assessment rating; assessment of the perineal area for any irritation, tears, or bleeding; and patient's reaction to the procedure.

Sample Documentation

> 7/22/25 1310 210-mL Sodium phosphate enema 197 mL given via rectum. Large amount of soft, brown stool returned. No irritation, tears, or bleeding noted in perineal area. Patient stated "stomach fullness" relieved when enema was released. Rates pain as 0 after evacuation of enema.
>
> —*K. Sanders, RN*

DEVELOPING CLINICAL REASONING AND CLINICAL JUDGMENT

UNEXPECTED SITUATIONS AND ASSOCIATED INTERVENTIONS

- *Patient cannot retain enema solution for adequate amount of time:* The patient may need to be placed on a bedpan in the supine position while receiving the enema. The head of the bed may be elevated 30 degrees for the patient's comfort.

SPECIAL CONSIDERATIONS

General Considerations

- Rectal agents should be avoided in patients at risk of thrombocytopenia, leukopenia, and/or mucositis, and manipulation of the rectum and anus, including administration of enemas, should be avoided in immunocompromised patients and/or patients at risk for myelosuppression and mucositis (NCI, 2020). These actions can lead to development of anal fissures or abscesses, which are portals for infection (NCI, 2020).
- If the enema has been prescribed to be given "until clear," check with the health care team before administering more than three enemas. Severe fluid and electrolyte imbalances may occur if the patient receives more than three cleansing enemas. Results are considered clear whenever there are no more pieces of stool in enema return. The solution may be colored but still considered a clear return.

Infant and Child Considerations

- Position the infant or toddler on their abdomen with knees bent. Position the child or adolescent on their left side with the right leg flexed toward chest (Cincinnati Children's, 2018).
- Insert the tubing into the rectum 2 to 3 inches (5 to 7.5 cm) for children (ages 2 to 10 years); 1 to 1.5 inches (2.5 to 4 cm) for infants (Cincinnati Children's, 2018).
- Hold the child's buttocks together for 5 to 10 minutes, if needed, to encourage retention of the enema (Kyle & Carman, 2021).

Older Adult Considerations

- If the older adult cannot retain the enema solution, administer the enema with the patient on the bedpan in the supine position. For comfort, elevate the head of the bed 30 degrees, if necessary, and use pillows appropriately.
- Phosphate enemas should not be used in older adults (Toughy & Jett, 2018). Sodium citrate enemas should be used with caution in older adults (NICE, 2017, a cited in Mitchell, 2019b).

Skill 13-3 ▶ Administering a Retention Enema

Retention enemas are prescribed for various reasons. *Oil-retention* enemas help to soften the stool and lubricate the intestinal mucosa, making defecation easier (Bauldoff et al., 2020). *Carminative* enemas help to expel **flatus** from the rectum and relieve distention secondary to flatus. *Medicated* enemas are used to administer a medication rectally.

DELEGATION CONSIDERATIONS

The administration of some types of enemas may be delegated to assistive personnel (AP) who have received appropriate training. The administration of a retention enema may be delegated to licensed practical/vocational nurses (LPN/LVNs). The decision to delegate must be based on careful analysis of the patient's needs and circumstances as well as the qualifications of the person to whom the task is being delegated. Refer to the Delegation Guidelines in Appendix A.

EQUIPMENT

- Enema solution (varies depending on reason for enema), usually prepackaged, commercially prepared solutions
- Nonsterile gloves
- Additional PPE, as indicated
- Waterproof pad

- Bath blanket
- Washcloth, skin cleanser, and towel
- Bedpan or commode
- Toilet tissue
- Water-soluble lubricant

ASSESSMENT

Ask the patient when they had their last bowel movement. Assess the patient's abdomen before and after the enema, including auscultating for bowel sounds and palpating. Assess the rectal area for any fissures, hemorrhoids, sores, or rectal tears. If present, added care should be taken while inserting the tube. Check the results of the patient's laboratory work, specifically the platelet count and white blood cell (WBC) count. Rectal agents should be avoided in patients at risk of thrombocytopenia, leukopenia, and/or mucositis, and manipulation of the rectum and anus, including administration of enemas, should be avoided in immunocompromised patients and/or patients at risk for myelosuppression and mucositis (NCI, 2020). Enemas are also contraindicated for patients with bowel obstruction or paralytic ileus (Mitchell, 2019b) and in situations in which administration could cause circulatory overload, mucosal damage, necrosis, perforation or hemorrhage or following any GI or gynecologic surgery in which sutures may be ruptured (Dougherty & Lister, 2015, as cited in Mitchell, 2019b, p. 154). Assess for dizziness, lightheadedness, diaphoresis, and clammy skin. The enema may stimulate a vagal response or stimulus, which increases parasympathetic stimulation, causing a decrease in heart rate.

(*continued on page 806*)

Skill 13-3 ▶ Administering a Retention Enema   *(continued)*

ACTUAL OR POTENTIAL HEALTH PROBLEMS AND NEEDS	Many actual or potential health problems or issues may require the use of this skill as part of related interventions. An appropriate health problem or issue may include: • Constipation • Acute pain • Injury risk
OUTCOME IDENTIFICATION AND PLANNING	The expected outcomes to achieve when administering a retention enema are that the patient retains the solution for the prescribed, appropriate length of time and experiences the expected therapeutic effect of the solution. Other appropriate outcomes may include that the patient verbalizes decreased discomfort, abdominal distention is absent, and the patient remains free of any evidence of trauma to the rectal mucosa or other adverse effect.

IMPLEMENTATION

ACTION	**RATIONALE**
1. Review the patient's health record for any limitations in physical activity. Verify the prescribed intervention for the enema. Gather equipment.	Physical limitations may require adaptations in performing the skill. Verifying the prescribed intervention ensures that the proper enema is administered to the right patient. Assembling equipment provides for an organized approach to the task.
2. Perform hand hygiene and put on PPE, if indicated.	Hand hygiene and PPE prevent the spread of microorganisms. PPE is required based on transmission precautions.
3. Identify the patient.	Identifying the patient ensures the right patient receives the intervention and helps prevent errors.
4. Explain the procedure to the patient and provide the rationale as to why the tube is needed. Discuss the associated discomforts that may be experienced and possible interventions that may allay this discomfort. Answer any questions, as needed.	Explanation facilitates patient engagement and reduces anxiety.
5. Assemble equipment on the overbed table or other surface within reach.	Arranging items nearby is convenient, saves time, and avoids unnecessary stretching and twisting of muscles on the part of the nurse.
6. Close the curtains around the bed and close the door to the room, if possible. Discuss where the patient will defecate. Have a bedpan, commode, or nearby bathroom ready for use.	This ensures the patient's privacy. Explanation relieves anxiety and facilitates patient engagement. The patient is better able to relax and participate if they are familiar with the procedure and know everything is in readiness if the urge to dispel the enema is felt.
7. Warm the enema solution to at or just above body temperature by placing the container with the enema solution in the amount prescribed in a container of warm water, and check the temperature with a thermometer, if available. If a thermometer is not available, warm and test on your inner wrist.	The enema solution should be at or just above body temperature and warmed, if necessary, by placing the container with the enema solution in a container of warm water (Dougherty & Lister, 2015, as cited in Mitchell, 2019b, p. 155). Warming the solution prevents chilling the patient, adding to the discomfort of the procedure. A cold solution could cause cramping; a too-warm solution could cause trauma to intestinal mucosa.
8. Adjust the bed to a comfortable working height (VHACEOSH, 2016). Position the patient on their left side (Sims position), with the upper thigh pulled toward the abdomen, if possible, or the knee–chest position, as dictated by patient comfort and condition. Fold the top linen back just enough to allow access to the patient's rectal area. Drape the patient with the bath blanket, as necessary, to maintain privacy and provide warmth. Place a waterproof pad under the patient's hip.	Having the bed at the proper height prevents back and muscle strain. The Sims or knee–chest position facilitates flow of solution via gravity into the rectum and colon, optimizing retention of the solution. Folding back the linen in this manner minimizes unnecessary exposure and promotes the patient's comfort and warmth. The waterproof pad will protect the bed.

ACTION	**RATIONALE**
9. Put on gloves.	Gloves prevent contact with blood and body fluids.
10. Remove the cap of the prepackaged enema solution. Apply a generous amount of lubricant to the end of the rectal tube 2 to 3 inches (5 to 7 cm). Purge the air from the enema nozzle, based on the manufacturer's guidance (Mitchell, 2019b).	Lubrication is necessary to minimize trauma on insertion. Introduction of air into the colon causes distention of the walls and unnecessary discomfort for the patient (Mitchell, 2019b).
11. Lift a buttock to expose the anus. Ask the patient to take several deep breaths. Slowly and gently insert the enema rectal tube 4 to 5 inches (10 to 12.5 cm) for an adult. Direct it at an angle pointing toward the umbilicus, not bladder (Figure 1). **Do not force entry of the tube.**	Good visualization of the anus helps prevent injury to tissues. Deep breathing helps relax the anal sphincters. The anal canal is about 1 to 2 inches (2.5 to 5 cm) long. Insertion 4 to 5 inches (10 to 12.5 cm) ensures the tube is inserted past the external and internal anal sphincters (Dougherty & Lister, 2015, as cited in Mitchell, 2019b, p. 155); further insertion may damage the intestinal mucous membrane. The suggested angle follows the normal intestinal contour, helping prevent perforation of the bowel. Slow insertion of the tube minimizes spasms of the intestinal wall and sphincters. Forcing a tube may injure the intestinal mucosa wall.

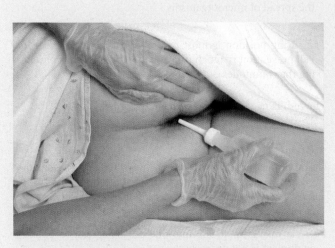

FIGURE 1. Inserting tube into rectum, directing toward umbilicus.

12. Compress the container with your hands (Figure 2). Roll the end of the enema container up on itself, from the bottom, toward the rectal tip. Administer all the solution in the container. Assess for dizziness, lightheadedness, nausea, diaphoresis, and clammy skin during administration. **If the patient experiences any of these symptoms, stop the procedure immediately, monitor the patient's heart rate and blood pressure, and notify the health care team.**	Rolling the container aids administration of all of the contents of the container. Assessment allows for detection of a vagal response. The enema may stimulate a vagal response, which increases parasympathetic stimulation, causing a decrease in heart rate.

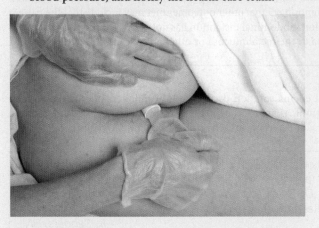

FIGURE 2. Compressing container.

(continued on page 808)

Skill 13-3 ▶ Administering a Retention Enema *(continued)*

ACTION	RATIONALE

13. After the solution has been given, remove the tube, **keeping the container compressed.** Have a paper towel ready to receive the tube as it is withdrawn.

If the container is released, a vacuum will form, allowing some of the enema solution to reenter the container.

14. Return the patient to a comfortable position. **Instruct the patient to retain the enema solution for at least 30 minutes or as indicated, per the manufacturer's direction.** Make sure the linens under the patient are dry. Remove gloves and ensure that the patient is covered. Perform hand hygiene.

The solution needs to dwell for at least 30 minutes, or per the manufacturer's direction, to allow for its optimal action. Covering the patient promotes comfort. Removing contaminated gloves and performing hand hygiene prevent the spread of microorganisms.

15. Raise the side rail. Lower the bed height and adjust the head of the bed to a comfortable position.

Positioning promotes patient safety.

16. Remove additional PPE, if used. Perform hand hygiene.

Proper removal of PPE reduces the risk for infection transmission and contamination of other items. Hand hygiene prevents the spread of microorganisms.

17. When the patient has a strong urge to dispel the solution, place them in a sitting position on the bedpan or assist them to the commode or bathroom. Stay with the patient or have the call bell readily accessible.

The sitting position is most natural and facilitates defecation. Fall prevention is a high priority due to the urgency of reaching the commode.

18. Remind the patient not to flush the commode before you inspect the results of the enema, if used for bowel evacuation. Record the character of stool, as appropriate, and the patient's reaction to the enema.

The results need to be observed and recorded.

19. Put on gloves and assist the patient, if necessary, with cleaning of the anal area. Offer washcloths, skin cleanser, and water for handwashing. Remove gloves. Perform hand hygiene.

Cleaning the anal area and proper hygiene deter the spread of microorganisms. Proper removal of PPE reduces the risk for infection transmission and contamination of other items. Hand hygiene prevents the spread of microorganisms.

20. Leave the patient clean and comfortable. Care for equipment properly.

Bacteria that grow in the intestine can be spread to others if equipment is not properly cleaned.

21. Perform hand hygiene.

Hand hygiene deters the spread of microorganisms.

EVALUATION

The expected outcomes have been met when the patient has retained the solution for the prescribed, appropriate length of time and experienced the expected therapeutic effect of the solution. Depending on the reason for the retention enema, other outcomes met may include that the patient has verbalized a decrease in discomfort, abdominal distention has not occurred, and the patient has remained free of evidence of trauma to the rectal mucosa or other adverse effect.

DOCUMENTATION

Guidelines

Document the amount and type of enema solution used; length of time retained by the patient; amount, consistency, and color of stool, as appropriate; pain assessment rating; assessment of the perineal area for any irritation, tears, or bleeding; and the patient's reaction to the procedure.

Sample Documentation

6/26/25 2030 100 mL of mineral oil administered as enema via rectum. Small amount of firm, black stool returned. Small (approx. 1 cm) tear noted at 2 o'clock position on anus. No erythema or bleeding noted. Dr. Zayer notified of tear and stool color. Reports pain as 2 on a 0-to-10 rating scale after enema evacuated.

—*K. Sanders, RN*

DEVELOPING CLINICAL REASONING AND CLINICAL JUDGMENT

UNEXPECTED SITUATIONS AND ASSOCIATED INTERVENTIONS

- *Solution does not flow into rectum:* Reposition the rectal tube; if the solution still will not flow, remove the tube and check for any fecal contents.
- *Patient cannot retain enema solution for adequate amount of time:* Place the patient on a bedpan in the supine position while receiving the enema. Elevate the head of the bed 30 degrees for the patient's comfort. If they are still unable to retain, notify the health care team.

SPECIAL CONSIDERATIONS

General Considerations

- Rectal agents should be avoided in patients at risk of thrombocytopenia, leukopenia, and/or mucositis, and manipulation of the rectum and anus, including administration of enemas, should be avoided in immunocompromised patients and/or patients at risk for myelosuppression and mucositis (NCI, 2020). These actions can lead to development of anal fissures or abscesses, which are portals for infection (NCI, 2020).
- Some retention enemas are retained overnight, to soften hard, impacted stool (Mitchell, 2019b).

Infant and Child Considerations

- Position the infant or toddler on their abdomen with knees bent. Position the child or adolescent on their left side with the right leg flexed toward chest (Cincinnati Children's, 2018).
- Insert the tubing into the rectum 2 to 3 inches (5 to 7.5 cm) for children (ages 2 to 10 years); 1 to 1.5 inches (2.5 to 4 cm) for infants (Cincinnati Children's, 2018).
- Hold the child's buttocks together for 5 to 10 minutes, if needed, to encourage retention of the enema (Kyle & Carman, 2021).

Skill 13-4 ▶ Digital Removal of Stool

Fecal impaction (prolonged retention or an accumulation of fecal material that forms a hardened mass in the rectum), most often caused by constipation, prevents the passage of normal stools. If a patient with a fecal impaction cannot expel the fecal mass voluntarily, and oil-retention and cleansing enemas fail to break up the mass, the impaction may need to be removed manually. Digital (manual) removal of feces is an invasive procedure that involves the manual removal of feces from the rectum using a gloved finger (Dougherty & Lister, 2015, as cited in Mitchell, 2019d, p. 430). Digital removal of stool is embarrassing and very uncomfortable and may cause great discomfort and pain to the patient as well as irritation of the rectal mucosa and bleeding (Mitchell, 2019d). Digital removal of stool is a prescribed intervention. The patient may be prescribed an oil-retention enema to be given before the procedure to soften stool (refer to Skill 13-3). In addition, many patients find that a sitz bath or tub bath after this procedure soothes the irritated perineal area.

DELEGATION CONSIDERATIONS

Digital removal of stool is not delegated to assistive personnel (AP). Depending on the state's nurse practice act and the organization's policies and procedures, the digital removal of stool may be delegated to licensed practical/vocational nurses (LPN/LVNs). The decision to delegate must be based on careful analysis of the patient's needs and circumstances as well as the qualifications of the person to whom the task is being delegated. Refer to the Delegation Guidelines in Appendix A.

EQUIPMENT

- Disposable gloves
- Additional PPE, as indicated
- Water-soluble lubricant
- Waterproof pad
- Bath blanket

- Bedpan
- Toilet paper, washcloth, skin cleanser, and towel
- Sitz bath (optional)
- Additional caregiver to assist with the procedure

(continued on page 810)

Skill 13-4 ▶ Digital Removal of Stool *(continued)*

ASSESSMENT

Ask the patient when they had their last bowel movement. Assess the patient's abdomen before and after the procedure, including auscultating for bowel sounds and palpating for tenderness and/or firmness. Inspect the rectal area for any fissures, hemorrhoids, sores, or rectal tears. If any of these are noted, consult the prescriber for the appropriateness of the intervention. Check the results of the patient's laboratory work, specifically the platelet count and white blood cell (WBC) count. A low platelet count may seriously compromise the patient's ability to clot blood. A low WBC count places the patient at risk for infection. Therefore, do not perform any unnecessary procedures that would place the patient at risk for bleeding or infection. Rectal agents and manipulation, such as digital removal of stool, should be avoided in patients at risk of thrombocytopenia, leukopenia, and/or mucositis, and manipulation of the rectum and anus, including administration of enemas, should be avoided in immunocompromised patients and/or patients at risk for myelosuppression and mucositis (NCI, 2020). Digital removal of stool may irritate or traumatize the GI mucosa, causing bleeding, bowel perforation, or infection. Assess for dizziness, lightheadedness, diaphoresis, and clammy skin. Assess pulse rate and blood pressure before and after the procedure. The procedure may stimulate a vagal response, which increases parasympathetic stimulation, causing a decrease in heart rate and blood pressure (Mitchell, 2019d). Do not perform digital removal of stool on patients who have bowel inflammation or bowel infection or after rectal, prostate, and colon surgery.

ACTUAL OR POTENTIAL HEALTH PROBLEMS AND NEEDS

Many actual or potential health problems or issues may require the use of this skill as part of related interventions. An appropriate health problem or issue may include:
- Fecal impaction
- Acute pain
- Injury risk

OUTCOME IDENTIFICATION AND PLANNING

The expected outcome to achieve when digitally removing stool is that the patient will expel feces with assistance. Other appropriate outcomes may include that the patient verbalizes decreased discomfort, abdominal distention is absent, and the patient remains free of any evidence of trauma to the rectal mucosa or other adverse effect.

IMPLEMENTATION

ACTION	RATIONALE
1. Review the patient's health record for any limitations in physical activity. Verify the prescribed intervention for digital removal of stool. Gather equipment.	Physical limitations may require adaptations in performing the skill. Verifying the prescribed intervention ensures that the correct intervention is administered to the right patient. Assembling equipment provides for an organized approach to the task.
2. Perform hand hygiene and put on PPE, if indicated.	Hand hygiene and PPE prevent the spread of microorganisms. PPE is required based on transmission precautions.
3. Identify the patient.	Identifying the patient ensures the right patient receives the intervention and helps prevent errors.
4. Explain the procedure to the patient and provide the rationale why the procedure is needed. Discuss the associated discomforts that may be experienced. Discuss signs and symptoms of a slow heart rate. Instruct the patient to alert you if any of these symptoms are felt during the procedure.	Explanation relieves anxiety and facilitates patient engagement. The patient is better able to relax and participate if they are familiar with the procedure.
5. Assemble equipment on the overbed table or other surface within reach.	Arranging items nearby is convenient, saves time, and avoids unnecessary stretching and twisting of muscles on the part of the nurse.

ACTION

6. Close the curtains around the bed and close the door to the room, if possible. Discuss where the patient will defecate, if necessary. Have a bedpan ready for use; have a commode or nearby bathroom ready for use, depending on the patient's abilities and circumstances.

7. Adjust the bed to a comfortable working height (VHACEOSH, 2016). Position the patient on their left side (Sims position), with the upper thigh pulled toward the abdomen, if possible, or the knee–chest position, as dictated by patient comfort and condition. Fold the top linen back just enough to allow access to the patient's rectal area. Drape the patient with the bath blanket, as necessary, to maintain privacy and provide warmth. Place a waterproof pad under the patient's hip. Position the additional health care provider close to the patient to provide reassurance and support to the patient during the procedure.

8. Put on nonsterile gloves. Assess the anal area for evidence of skin soreness, swelling, bleeding, discharge, prolapse, excoriation, and hemorrhoids. If any abnormalities are present, do not continue with the procedure (Mitchell, 2019d). Confer with the health care team.

9. Generously lubricate the index finger of your dominant hand with water-soluble lubricant and insert your finger gently into the anal canal, pointing toward the umbilicus (Figure 1).

10. Slowly and gently work the finger around in circular movements and into the hardened mass to break it up (Figure 2) and then remove pieces of it. Instruct the patient to bear down, if possible, while extracting feces to ease in removal. Avoid using a hooked finger to remove feces (Mitchell, 2019d). Place the extracted stool in the bedpan.

RATIONALE

This ensures the patient's privacy. Explanation relieves anxiety and facilitates patient engagement. The patient is better able to relax and participate if they are familiar with the procedure and know everything is in readiness if the urge to defecate is felt.

Having the bed at the proper height prevents back and muscle strain. The Sims or knee–chest position facilitates access into the rectum and colon. Folding back the linen in this manner minimizes unnecessary exposure and promotes the patient's comfort and warmth. The waterproof pad will protect the bed.

Gloves prevent contact with blood and body fluids as well as feces. Collaboration with the health care team provides for planning and alterations in plan of care based on patient circumstances.

Lubrication reduces irritation of the rectum. The presence of the finger added to the mass tends to cause discomfort for the patient if the work is not done slowly and gently.

The fecal mass may be large and may need to be removed in smaller pieces. Use of a hooked finger to remove feces may cause damage to the rectal mucosa and anal sphincter (Mitchell, 2019d).

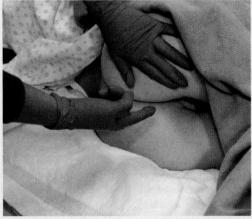

FIGURE 1. Inserting lubricated forefinger of dominant hand into anal canal.

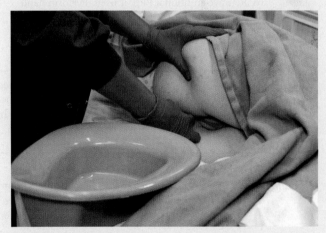

FIGURE 2. Gently working finger around to break up stool mass.

11. Remove impaction at intervals if it is severe. **Observe the patient throughout for any signs of distress and stop if the patient reports pain or asks you to stop (Mitchell, 2019d). Remind the patient to alert you if they begin to feel lightheaded or nauseated. If the patient reports either symptom, stop removal and assess the patient, including the patient's heart rate and blood pressure.**

Removal of stool in intervals helps to prevent discomfort, irritation, and vagal nerve stimulation. Assessment allows for detection of a vagal response. Digital removal of a fecal mass can stimulate the vagus nerve, resulting in a slowed heart rate (Mitchell, 2019d). If this occurs, stop the procedure immediately, monitor the patient's heart rate and blood pressure, and notify the health care team.

(continued on page 812)

Skill 13-4 ▶ Digital Removal of Stool *(continued)*

ACTION	RATIONALE
12. When the procedure is completed, put on clean gloves. Assist the patient, if necessary, with cleaning of the anal area (Figure 3). Offer a washcloth, skin cleanser, and water for handwashing. If the patient is able, offer a sitz bath.	Cleaning deters the transmission of microorganisms and promotes hygiene. A sitz bath may relieve the irritated perianal area.

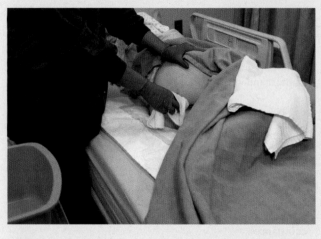

FIGURE 3. Cleaning anal area with washcloth and skin cleanser.

ACTION	RATIONALE
13. Remove gloves. Perform hand hygiene. If the patient verbalizes the need to defecate, assist the patient to the commode or the bathroom, as appropriate.	Removing contaminated gloves prevents the spread of microorganisms. Hand hygiene prevents the spread of microorganisms. The other actions promote patient comfort.
14. Return the patient to a comfortable position. Make sure the linens under the patient are dry. Ensure that the patient is covered.	These actions promote patient comfort.
15. Raise the side rail. Lower the bed height and adjust the head of the bed to a comfortable position.	Positioning promotes patient comfort and safety.
16. Remove additional PPE, if used. Perform hand hygiene.	Proper removal of PPE reduces the risk for infection transmission and contamination of other items. Hand hygiene prevents the spread of microorganisms.

EVALUATION

The expected outcomes have been met when the fecal impaction has been removed and the patient has expelled feces with assistance, the patient has verbalized decreased discomfort, abdominal distention has not occurred, and the patient has remained free of any evidence of trauma to the rectal mucosa or other adverse effect.

DOCUMENTATION

Guidelines

Document the following: abdominal assessment; color, consistency, and amount of stool removed; condition of perianal area after the procedure; pain assessment rating; heart rate and blood pressure, if measured; and the patient's reaction to the procedure.

Sample Documentation

> 6/29/25 1030 Digital removal of large amount of hard, brown stool. Abdomen soft, nondistended. Perineal area remains free from tears, erythema, or bleeding. Patient denied any lightheadedness or nausea during the procedure. Rates pain as 1 on a 0-to-10 scale.
>
> —K. Sanders, RN

DEVELOPING CLINICAL REASONING AND CLINICAL JUDGMENT

UNEXPECTED SITUATIONS AND ASSOCIATED INTERVENTIONS

- *Patient reports feeling dizzy, lightheaded, or nauseated; begins to vomit; or has pain:* Stop digital stimulation immediately. The vagal nerve might have been stimulated. Assess heart rate and blood pressure. Consult with the health care team.
- *Patient experiences significant pain during the procedure:* Stop the procedure and consult with the health care team.

SPECIAL CONSIDERATIONS

- Rectal agents and manipulation, such as digital removal of stool, should be avoided in patients at risk of thrombocytopenia, leukopenia, and/or mucositis, and manipulation of the rectum and anus, including administration of enemas, should be avoided in immunocompromised patients and/or patients at risk for myelosuppression and mucositis (NCI, 2020). These actions can lead to development of anal fissures or abscesses, which are portals for infection (NCI, 2020).
- Recurrence of fecal impaction is common. It is important to help prevent and manage this condition by increasing dietary fiber content to 25 to 38 g/day (USDA & USDHHS, 2020), ensuring a daily fluid intake of at least 2,000 mL/day (Dudek, 2022), and evaluating medications that can contribute to colonic hypomotility (Obokhare, 2012).

Skill 13-5 ▶ Applying an External Anal Pouch

Fecal collection devices are intended to collect stool as it passes from the rectum and are mainly useful for patients who are very ill or confined to bed and who are experiencing bowel management problems (Continence Product Advisor, 2021). An external anal pouch is an external collection system used to protect the perianal and perineal skin from excoriation due to repeated exposure to very loose stool. This device reduces skin damage by diverting liquid stool into a collection container (Palmer, 2019). A flexible wafer that has an opening at its center adheres to the skin around the anus, and the other side is connected to a collection bag (pouch) (Palmer, 2019). The bag has a re-sealable port at the lower end through which the stool can be emptied or connected to a larger drainage bag (Continence Product Advisor, 2021). A skin barrier may be applied to the skin before the device to protect the patient's skin and improve adhesion. If excoriation is already present, application of a skin barrier prior to applying the pouch may be helpful. Disadvantages of these devices include the risk of skin damage from the adhesive on the perianal skin (Continence Product Advisor, 2021).

DELEGATION CONSIDERATIONS

Application of a fecal incontinence collection device may be delegated to assistive personnel (AP) who have received appropriate training. Application of a fecal incontinence collection device may be delegated to licensed practical/vocational nurses (LPN/LVNs). The decision to delegate must be based on careful analysis of the patient's needs and circumstances as well as the qualifications of the person to whom the task is being delegated. Refer to the Delegation Guidelines in Appendix A.

EQUIPMENT

- External anal pouch
- Disposable gloves
- Additional PPE, as indicated
- Washcloth and skin cleanser or disposable bathing cloths and towel
- Drainage (Foley) bag
- Scissors (optional)
- Skin protectant or barrier
- Bath blanket

ASSESSMENT

Assess the amount and consistency of stool being passed. Assess the frequency of bowel movements. Assess the integrity of the perianal skin; assess for alterations in skin integrity, wounds, or hemorrhoids.

(continued on page 814)

Skill 13-5 ▶ Applying an External Anal Pouch *(continued)*

ACTUAL OR POTENTIAL HEALTH PROBLEMS AND NEEDS	Many actual or potential health problems or issues may require the use of this skill as part of related interventions. An appropriate health problem or issue may include: • Bowel incontinence • Altered skin integrity risk • Altered skin integrity
OUTCOME IDENTIFICATION AND PLANNING	The expected outcomes to achieve when applying an external anal pouch are that the patient expels feces into the device and maintains intact perianal skin. Other outcomes may include that the patient demonstrates a decrease in the amount and severity of excoriation, and the patient verbalizes decreased discomfort.

IMPLEMENTATION

ACTION	RATIONALE
1. Gather equipment.	Assembling equipment provides for an organized approach to the task.
2. Perform hand hygiene and put on PPE, if indicated.	Hand hygiene and PPE prevent the spread of microorganisms. PPE is required based on transmission precautions.
3. Identify the patient.	Identifying the patient ensures the right patient receives the intervention and helps prevent errors.
4. Close the curtains around the bed and close the door to the room, if possible. Explain to the patient what you are going to do and why.	This ensures the patient's privacy. Discussion promotes patient engagement and helps to minimize anxiety.
5. Assemble equipment on the overbed table or other surface within reach.	Arranging items nearby is convenient, saves time, and avoids unnecessary stretching and twisting of muscles on the part of the nurse.
6. Adjust the bed to a comfortable working height (VHACEOSH, 2016). Position the patient on their left side (Sims position), as dictated by patient comfort and condition. Fold the top linen back just enough to allow access to the patient's rectal area. Drape the patient with the bath blanket, as necessary, to maintain privacy and provide warmth. Place a waterproof pad under the patient's hip.	Having the bed at the proper height prevents back and muscle strain. The Sims position facilitates access into the rectum. Folding back the linen in this manner minimizes unnecessary exposure and promotes the patient's comfort and warmth. The waterproof pad will protect the bed.
7. Put on gloves. Cleanse the perianal area, and pat it dry thoroughly.	Gloves protect the nurse from microorganisms in feces. The skin must be dry for the device to adhere securely.
8. Trim perianal hair with scissors, if needed.	It may be uncomfortable for the patient if the perianal hair is pulled by the adhesive from the fecal device; excess hair can interfere with adhesion (Hollister, 2021). Trimming with scissors minimizes the risk for infection compared with shaving.
9. Apply the skin protectant or barrier and allow it to dry. Skin protectant may be contraindicated for use with some devices. Check the manufacturer's recommendations before use.	The skin protectant aids in device adhesion and protects the skin from irritation and injury from the adhesive. The skin must be dry for the device to adhere securely.
10. If necessary, enlarge the opening in the adhesive skin barrier to fit the patient's anatomy (Hollister, 2021). Do not cut beyond the printed line on the barrier. Remove the paper backing from the adhesive of device (Figure 1).	Cutting away too much of the adhesive backing will result in poor adhesion to the patient's skin. Removing the paper backing is necessary so that the device can adhere to the skin.

ACTION

11. Fold the adhesive skin barrier in half, with the adhesive side facing out; hold it in your dominant hand. With your non-dominant hand, separate the patient's buttocks. Apply the fecal device to the anal area with your dominant hand, ensuring that the bag opening is over anus (Figure 2). Hold the device in place for 30 seconds to achieve good adhesion. For patients with female anatomy, check to ensure the skin barrier does not cover the labia or vaginal opening (Hollister, 2021).

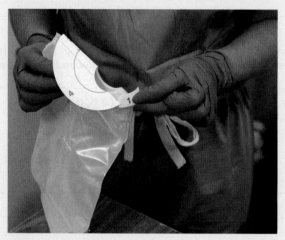

FIGURE 1. Removing paper backing from adhesive of rectal device.

12. Release the buttocks. Close the drainage cap on the bag or attach the connector of the fecal incontinence device to the drainage bag (Figure 3). Hang the drainage bag below the level of the patient (Figure 4).

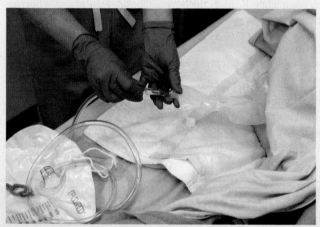

FIGURE 3. Attaching connector of fecal device to tubing of drainage bag.

13. Remove gloves. Perform hand hygiene. Return the patient to a comfortable position. Make sure the linens under the patient are dry. Ensure that the patient is covered.

14. Raise the side rail. Lower the bed height and adjust the head of the bed to a comfortable position.

RATIONALE

The opening should be over the anus so that stool empties into the bag and does not stay on the patient's skin, which could lead to skin breakdown. The device is effective only if it is properly positioned and adhered securely. The warmth of your hand pressing on the skin barrier activates the adhesive bond (Hollister, 2021).

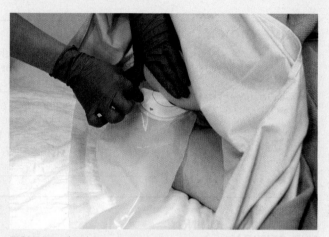

FIGURE 2. Applying device over anal opening.

The bag must be dependent for stool to drain into the bag.

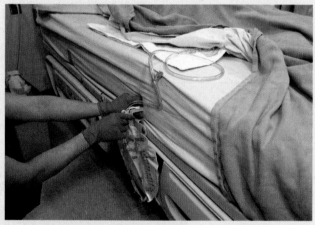

FIGURE 4. Hanging drainage bag below level of patient.

Removing contaminated gloves and hand hygiene prevent spread of microorganisms. Covering the patient promotes patient comfort.

Positioning promotes patient comfort and safety.

(*continued on page 816*)

Skill 13-5 ▶ Applying an External Anal Pouch *(continued)*

ACTION	RATIONALE

 15. Remove additional PPE, if used. Perform hand hygiene.

Proper removal of PPE reduces the risk for infection transmission and contamination of other items. Hand hygiene prevents the spread of microorganisms.

EVALUATION

The expected outcomes have been met when the patient has expelled feces into the device, has maintained intact perianal skin, has demonstrated a decrease in the amount and severity of excoriation, has verbalized decreased discomfort.

DOCUMENTATION

Guidelines

Document the date and time the external anal pouch was applied; appearance of perianal area; color of stool; intake and output (amount of stool out); and the patient's reaction to the procedure.

Sample Documentation

8/13/25 1210 Perianal area slightly erythematous. Fecal incontinence bag applied due to incontinence of large amounts of liquid stool and potential skin breakdown; skin barrier applied to area prior to use of pouch. Approximately 90 mL of liquid brown stool noted in drainage bag.

—*K. Sanders, RN*

DEVELOPING CLINICAL REASONING AND CLINICAL JUDGMENT

UNEXPECTED SITUATIONS AND ASSOCIATED INTERVENTIONS

- *Perianal area becomes excoriated:* Remove the device. Thoroughly cleanse the skin and apply a skin barrier. Allow it to dry completely. Reapply the device. Monitor device adhesion and change the device as soon as there is a break in adhesion. Confer with the health care team for a wound, ostomy, and continence nurse consult to manage these issues.
- *Stool is leaking from around sides of device:* Remove the device. Thoroughly cleanse the skin and apply a skin barrier. Allow it to dry completely. Reapply the device. Consider use of a skin barrier paste; apply the paste around the opening of the skin barrier on the adhesive side of the barrier. Use of the skin barrier paste enhances the seal of the skin barrier and helps to fill in uneven skin surfaces to help prevent leakage of feces under the skin barrier (Holllister, 2021). Monitor device adhesion and change the device as soon as there is a break in adhesion.

SPECIAL CONSIDERATIONS

- The fecal collector may be left in place for up to 7 days as long as the skin barrier is intact and adherent (Hollister, 2005). Remove the fecal device based on the manufacturer's recommendations.
- Make sure the patient's perianal skin is clean and completely dry and free from powders, lotions, ointments, or oily residue to support sufficient adhesion of the skin barrier (Hollister, 2021).

Skill 13-6 ▶ Emptying and Changing an Ostomy Appliance

Skill Variation: *Applying a Two-Piece Ostomy Appliance*

Patients sometimes undergo a bowel diversion (surgical procedure) to create an opening into the abdominal wall for fecal elimination. The word **ostomy** is a term for a surgically formed opening in an organ of the body. In the case of the GI tract, the intestinal mucosa is brought out to the abdominal wall, and a **stoma**, the part of the ostomy that is attached to the skin, is formed by suturing the mucosa to the skin. An **ileostomy** allows liquid fecal content from the ileum of the small intestine to be eliminated through the stoma. A **colostomy** permits formed feces in the colon to exit through the stoma. Colostomies are further classified by the part of the colon from which they originate.

Ostomy appliances or pouches are applied to the opening to collect stool. Empty an ostomy appliance before it is half-full to reduce the risk of separation from the skin and leakage (Blevins,

2019; WOCN, 2018); remove and change nondrainable pouches when they are half-full. Ostomy appliances are available in a one-piece (barrier backing already attached to the pouch) or two-piece (separate pouch that fastens to the barrier backing) system. How frequently a drainable appliance should be changed depends on the type being used and specific patient circumstances, but usually every 3 to 7 days (Berti-Hearn & Elliott, 2019; O'Flynn, 2018; Stelton, 2019). Proper application minimizes the risk for skin breakdown around the stoma. The skill outlined below addresses changing a one-piece appliance. A one-piece appliance consists of a pouch with an integral adhesive section that adheres to the patient's skin. The adhesive flange is generally made from hydrocolloid. The accompanying Skill Variation addresses changing a two-piece appliance. Box 13-1 summarizes guidelines for care of the patient with a bowel diversion.

Box 13-1 Guidelines for Ostomy Care

The patient with an ostomy needs physical and psychological support both preoperatively and postoperatively (Wasserman & McGee, 2017). Support can come from the patient's family/caregivers, significant others, members of the health care team, and people who have had similar experiences. Patients who receive consultation preoperatively and care postoperatively from an enterostomal therapy nurse or a wound ostomy continence nurse (WOCN) experience better long-term outcomes (Schreiber, 2016). Use the following guidelines to help promote the physical and psychological comfort of the patient with an ostomy:

- Keep the patient as free of odors as possible. Empty an ostomy appliance before it is half-full to reduce the risk of separation from the skin and leakage (Blevins, 2019; WOCN, 2018).
- Inspect the patient's stoma regularly. Note the size of the stoma, which usually stabilizes within 6 to 8 weeks (Stelton, 2019). It should ideally protrude about 1 to 3 cm above skin level and be dark pink to red in color and moist (Stelton, 2019). A pale stoma may indicate anemia and a dark or purple-blue stoma may reflect compromised circulation or ischemia and may initially appear swollen and edematous. After 6 weeks, the edema has usually subsided. Bleeding around the stoma and its stem should be minimal. The edges of the stoma should appear secure to the surrounding skin (Stelton, 2019). The pulling away of the stoma from the peristomal skin is called mucocutaneous separation or stoma dehiscence (Stelton, 2019) and occurs more often in patients who are at risk for impaired healing, including patients with diabetes, poor nutritional status or who received high-dose steroid therapy or chemotherapy before surgery (Butler, 2009). Notify the health care team promptly if bleeding persists or is excessive, or if color changes occur in the stoma or if it appears the stoma is separating from the peristomal skin (Stelton, 2019).
- Depending on the surgical technique, the final stoma may be flush with the skin. Erosion of skin around the stoma area can also lead to a flush stoma. If an abdominal dressing is in place at the surgical incision, check it frequently for drainage and bleeding. The dressing is usually removed after 24 hours.
- Keep the skin around the stoma site (peristomal area) clean and dry. Assess the peristomal (around the stoma)

skin; peristomal skin should be intact and appear consistent with that of the rest of the abdomen, without pain or discomfort (Burch, 2018). In patients with light skin tones, the peristomal skin should not be reddened; in patients with darker skin tones, the skin should not have darker discolorations (Stelton, 2019). A leaking or ill-fitted stoma appliance will cause moisture-associated skin damage (Berti-Hearn & Elliott, 2019) (refer to the discussion earlier in the chapter). *Candida* or yeast infections can also occur around the stoma if the area is not kept dry.

- Measure the patient's fluid intake and output. Check the ostomy appliance for the quality and quantity of discharge. Initially after surgery, peristalsis may be inhibited. As peristalsis returns, stool will be eliminated from the stoma. Record intake and output every 4 hours for the first 3 days after surgery. If the patient's output decreases while intake remains stable, report the condition promptly.
- Explain each aspect of care to the patient and explain what their role will be when beginning self-care. Patient teaching is one of the most important aspects of ostomy care and should include family members, caregivers, and/or people identified by the patient to include in care, when appropriate. Teaching can begin before surgery, if possible, so that the patient has adequate time to absorb the information.
- Encourage the patient to participate in care and to look at the ostomy. Patients normally experience emotional depression during the early postoperative period. Help the patient cope by listening, explaining, and being available and supportive. A visit from a representative of the local ostomy support group may be helpful. Patients usually begin to accept their altered body image when they are willing to look at the stoma, make neutral or positive statements concerning the ostomy, and express interest in learning self-care.
- Provide support for the patient's physical, psychological, and social activities. Coping strategies need to address body image concerns, permanent body changes, and underlying health issue(s) that resulted in the surgery (Berti-Hearn & Elliott, 2019; Díaz et al., 2018). Encourage patients and their partner/family/caregiver to discuss concerns and to seek help and support (Berti-Hearn & Elliott, 2019; Chandler, 2020; Hill, 2020).

(continued on page 818)

Skill 13-6 ▶ Emptying and Changing an Ostomy Appliance (continued)

DELEGATION CONSIDERATIONS

Emptying a stoma appliance on an ostomy may be delegated to assistive personnel (AP) as well as to licensed practical/vocational nurses (LPN/LVNs). Changing a stoma appliance on an ostomy may be delegated to an LPN/LVN. The decision to delegate must be based on careful analysis of the patient's needs and circumstances as well as the qualifications of the person to whom the task is being delegated. Refer to the Delegation Guidelines in Appendix A.

EQUIPMENT

- Premoistened disposable washcloths or
  - Basin with warm water
  - Skin cleanser, towel, washcloth
- Toilet tissue or paper towel
- Silicone-based adhesive remover
- Gauze squares
- Skin protectant, such as Skin-Prep™
- One-piece ostomy appliance
- Closure clamp, if required, for appliance
- Stoma measuring guide
- Graduated container, toilet, or bedpan
- Ostomy belt (optional)
- Disposable gloves
- Additional PPE, as indicated
- Small plastic trash bag
- Waterproof disposable pad

ASSESSMENT

Assess the current appliance, looking at product style, condition of appliance, and stoma (if the bag is clear). Note the length of time the appliance has been in place. Determine the patient's knowledge of ostomy care, including their level of self-care and ability to manipulate the equipment. After removing the appliance, assess the stoma and the skin surrounding the fecal diversion. The stoma should ideally protrude about 1 to 3 cm above skin level and be dark pink to red in color and moist (Berti-Hearn & Elliott, 2019; Stelton, 2019). The peristomal skin should look like the skin on the rest of the abdomen (Stelton, 2019). If an abdominal dressing is in place at the surgical incision, check it frequently for drainage and bleeding. The dressing is usually removed after 24 hours. Assess the condition of any abdominal scars or incisional areas, if surgery to create the diversion was recent. Assess the amount, color, consistency, and odor of stool from the ostomy.

ACTUAL OR POTENTIAL HEALTH PROBLEMS AND NEEDS

Many actual or potential health problems or issues may require the use of this skill as part of related interventions. An appropriate health problem or issue may include:
- Altered skin integrity risk
- Knowledge deficiency
- Altered body image perception

OUTCOME IDENTIFICATION AND PLANNING

The expected outcome to be met when changing and emptying a bowel diversion appliance is that the stoma appliance is applied correctly to the skin to allow stool to drain freely and without leakage. Other outcomes may include that the patient exhibits a moist red stoma with intact skin surrounding the stoma, demonstrates knowledge of how to apply the appliance, demonstrates positive coping skills, expels stool that is appropriate in consistency and amount for the ostomy location, verbalizes positive self-image.

IMPLEMENTATION

ACTION	RATIONALE
1. Gather equipment.	Assembling equipment provides for an organized approach to the task.
2. Perform hand hygiene and put on PPE, if indicated.	Hand hygiene and PPE prevent the spread of microorganisms. PPE is required based on transmission precautions.
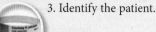 3. Identify the patient.	Identifying the patient ensures the right patient receives the intervention and helps prevent errors.

ACTION

4. Close the curtains around the bed and close the door to the room, if possible. Explain to the patient what you are going to do and why. Encourage the patient to observe or participate, if possible and as appropriate.

5. Assemble equipment on the overbed table or other surface within reach.

6. Assist the patient to a comfortable sitting or lying position in bed or a standing or sitting position in the bathroom. If the patient is in bed, adjust the bed to a comfortable working height (VHACEOSH, 2016). Place a waterproof pad under the patient at the stoma site.

Emptying an Appliance

7. Put on gloves. Remove the clamp (Figure 1) and fold the end of the appliance or pouch upward like a cuff.

8. Empty the contents into a bedpan, toilet, or measuring device (Figure 2).

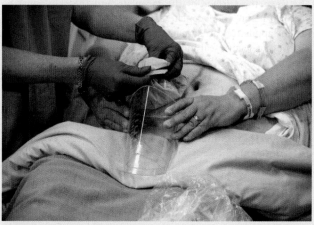

FIGURE 1. Removing clamp, getting ready to empty pouch.

9. Wipe the lower 2 inches of the appliance or pouch with toilet tissue or a paper towel (Figure 3).

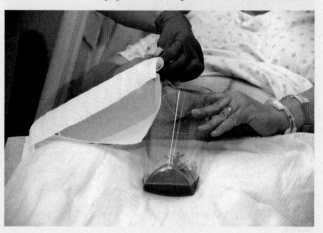

FIGURE 3. Wiping lower 2 inches of pouch with paper towel.

RATIONALE

This ensures the patient's privacy. Explanation relieves anxiety and facilitates engagement. Having the patient observe or assist encourages self-acceptance and helps patient develop self-care skills.

Arranging items nearby is convenient, saves time, and avoids unnecessary stretching and twisting of muscles on the part of the nurse.

Either position should allow the patient to view the procedure in preparation to learn to perform it independently. Lying flat or sitting upright facilitates smooth application of the appliance. Having the bed at the proper height prevents back and muscle strain. A waterproof pad protects linens and the patient from moisture.

Gloves prevent contact with blood, body fluids, and microorganisms. Creating a cuff before emptying prevents additional soiling and odor.

Appliances do not need rinsing because rinsing may reduce the appliance's odor barrier.

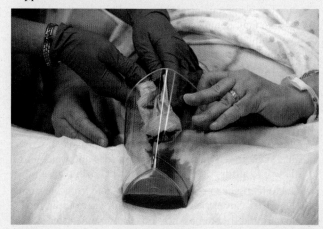

FIGURE 2. Emptying contents of appliance into a measuring device.

Drying the lower section removes any additional fecal material, thus decreasing odor problems.

(*continued on page 820*)

Skill 13-6 ▶ Emptying and Changing an Ostomy Appliance *(continued)*

ACTION	**RATIONALE**
10. Uncuff the edge of the appliance or pouch and apply a clip or clamp, or secure the Velcro closure. Ensure the curve of the clamp follows the curve of the patient's body. Remove gloves. Perform hand hygiene. Assist the patient to a comfortable position.	The edge of the appliance or pouch should remain clean. The clamp secures closure. Hand hygiene deters spread of microorganisms. Positioning ensures patient comfort.
11. If the appliance is not to be changed, place the bed in the lowest position. Remove additional PPE, if used. Perform hand hygiene.	Proper removal of PPE reduces the risk for infection transmission and contamination of other items. Hand hygiene prevents the spread of microorganisms.

Changing an Appliance

ACTION	**RATIONALE**
12. Place a disposable pad on the work surface. Open the premoistened disposable washcloths or set up the washbasin with warm water and the rest of the supplies. Place a trash bag within reach.	The pad protects the work surface. Organization facilitates performance of the procedure.
13. Put on clean gloves. Place a waterproof pad under the patient at the stoma site. Empty the appliance as described in Steps 7–10.	The pad protects linens and the patient from moisture. Emptying the contents before removal prevents accidental spillage of fecal material.
14. Put on gloves. Use two hands to gently remove the appliance faceplate, starting at the top and keeping the abdominal skin taut. Remove the appliance faceplate from the skin by pushing the skin from the appliance rather than pulling the appliance from the skin (Figure 4). Apply a silicone-based adhesive remover by spraying or wiping with the remover wipe, as indicated.	Gloves prevent contact with blood and body fluids. The seal between the surface of the faceplate and the skin must be broken before the faceplate can be removed. Harsh handling of the appliance can damage the skin and impair the development of a secure seal in the future. A silicone-based adhesive remover loosens the adhesive bond to make removal easier and less likely to damage the skin and is particularly beneficial for patients with fragile skin and those at increased risk for medical adhesive–related skin injury/stripping (Collier, 2019; LeBlanc et al., 2019; Swift et al., 2020).
15. Place the appliance in the trash bag, if disposable. If reusable, set it aside to wash in lukewarm soap and water and allow it to air dry after the new appliance is in place.	Thorough cleaning and airing of the appliance reduces odor and deterioration of the appliance. For aesthetic and infection control purposes, discard used appliances appropriately.
16. Use toilet tissue to remove any excess stool from the stoma (Figure 5). Cover the stoma with a gauze pad. Clean the skin around the stoma with skin cleanser and water or a cleansing agent and a washcloth. Remove all old adhesive from the skin; use an adhesive remover, as necessary. Do not apply lotion to the peristomal area.	Toilet tissue, used gently, will not damage the stoma. The gauze absorbs any drainage from the stoma while the skin is being prepared. Cleaning the skin removes excretions, old adhesive, and skin protectant. Excretions or a buildup of other substances can irritate and damage the skin. Lotion will prevent a tight adhesive seal.

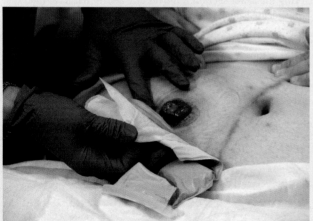

FIGURE 4. Gently removing appliance.

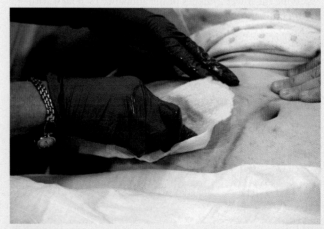

FIGURE 5. Using toilet tissue to remove excess stool from the stoma.

ACTION

17. Gently pat the area dry. **Make sure the skin around the stoma is thoroughly dry.** Assess the stoma and the condition of the surrounding skin (Figure 6).

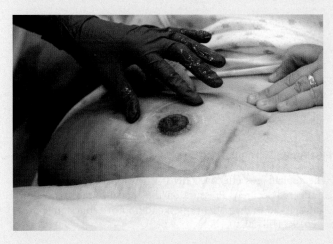

FIGURE 6. Assessing stoma and peristomal skin.

18. Apply skin protectant/barrier film to a 2-inch (5 cm) radius around the stoma, and allow it to dry completely, which takes about 30 seconds.

19. Lift the gauze squares for a moment and measure the stoma opening, using the measurement guide (Figure 7). Replace the gauze. Trace the same-sized opening on the back center of the appliance (Figure 8). Cut the opening 1/8 inch (2 to 3 mm) larger than the stoma size (Hill, 2020) (Figure 9). Using a finger, gently smooth the wafer edges after cutting.

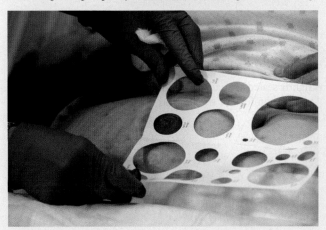

FIGURE 7. Using measurement guide to measure size of stoma.

RATIONALE

Careful drying prevents trauma to the skin and stoma. An intact, properly applied fecal collection device protects skin integrity. Any change in color and size of the stoma may indicate circulatory problems. Refer to Box 13-1 on page 817.

The skin needs protection from the excoriating effect of the excretion and potentially from the appliance adhesive (WOCN, 2018). The skin must be perfectly dry before the appliance is placed to get good adherence and to prevent leaks.

The appliance should fit snugly around the stoma, with only 1/8 inch of skin visible around the opening. A faceplate opening that is too small can cause trauma to the stoma. If the opening is too large, exposed skin will be irritated by stool. The wafer edges may be uneven after cutting and could cause irritation to, and/or pressure on, the stoma.

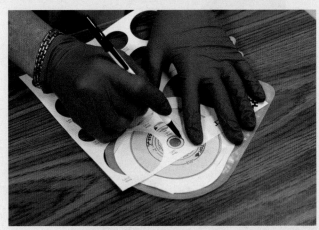

FIGURE 8. Tracing the same-sized circle on back and center of skin barrier.

(*continued on page 822*)

Skill 13-6 ▶ Emptying and Changing an Ostomy Appliance *(continued)*

ACTION	RATIONALE

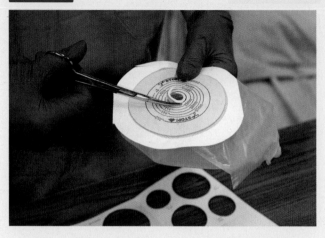

FIGURE 9. Cutting the opening 1/8 inch larger than stoma size.

20. Remove the paper backing from the appliance faceplate (Figure 10). Quickly remove the gauze squares and ease the appliance over the stoma (Figure 11). Gently press it onto the skin while smoothing over the surface. Apply gentle, even pressure to the appliance for approximately 30 seconds (Burch, 2019a; Hill, 2020).

The appliance is effective only if it is properly positioned and adhered securely. Pressure on the appliance faceplate allows it to mold to the patient's skin and improve adhesion (Burch, 2019a; Hill, 2020).

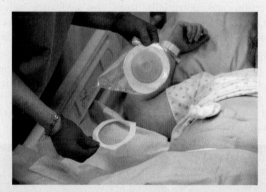

FIGURE 10. Removing paper backing on faceplate.

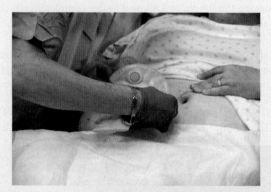

FIGURE 11. Easing appliance over stoma.

21. Close the bottom of the appliance or pouch by folding the end upward and using the clamp or clip that comes with the product (Figure 12), or secure the Velcro closure. Ensure the curve of the clamp follows the curve of the patient's body.

A tightly sealed appliance will not leak and cause embarrassment and discomfort for the patient.

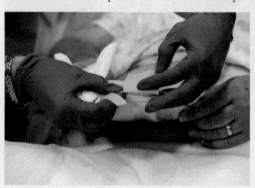

FIGURE 12. Using clip to close bottom of appliance.

ACTION	**RATIONALE**
22. Remove gloves. Perform hand hygiene. Assist the patient to a comfortable position. Cover the patient with bed linens. Place the bed in the lowest position.	Removing gloves reduces risk of transmission of microorganisms. Hand hygiene prevents the spread of microorganisms. Covering provides warmth and promotes patient comfort and safety. The bed in the lowest position promotes patient safety.
23. Put on clean gloves. Remove or discard equipment and assess the patient's response to the procedure.	Gloves prevent contact with blood, body fluids, and microorganisms that contaminate the used equipment. The patient's response may indicate acceptance of the ostomy as well as the need for health teaching.
24. Remove gloves and additional PPE, if used. Perform hand hygiene.	Proper removal of PPE reduces the risk for infection transmission and contamination of other items. Hand hygiene prevents the spread of microorganisms.

EVALUATION

The expected outcomes have been met when the stoma appliance has been applied correctly to the skin to allow stool to drain freely and without leakage, and the patient has exhibited a moist red stoma with intact skin surrounding the stoma, has demonstrated knowledge of how to apply the appliance, has demonstrated positive coping skills, has expelled stool appropriate in consistency and amount for the ostomy location, and has verbalized a positive self-image.

DOCUMENTATION

Guidelines

Document the appearance of the stoma, the condition of the peristomal skin, characteristics of drainage (amount, color, consistency, unusual odor), the patient's reaction to the procedure, and pertinent patient teaching.

Sample Documentation

Lippincott

DocuCare

Practice documenting changing and emptying an ostomy appliance in *Lippincott DocuCare.*

> <u>7/22/25</u> 1630 Colostomy appliance changed due to leakage. Stoma is pink, moist, and flat against abdomen. No erythema or excoriation of surrounding skin. Moderate amount of pasty, brown stool noted in bag. Patient asking appropriate questions during appliance application; states, "I'm ready to try changing the next one."
>
> —*B. Clapp, RN*

DEVELOPING CLINICAL REASONING AND CLINICAL JUDGMENT

UNEXPECTED SITUATIONS AND ASSOCIATED INTERVENTIONS

- *Peristomal skin is excoriated or irritated:* Make sure that the appliance is not cut too large. Skin that is exposed inside of the ostomy appliance will become excoriated. Assess for the presence of a fungal skin infection. If present, consult with the health care team to obtain appropriate treatment. Thoroughly cleanse and dry the skin and apply a product made for excoriated skin before reapplication of the appliance. Allow it to dry completely. Reapply the pouch. Monitor pouch adhesion and change the pouch as soon as there is a break in adhesion. Confer with the health care team for a wound, ostomy, and continence nurse consult to manage these issues. Document the assessment findings and related interventions in the patient's health record.
- *Patient continues to notice odor:* Check the system for any leaks or poor adhesion. Clean the outside of the bag thoroughly when emptying.
- *Bag continues to come loose or fall off:* Thoroughly cleanse the skin and apply a skin barrier. Allow it to dry completely. Reapply the pouch. Monitor pouch adhesion and change the pouch as soon as there is a break in adhesion.

(continued on page 824)

Skill 13-6 ▶ Emptying and Changing an Ostomy Appliance *(continued)*

- *Stoma is protruding into bag:* This is called a prolapse. Have the patient rest for 30 minutes. If the stoma is not back to normal size within that time, notify the health care team. If the stoma stays prolapsed, it may twist, resulting in impaired circulation to the stoma.
- *Stoma is dark brown or black:* Stoma should appear pink to red, shiny, and moist. Alterations indicate compromised circulation. If the stoma is dark brown or black, suspect ischemia and necrosis. Notify the health care team immediately.

Skill Variation ▶ Applying a Two-Piece Ostomy Appliance

A two-piece colostomy appliance is composed of a pouch and a separate adhesive faceplate that attach together (Figure A). The faceplate is left in place for a period of time, depending on the type being used and specific patient circumstances, but usually every 3 to 7 days (American Cancer Society, 2019; Berti-Hearn & Elliott, 2019; O'Flynn, 2018; Stelton, 2019). The pouch/bag may be replaced as needed during this time. The two main types of two-piece appliances are (1) those that "click" together, and (2) those that "adhere" together. The clicking Tupperware-type joining action provides extra security because there is a sensation when the appliance is secured, which the patient can feel. One problem with this type of system is that those with reduced manual dexterity may find it difficult to secure. Another disadvantage is that it is less discreet because the parts of the appliance that click together are bulkier than that of the one-piece system. Two-piece appliances with an adhesive system have the advantage of being more discreet than conventional two-piece systems. They may also be simpler to use for those with poor manual dexterity. A potential disadvantage is that if the adhesive is not joined correctly and forms a crease, feces or flatus may leak out, causing odor and embarrassment. Regardless of the type of two-piece appliance in use, the procedure to change it is basically the same.

1. Gather necessary equipment.

2. Perform hand hygiene and put on PPE, if indicated.

3. Identify the patient.

4. Close the curtains around the bed and close the door to the room, if possible. Explain to the patient what you are going to do and why. Encourage the patient to observe or participate, if possible and as appropriate.

5. Assemble equipment on the overbed table or other surface within reach.

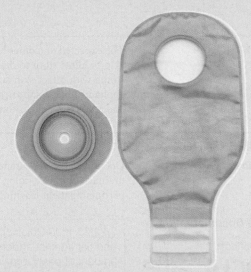

FIGURE A. Two-piece appliances. (*Source:* Courtesy of Hollister, Incorporated, Libertyville, Illinois.)

6. Assist the patient to a comfortable sitting or lying position in bed or a standing or sitting position in the bathroom.

7. Place a disposable pad on the work surface. Set up the washbasin with warm water and the rest of the supplies. Place a trash bag within reach.

8. Put on gloves. Place waterproof pad under the patient at the stoma site. Empty the appliance as described previously in Skill 13-6.

9. Use two hands to gently remove the pouch faceplate from the skin by pushing the skin from the appliance rather than pulling the appliance from the skin. Start at the top of the appliance, while keeping the abdominal skin taut. Apply a silicone-based adhesive remover by spraying or wiping with the remover wipe, as indicated.

10. Place the appliance in the trash bag, if disposable. If it is reusable, set it aside to wash in lukewarm soap and water and allow it to air dry after the new appliance is in place.

11. Use toilet tissue to remove any excess stool from the stoma. Cover the stoma with a gauze pad. Clean the

skin around the stoma with skin cleanser and water or a cleansing agent and a washcloth. Remove all old adhesive from the skin; use an adhesive remover as necessary. Do not apply lotion to the peristomal area.

12. Gently pat the area dry. Make sure the skin around the stoma is thoroughly dry. Assess the stoma and the condition of surrounding skin.

13. Apply a skin protectant/barrier film to a 2-inch (5-cm) radius around the stoma, and allow it to dry completely, which takes about 30 seconds.

14. Lift the gauze squares for a moment and measure the stoma opening, using the measurement guide. Replace the gauze. Trace the same-sized opening on the back center of the appliance faceplate. Cut the opening 1/8 inch (2 to 3 mm) larger than the stoma size (Hill, 2020). Use a finger to gently smooth the wafer edges after cutting.

15. Remove the backing from the faceplate. Quickly remove the gauze squares and ease the faceplate over the stoma. Gently press it onto the skin while smoothing over the surface. Apply gentle pressure to the faceplate for approximately 30 seconds (Burch, 2019a; Hill, 2020) (Figure B).

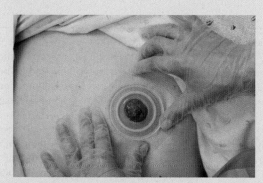

FIGURE B. Gently press faceplate to skin.

16. Apply the appliance pouch to the faceplate following the manufacturer's directions. If using a "click" system, lay the ring on the pouch over the ring on the faceplate. Ask the patient to tighten their stomach muscles, if possible. Beginning at one edge of the ring, push the pouch ring onto the faceplate ring (Figure C). A "click" should be heard when the pouch is secured onto the faceplate.

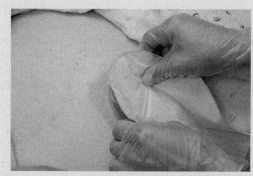

FIGURE C. Applying appliance pouch to faceplate.

17. If using an "adhere" system, remove the paper backing from the faceplate and pouch. Starting at one edge, carefully match the pouch adhesive with the faceplate adhesive. Press firmly and smooth the pouch onto the faceplate, taking care to avoid creases.

18. Close the bottom of the pouch by folding the end upward and using the clamp or clip that comes with the product, or secure the Velcro closure. Ensure the curve of the clamp follows the curve of the patient's body.

19. Remove gloves. Perform hand hygiene. Assist the patient to a comfortable position. Cover the patient with bed linens. Place the bed in the lowest position.

20. Put on clean gloves. Remove or discard equipment and assess the patient's response to the procedure.

21. Remove gloves and additional PPE, if used. Perform hand hygiene.

EVIDENCE FOR PRACTICE ▶

EVIDENCE-BASED PRACTICE GUIDELINE
Providing Care for Patients With Ostomies
Goldberg, M., Colwell, J., Burns, S., Carmel, J., Fellows, J., Hendren, S., Livingston, V., Nottingham, C. U., Pittman, J., Rafferty, J., Salvadalena, G., Steinberg, G., Wound, Ostomy and Continence Nurses Society, & Guideline Development Task Force. (2018). WOCN Society Clinical Guideline: Management of the adult patient with a fecal or urinary ostomy–An executive summary. *Journal of Wound, Ostomy and Continence Nursing, 45*(1), 50–58. https://doi.org/10.1097/WON.0000000000000396

These guidelines provide evidence-based recommendations to guide care for patients with ostomies, prevent or decrease complications, and improve patient outcomes.

Skill 13-7 ▶ Irrigating a Colostomy

Colostomy irrigation is a way of achieving fecal continence and control (Kent et al., 2015). Irrigations are used to stimulate the colon to empty to promote regular evacuation of stool (up to 24 to 48 hours) from distal colostomies, resulting in reduction or elimination of the need for the patient to use a pouch to collect stool (Cleveland Clinic, 2016; Kent et al., 2015). Colostomy irrigation may be indicated in patients who have a left-sided end colostomy in the descending or sigmoid colon, are mentally alert, have adequate vision, and have adequate manual dexterity needed to perform the procedure (Goldberg et al., 2018; Kent et al., 2015). Contraindications to colostomy irrigation include irritable bowel syndrome (IBS), peristomal hernia, postradiation damage to the bowel, diverticulitis, and Crohn disease (Kent et al., 2015). Ileostomies are not irrigated because the fecal content of the ileum is liquid and cannot be controlled.

The patient establishes a routine by repeating this process regularly, once a day or once every second day; the colon can be trained to empty with minimal spillage of stool in between irrigations (Cleveland Clinic, 2016). Once the patient has established a routine and bowel continence has been established, a small appliance can be worn over the stoma. These "stoma caps" are small-capacity coverings with a pad to soak up discharge and a flatus filter (Kent et al., 2015; Palmer, 2020). If a colostomy irrigation is to be implemented, the nurse should consult facility policy regarding the accepted procedure and, ideally, consult with a wound, ostomy, and continence nurse (WOCN) for patient education, supervision, and support (Boutry et al., 2021).

DELEGATION CONSIDERATIONS

Colostomy irrigation is not delegated to assistive personnel (AP). Depending on the state's nurse practice act and the organization's policies and procedures, the administration of a colostomy irrigation may be delegated to licensed practical/vocational nurses (LPN/LVNs). The decision to delegate must be based on careful analysis of the patient's needs and circumstances as well as the qualifications of the person to whom the task is being delegated. Refer to the Delegation Guidelines in Appendix A.

EQUIPMENT

- Disposable irrigation system and irrigation sleeve
- Waterproof pad
- Bedpan or toilet
- Water-soluble lubricant
- IV pole
- Disposable gloves
- Additional PPE, as indicated
  - Warmed irrigation solution (usually tap water) at or just above body temperature (Dougherty & Lister, 2015, as cited in Mitchell, 2019b, p. 155; Memorial Sloan Kettering Cancer Center, 2021)
  - First day of irrigation: 250 mL of water (Memorial Sloan Kettering Cancer Center, 2021)
  - Second day: 500 mL of water (Memorial Sloan Kettering Cancer Center, 2021)
  - Third day: 750 mL of water (Memorial Sloan Kettering Cancer Center, 2021)

- Fourth day:
  - If patient is having a large bowel movement when using 750 mL and no bowel movements between irrigations, continue with use of 750 mL (Memorial Sloan Kettering Cancer Center, 2021).
  - If patient is having bowel movements between irrigations, use 100 mL of water. Do not use more than 1,000 mL of water (Memorial Sloan Kettering Cancer Center, 2021).
- Premoistened disposable washcloths or
- Basin with warm water
- Skin cleanser, towel, washcloth
- Paper towel
- New ostomy appliance, if needed, or stoma cover

ASSESSMENT

Ask the patient when they had their last bowel movement. Determine the patient's knowledge of ostomy care, including their level of self-care and ability to manipulate the equipment. Assess the patient's abdomen, including auscultating for bowel sounds and palpating for tenderness and/or firmness. Ask the patient if they have been experiencing any abdominal discomfort. Ask the patient about the date of the last irrigation and whether there have been any changes in stool pattern or consistency. If the patient irrigates their colostomy at home, ask if they have any special routines during irrigation, such as reading the newspaper or listening to music. Also determine how much solution the patient typically uses for irrigation. The normal amount of irrigation fluid varies but is usually around 750 to 1,000 mL for an adult (Memorial Sloan Kettering Cancer Center, 2021). Assess the ostomy, ensuring that the diversion is a colostomy. Note the placement of the colostomy on the abdomen, color and size of the ostomy, color and condition of the stoma, and amount and consistency of stool. The stoma should ideally protrude about 1 to 3 cm above skin level and be dark pink to red in color and moist (Berti-Hearn & Elliott, 2019; Stelton, 2019). The peristomal skin should look like the skin on the rest of the abdomen (Stelton, 2019).

ACTUAL OR POTENTIAL HEALTH PROBLEMS AND NEEDS	Many actual or potential health problems or issues may require the use of this skill as part of related interventions. An appropriate health problem or issue may include: • Knowledge deficiency • Impaired ability to manage stoma care • Altered body image perception
OUTCOME IDENTIFICATION AND PLANNING	The expected outcome to be met when irrigating a colostomy is that the patient expels soft, formed stool. Other appropriate outcomes include that the patient remains free of any evidence of trauma to the stoma and intestinal mucosa, demonstrates the ability to participate in care, and voices increased confidence with ostomy care.

IMPLEMENTATION

ACTION	**RATIONALE**
1. Verify the prescribed intervention for an irrigation. Gather equipment (Figure 1).	Verifying the prescribed intervention is crucial to ensuring that the proper treatment is administered to the right patient. Assembling equipment provides for an organized approach to the task.

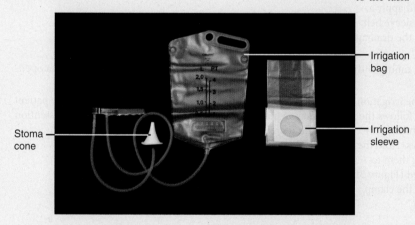

FIGURE 1. Irrigation sleeve and bag.

ACTION	**RATIONALE**
2. Perform hand hygiene and put on PPE, if indicated.	Hand hygiene and PPE prevent the spread of microorganisms. PPE is required based on transmission precautions.
3. Identify the patient.	Identifying the patient ensures the right patient receives the intervention and helps prevent errors.
4. Close the curtains around the bed and close the door to the room, if possible. Explain to the patient what you are going to do and why. Plan where the patient will receive irrigation. Assist the patient onto a bedside commode or into a nearby bathroom. If administering in the bathroom, assist the patient to sit on the toilet or a chair next to the toilet.	Closing the curtains and door ensures the patient's privacy. Discussion and explanation promote patient engagement and help to minimize anxiety. The patient cannot hold the irrigation solution. A large immediate return of irrigation solution and stool usually occurs.

(continued on page 828)

Skill 13-7 ▶ Irrigating a Colostomy (continued)

ACTION

5. Assemble equipment on the overbed table or other surface within reach.

6. Warm the irrigation solution to at or just above body temperature by placing the container with the solution in the amount prescribed in another container of warm water, and check the temperature with a thermometer, if available. If a thermometer is not available, warm and test on your inner wrist. If tap water is used, adjust the temperature as it flows from the faucet.

7. Add the irrigation solution to the container. Release the clamp and allow fluid to progress through the tube before reclamping.

8. Hang the container on the IV pole so that bottom of bag will be at the patient's shoulder level when seated. As a result, the bag should be about 18 inches above the stoma (Memorial Sloan Kettering Cancer Center, 2021).

9. Put on gloves.

10. Unsnap and remove the ostomy cover or the bag from the back plate of a two-piece appliance and snap on the irrigation sleeve (Figure 2). Alternatively, if the patient uses a one-piece appliance, remove the appliance, and apply a disposable irrigation sleeve. Use an irrigation sleeve belt, depending on type of device (Figure 2). Place the drainage end into the toilet bowl or commode.

11. Cover the cone tip at the end of the irrigation tubing with water-soluble lubricant.

12. Insert the cone through the top open end of the irrigation sleeve and into the stoma, angling the tip so it follows the natural direction of the colon (Figure 3A). Introduce the solution slowly over a period of 5 to 10 minutes. Hold the cone and tubing (or if the patient is able, allow them to hold) all the time that solution is being instilled (Figure 3B). Control the rate of flow by closing or opening the clamp.

RATIONALE

Arranging items nearby is convenient, saves time, and avoids unnecessary stretching and twisting of muscles on the part of the nurse.

The irrigation solution should be at or just above body temperature and warmed if necessary (Dougherty & Lister, 2015, as cited in Mitchell, 2019b, p. 155; Memorial Sloan Kettering Cancer Center, 2021). Warming the solution prevents chilling the patient, which would add to the discomfort of the procedure. A cold solution could cause cramping; a too-warm solution could cause trauma to intestinal mucosa.

This process causes any air to be expelled from the tubing. Although allowing air to enter the intestine is not harmful, it may further distend the intestine.

Gravity forces the solution to enter the intestine. The amount of pressure determines the rate of flow and pressure exerted on the intestinal wall.

Gloves prevent contact with blood, body fluids, and microorganisms.

The irrigation sleeve directs all irrigation fluid and stool into the toilet or commode for easy disposal.

The lubricant facilitates passage of the cone into the stoma opening.

If the irrigation solution is administered too quickly, the patient may experience nausea and cramps due to rapid distention and increased pressure in the intestine.

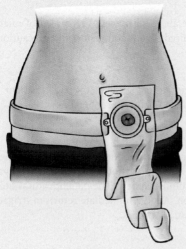

FIGURE 2. Positioning of irrigation sleeve on abdomen.

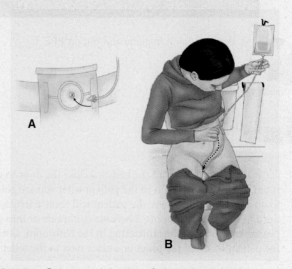

FIGURE 3. Colostomy irrigation. A. Inserting irrigation cone. B. Instilling irrigating fluid with sleeve in place.

ACTION	**RATIONALE**
13. Once the irrigation bag is empty, close the clamp on the tubing. Remove the cone and close the tip of the irrigation sleeve.	Once the irrigation solution has been completely instilled, the irrigation bag is no longer needed.
14. The patient should remain seated on the toilet or bedside commode.	An immediate return of solution and stool will usually occur, followed by a return in spurts for 30 to 45 more minutes.
15. After the majority of solution has returned, assist the patient to clip (close) the bottom of the irrigating sleeve and continue with daily activities.	Leaving the sleeve in place allows the patient to continue with daily activities until the return of solution is complete. Solution may return in spurts for 30 to 45 minutes.
16. After solution has stopped flowing from the stoma (about an hour after the start of the irrigation), put on clean gloves. Empty the contents of the sleeve into the toilet. Remove the irrigating sleeve and cleanse the skin around the stoma opening with skin cleanser and water. Gently pat the peristomal skin dry.	Gloves prevent contact with blood and body fluids. Peristomal skin must be clean and free of any liquid or stool before application of a new appliance.
17. Attach a new appliance to the stoma or stoma cover (see Skill 13-6), as needed.	Some patients will not require an appliance but may use a stoma cover. This protects the stoma.
18. Remove gloves. Perform hand hygiene. Return the patient to a comfortable position. Make sure the linens under the patient are dry, if appropriate. Ensure that the patient is covered.	Removing gloves prevents the spread of microorganisms. Hand hygiene prevents the spread of microorganisms. Dry linens promote patient comfort.
19. Raise the side rail, lower the bed height, and adjust the head of the bed to a comfortable position, as necessary.	Positioning promotes patient comfort. The bed in the lowest position promotes patient safety.
20. Clean reusable irrigation equipment; rinse it with water to remove any stool and use a paper towel or washcloth to wash it with mild soap and water. Dry the inside and outside and leave out to finish air drying; alternatively, clean it according to the manufacturer's directions. Dispose of a disposable irrigation sleeve in an appropriate trash receptacle.	Cleaning the equipment reduces the risk of transmission of microorganisms and leaves equipment ready for future use.
21. Remove additional PPE, if used. Perform hand hygiene.	Proper removal of PPE reduces the risk for infection transmission and contamination of other items. Hand hygiene prevents the spread of microorganisms.

EVALUATION

The expected outcomes have been met when the irrigation solution has flowed easily into the stoma opening, and the patient has expelled soft, formed stool; has remained free of any evidence of trauma to the stoma and intestinal mucosa; has demonstrated the ability to participate in care; and has voiced increased confidence with ostomy care.

DOCUMENTATION

Guidelines

Document the procedure, including the amount of irrigating solution used; color, amount, and consistency of stool returned; condition of the stoma; degree of patient participation; and the patient's reaction to irrigation.

Sample Documentation

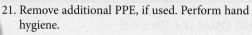

8/1/25 0945 1,000 mL of warmed tap water used to irrigate colostomy. Large amount of soft, dark brown stool returned. Patient performed procedure with small amount of assistance from nurse. Stoma is pink and moist with no signs of bleeding. Patient tolerated procedure without incident. New ostomy appliance applied.

—*B. Clapp, RN*

(continued on page 830)

Skill 13-7 ▶ Irrigating a Colostomy *(continued)*

DEVELOPING CLINICAL REASONING AND CLINICAL JUDGMENT

UNEXPECTED SITUATIONS AND ASSOCIATED INTERVENTIONS

- *Irrigation solution is not flowing or is flowing at a slow rate:* Check the clamp on the tubing to make sure that the tubing is open. Gently manipulate the cone in the stoma to alter the direction of the cone; if stool or tissue is blocking the cone opening, this may block the flow of fluid. Remove the cone from the stoma, clean the area, and gently reinsert. Alternatively, assist the patient to a side-lying or sitting position in bed. Place a waterproof pad under the irrigation sleeve. Place the drainage end of the sleeve in a bedpan.
- *Patient experiences abdominal cramping:* Stop the flow of the water; encourage the patient to take some slow deep breaths and gently rub their abdomen to help the muscles relax (Memorial Sloan Kettering Cancer Center, 2021). Check the height of the irrigation bag; adjust the height if it is too high, as the increased pressure may cause cramping. Restart the irrigation at a decreased rate to reduce risk of cramping.
- *Patient experiences breakthrough evacuation of stool:* This is not uncommon in the beginning. The bowel needs to get used to the procedure over a period of 2 or 3 weeks (Clow et al., 2015). Once irrigation is established, irrigate at approximately the same time on each occasion and do not hurry the procedure (Clow et al., 2015; Memorial Sloan Kettering Cancer Center, 2021).

SPECIAL CONSIDERATIONS

- Irrigation and manipulation of the stoma should be avoided in patients who are myelosuppressed and/or in patients at risk for myelosuppression and mucositis (NCI, 2020).
- Patients should irrigate their colostomy close to the same time every day to decrease the risk for bowel movements between irrigations (Memorial Sloan Kettering Cancer Center, 2021). Patients may consider timing irrigation after having a meal or hot drink (Memorial Sloan Kettering Cancer Center, 2021).
- Inform patients that it is important not to rush an irrigation; irrigation of a colostomy will take 1 to 1.5 hours (Memorial Sloan Kettering Cancer Center, 2021).

EVIDENCE FOR PRACTICE ▶

COLOSTOMY IRRIGATION AND QUALITY OF LIFE

Colostomy irrigation stimulates emptying of the colon at regularly scheduled times and offers the patient some control over bowel function. The presence of a colostomy often has a major impact on quality of life; colostomy irrigation has the potential to positively impact the quality of life for patients with a descending or sigmoid colostomy (Boutry et al., 2021). Is this an intervention that should be considered an important part of patient care?

Related Research

Boutry, E., Bertrand, M. M., Ripoche, J., Alonso, S., Bastide, S., Prudhomme, M., & French Federation of Ostomy. (2021). Quality of life in colostomy patients practicing colonic irrigation: An observational study. *Journal of Visceral Surgery, 158*(1), 4–10. https://doi.org/10.1016/j.jviscsurg.2020.07.003

The purpose of this study was to assess the impact of colostomy irrigation on the quality of life of patients with a colostomy. The study evaluated patients with a colostomy who utilized irrigation versus patients with a colostomy who did not practice irrigation. Patients with colostomies who were members of the French Federation of Ostomy members were eligible to participate. Data were collected from participants using a self-questionnaire that assessed their experience of colostomy irrigation (CI), including habits related to CI, difficulties encountered, if help was required, who trained the participant, whether they had a referent nurse, time required, frequency of stools, position when irrigating, consistency of stools, liquid used, product used to cover stoma, occurrence of leaks, whether they would recommend CI, and if they were satisfied with the procedure. In addition, participants completed the Stoma-QOL (quality of life) questionnaire. A total of 2,673 questionnaires were sent to members, and 1,120 were returned; 371 were excluded for several reasons, including incomplete data and indeterminable stoma type, resulting in the analysis of 749 questionnaires. Forty-one percent (41%) of the participants practiced CI. The median quality-of-life score as measured by the Stoma-QOL score was significantly higher for the patients practicing CI ($p < .001$). The majority of patients practicing CI (99.3%) would recommend it to other patients. Almost 99% (98.9%) of participants using CI expressed satisfaction with the procedure and a desire to continue with the practice. Risk factors for not performing CI included age, obesity, the presence of the colostomy for less than 6 years, and a nononcologic indication for the surgery. The researchers concluded CI appeared to improve the quality of life of patients with a colostomy and suggested education about this intervention should be offered to all patients. The researchers also suggested that supervision by an enterostomal nurse is recommended, especially for patients with a high risk of failure.

Relevance to Nursing Practice
Nurses have a responsibility to update and maintain relevant knowledge and skills to maintain competence in providing care options to patients. The creation of a bowel diversion can negatively affect every aspect of a person's life, including overall quality of life. Nurses need to consider the effect of this treatment on patients' lifestyles and health-related quality of life in order to provide thoughtful, person-centered nursing care. Colostomy irrigation provides a management option that has the potential to contribute to patient-focused and thoughtful, person-centered care.

EVIDENCE FOR PRACTICE ▶

EVIDENCE-BASED PRACTICE GUIDELINE
Providing Care for Patients With Ostomies
Goldberg, M., Colwell, J., Burns, S., Carmel, J., Fellows, J., Hendren, S., Livingston, V., Nottingham, C. U., Pittman, J., Rafferty, J., Salvadalena, G., Steinberg, G., Wound, Ostomy and Continence Nurses Society, & Guideline Development Task Force. (2018). WOCN Society Clinical Guideline: Management of the adult patient with a fecal or urinary ostomy—An executive summary. *Journal of Wound, Ostomy and Continence Nursing, 45*(1), 50–58. https://doi.org/10.1097/WON.0000000000000396

These guidelines provide evidence-based recommendations to guide care for patients with ostomies, prevent or decrease complications, and improve patient outcomes.

Skill 13-8 ▶ Inserting a Nasogastric Tube

A nasogastric (NG) tube is a pliable single- or double-lumen (inner open space) plastic tube that is hollow and is passed through the nose and into the stomach. Double-lumen tubes are used for gastric decompression (Sigmon & An, 2020) (Figure 1). One larger lumen empties the stomach via suction, and the other provides for a continuous flow of air (acting as a sump) (Sigmon & An, 2020). The airflow lumen controls suction by preventing the drainage lumen from pulling stomach mucosa into the tube's openings and irritating the stomach lining. A one-way antireflux valve may be used in the airflow lumen to prevent reflux of gastric contents through the airflow lumen (Figure 1). When pressure from gastric contents enters the airflow tubing, the valve closes to prevent secretions from exiting the tube.

NG tubes may be used to decompress or drain the stomach of fluid or unwanted stomach contents such as poison or medication and air (Burns & Delgado, 2019) and may be used when conditions are present in which peristalsis is absent. Examples include paralytic ileus and intestinal obstruction by tumor or hernia and adhesive small bowel obstruction (ten Broek et al., 2018). NG tubes may also be used to allow the gastrointestinal tract to rest before or after abdominal surgery to promote healing

(*continued on page 832*)

Skill 13-8 ▶ Inserting a Nasogastric Tube *(continued)*

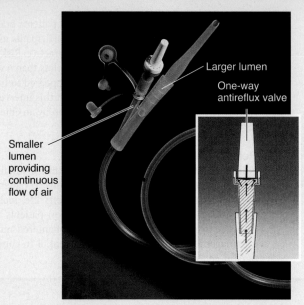

Larger lumen
One-way antireflux valve
Smaller lumen providing continuous flow of air

FIGURE 1. Double-lumen nasogastric tube with a one-way antireflux valve in the airflow lumen.

(Bauldoff et al., 2020). Historically, an NG tube was often used postoperatively as a routine part of care after major abdominal surgery, to rest the intestinal tract and promote healing. Research now shows the routine use of NG tubes after abdominal surgery may serve no beneficial purpose and may actually delay the patient's progress, increasing the time required for flatus to occur and increasing pulmonary complications (Hodin & Bordeianou, 2020; Kantrancha & George, 2014; Sigmon & An, 2020; Venara et al., 2020). Decompression should be reserved for patients with conditions such as a prolonged postoperative ileus or a small bowel obstruction (Hodin & Bordeianou, 2020). Tubes for decompression typically are attached to suction. Suction can be applied intermittently or continuously. When the underlying condition has been resolved and/or the NG tube is no longer indicated, the tube is removed (refer to Skill 13-10).

NG tubes may also be used to administer medications or to provide short-term nutrition, using the stomach as a natural reservoir for food. The use of NG tubes for nutritional purposes is discussed in Chapter 11. Administration of medications via an NG tube is discussed in Chapter 5.

Radiographic examination, measurement of tube length and measurement of tube marking, measurement of aspirate pH, and monitoring of carbon dioxide have been suggested to confirm tube placement in the stomach. The use of two or more of these techniques in conjunction with each other increases the likelihood of correct tube placement (AACN, 2020; Anderson, 2019; Dias et al., 2019; Irving et al., 2018; Methany et al., 2019; Rahimi et al., 2015). Recommendations for use of visual inspection of gastric aspirate are conflicting; this method should be used cautiously if part of policy and procedure guidelines and with consideration to the potential for inaccuracy (AACN, 2020; Dias et al., 2019; Mak & Tam, 2020; Metheny et al., 2019). When bedside methods to check placement suggest the tube has been displaced, a radiograph should be requested to determine the tube's location (AACN, 2020). An old technique of auscultation of air injected into a tube has been proved unreliable and should not be used (AACN, 2020; Boeykens et al., 2014; Boullata et al., 2017; Irving et al., 2018; Metheny et al., 2019). A detailed discussion of each of these methods to confirm placement is provided in Chapter 11, Nutrition.

DELEGATION CONSIDERATIONS

The insertion of an NG tube is not delegated to assistive personnel (AP). Depending on the state's nurse practice act and the organization's policies and procedures, insertion of an NG tube may be delegated to licensed practical/vocational nurses (LPN/LVNs). The decision to delegate must be based on careful analysis of the patient's needs and circumstances as well as the qualifications of the person to whom the task is being delegated. Refer to the Delegation Guidelines in Appendix A.

EQUIPMENT

- NG tube of appropriate size (8 to 18F)
- Stethoscope
- Water-soluble lubricant
- Normal saline solution or sterile water, for irrigation, depending on facility policy
- Tongue blade
- Irrigations set, including a large syringe (20 to 50 mL)
- Flashlight
- Nonallergenic tape (1 inch wide)
- Tissues
- Glass of water with straw
- Topical anesthetic—lidocaine spray or gel (optional)

- Clamp
- Suction apparatus (if prescribed)
- Bath towel or disposable pad
- Emesis basin
- Safety pin and rubber band
- Nonsterile, disposable gloves
- Additional PPE, as indicated
- Tape measure, or other measuring device
- Skin barrier
- pH test strip (calibrated in units of 0.5 and approved for use with human secretions)

ASSESSMENT

Assess the patency of the patient's nares by asking the patient to occlude one nostril and breathe normally through the other. Select the nostril through which air passes more easily. Also, assess the patient's history for any recent facial trauma, polyps, blockages, or surgeries. Patients with facial fractures or facial surgeries present a higher risk for misplacement of the tube into the brain. Many facilities require a health care provider to place NG tubes in these patients. Inspect the abdomen for distention and firmness; auscultate for bowel sounds or peristalsis and palpate the abdomen for distention and tenderness. If the abdomen is distended, consider measuring the abdominal girth at the umbilicus to establish a baseline.

ACTUAL OR POTENTIAL HEALTH PROBLEMS AND NEEDS

Many actual or potential health problems or issues may require the use of this skill as part of related interventions. An appropriate health problem or issue may include:
- Impaired gastrointestinal system function
- Knowledge deficiency
- Risk for impaired gastrointestinal system function

OUTCOME IDENTIFICATION AND PLANNING

The expected outcome to achieve when inserting an NG tube is that the tube is passed into the patient's stomach without any complications. Other outcomes may include that the patient exhibits no signs and symptoms of aspiration, rates pain as decreased from prior to insertion, and verbalizes an understanding of the reason for NG tube insertion.

IMPLEMENTATION

ACTION	RATIONALE
1. Verify the prescribed intervention for insertion of an NG tube. Gather equipment, including selection of the appropriate NG tube.	This ensures the patient receives the correct treatment. Assembling equipment provides for an organized approach to the task. NG tubes should be radiopaque, contain clearly visible markings for measurement, and may have multiple ports for aspiration.
2. Perform hand hygiene and put on PPE, if indicated.	Hand hygiene and PPE prevent the spread of microorganisms. PPE is required based on transmission precautions.
3. Identify the patient.	Identifying the patient ensures the right patient receives the intervention and helps prevent errors.

(continued on page 834)

Skill 13-8 ▶ Inserting a Nasogastric Tube *(continued)*

ACTION	**RATIONALE**
4. Explain the procedure to the patient, including the rationale for why the tube is needed. Discuss the associated discomforts that may be experienced and possible interventions that may allay this discomfort. Answer any questions, as needed.	Explanation facilitates patient engagement and reduces anxiety.
5. Assemble equipment on the overbed table or other surface within reach.	Arranging items nearby is convenient, saves time, and avoids unnecessary stretching and twisting of muscles on the part of the nurse.
6. Close the patient's bedside curtain or door. Raise the bed to a comfortable working position (VHACEOSH, 2016). Assist the patient to high-Fowler position or elevate the head of the bed 45 degrees if the patient is unable to maintain an upright position. Drape their chest with a bath towel or disposable pad. Have an emesis basin and tissues within reach.	Closing the curtains or the door provides for patient privacy. Having the bed at the proper height prevents back and muscle strain. The upright position is more natural for swallowing and reduces the risk for aspiration if the patient should vomit. Passage of the tube may stimulate gagging and tearing of the eyes.
7. **Refer to facility policy regarding method(s) to determine insertion length.** Measure the distance to insert the tube by placing the tube tip at the patient's nostril and extending it to the tip of the earlobe and then to the point midway between the xiphoid process and umbilicus. Alternatively, measure from the xiphisternum (xiphoid process) to the earlobe, to the nose and add 10 cm (Fan et al., 2019). **Refer to facility policy. Mark the tube with an indelible marker.**	The NEMU (nose-ear-mid-umbilicus) has been suggested as an accurate method of measurement in infants and children (Ellett et al., 2012; Irving et al., 2018). Another method, the xiphisternum-earlobe-nose +10 cm, has been suggested as the best estimate for the length of NG tube required (Fan et al., 2019). Correct positioning results in tip positioning between 3 and 10 cm under the lower esophageal sphincter (Torsy et al., 2018). Determination of NG tube insertion length is controversial, and recommendations are conflicting; most evidence for practice identifies the need for more research to determine more accurate and reliable ways to determine tube insertion depth (Boeykens, 2018; Fan et al., 2019; Mak & Tam, 2020; Parker et al., 2018; Taylor, 2020; Torsy et al., 2018).
8. Put on gloves. Lubricate the tip of the tube (at least 2 to 4 inches) with water-soluble lubricant. Apply topical anesthetic to the nostril and oropharynx, as appropriate.	Lubrication reduces friction and facilitates passage of the tube into the stomach. Water-soluble lubricant will not cause pneumonia if the tube accidentally enters the lungs. Topical anesthetics act as local anesthetics, reducing discomfort. Consult the health care team for an order for a topical anesthetic, such as lidocaine gel or spray, if needed.
9. After selecting the appropriate nostril, ask the patient to flex their head slightly back against the pillow. Gently insert the tube into the nostril while directing the tube upward and backward along the floor of the nose (Figure 2). The patient may gag when the tube reaches the pharynx. Provide tissues for tearing or watering of the eyes. Offer comfort and reassurance to the patient.	Following the normal contour of the nasal passage while inserting the tube reduces irritation and the likelihood of mucosal injury. The tube stimulates the gag reflex readily. Tears are a natural response as the tube passes into the nasopharynx. Many patients report that gagging and throat discomfort can be more painful than the tube passing through the nostrils.

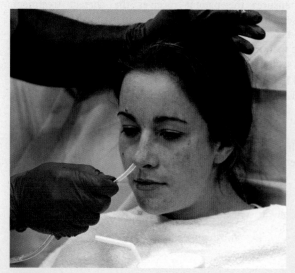

FIGURE 2. Beginning insertion with patient positioned with head slightly flexed back.

ACTION

10. When the pharynx is reached, instruct the patient to touch their chin to their chest. Encourage the patient to sip water through a straw or swallow (Figure 3). Advance the tube in a downward and backward direction when the patient swallows. Stop when the patient breathes. **If gagging and coughing persist, stop advancing the tube and check placement of the tube with a tongue blade and flashlight.** If the tube is curled, straighten the tube and attempt to advance it again. Keep advancing the tube until the pen marking is reached. **Do not use force.** Rotate the tube if it meets resistance.

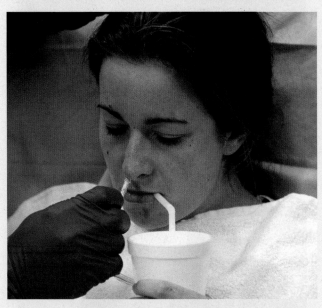

FIGURE 3. Advancing tube after patient drops chin to chest and while swallowing.

11. **Discontinue the procedure and remove the tube if there are signs of distress, such as gasping, coughing, cyanosis, and inability to speak or hum.**

12. Secure the tube loosely to the nose or cheek with tape until placement is verified. Confirm placement of the NG tube in the patient's stomach using at least two methods. Refer to Skill 11-2 in Chapter 11.

13. After confirmation of tube placement, secure the tube. Apply a skin barrier to the tip and end of the nose and allow it to dry. Remove gloves and secure the tube with a commercially prepared securement device (Figure 4) (follow the manufacturer's directions) or tape it to the patient's nose. To secure with tape:

    a. Cut a 4-inch piece of tape and split the bottom 2 inches (Figure 5) or use packaged nose tape for NG tubes.

RATIONALE

Bringing the head forward helps close the trachea and open the esophagus. Swallowing helps advance the tube, causes the epiglottis to cover the opening of the trachea, and helps to eliminate gagging and coughing. Excessive coughing and gagging may occur if the tube has curled in the back of the throat. Forcing the tube may injure mucous membranes.

The tube is in the airway if the patient shows signs of distress and cannot speak or hum. If, after three attempts, NG insertion is unsuccessful, another nurse may try, or the patient should be referred to another health care professional.

Verify correct placement of the NG tube after the initial insertion, before beginning a feeding or instilling medications or liquids, and at regular intervals during continuous feedings (Metheny et al., 2019). A misplaced tube in the lungs or pulmonary tissue places the patient at risk for aspiration, pneumonia, and even death (Lamont et al., 2011, as cited in Anderson, 2018). With the exception of radiographic examination, which is usually done immediately after insertion to verify initial tube placement, the use of two or more techniques in conjunction with each other increases the likelihood of correct tube placement (AACN, 2020; Anderson, 2019; Anderson, 2018; Dias et al., 2019; Rahimi et al., 2015).

Securing the tube prevents migration of the tube inward and outward. The skin barrier improves adhesion and protects skin. Constant pressure of the tube against the skin and mucous membranes may cause pressure injury (Powers, 2019).

(continued on page 836)

Skill 13-8 ▶ Inserting a Nasogastric Tube *(continued)*

ACTION

b. Place the unsplit end over the bridge of the patient's nose (Figure 6).

c. Wrap the split ends under and around the NG tube (Figure 7). **Be careful not to pull the tube too tightly against the nose** (Powers, 2019).

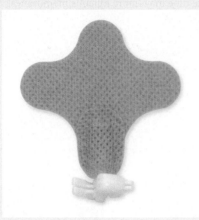

FIGURE 4. Example of a commercially prepared securement device. (*Source:* Courtesy of Hollister, Incorporated, Libertyville, Illinois.)

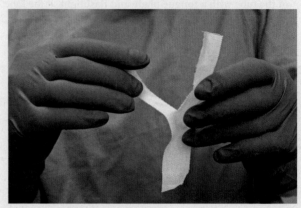

FIGURE 5. Making a 2-inch cut into a 4-inch strip of tape.

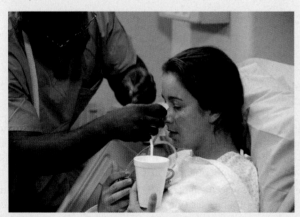

FIGURE 6. Applying tape to patient's nose.

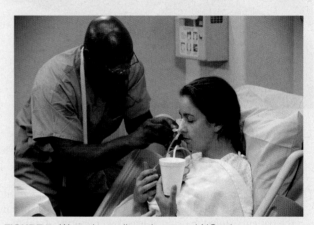

FIGURE 7. Wrapping split ends around NG tube.

14. Put on gloves. Clamp the tube and remove the syringe. Cap or attach the tube to suction (Figure 8), according to the prescribed interventions. Remove gloves. Perform hand hygiene.

15. Measure the length of the exposed tube. Reinforce the marking on the tube at the nostril with indelible ink. Ask the patient to turn their head to the side opposite the nostril in which the tube is inserted. Secure the tube to the patient's gown by using rubber band or tape and a safety pin. For additional support, tape the tube onto the patient's cheek using a piece of tape. **Secure the vent of the double-lumen tube above stomach level.** Attach the vent at shoulder level (Figure 9).

RATIONALE

Gloves prevent contact with blood and body fluids and transfer of microorganisms. Suction provides for decompression of the stomach and drainage of gastric contents. Removing gloves properly and using hand hygiene reduces the risk for infection transmission and contamination of other items.

The tube should be marked with an indelible marker at the nostril. This marking should be assessed each time the tube is used to ensure the tube has not become displaced. Tube length should be checked and compared with this initial measurement, in conjunction with pH measurement and visual assessment of aspirate, at regular intervals. An increase in the length of the exposed tube may indicate dislodgement (AACN, 2020; Boullata et al., 2017). Securing prevents tension and tugging on the tube. Turning the head ensures adequate slack in the tubing to prevent tension when the patient turns the head. Securing the double-lumen tube above stomach level prevents seepage of gastric contents and keeps the lumen clear for venting air.

ACTION

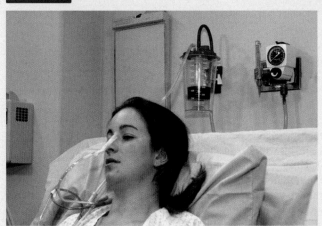

FIGURE 8. NG tube attached to wall suction.

RATIONALE

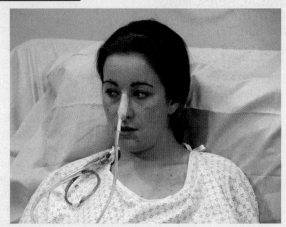

FIGURE 9. Patient with Salem sump tube (NG) secured. Note blue vent at patient's shoulder.

16. Put on gloves. Assist with or provide oral hygiene at 2- to 4-hour intervals. Lubricate the lips generously and clean nares and lubricate, as needed. Offer analgesic throat lozenges or anesthetic spray for throat irritation, if needed.

Gloves prevent contact with blood and body fluids and transfer of microorganisms. Oral hygiene keeps the mouth clean and moist, promotes comfort, and reduces thirst.

17. Remove and reapply the NG tube securement device every 24 hours; assess, clean, and apply a skin barrier to the skin beneath or in contact with the NG tube prior to replacement. Reposition the tube to alleviate pressure. Provide nares hygiene as needed (Schroeder & Sitzer, 2019).

Pressure from the tube can create pressure damage; these actions help prevent development of pressure injury (Baranoski & Ayello, 2020; EPUAP, NPIAP, & PPPIA, 2019; Schroeder & Sitzer, 2019).

18. Remove equipment and return the patient to a position of comfort. Remove gloves. Perform hand hygiene. Raise the side rail and lower the bed.

Positioning promotes patient comfort and safety. Removing gloves properly and using hand hygiene reduces the risk for infection transmission and contamination of other items.

19. Remove additional PPE, if used. Perform hand hygiene.

Proper removal of PPE reduces the risk for infection transmission and contamination of other items. Hand hygiene prevents transmission of microorganisms.

EVALUATION

The expected outcomes have been met when the tube has been passed into the patient's stomach without any complications, and the patient has exhibited no signs and symptoms of aspiration, has rated pain as decreased from prior to insertion, and has verbalized an understanding of the reason for NG tube insertion.

DOCUMENTATION

Guidelines

Document the size and type of the NG tube that was inserted and the postinsertion measurement of the length of the tube from the tip of the nose to the end of the exposed tube. Also, document the results of the x-ray that was taken to confirm the tube position, if applicable. Record the pH of the aspirated gastric contents. Document the naris where the tube was placed and the patient's response to the procedure. Include assessment data related to the abdomen. Record the patient teaching that was discussed.

Sample Documentation

Lippincott
DocuCare

Practice documenting NG tube insertion in *Lippincott DocuCare*.

10/4/25 0945 Abdomen slightly distended and taut; hypoactive bowel sounds. Patient reports transient nausea. 14F double-lumen nasogastric tube inserted via right naris, 20 cm of tube from naris to end of tube post insertion; aspirate pH 4; patient tolerated without incident.

—*S. Essner, RN*

(*continued on page 838*)

Skill 13-8 ▶ Inserting a Nasogastric Tube   *(continued)*

DEVELOPING CLINICAL REASONING AND CLINICAL JUDGMENT

UNEXPECTED SITUATIONS AND ASSOCIATED INTERVENTIONS

- *As tube is passing through the pharynx, patient begins to retch and gag:* This is common during placement of an NG tube. Ask the patient if they want to stop the procedure, which will allow the patient to gain composure from the gagging episode. Continue to advance the tube when the patient relates that they are ready. Have the emesis basin nearby in case the patient begins to vomit.
- *You are unable to pass the tube after trying a second time down the one nostril:* If the patient's condition permits, inspect the other nostril and attempt to pass the NG tube down this nostril. If unable to pass down this nostril, consult with the health care team.
- *As the tube is passing through the pharynx, the patient begins to cough and shows signs of respiratory distress:* **Stop advancing the tube.** The tube is most likely entering the trachea. Pull the tube back into the nasal area. Support the patient as they regain normal breathing ability and composure. If the patient feels that they can tolerate another attempt, ask the patient to keep their chin on their chest and swallow as the tube is advanced to help prevent the tube from entering the trachea. Begin to advance the tube, watching for any signs of respiratory distress.
- *No gastric contents can be aspirated:* Reposition the patient and flush the tube with 30 mL of air in a large syringe. Slowly apply negative pressure to withdraw fluid.

SPECIAL CONSIDERATIONS

General Considerations

- A nasal bridle (Figure 10) is another type of commercial device that has been suggested to secure NG tubes (Stabler et al., 2018; Taylor et al., 2018).
- Check tube placement before administering any fluids, medications, or feeding, using multiple techniques: x-ray, external length, external verification marking, pH testing, and carbon dioxide monitoring (if available). Consistent inability to withdraw fluid from tube may indicate displacement of the tube from the stomach into the esophagus (AACN, 2020).
- Signs of respiratory distress may be absent in patients with an impaired level of consciousness when NG tubes are inadvertently positioned in the airway (AACN, 2020).
- Sterile water should be used for tube flushes in immunocompromised or critically ill patients (Allen, 2015; Boullata et al., 2017).
- Gastric pH ≥6 is of no benefit in predicting tube location in the GI tract or in ruling out tracheopulmonary placement (Boullata et al., 2017).

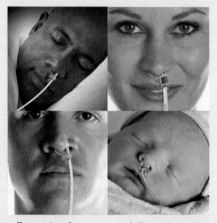

FIGURE 10. Example of a commercially prepared nasal bridle. (*Source:* Images courtesy of Applied Medical Technology, Inc. [AMT] | www.AppliedMedical.net)

Infant and Child Considerations

- Infants are obligate nose breathers; tubes are usually inserted via the mouth (orogastric tube). Insertion through a nostril is usually more comfortable for older children (Silbert-Falgg & Pillitteri, 2018).

Skill 13-9 ▶ Irrigating a Nasogastric Tube Connected to Suction

Nasogastric (NG) tubes may be used to decompress or drain the stomach of fluid or unwanted stomach contents such as poison or medication and air (Burns & Delgado, 2019) and may be used when conditions are present in which peristalsis is absent. Tubes for decompression typically are attached to suction or the tube may be clamped. Suction can be applied intermittently or continuously. When the underlying condition has been resolved and/or the NG tube is no longer indicated, the tube is removed (refer to Skill 13-10). The tube must be kept free from obstruction or clogging and is usually irrigated every 4 to 8 hours.

To promote patient safety, NG tube placement must be verified after the initial insertion, before beginning a feeding or instilling medications or liquids, and at regular intervals during continuous feedings (Metheny et al., 2019). This increases the likelihood that the tip of the tube is situated in the stomach or intestine, preventing inadvertent administration of substances into the wrong place. A misplaced tube in the lungs or pulmonary tissue places the patient at risk for aspiration, pneumonia, and even death (AACN, 2020; Metheny et al., 2019). Radiographic examination, measurement of tube length and measurement of tube marking, measurement of aspirate pH, and monitoring of carbon dioxide have been suggested to confirm tube placement (Irving et al., 2018; Metheny et al., 2019). The use of two or more of these techniques in conjunction with each other increases the likelihood of correct tube placement (AACN, 2020; Anderson, 2019; Anderson, 2018; Dias et al., 2019; Rahimi et al., 2015). An old technique of auscultation of air injected into a tube has been proved unreliable and is not suggested for use (AACN, 2020; Anderson, 2018; Boeykens et al., 2014; Boullata et al., 2017; Irving et al., 2018; Metheny et al., 2019). Recommendations for use of visual inspection of gastric aspirate are conflicting; this method should be used cautiously if part of policy and procedure guidelines and with consideration to the potential for inaccuracy (AACN, 2020; Dias et al., 2019; Mak & Tam, 2020; Metheny et al., 2019). When bedside methods to check placement suggest the tube has been displaced, a radiograph should be requested to determine the tube's location (AACN, 2020).

NG tubes may also be used to administer medications or to provide short-term nutrition, using the stomach as a natural reservoir for food. The use of NG tubes for nutritional purposes is discussed in Chapter 11. Administration of medications via an NG tube is discussed in Chapter 5.

DELEGATION CONSIDERATIONS	The irrigation of an NG tube is not delegated to assistive personnel (AP). Depending on the state's nurse practice act and the organization's policies and procedures, irrigation of an NG tube may be delegated to licensed practical/vocational nurses (LPN/LVNs). The decision to delegate must be based on careful analysis of the patient's needs and circumstances as well as the qualifications of the person to whom the task is being delegated. Refer to the Delegation Guidelines in Appendix A.

EQUIPMENT

- Water, sterile water, or normal saline solution for irrigation (based on facility policy)
- Nonsterile gloves
- Additional PPE, as indicated
- Irrigation set, including a large syringe (20 to 50 mL)
- Clamp
- Disposable waterproof pad or bath towel
- Emesis basin
- Tape measure, or other measuring device
- pH test strip (calibrated in units of 0.5 and approved for use with human secretions)
- Stethoscope (for abdominal assessment)

ASSESSMENT	Assess for signs of respiratory distress; coughing, choking, dyspnea may occur when a tube is inadvertently positioned in the airway (AACN, 2020). Inspect the abdomen for distention and firmness; auscultate for bowel sounds or peristalsis and palpate the abdomen for distention and tenderness. If the abdomen is distended, consider measuring the abdominal girth at the umbilicus. If the patient reports any tenderness or nausea or exhibits any rigidity or firmness of the abdomen, confer with the health care team. If the NG tube is attached to suction, assess suction to ensure that it is set at the prescribed pressure. Also, inspect drainage from NG tube, including color, consistency, and amount.

ACTUAL OR POTENTIAL HEALTH PROBLEMS AND NEEDS	Many actual or potential health problems or issues may require the use of this skill as part of related interventions. An appropriate health problem or issue may include: • Impaired gastrointestinal system function • Aspiration risk • Risk for impaired gastrointestinal system function

(continued on page 840)

Skill 13-9 ▶ Irrigating a Nasogastric Tube Connected to Suction *(continued)*

OUTCOME IDENTIFICATION AND PLANNING

The expected outcome to achieve when irrigating a patient's NG tube is that the tube is successfully irrigated and maintains patency. In addition, the patient will not experience any trauma or injury.

IMPLEMENTATION

ACTION

1. Gather equipment. Verify the prescribed intervention or facility policy and procedure regarding frequency of irrigation, solution type, and amount of irrigant. Check expiration dates on the irrigating solution and irrigation set.

 2. Perform hand hygiene and put on PPE, if indicated.

 3. Identify the patient.

4. Explain the procedure to the patient and why this intervention is needed. Answer any questions, as needed. Perform key assessments as described above.

5. Assemble equipment on the overbed table or other surface within reach.

6. Pull the patient's bedside curtain. Raise the bed to a comfortable working position (VHACEOSH, 2016). Assist the patient to 30- to 45-degree position, unless this is contraindicated. Pour the irrigating solution into container.

7. Put on gloves. Place a waterproof pad on the patient's chest, under the connection of the NG tube and suction tubing. **Check placement of the NG tube.** Refer to Skill 11-2 in Chapter 11.

8. Draw up 30 mL of irrigation solution (or amount indicated in the order or policy) into the irrigation syringe (Figure 1).

RATIONALE

Assembling equipment provides for an organized approach to the task. Verification ensures the patient receives the correct intervention. Facility policy dictates safe interval for reuse of equipment.

Hand hygiene and PPE prevent the spread of microorganisms. PPE is required based on transmission precautions.

Identifying the patient ensures the right patient receives the intervention and helps prevent errors.

Explanation facilitates patient engagement. Due to potential changes in a patient's condition, assessment is vital before initiating an intervention.

Organization facilitates performance of the task.

This provides for privacy. An appropriate working height facilitates comfort and proper body mechanics for the nurse. This position minimizes risk for aspiration. Preparing the irrigation provides for an organized approach to the task.

Gloves prevent contact with body fluids. The waterproof pad protects the patient's clothing and bed linens from accidental leakage of gastric fluid. Checking placement before the instillation of fluid is necessary to prevent accidental instillation into the respiratory tract if the tube has become dislodged.

This delivers measured amount of irrigant through the tube. Flushing the tube prevents occlusion (Bischoff et al., 2020; Boullata et al., 2017).

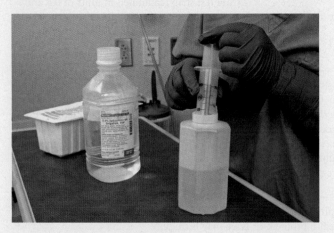

FIGURE 1. Preparing syringe with 30 mL of irrigation solution.

ACTION

RATIONALE

9. Clamp the NG tube near the connection site using a clamp, or double the tube on itself. Disconnect the tube from the suction apparatus (Figure 2) and lay it on a disposable pad or towel, or hold both tubes upright in your nondominant hand (Figure 3).

Clamping prevents leakage of gastric fluid.

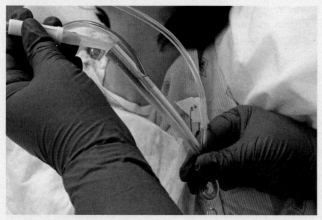

FIGURE 2. Clamping nasogastric tube while disconnecting.

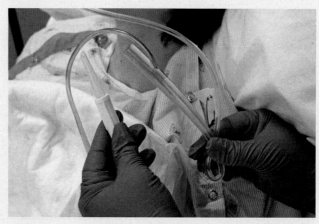

FIGURE 3. Keeping both tubes upright to prevent leakage of gastric fluid.

10. Place tip of the syringe in the tube. **If a double-lumen tube is used, make sure that the syringe tip is placed in the drainage port and not in the blue air vent.** Hold the syringe upright and gently insert the irrigant (Figure 4) (or allow solution to flow in by gravity if facility policy or prescribed intervention indicates). **Do not force solution into the tube.**

Gentle insertion of saline solution (or gravity insertion) is less traumatic to gastric mucosa.

The blue air vent acts to decrease pressure built up in the stomach when the Salem sump is attached to suction. It is not to be used for irrigation. Flushing the tube prevents occlusion (Bischoff et al., 2020; Boullata et al., 2017).

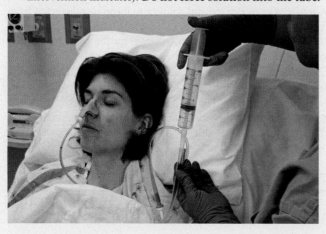

FIGURE 4. Gently instilling irrigation.

11. If you are unable to irrigate the tube, reposition the patient and attempt irrigation again. Inject 10 to 20 mL of air and aspirate again. **If repeated attempts to irrigate the tube fail, consult with the health care team or follow facility policy.**

The tube may be positioned against gastric mucosa, making it difficult to irrigate. Injection of air may reposition the end of the tube.

12. After irrigant has been instilled, hold the end of the NG tube over the irrigation tray or emesis basin. Observe for return flow of NG drainage into the container. Alternatively, you may reconnect the NG tube to suction and observe the return drainage as it drains into the suction container.

Return flow may be collected in an irrigating tray or other available container and measured. This amount will need to be subtracted from the irrigant to record the true NG drainage. A second method involves subtracting the total irrigant from the shift from the total NG drainage emptied over the entire shift to find the true NG drainage. Check facility policy for guidelines.

(continued on page 842)

Skill 13-9 ▶ Irrigating a Nasogastric Tube Connected to Suction *(continued)*

ACTION	**RATIONALE**
13. If not already done, reconnect the drainage port to suction, if prescribed.	This allows for continued removal of gastric contents, as prescribed.
14. Inject air into the blue air vent after irrigation is complete. Position the blue air vent above the patient's stomach.	Following irrigation, the blue air vent is injected with air to keep it clear. Positioning the blue air vent above the stomach prevents the stomach contents from leaking from the NG tube.
15. Remove gloves. Perform hand hygiene. Lower the bed and raise the side rails, as necessary. Assist the patient to a position of comfort.	Proper removal of gloves and hand hygiene prevent transmission of microorganisms. Lowering the bed and assisting the patient to a comfortable position promote safety and comfort.
16. Put on gloves. Measure returned solution, if collected outside of the suction apparatus. Rinse equipment if it will be reused. Label equipment with the date, patient's name, room number, and purpose (for NG tube/irrigation).	Gloves prevent contact with blood and body fluids. The irrigant placed in the tube is considered intake; solution returned is recorded as output. Record on the intake and output record. Rinsing promotes cleanliness, infection control, and prepares equipment for the next irrigation.
17. Remove gloves and additional PPE, if used. Perform hand hygiene.	Proper removal of PPE reduces the risk for infection transmission and contamination of other items. Hand hygiene prevents transmission of microorganisms.

EVALUATION

The expected outcomes have been met the NG tube has successfully irrigated and maintained patency, and the patient has not experienced any trauma or injury.

DOCUMENTATION

Guidelines

Document assessment of the patient's abdomen. Record if the patient's NG tube is clamped or connected to suction, including the type of suction. Document the color and consistency of the NG drainage. Record the solution type and amount used to irrigate the NG tube as well as ease of irrigation or any difficulty related to the procedure. Record the amount of returned irrigant, if collected outside of the suction apparatus. Alternatively, record irrigant amount so it can be subtracted from the total NG drainage amount at the end of the shift. Record the patient's response to the procedure and any pertinent teaching points that were reviewed, such as instructions for the patient to contact the nurse for any feelings of nausea, bloating, or abdominal pain.

Sample Documentation

> 10/15/25 1100 Abdomen slightly distended but soft; absent bowel sounds, denies nausea. NG tube placement confirmed; aspirate pH 4; exposed NG tube 20 cm, consistent with documented length. NG tube irrigated with 30 mL of normal saline. NG tube reconnected to low intermittent suction. Clear drainage with brown flecks noted from tube. Patient tolerated irrigation without incident.
> —S. Essner, RN

DEVELOPING CLINICAL REASONING AND CLINICAL JUDGMENT

UNEXPECTED SITUATIONS AND ASSOCIATED INTERVENTIONS

- *Flush solution is meeting a lot of force when plunger is pushed:* Inject 20 to 30 mL of free air through the NG tube into the stomach in an attempt to reposition the tube and enable flushing of the tube.
- *Tube is connected to suction as prescribed, but nothing is draining from the tube:* First, check the suction canister to ensure that the suction is working appropriately. Disconnect the NG tube from suction and place your gloved thumb over the end of the suction tubing. If there is suction present, the problem lies in the tube itself. Next, attempt to flush the tube to ensure its patency.
- *After flushing the tube, the tube is not reconnected to suction as prescribed:* Reconnect the tube to suction as soon as the error is noticed. Assess the abdomen for distention and ask the patient if they are experiencing any nausea or any abdominal discomfort. Complete any paperwork per institutional policy, such as a variance report.

SPECIAL CONSIDERATIONS

General Considerations

- A one-way, antireflux valve may be used in the airflow lumen to prevent reflux of gastric contents through the airflow lumen (refer to Figure 1 in Skill 13-8). When pressure from gastric contents enters the airflow tubing, the valve closes to prevent secretions from exiting the tube. This valve is removed before flushing the lumen with air and then replaced.
- Check tube placement before administering any fluids, medications, or feeding, using multiple techniques: x-ray, external length, external verification marking, pH testing, and carbon dioxide monitoring (if available). Consistent inability to withdraw fluid from tube may indicate displacement of the tube from the stomach into the esophagus (AACN, 2020).

Signs of respiratory distress may be absent in patients with an impaired level of consciousness when NG tubes are inadvertently positioned in the airway (AACN, 2020).

- Sterile water should be used for tube flushes in immunocompromised or critically ill patients (Allen, 2015; Boullata et al., 2017).
- Gastric pH ≥6 is of no benefit in predicting tube location in the GI tract or in ruling out tracheopulmonary placement (Boullata et al., 2017).
- Monitoring for carbon dioxide to determine NG tube position and/or dislodgement has been investigated (Hess et al., 2021). This involves the use of a colorimetric end-tidal CO_2 detector to detect the presence of carbon dioxide, which would indicate tube positioning in the patient's airway (Hess et al., 2021). Monitoring for carbon dioxide may be helpful to detect placement of a feeding tube in the tracheobronchial tree (AACN, 2020; Boullata et al., 2017; Hess et al., 2021). However, this technique may be unreliable, as it cannot differentiate placement in the mouth, and carbon dioxide may not be detected when the tube is in the patient's airway if the ports in the tube are occluded (Gilbert & Burns, 2010, as cited in AACN, 2020).

Skill 13-10 ▶ Removing a Nasogastric Tube

When the nasogastric (NG) tube is no longer necessary for treatment, removal of the tube will be prescribed. The NG tube is removed as carefully as it was inserted, to provide as much comfort as possible for the patient and to prevent complications. When the tube is removed, the patient should hold their breath to prevent aspiration of any secretions or fluid left in the tube as it is removed.

DELEGATION CONSIDERATIONS

The removal of an NG tube is not delegated to assistive personnel (AP). Depending on the state's nurse practice act and the organization's policies and procedures, removal of an NG tube may be delegated to licensed practical/vocational nurses (LPN/LVNs). The decision to delegate must be based on careful analysis of the patient's needs and circumstances as well as the qualifications of the person to whom the task is being delegated. Refer to the Delegation Guidelines in Appendix A.

EQUIPMENT

- Tissues
- 50-mL syringe
- Nonsterile gloves
- Additional PPE, as indicated
- Stethoscope
- Disposable plastic bag
- Bath towel or disposable pad
- Normal saline solution for irrigation (optional)
- Emesis basin

ASSESSMENT

Perform an abdominal assessment by inspecting for presence of distention, auscultating for bowel sounds, and palpating the abdomen for firmness or tenderness. If the abdomen is distended, consider measuring the abdominal girth at the umbilicus. If the patient reports any tenderness or nausea, exhibits any rigidity or firmness with distention, and if bowel sounds are absent, confer with the health care team before discontinuing the NG tube. Assess any output from the NG tube, noting amount, color, and consistency.

(continued on page 844)

Skill 13-10 ▶ Removing a Nasogastric Tube (continued)

ACTUAL OR POTENTIAL HEALTH PROBLEMS AND NEEDS	Many actual or potential health problems or issues may require the use of this skill as part of related interventions. An appropriate health problem or issue may include: • Knowledge deficiency • Aspiration risk • Risk for impaired gastrointestinal system function
OUTCOME IDENTIFICATION AND PLANNING	The expected outcomes to achieve when removing an NG tube is that the tube is removed with minimal discomfort to the patient, and the patient does not aspirate.

IMPLEMENTATION

ACTION	**RATIONALE**
1. Check the health record for the prescribed intervention for removal of the NG tube. Gather equipment.	This ensures the patient receives the correct treatment. Gathering equipment provides for an organized approach to the task.
2. Perform hand hygiene and put on PPE, if indicated.	Hand hygiene and PPE prevent the spread of microorganisms. PPE is required based on transmission precautions.
3. Identify the patient.	Identifying the patient ensures the right patient receives the intervention and helps prevent errors.
4. Explain the procedure to the patient and why this intervention is warranted. Describe that it will entail a few moments of discomfort. Perform key abdominal assessments as described above.	Patient engagement is facilitated when explanations are provided. Due to potential changes in a patient's condition, assessment is vital before initiating intervention.
5. Pull the patient's bedside curtain. Raise the bed to a comfortable working position (VHACEOSH, 2016). Assist the patient to a 30- to 45-degree position. Place a towel or disposable pad across the patient's chest (Figure 1). Give tissues and an emesis basin to the patient.	This provides for privacy. An appropriate working height facilitates comfort and proper body mechanics for the nurse. A towel or pad protects the patient from contact with gastric secretions. An emesis basin is helpful if the patient vomits or gags. Tissues are necessary if the patient wants to blow their nose when the tube is removed.
6. Put on gloves. Discontinue suction and separate the tube from suction. Detach the tube from any securement to patient's gown and/or face and carefully remove the securement device or adhesive tape from the patient's nose.	Gloves prevent contact with blood and body fluids. Disconnecting the tube from suction and the patient allows for its unrestricted removal.
7. Check placement (refer to Skill 11-2 in Chapter 11) and flush the tube with 10 mL of water or normal saline solution (optional) or clear with 30 to 50 mL of air (Figure 2) (refer to Skill 13-9).	Air or saline solution clears the tube of secretions or debris.

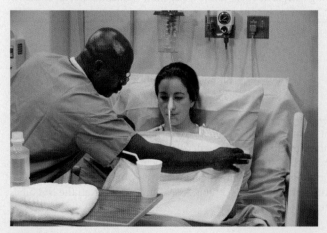

FIGURE 1. Placing towel or disposable pad across patient's chest.

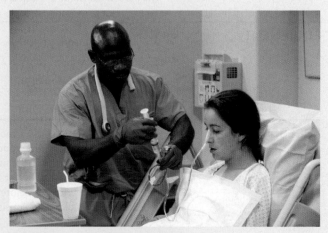

FIGURE 2. Flushing NG tube with 10-mL water.

ACTION	**RATIONALE**

8. Clamp the tube with your fingers by doubling the tube on itself (Figure 3). **Instruct the patient to take a deep breath and hold it. Quickly and carefully remove the tube while the patient holds their breath.** Coil the tube in the disposable pad as you remove it from the patient.

Clamping prevents drainage of gastric contents into the pharynx and esophagus. The patient holds their breath to prevent accidental aspiration of gastric secretions in the tube. Careful removal minimizes trauma and discomfort for the patient. Containing the tube in a towel while removing it prevents leakage onto the patient.

9. Dispose of the tube per facility policy. Remove gloves. Perform hand hygiene.

This prevents contamination with microorganisms.

10. Offer mouth care to the patient and facial tissue to blow their nose. Assist the patient to a position of comfort, as needed.

These interventions promote patient comfort.

11. Remove equipment, raise the side rail, and lower the bed.

Positioning promotes patient comfort and safety.

12. Put on gloves and measure the amount of NG drainage in the collection device. Record the measurement on the output flow record, subtracting irrigant fluids if necessary (Figure 4). Add solidifying agent to the NG drainage and dispose of the drainage according to facility policy.

Irrigation fluids are considered intake. To obtain the true NG drainage, irrigant fluid amounts are subtracted from the total NG drainage. NG drainage is recorded as part of the output of fluids from the patient. Solidifying agents added to liquid NG drainage facilitate safe biohazard disposal.

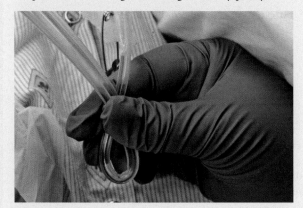

FIGURE 3. Doubling tube on itself.

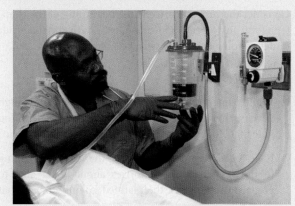

FIGURE 4. Measuring the amount of nasogastric drainage in collection device.

13. Remove gloves and additional PPE, if used. Perform hand hygiene.

Proper removal of PPE reduces the risk for infection transmission and contamination of other items. Hand hygiene prevents transmission of microorganisms.

EVALUATION

The expected outcomes have been met when the tube has been removed with minimal discomfort to the patient, and the patient has not aspirated.

DOCUMENTATION

Guidelines

Document assessment of the abdomen. If an abdominal girth reading was obtained, record this measurement. Document the removal of the NG tube from the naris where it had been placed. Note if there is any irritation to the skin of the naris. Record the amount of NG drainage in the suction container on the patient's intake-and-output record as well as the color of the drainage. Record any pertinent teaching, such as instructions to the patient to notify the nurse if they experience any nausea, abdominal pain, or bloating.

(continued on page 846)

Skill 13-10 ▶ Removing a Nasogastric Tube *(continued)*

Sample Documentation

<u>10/29/25</u> 1320 NG tube removed from L naris without incident. 300 mL of dark brown liquid emptied from NG tube. Patient's abdomen is 66 cm; abdomen is soft, nontender with hypoactive bowel sounds in all four quadrants.

—*S. Essner, RN*

DEVELOPING CLINICAL REASONING AND CLINICAL JUDGMENT

UNEXPECTED SITUATIONS AND ASSOCIATED INTERVENTIONS

- *Within 2 hours after NG tube removal, the patient's abdomen is showing signs of distention:* Notify the health care team. Anticipate an order to reinsert the NG tube.
- *Epistaxis occurs with removal of the NG tube:* Occlude both nares until bleeding has subsided. Ensure that patient is in upright position. Document the epistaxis in the patient's health record.

Enhance Your Understanding

Focusing on Patient Care: Developing Clinical Reasoning and Clinical Judgment

Consider the case scenarios at the beginning of the chapter as you answer the following questions to enhance your understanding and apply what you have learned.

QUESTIONS

1. While you are digitally removing feces from Hugh Levens, they suddenly report feeling lightheaded. You note that Hugh is now diaphoretic. What should you do?

2. Isaac Greenberg is afraid that the enema is going to hurt. Their mother worries about being able to prepare properly for the planned colonoscopy. What information should you include when teaching the steps to administer a small-volume enema? What interventions should you include to promote Isaac's comfort and safety?

3. Maria Blakely has noted that an area of peristomal skin is becoming erythematous and excoriated. They ask you whether the ostomy bag opening should be cut bigger so that the adhesive does not irritate this skin. How should you reply?

You can find suggested answers after the Bibliography at the end of this chapter.

Integrated Case Study Connection

The case studies in the back of the book focus on integrating concepts. Refer to the following case studies to enhance your understanding of the concepts and skills in this chapter.

- Intermediate Case Studies: Victoria Holly, page 1211.

Bibliography

Allen, S. M. (2015). As a flushing agent for enteral nutrition, does sterile water compared to tap water affect the associated risk of infection in critically ill patients? *The Alabama Nurse, 42*(1), 5–6.

American Association of Critical Care Nurses (AACN). (2020, January 29). *AACN practice alert. Initial and ongoing verification of feeding tube placement in adults.* https://www.aacn.org/

Anderson, L. (2018). Fine-bore nasogastric tube feeding: Reducing the risks. *British Journal of Nursing, 27*(12), 674–675.

Anderson, L. (2019). Enteral feeding tubes: An overview of nursing care. *British Journal of Nursing, 28*(12), 748–754. https://doi.org/10.12968/bjon.2019.28.12.748

Baranoski, S., & Ayello, E. A. (2020). *Wound care essentials. Practice principles* (5th ed.). Wolters Kluwer.

Bauldoff, G., Gubrud, P., & Carno, M. A. (2020). *LeMone and Burke's medical-surgical nursing: Clinical reasoning in patient care* (7th ed.). Pearson.

Berti-Hearn, L., & Elliott, B. (2019). Ileostomy care: A guide for home care clinicians. *Home Healthcare Now, 37*(3), 136–144. https://doi.org/10.1097/NHH.0000000000000776

Blevins, S. (2019). Colostomy care. *MEDSURG Nursing, 28*(2), 125–126.

Boeykens, K. (2018). Verification of blindly inserted nasogastric feeding tubes: A review of different test methods. *Journal of Perioperative & Critical Intensive Care Nursing, 4*(3). https://doi.org/10.4172/2471-9870.10000145

Boeykens, K., Steeman, E., & Dyusburgh, I. (2014). Reliability of pH measurement and the auscultatory method to confirm the position of a nasogastric tube. *International Journal of Nursing Studies, 51*(11), 1427–1433. https://doi.org/10.1016/j.ijnurstu.2014.03.004

Boullata, J. I., Carrera, A. L., Harvey, L., Escuro, A. A., Hudson, L., Mays, A., McGinnis, C., Wessel, J. J., Bajpai, S., Beebe, M. L., Kinn, T. J., Klang, M. G., Lord, L., Martin, K., Pompeii-Wolfe, C., Sullivan, J., Wood, A., Malone, A., Guenter, P., & ASPEN Safe Practices for Enteral Nutrition Therapy, American Society for Parenteral and Enteral Nutrition. (2017). ASPEN safe practices for enteral nutrition therapy. *Journal of Parenteral and Enteral Nutrition, 41*(1), 15–103. https://doi.org/10.1177/0148607116673053

Boutry, E., Bertrand, M. M., Ripoche, J., Alonso, S., Bastide, S., Prudhomme, M., & French Federation of Ostomy. (2021). Quality of life in colostomy patients practicing colonic irrigation: An observational study. *Journal of Visceral Surgery, 158*(1), 4–10. https://doi.org/10.1016/j.jviscsurg.2020.07.003

Burch, J. (2018). Stoma-related complications and treatments. *Nursing & Residential Care, 20*(9), 430–433. https://doi.org/10.12968/nrec.2018.20.9.430

Burch, J. (2019a). Supporting residents to care for a stoma independently. *Nursing and Residential Care, 21*(5), 276–280. https://doi.org/10.12968/nrec.2019.21.5.276

Burch, J. (2019b). Peristomal skin care considerations for community nurses. *British Journal of Community Nursing, 24*(9), 414–418. https://doi.org/10.12968/bjcn.2019.24.9.414

Burns, S. M., & Delgado, S. A. (2019). *AACN essentials of critical care nursing* (4th ed.). McGraw Hill Education.

Butler, D. L. (2009). Early postoperative complications following ostomy surgery: A review. *Journal of Wound, Ostomy and Continence Nursing, 36*(5), 513–519.

Chandler, P. (2020). Lesbian, gay, bisexual and transgender (LGBT) inclusion in nursing services: A reflective case study from stoma care. *European Wound, Ostomy and Continence, 18*(Sup9), S26–S32. https://doi.org/10.12968/gasn.2020.18.Sup9.S26

Cincinnati Children's. (2018, July). *Enema administration.* https://www.cincinnatichildrens.org/health/e/enema

Cleveland Clinic. (2016, November 7). *Colostomy irrigation.* https://my.clevelandclinic.org/health/treatments/10747-colostomy-irrigation

Clow, T., Disley, H., Greening, L., & Harker, G. (2015). Professional guidance for teaching colostomy irrigation. *World Council of Enterostomal Therapists Journal, 35*(2), 15–19.

Collier, M. (2019). Minimising pain and medical adhesive related skin injuries in vulnerable patients. *British Journal of Nursing, 28*(15), S26–S32. https://doi.org/10.12968/bjon.2019.28.15.S26

Colwell, J. C., Bain, K. A., Hansen, A. S., Droste, W., Vendelbo, G., & James-Reid, S. (2019). International consensus results: Development of practice guidelines for assessment of peristomal body and stoma profiles, patient engagement, and patient follow-up. *Journal of Wound, Ostomy and Continence Nursing, 46*(6), 497–504. https://doi.org/10.1097/WON.0000000000000599

Continence Product Advisor. (2021). *Faecal devices. Products for faecal incontinence.* https://www.continenceproductadvisor.org/faecaldevices

de Souza Barbosa Dias, F., de Almeida, B. P., Alvares, B. R., Jales, R. M., de Siqueira Caldas, J. P., & Carmona, E. V. (2019). Use of pH reagent strips to verify gastric tube placement in newborns. *Revista Latino-Americana de Enfermagem, 27*, e3227. https://doi.org/10.1590/1518-8345.3150.3227

Díaz, C. C., Zambrano, S. M. H., Muñoz, B. M., Crisol, I. S., Marfil, M. N. P., Montoya-Juárez, R., & Montoro, C. H. (2018). Stoma care nurses' perspectives on the relative significance of factors influencing ostomates' quality of life. *Gastrointestinal Nursing, 16*(3), 28–33. https://doi.org/10.12968/gasn.2018.16.3.28

Dudek, S. (2022). *Nutrition essentials for nursing practice* (9th ed.). Wolters Kluwer.

Eliopoulos, C. (2018). *Gerontological nursing* (9th ed.). Wolters Kluwer.

Ellett, M. L. C., Cohen, M. D., Perkins, S. M., Croffie, J. M. B., Lane, K. A., & Austin, J. K. (2012). Comparing methods of determining insertion length for placing gastric tubes in children 1 month to 17 years of age. *Journal for Specialists in Pediatric Nursing, 17*(1), 19–32. https://doi.org/10.1111/j.1744-6155.2011.00302.x

European Pressure Ulcer Advisory Panel (EPUAP), National Pressure Injury Advisory Panel (NPIAP), and Pan Pacific Pressure Injury Alliance (PPPIA), & Haesler, E. (Ed). (2019). *Prevention and treatment of pressure ulcers/injuries: Clinical practice guideline. The international guideline.* http://www.internationalguideline.com/

Fan, P. E. M., Tan, S. B., Farah, G. I., Cheok, P. G., Chock, W. T., Sutha, W., Xu, D., Chua, W., Kwan, X. L., Li, C. L., Teo, W. Q., & Ang, S. Y. (2019). Adequacy of different measurement methods in determining nasogastric tube insertion lengths: An observational study. *International Journal of Nursing Studies, 92*, 73–78. https://doi.org/10.1016/j.ijnurstu.2019.01.003

Fischbach, F. T., & Fischbach, M. A. (2018). *A manual of laboratory and diagnostic tests* (10th ed.). Wolters Kluwer.

Fisher, P., & Himan, C. (2020). Moisture-associated skin damage: A skin issue more prevalent than pressure ulcers. *Wounds UK, 16*(1), 58–63.

Francis, K. (2018). Incontinence-associated dermatitis: Management update. *American Nurse Today, 13*(1), 25–27.

Goldberg, M., Colwell, J., Burns, S., Carmel, J., Fellows, J., Hendren, S., Livingston, V., Northington, C. U., Pittman, J., Rafferty, J., Salvadalena, G., Steinberg, G., Wound, Ostomy and Continence Nurses Society, & Guideline Development Task Force. (2018). WOCN Society Clinical Guideline: Management of the adult patient with a fecal or urinary ostomy–An executive summary. *Journal of Wound, Ostomy and Continence Nursing, 45*(1), 50–58. https://doi.org/10.1097/WON.0000000000000396

Hess, D. R., MacIntyre, N. R., Galvin, W. F., & Mishoe, S. C. (2021). *Respiratory care. Principles and practice* (4th ed.). Jones & Bartlett Learning.

Hill, B. (2020). Stoma care: Procedures, appliances and nursing considerations. *British Journal of Nursing, 29*(22), S14–S19. https://doi.org/10.12968/bjon.2020.29.22.s14

Hinkle, J. L., Cheever, K. H., & Overbaugh, K. J. (2022). *Brunner & Suddarth's Textbook of medical-surgical nursing* (15th ed.). Wolters Kluwer.

Hodin, R. A., & Bordeianou, L. (2020). *UpToDate. Inpatient placement and management of nasogastric and nasoenteric tubes in adults.* Wolters Kluwer. https://www.uptodate.com/contents/inpatient-placement-and-management-of-nasogastric-and-nasoenteric-tubes-in-adults

Hollister. (2005). *Drainable fecal incontinence collector. Protocol.* https://www.hollister.com/-/media/files/pdfs-for-download/critical-care/fecal_collector_care_tips_1907278-405.ashx

Hollister. (2021). *Fecal collectors. Fecal collectors instructions for use video.* [Video]. http://www.hollister.com/en/products/critical-care-products/bowel-care/fecal-collectors/fecal-collector

International Continence Society (ICS). (2015, August). *Fact sheets. A background to urinary and faecal incontinence.* https://www.ics.org/search?q=fact%20sheet

International Council of Nurses (ICN). (2019). *Nursing diagnosis and outcome statements.* https://www.icn.ch/sites/default/files/inline-files/ICNP2019-DC.pdf

Irving, S. Y., Rempel, G., Lyman, B., Sevilla, W. M. A., Northington, L., Guenter, P., & The American Society for Parenteral and Enteral Nutrition. (2018). Pediatric nasogastric tube placement and verification: Best practice recommendations from the NOVEL Project. *Nutrition in Clinical Practice, 33*(6), 921–927. https://doi.org/10.1002/ncp.10189

Jarvis, C., & Echkardt, A. (2020). *Physical examination & health assessment* (8th ed.). Elsevier.

Jensen, S. (2019). *Nursing health assessment. A best practice approach* (3rd ed.). Wolters Kluwer.

Jones, T., Springfield, T., Brudwich, M., & Ladd, A. (2011). Fecal ostomies: Practical management for the home health clinician. *Home Healthcare Nurse, 29*(5), 306–317.

Judd, M. (2020). Confirming nasogastric tube placement in adults. *Nursing, 50*(4), 43–46.

Kantrancha, E. D., & George, N. M. (2014). Postoperative ileus. *MedSurg Nursing, 23*(6), 387-390, 413.

Karch, A. M. (2020). *Focus on nursing pharmacology* (8th ed.). Wolters Kluwer.

Kent, D. J., Long, M. A., & Bauer, C. (2015). Does colostomy irrigation affect functional outcomes and quality of life in persons with a colostomy? *Journal of Wound, Ostomy and Continence Nursing, 42*(2), 155–161.

Kyle, T., & Carman, S. (2021). *Essentials of pediatric nursing* (4th ed.). Wolters Kluwer.

Landmann, R. G., & Cashman, A. L. (2020, June 9). UpToDate. *Ileostomy or colostomy care and complications.* Wolters Kluwer. https://www.uptodate.com/contents/ileostomy-or-colostomy-care-and-complications

LeBlanc, K., Whiteley, I., McNichol, L., Salfadalena, G., & Gray, M. (2019). Peristomal medical adhesive-related skin injury. Results of an international consensus meeting. *Journal of Wound, Ostomy and Continence Nursing, 46*(2), 125–136. https://doi.org/10.1097/WON.0000000000000513

Lyman, B., Peyton, C., & Healey, F. (2018). Reducing nasogastric tube misplacement through evidence-based practice. Is your practice up-to-date? *American Nurse Today, 13*(11), 610.

Mak, M. Y., & Tam, G. (2020). Ultrasonography for nasogastric tube placement verification: An additional reference. *British Journal of Community Nursing, 25*(7), 328–334. https://doi.org/10.12968/bjcn.2020.25.7.328

Mayo Foundation for Medical Education and Research (MFMER). (2019, October 10). *Diseases and conditions. Constipation.* https://www.mayoclinic.org/diseases-conditions/constipation/symptoms-causes/syc-20354253

Mayo Foundation for Medical Education and Research (MFMER). (2020, February 25). *Stool color: When to worry.* https://www.mayoclinic.org/stool-color/expert-answers/faq-20058080

Memorial Sloan Kettering Cancer Center. (2021). *Patient & caregiver education. Irrigating your sigmoid or descending colostomy.* https://www.mskcc.org/cancer-care/patient-education/colostomy-irrigation-instructions-sigmoid-descending-colostomy

Metheny, N. A., Krieger, M. M., Healey, F., & Meert, K. L. (2019). A review of guidelines to distinguish between gastric and pulmonary placement of nasogastric tubes. *Heart & Lung, 48*(3), 226–235. https://doi.org/10.1016/j.hrtlng.2019.01.003

Mitchell, A. (2019a). Carrying out a holistic assessment of a patient with constipation. *British Journal of Nursing, 28*(4), 230–232. https://doi.org/10.12968/bjon.2019.28.4.230

Mitchell, A. (2019b). Administering an enema: Indications, types, equipment and procedure. *British Journal of Nursing, 28*(3), 154–156. https://doi.org/10.12968/bjon.2019.28.3.154

Mitchell, A. (2019c). Administering a suppository: Types, considerations and procedure. *British Journal of Nursing, 28*(5), 288–289. https://doi.org/10.12968/bjon.2019.28.5.288

Mitchell, A. (2019d). Rationale and procedure for performing digital removal of faeces. *British Journal of Nursing, 28*(7), 430–433. https://doi.org/10.12968/bjon.2019.28.7.430

Morton, P. G., & Fontaine, D. K. (2018). *Critical care nursing. A holistic approach* (11th ed.). Wolters Kluwer.

National Cancer Institute (NCI). (2020, April 22). *Gastrointestinal complications (PDQ®)-health professional version. Constipation.* https://www.cancer.gov/about-cancer/treatment/side-effects/constipation/gi-complications-hp-pdq#_8

National Institute of Diabetes and Digestive and Kidney Diseases (NIDDK). (2014, August). *Ostomy surgery of the bowel.* https://www.niddk.nih.gov/health-information/digestive-diseases/ostomy-surgery-bowel#ileonalReservoir

Norris, T. L. (2020). *Porth's essentials of pathophysiology* (5th ed.). Wolters Kluwer.

Obokhare, I. (2012). Fecal impaction: A cause for concern? *Clinics in Colon and Rectal Surgery, 25*(1), 53–58.

O'Flynn, S. K. (2018). Care of the stoma: Complications and treatments. *British Journal of Community Nursing, 23*(8), 382–387. https://doi.org/10.12968/bjcn.2018.23.8.382

Palmer, S. J. (2019). Faecal incontinence in palliative and end-of-life care. *British Journal of Community Nursing, 24*(11), 528–532. DOI: 10.12968/bjcn.2019.24.11.528

Palmer, S. J. (2020). Overview of stoma care for community nurses. *British Journal of Community Nursing, 25*(7), 340–344. https://doi.org/10.12968/bjcn.2020.25.7.340

Parker, L. A., Withers, J. H., & Talaga, E. (2018). Comparison of neonatal nursing practices for determining feeding tube insertion length and verifying gastric placement with current best evidence. *Advances in Neonatal Care, 18*(4), 307–317. https://doi.org/10.1097/ANC.0000000000000526

Patient Safety Movement Foundation. (2021). *Actionable patient safety solutions (APSS). Nasogastric tube placement and verification.* https://patientsafetymovement.org/clinical/enteral-tube-safety/enteral-tube-safety-nasogastric-tube-ngt-placement-and-verification/#gf_111

Powers, J. (2019). Securing orogastic and nasogastric tubes in intubated patients. *Critical Care Nurse, 39*(4), 61–63. https://doi.org/10.4037/ccn2019542

Rahimi, M., Farhadi, K., Ashtarian, H., & Changaei, F. (2015). Confirming nasogastric tube position: Methods and restrictions. A narrative review. *Journal of Nursing and Midwifery Sciences, 2*(1), 55–62. https://doi.org/10.4103/2345-5756.231420

Schreiber, M. L. (2016). Ostomies: Nursing care and management. *MEDSURG Nursing, 25*(2), 127–130, 124.

Schroeder, J., & Sitzer, V. (2019). Nursing care guidelines for reducing hospital-acquired nasogastric tube-related pressure injuries. *Critical Care Nurse, 39*(6), 54–63. https://doi.org/10.4037/ccn2019872

Sigmon, D. F., & An, J. (2020, July 31). StatPearls. *Nasogastric tube.* National Center for Biotechnology Information. U.S. National Library of Medicine. https://www.ncbi.nlm.nih.gov/books/NBK556063/#:~:text=Nasogastric%20tubes%20are%20typically%20used,unable%20to%20tolerate%20oral%20intake

Silbert-Flagg, J., & Pillitteri, A. (2018). *Maternal and child health nursing* (8th ed.). Wolters Kluwer.

Stabler, S. N., Ku, J., Brooks, L., Gellatley, R., & Halijan, G. (2018). Implementation of a nasogastric tube securement device in a tertiary care intensive care unit. *The Canadian Journal of Critical Care Nursing, 29*(1), 14–16.

Stelton, S. (2019). Stoma and peristomal skin care: A clinical review. *American Journal of Nursing, 119*(6), 38–45. https://doi.org/10.1097/01.NAJ.0000559781.86311.64

Swift, T., Westgate, G., Van Onselen, J., & Lee, S. (2020). Developments in silicone technology for use in stoma care. *British Journal of Nursing, 29*(6), S6–S15. https://doi.org/10.12968/bjon.2020.29.6.S6

Taylor, S. J. (2020). Methods of estimating nasogastric tube length: All, including "NEX", are unsafe. *Nutrition in Clinical Practice, 35*(5), 864–870. https://doi.org/10.1002/ncp.10497

Taylor, S. J., Allan, K., Clemente, R., Marsh, A., & Toher, D. (2018). Feeding tube securement in critical illness: Implications for safety. *British Journal of Nursing, 27*(18), 1036–1041.

Taylor, C., Lynn, P., & Bartlett, J. (2023). *Fundamentals of nursing: The art and science of person-centered care* (10th ed.). Wolters Kluwer.

Ten Broek, R. P. G., Krielen, P., Di Saverio, S., Coccolini, F., Biffl, W. L., Ansolani, L., Velmahos, G. C., Sartelli, M., Fraga, G. P., Kelly, M. D., Moore, F. A., Peitzman, A. B., Leppaniemi, A., Moore, E. E., Jeekel, J., Kluger, Y., Sugrue, M., Balogh, Z. J., Bendinelli, C., …. Van Goor, H. (2018). Bologna guidelines for diagnosis and management of adhesive small bowel obstruction (ASBO): 2017 update of the evidence-based guidelines from the World Society of Emergency Surgery ASBO working group. *World Journal of Emergency Surgery, 13*, 24. https://doi.org/10.1186/s13017-018-0185-2

Torsy, T., Saman, R., Boeykens, K., Duysburgh, I., Van Damme, N., & Beeckman, D. (2018). Comparison of two methods for estimating the tip position of a nasogastric feeding tube: A randomized controlled trial. *Nutrition in Clinical Practice, 33*(6), 843–850. https://doi.org/10.1002/ncp.10112

Toughy, T. A., & Jett, K. (2018). *Ebersol and Hess' gerontological nursing & healthy aging* (5th ed.). Elsevier.

U.S. Department of Agriculture (USDA) and U. S. Department of Health and Human Services (USDHHS). (2020, December). *Dietary guidelines for Americans, 2020–2025* (9th ed.). DietaryGuidelines.gov

Venara, A., Hamel, J. F., Cotte, E., Meillat, H., Sage, P. Y., Slim, K., the GRACE Group, Arimont, J., M., Arnalsteen, L., Atger, J., Auvray, S., Beguinot-Holtzscherer, S., Belouard, A., Heda, B., Blehaut, D., Bonnet, M., Boret, H., Buisset-Suiran, C., Massa, D., … Wolthuis, A. (2020). Intraoperative nasogastric tube during colorectal surgery may not be mandatory: A propensity score analysis of a prospective database. *Surgical Endoscopy, 34*(12), 5583–5592. https://doi.org/10.1007/s00464-019-07359-9

VHA Center for Engineering & Occupational Safety and Health (CEOSH). (2016). *Safe patient handling and mobility guidebook.* http://www.tnpatientsafety.com/pubfiles/Initiatives/workplace-violence/sphm-pdf.pdf

Voegeli, D. (2018). Incontinence-associated dermatitis: Management. *Nursing & Residential Care, 20*(10), 506–512. https://doi.org/10.12968/nrec.2018.20.10.506

Wangui-Verry, J., Farrington, M., Matthews, G., & Tucker, S. J. (2019). CE: Original Research: Are milk and molasses enemas safe for hospitalized adults? A retrospective electronic health record review. *American Journal of Nursing, 119*(9), 24–28. https://doi.org/10.1097/01.NAJ.0000580148.43193.76

Wasserman, M. A., & McGee, M. F. (2017). Preoperative considerations for the ostomate. *Clinics in Colon and Rectal Surgery, 30*(3), 157–161. DOI https://doi.org/ 10.1055/s-0037-1598155

Wolters Kluwer. (2022). Problem-based care plans. In *Lippincott Advisor.* Wolters Kluwer.

Wound, Ostomy and Continence Nurses Society (WOCN). (2018). *Basic ostomy skin care: A guide for patients and health care providers.* https://www.ostomy.org/wp-content/uploads/2018/11/wocn_basic_ostomy_skin_care_2018.pdf

Yates, A. (2018a). Incontinence-associated dermatitis in older people: prevention and management. *British Journal of Community Nursing, 23*(5), 218–224. https://doi.org/10.12968/bjcn.2018.23.5.218

Yates, A. (2018b). Incontinence-associated dermatitis: What nurses need to know. *British Journal of Nursing, 27*(19), 1094–1100. https://doi.org/10.12968/bjon.2018.27.19.1094

Yates, A. (2019). Basic continence assessment: What community nurses should know. *Journal of Community Nursing, 33*(3), 52–55.

SUGGESTED ANSWERS FOR FOCUSING ON PATIENT CARE: DEVELOPING CLINICAL REASONING AND CLINICAL JUDGMENT

1. This procedure is very uncomfortable and may cause great discomfort to the patient as well as irritation of the rectal mucosa and bleeding. Digital removal of a fecal mass can stimulate the vagus nerve, resulting in a slowed heart rate, as well as nausea, diaphoresis, lightheadedness, and/or dizziness. If the patient experiences any of these symptoms, stop the procedure immediately; monitor the patient's heart rate, blood pressure, and symptoms. Maintain the patient in a supine position, provide reassurance, and notify the health care team.

2. Hypertonic (phosphate and sodium citrate) solution preparations are available commercially and are administered in smaller volumes (adult: 118 to 197 mL). These solutions draw water into the colon, which stimulates the defecation reflex. This enema is packaged in a flexible bottle containing hypertonic solution with an attached prelubricated firm tip about 2 to 3 inches (5 to 7.5 cm) long and is easy to use. Explain the purpose and what they can expect. Use developmentally appropriate terms for a 9-year-old. Isaac and his mother should plan to administer the enema in or near the bathroom, so Isaac is not worried about being incontinent or getting to the toilet in time. Reinforce that the procedure will not hurt. Isaac will feel some pressure from the tube in his rectum, and in his belly. Explain that a child or adolescent should be positioned on the left side with the right leg flexed toward chest (Cincinnati Children's, 2018). Explain to Isaac's mother that she should generously lubricate the end of the rectal tube 2 to 3 inches before administering. She should direct it at an angle pointing toward the umbilicus, not the bladder. She should ask Isaac to take several deep breaths when inserting it to help relax the anal sphincter. She should encourage Isaac to hold the solution until the urge to defecate is strong. Finally, the mother should hold the child's buttocks together, if needed, to encourage retention of the enema.

3. Explain that Maria should cut the opening only 1/8 inch larger than the stoma size. Creating a larger opening will expose the already irritated peristomal skin to further irritation from stool. Advise Maria to contact her ostomy nurse specialist or her health care provider to rule out a superimposed fungal infection, which would require treatment with an antifungal medication. Reinforce basic teaching with Maria. Ensure she understands the routine care of her ostomy. Explain that she should empty the ostomy appliance frequently. This prevents excess pressure on the adhesive that could pull the adhesive plate off her skin and allow fecal material to come in contact with peristomal skin. Instruct Maria to keep the skin around the stoma site (peristomal area) clean and dry. If care is not taken to protect the skin around the stoma, irritation or infection may occur. A leaking appliance frequently causes skin erosion. Candida or yeast infections can also occur around the stoma if the area is not kept dry. If an appliance is leaking from underneath the skin barrier, ring, or wafer, the bag will have to be removed, the skin cleaned, and a new bag applied. The act of removing an appliance from the skin can result in skin stripping, removal of the outer, loosely bound, epidermal cell layers. This can be uncomfortable for the patient or, at worst, very painful. The cumulative effects of skin stripping over time can result in peristomal skin breakdown. The use of silicone-based adhesive remover loosens the adhesive bond to make removal easier and less likely to damage the skin and is particularly beneficial for patients with fragile skin/those at increased risk for medical adhesive-related skin injury/stripping (Collier, 2019; LeBlanc et al., 2019; Swift et al., 2020). Instruct Maria to use adhesive remover when removing her appliance, to prevent further skin damage. Explain that she should thoroughly cleanse the peristomal skin with a gentle cleanser, and then thoroughly dry it. The use of a skin barrier is important, as well as ensuring good adhesion when the appliance is replaced.

14

Oxygenation

Focusing on Patient Care

This chapter will help you develop some of the skills related to oxygenation necessary to care for the following patients:

Scott Mingus, age 35, who has a chest drain after thoracic surgery.

Saranam Srivastava, age 58, with a history of smoking, who is scheduled for a bowel resection and needs preoperative teaching regarding an incentive spirometer.

Paula Cunningham, age 72, who is intubated and requires suctioning through her endotracheal tube.

Refer to Focusing on Patient Care: Developing Clinical Reasoning and Clinical Judgment at the end of the chapter to apply what you learn.

Learning Outcomes

After completing the chapter, you will be able to accomplish the following:

1. Use a pulse oximeter.
2. Teach a patient to use a peak flow meter.
3. Teach a patient to use an incentive spirometer.
4. Administer oxygen by nasal cannula.
5. Administer oxygen by mask.
6. Care for a patient receiving noninvasive continuous positive pressure.
7. Suction the oropharynx and nasopharynx.
8. Perform nasotrachaeal suctioning.
9. Insert an oropharyngeal airway.
10. Insert a nasopharyngeal airway.
11. Suction the airway via an endotracheal tube using an open system.
12. Suction the airway via an endotracheal tube using a closed system.
13. Secure an endotracheal tube.
14. Suction the airway via a tracheostomy using an open system.
15. Provide care of a tracheostomy tube and site.
16. Provide care of a chest drainage system.
17. Assist with chest tube removal.
18. Use a manual resuscitation bag and mask to deliver oxygen.

Nursing Concepts

- Assessment
- Cellular Regulation
- Clinical Decision Making/Clinical Judgment
- Oxygenation/Gas Exchange
- Perfusion
- Safety

Life depends on a constant supply of oxygen. This demand for oxygen is met by the function of the respiratory and cardiovascular systems, together known as the **cardiopulmonary system**. Gas exchange, the intake of oxygen and the release of carbon dioxide, is made possible by the respiratory system (Fig. 14-1). The cardiovascular system (Fig. 14-2) delivers oxygen to the cells. Oxygenation and perfusion of body tissues depend on essentially three factors:

- Integrity of the airway system to transport air to and from the lungs.
- A properly functioning alveolar system in the lungs to oxygenate venous blood and to remove carbon dioxide from the blood.
- A properly functioning cardiovascular system and blood supply to carry nutrients and wastes to and from body cells.

Any condition that interferes with normal functioning must be minimized or eliminated to prevent cardiopulmonary distress, which could lead to death. This chapter covers the skills necessary for the nurse to promote oxygenation. While performing skills related to oxygenation, keep in mind factors that affect cardiopulmonary function which may result in impaired oxygenation, and how these factors might affect a particular patient (Fundamentals Review 14-1). Chapter 15 presents select skills necessary for the nurse to promote perfusion.

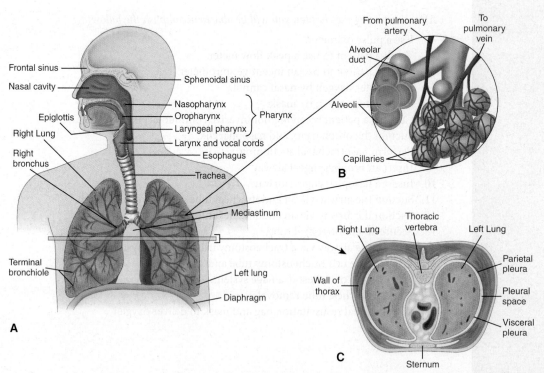

FIGURE 14-1. Organs of respiratory tract. **A.** Overview. **B.** Alveoli (air sacs) of lungs and blood capillaries. **C.** Transverse section through lungs.

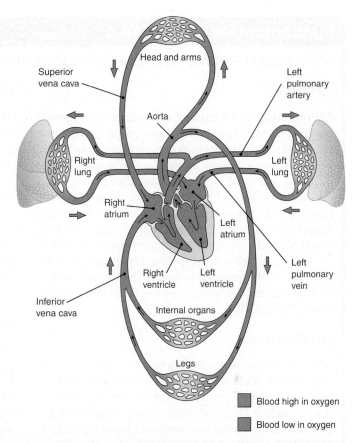

FIGURE 14-2. The right side of the heart pumps deoxygenated blood to the lungs, where oxygen is picked up and carbon dioxide is released. The left side of the heart pumps oxygenated blood out to all other parts of the body.

■ Blood high in oxygen
■ Blood low in oxygen

Fundamentals Review 14-1

FACTORS AFFECTING OXYGENATION AND PERFUSION

A variety of factors can affect cardiopulmonary functioning. This display reviews common factors.

LEVEL OF HEALTH

Acute and chronic illness can dramatically affect a person's cardiopulmonary function. Body systems (e.g., the cardiovascular system and respiratory system or the musculoskeletal system and the respiratory system) work together, so alterations in one may affect the other. For example,

alterations in muscle function contribute to inadequate pulmonary **ventilation** and **respiration**, as well as to inadequate functioning of the heart.

DEVELOPMENTAL LEVEL

Respiratory function varies across the life span. The table below summarizes variations. Age-related variations in pulse rate and blood pressure can be found in Chapter 2, Fundamentals Review 2-1.

	Infant (Birth–1 year)	Early Childhood (1–5 years)	Late Childhood (6–12 years)	Adolescent and Adult (18+ years)
Respiratory rate	30–60 breaths/min	20–40 breaths/min	15–25 breaths/min	12–20 breaths/min
Respiratory pattern	Abdominal breathing, irregular in rate and depth	Abdominal breathing, irregular	Thoracic breathing, regular	Thoracic, regular
Shape of thorax	Round	Elliptical	Elliptical	Elliptical or barrel-shaped

MEDICATIONS

Many medications affect the function of the cardiopulmonary system. Patients receiving drugs that affect the central nervous system need to be monitored carefully for respiratory complications. The nurse should monitor

rate and depth of respirations in patients who are taking certain medications, such as opioids or sedatives. Other medications decrease heart rate, with associated decreased cardiac output, and the potential to alter the flow of blood to body tissues.

(continued)

Fundamentals Review 14-1   continued

FACTORS AFFECTING OXYGENATION AND PERFUSION

LIFESTYLE

Activity levels and habits can dramatically affect a person's cardiopulmonary status. For example, people who exercise can better respond to stressors to cardiopulmonary health. Regular physical activity provides many health benefits, including increased heart and lung fitness, improved muscle fitness, and reduced risk of heart disease. Cigarette smoking (active or passive) is a major contributor to lung disease and respiratory distress, heart disease, and lung cancer. Cigarette smoking is the most important risk factor for chronic obstructive pulmonary disease (COPD) (NHLBI, 2019). Smoking is one of the key risk factors for heart disease, the leading cause of death in the United States (CDC, 2021).

ENVIRONMENT

Research indicates that there is a high correlation between air pollution (Kurt et al., 2016; Turner, Anderson et al., 2020) and occupational exposure to certain chemicals (Johns Hopkins Medicine, 2021) and cancer and lung disease and cardiovascular risk factors (Al-Kindi et al., 2020). In addition, people who have experienced an alteration in respiratory functioning often have difficulty continuing to perform self-care activities in a polluted environment.

OLDER ADULTS

The tissues and airways of the respiratory tract (including the **alveoli**) become less elastic with age. The power of the respiratory and abdominal muscles is reduced, and therefore the diaphragm moves less efficiently. Airways collapse more easily. These alterations increase the risk for disease, especially pneumonia and other chest infections. The normal aging heart can maintain adequate cardiac output under ordinary circumstances but may have a limited ability to respond to situations that cause physical or emotional stress, when the demands on the heart are increased (Eliopoulos, 2018; Hinkle et al., 2022). Decreased physical activity, physical deconditioning, decreased elasticity of the blood vessels, and stiffening of the heart valves can lead to a decrease in the overall function of the heart, leading to decreased oxygenation of body tissues.

PSYCHOLOGICAL HEALTH

Many psychological factors can have an impact on the respiratory system. People responding to stress or anxiety may experience **hyperventilation**. In addition, patients with respiratory problems often develop some anxiety as a result of the **hypoxia** caused by the respiratory problem.

Skill 14-1 ▶ Using a Pulse Oximeter

Pulse oximetry is a noninvasive technique that measures the peripheral arterial oxyhemoglobin saturation (SpO$_2$) of arterial blood. The reported result is a ratio, expressed as a percentage, between the actual oxygen content of the hemoglobin and the potential maximum oxygen-carrying capacity of the hemoglobin (Fischbach & Fischbach, 2018). A sensor, or probe, uses a beam of red and infrared light that travels through tissue and blood vessels. One part of the sensor emits the light, and another part receives the light. The oximeter then calculates the amount of light that has been absorbed by arterial blood. Oxygen saturation is determined by the amount of each light absorbed; nonoxygenated hemoglobin absorbs more red light and oxygenated hemoglobin absorbs more infrared light.

Sensors are available for use on a finger, a toe, a foot (infants), an earlobe, and forehead (Hess et al., 2021). It is important to use the appropriate sensor for the intended site and that it is fitted correctly (Hess et al., 2021); use of a sensor on a site other than what it is intended can result in inaccurate or unreliable readings. Circulation to the sensor site must be adequate to ensure accurate readings. Pulse oximeters also display a measured pulse rate.

It is important to know the patient's hemoglobin level before evaluating oxygen saturation because the test measures only the percentage of oxygen carried by the available hemoglobin. Thus, even a patient with a low hemoglobin level could appear to have a normal SpO$_2$ because most of that hemoglobin is saturated. However, the patient may not have enough oxygen to meet body needs (Morton & Fontaine, 2018).

A range of 90% to 100% is considered the normal SpO$_2$ (Bauldoff et al., 2020), depending on the patient's health status and health problems and needs; values <90% are considered low (American Thoracic Society, 2021; MFMER, 2018b), indicate that oxygenation to the tissues may be inadequate, and should be investigated for potential hypoxia or technical error (Hinkle et al., 2022). When administering supplemental oxygen, most patients will have a target oxygen saturation of 94% to 98% (O'Driscoll et al., 2017). Patients with chronic obstructive pulmonary disease (COPD) and other risk factors for hypercapnia may have a target oxygen saturation of 88% to 92% (Mirza et al., 2018; Mitchell, 2015; O'Driscoll et al., 2017). Be aware of any prescribed interventions regarding acceptable ranges and/or check with the patient's health care team.

Pulse oximetry is useful for monitoring patients receiving oxygen therapy, titrating oxygen therapy, monitoring those at risk for hypoxia, monitoring those at risk of hypoventilation (opioids use, neurologic compromise), and postoperative patients. Pulse oximeter measurements are less accurate at SpO_2 less than 80%, but the clinical importance of this is questionable (Hess et al., 2021, p. 25). In addition, a patient's SpO_2 may remain relatively normal initially due to an increase in respiratory rate compensating for inadequate oxygen delivery (Dix, 2018; Elliott & Baird, 2019). Pulse oximetry does not replace arterial blood gas analysis. Desaturation (decreased level of SpO_2) indicates gas exchange abnormalities. Oxygen desaturation is considered a late sign of respiratory compromise in patients with reduced rate and depth of breathing.

DELEGATION CONSIDERATIONS	The measurement of oxygen saturation using a pulse oximeter may be delegated to assistive personnel (AP) as well as to licensed practical/vocational nurses (LPN/LVNs). The decision to delegate must be based on careful analysis of the patient's needs and circumstances as well as the qualifications of the person to whom the task is being delegated. Refer to the Delegation Guidelines in Appendix A.
EQUIPMENT	• Pulse oximeter with an appropriate sensor or probe • Disposable cleansing cloth or skin cleanser and water • Nail polish remover (if necessary) • PPE, as indicated
ASSESSMENT	Assess for the presence of health problems that may impact oxygenation. Assess the patient's respiratory rate, rhythm, and depth and their mental status. Significant changes from baseline may indicate an alteration in oxygenation. Assess the patient's skin temperature and color, including the color of the nail beds. Temperature is a good indicator of blood flow. Warm skin indicates adequate circulation. Pallor (lack of color) of skin and mucous membranes can indicate less than optimal oxygenation. Cyanosis (bluish discoloration) and/or coolness or decreased temperature may indicate decreased blood flow or poor blood oxygenation. Check capillary refill; prolonged capillary refill indicates a reduction in blood flow. Assess the quality of the pulse proximal to the sensor application site. Assess for edema of the sensor site. Avoid placing a sensor on edematous tissue; the presence of edema can interfere with readings. Auscultate the lungs (see Skill 3-5). Note the amount of oxygen and delivery method if the patient is receiving supplemental oxygen.
ACTUAL OR POTENTIAL HEALTH PROBLEMS AND NEEDS	Many actual or potential health problems or issues may require the use of this skill as part of related interventions. An appropriate health problem or issue may include: • Impaired gas exchange • Ineffective airway clearance • Activity intolerance
OUTCOME IDENTIFICATION AND PLANNING	The expected outcomes to achieve when measuring oxygen saturation with a pulse oximeter is that the patient will exhibit oxygen saturation within their specified target range and based on their clinical status, and the heart rate displayed on the oximeter will correlate with the pulse measurement.

IMPLEMENTATION

ACTION	RATIONALE
1. Review the patient's health record for any health problems that would affect the patient's oxygenation status. Gather equipment.	Identifying influencing factors aids in interpretation of results. Assembling equipment provides for an organized approach to the task.

(continued on page 854)

Skill 14-1 ► Using a Pulse Oximeter *(continued)*

ACTION

2. Perform hand hygiene and put on PPE, if indicated.

3. Identify the patient.

4. Assemble equipment on the bedside stand or overbed table or other surface within reach.

5. Close the curtains around the bed and close the door to the room, if possible. Explain to the patient what you are going to do and why.

6. Select an appropriate site for application of the sensor.

   a. Use the patient's index, middle, or ring finger (Figure 1).

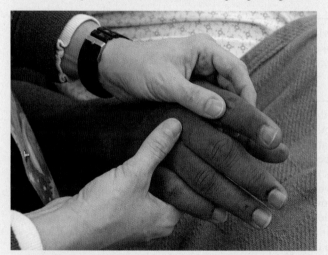

FIGURE 1. Selecting an appropriate finger.

   b. Check the proximal pulse (Figure 2) and capillary refill (Figure 3) closest to the site.

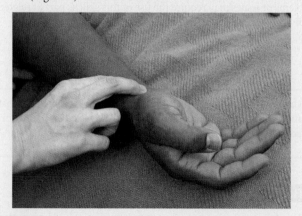

FIGURE 2. Assessing pulse.

RATIONALE

Hand hygiene and PPE prevent the spread of microorganisms. PPE is required based on transmission precautions.

Identifying the patient ensures the right patient receives the intervention and helps prevent errors.

Bringing everything to the bedside conserves time and energy. Arranging items nearby is convenient, saves time, and avoids unnecessary stretching and twisting of muscles on the part of the nurse.

This ensures the patient's privacy. Explanation relieves anxiety and facilitates engagement with care.

Inadequate circulation can interfere with the oxygen saturation (SpO_2) reading.

Fingers are easily accessible.

Brisk capillary refill and a strong pulse indicate adequate circulation to the site.

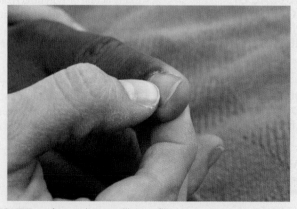

FIGURE 3. Assessing capillary refill.

ACTION

  c. If circulation to the site is inadequate, consider using the earlobe or forehead. Use the appropriate oximetry sensor for the chosen site.

  d. Use a toe only if lower extremity circulation is not compromised.

7. Select the proper equipment:

  a. If one finger is too large for the probe, use a smaller finger.

  b. Use probes appropriate for the patient's age and size. Use a pediatric probe for a small adult, if necessary.

  c. Check if the patient is allergic to the adhesive. A nonadhesive finger clip or reflectance sensor is available.

8. Prepare the monitoring site. Cleanse the selected area with a disposable cleansing cloth, as necessary; alternatively, have the patient wash their hands. Allow the area to dry. If necessary, remove any nail polish and artificial nails after checking the pulse oximeter's manufacturer's instructions.

9. Attach the probe securely to the skin (Figure 4). **Make sure that the light-emitting sensor and the light-receiving sensor are aligned opposite each other (not necessary to check if placed on the forehead).**

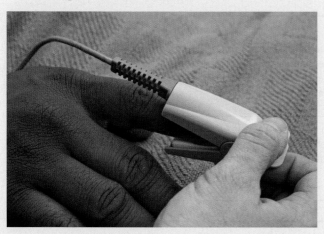

FIGURE 4. Attaching probe to patient's finger.

10. Connect the sensor probe to the pulse oximeter (Figure 5), turn the oximeter on, and check operation of the equipment (audible beep and fluctuation of the bar of light or waveform on the face of the oximeter).

11. Set alarms on the pulse oximeter. Check the manufacturer's alarm limits for high and low pulse rate settings (Figure 6).

12. Check oxygen saturation at regular intervals, as prescribed, as per nursing assessment, and as signaled by alarms. Monitor the hemoglobin level.

13. Remove the sensor on a regular basis and check for skin irritation or signs of pressure (every 2 hours for a spring-tension sensor and every 4 hours for an adhesive finger or toe sensor).

RATIONALE

These alternative sites are highly vascular. Correct use of appropriate equipment is vital for accurate results.

Peripheral vascular disease is common in lower extremities.

Inaccurate readings can result if the probe or sensor is not attached correctly.

Probes come in adult, pediatric, and infant sizes.

A reaction may occur if the patient is allergic to an adhesive substance.

Skin oils, dirt, or grime on the site can interfere with the passage of light waves. Research is conflicting regarding the effect of dark color nail polish and artificial nails. However, it is prudent to remove the nail polish (American Thoracic Society, 2021; USFDA, 2021; World Health Organization [WHO], 2011; Yönt et al., 2014). Refer to facility policy and the pulse oximeter's manufacturer's instructions regarding nail polish and artificial nails for additional information.

Secure attachment and proper alignment promote satisfactory operation of the equipment and an accurate recording of the SpO_2.

An audible beep represents the arterial pulse, and a fluctuating waveform or light bar indicates the strength of the pulse. A weak signal will produce an inaccurate recording of the SpO_2. The tone of the beep reflects the SpO_2 reading. If SpO_2 drops, the tone becomes lower in pitch.

The alarm provides an additional safeguard and signals when high or low limits have been surpassed.

Monitoring SpO_2 provides ongoing assessment of the patient's condition. A low hemoglobin level may be satisfactorily saturated yet inadequate to meet a patient's oxygen needs.

Prolonged pressure may lead to tissue necrosis. An adhesive sensor may cause skin irritation.

(*continued on page 856*)

Skill 14-1 ▶ Using a Pulse Oximeter *(continued)*

ACTION	RATIONALE

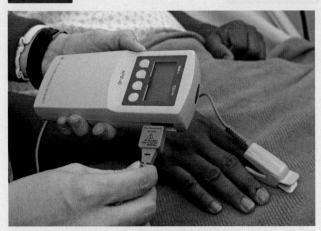

FIGURE 5. Connecting sensor probe to unit.

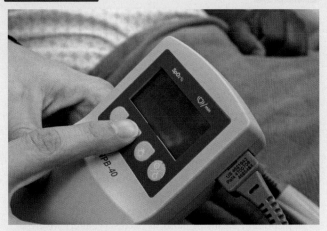

FIGURE 6. Checking alarms.

14. Clean nondisposable sensors according to the manufacturer's directions. Remove PPE, if used. Perform hand hygiene.

Cleaning equipment between each patient use reduces the spread of microorganisms. Proper removal of PPE reduces the risk for infection transmission and contamination of other items. Hand hygiene prevents the spread of microorganisms.

EVALUATION

The expected outcomes have been met when the patient has exhibited an oxygen saturation within their specified target range and based on their clinical status, and the heart rate displayed on the oximeter has correlated with the pulse measurement.

DOCUMENTATION

Guidelines

Documentation should include the type of sensor and location used, assessment of the proximal pulse and capillary refill, the pulse oximeter reading, the amount of oxygen, and delivery method if the patient is receiving supplemental oxygen, respiratory status, and any other relevant interventions required as a result of the reading.

Sample Documentation

> 9/03/25 Pulse oximeter placed on patient's index finger on right hand. Radial pulse presents with brisk capillary refill. Pulse oximeter reading 98% on oxygen at 2 L/min via nasal cannula. Heart rate measured by oximeter correlates with the radial pulse measurement.
>
> —C. Bausler, RN

DEVELOPING CLINICAL REASONING AND CLINICAL JUDGMENT

UNEXPECTED SITUATIONS AND ASSOCIATED INTERVENTIONS

- *Absent or weak signal:* Check vital signs and patient condition. If satisfactory, check connections and circulation to site. Hypotension and other conditions that result in low blood flow make an accurate recording difficult (Hess et al., 2021). Equipment such as a restraint or blood pressure cuff may compromise circulation to the site and cause venous blood to pulsate, giving an inaccurate reading. If the extremity is cold, cover it with a warm blanket and/or use another site.
- *Potentially inaccurate reading:* Check prescribed medications and history of circulatory disorders. Try the device on another person to see if the problem is equipment related or patient related. Drugs that cause vasoconstriction interfere with accurate recording of the oxygen saturation.

SPECIAL CONSIDERATIONS

General Considerations

- Review facility procedures for obtaining pulse oximetry readings if the patient's fingers are not suitable. Correct use of appropriate equipment is vital for accurate results. The appropriate ear oximetry sensor should be used to obtain measurements from a patient's ear. A finger sensor should be limited to use on the finger. The oximetry measurement obtained during clinical assessment should include a record of the type of sensor used.
- Accuracy of readings can be influenced by conditions that decrease arterial blood flow, such as peripheral edema, hypotension, and peripheral vascular disease. Bradycardia and irregular cardiac rhythms may also cause inaccurate readings.
- Accuracy of readings may also be affected by skin pigmentation (deeply pigmented skin) (Hess et al., 2021; Sjoding et al., 2020; USFDA, 2021), nail polish, and intravascular dyes (methylene blue and indocyanine green) (Hess et al., 2021; USFDA, 2021).
- Pulse oximetry may be less reliable in patients with chronic bronchitis and emphysema (Amalakanti & Pentakota, 2016).
- Inexpensive, portable over-the-counter pulse oximeters may be less reliable and are not intended for medical purposes, do not undergo FDA review, and should not be used for medical purposes (USFDA, 2021).
- Correlate the pulse reading on the pulse oximeter with the patient's heart rate (American Thoracic Society, 2021). Variation between pulse and heart rate may indicate that not all pulsations are being detected, and another sensor site may be required.
- Excessive motion of the sensor probe site, such as with extremity tremors or shivering, can also interfere with obtaining an accurate reading.
- In patients with low cardiac output, the forehead or ear sensor may be better than the digit sensor for pulse oximetry.

Infant and Child Considerations

- For infants, the oximeter probe may be placed on the toe or foot (Figure 7).

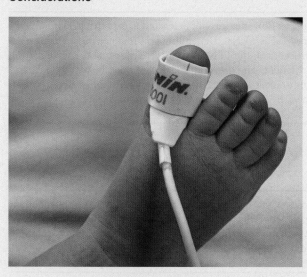

FIGURE 7. Oximetry probe on infant's toe.

Older Adult Considerations

- Careful attention to the patient's skin integrity and condition is necessary to prevent injury. Pressure or tension from the probe, as well as any adhesive used, can damage older, dry, thin skin.

Community-Based Care Considerations

- Portable prescription units are available for use in the home or in an outpatient setting (USFDA, 2021).

Skill 14-2 ▶ Teaching a Patient to Use a Peak Flow Meter

Peak expiratory flow rate (PEFR) refers to the point of highest flow during forced expiration, measured in liters per minute (LPM). PEFR reflects changes in the size of pulmonary airways and is measured using a **peak flow meter** (Figure 1). A peak flow meter can be an important part of an asthma management plan as well as management of chronic bronchitis and emphysema (American Lung Association, 2020a). Peak flow measurements can provide information about day-to-day changes in the patient's breathing to guide care decisions, including treatment and medication, as well as measure the severity of the disease, degree of disease management, and disease exacerbations (MFMER, 2020). In order to obtain consistent readings, the patient should use the same peak flow meter on a routine basis (Hess et al., 2021). There are many commercially available peak flow meters; refer to the manufacturer's guidelines for the specific device in use.

The individual patient's personal best peak flow provides the benchmark value for their asthma management plan (Hess et al., 2021; MFMER, 2020). The personal best peak flow is identified by measuring the daily peak flow rate over a 2- to 3-week period; the highest peak flow rate over this period is the patient's personal best (AAFA, 2017; MFMER, 2020).

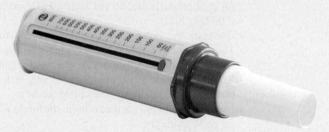

FIGURE 1. Example of a commercially available peak flow meter. (Courtesy of Clement Clarke International Ltd.)

DELEGATION CONSIDERATIONS	Patient teaching related to the use of a peak flow meter is not delegated to assistive personnel (AP) or to licensed practical/vocational nurses (LPN/LVNs). Depending on the state's nurse practice act and the organization's policies and procedures, the LPN/LVN may reinforce and encourage the use of the incentive spirometer by the patient. The decision to delegate must be based on careful analysis of the patient's needs and circumstances as well as the qualifications of the person to whom the task is being delegated. Refer to the Delegation Guidelines in Appendix A.
EQUIPMENT	• Peak flow meter • Stethoscope • PPE, as indicated
ASSESSMENT	Auscultate the lungs (see Skill 3-5). Assess vital signs and oxygen saturation. Ask the patient about symptoms, including shortness of breath, wheezing, coughing, chest tightness, and ability to complete activities of daily living. Ask the patient about their use of prescribed medications, including inhaled and oral. Assess the patient's understanding of the use of a peak flow meter.
ACTUAL OR POTENTIAL HEALTH PROBLEMS AND NEEDS	Many actual or potential health problems or issues may require the use of this skill as part of related interventions. An appropriate health problem or issue may include: • Impaired gas exchange • Activity intolerance • Knowledge deficiency
OUTCOME IDENTIFICATION AND PLANNING	The expected outcome to achieve when teaching a patient to use a peak flow meter is that the patient accurately demonstrates the procedure for using the meter. Other outcomes that may be appropriate include that the patient verbalizes an understanding of and engages in the plan of care.

IMPLEMENTATION

ACTION

1. Review the patient's health record for any health problems that would affect their oxygenation status. Gather equipment.

2. Perform hand hygiene and put on PPE, if indicated.

3. Identify the patient.

4. Assemble equipment on the overbed table or other surface within reach.

5. Close the curtains around the bed and close the door to the room, if possible. Explain to the patient what you are going to do and why.

6. Assist the patient to a standing position if they are able, otherwise, to an upright position, if possible.

7. Move the marker on the meter to the bottom of the numbered scale. Connect the mouthpiece to the meter if it is not already connected.

8. Instruct the patient to take a deep breath, filling their lungs completely, and then hold their breath. Have the patient place the meter in their mouth, between their teeth with their tongue under the mouthpiece, and then close their lips tightly around the mouthpiece (Figure 2).

RATIONALE

Identifying influencing factors aids in interpretation of results. Assembling equipment provides for an organized approach to the task.

Hand hygiene and PPE prevent the spread of microorganisms. PPE is required based on transmission precautions.

Identifying the patient ensures the right patient receives the intervention and helps prevent errors.

Bringing everything to the bedside conserves time and energy. Arranging items nearby is convenient, saves time, and avoids unnecessary stretching and twisting of muscles on the part of the nurse.

This ensures the patient's privacy. Explanation relieves anxiety and facilitates engagement.

An upright position facilitates lung expansion.

This starts the measurement at "0" and allows for an accurate reading. The mouthpiece is required to use the meter.

The patient should fully fill their lungs so that the maximum volume may be exhaled. The tongue under the mouthpiece prevents the tongue from blocking the hole in the mouthpiece (AAFA, 2017). A tight seal allows for maximum use of the device.

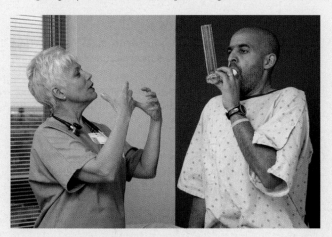

FIGURE 2. Patient placing meter in mouth. (Used with permission from Hinkle, J. L., Cheever, K. H., & Overbaugh, K. J. (2022). *Brunner & Suddarth's Textbook of medical-surgical nursing* (15th ed.). Wolters Kluwer; Fig. 20.12A.)

(continued on page 860)

Skill 14-2 ▶ Teaching a Patient to Use a Peak Flow Meter *(continued)*

ACTION	RATIONALE
9. **Instruct the patient to blow out as hard and as fast as they can in a single blow (Figure 3).**	The meter measures the force of the air coming out of the lungs, indicating how open the airways are in the lungs (Cleveland Clinic, 2020).

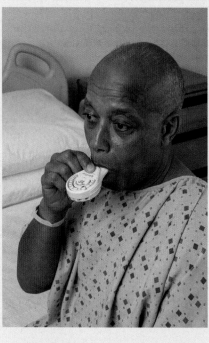

FIGURE 3. Patient blowing out has hard and fast as they can in a single blow.

ACTION	RATIONALE
10. Note the final position of the marker on the gauge on the meter and write it down.	The marker on the meter moves during exhalation, to gauge the point of highest flow.
11. Instruct the patient to remove their lips from mouthpiece and breathe normally. **If the patient coughs when using the meter or makes a mistake in the steps, instruct them to not record the number and to repeat the reading** (AAFA, 2017).	Coughing or other mistakes in the process may result in inaccurate readings.
12. Instruct the patient to blow into the meter two more times. The highest number of the three should be recorded in the patient's asthma diary.	Use of the highest of three measurements takes patient effort into consideration and provides more accurate representation of the patient's status.
13. Remove PPE, if used. Perform hand hygiene.	Proper removal of PPE reduces the risk for infection transmission and contamination of other items. Hand hygiene prevents the spread of microorganisms.
14. Clean the peak flow meter weekly with warm water and a mild detergent or according to the manufacturer's instructions (MFMER, 2020).	Cleaning the equipment deters the spread of microorganisms and contaminants (American Lung Association, 2020a).

EVALUATION

The expected outcomes have been met when the patient has correctly demonstrated the procedure for use of the peak flow meter has verbalized an understanding of the importance of and rationale for use of the meter.

DOCUMENTATION

Guidelines

Document that the peak flow meter was used by the patient, the number of repetitions, and the highest measurement. Document patient teaching and patient response, if appropriate. If the patient reports signs and/or symptoms of cough, document whether the cough is productive or nonproductive. If productive cough is present, include the characteristics of the sputum, including consistency, amount, and color.

Sample Documentation

9/8/25 1400 Patient education related to use of peak flow meter provided. Peak flow reading = 400 LPM (highest reading of three). Patient verbalized and demonstrated an understanding of steps for use of the meter, needs reinforcement about use of the Asthma Action Plan.

—C. Bausler, RN

DEVELOPING CLINICAL REASONING AND CLINICAL JUDGMENT

UNEXPECTED SITUATIONS AND ASSOCIATED INTERVENTIONS

- *Patient attempts to inhale on the meter:* Remind the patient that they are exhaling into the meter. They should blow a fast, hard blast to empty their lungs (American Lung Association, 2020a).
- *Each of three measurements at one use are very different:* Assess the patient's effort and technique in using the device. Remind the patient that it is important to inhale completely and blow out has hard and fast as they are able in a single burst of air. Check that the patient is not spitting or thrusting their tongue when blowing out.

SPECIAL CONSIDERATIONS

General Considerations

- It is important for the patient to know their peak flow reading, but it is even more important for them to know what to do based on that reading (American Lung Association, 2020a). The patient should refer to the Asthma Action Plan developed with their health care team (American Lung Association, 2020a).
- A decrease in peak flow of 20% to 30% of a person's personal best may indicate the start of an asthma episode (AAFA, 2017).
- The American Lung Association (2020a) provides a video showing patients how to use a peak flow meter at https://www.lung.org/lung-health-diseases/lung-disease-lookup/asthma/living-with-asthma/managing-asthma/measuring-your-peak-flow-rate.
- In order to obtain consistent readings, the patient should use the same peak flow meter on a routine basis (AAFA, 2017; Hess et al., 2021).
- Patients should collaborate with their health care team regarding the frequency of checking their peak flow (MFMER, 2020).
- Peak flow readings can be artificially high if the patient thrusts their tongue or spits during the measurement. Peak flow readings can be artificially low due to not enough effort or poor technique (AAFA, 2017).
- A common mistake is to attribute low measurements to poor effort or lack of cooperation when airway obstruction is actually present (Hess et al., 2021).

Infant and Child Considerations

- Children ages 5 years and older are usually able to use a peak flow meter to help manage their asthma (American Lung Association, 2020a).
- Meters come in two ranges to measure the air pushed out of the lungs; small children need to have a low-range peak flow meter (American Lung Association, 2020a).

Skill 14-3 ▶ Teaching a Patient to Use an Incentive Spirometer

Incentive spirometry provides visual reinforcement for deep breathing by the patient (Hess et al., 2021). It assists the patient to breathe slowly and deeply, and to sustain maximal **inspiration** (Eltorai et al., 2019), while providing immediate positive reinforcement. Use of an incentive spirometer encourages the patient to maximize lung inflation and prevent or reduce respiratory complications (Kotta & Ali, 2021). Evidence is conflicting in regard to the actual effectiveness of routine use of incentive spirometry, including routine postoperative use; deep breathing without mechanical aids may be as beneficial (Adams, 2018; Eltorai et al., 2018; Moore et al., 2018). Use of incentive spirometers is not recommended for routine use in postoperative care (Adams, 2018; Eltorai et al., 2018; Hess et al., 2021) but may be of more benefit in higher-risk patient populations (Kotta & Ali, 2021). If the use of incentive spirometry is prescribed for a patient, before use, the patient needs instructions on using the equipment properly. Validate the patient's correct use of this equipment in both health care and community-care environments.

DELEGATION CONSIDERATIONS	Patient teaching related to the use of an incentive **spirometer** is not delegated to assistive personnel (AP) or to licensed practical/vocational nurses (LPN/LVNs). Depending on the state's nurse practice act and the organization's policies and procedures, the LPN/LVN may reinforce and encourage the use of the incentive spirometer by the patient. The decision to delegate must be based on careful analysis of the patient's needs and circumstances as well as the qualifications of the person to whom the task is being delegated. Refer to the Delegation Guidelines in Appendix A.
EQUIPMENT	• Incentive spirometer • Stethoscope • Folded blanket or pillow for splinting of chest or abdominal incision, if appropriate • PPE, as indicated
ASSESSMENT	Assess the patient for pain and administer pain medication, as prescribed, if deep breathing may cause pain. The presence of pain may interfere with learning and performing the required activities. Assess lung sounds before and after use to establish a baseline and to determine the effectiveness of incentive spirometry. Incentive spirometry encourages patients to take deep breaths, and lung sounds may be diminished before using the incentive spirometer. Assess vital signs and oxygen saturation to provide baseline data to evaluate patient response. Oxygen saturation may increase due to reinflation of alveoli. Assess the patient's understanding of the use of an incentive spirometer.
ACTUAL OR POTENTIAL HEALTH PROBLEMS AND NEEDS	Many actual or potential health problems or issues may require the use of this skill as part of related interventions. An appropriate health problem or issue may include: • Impaired gas exchange • Altered breathing pattern • Knowledge deficiency
OUTCOME IDENTIFICATION AND PLANNING	The expected outcome to achieve when teaching a patient to use an incentive spirometer is that the patient accurately demonstrates the procedure for using the spirometer. Other outcomes that may be appropriate include that the patient demonstrates increased oxygen saturation level, reports adequate control of pain during use; demonstrates increased lung expansion with clear breath sounds, and verbalizes an understanding of and engages in the plan of care.

IMPLEMENTATION

ACTION	**RATIONALE**
1. Review the patient's health record for any health problems that would affect their oxygenation status. Gather equipment.	Identifying influencing factors aids in interpretation of results. Assembling equipment provides for an organized approach to the task.

ACTION

2. Perform hand hygiene and put on PPE, if indicated.

3. Identify the patient.

4. Assemble equipment on the overbed table or other surface within reach.

5. Close the curtains around the bed and close the door to the room, if possible. Explain to the patient what you are going to do and why. Using the chart provided with the device by the manufacturer, note the patient's inspiration target based on their height and age and/or volume of flow they generated preoperatively or prior to their change in health status (Hess et al., 2021).

6. Assist the patient to an upright or semi-Fowler position, if possible. Remove any dentures present if they fit poorly. Assess the patient's level of pain. Administer pain medication, as prescribed, if needed. Wait the appropriate amount of time for the medication to take effect. **If the patient has recently undergone abdominal or chest surgery, place a pillow or folded blanket over a chest or abdominal incision for splinting.**

7. Place the spirometer on a flat surface, like the overbed table, or have the patient hold it in an upright position. Have the patient hold the device steady with one hand and hold the mouthpiece with the other hand (Figure 1). If the patient cannot use their hands, assist the patient with the incentive spirometer.

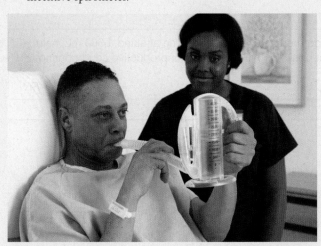

FIGURE 1. Patient using incentive spirometer.

8. Instruct the patient to exhale normally and then place their lips securely around the mouthpiece.

RATIONALE

Hand hygiene and PPE prevent the spread of microorganisms. PPE is required based on transmission precautions.

Identifying the patient ensures the right patient receives the intervention and helps prevent errors.

Bringing everything to the bedside conserves time and energy. Arranging items nearby is convenient, saves time, and avoids unnecessary stretching and twisting of muscles on the part of the nurse.

This ensures the patient's privacy. Explanation relieves anxiety and facilitates engagement with care. The target for inspiration is based on the patient's height and age and/or returning to preoperative/preprocedure volume (Hess et al., 2021) and provides an individualized target for each patient.

An upright position facilitates lung expansion. Dentures may inhibit the patient from taking deep breaths if the patient is concerned that dentures may fall out. Pain may decrease the patient's ability to take deep breaths. Deep breaths may cause the patient to cough. Splinting the incision supports the area and helps reduce pain from the incision (refer to Chapter 6, Skill 6-1).

This allows the patient to remain upright, visualize the volume of each breath, and stabilize the device.

The patient should fully empty their lungs so that the maximum volume may be inhaled. A tight seal allows for maximum use of the device.

(continued on page 864)

Skill 14-3 ▶ Teaching a Patient to Use an Incentive Spirometer *(continued)*

ACTION	**RATIONALE**
9. Instruct the patient not to breathe through the nose. Use a nose clip if necessary. **Instruct the patient to inhale slowly and as deeply as possible through the mouthpiece without using their nose.** Note the movement of the inhalation indicator on the spirometer.	Inhaling through the nose would provide an inaccurate measurement of inhalation volume. The inhalation indicator on the spirometer moves during inhalation, to gauge lung expansion.
10. When the patient cannot inhale anymore, **the patient should hold their breath for 3 to 5 seconds** (Hess et al., 2021). Check the position of the gauge to determine progress and level attained. If the patient begins to cough, splint an abdominal or chest incision.	Holding the breath for 3 to 5 seconds helps the alveoli to reexpand. The volume on the incentive spirometry should increase with practice.
11. Instruct the patient to remove their lips from the mouthpiece and exhale normally. **If the patient becomes lightheaded during the process, tell them to stop and take a few normal breaths before resuming incentive spirometry.**	Deep breaths may change the CO_2 level, leading to lightheadedness.
12. Encourage the patient to perform incentive spirometry 5 to 10 times every 1 to 2 hours, if possible.	This helps to reinflate the alveoli and prevent atelectasis due to **hypoventilation**.
13. Clean the mouthpiece with water and shake to dry. Remove PPE, if used. Perform hand hygiene.	Cleaning the equipment deters the spread of microorganisms and contaminants. Proper removal of PPE reduces the risk for infection transmission and contamination of other items. Hand hygiene prevents the spread of microorganisms.

EVALUATION

The expected outcomes have been met when the patient has demonstrated the steps for use of the incentive spirometer correctly and exhibited clear lung sounds and equal in all lobes, has demonstrated an increase in oxygen saturation levels, has verbalized adequate pain control and an understanding of the plan of care, and has engaged in the plan of care.

DOCUMENTATION

Guidelines

Document that the incentive spirometer was used by the patient, the number of repetitions, the average volume reached, length of time the breaths were held, and how many times the patient succeeded in meeting their volume goal (Hess et al., 2021). Document patient teaching and patient response, if appropriate. If the patient coughs, document whether the cough is productive or nonproductive. If productive cough is present, include the characteristics of the sputum, including consistency, amount, and color.

Sample Documentation

> 9/8/25 Incentive spirometry performed × 10, average volume attained 1,500 mL, held breath average 3 seconds, met goal 10/10. Patient with nonproductive cough during incentive spirometry.
>
> —C. Bausler, RN

DEVELOPING CLINICAL REASONING AND CLINICAL JUDGMENT

UNEXPECTED SITUATIONS AND ASSOCIATED INTERVENTIONS

- *Volume inhaled is decreasing:* Assess the patient's pain and anxiety level. The patient may have pain and not be inhaling fully, or they may have experienced pain previously during incentive spirometry and have an increased anxiety level. If prescribed, medicate the patient when pain is present. Discuss fears with the patient and encourage them to inhale fully or to strive to increase the volume by 100 each time incentive spirometry is performed.
- *Patient attempts to blow into incentive spirometer:* Compare the incentive spirometer to a straw. Remind the patient to exhale before beginning each time.

SPECIAL CONSIDERATIONS

General Considerations
- Incentive spirometers are not recommended for routine prophylactic use in postoperative adult and pediatric patients (Adams, 2018; Eltorai et al., 2018).
- The use of an incentive spirometer is not a viable therapeutic option for the obtunded, confused, or uncooperative patient because it requires patient engagement and the ability to understand and demonstrate proper use of the device (Hess et al., 2021).

Older Adult Considerations
- Older adults have decreased muscle function and fatigue more easily (Eliopoulos, 2018). Encourage rest periods between repetitions.

Skill 14-4 ▶ Administering Oxygen by Nasal Cannula

A variety of devices are available for delivering oxygen to the patient. Each has a specific function and provides an associated concentration of oxygen. Device selection is based on the patient's condition and oxygen needs. A **nasal cannula**, also called nasal prongs, is the most commonly used oxygen delivery device for administering low-flow oxygen to infants, children, and adults in the hospital and community settings (Hess et al., 2021). Oxygen may be administered using a nasal cannula by a low- or high-flow system. A low-flow nasal cannula can be set to deliver oxygen flows of 1 to 6 L/min in usual circumstances and to deliver an increased flow of 10 to 15 L/min for short-term use (Hess et al., 2021). High-flow systems deliver oxygen flow greater than 30 L/min (up to 60 L/min) and up to 100% humidified oxygen (Hernández et al., 2017; Lu et al., 2019; Zemach et al., 2019).

The cannula is a disposable plastic delivery tubing with two protruding prongs for insertion into the nostrils. The delivery tubing connects to an oxygen source with a flow meter and, as appropriate, a humidifier. Table 14-1 compares various oxygen delivery systems.

Table 14-1 Oxygen Delivery Systems

METHOD	AMOUNT DELIVERED FiO$_2$ (FRACTION OF INSPIRED OXYGEN)	PRIORITY NURSING INTERVENTIONS
Nasal cannula	Low flow 1–2 L/min = 24–28% 3–5 L/min = 32–40% 6 L/min = 44%	Check frequently that both prongs are in the patient's nares. For patients with chronic lung disease, limit rate to the minimum needed to raise arterial oxygen saturation to maintain a level of 88–92% (Mitchell, 2015).
Nasal cannula	High flow Maximum flow 60 L/min 10 L/min = 65% 15 L/min = 90%	Closely monitor the patient's respiratory status for changes indicating impending respiratory failure. Pharyngeal pressure is affected by mouth opening or closing, delivered flow, and size of nasal prongs (Nishimura, 2016). High-flow nasal cannula oxygen delivery is often better tolerated by children than other noninvasive delivery methods (Mayfield et al., 2014).
Simple mask	Low flow 5–8 L/min = 40–60% (5 L/min is minimum setting)	Monitor patient frequently to check mask placement. Support patient if claustrophobia is a concern. Secure a prescribed intervention to replace mask with nasal cannula during mealtime.
Nonrebreather mask	Low flow 10–15 L/min = 80–95%	Maintain flow rate so reservoir bag collapses only slightly during inspiration. Check that valves and rubber flaps are functioning properly (open during **expiration** and closed during inhalation). Monitor SaO$_2$ with pulse oximeter.
Venturi mask	High flow 4–10 L/min = 24–40%	Requires careful monitoring to verify FiO$_2$ at prescribed flow rate. Check that air intake valves are not blocked.

Source: Reprinted with permission from Hinkle, J. L., Cheever, K. H., & Overbaugh, K. (2022). *Brunner & Suddarth's Textbook of medical–surgical nursing* (15th ed.). Wolters Kluwer; additional information adapted from Nishimura, M. (2016). High-glow nasal cannula oxygen therapy in adults: Physiological benefits, indication, clinical benefits and adverse effects. *Respiratory Care, 61*(4), 529–541. https://doi.org/10.4187/respcare.04577

(continued on page 866)

Skill 14-4 ▶ Administering Oxygen by Nasal Cannula *(continued)*

DELEGATION CONSIDERATIONS

The administration of oxygen by nasal cannula is not delegated to assistive personnel (AP). Reapplication of the nasal cannula during nursing care activities, such as during bathing, may be performed by assistive personnel (AP). Depending on the state's nurse practice act and the organization's policies and procedures, administration of oxygen by nasal cannula may be delegated to licensed practical/vocational nurses (LPN/LVNs). The decision to delegate must be based on careful analysis of the patient's needs and circumstances as well as the qualifications of the person to whom the task is being delegated. Refer to the Delegation Guidelines in Appendix A.

EQUIPMENT

- Flow meter connected to oxygen supply
- Humidifier with sterile, distilled water (based on circumstances, system, and facility policy)
- Nasal cannula and tubing
- Gauze to pad tubing over ears or commercial padding (optional)
- PPE, as indicated

ASSESSMENT

Assess the patient's oxygen saturation level before starting oxygen therapy to provide a baseline for evaluating the effectiveness of oxygen therapy. Assess the patient's respiratory status, including respiratory rate, rhythm, effort, and lung sounds. Note any signs of respiratory distress, such as **tachypnea**, nasal flaring, use of accessory muscles, or **dyspnea**.

ACTUAL OR POTENTIAL HEALTH PROBLEMS AND NEEDS

Many actual or potential health problems or issues may require the use of this skill as part of related interventions. An appropriate health problem or issue may include:
- Impaired gas exchange
- Altered breathing pattern
- Activity intolerance

OUTCOME IDENTIFICATION AND PLANNING

The expected outcome to achieve when administering oxygen by nasal cannula is that the patient will exhibit an oxygen saturation level within acceptable parameters. Other outcomes that may be appropriate include that the patient will not experience dyspnea and will demonstrate effortless respirations within an acceptable and appropriate range, without evidence of nasal flaring or use of accessory muscles.

IMPLEMENTATION

ACTION	RATIONALE
1. Review the prescribed intervention to verify the use of the nasal cannula, flow rate, and administration parameters. Gather equipment.	Verifying the prescribed intervention ensures the patient receives the prescribed amount of oxygen. Assembling equipment provides for an organized approach to the task.
2. Perform hand hygiene and put on PPE, if indicated.	Hand hygiene and PPE prevent the spread of microorganisms. PPE is required based on transmission precautions.
3. Identify the patient.	Identifying the patient ensures the right patient receives the intervention and helps prevent errors.
4. Assemble equipment on the overbed table or other surface within reach.	Bringing everything to the bedside conserves time and energy. Arranging items nearby is convenient, saves time, and avoids unnecessary stretching and twisting of muscles on the part of the nurse.
5. Close the curtains around the bed and close the door to the room, if possible.	This ensures the patient's privacy.
6. Explain to the patient what you are going to do and why. Review safety precautions necessary when oxygen is in use.	Explanation relieves anxiety and facilitates engagement with care. Oxygen supports combustion; a small spark could cause a fire.

ACTION

7. Connect the nasal cannula to the oxygen source (Figure 1), with humidification, if appropriate. Adjust the flow rate as prescribed (Figure 2). Check that oxygen is flowing out of prongs.

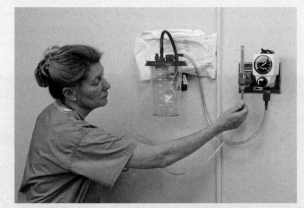

FIGURE 1. Connecting cannula to oxygen source.

8. Place the prongs in the patient's nostrils (Figure 3). Place the tubing over and behind each ear with the adjuster comfortably under the chin. Alternatively, the tubing may be placed around the patient's head, with the adjuster at the back or base of the head. Place the gauze (Figure 4) or commercially available pads at the ear beneath the tubing, as necessary.

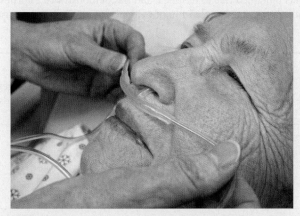

FIGURE 3. Putting the prongs in the patient's nostrils.

9. Adjust the fit of the cannula, as necessary (Figure 5). The tubing should be snug but not tight against the skin.

10. Reassess the patient's respiratory status, including the respiratory rate, effort, and lung sounds. Note any signs of respiratory distress, such as tachypnea, nasal flaring, use of accessory muscles, or dyspnea.

RATIONALE

Oxygen forced through a water reservoir is humidified before it is delivered to the patient, thus preventing dehydration of the mucous membranes. Low-flow oxygen does not require humidification.

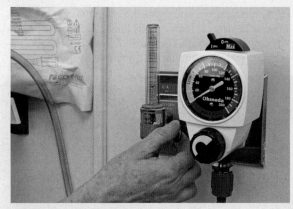

FIGURE 2. Adjusting flow rate.

Correct placement of the prongs and fastener facilitates oxygen administration and patient comfort. Pads reduce irritation and pressure and protect the skin. Pressure injuries may be related to a medical device or other object (EPUAP, NPIAP, & PPPIA, 2019, p. 16; Joint Commission, 2018). Any tube, electrode, sensor, or other rigid or stiff device element under pressure can create pressure damage (Baranoski & Ayello, 2020; EPUAP, NPIAP, & PPPIA, 2019).

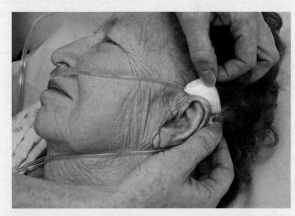

FIGURE 4. Placing gauze pad at ears.

Proper adjustment maintains the prongs in the patient's nose. Excessive pressure from the tubing could cause irritation and pressure to the skin. Nasal cannulas may cause pressure injuries behind the ears, around the nostril, or in the nasal vestibule (Camacho-Del Rio, 2018).

This assesses the effectiveness of oxygen therapy.

(continued on page 868)

Skill 14-4 ▶ Administering Oxygen by Nasal Cannula *(continued)*

ACTION

11. Remove PPE, if used. Perform hand hygiene.

12. Put on clean gloves. Remove and clean the cannula and assess the nares at least every 8 hours, or according to facility recommendations (Figure 6). Assess the areas of skin contact with the cannula for alterations in skin integrity.

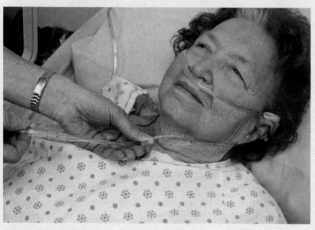

FIGURE 5. Adjusting the fit of the cannula.

RATIONALE

Proper removal of PPE reduces the risk for infection transmission and contamination of other items. Hand hygiene prevents the spread of microorganisms.

The continued presence of the cannula causes irritation and dryness of the mucous membranes. Nasal cannulas may cause pressure injuries behind the ears, around the nostril, or in the nasal vestibule (Camacho-Del Rio, 2018).

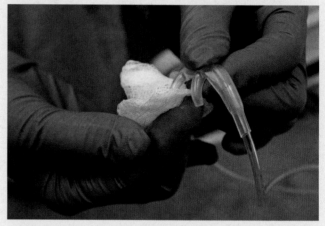

FIGURE 6. Cleaning cannula, when indicated.

EVALUATION

The expected outcomes have been met when the patient has demonstrated an oxygen saturation level within acceptable parameters; has remained free of dyspnea; and has demonstrated effortless respirations within an acceptable and appropriate range, without evidence of nasal flaring or use of accessory muscles.

DOCUMENTATION

Guidelines

Document your assessment before and after intervention. Document the amount of oxygen applied; the delivery method; and the patient's respiratory rate, oxygen saturation, and lung sounds.

Sample Documentation

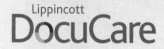

Practice documenting the administration of oxygen by nasal cannula in *Lippincott DocuCare*.

> 9/17/25 1300 Oxygen via nasal cannula applied at 2 L/min. Humidification in place. Pulse oximeter before placing oxygen 92%; after oxygen at 2 L/min 98%. Respirations even and unlabored. Chest rises symmetrically. No nasal flaring or retractions noted. Lung sounds clear and equal in all lobes.
>
> —C. Bausler, RN

DEVELOPING CLINICAL REASONING AND CLINICAL JUDGMENT

UNEXPECTED SITUATIONS AND ASSOCIATED INTERVENTIONS

- *Patient was fine on oxygen delivered by nasal cannula but now states they are short of breath, and the pulse oximeter reading is less than 93%:* Check to see that the oxygen tubing is still connected to the flow meter and the flow meter is still on the previous setting. Someone may have stepped on the tubing, pulling it from the flow meter, or the oxygen may have accidentally been turned off. Assess the patient's respiratory status, including respiratory rate, rhythm, effort, and lung sounds. Note any additional signs of respiratory distress. Collaborate with the health care team regarding any changes and assessment findings.

- *Areas over ear or back of head are reddened:* Ensure that areas are adequately padded and that the tubing is not pulled too tight. Consider consultation with the skin care team or wound nurse specialist.

SPECIAL CONSIDERATIONS

General Considerations

- Soft nasal cannulas have been shown to decrease the incidence of pressure injuries (Camacho-Del Rio, 2018).
- When providing oxygen via high-flow nasal cannula, protect the back of the ears with a hydrocolloid or foam dressing (Camacho-Del Rio, 2018).
- There is no evidence that mouth breathing influences the efficiency of oxygen delivery; even when the patient inspires through the mouth, oxygen still flows through the nose into the pharynx (Hess et al., 2021; O'Driscoll et al., 2017).

Community-Based Care Considerations

- Oxygen administration may need to be continued in the home setting. Liquid oxygen in a tank and oxygen concentrators are used frequently in home situations, including portable versions of both sources. Instruct caregivers about safety precautions with oxygen use and make sure they understand the rationale for the specific liter flow of oxygen.
- Oxygen supports combustion. To prevent fires and injuries, patients and families/caregivers should take the following precautions:
  - Do not smoke in a home where oxygen is in use. Place "No Smoking" signs in conspicuous places in the patient's home. Instruct the patient and family/caregivers about the hazard of smoking when oxygen is in use.
  - Keep oils, grease, alcohol, and other liquids that can burn away from the oxygen.
  - Keep the oxygen at least 6 ft away from any source of fire, such as a stove, fireplace, or candle (MedlinePlus, 2020).
  - Keep the oxygen 6 ft away from toys with electric motors, electric baseboard or space heaters, hairdryers, electric razors, and electric toothbrushes (MedlinePlus, 2020).
  - Do not use electrical equipment near oxygen administration set (e.g., electric blanket; see also above).
  - Use caution with gas or electric appliances.
  - Ground oxygen concentrators.
  - Secure the oxygen tank in a holder and away from direct sunlight or heat.
  - Allow adequate airflow around the oxygen concentrator (avoid placing it flush against the wall).
  - Notify the local fire department of the use of oxygen in the home.
  - Have working smoke detectors and a working fire extinguisher in the home (MedlinePlus, 2020).

EVIDENCE FOR PRACTICE ▶

HOME OXYGEN THERAPY FOR CHILDREN
Related Guideline

Hayes, D. Jr, Wilson, K. C., Krivchenia, K., Hawkins, S. M., Balfour-Lynn, I. M., Gozal, D., Panitch, H. B., Splaingard, M. L., Rhein, L. M., Kurland, G., Abman, S. H., Hoffman, T. M., Carroll, C. L., Cataletto, M. E., Tumin, D., Oren, E., Martin, R. J., Baker, J., Porta, G. R.,...on behalf of the American Thoracic Society Assembly on Pediatrics. (2019). Home oxygen therapy for children. An official American Thoracic Society Clinical Practice Guideline. *American Journal of Respiratory and Critical Care Medicine, 199*(3), e5–e23. https://doi.org/10.1164/rccm.201812-2276ST

The American Thoracic Society's *Home Oxygen Therapy for Children* provides recommendations based on the available evidence and expert consensus for safe practices for pediatric patients receiving home oxygen therapy, including defining hypoxemia, indications for and provision of home oxygen therapy, and discontinuation of therapy in this patient population.

(continued on page 870)

Skill 14-4 ▶ Administering Oxygen by Nasal Cannula *(continued)*

EVIDENCE FOR PRACTICE ▶

HOME OXYGEN THERAPY FOR ADULTS WITH CHRONIC LUNG DISEASE
Related Guideline
Jacobs, S. S., Krishnan, J. A., Lederer, D. J., Ghazipura, M., Hossain, T., Tan, A. Y. M., Carlin, B., Drummond, M. B., Ekström, M., Garvey, C., Graney, B. A., Jackson, B., Kallstrom, T., Knight, S. L., Lindell, K., Prieto-Centurion, V., Renzoni, E. A., Ryerson, C. J., Schneidman, A.,...on behalf of the American Thoracic Society Assembly on Nursing. (2020). Home oxygen therapy for adults with chronic lung disease. An official American Thoracic Society Clinical Practice Guideline. *American Journal of Respiratory and Critical Care Medicine, 202*(10), e121–e141. https://doi.org/10.1164/rccm.202009-3608ST
The American Thoracic Society's *Home Oxygen Therapy for Adults with Chronic Lung Disease* provides recommendations based on the available evidence and expert consensus for safe practices for adult patients with chronic obstructive pulmonary disease and interstitial lung disease.

Skill 14-5 ▶ Administering Oxygen by Mask

When a patient requires a higher concentration of oxygen than can be attained with a nasal cannula or when a cannula is not appropriate, such as with nasal obstruction (Hess et al., 2021), an oxygen mask may be used (see Table 14-1 in Skill 14-4 for a comparison of different types of oxygen delivery systems). Fit the mask carefully to the patient's face to avoid oxygen leakage. The mask should be comfortably snug but not tight against the face. The most commonly used types of masks are the simple face mask, the partial rebreather mask, the nonrebreather mask, and the Venturi mask. Figure 1 illustrates different types of oxygen masks.

Implement medical device–related pressure injury prevention strategies, including appropriate selection, fitting and securing of the mask, pressure redistribution by frequent repositioning or rotation, and use of a prophylactic cushioning/proactive dressing between the skin and mask (Pittman & Gillespie, 2020). Masks for oxygen delivery may cause injuries to the cheeks, chin, or

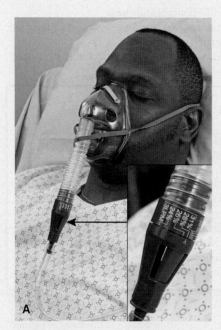
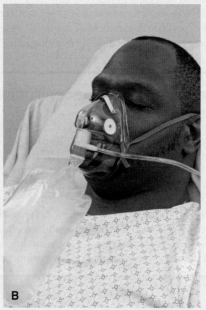
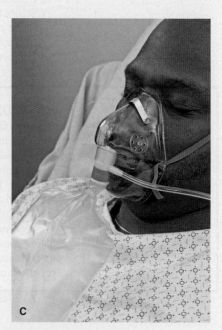

FIGURE 1. Types of oxygen masks. **A.** Venturi mask. **B.** Nonrebreather mask. **C.** Partial rebreather mask.

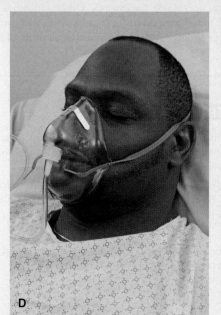
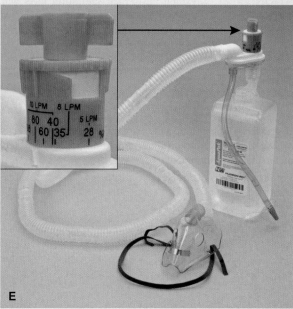

FIGURE 1. (*Continued*) **D.** Simple face mask. **E.** High-flow oxygen face mask and bottle.

bridge of the nose; place a silicone border or hydrocolloid dressings over bony prominences or other areas that come in contact with the device and between the device and the skin (Camacho-Del Rio, 2018).

DELEGATION CONSIDERATIONS	The administration of oxygen by a mask is not delegated to assistive personnel (AP). Reapplication of the mask during nursing care activities, such as during bathing, may be performed by AP. Depending on the state's nurse practice act and the organization's policies and procedures, administration of oxygen by a mask may be delegated to licensed practical/vocational nurses (LPN/LVNs). The decision to delegate must be based on careful analysis of the patient's needs and circumstances as well as the qualifications of the person to whom the task is being delegated. Refer to the Delegation Guidelines in Appendix A.
EQUIPMENT	• Flow meter connected to oxygen supply • Humidifier with sterile distilled water, if necessary, for the type of mask prescribed (based on circumstances, system, and facility policy) • Face mask, as prescribed or indicated based on the patient's condition and circumstances • Gauze to pad elastic band or commercial padding; silicone border or hydrocolloid dressing (optional) • PPE, as indicated
ASSESSMENT	Assess the patient's oxygen saturation level before starting oxygen therapy to provide a baseline for determining the effectiveness of therapy. Assess the patient's respiratory status, including respiratory rate, rhythm, effort, and lung sounds. Note any signs of respiratory distress, such as tachypnea, nasal flaring, use of accessory muscles, or dyspnea.
ACTUAL OR POTENTIAL HEALTH PROBLEMS AND NEEDS	Many actual or potential health problems or issues may require the use of this skill as part of related interventions. An appropriate health problem or issue may include: • Impaired gas exchange • Altered breathing pattern • Activity intolerance

(*continued on page 872*)

Skill 14-5 ▶ Administering Oxygen by Mask *(continued)*

OUTCOME IDENTIFICATION AND PLANNING

The expected outcome to achieve when administering oxygen by mask is that the patient will exhibit an oxygen saturation level within acceptable parameters. Other outcomes that may be appropriate include that the patient will not experience dyspnea and will demonstrate effortless respirations within an acceptable and appropriate range, without evidence of nasal flaring or use of accessory muscles.

IMPLEMENTATION

ACTION	RATIONALE
1. Review the prescribed intervention to verify the use of the particular mask, flow rate/concentration, and administration parameters. Gather equipment.	Verifying the prescribed intervention ensures the patient receives prescribed amount of oxygen. Assembling equipment provides for an organized approach to the task.
2. Perform hand hygiene and put on PPE, if indicated.	Hand hygiene and PPE prevent the spread of microorganisms. PPE is required based on transmission precautions.
3. Identify the patient.	Identifying the patient ensures the right patient receives the intervention and helps prevent errors.
4. Assemble equipment on the overbed table or other surface within reach.	Bringing everything to the bedside conserves time and energy. Arranging items nearby is convenient, saves time, and avoids unnecessary stretching and twisting of muscles on the part of the nurse.
5. Close the curtains around the bed and close the door to the room, if possible.	This ensures the patient's privacy.
6. Explain to the patient what you are going to do and why. Review safety precautions necessary when oxygen is in use.	Explanation relieves anxiety and facilitates engagement with care. Oxygen supports combustion; a small spark could cause a fire.
7. Attach the face mask to the oxygen source (with humidification, if appropriate, for the specific mask) (Figure 2). Start the flow of oxygen at the specified rate. For a mask with a reservoir, be sure to allow oxygen to fill the bag (Figure 3) before proceeding to the next step.	Oxygen forced through a water reservoir is humidified before it is delivered to the patient, thus preventing dehydration of the mucous membranes. A reservoir bag must be inflated with oxygen because the bag is the oxygen supply source for the patient.

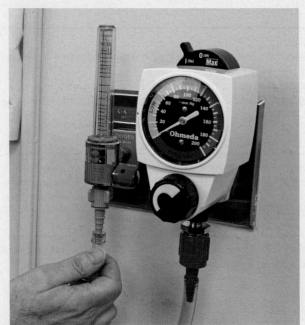

FIGURE 2. Connecting face mask to oxygen source.

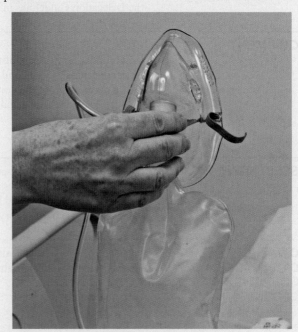

FIGURE 3. Allowing oxygen to fill bag.

ACTION

8. Position face mask over the patient's nose and mouth (Figure 4). **Adjust the elastic strap so that the mask fits snugly but comfortably on the face (Figure 5).** Adjust to the prescribed flow rate (Figure 6).

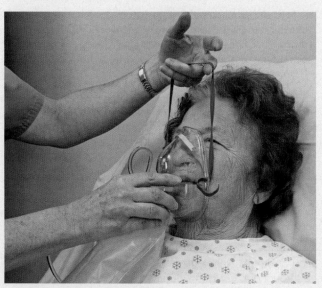

FIGURE 4. Applying face mask over nose and mouth.

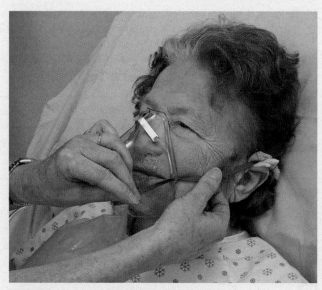

FIGURE 5. Adjusting elastic straps.

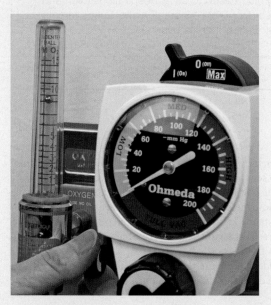

FIGURE 6. Adjusting flow rate.

9. If the patient reports irritation or you note any alteration in skin integrity, use gauze pads under the elastic strap at pressure points to reduce irritation to the ears and scalp. Consider use of a silicone border or hydrocolloid dressings over bony prominences or other areas that come in contact with the device and between the device and the skin (Camacho-Del Rio, 2018).

10. Reassess the patient's respiratory status, including respiratory rate, effort, and lung sounds, and their oxygen saturation. Note any signs of respiratory distress, such as tachypnea, nasal flaring, use of accessory muscles, or dyspnea.

RATIONALE

A loose or poorly fitting mask will result in oxygen loss and decreased therapeutic value. Masks may cause a feeling of suffocation, so the patient needs frequent attention and reassurance.

Pressure injuries may be related to a medical device or other object (EPUAP, NPIAP, & PPPIA, 2019, p. 16; Joint Commission, 2018). Any tube, electrode, sensor, or other rigid or stiff device element under pressure can create pressure damage (Baranoski & Ayello, 2020; EPUAP, NPIAP, & PPPIA, 2019). Pads reduce irritation and pressure and protect the skin.

This helps assess the effectiveness of oxygen therapy.

(*continued on page 874*)

Skill 14-5 ▶ Administering Oxygen by Mask *(continued)*

ACTION

11. Remove PPE, if used. Perform hand hygiene.

12. **Remove the mask and dry the skin under the mask every 2 to 3 hours if the oxygen is running continuously. Do not use powder around the mask.** Assess the areas of skin contact with the mask for alterations in skin integrity at least every 8 hours or according to facility recommendations.

RATIONALE

Proper removal of PPE reduces the risk for infection transmission and contamination of other items. Hand hygiene prevents the spread of microorganisms.

The tight-fitting mask and moisture from condensation can irritate the skin on the face. There is a danger of inhaling powder if it is placed on the mask. Masks may cause pressure injuries behind the ears, and to the cheeks, chin, or bridge of the nose (Camacho-Del Rio, 2018).

EVALUATION

The expected outcomes have been met when the patient has demonstrated an oxygen saturation level within acceptable parameters; has remained free of dyspnea; and has demonstrated effortless respirations within an acceptable and appropriate range, without evidence of nasal flaring or use of accessory muscles.

DOCUMENTATION

Guidelines

Document the type of mask used, the amount of oxygen used, oxygen saturation level, lung sounds, and rate/pattern of respirations. Document your assessment before and after the intervention.

Sample Documentation

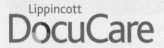

Practice documenting the administration of oxygen by mask in *Lippincott DocuCare*.

9/22/25 Patient reports feeling short of breath. Respirations 30 breaths/min and labored. Lung sounds decreased throughout. Oxygen saturation via pulse oximeter 88%. Findings reported to Dr. Lu. Oxygen via nonrebreather face mask applied at 12 L/min as prescribed. Oxygen saturation increased to 98%. Respirations even and unlabored. Chest rises symmetrically. Respiratory rate 18 breaths/min. Lungs remain with decreased breath sounds throughout. Patient denies dyspnea.

—C. Bausler, RN

DEVELOPING CLINICAL REASONING AND CLINICAL JUDGMENT

UNEXPECTED SITUATIONS AND ASSOCIATED INTERVENTIONS

- *Patient was previously fine on oxygen delivered by mask but is now short of breath, and the pulse oximeter reading is less than 93%:* Check to see that the oxygen tubing for the mask is still connected to the flow meter and the flow meter is still on the previous setting. Someone may have stepped on the tubing, pulling it from the flow meter, or the oxygen may have accidentally been turned off. Assess the patient's respiratory status, including respiratory rate, rhythm, effort, and lung sounds. Note any additional signs of respiratory distress. Collaborate with the health care team regarding any changes and assessment findings.
- *Areas over ear, face, or back of head are reddened:* Ensure that areas are adequately padded and that the elastic band for the mask is not pulled too tight. Consider consultation with the skin care team or wound nurse specialist.

SPECIAL CONSIDERATIONS

General Considerations

- Different types of face masks are available for use (refer to Table 14-1 in Skill 14-4 for more information).
- It is important to ensure the mask fits snugly around the patient's face. If it is loose, it will not effectively deliver the right amount of oxygen.
- The mask may be removed for the patient to eat, drink, and take medications. If appropriate, consult with the health care team regarding the use of oxygen via nasal cannula for use during mealtimes and limit the number of times the mask is removed to maintain adequate oxygenation.

Community-Based Care Considerations

- Oxygen administration may need to be continued in the home setting. Liquid oxygen in a tank and oxygen concentrators are used frequently in home situations, including portable versions of both sources. Instruct caregivers about safety precautions with oxygen use and make sure they understand the rationale for the specific liter flow of oxygen.
- Oxygen supports combustion. To prevent fires and injuries, patients and families/caregivers should take the following precautions:
  - Do not smoke in a home where oxygen is in use. Place "No Smoking" signs in conspicuous places in the patient's home. Instruct the patient and family/caregivers about the hazard of smoking when oxygen is in use.
  - Keep oils, grease, alcohol, and other liquids that can burn away from the oxygen.
  - Keep the oxygen at least 6 ft away from any source of fire, such as a stove, fireplace, or candle (MedlinePlus, 2020).
  - Keep the oxygen 6 ft away from toys with electric motors, electric baseboard or space heaters, hairdryers, electric razors, and electric toothbrushes (MedlinePlus, 2020).
  - Do not use electrical equipment near oxygen administration set (e.g., electric blanket; see also above).
  - Use caution with gas or electric appliances.
  - Ground oxygen concentrators.
  - Secure the oxygen tank in a holder and away from direct sunlight or heat.
  - Allow adequate airflow around the oxygen concentrator (avoid placing it flush against the wall).
  - Notify the local fire department of the use of oxygen in the home.
  - Have working smoke detectors and a working fire extinguisher in the home (MedlinePlus, 2020).

EVIDENCE FOR PRACTICE ▶

HOME OXYGEN THERAPY FOR CHILDREN
Related Guideline

Hayes, D. Jr, Wilson, K. C., Krivchenia, K., Hawkins, S. M., Balfour-Lynn, I. M., Gozal, D., Panitch, H. B., Splaingard, M. L., Rhein, L. M., Kurland, G., Abman, S. H., Hoffman, T. M., Carroll, C. L., Cataletto, M. E., Tumin, D., Oren, E., Martin, R. J., Baker, J., Porta, G. R.,...on behalf of the American Thoracic Society Assembly on Pediatrics. (2019). Home oxygen therapy for children. An official American Thoracic Society Clinical Practice Guideline. *American Journal of Respiratory and Critical Care Medicine, 199*(3), e5–e23. https://doi.org/10.1164/rccm.201812-2276ST.

Refer to details about this clinical practice guideline in Skill 14-4, Evidence for Practice.

EVIDENCE FOR PRACTICE ▶

HOME OXYGEN THERAPY FOR ADULTS WITH CHRONIC LUNG DISEASE
Related Guideline

Jacobs, S. S., Krishnan, J. A., Lederer, D. J., Ghazipura, M., Hossain, T., Tan, A. Y. M., Carlin, B., Drummond, M. B., Ekström, M., Garvey, C., Graney, B. A., Jackson, B., Kallstrom, T., Knight, S. L., Lindell, K., Prieto-Centurion, V., Renzoni, E. A., Ryerson, C. J., Schneidman, A.,...on behalf of the American Thoracic Society Assembly on Nursing. (2020). Home oxygen therapy for adults with chronic lung disease. An official American Thoracic Society Clinical Practice Guideline. *American Journal of Respiratory and Critical Care Medicine, 202*(10), e121–e141. https://doi.org/10.1164/rccm.202009-3608ST.

Refer to details about this clinical practice guideline in Skill 14-4, Evidence for Practice.

Skill 14-6 ▶ Caring for a Patient Receiving Noninvasive Continuous Positive Airway Pressure

Noninvasive positive airway pressure (PAP) therapy uses mild air pressure to keep airways open delivered via a mask. This treatment can help the body to maintain better carbon dioxide and oxygen levels in the blood. PAP therapy may be used to treat many adult disorders, such as sleep apnea, obstructive sleep apnea, obesity hypoventilation syndrome, acute cardiogenic pulmonary edema, heart failure, COPD, and acute hypoxemic respiratory failure (Hess et al., 2021; Martin, 2020; Medline Plus, 2021). It also may be used to treat disorders in infants and children, such as respiratory distress syndrome in preterm infants (Stanford Children's Health, 2021), infants with bronchiolitis (Franklin et al., 2019), and obstructive sleep apnea in children (Al-lede et al., 2018).

Continuous positive airway pressure (CPAP) provides continuous mild air pressure to keep airways open. *Bilevel positive airway pressure (BiPAP)* changes the air pressure while the patient breathes in and out. *Autotitrating (adjustable) positive airway pressure (APAP)* changes pressure throughout the therapy, based on the patient's breathing patterns (Medline Plus, 2021). All therapies use a mask or other device that fits over the nose or nose and mouth. Straps keep the mask in place. A tube connects the mask to the machine, which blows air into the tube.

This skill addresses noninvasive CPAP, the use of continuous mild air pressure applied throughout the respiratory cycle in a spontaneously breathing patient to promote alveolar and airway stability and increase functional residual capacity (Hinkle et al., 2022). CPAP is an effective treatment of obstructive sleep apnea; the air pressure holds the upper airway and trachea open during sleep (Bauldoff et al., 2020). CPAP may also be used as an adjunct to mechanical ventilation with an **endotracheal tube** or **tracheostomy tube** (Hinkle et al., 2022). Use of CPAP is contraindicated for patients with poor inspiratory drive and those who are not spontaneously breathing (Pinto & Sharma, 2021). Additional contraindications are identified in the Special Considerations discussion at the end of the Skill.

Nurses also play an important role in assisting with adherence to the prescribed CPAP intervention; nurses can assist patients by reinforcing accurate information about treatment and providing support and encouragement (López-López et al., 2020). If the device is used in the hospital or other facility or in the community, nursing responsibilities also may include monitoring the settings, ensuring correct use by the patient, and assessment of respiratory status. Initial use of CPAP may be difficult while patients acclimate to the device (Pinto & Sharma, 2021). Box 14-1 presents tips to avoid/address common problems encountered with CPAP.

Careful assessment of the patient's skin on the face, in the areas where the mask or nosepiece sits, and on the head where the straps sit is an important part of care. Pressure and moisture from the mask or nosepiece can cause alterations in skin integrity (Alqahtani et al., 2018). There are many kinds of CPAP machines and masks/nosepieces. Refer to the manufacturer's information for details for the specific equipment in use.

DELEGATION CONSIDERATIONS

The application of noninvasive CPAP is not delegated to assistive personnel (AP). Depending on the state's nurse practice act and the organization's policies and procedures, the application of noninvasive CPAP may be delegated to licensed practical/vocational nurses (LPN/LVNs). The decision to delegate must be based on careful analysis of the patient's needs and circumstances as well as the qualifications of the person to whom the task is being delegated. Refer to the Delegation Guidelines in Appendix A.

EQUIPMENT

- CPAP machine with tube/hose
- Prescribed mask or nosepiece (Figure 1)
- Distilled or sterile water for humidification, as indicated or prescribed; heated humidification may be built into CPAP machine
- Pressure injury prevention cushioning/proactive dressings, as indicated
- PPE, as indicated

ASSESSMENT

Assess respiratory status. Assess vital signs and oxygen saturation. Ask the patient about symptoms, including loud, ongoing snoring; daytime sleepiness; snorting/gasping during sleep; morning headaches; and waking up with a dry mouth or sore throat. Assess the patient's skin on the areas that come in contact with the CPAP headgear. Assess the patient's understanding of the use of CPAP.

Box 14-1	Tips to Address Common Problems Patients Encounter When Using CPAP and Possible Interventions	

Problem	Cause	Possible Solution
Congestion, nasal irritation, runny nose, nosebleed	Dry air	Addition of heated humidification
Dry throat and/or mouth	Dry air, improperly fitting mask	Addition of heated humidification; check fit of mask/nosepiece; tighten straps on mask/nosepiece
Trouble getting used to wearing the CPAP device	Feeling claustrophobic, sensitization to new device	• Gradually increase time wearing equipment; practice using the mask while awake. First just hold the mask to their face, then try wearing just the mask with the straps. Then, put the hose on the mask and hold the mask on their face, then try wearing with the straps. Finally, turn on the machine while wearing • Try wearing just the mask for short periods of time during the day while relaxing • Use every time during sleep, including naps
Patient has a hard time falling asleep or staying sleeping	Noise from motor	• Try using earplugs while sleeping • Consult with health care provider to consider use of ramp or delay • Follow good general sleep habits, regular exercise, avoid caffeine • Use relaxation techniques • Check/replace filter in device
Abdominal distention or a sensation of bloating	High airway pressure	Decrease CPAP pressure
Poorly fitting/leaking mask/nosepiece	Wrong size or style CPAP mask/nosepiece Excessive facial hair	Try a different mask or nosepiece Check sizing Check fit/adjustment of straps Shave facial hair
Difficulty tolerating forced air	High air flow/pressure Sensitization to new device	Consult with health care provider to consider use of ramp or delay Consult with health care provider to consider use of bi-level positive airway pressure
Irritation or redness of the skin that comes in contact with equipment	Incorrect size/type of mask/nosepiece Incorrect fit Sensitivity to mask/nosepiece Heated humidification	Check size/fit of mask/nosepiece Consider use of padding on straps Readjust straps Clean mask/nosepiece and tubing regularly and replace as directed Lower temperature on humidifier Wash face before putting on the mask

Source: Adapted from American Sleep Association (ASA). (2021). *CPAP user guide.* https://www.sleepassociation.org/sleep-apnea/cpap-treatment/cpap-user-guide/; Hess, D. R., MacIntyre, N. R., Galvin, W. F., & Mishoe, S. C. (2021). *Respiratory care: Principles and practice* (4th ed.). Jones & Bartlett Learning; Mayo Foundation for Medical Education and Research (MFMER). (2018, May 17). *CPAP machines: Tips for avoiding 10 common problems.* https://www.mayoclinic.org/diseases-conditions/sleep-apnea/in-depth/cpap/art-20044164; Pinto, V. L., & Sharma, S. (2021, May 7). *Continuous positive airway pressure.* StatPearls. https://www.ncbi.nlm.nih.gov/books/NBK482178; and Suni, E. (2020, September 11). *How to use a CPAP machine for better sleep.* Sleep Foundation. https://www.sleepfoundation.org/cpap/how-to-use-cpap-machine

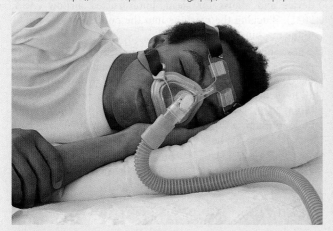
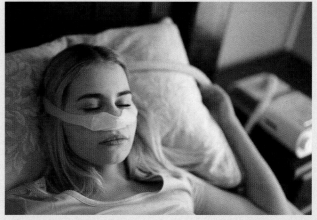

FIGURE 1. Examples of CPAP face mask/nosepiece.

(continued on page 878)

Skill 14-6 ▶ Caring for a Patient Receiving Noninvasive Continuous Positive Airway Pressure *(continued)*

ACTUAL OR POTENTIAL HEALTH PROBLEMS AND NEEDS	Many actual or potential health problems or issues may require the use of this skill as part of related interventions. An appropriate health problem or issue may include: • Altered breathing pattern • Fatigue • Knowledge deficiency
OUTCOME IDENTIFICATION AND PLANNING	The expected outcomes to achieve when implementing CPAP are that the headgear fits properly and is comfortable for the patient, there is no air leakage from the headgear during use, and the CPAP remains in place during sleep. Other outcomes that may be appropriate include that the patient experiences restful sleep and symptom improvement and verbalizes an understanding of and engages in the plan of care.

IMPLEMENTATION

ACTION	RATIONALE
1. Review the health care record for contraindications to the use of CPAP. Review the health record to verify the prescribed intervention, including the use of CPAP, pressure settings, and administration parameters. Gather equipment.	Verifying the prescribed intervention and the absence of contraindications ensures the patient appropriately receives the prescribed intervention. Assembling equipment provides for an organized approach to the task.
2. Perform hand hygiene and put on PPE, if indicated.	Hand hygiene and PPE prevent the spread of microorganisms. PPE is required based on transmission precautions.
3. Identify the patient.	Identifying the patient ensures the right patient receives the intervention and helps prevent errors.
4. Assemble equipment on the overbed table or other surface within reach.	Bringing everything to the bedside conserves time and energy. Arranging items nearby is convenient, saves time, and avoids unnecessary stretching and twisting of muscles on the part of the nurse.
5. Close the curtains around the bed and close the door to the room, if possible. Explain to the patient what you are going to do and why.	This ensures the patient's privacy. Explanation relieves anxiety and facilitates engagement.
6. Assist the patient to a comfortable sleeping position in the bed.	Comfort supports relaxation and sleep.
7. If it is the first time the CPAP machine is being used, install the CPAP machine filter as directed by the manufacturer.	Room air is drawn into the machine through a filter to remove dust, lint, and other large airborne matter (Hess et al., 2021).
8. Place the CPAP machine on a flat, stable surface near the bed (Figure 2). Position the vents of the machine at least 12 inches away from the wall, curtains, and other objects. Plug the electric cord into the electric outlet.	Proper positioning is necessary for optimal functioning of the device and allows for clean, unobstructed airflow (ASA, 2021). Plugging the machine into the outlet provides power to the machine.
9. Attach the CPAP hose and mask/nosepiece (Figure 3). Add distilled or sterile water to the humidifier compartment of the machine; fill to the "MAX" fill line.	The hose and mask provide the means for delivery of the positive pressure. Some CPAP machines have a humidifier built into the device; water provides humidification to moisturize the air to reduce the risk of drying of the mouth, nose, and throat (Suni, 2020). Use of distilled or sterile water prevents mineral buildup (Suni, 2020). Overfilling of the humidifier can cause water to enter the hose (Suni, 2020).
10. Enter the prescribed pressure setting (5 to 10 cm H_2O) into the CPAP machine, if not already programmed into the device.	Most CPAP machines have a pressure setting range from 4 to 25 cm H_2O (Fountain, 2021a); the usual pressure range is between 5 and 10 cm H_2O (Pacheco, 2021).

ACTION

RATIONALE

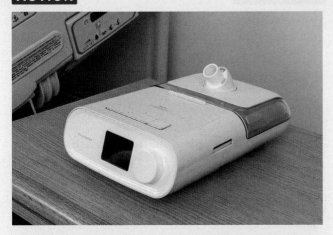

FIGURE 2. Placing the CPAP machine on a stable surface near the bed.

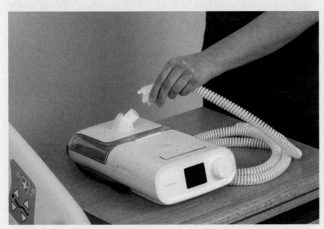

FIGURE 3. Attaching the CPAP hose and mask/nosepiece.

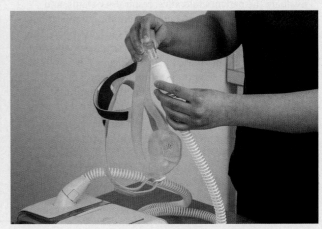

11. Assist the patient to put on the mask or nosepiece. Position the mask/nosepiece on the face and attach or pull the straps to secure it. The mask/nosepiece should form a seal against the face/nose but should not pinch or press deeply into the skin (Figure 4). Adjust the straps for a comfortable fit.

A proper fit is necessary to ensure optimal delivery of pressure but reduce the risk for pressure injury (Pinto & Sharma, 2021; Suni, 2020). A properly fitting mask should not be uncomfortable or cause pain (MFMER, 2018a).

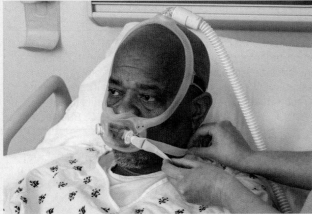

FIGURE 4. CPAP mask/nosepiece properly fitted on the patient's face.

(*continued on page 880*)

Skill 14-6 ▶ Caring for a Patient Receiving Noninvasive Continuous Positive Airway Pressure *(continued)*

ACTION	RATIONALE
12. Turn the machine on. The patient should experience pressurized air coming through the mask/nosepiece. Assess for air escaping/leaking from the mask/nosepiece. Adjust the straps as needed for a tighter seal.	A proper fit is necessary to ensure optimal delivery of pressure but reduce the risk for pressure injury (Pinto & Sharma, 2021; Suni, 2020).
13. Assist the patient to adjust their sleeping position, as necessary, to attain comfort without interfering with wearing of the mask/nosepiece or pinching or blocking the machine's hose (Suni, 2020).	This positioning supports optimal sleep and functioning of the device.
14. Remove PPE, if used. Perform hand hygiene.	Proper removal of PPE reduces the risk for infection transmission and contamination of other items. Hand hygiene prevents the spread of microorganisms.
15. Monitor the patient's use of the CPAP during sleep. Assist the patient to remove the CPAP upon waking, as needed. Evaluate the patient's tolerance, respiratory status, and symptom management. Assess for possible complications from use, such as discomfort, feelings of claustrophobia or embarrassment, dry mouth, nosebleeds, nasal congestion, and skin irritation (MFMER, 2018a). Provide interventions as necessary to assist with transition to the use of CPAP. Refer to Box 14-1 for tips to avoid/address common problems with CPAP.	Monitoring and evaluation after use supports effective use and provides information to guide adjustments to use and maintain compliance. Initial use of CPAP maybe difficult while patients acclimate to the device (Pinto & Sharma, 2021).
16. Clean the CPAP tubing and mask/nosepiece regularly, at least weekly and preferably daily with warm water and a mild detergent, or according to the manufacturer's instructions (ASA, 2021; Fountain, 2021b). Refer to suggested cleaning guidelines in the Community-Based Care Considerations section below.	Cleaning the equipment removes contaminants, microorganisms, mold, dust, and debris (Fountain, 2021b; Pinto & Sharma, 2021). Rinsing removes soap. Components must be in good working order to support optimal functioning of the device.

EVALUATION

The expected outcomes have been met when the headgear has fit properly and was comfortable for the patient, no air has leaked from the headgear during use, the CPAP has remained in place during sleep, the patient has experienced restful sleep and symptom improvement, and the patient has verbalized an understanding of and has engaged in the plan of care.

DOCUMENTATION

Guidelines

Document that the CPAP was used by the patient and the pressure setting. Document assessment findings. Document patient teaching and patient response, if appropriate.

Sample Documentation

06/6/25 1400 Patient verbalized accurate understanding on use of CPAP; reinforcement of necessity and importance of daily cleaning and other maintenance of device provided. Patient denies adverse issues related to CPAP use; states "I was having some trouble with my mask, but I now have a different kind, and it's much more comfortable. I can't believe how much better I feel since I started using this thing!"

—C. Bausler, RN

DEVELOPING CLINICAL REASONING AND CLINICAL JUDGMENT

UNEXPECTED SITUATIONS AND ASSOCIATED INTERVENTIONS

- *Patient does not want to wear the CPAP and reports that exhaling against the CPAP is difficult and uncomfortable, and they feel anxious:* Remind the patient that sleeping with the CPAP may take some time to get used to (ASA, 2021; MFMER, 2018a) and that there are some strategies for helping them get used to wearing the device. Box 14-1 describes some strategies to help address this issue. Check if the CPAP device in use has a timed pressure ramp or delay setting (refer to the discussion of the ramp setting in the Special Considerations section below). Collaborate with the health care team to consider if a CPAP with this setting is appropriate for the patient.
- *Air leaks loudly from around the mask/nosepiece when the CPAP is turned on:* Assess the fit of the mask/nosepiece. Readjust the straps. If the patient has facial hair, check for facial hair interference and the need for shaving. Check the timing of replacement of the mask/nosepiece and consider replacing with a new one. Check the pressure setting to ensure it is set at the prescribed pressure. If the leaking persists, consider collaboration with the health care team to evaluate the need for a trial of a different type of mask/nosepiece.

SPECIAL CONSIDERATIONS

General Considerations

- CPAP cannot be used in patients who are not spontaneously breathing (Pinto & Sharma, 2021).
- Contraindications to the use of CPAP include uncooperative or extremely anxious patients; patients with reduced consciousness and inability to protect their airway; unstable cardiorespiratory status or respirator arrest; trauma or burns involving the face; facial, esophageal, or gastric surgery; copious respiratory secretions; severe nausea with vomiting; and severe air trapping diseases with hypercarbia asthma or COPD (Pinto & Sharma, 2021).
- Getting used to using a CPAP often takes time and patience; the settings may have to be adjusted by the prescriber, several mask/nosepieces may have to be tried, and/or the individual patient may need to try several different types of CPAP machines in order to identify the optimal system for them (NHLBI, n.d.). Box 14-1 identifies some common problems patients encounter when using CPAP and provides some possible interventions to address the problems.
- Patient education can increase CPAP adherence (López-López et al., 2020). Refer to the information provided in the Evidence for Practice box and the end of this skill.
- Most CPAP machines have an adjustable ramp or delay setting that may be helpful when the prescribed CPAP pressure exceeds 10 cm H_2O, as some patients are bothered by the high flow (Hess et al., 2021). After the patient puts on the mask/nosepiece and adjusts for any leaks, the ramp/delay setting can be activated, which causes the pressure to drop to 4 to 6 cm H_2O, a level that may make it more comfortable and easier to become accustomed to the CPAP and more tolerable while the patient falls asleep (ASA, 2021; Hess et al., 2021; Pinto & Sharma, 2021). The ramp/delay setting can be preset to a range of 5 to 45 minutes, during which time the machine divides the set prescribed pressure by the number of ramp/delay minutes and delivers an increasing pressure until the prescribed level is reached (Hess et al., 2021).

Infant and Child Considerations

- CPAP may be used to treat preterm infants/newborns who have underdeveloped lungs (NHLBI, n.d.; Silbert-Flagg & Pillitteri, 2018).
- Infants with frequent or difficult-to-correct apneic episodes may be treated with CPAP (Silbert-Flagg & Pillitteri, 2018).

Community-Based Care Considerations

- Reinforce accurate information about treatment and provide support and encouragement for patients using CPAP in the community.
- Educate patients about possible side effects and ways to manage any effects. Refer to Box 14-1.
- Instruct patients to clean the CPAP tubing and mask/nosepiece regularly, at least weekly and preferably daily with warm water and a mild detergent, or according to the manufacturer's instructions (ASA, 2021; Fountain, 2021b). Use warm water and white vinegar to soak and clean the humidifier tank. Thoroughly rinse all components with cool clean water after washing and

(continued on page 882)

Skill 14-6 ▶ Caring for a Patient Receiving Noninvasive Continuous Positive Airway Pressure *(continued)*

allow to air dry. Reassemble the CPAP machine once components are fully dry. Inspect the components and replace as necessary; the mask and tube should be replaced as indicated by the manufacturer, usually every 3 to 12 months (ASA, 2021; Pinto & Sharma, 2021).
- Replace the CPAP machine filter every 4 weeks or according to the manufacturer's guidelines (ASA, 2021).

EVIDENCE FOR PRACTICE ▶

IMPROVING ADHERENCE WITH CPAP

When used as prescribed, CPAP reduces daytime sleepiness, normalizes sleep architecture, and improves numerous health outcomes related to obstructive sleep apnea. Adherence to the prescribed use of CPAP is critical to achieve optimal effect of the therapy. However, a significant number of patients experience difficulties associated with use with resulting lack of adherence and compliance with the therapy (Pinto & Sharma, 2021). What can nurses do to help improve patient adherence to CPAP?

Related Research

López-López, L., Torres-Sánchez, I., Cabrera-Martos, I., Ortíz-Rubio, A., Granados-Santiago, M., & Valenza, M. C. (2020). Nursing interventions improve continuous positive airway pressure adherence in obstructive sleep apnea with excessive daytime sleepiness: A systematic review. *Rehabilitation Nursing, 45*(3), 140–146. https://doi.org/10.1097/rnj.0000000000000190.

The purpose of this systematic review was to summarize the effectiveness of interventions in the literature to improve adherence to continuous positive airway pressure (CPAP) treatment in patients with excessive daytime sleepiness. Three data bases (MEDLINE, ScienceDirect, and Google Scholar) were systematically searched for randomized controlled trials published between January 2005 and May 2018 that included interventions to improve CPAP adherence in adult obstructive sleep apnea patients with high daytime sleepiness. Key words included *apnea, compliance, CPAP, adherence,* and *somnolence.* Eight trials were identified to meet the criteria. The methodologic quality of the included studies was classified according to the Jadad Scale (Jadad or Oxford score). Three trials had scores below 3 points, indicating lack of rigor; five trials had scores of 3, indicating rigor. The reviewed studies identified four categories of interventions to improve adherence to CPAP: educational (five studies), technological (one study), pharmacologic (one study) and multidimensional interventions, including patient education (one study). The majority of the trials reviewed examined the impact of patient education on CPAP adherence, and the results suggested that educational interventions are the most effective at improving adherence to CPAP. The researchers concluded that patient education strategies alone and in combination with other modalities, such as relaxation, improve patient adherence to CPAP.

Relevance to Nursing Practice

Nurses play a large role in designing interventions to positively impact patient outcomes. Nurses can support and encourage adherence to a prescribed CPAP intervention. Patient education can increase CPAP adherence. Nurses can also use therapeutic strategies to improve CPAP adherence and should consider multidimensional interventions to enhance compliance.

Skill 14-7 ▶ Suctioning the Oropharyngeal and Nasopharyngeal Airways

Skill Variation: *Oropharyngeal Suctioning using a Yankauer Device*

Skill Variation: *Performing Nasotracheal Suctioning*

Suctioning of the pharynx is indicated to maintain a patent airway and to remove saliva, pulmonary secretions, blood, vomitus, and foreign material from the pharynx. Suctioning of the oropharynx or nasopharynx may be indicated if the patient is able to raise secretions from the airways but unable to clear from the mouth. Nasotracheal suctioning may be indicated to help a patient who cannot clear their airway by coughing or is unable to raise secretions from the airways. The frequency of suctioning varies with the amount of secretions present but should be done often enough to keep ventilation effective and as effortless as possible. Suctioning should be performed only when clinically indicated based on assessment and not routinely (Burns & Delgado, 2019; Hess et al., 2021; Morton & Fontaine, 2018). Anticipate the administration of pharmacologic (analgesic medication) and use of nonpharmacologic interventions for the patient before suctioning.

A Yankauer device (tonsil-tip suction apparatus) may be used when performing oral suctioning and when secretions are visible in the oral cavity (Hess et al., 2021; Morton & Fontaine, 2018). A suction catheter may be used for oropharyngeal suctioning; a suction catheter is used for nasopharyngeal and nasotracheal suctioning.

When performing suctioning, position yourself on the appropriate side of the patient. If you are right-handed, stand on the patient's right side; if you are left-handed, stand on the patient's left side. This allows for comfortable use of your dominant hand to manipulate the suction catheter.

The following skill describes suctioning of the **oropharyngeal and nasopharyngeal airways** using a suction catheter. See the accompanying Skill Variation for a description of oropharyngeal suctioning using a Yankauer device. Suctioning of the **nasotracheal airway** is outlined in the subsequent accompanying Skill Variation. Suctioning of the airway in patients with artificial airways (endotracheal and tracheostomy tubes) is discussed in Skills 14-9, 14-10, and 14-12.

DELEGATION CONSIDERATIONS	Suctioning of the oropharyngeal airway may be delegated to assistive personnel (AP) who have received appropriate training. Depending on the state's nurse practice act and the organization's policies and procedures, the suctioning of the oropharyngeal and nasopharyngeal airways may be delegated to licensed practical/vocational nurses (LPN/LVNs). The decision to delegate must be based on careful analysis of the patient's needs and circumstances as well as the qualifications of the person to whom the task is being delegated. Refer to the Delegation Guidelines in Appendix A.

EQUIPMENT

- Portable or wall suction unit with tubing
- A commercially prepared suction kit with an appropriate-size catheter or
  - Sterile suction catheter with Y-port in the appropriate size (adult: 10 to 16 Fr)
  - Sterile disposable container
  - Sterile gloves
- Sterile water or saline

- Towel or waterproof pad
- Goggles and mask or face shield; N95 mask or equivalent, based on patient's health status
- Disposable, clean gloves
- Water-soluble lubricant (nasopharyngeal and nasotracheal suctioning)
- Additional PPE, as indicated

ASSESSMENT

Assess lung sounds. Patients who need to be suctioned may have coarse crackles or gurgling present and/or reduced breath sounds. Assess the oxygen saturation level. Oxygen saturation usually decreases when a patient needs to be suctioned. Assess respiratory status, including respiratory rate, rhythm, and depth. Patients may become tachypneic when they need to be suctioned. Assess the patient for signs of respiratory distress, such as nasal flaring, retractions, or grunting. Assess effectiveness of coughing and expectoration. Suctioning of the airway may be necessary for patients with an ineffective cough who are unable to expectorate secretions. Assess for history of a deviated septum, nasal polyps, nasal obstruction, nasal injury, epistaxis (nasal bleeding), or nasal swelling, which may influence the use of one or the other naris. Assess for pain. Assess the characteristics and amount of secretions while suctioning.

(continued on page 884)

Skill 14-7 ▶ Suctioning the Oropharyngeal and Nasopharyngeal Airways *(continued)*

ACTUAL OR POTENTIAL HEALTH PROBLEMS AND NEEDS

Many actual or potential health problems or issues may require the use of this skill as part of related interventions. An appropriate health problem or issue may include:
- Ineffective airway clearance
- Altered breathing pattern
- Risk for aspiration

OUTCOME IDENTIFICATION AND PLANNING

The expected outcome to achieve when suctioning the patient's oropharyngeal or nasopharyngeal airway is that the patient will exhibit improved breath sounds and a clear, patent airway. Other outcomes that may be appropriate include that the patient will exhibit an oxygen saturation level within acceptable parameters and will demonstrate effortless respirations within an acceptable and appropriate range, without evidence of respiratory distress.

IMPLEMENTATION

ACTION	RATIONALE
1. Gather equipment.	Assembling equipment provides for an organized approach to the task.
2. Perform hand hygiene and put on PPE, if indicated.	Hand hygiene and PPE prevent the spread of microorganisms. PPE is required based on transmission precautions.
3. Identify the patient.	Identifying the patient ensures the right patient receives the intervention and helps prevent errors.
4. Assemble equipment on the overbed table or other surface within reach.	Bringing everything to the bedside conserves time and energy. Arranging items nearby is convenient, saves time, and avoids unnecessary stretching and twisting of muscles on the part of the nurse.
5. Close the curtains around the bed and close the door to the room, if possible.	This ensures the patient's privacy.
6. Perform assessments to determine the need for suctioning. Verify the prescribed suctioning intervention in the patient's health record, if necessary. Anticipate the administration of pharmacologic (analgesic medication) and use of nonpharmacologic interventions for the patient before suctioning. **Assess for pain or the potential to cause pain. Administer pain medication, as prescribed, before suctioning.**	Suctioning should be performed only when clinically indicated based on assessment and not routinely (AARC, 2010; Burns & Delgado, 2019; Hess et al., 2021; Morton & Fontaine, 2018). Some facilities require that naso- and oropharyngeal suctioning are a prescribed intervention. At a minimum, suctioning is an uncomfortable procedure, and it can be a very painful and/or distressing experience. Individualized pain management must be performed in response to the patient's needs (Arroyo-Novoa et al., 2008; Chaseling et al., 2014; Wrona et al., 2021; Düzkaya & Kuğuoğlu, 2015).
7. Explain to the patient what you are going to do and why, even if the patient does not appear to be alert. Reassure the patient that you will interrupt the procedure if they indicate respiratory difficulty.	Explanation alleviates fears. Even if the patient appears unconscious, explain what is happening. Any procedure that compromises respiration is frightening for the patient.
8. Adjust the bed to a comfortable working height (VHACEOSH, 2016). Lower the side rail closest to you. **If the patient is conscious, place them in a semi-Fowler position. If the patient is unconscious, place them in the lateral position, facing you.** Move the bedside table close to your work area and raise it to waist height.	Having the bed at the proper height prevents back and muscle strain. A sitting position helps the patient to cough and makes breathing easier. Gravity also facilitates catheter insertion. The lateral position prevents the airway from becoming obstructed and promotes drainage of secretions. The bedside table provides a work surface and helps maintain sterility of objects on the work surface.

ACTION

9. Place a towel or waterproof pad across the patient's chest.

10. **Adjust suction to the appropriate pressure** (Hess et al., 2021) (Figure 1):
    - No more than 150 mm Hg for adults and adolescents
    - No more than 125 mm Hg for children
    - No more than 100 mm Hg for infants
    Put on a disposable, clean glove and occlude the end of the connecting tubing to check suction pressure. Place the connecting tubing in a convenient location.

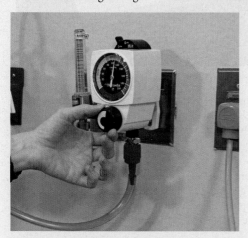

FIGURE 1. Adjusting wall suction.

11. Open the sterile suction package using aseptic technique. The open wrapper or container becomes a sterile field to hold other supplies. Carefully remove the sterile container, touching only the outside surface. Set it up on the work surface and pour sterile saline into it.

12. Place a small amount of water-soluble lubricant on the sterile field, taking care to avoid touching the sterile field with the lubricant package.

13. Increase the patient's supplemental oxygen level, or apply supplemental oxygen per facility policy or prescribed intervention.

14. Put on a face shield or goggles and mask. Put on sterile gloves. Your dominant hand will manipulate the catheter and must remain sterile. The nondominant hand is considered clean rather than sterile and will control the suction valve (Y-port) on the catheter. In the home setting and other community-based settings, maintenance of sterility is not necessary.

15. With your dominant gloved hand, pick up the sterile catheter. Pick up the connecting tubing with the nondominant hand and connect the tubing and suction catheter (Figure 2).

16. Moisten the catheter by dipping it into the container of sterile saline (Figure 3). Occlude the Y-tube to check suction.

17. Encourage the patient to take several deep breaths.

18. Apply lubricant to the first 2 to 3 inches of the catheter, using the lubricant that was placed on the sterile field.

RATIONALE

This protects bed linens.

Higher pressures can cause excessive trauma, hypoxemia, and atelectasis.

Sterile normal saline or water is used to lubricate the outside of the catheter, minimizing irritation of the mucosa during introduction. It is also used to clear the catheter between suction attempts.

Lubricant facilitates passage of the catheter and reduces trauma to mucous membranes.

Suctioning removes air from the patient's airway and can cause hypoxemia. Hyperoxygenation can help prevent suction-induced hypoxemia (Morton & Fontaine, 2018).

Gloves and other PPE protect the nurse from microorganisms. Handling the sterile catheter using a sterile glove helps prevent introducing organisms into the respiratory tract. In the home setting and other community-based settings, clean (instead of sterile) technique is used because the patient is not exposed to disease-causing organisms that may be found in health care settings, such as hospitals.

Sterility of the suction catheter is maintained.

Lubricating the inside of the catheter with saline helps move secretions in the catheter. Checking suction ensures equipment is working properly.

Hyperventilation can help prevent suction-induced hypoxemia (Hess et al., 2021).

Lubricant facilitates passage of the catheter and reduces trauma to mucous membranes.

(*continued on page 886*)

Skill 14-7 ▶ Suctioning the Oropharyngeal and Nasopharyngeal Airways *(continued)*

ACTION

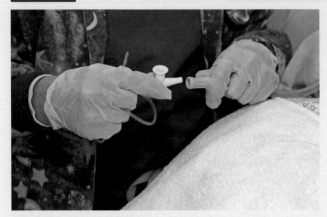

FIGURE 2. Connecting suction catheter to tubing.

19. Remove the oxygen delivery device, if appropriate. Do not apply suction as the catheter is inserted. Hold the catheter between your thumb and forefinger.

20. Insert the catheter:
    a. **For nasopharyngeal suctioning**, gently insert the catheter through the naris and along the floor of the nostril toward the trachea (Figure 4). Roll the catheter between your fingers to help advance it. Advance the catheter approximately 6 to 8 inches to reach the pharynx (Hinkle et al., 2022) (for guidelines for nasotracheal suctioning, see the accompanying Skill Variation).
    b. **For oropharyngeal suctioning**, insert the catheter through the mouth, along the side of the mouth toward the trachea. Advance the catheter 3 to 4 inches to reach the pharynx (for nasotracheal suctioning, see the accompanying Skill Variation).

21. **Apply suction by intermittently occluding the Y-port on the catheter with the thumb of your nondominant hand and gently rotating the catheter as it is being withdrawn (Figure 5). Do not suction for more than 15 seconds at a time** (AARC, 2010; Hess et al., 2021).

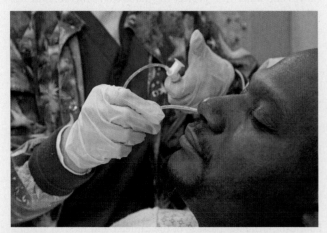

FIGURE 4. Inserting catheter into naris.

RATIONALE

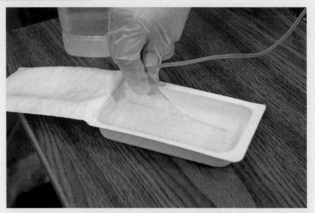

FIGURE 3. Dipping catheter into sterile saline.

Suctioning removes air from the patient's airway and can cause hypoxemia. Using suction while inserting the catheter can cause trauma to the mucosa and remove excessive oxygen from the respiratory tract.

The correct distance for insertion ensures proper placement of the catheter. The general guideline for determining insertion distance for nasopharyngeal suctioning for an individual patient is to estimate the distance from the patient's earlobe to the nose.

Turning the catheter as it is withdrawn minimizes trauma to the mucosa. Suctioning for longer than 15 seconds robs the respiratory tract of oxygen, which may result in hypoxemia. Suctioning too quickly may be ineffective at clearing all secretions.

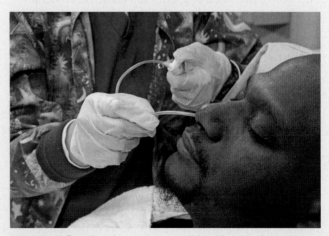

FIGURE 5. Rotating the catheter as it is withdrawn to suction the nasopharynx.

ACTION

22. Replace the oxygen delivery device using your nondominant hand, if appropriate, and have the patient take several deep breaths.

23. Flush the catheter with saline (Figure 6). Assess the effectiveness of suctioning and repeat, as needed, and according to the patient's tolerance. Wrap the suction catheter around your dominant hand between attempts.

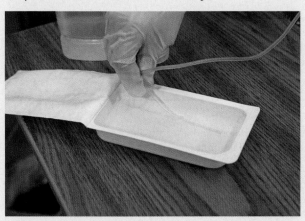

FIGURE 6. Rinsing catheter.

24. **Allow at least a 30-second interval if additional suctioning is needed. Alternate the naris, unless contraindicated, if repeated suctioning is required.** No more than three suction passes should be made per suctioning episode. Do not force the catheter through the naris. Encourage the patient to cough and deep breathe between suctioning. **Suction the oropharynx after suctioning the nasopharynx.**

25. When suctioning is complete, remove the glove from your dominant hand over the coiled catheter, pulling it off inside out. Remove the glove from your nondominant hand, and dispose of gloves, catheter, and the container with the solution in the appropriate receptacle. Perform hand hygiene.

26. Assist the patient to a comfortable position. Raise the bed rail and place the bed in the lowest position.

27. Turn off the suction. Remove the supplemental oxygen placed for suctioning, if appropriate. Remove the face shield or goggles and mask. Perform hand hygiene.

28. Perform oral hygiene after suctioning. Oral hygiene measures are discussed in Chapter 7.

RATIONALE

Suctioning removes air from the patient's airway and can cause hypoxemia. Hyperventilation can help prevent suction-induced hypoxemia.

Flushing clears the catheter and lubricates it for next insertion. Reassessment determines the need for additional suctioning. Wrapping prevents inadvertent contamination of the catheter.

The interval allows for reventilation and reoxygenation of airways. Excessive suction passes contribute to complications. Alternating the naris reduces trauma. Suctioning the oropharynx after the nasopharynx clears the mouth of secretions. More microorganisms are usually present in the mouth, so it is suctioned last to prevent transmission of contaminants.

This technique of glove removal and hand hygiene reduces transmission of microorganisms.

Proper positioning with raised side rails and the proper bed height provides for patient comfort and safety.

Proper removal of PPE and hand hygiene reduce the risk of transmission of microorganisms.

Respiratory secretions that are allowed to accumulate in the mouth are irritating to mucous membranes, pose a risk for aspiration, and are unpleasant for the patient. Diligent oral hygiene care can improve oral health and limit the growth of pathogens in the oropharyngeal secretions, decreasing the incidence of aspiration pneumonia, community-acquired pneumonia, non-ventilator health care–associated pneumonia (NV-HAP), and ventilator-associated pneumonia (VAP) (AACN, 2017; Chick & Wynne, 2020; Jenson et al., 2018; Quinn et al., 2020).

(continued on page 888)

Skill 14-7 ▶ Suctioning the Oropharyngeal and Nasopharyngeal Airways *(continued)*

ACTION	**RATIONALE**
29. Reassess the patient's respiratory status, including respiratory rate, effort, oxygen saturation, and lung sounds, and their response to suctioning.	This assesses effectiveness of suctioning and the presence of complications.
30. Remove additional PPE, if used. Perform hand hygiene.	Proper removal of PPE reduces the risk for infection transmission and contamination of other items. Hand hygiene prevents the spread of microorganisms.

EVALUATION

The expected outcomes have been met when the patient has demonstrated improved breath sounds and a clear, patent airway; has exhibited an oxygen saturation level within acceptable parameters; and has demonstrated effortless respirations within an acceptable and appropriate range, without evidence of respiratory distress.

DOCUMENTATION

Guidelines

Document the time of suctioning, assessments before and after the intervention, the reason for suctioning, route used, and the characteristics and amount of secretions.

Sample Documentation

> 9/17/25 1440 Patient with gurgling on inspiration and weak cough; unable to clear secretions. Lungs with rhonchi (sonorous wheezes) in upper airways. Nasopharyngeal suction completed with 12-Fr catheter. Large amount of thick, yellow secretions obtained. After suctioning, lung sounds clear in all lobes, respirations 18 breaths/min, no gurgling noted.
>
> —*C. Bausler, RN*

DEVELOPING CLINICAL REASONING AND CLINICAL JUDGMENT

UNEXPECTED SITUATIONS AND ASSOCIATED INTERVENTIONS

- *Patient vomits during suctioning:* If the patient gags or becomes nauseated, remove the catheter; it has probably entered the esophagus inadvertently. If the patient needs to be suctioned again, change the catheter, because it is probably contaminated. Turn the patient to the side and elevate the head of the bed to prevent aspiration.
- *Epistaxis (bleeding) is noted with continued suctioning:* Notify the health care team and anticipate the need for a nasal trumpet (see the Skill Variation in Skill 14-8: Inserting a Nasopharyngeal Airway). The nasal trumpet will protect the nasal mucosa from further trauma related to suctioning (Morton& Fontaine, 2018).

SPECIAL CONSIDERATIONS

General Considerations

- The use of suction pressure higher than the pressure guidelines presented in the skill have been suggested by some researchers (Maras et al., 2020; Yazdannik et al., 2019).

Infant and Child Considerations

- For infants, use a 5- to 6-Fr catheter.
- For children, use a 6- to 10-Fr catheter.

Skill Variation ▷ Oropharyngeal Suctioning Using a Yankauer Device

A Yankauer device (tonsil-tip suction apparatus) (Figure A) may be used when performing oral suctioning and when secretions are visible in the oral cavity (Hess et al., 2021; Morton & Fontaine, 2018). This device is angled to allow it to follow the contour of the oral cavity along the palate to facilitate suctioning in the posterior oropharynx and the buccal pouches (Morton & Fontaine, 2018). The larger openings on the Yankauer tip allow for suctioning of thick or copious secretions better than other suction catheters designed for suctioning through the endotracheal or nasotracheal tubes, which are smaller in diameter (Morton & Fontaine, 2018). Alternatively, a suction catheter may be used for oropharyngeal suctioning (refer to Skill 14-7). The frequency of suctioning varies with the amount of secretions present but should be done often enough to keep ventilation effective and as effortless as possible. Suctioning should be performed only when clinically indicated based on assessment and not routinely (Burns & Delgado, 2019; Hess et al., 2021; Morton & Fontaine, 2018).

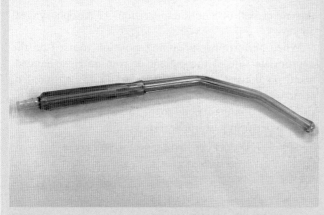

FIGURE A. Yankauer suction device. (Used with permission from Dorsch, J. A. & Dorsch, S. E. (2008). *Understanding anesthesia equipment.* Wolters Kluwer; Fig. 3.13.)

When performing suctioning, position yourself on the appropriate side of the patient. If you are right-handed, stand on the patient's right side; if you are left-handed, stand on the patient's left side. This allows for comfortable use of your dominant hand to manipulate the suction catheter. To perform oropharyngeal suctioning using a Yankauer device:

1. Perform hand hygiene. Put on PPE, as indicated.

2. Identify the patient.

3. Assemble equipment on the bedside stand or overbed table or other surface within reach.

4. Close the curtains around the bed and close the door to the room, if possible.

5. Perform assessments to determine the need for suctioning. Verify the prescribed suctioning intervention in the patient's health record, if necessary. Anticipate the administration of pharmacologic (analgesic medication) and use of nonpharmacologic interventions for the patient before suctioning. **Assess for pain or the potential to cause pain. Administer pain medication, as prescribed, before suctioning.**

6. Explain to the patient what you are going to do and why, even if the patient does not appear to be alert.

7. Adjust the bed to a comfortable working position. Lower the side rail closest to you. **If the patient is conscious, place them in a semi-Fowler position. If the patient is unconscious, place them in the lateral position, facing you.** Move the overbed table close to your work area and raise it to waist height.

8. Place a towel or waterproof pad across the patient's chest.

9. **Turn the suction to the appropriate pressure. Put on a disposable, clean glove and occlude the end of the connecting tubing to check suction pressure.** Place the connecting tubing in a convenient location.

10. Open the sterile suction package and carefully remove the sterile container, touching only the outside surface. Set it up on the work surface and pour saline into it.

11. Increase the patient's supplemental oxygen level, or apply supplemental oxygen per facility policy or prescribed intervention.

12. Put on a face shield or goggles and a mask (put on an N95 mask or equivalent, based on the patient's health status). Peel open the Yankauer device package and place it on the work surface with the Yankauer device sitting in the wrapper with the top side peeled back. Put on gloves.

13. With your dominant gloved hand, pick up the Yankauer device. Pick up the connecting tubing with your nondominant hand and connect the tubing and Yankauer device.

14. Moisten the catheter by dipping it into the container of sterile saline.

15. Remove the oxygen delivery device, if appropriate. Gently insert the Yankauer device into the oral cavity and move it along the contour of the oral cavity and the palate to suction the posterior oropharynx and the buccal pouches (Morton & Fontaine, 2018). **Do not suction for more than 10 to 15 seconds at a time.**

(continued)

Skill 14-7 ▶ Suctioning the Oropharyngeal and Nasopharyngeal Airways *(continued)*

Skill Variation ▶ Oropharyngeal Suctioning Using a Yankauer Device *(continued)*

16. Replace the oxygen delivery device using your non-dominant hand, and have the patient take several deep breaths.
17. Flush the Yankauer device with saline. Assess effectiveness of the suctioning and repeat, as needed, and according to the patient's tolerance. Encourage the patient to cough and deep breathe between suctioning.
18. When suctioning is complete, rinse the Yankauer device and store it for reuse as directed by facility policy. The outer wrapper may be used to store the Yankauer device between use. Replace the Yankauer device every 24 hours. Dispose of the waterproof pad and saline container.

19. Remove gloves. Remove the face shield or goggles and mask. Perform hand hygiene.

20. Turn off the suction. Remove the supplemental oxygen placed for suctioning, if appropriate. Assist the patient to a comfortable position.
21. Offer oral hygiene after suctioning.
22. Reassess the patient's respiratory status, including respiratory rate, effort, oxygen saturation, and lung sounds.

23. Remove additional PPE, if used. Perform hand hygiene.

24. Document the time of suctioning, your assessments before and after intervention, the reason for suctioning, the route used, the characteristics and amount of secretions, and the patient's response to the intervention.

Skill Variation ▶ Performing Nasotracheal Suctioning

Nasotracheal suctioning is indicated to maintain a patent airway and remove saliva, pulmonary secretions, blood, vomitus, and foreign material from the trachea. Tracheal suctioning can lead to hypoxemia, cardiac dysrhythmias, trauma, atelectasis, infection, bleeding, and pain. The frequency of suctioning varies with the amount of secretions present but should be done often enough to keep ventilation effective and as effortless as possible. Suctioning should be performed only when clinically indicated based on assessment and not routinely (Burns & Delgado, 2019; Hess et al., 2021; Morton & Fontaine, 2018). Anticipate the administration of pharmacologic (analgesic medication) and use of nonpharmacologic interventions for the patient before suctioning. A suction catheter is used for nasotracheal suctioning.

It is imperative to be diligent in maintaining aseptic technique and following facility guidelines and procedures to prevent potential hazards. In the home setting and other community-based settings, clean technique is used because the patient is not exposed to disease-causing organisms that may be found in health care settings, such as hospitals.

A suction catheter is used for nasopharyngeal and nasotracheal suctioning. In patients who require frequent nasotracheal suctioning, a nasopharyngeal airway may be used to prevent patient discomfort and minimize trauma from repeated introduction of the suction catheter through the nares (Morton & Fontaine, 2018). The Skill Variation at the end of Skill 14-8 outlines insertion of a nasopharyngeal airway.

When performing suctioning, position yourself on the appropriate side of the patient. If you are right-handed, stand on the patient's right side; if you are left-handed, stand on the patient's left side. This allows for comfortable use of your dominant hand to manipulate the suction catheter. To perform nasotracheal suctioning:

1. Perform hand hygiene. Put on PPE, as indicated.

2. Identify the patient.

3. Assemble equipment on the bedside stand or overbed table or other surface within reach.
4. Close the curtains around the bed and close the door to the room, if possible.
5. Perform assessments to determine the need for suctioning. Verify the prescribed suctioning intervention in the patient's health record, if necessary. Anticipate the administration of pharmacologic (analgesic medication) and use of nonpharmacologic interventions for the patient before suctioning. **Assess for pain or the potential to cause pain. Administer pain medication, as prescribed, before suctioning.**

6. Explain to the patient what you are going to do and why, even if the patient does not appear to be alert.

7. Adjust the bed to a comfortable working position. Lower the side rail closest to you. **If the patient is conscious, place them in a semi-Fowler position. If the patient is unconscious, place them in the lateral position, facing you.** Move the overbed table close to your work area and raise it to waist height.

8. Place a towel or waterproof pad across the patient's chest.

9. **Turn the suction to the appropriate pressure. Put on a disposable, clean glove and occlude the end of the connecting tubing to check suction pressure.** Place the connecting tubing in a convenient location.

10. Open the sterile suction package using aseptic technique. The open wrapper becomes a sterile field to hold other supplies. Carefully remove the sterile container, touching only the outside surface. Set it up on the work surface and pour sterile saline into it.

11. Place a small amount of water-soluble lubricant on the sterile field, taking care to avoid touching the sterile field with the lubricant package.

12. Increase the patient's supplemental oxygen level, or apply supplemental oxygen per facility policy or prescribed intervention.

13. Put on a face shield or goggles and a mask (put on an N95 mask or equivalent, based on the patient's health status). Put on sterile gloves. **Your dominant hand will manipulate the catheter and must remain sterile.** The nondominant hand is considered clean rather than sterile and will control the suction valve.

14. With your dominant gloved hand, pick up the sterile catheter. Pick up the connecting tubing with your nondominant hand and connect the tubing and suction catheter.

15. Moisten the catheter by dipping it into the container of sterile saline. Occlude the Y-tube to check suction.

16. Encourage the patient to take several deep breaths.

17. Apply lubricant to the first 2 to 3 inches of the catheter, using the lubricant that was placed on the sterile field.

18. Remove the oxygen delivery device, if appropriate. Do not apply suction as the catheter is inserted. Hold the catheter in your thumb and forefinger. Gently insert the catheter through the naris and along the floor of the nostril toward the trachea. Roll the catheter between your fingers to help advance it. Advance the catheter approximately 8 to 9 inches to reach the trachea. Resistance should not be met. If resistance is met, the carina or tracheal mucosa has been hit. Withdraw the catheter at least 1 to 2 inches before applying suction.

19. Apply suction by intermittently occluding the Y-port on the catheter with the thumb of your nondominant hand and gently rotating the catheter as it is being withdrawn. **Do not suction for more than 10 to 15 seconds at a time** (AARC, 2010; Hess et al., 2021).

20. Replace the oxygen delivery device using your nondominant hand, and have the patient take several deep breaths.

21. Flush the catheter with saline. Assess effectiveness of the suctioning and repeat, as needed, and according to the patient's tolerance. Wrap the suction catheter around your dominant hand between attempts.

22. **Allow at least a 30-second to 1-minute interval if additional suctioning is needed. No more than three suction passes should be made per suctioning episode.** Alternate the naris, unless contraindicated, if repeated suctioning is required. Do not force the catheter through the naris. Encourage the patient to cough and deep breathe between suctioning. Suction the oropharynx after suctioning the trachea.

23. When suctioning is completed, remove the glove from your dominant hand over the coiled catheter, pulling it off inside out. Remove the glove from your nondominant hand and dispose of gloves, catheter, and the container with the solution in the appropriate receptacle. Remove the face shield or goggles and mask. Perform hand hygiene.

24. Turn off the suction. Remove the supplemental oxygen placed for suctioning, if appropriate. Assist the patient to a comfortable position.

25. Offer oral hygiene after suctioning.

26. Reassess the patient's respiratory status, including respiratory rate, effort, oxygen saturation, and lung sounds.

27. Remove additional PPE, if used. Perform hand hygiene.

28. Document the time of suctioning, your assessments before and after intervention, the reason for suctioning, the route used, the characteristics and amount of secretions, and the patient's response to the intervention.

Skill 14-8

Inserting an Oropharyngeal Airway
Skill Variation: *Inserting a Nasopharyngeal Airway*

An oropharyngeal airway is a semicircular tube of plastic inserted into the back of the pharynx through the mouth in an unconscious patient who is breathing spontaneously (Hinkle et al., 2022). The oropharyngeal airway can help protect the airway of an unconscious patient by preventing the tongue from falling back against the posterior pharynx and blocking it. Once the patient regains consciousness, the oropharyngeal airway is removed. Tape is not used to hold the airway in place because the patient should be able to expel the airway once they become alert. The nurse can insert this device at the bedside with little to no trauma to the unconscious patient. Oropharyngeal airways may also be used to aid in ventilation during a code situation and to facilitate suctioning an unconscious or semiconscious patient. Alternatively, airway support may be provided with a nasopharyngeal airway (refer to the accompanying Skill Variation).

DELEGATION CONSIDERATIONS

The insertion of an oropharyngeal airway is not delegated to assistive personnel (AP). Depending on the state's nurse practice act and the organization's policies and procedures, the insertion of an oropharyngeal airway may be delegated to licensed practical/vocational nurses (LPN/LVNs). The decision to delegate must be based on careful analysis of the patient's needs and circumstances as well as the qualifications of the person to whom the task is being delegated. Refer to the Delegation Guidelines in Appendix A.

EQUIPMENT

- Oropharyngeal airway of appropriate size
- Disposable gloves
- Suction equipment
- Goggles and mask or face shield (optional)
- Flashlight (optional)
- Additional PPE, as indicated

ASSESSMENT

Assess the patient's level of consciousness and ability to protect the airway. Assess amount and consistency of oral secretions. Auscultate lung sounds. If the tongue is occluding the airway, lung sounds may be diminished. Assess for loose teeth or recent oral surgery, which may contraindicate the use of an oropharyngeal airway.

ACTUAL OR POTENTIAL HEALTH PROBLEMS AND NEEDS

Many actual or potential health problems or issues may require the use of this skill as part of related interventions. An appropriate health problem or issue may include:
- Aspiration risk
- Ineffective airway clearance
- Injury risk

OUTCOME IDENTIFICATION AND PLANNING

The expected outcome to achieve is that the patient will maintain a patent airway and exhibit oxygen saturation within acceptable parameters. Another outcome that may be appropriate is that the patient remains free from aspiration and injury.

IMPLEMENTATION

ACTION	RATIONALE
1. Gather equipment.	Assembling equipment provides for an organized approach to the task.
2. Perform hand hygiene and put on PPE, if indicated.	Hand hygiene and PPE prevent the spread of microorganisms. PPE is required based on transmission precautions.
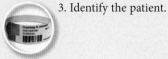 3. Identify the patient.	Identifying the patient ensures the right patient receives the intervention and helps prevent errors.

ACTION

4. Assemble equipment on the overbed table or other surface within reach.

5. Close the curtains around the bed and close the door to the room, if possible.

6. Explain to the patient what you are going to do and why, even if the patient does not appear to be alert.

7. Put on disposable gloves; put on goggles and a mask or face shield, as indicated.

8. Measure the oropharyngeal airway for the correct size (Figure 1). Measure the oropharyngeal airway by holding the airway on the side of the patient's face. The airway should reach from the opening of the mouth to the back angle of the jaw, and the tip of the airway should reach no farther than the pinna of the ear (Hess et al., 2021).

9. Adjust the bed to a comfortable working level (VHACEOSH, 2016). **Check the patient's mouth for any loose teeth, dentures, or other foreign material. Remove dentures or material, if present.**

10. Position the patient in the semi-Fowler position.

11. Suction the patient, if necessary.

12. Open the patient's mouth by using your thumb and index finger to gently pry the teeth apart. **Insert the airway with the curved tip pointing up toward the roof of the mouth (Figure 2).**

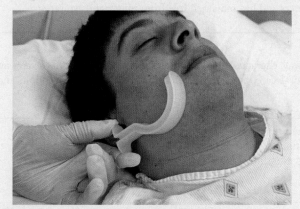

FIGURE 1. Measuring for oropharyngeal airway.

13. Slide the airway across the tongue to the back of the mouth. Rotate the airway 180 degrees as it passes the uvula (Figure 3). The tip should point down, and the curvature should follow the contour of the roof of the mouth. Use a flashlight to confirm the position of the airway with the curve fitting over the tongue.

14. Ensure accurate placement and adequate ventilation by auscultating breath sounds (Figure 4).

RATIONALE

Arranging items nearby is convenient, saves time, and avoids unnecessary stretching and twisting of muscles on the part of the nurse.

This ensures the patient's privacy.

Explanation alleviates fears. Even if a patient appears unconscious, the nurse should explain what is happening.

Gloves and other PPE prevent contact with contaminants and body fluids.

The correct size ensures correct insertion and fit, allowing for conformation of the airway to the curvature of the palate.

Having the bed at the proper height prevents back and muscle strain. Checking for these materials prevents aspiration or swallowing of objects. During insertion, the airway may push any foreign objects in the mouth to the back of the throat.

This position facilitates airway insertion and helps prevent the tongue from moving back against the posterior pharynx.

This removes excess secretions and helps maintain a patent airway.

This is done to advance the tip of the airway past the tongue, toward the back of the throat.

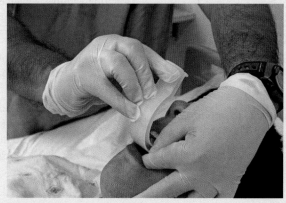

FIGURE 2. Inserting airway with curved tip pointing toward the roof of the mouth.

This is done to shift the tongue anteriorly, thereby allowing the patient to breathe through and around the airway.

If the airway is placed correctly, lung sounds should be audible and equal in all lobes.

(continued on page 894)

Skill 14-8 ▶ Inserting an Oropharyngeal Airway *(continued)*

ACTION

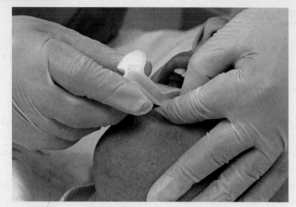

FIGURE 3. Rotating the airway so the tip points down.

15. Position the patient on their side when the airway is in place.

 16. Remove gloves and additional PPE, if used. Perform hand hygiene.

17. Remove the airway for a brief period every 4 hours, or according to facility policy. Suction the oropharynx prior to removal of the airway. Assess the mouth; provide mouth care and clean the airway according to facility policy before reinserting it.

RATIONALE

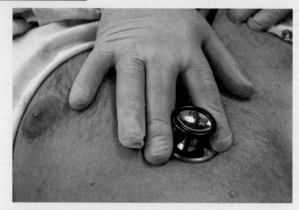

FIGURE 4. Auscultating breath sounds.

This position helps keep the tongue out of the posterior pharynx area and helps to prevent aspiration if the unconscious patient should vomit.

Proper removal of PPE reduces the risk for infection transmission and contamination of other items. Hand hygiene prevents the spread of microorganisms.

Tissue irritation and ulceration can result from prolonged use of an airway. Mouth care provides moisture to mucous membranes and helps maintain tissue integrity.

EVALUATION

The expected outcomes have been met when the patient has exhibited a patent airway with oxygen saturation within acceptable parameters and has remained free from injury and aspiration.

DOCUMENTATION

Guidelines

Document the suctioning of the airway, characteristics of any secretions, placement of the airway, airway size, removal/cleaning and oral care, assessment before and after the intervention, and oxygen saturation level.

Sample Documentation

9/22/25 1210 Patient noted to have gurgling with respirations, tongue back in posterior pharynx. Difficult to suction oropharynx. Size 4 oropharyngeal airway inserted. Patient placed on left side. Lung sounds clear and equal in all lobes. Pulse oximeter 98% on room air.

—C. Bausler, RN

DEVELOPING CLINICAL REASONING AND CLINICAL JUDGMENT

UNEXPECTED SITUATIONS AND ASSOCIATED INTERVENTIONS

- *Patient awakens:* Remove the oral airway once the patient is awake because it may be uncomfortable and cause vomiting. Conscious patients can usually protect their airway.
- *Patient's tongue is sliding back into the posterior pharynx, causing respiratory difficulties:* Put on disposable gloves and remove the airway. Make sure the airway is the appropriate size for the patient.
- *Patient vomits as oropharyngeal airway is inserted:* Quickly position the patient onto their side to prevent aspiration. Remove the oral airway. Suction the mouth and oropharynx as indicated.

SPECIAL
CONSIDERATIONS
General Considerations

- Wearing gloves, remove the airway briefly every 4 hours to provide oral hygiene. Assess the mouth and tongue for tissue irritation, tooth damage, bleeding, and ulceration. Ensure that the lips and tongue are not between the teeth and the airway to prevent injury.
- When reinserting the oropharyngeal airway, attempt to insert it on the other side of the patient's mouth. This helps to prevent irritation to the tongue and mouth.
- Suction secretions, as needed, by manipulating around and through the oropharyngeal airway.

Skill Variation ▶ Inserting a Nasopharyngeal Airway

Nasopharyngeal airways (nasal trumpets) are curved, uncuffed, soft, plastic tubes inserted into the back of the pharynx through the nose in patients who are breathing spontaneously. The nasal trumpet provides a route from the nares to the pharynx to help maintain a patent airway. These airways may be indicated if the patient's teeth are clenched, the patient's tongue is enlarged, or the patient needs frequent nasopharyngeal suctioning. This airway may be left in place, without much discomfort, in the patient who is alert and conscious.

The appropriate-size range for a nasal trumpet for adolescents to adults is 24 to 36 Fr. Additional assessments include assessing for the presence of nasal conditions, such as a deviated septum or recent nasal or oral surgery; traumatic brain injury; central facial fractures; basilar skull or cribriform fractures; and increased risk for bleeding, such as from anticoagulant therapy, which would contraindicate the use of a nasopharyngeal airway.

1. Perform hand hygiene and put on PPE, if indicated.

2. Identify the patient.

3. Assemble equipment on the overbed table or other surface within reach.
4. Close the curtains around the bed and close the door to the room, if possible.
5. Explain to the patient what you are going to do and why, even if the patient does not appear to be alert.
6. Put on disposable gloves. If the patient is coughing or has copious secretions, also wear a mask and goggles.
7. Measure the nasopharyngeal airway for the correct size (Figure A). Measure the nasopharyngeal airway length by holding the airway on the side of the patient's face. The airway should reach from the tip of the nose to the earlobe. The airway with the largest outer diameter that fits the patient's nostril should be used (Morton & Fontaine, 2018).

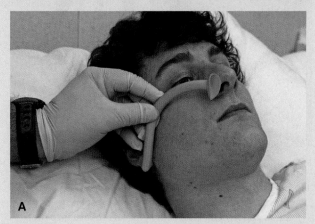

FIGURE A. Measuring nasopharyngeal airway.

8. Adjust the bed to a comfortable working level (VHACEOSH, 2016). **If the patient is awake and alert, position them in semi-Fowler position. If the patient is not conscious or alert, position them in a side-lying position.**
9. Suction the patient, if necessary.
10. Lubricate the nasopharyngeal airway generously with the water-soluble lubricant, covering the airway from the tip to the guard rim (Figure B).

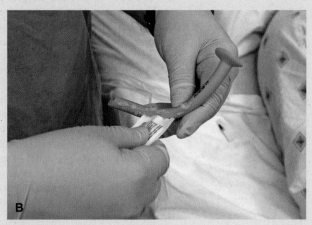

FIGURE B. Lubricating nasopharyngeal airway.

(continued)

Skill 14-8 ▶ Inserting an Oropharyngeal Airway *(continued)*

Skill Variation ▶ Inserting a Nasopharyngeal Airway *(continued)*

11. Gently insert the airway into the naris (Figure C), the narrow end first, pointing it down and toward the back of the throat, until the rim is touching the naris (Figure D). If **resistance is met, stop and try the other naris.**

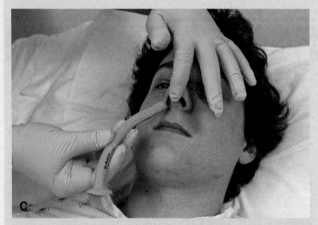

FIGURE C. Inserting nasopharyngeal airway.

12. Check placement by closing the patient's mouth and placing your fingers in front of the tube opening to check for air movement. Assess the pharynx to visualize the tip of the airway behind the uvula. Assess the nose for blanching or skin stretching.

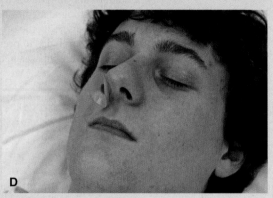

FIGURE D. Nasopharyngeal airway inserted until the rim is touching the naris.

13. Remove gloves and perform hand hygiene. Place the bed in the lowest position. Remove additional PPE, if used. Perform hand hygiene.

14. Remove the airway, clean it in warm soapy water, and place in the other naris at least every 8 hours, or according to facility policy. Assess for evidence of alterations in skin integrity. If the patient coughs or gags on insertion, the nasal trumpet may be too long. Assess the pharynx. You should be able to visualize the tip of the airway behind the uvula.

Skill 14-9 ▶ Suctioning an Endotracheal Tube: Open System

The purpose of suctioning is to maintain a patent airway and remove pulmonary secretions, blood, vomitus, or foreign material from the airway. When suctioning via an endotracheal tube, the goal is to remove secretions that are not accessible to **cilia** bypassed by the tube itself. Tracheal suctioning can lead to hypoxemia, cardiac dysrhythmias, airway trauma, atelectasis, hyperinflation, infection, bleeding, and pain. Therefore, it is imperative to be diligent in maintaining aseptic technique and in following best practice and facility guidelines and procedures to prevent potential hazards. Tracheal suctioning should be performed only when clinically indicated based on assessment and not routinely (AARC, 2010; Burns & Delgado, 2019; Hess et al., 2021; Morton & Fontaine, 2018). Indications for the need for suctioning include audible and/or visible secretions, reduced oxygen saturation, presence of coarse crackles over the trachea, deterioration of arterial blood gas values, reduced breath sounds, the patient's inability to generate an effective spontaneous cough, acute respiratory distress, and suspected aspiration of secretions (AARC, 2010; Patton, 2019).

Because suctioning removes secretions not accessible to bypassed cilia, the recommendation is to insert the catheter only as far as the end of the endotracheal tube. Catheter contact and suction can cause tracheal mucosal damage, loss of cilia, edema, and fibrosis and increase the risk of infection and bleeding. Insertion of the suction catheter to a predetermined distance, no more than the tip of the artificial airway to no more than 1 cm past the length of the endotracheal tube (adults) and 0.5 cm (pediatric patients) (Boroughs & Dougherty, 2015; Hess et al., 2021; Kendrick, 2020), avoids contact with the trachea and carina, reducing the effects of tracheal mucosal damage (Boroughs & Dougherty, 2015; Hahn, 2010; Ireton, 2007; Pasrija & Hall, 2020; Pate & Zapata, 2002). Box 14-2 outlines several methods for determining the appropriate suction catheter depth. The suction catheter should be small enough not to occlude the airway being suctioned but large enough to remove secretions; use a suction catheter that occludes less than 50% of the lumen of the endotracheal tube (AARC, 2010; Pasrija & Hall, 2020).

Tracheal suctioning is an uncomfortable procedure at a minimum, and it can be a very painful and/or distressing experience. Individualized pain management must be performed in response to the patient's needs (Arroyo-Novoa et al., 2008; Chaseling et al., 2014; Wrona et al., 2021; Düzkaya & Kuğuoğlu, 2015). Anticipate the administration of pharmacologic (analgesic medication) and use of nonpharmacologic interventions for the patient before suctioning. As mentioned previously, perform suctioning only when clinically necessary because of the many potential risks, including hypoxia, infection, tracheal tissue damage, dysrhythmias, and atelectasis.

Open-system suctioning and closed-system suctioning are equally effected at secretion clearance (Hess et al., 2021). The open suctioning system requires disconnection of the endotracheal or tracheostomy tube from the ventilator or oxygen therapy source and insertion of a suction catheter each time the patient requires suctioning (Burns & Delgado, 2019), but it is associated with gas exchange deterioration and hypoxia (Burns & Delgado, 2019), potential contamination (Hess et al., 2021), and bioaerosol exposure risk for caregivers (Imbriaco & Monesi, 2021). In closed-system suction, a sterile multiple-use catheter enclosed in a plastic sheath is connected to the ventilation circuit and allows periodic insertion of the suction catheter without disconnection of the endotracheal or tracheostomy tube from the ventilator or oxygen therapy source (Burns & Delgado, 2019; Hess et al., 2021; Pasrija & Hall, 2020). Closed-system suctioning prevents gas exchange deterioration, atelectasis, and hypoxia; is cost-effective because only one catheter is used daily; and reduces bioaerosol exposure risk for caregivers and contamination of the surrounding environment (Hess et al., 2021; Imbriaco & Monesi, 2021; Yazdannik et al., 2019). Closed-system suctioning is recommended for use with patients who are mechanically ventilated; refer to facility policies for specifics of use (AARC, 2010; Morton & Fontaine, 2018; Pasrija & Hall, 2020; Raimundo et al., 2021). Refer to Skill 14-10 for guidelines related to closed-system suctioning.

Box 14-2 | Methods to Determine Suction Catheter Depth

Open Suction System

Method 1 (Endotracheal Tubes)
- Using a suction catheter with centimeter increments on it, insert the suction catheter into the endotracheal tube until the centimeter markings on both the endotracheal tube and catheter align.
- Insert the suction catheter no further than an additional 1 cm.

Method 2 (Endotracheal Tubes)
- Combine the length of the endotracheal tube and any adapter being used, and add an additional 1 cm.
- Document the determined length at the bedside or on the plan of care, according to facility policy.

Method 3 (Endotracheal and Tracheostomy Tubes)
- Using a spare endotracheal or tracheostomy tube of the same size as being used for the patient, insert the suction catheter to the end of the tube.

- Note the length of catheter used to reach the end of the tube.
- Document the determined length at the bedside or on the plan of care. Alternatively, mark the distance on the suction catheter with permanent ink or tape and place the catheter at the bedside for reference. Refer to facility policy.

Closed Suction System (Endotracheal and Tracheostomy Tubes)
- Combine the length of the endotracheal or **tracheostomy tube** and any adapter being used, and add an additional 1 cm.
- Advance the catheter until the appropriate length can be seen through the catheter sheath or window.
- Document the depth of the catheter at the bedside or on the plan of care.

Source: Adapted from Hahn, M. (2010). 10 considerations for endotracheal suctioning. *The Journal for Respiratory Care Practitioners, 23*(7), 32–33; Republished with permission of American Association of Critical Care Nurses from Pate, M., & Zapata, T. (2002). Ask the experts: How deeply should I go when I suction an endotracheal or tracheostomy tube? *Critical Care Nurse, 22*(2), 130–131, permission conveyed through Copyright Clearance Center, Inc.

(continued on page 898)

Skill 14-9 ▶ Suctioning an Endotracheal Tube: Open System *(continued)*

DELEGATION CONSIDERATIONS

Suctioning an endotracheal tube is not delegated to assistive personnel (AP). Depending on the state's nurse practice act and the organization's policies and procedures, suctioning of an endotracheal tube in a stable situation, such as long-term care and other community-based care settings, may be delegated to licensed practical/vocational nurses (LPN/LVNs). The decision to delegate must be based on careful analysis of the patient's needs and circumstances as well as the qualifications of the person to whom the task is being delegated. Refer to the Delegation Guidelines in Appendix A.

EQUIPMENT

- Portable or wall suction unit with tubing
- A commercially prepared suction kit with an appropriate-size catheter (see General Considerations) or
  - Sterile suction catheter with Y-port in the appropriate size
- Sterile, disposable container
- Sterile gloves
- Towel or waterproof pad
- Goggles and mask or face shield; N95 mask or equivalent, based on patient's health status
- Additional PPE, as indicated
- Disposable, clean gloves
- Resuscitation bag connected to 100% oxygen
- Assistant (optional)

ASSESSMENT

Assess for indications for the need for suctioning: audible and/or visible secretions, reduced oxygen saturation, presence of coarse crackles over the trachea, deterioration of arterial blood gas values, reduced breath sounds, the patient's inability to generate an effective spontaneous cough, acute respiratory distress, or suspected aspiration of secretions (AARC, 2010; Patton, 2019; Sole et al., 2015). Assess lung sounds. Wheezes, coarse crackles, gurgling or diminished breath sounds may indicate the need for suctioning. Assess for the presence of visualized secretions in the artificial airway, audible secretions, and ineffective coughing (Morton & Fontaine, 2018; Sole et al., 2015). Assess the oxygen saturation level. Deterioration in oxygen desaturation may be an indication of the need for suctioning (AARC, 2010). Assess respiratory status, including respiratory rate and depth. Patients may become tachypneic when they need to be suctioned. Assess the patient for signs of respiratory distress, such as nasal flaring, retractions, or grunting. Assess for pain and the potential to cause pain during the intervention (Arroyo-Novoa et al., 2008; Chaseling et al., 2014; Wrona et al., 2021; Düzkaya & Kuğuoğlu, 2015). Anticipate the administration of pharmacologic (analgesic medication) and use of nonpharmacologic interventions for the patient before suctioning (Arroyo-Novoa et al., 2008; Düzkaya & Kuğuoğlu, 2015). Assess the appropriate suction catheter depth. Refer to Box 14-2. Assess the characteristics and amount of secretions while suctioning.

ACTUAL OR POTENTIAL HEALTH PROBLEMS AND NEEDS

Many actual or potential health problems or issues may require the use of this skill as part of related interventions. An appropriate health problem or issue may include:
- Ineffective airway clearance
- Altered breathing pattern
- Impaired gas exchange

OUTCOME IDENTIFICATION AND PLANNING

The expected outcome to achieve is that the patient will exhibit a clear, patent airway. Other outcomes that may be appropriate include that the patient will exhibit an oxygen saturation level within acceptable parameters, will demonstrate a respiratory rate and depth within acceptable parameters, and will remain free from any signs of respiratory distress and adverse effect.

IMPLEMENTATION

ACTION	RATIONALE
1. Gather equipment.	Assembling equipment provides for an organized approach to the task.
2. Perform hand hygiene and put on PPE, if indicated.	Hand hygiene and PPE prevent the spread of microorganisms. PPE is required based on transmission precautions.

ACTION

3. Identify the patient.

4. Assemble equipment on the overbed table or other surface within reach.

5. Close the curtains around the bed and close the door to the room, if possible.

6. Perform assessments to determine the need for suctioning. Verify the prescribed suctioning intervention in the patient's health record, if necessary. Anticipate the administration of pharmacologic (analgesic medication) and use of nonpharmacologic interventions for the patient before suctioning. **Assess for pain or the potential to cause pain. Administer pain medication, as prescribed, before suctioning**.

7. Explain to the patient what you are going to do and why, even if the patient does not appear to be alert. Reassure the patient that you will interrupt the procedure if they indicate respiratory difficulty.

8. Adjust the bed to a comfortable working position (VHACEOSH, 2016). Lower the side rail closest to you. **If the patient is conscious, place them in a semi-Fowler position. If the patient is unconscious, place them in the lateral position, facing you.** Move the overbed table close to your work area and raise it to waist height.

9. Place a towel or waterproof pad across the patient's chest.

10. **Adjust suction to the appropriate pressure** (Hess et al., 2021) (Figure 1):
    - No more than 150 mm Hg for adults and adolescents
    - No more than 125 mm Hg for children
    - No more than 100 mm Hg for infants.

RATIONALE

Identifying the patient ensures the right patient receives the intervention and helps prevent errors.

Arranging items nearby is convenient, saves time, and avoids unnecessary stretching and twisting of muscles on the part of the nurse.

This ensures the patient's privacy.

Suctioning should be performed only when clinically indicated based on assessment and not routinely (AARC, 2010; Burns & Delgado, 2019; Hess et al., 2021; Morton & Fontaine, 2018). At a minimum, suctioning is an uncomfortable procedure, and it can be a very painful and/or distressing experience. Individualized pain management must be performed in response to the patient's needs (Arroyo-Novoa et al., 2008; Chaseling et al., 2014; Wrona et al., 2021; Düzkaya & Kuğuoğlu, 2015).

Explanation alleviates fears. Even if the patient appears unconscious, the nurse should explain what is happening. Any procedure that compromises respiration is frightening for the patient.

Having the bed at the proper height prevents back and muscle strain. A sitting position helps the patient to cough and makes breathing easier. Gravity also facilitates catheter insertion. The lateral position prevents the airway from becoming obstructed and promotes drainage of secretions. The overbed table provides a work surface and maintains sterility of the objects on the work surface.

This protects bed linens and the patient.

Higher pressures can cause excessive trauma, hypoxemia, and atelectasis.

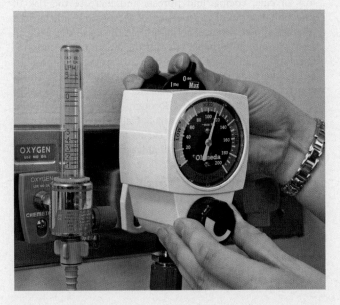

FIGURE 1. Turning suction unit to appropriate pressure.

(*continued on page 900*)

Skill 14-9 ▶ Suctioning an Endotracheal Tube: Open System *(continued)*

ACTION	RATIONALE
11. **Put on a disposable, clean glove and occlude the end of the connecting tubing to check suction pressure.** Place the connecting tubing in a convenient location. Place the resuscitation bag connected to oxygen within convenient reach, if using.	The glove prevents contact with blood and body fluids. Checking pressure ensures the equipment is working properly. Having the resuscitation bag within easy reach allows for an organized approach to the procedure.
12. Open the sterile suction package using aseptic technique. The open wrapper becomes a sterile field to hold other supplies. Carefully remove the sterile container, touching only the outside surface. Set it up on the work surface and pour sterile saline into it.	Sterile normal saline or water is used to lubricate the outside of the catheter, minimizing irritation of mucosa during introduction. It is also used to clear the catheter between suction attempts.
13. Put on a face shield or goggles and a mask. Put on sterile gloves. Your dominant hand will manipulate the catheter and must remain sterile. The nondominant hand is considered clean rather than sterile and will control the suction valve (Y-port) on the catheter.	Handling the sterile catheter using a sterile glove helps prevent introducing organisms into the respiratory tract; the clean glove protects the nurse from microorganisms.
14. With your dominant gloved hand, pick up the sterile catheter. Pick up the connecting tubing with your nondominant hand and connect the tubing and suction catheter.	Sterility of the suction catheter is maintained.
15. Moisten the catheter by dipping it into the container of sterile saline, unless it is a silicone catheter. Occlude the Y-tube to check suction.	Lubricating the inside of the catheter with saline helps move secretions in the catheter. Silicone catheters do not require lubrication. Checking suction ensures the equipment is working properly.
16. Using your nondominant hand, remove the ventilator tubing or oxygen source from the endotracheal tube and attach the manual resuscitation bag. Hyperoxygenate the patient using your nondominant hand and the manual resuscitation bag for a minimum of 30 seconds (Burns & Delgado, 2019). Alternatively, use the sigh mechanism on a mechanical ventilator.	Hyperoxygenation aids in preventing hypoxemia during suctioning.
17. Using your nondominant hand, remove the manual resuscitation bag from the endotracheal tube. Alternatively, open the adapter on the mechanical ventilator tubing.	This exposes the endotracheal tube without contaminating your sterile gloved hand.
18. Using your dominant hand, gently and quickly insert the catheter into the endotracheal tube (Figure 2). **Advance the catheter to the predetermined length. Do not occlude the Y-port when inserting the catheter.**	Catheter contact and suction cause tracheal mucosal damage, loss of cilia, edema, and fibrosis and increase the risk of infection and bleeding. Insertion of the suction catheter to a predetermined distance, no more than the tip of the artificial airway to no more than 1 cm past the length of the endotracheal tube (adults) and 0.5 cm (pediatric patients) (Boroughs & Dougherty, 2015; Hess et al., 2021; Kendrick, 2020) avoids contact with the trachea and carina, reducing the effects of tracheal mucosal damage (Boroughs & Dougherty, 2015; Hahn, 2010; Ireton, 2007; Pasrija & Hall, 2020; Pate & Zapata, 2002). If resistance is met, the carina or tracheal mucosa has been hit. Withdraw the catheter at least 0.5 inch before applying suction. Occluding the Y-port (i.e., suctioning) when inserting the catheter increases the risk for trauma to the airway mucosa and increases the risk of hypoxemia.
19. Apply suction by intermittently occluding the Y-port on the catheter with the thumb of your nondominant hand, and gently rotate the catheter as it is being withdrawn (Figure 3). **Do not suction for more than 10 to 15 seconds at a time** (AARC, 2010; Burns & Delgado, 2019; Hess et al., 2021; Pasrija & Hall, 2020).	Turning the catheter as it is withdrawn minimizes trauma to the mucosa. Suctioning for longer than 15 seconds robs the respiratory tract of oxygen, which may result in hypoxemia (AARC, 2010; Pasrija & Hall, 2020). Suctioning too quickly may be ineffective at clearing all secretions.

ACTION

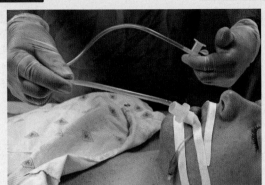

FIGURE 2. Inserting suction catheter into endotracheal tube.

20. Hyperoxygenate the patient using your nondominant hand and a manual resuscitation bag for a minimum of 30 seconds (Burns & Delgado, 2019). Replace the oxygen delivery device, if applicable, using your nondominant hand, and have the patient take several deep breaths. If the patient is mechanically ventilated, close the adapter on the mechanical ventilator tubing, or replace the ventilator tubing and use the sigh mechanism on a mechanical ventilator.

21. Flush the catheter with saline. Assess the effectiveness of suctioning and repeat, as needed, and according to the patient's tolerance. Wrap the suction catheter around your dominant hand between attempts.

22. **Allow at least a 30-second interval if additional suctioning is needed** (Burns & Delgado, 2019). Do not make more than three suction passes per suctioning episode. Suction the oropharynx after suctioning the trachea (refer to Skill 14-7). Do not reinsert it in the endotracheal tube after suctioning the mouth.

23. Perform oral hygiene after tracheal suctioning. Oral hygiene measures are discussed in Chapter 7.

 24. When suctioning is complete, remove the glove from your dominant hand over the coiled catheter, pulling it off inside out. Remove the glove from your nondominant hand, and dispose of gloves, catheter, and the container with the solution in the appropriate receptacle. Perform hand hygiene. Assist the patient to a comfortable position. Raise the bed rail and place the bed in the lowest position.

RATIONALE

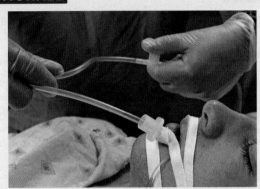

FIGURE 3. Withdrawing suction catheter and intermittently occluding Y-port with thumb to apply suction.

Suctioning removes air from the patient's airway and can cause hypoxemia. Hyperoxygenation can help prevent suction-induced hypoxemia.

Flushing clears the catheter and lubricates it for the next insertion. Reassessment determines the need for additional suctioning. Wrapping the catheter prevents inadvertent contamination of the catheter.

The interval allows for reventilation and reoxygenation of airways. Excessive suction passes contribute to complications. Suctioning the oropharynx clears the mouth of secretions. Routine oral suctioning to aspirate secretions that accumulate above the cuff of the tube is also necessary to reduce the risk of pneumonia and provide patient comfort (AACN, 2018; Hess et al., 2021; Morton & Fontaine, 2018). More microorganisms are usually present in the mouth, so it is suctioned last to prevent transmission of contaminants.

Respiratory secretions that are allowed to accumulate in the mouth are irritating to mucous membranes, pose a risk for aspiration, are unpleasant for the patient, and contribute to the colonization of the oropharyngeal secretions by respiratory pathogens. Diligent oral hygiene care can improve oral health and limit the growth of pathogens in the oropharyngeal secretions, decreasing the incidence of aspiration pneumonia, community-acquired pneumonia, nonventilator health care–associated pneumonia (NV-HAP), and ventilator-associated pneumonia (VAP) (AACN, 2017; Chick & Wynne, 2020; Jenson et al., 2018; Quinn et al., 2020).

This technique of glove removal, disposal of equipment, and hand hygiene reduces transmission of microorganisms. Proper positioning with raised side rails and the proper bed height provides for patient comfort and safety.

(continued on page 902)

Skill 14-9 ▶ Suctioning an Endotracheal Tube: Open System (continued)

ACTION

25. Turn off the suction. Remove the face shield or goggles and mask. Perform hand hygiene.

26. Reassess the patient's respiratory status, including respiratory rate, effort, oxygen saturation, lung sounds, tracheal sounds, and the presence/absence of secretions in artificial airway, and the patient's response to the intervention.

27. Remove additional PPE, if used. Perform hand hygiene.

RATIONALE

Removing the face shield or goggles and mask properly reduces the risk for infection transmission and contamination of other items. Hand hygiene prevents transmission of microorganisms.

These assess effectiveness of suctioning and the presence of complications.

Proper removal of PPE reduces the risk for infection transmission and contamination of other items. Hand hygiene prevents the spread of microorganisms.

EVALUATION

The expected outcomes have been met when the patient has exhibited a clear, patent airway; an oxygen saturation level within acceptable parameters; and a respiratory rate and depth within acceptable parameters; and the patient has remained free from any signs of respiratory distress and adverse effect.

DOCUMENTATION

Guidelines

Document the time of suctioning, assessments before and after interventions, the reason for suctioning, oxygen saturation levels, and the characteristics and amount of secretions.

Sample Documentation

9/1/25 1850 Tan secretions noted in ET tube; coarse crackles noted to auscultation over trachea. Lung sounds coarse in lower lobes. Respirations 24 breaths/min, regular rhythm. Intercostal retractions noted. Endotracheal tube suctioning completed with 12-Fr catheter. Small amount of thin, tan secretions obtained. Specimen for culture collected and sent. After suctioning, no secretions noted in ET tube, auscultation over trachea clear, lung sounds clear, respirations 18 breaths/min, no intercostal retractions noted.
—C. Bausler, RN

DEVELOPING CLINICAL REASONING AND CLINICAL JUDGMENT

UNEXPECTED SITUATIONS AND ASSOCIATED INTERVENTIONS

- *Catheter or sterile glove is contaminated:* Reconnect the patient to the ventilator or oxygen supply. Discard gloves and the suction catheter. Gather supplies and begin the procedure again.
- *When suctioning, your eye becomes contaminated with respiratory secretions:* After attending to the patient, perform hand hygiene and flush your eye with a large amount of sterile water. Contact employee health or your supervisor immediately for further treatment and complete adverse event documentation as per facility policy. Wear goggles or a face shield when suctioning to prevent exposure to body fluids.
- *Patient is extubated during suctioning:* Remain with the patient. Call for help to notify the health care team. Assess the patient's vital signs, ability to breathe without assistance, and oxygen saturation. Be ready to deliver assisted breaths with a bag-valve mask (see Skill 14-16) or administer oxygen. Anticipate the need for reintubation.
- *Oxygen saturation level decreases after suctioning:* Hyperoxygenate the patient. Auscultate lung sounds. If lung sounds are absent over one lobe, notify the health care team. Remain with the patient. The patient may have **pneumothorax** or a misplaced endotracheal tube. Anticipate a prescribed intervention for a stat chest x-ray and possible chest tube placement or reintubation.
- *Patient develops signs of intolerance to suctioning; oxygen saturation level decreases and remains low after hyperoxygenation; patient becomes cyanotic; or patient becomes bradycardic:* Stop

suctioning. Auscultate lung sounds. Consider hyperventilating the patient with a manual resuscitation device. Remain with the patient. Alert staff to notify the health care team of the change in the patient's status.

SPECIAL CONSIDERATIONS

General Considerations

- Determine the size of catheter to use by the size of the endotracheal tube. The suction catheter should be small enough not to occlude the airway being suctioned but large enough to remove secretions; use a suction catheter that occludes less than 50% of the lumen of the endotracheal tube (AARC, 2010; Pasrija & Hall, 2020). Larger catheters can contribute to trauma and hypoxemia.
- The practice of instillation of saline solution directly into the airway during tracheal suctioning is not supported by evidence and is not recommended for inclusion as part of evidence-based practice and suctioning (AARC, 2010; Boroughs & Dougherty, 2015; Burns & Delgado, 2019; Leddy & Wilkinson, 2015; Owen et al., 2016; Wang et al., 2017).
- Keep emergency equipment easily accessible at the bedside. Keep a bag-valve mask, oxygen, and suction equipment at the bedside of a patient with an endotracheal tube at all times.
- Higher values of suction pressure have been suggested by some evidence for practice. The use of suction pressure of 250 mm Hg has been suggested as more effective for open-system suctioning and equally safe in comparison to the use of 80 to 150 mm Hg suction pressure (Maraş et al., 2020). Yazdannik et al. (2019) suggest the use of 200 mm Hg pressure during closed-system suctioning for mechanically ventilated patients to improve the efficacy of secretion removal.

Infant and Child Considerations

- Insertion of the suction catheter to a predetermined distance, no more than the tip of the artificial airway to no more than 0.5 cm past the length of the endotracheal tube avoids contact with the trachea and carina, reducing the effects of tracheal mucosal damage (Boroughs & Dougherty, 2015; Kendrick, 2020).
- The maximal time for application of negative pressure (suction) for neonates, children, and adolescents should be less than 5 to 10 seconds (Boroughs & Dougherty, 2015; Dawson et al., 2012, as cited in Edwards, 2018, p. 51; Hockenberry et al., 2019).

EVIDENCE FOR PRACTICE ▶

ENDOTRACHEAL TUBES AND PATIENT COMMUNICATION

Placement of an endotracheal tube results in the inability to speak, which can be frightening and frustrating for the patient and may contribute to ineffective responses to patient concerns and needs.

Related Evidence

Karlsen, M. M. W., Ølnes, M. A., & Heyn, L. G. (2019). Communication with patients in intensive care units: A scoping review. *Nursing in Critical Care, 24*(3), 115–131. https://doi.org/10.1111/nicc.12377

The purpose of this literature review was to assess knowledge about interaction and communication between health care personnel and conscious and alert mechanically ventilated patients in intensive care units. A search from 1998 to 2017 in five databases was completed for empirical studies or literature reviews of studies related to interactions between health care personnel and patients older than 18 years on mechanical ventilation. Exclusions included case studies or studies with a focus on end-of-life care, weaning from mechanical ventilation and symptom management, or using only health care personnel as participants. There were 82 studies identified with 46 matching the inclusion criteria. Studies were collected by the design used, then described, and the topics of all the studies across the different types of design were compared. The relevant studies were summarized in a standardized data-charting sheet. No data were extracted for statistical meta-analyses or qualitative meta-syntheses. Of the 46 articles, 16 used a qualitative design, 17 used a quantitative design, 6 were mixed-methods studies, and 7 were pilot and feasibility studies. Most of the studies (37 of 46; 80%) were published between 2006 and 2017. The most prominent research topics in the studies were identified as "experiences with communication while on mechanical ventilation" (patients' experiences, experiences of health care personnel, the shared experiences) and "communication exchanges" (descriptions

(continued)

Skill 14-9 ▶ Suctioning an Endotracheal Tube: Open System *(continued)*

of communication exchanges, communication aids). The use of communication aids was identified to positively influence the patient experience; however, there is gap in the research on comparison of communication aids. The authors concluded a variety of communication aids that appear to have some effect on patients should be made available in intensive care units. The authors suggest that health care personnel in intensive care units should be provided educational interventions on the use of communication aids and that a variety of communication aids should be implemented as part of patient care in intensive care setting.

Relevance for Nursing Practice

Effective communication is a cornerstone of professional nursing care. Communication strategies for patients who are unable to communicate verbally are a critical part of the provision of care. Good communication enables nurses to provide appropriate and person-centered nursing care. Nurses have a responsibility to develop and implement communication strategies to meet the needs of all patients in their care.

EVIDENCE FOR PRACTICE ▶

SUCTION PRESSURE FOR ENDOTRACHEAL SUCTIONING
Related Research
Yazdannik, A., Saghaei, M., Haghighat, S., & Eghbali-Babadi, M. (2019). Efficacy of closed endotracheal suctioning in critically ill patients: A clinical trial of comparing two levels of negative suctioning pressure. *Journal of Nursing Practice Today, 6*(2), 60–67.
Refer to details in Skill 14-10, Evidence for Practice.

Skill 14-10 ▶ Suctioning an Endotracheal Tube: Closed System

The purpose of suctioning is to maintain a patent airway and remove pulmonary secretions, blood, vomitus, or foreign material from the airway. When suctioning via an endotracheal tube, the goal is to remove secretions that are not accessible to cilia bypassed by the tube itself. Tracheal suctioning can lead to hypoxemia, cardiac dysrhythmias, airway trauma, atelectasis, hyperinflation, infection, bleeding, and pain. Therefore, it is imperative to be diligent in maintaining aseptic technique and in following best practice and facility guidelines and procedures to prevent potential hazards. Tracheal suctioning should be performed only when clinically indicated based on assessment and not routinely (AARC, 2010; Burns & Delgado, 2019; Hess et al., 2021; Morton & Fontaine, 2018). Indications for the need for suctioning include audible and/or visible secretions, reduced oxygen saturation, presence of coarse crackles over the trachea, deterioration of arterial blood gas values, reduced breath sounds, the patient's inability to generate an effective spontaneous cough, acute respiratory distress, and suspected aspiration of secretions (AARC, 2010; Patton, 2019).

Because suctioning removes secretions not accessible to bypassed cilia, the recommendation is to insert the catheter only as far as the end of the endotracheal tube. Catheter contact and suction can cause tracheal mucosal damage, loss of cilia, edema, and fibrosis and increase the risk of infection and bleeding. Insertion of the suction catheter to a predetermined distance, no more than the tip of the artificial airway to no more than 1 cm past the length of the endotracheal tube (adults) and 0.5 cm (pediatric patients) (Boroughs & Dougherty, 2015; Hess et al., 2021; Kendrick, 2020) avoids contact with the trachea and carina, reducing the effects of tracheal mucosal damage (Boroughs & Dougherty, 2015; Hahn, 2010; Ireton, 2007; Pasrija & Hall, 2020; Pate & Zapata, 2002). Box 14-2 in

Skill 14-9 outlines several methods for determining appropriate suction catheter depth. The suction catheter should be small enough not to occlude the airway being suctioned but large enough to remove secretions; the suction catheter should be small enough not to occlude the airway being suctioned but large enough to remove secretions; use a suction catheter that occludes less than 50% of the lumen of the endotracheal tube (AARC, 2010; Pasrija & Hall, 2020).

Tracheal suctioning is an uncomfortable procedure at a minimum, and it can be a very painful and/or distressing experience. Individualized pain management must be performed in response to the patient's needs (Arroyo-Novoa et al., 2008; Chaseling et al., 2014; Wrona et al., 2021; Düzkaya & Kuğuoğlu, 2015). Anticipate the administration of pharmacologic (analgesic medication) and use of nonpharmacologic interventions for the patient before suctioning. As mentioned previously, perform suctioning only when clinically necessary because of the many potential risks, including hypoxia, infection, tracheal tissue damage, dysrhythmias, and atelectasis.

Open-system suctioning and closed-system suctioning are equally effected at secretion clearance (Hess et al., 2021). In closed-system suction, a sterile multiple-use catheter enclosed in a plastic sheath is connected to the ventilation circuit and allows periodic insertion of the suction catheter without disconnection of the endotracheal or tracheostomy tube from the ventilator or oxygen therapy source (Figure 1) (Burns & Delgado, 2019; Hess et al., 2021; Pasrija & Hall, 2020). Closed-system suction prevents gas exchange deterioration, atelectasis, and hypoxia; is cost-effective because only one catheter is used daily; and reduces bioaerosol exposure risk for caregivers and contamination of the surrounding environment (Hess et al., 2021; Imbriaco & Monesi, 2021; Yazdannik et al., 2019). Closed-system suctioning is recommended for use with patients who are mechanically ventilated; refer to facility policies for specifics of use (AARC, 2010; Morton & Fontaine, 2018; Pasrija & Hall, 2020; Raimundo et al., 2021). Refer to Skill 14-10 for guidelines related to closed-system suctioning. One drawback of closed suctioning may be the hindrance of the sheath when rotating the suction catheter upon removal.

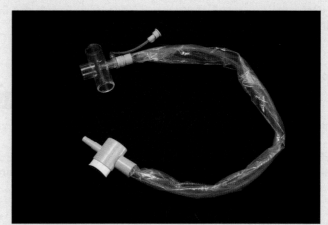

FIGURE 1. Closed suction device.

DELEGATION CONSIDERATIONS

Suctioning an endotracheal tube is not delegated to assistive personnel (AP). Depending on the state's nurse practice act and the organization's policies and procedures, suctioning of an endotracheal tube in a stable situation, such as long-term care and other community-based care settings, may be delegated to licensed practical/vocational nurses (LPN/LVNs). The decision to delegate must be based on careful analysis of the patient's needs and circumstances as well as the qualifications of the person to whom the task is being delegated. Refer to the Delegation Guidelines in Appendix A.

EQUIPMENT

- Portable or wall suction unit with tubing
- Closed suction device of appropriate size for patient
- 3- or 5-mL normal saline solution in dosette or syringe
- Sterile gloves
- Additional PPE, as indicated

(*continued on page 906*)

Skill 14-10 ▶ Suctioning an Endotracheal Tube: Closed System *(continued)*

ASSESSMENT

Assess for indications for the need for suctioning: audible and/or visible secretions, reduced oxygen saturation, presence of coarse crackles over the trachea, deterioration of arterial blood gas values, reduced breath sounds, the patient's inability to generate an effective spontaneous cough, acute respiratory distress, and suspected aspiration of secretions (AARC, 2010; Patton, 2019; Sole et al., 2015). Assess lung sounds. Wheezes, coarse crackles, gurgling, or diminished breath sounds may indicate the need for suctioning. Assess for the presence of visualized secretions in the artificial airway, audible secretions, and ineffective coughing (Morton & Fontaine, 2018; Sole et al., 2015). Assess the oxygen saturation level. Deterioration in oxygen desaturation may be an indication of the need for suctioning (AARC, 2010). Assess respiratory status, including respiratory rate and depth. Patients may become tachypneic when they need to be suctioned. Assess the patient for signs of respiratory distress, such as nasal flaring, retractions, or grunting. Assess for pain and the potential to cause pain during the intervention (Arroyo-Novoa et al., 2008; Chaseling et al., 2014; Wrona et al., 2021; Düzkaya & Kuğuoğlu, 2015). Anticipate the administration of pharmacologic (analgesic medication) and use of nonpharmacologic interventions for the patient before suctioning (Arroyo-Novoa et al., 2008; Düzkaya & Kuğuoğlu, 2015). Assess the appropriate suction catheter depth. Refer to Box 14-2 in Skill 14-9. Assess the characteristics and amount of secretions while suctioning.

ACTUAL OR POTENTIAL HEALTH PROBLEMS AND NEEDS

Many actual or potential health problems or issues may require the use of this skill as part of related interventions. An appropriate health problem or issue may include:
- Ineffective airway clearance
- Altered breathing pattern
- Impaired gas exchange

OUTCOME IDENTIFICATION AND PLANNING

The expected outcome to achieve is that the patient will exhibit a clear, patent airway. Other outcomes that may be appropriate include that the patient will exhibit an oxygen saturation level within acceptable parameters, will demonstrate a respiratory rate and depth within acceptable parameters, and will remain free from any signs of respiratory distress and adverse effect.

IMPLEMENTATION

ACTION	RATIONALE
1. Gather equipment.	Assembling equipment provides for an organized approach to the task.
2. Perform hand hygiene and put on PPE, if indicated.	Hand hygiene and PPE prevent the spread of microorganisms. PPE is required based on transmission precautions.
3. Identify the patient.	Identifying the patient ensures the right patient receives the intervention and helps prevent errors.
4. Assemble equipment on the overbed table or other surface within reach.	Arranging items nearby is convenient, saves time, and avoids unnecessary stretching and twisting of muscles on the part of the nurse.
5. Close the curtains around the bed and close the door to the room, if possible.	This ensures the patient's privacy.
6. Perform assessments to determine the need for suctioning. Verify the prescribed suctioning intervention in the patient's health record, if necessary. Anticipate the administration of pharmacologic (analgesic medication) and use of nonpharmacologic interventions for the patient before suctioning. **Assess for pain or the potential to cause pain. Administer pain medication, as prescribed, before suctioning.**	Suctioning should be performed only when clinically indicated based on assessment and not routinely (AARC, 2010; Burns & Delgado, 2019; Hess et al., 2021; Morton & Fontaine, 2018). At a minimum, suctioning is an uncomfortable procedure, and it can be a very painful and/or distressing experience. Individualized pain management must be performed in response to the patient's needs (Arroyo-Novoa et al., 2008; Chaseling et al., 2014; Wrona et al., 2021; Düzkaya & Kuğuoğlu, 2015).

ACTION

7. Explain to the patient what you are going to do and why, even if the patient does not appear to be alert. Reassure the patient that you will interrupt the procedure if they indicate respiratory difficulty.

8. Adjust the bed to a comfortable working position (VHACEOSH, 2016). Lower the side rail closest to you. **If the patient is conscious, place them in a semi-Fowler position. If the patient is unconscious, place them in an appropriate position based on assessment of individual circumstances.** Move the overbed table close to your work area and raise it to waist height.

9. **Adjust suction to the appropriate pressure** (Hess et al., 2021) (Figure 2):
   - No more than 150 mm Hg for adults and adolescents
   - No more than 125 mm Hg for children
   - No more than 100 mm Hg for infants.

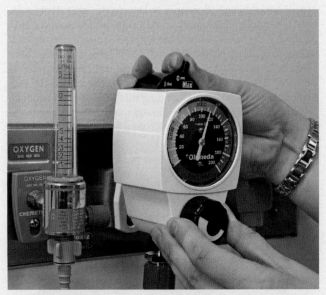

10. **Put on a disposable, clean glove and occlude the end of the connecting tubing to check suction pressure.** Place the connecting tubing in a convenient location.

11. Open the package of the closed suction device using aseptic technique. Make sure that the device remains sterile.

12. Put on sterile gloves.

13. If a closed suctioning device is not in place, continue with Step 14. If this device is already in place, continue with Step 17.

14. Using your nondominant hand, disconnect the ventilator from the endotracheal tube. Place the ventilator tubing in a convenient location so that the inside of the tubing remains sterile, or continue to hold the tubing in your nondominant hand.

15. **Using your dominant hand and keeping the device sterile, connect the closed suctioning device so that the suctioning catheter is in line with the endotracheal tube.**

RATIONALE

Explanation alleviates fears. Even if the patient appears unconscious, the nurse should explain what is happening. Any procedure that compromises respiration is frightening for the patient.

Having the bed at the proper height prevents back and muscle strain. A sitting position helps the patient to cough and makes breathing easier. Gravity also facilitates catheter insertion. Positioning of the unconscious patient is based on the circumstances of the individual patient; health status, health problems, presence of drains and/or monitoring devices, etc. The overbed table provides a work surface and maintains sterility of the objects on the work surface.

Higher pressures can cause excessive trauma, hypoxemia, and atelectasis.

FIGURE 2. Turning suction device to appropriate pressure.

The glove prevents contact with blood and body fluids. Checking pressure ensures the equipment is working properly.

The device must remain sterile to prevent a nosocomial infection.

Gloves deter the spread of microorganisms.

This provides access to the endotracheal tube while keeping one hand sterile. The inside of the ventilator tubing should remain sterile to prevent a nosocomial infection.

Keeping the device sterile decreases the risk for a nosocomial infection.

(continued on page 908)

Skill 14-10 ▶ Suctioning an Endotracheal Tube: Closed System *(continued)*

ACTION	RATIONALE
16. **Keeping the inside of the ventilator tubing sterile, attach the ventilator tubing to the port perpendicular to the endotracheal tube.** Attach the suction connecting tubing to the suction catheter.	The inside of the ventilator tubing must remain sterile to prevent a nosocomial infection. By connecting the ventilator tubing to the port, the patient does not need to be disconnected from the ventilator to be suctioned.
17. Pop the top off the sterile normal saline dosette. Open the plug to the port by the suction catheter and insert the saline dosette or syringe.	The saline will help to clean the catheter between suctioning.
18. Hyperoxygenate the patient by using the sigh button on the ventilator before suctioning. Turn the safety cap on the suction button of the catheter so that the button is depressed easily.	Hyperoxygenating before suctioning helps to decrease the effects of oxygen removal during suctioning. The safety button keeps the patient from accidentally depressing the button and decreasing the oxygen saturation.
19. Grasp the suction catheter through the protective sheath, about 6 inches (15 cm) from the endotracheal tube. Gently insert the catheter into the endotracheal tube (Figure 3). Release the catheter while holding on to the protective sheath. Move your hand farther back on the catheter. **Grasp the catheter through the sheath and repeat the movement, advancing the catheter to the predetermined length. Do not occlude the Y-port when inserting the catheter.**	The sheath keeps the suction catheter sterile. Catheter contact and suction cause tracheal mucosal damage, loss of cilia, edema, and fibrosis and increase the risk of infection and bleeding. Insertion of the suction catheter to a predetermined distance, no more than the tip of the artificial airway to no more than 1 cm past the length of the endotracheal tube (adults) and 0.5 cm (pediatric patients) (Boroughs & Dougherty, 2015; Hess et al., 2021; Kendrick, 2020) avoids contact with the trachea and carina, reducing the effects of tracheal mucosal damage (Boroughs & Dougherty, 2015; Hahn, 2010; Ireton, 2007; Pasrija & Hall, 2020; Pate & Zapata, 2002). If resistance is met, the carina or tracheal mucosa has been hit. Withdraw the catheter at least 0.5 inch before applying suction. Occluding the Y-port (i.e., suctioning) when inserting the catheter increases the risk for trauma to the airway mucosa and increases the risk of hypoxemia.
20. Apply intermittent suction by depressing the suction button with the thumb of your nondominant hand (Figure 4). Gently rotate the catheter with the thumb and index finger of your dominant hand as the catheter is being withdrawn. **Do not suction for more than 10 to 15 seconds at a time** (AARC, 2010; Burns & Delgado, 2019; Hess et al., 2021; Pasrija & Hall, 2020). Hyperoxygenate with the sigh button on the ventilator (as prescribed or as identified in facility policy) for a minimum of 30 seconds (Burns & Delgado, 2019).	Turning the catheter while withdrawing it helps clean the surfaces of the respiratory tract and prevents injury to the tracheal mucosa. Suctioning for longer than 15 seconds robs the respiratory tract of oxygen, which may result in hypoxemia (AARC, 2010; Pasrija & Hall, 2020). Suctioning too quickly may be ineffective at clearing all secretions. Hyperoxygenation reoxygenates the lungs and helps prevent suction-induced hypoxemia.

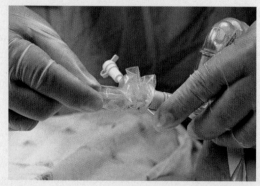

FIGURE 3. Grasping the catheter through the protective sheath and inserting into endotracheal tube.

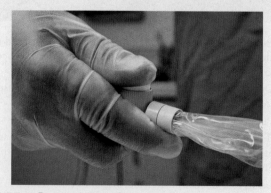

FIGURE 4. Depressing suction button.

ACTION

RATIONALE

21. Once the catheter is withdrawn back into the sheath (Figure 5), depress the suction button while gently squeezing the normal saline dosette until the catheter is clean. **Allow at least a 30-second to 1-minute interval if additional suctioning is needed** (Burns & Delgado, 2019). Do not make more than three suction passes per suctioning episode.

Flushing cleans and clears the catheter and lubricates it for the next insertion. Allowing a time interval and replacing the oxygen delivery setup help compensate for hypoxia induced by the suctioning. Excessive suction passes contribute to complications.

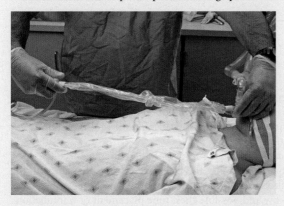

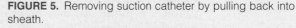
FIGURE 5. Removing suction catheter by pulling back into sheath.

22. When the procedure is completed, **ensure that the catheter is withdrawn into the sheath** and turn the safety button. Remove the normal saline dosette and apply the cap to the port.

By turning the safety button, the suction is blocked at the catheter so the suction cannot remove oxygen from the endotracheal tube.

23. Suction the oropharynx with a separate single-use, disposable catheter (Skill 14-7) and perform oral hygiene (oral hygiene measures are discussed in Chapter 7). Remove gloves. Perform hand hygiene. Turn off suction.

Suctioning the oropharynx clears the mouth of secretions. Routine oral suctioning to aspirate secretions that accumulate above the cuff of the tube is also necessary to reduce the risk of pneumonia and provide patient comfort (AACN, 2018; Hess et al., 2021; Morton & Fontaine, 2018). More microorganisms are usually present in the mouth, so it is suctioned last to prevent transmission of contaminants. Proper removal of PPE and hand hygiene reduce transmission of microorganisms and contamination of other items.

24. Assist the patient to a comfortable position. Raise the bed rail and place the bed in the lowest position.

This ensures patient comfort. Proper positioning with raised side rails and the proper bed height provides for patient comfort and safety.

25. Reassess the patient's respiratory status, including respiratory rate, effort, oxygen saturation, lung sounds, tracheal sounds, and presence/absence of secretions in artificial airway, and the patient's response to the intervention.

These assess effectiveness of suctioning and the presence of complications.

26. Remove additional PPE, if used. Perform hand hygiene.

Proper removal of PPE reduces the risk for infection transmission and contamination of other items. Hand hygiene prevents the spread of microorganisms.

EVALUATION

The expected outcomes have been met when the patient has exhibited a clear, patent airway; an oxygen saturation level within acceptable parameters; and a respiratory rate and depth within acceptable parameters; and the patient has remained free from any signs of respiratory distress and adverse effect.

DOCUMENTATION

Guidelines

Document the time of suctioning, your assessments before and after the intervention, the reason for suctioning, oxygen saturation levels, and the characteristics and amount of secretions.

(continued on page 910)

Skill 14-10 ▶ Suctioning an Endotracheal Tube: Closed System (continued)

Sample Documentation

> <u>9/1/25</u> 1850 Tan secretions noted in ET tube; coarse crackles noted to auscultation over trachea. Lung sounds coarse in lower lobes. Respirations 24 breaths/min, regular rhythm. Intercostal retractions noted. Endotracheal tube suctioning completed with 12-Fr catheter. Small amount of thin, tan secretions obtained. Specimen for culture collected and sent. After suctioning, no secretions noted in ET tube, auscultation over trachea clear, lung sounds clear, respirations 18 breaths/min, no intercostal retractions noted.
>
> —*C. Bausler, RN*

DEVELOPING CLINICAL REASONING AND CLINICAL JUDGMENT

UNEXPECTED SITUATIONS AND ASSOCIATED INTERVENTIONS

- *Patient is extubated during suctioning:* Remain with the patient. Call for help to notify the health care team. Assess the patient's vital signs, ability to breathe without assistance, and oxygen saturation. Be ready to deliver assisted breaths with a bag-valve mask (see Skill 14-16) or administer oxygen. Anticipate the need for reintubation.
- *Oxygen saturation level decreases after suctioning:* Hyperoxygenate the patient. Auscultate lung sounds. If lung sounds are absent over one lobe, notify the health care team. Remain with the patient. The patient may have pneumothorax or a misplaced endotracheal tube. Anticipate a prescribed intervention for a stat chest x-ray and possible chest tube placement or reintubation.
- *Patient develops signs of intolerance to suctioning; oxygen saturation level decreases and remains low after hyperoxygenation; patient becomes cyanotic; or patient becomes bradycardic:* Stop suctioning. Auscultate lung sounds. Consider hyperventilating the patient with a manual resuscitation device. Remain with the patient. Alert staff to notify the health care team of the change in the patient's status.

SPECIAL CONSIDERATIONS

General Considerations

- The practice of instillation of saline solution directly into the airway during tracheal suctioning is not supported by evidence and is not recommended for inclusion as part of evidence-based practice and suctioning (AARC, 2010; Boroughs & Dougherty, 2015; Burns & Delgado, 2019; Leddy & Wilkinson, 2015; Owen et al., 2016; Wang et al., 2017).
- Determine the size of catheter to use by the size of the endotracheal tube. The suction catheter should be small enough not to occlude the airway being suctioned but large enough to remove secretions; use a suction catheter that occludes less than 50% of the lumen of the endotracheal tube (AARC, 2010; Pasrija & Hall, 2020). Larger catheters can contribute to trauma and hypoxemia.
- Make sure emergency equipment is easily accessible at the bedside. Keep a bag-valve mask, oxygen, and suction equipment at the bedside of a patient with an endotracheal tube at all times.
- Higher values of suction pressure have been suggested by some evidence for practice. The use of suction pressure of 250 mm Hg has been suggested as more effective for open-system suctioning and equally safe in comparison to the use of 80 to 150 mmHg suction pressure (Maraş et al., 2020). Yazdannik et al. (2019) suggest the use of 200 mm Hg pressure during closed-system suctioning for mechanically ventilated patients to improve the efficacy of secretion removal.

Infant and Child Considerations

- Insertion of the suction catheter to a predetermined distance, no more than the tip of the artificial airway to no more than 0.5 cm past the length of the endotracheal tube avoids contact with the trachea and carina, reducing the effects of tracheal mucosal damage (Boroughs & Dougherty, 2015; Kendrick, 2020).
- The maximal time for application of negative pressure (suction) for neonates, children, and adolescents should be less than 5 to 10 seconds (Boroughs & Dougherty, 2015; Dawson et al., 2012, as cited in Edwards, 2018, p. 51; Hockenberry et al., 2019).

EVIDENCE FOR PRACTICE ▶

SUCTION PRESSURE FOR ENDOTRACHEAL SUCTIONING

Evidence suggests that pressure related to suctioning of the endotracheal airway could potentially lead to complications including hypoxia, tracheal mucosal damage, and bleeding (AARC, 2010; Gilder et al., 2020). The American Association of Respiratory Care (AARC) (2010) and other sources suggest a maximum suction pressure of 150 mm Hg for adults (Hess et al., 2021). Higher values of suction pressure have been suggested as safe and more effective in removing tracheal secretions by some evidence for practice (Maraş et al., 2020; Yazdannik et al., 2019).

Related Research

Yazdannik, A., Saghaei, M., Haghighat, S., & Eghbali-Babadi, M. (2019). Efficacy of closed endotracheal suctioning in critically ill patients: A clinical trial of comparing two levels of negative suctioning pressure. *Journal of Nursing Practice Today*, 6(2), 60–67.

The purpose of this study was to compare the effectiveness of two levels of negative suctioning pressure in airway secretion removal during closed-system suctioning in mechanically ventilated adult intensive care unit patients. Participants were randomly assigned to one of two intervention groups (AB and BA). Each group had 20 participants. Participants in group AB were suctioned with 100 mm Hg first and after 2 hours with 200 mm Hg, followed by a second round of suctioning with reversed suction pressures. Suctioning for participants in group BA was reversed, starting with 200 mm Hg and then 100 mm Hg. Each participant received suctioning using 100 mm Hg and 200 mm Hg suction pressure in the order determined by group assignment. Each round of suctioning was separated by 2 hours. The level of suction pressure was controlled and set by a researcher; the person who performed the suctioning procedure was not aware of the level of suction pressure or the patient's group assignment. The same suctioning procedure was used for all participants, including timing of hyperoxygenation and suctioning. Efficacy of the suctioning was measured by the absence of secretion flow at the end of suctioning. Volume of the secretions was measured and compared in each suctioning. Results indicated closed-system suctioning using 200 mm Hg resulted in an efficacy of 96% for removing secretions, compared to 34% for 100 mm Hg ($p < .0001$). Suctioning volume was significantly increased with 200 mm Hg pressure compared to values with 100 mm Hg pressure ($p < .0001$). The researchers concluded the use of closed-system suctioning with a pressure of 200 mm Hg resulted in nearly complete clearance of respiratory secretions. The researchers suggested 200 mm Hg suction pressure should be used for trachea-bronchial suctioning in mechanically ventilated patients.

Relevance for Nursing Practice

Tracheal suctioning should be performed only when clinically indicated and not routinely (AARC, 2010; Morton & Fontaine, 2018; Sole et al., 2015). Use of the best evidence, including appropriate suction pressure, can lead to a decrease in the required number of suction attempts and fewer adverse effects. Nurses have a responsibility to use evidence to support clinical decision making and evidence-based strategies to meet the needs of patients in their care.

EVIDENCE FOR PRACTICE ▶

ENDOTRACHEAL TUBES AND PATIENT COMMUNICATION
Related Evidence

Karlsen, M. M. W., Ølnes, M. A., & Heyn, L. G. (2019). Communication with patients in intensive care units: A scoping review. *Nursing in Critical Care*, 24(3), 115–131. https://doi.org/10.1111/nicc.12377

Refer to details in Skill 14-9, Evidence for Practice.

Skill 14-11 ▶ Securing an Endotracheal Tube

Endotracheal tubes provide an airway for patients who cannot maintain a sufficient airway on their own. A tube is passed through the mouth or nose into the trachea. The endotracheal tube is often held in place with adhesive tape and should be retaped every 24 hours to prevent skin breakdown and to ensure that the tube is secured properly. Retaping an endotracheal tube requires two people.

There are other ways of securing an endotracheal tube besides using tape. Knotted twill tape can be used to secure an endotracheal tube (Hess et al., 2021; Walters et al., 2018) but may result in excessive pressure over time with resulting alterations in skin integrity. Commercial devices specifically designed to hold an endotracheal tube in place are available. Figure 1 shows an example of a commercially available endotracheal tube holder. Follow the manufacturer's recommendations for application when using commercial tube holders. Some potential drawbacks to use of these devices include that the size of the holder can interfere with provision of oral and facial care and that they are more costly than the use of tape or twill (Hess et al., 2021).

Any tube, electrode, sensor, or other rigid or stiff device element under pressure can create pressure damage (Baranoski & Ayello, 2020; EPUAP, NPIAP, & PPPIA, 2019). Patients who have an endotracheal tube have a high risk for skin and mucosal breakdown related to pressure from the tube and the securing of the endotracheal tube and moisture, compounded by the risk of increased secretions (Camacho-Del Rio, 2018). Careful assessment of the skin on the patient's face, the lips and tongue, and the skin on the patient's head in the areas where the securement device and the endotracheal tube sit are an important part of care (Mussa et al., 2018). Implement medical device–related pressure injury prevention strategies to reduce the risk for alterations in skin integrity. Interventions may include the use of a prophylactic cushioning/proactive dressings between the skin and securement device, an endotracheal tube repositioning schedule, routine skin and oral assessments, and provision of scheduled skin and oral hygiene interventions (Gupta et al., 2020; Holdman et al., 2020).

One example of a method of taping an endotracheal tube is provided below, but this skill might be performed differently in your facility. Always refer to specific facility policy.

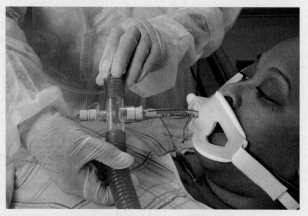

FIGURE 1. Commercially available endotracheal tube holder.

DELEGATION CONSIDERATIONS	Securing an endotracheal tube is not delegated to assistive personnel (AP). Depending on the state's nurse practice act and the organization's policies and procedures, securing of an endotracheal tube in a stable situation, such as long-term care and other community-based care settings, may be delegated to licensed practical/vocational nurses (LPN/LVNs). The decision to delegate must be based on careful analysis of the patient's needs and circumstances as well as the qualifications of the person to whom the task is being delegated. Refer to the Delegation Guidelines in Appendix A.

EQUIPMENT	• Assistant (nurse or respiratory therapist) • Portable or wall suction unit with tubing • Sterile suction catheter with Y-port • 1-inch tape (adhesive or waterproof tape) • Disposable gloves • Mask and goggles or face shield	• Additional PPE, as indicated • Sterile suctioning kit • Oral suction catheter • Two 3-mL syringes or tongue blade • Scissors • Washcloth and cleaning agent

- Skin barrier (e.g., 3M® or Skin-Prep™)
- Cushioning/proactive pressure reducing dressing, such as hydrocolloid/silicone dressing
- Adhesive remover swab

- Towel
- Razor (optional)
- Shaving cream (optional)
- Sterile saline or water
- Handheld pressure gauge

ASSESSMENT	Assess for the need for retaping, which may include loose or soiled tape, pressure on mucous membranes, and repositioning of the tube. Assess endotracheal tube length. The tube has markings on the side to ensure it is not moved during the retaping. Note the centimeter (cm) marking at the patient's lip or naris. Assess the patient's respiratory status, including respiratory rate, rhythm, and effort. Assess lung sounds to obtain a baseline. Ensure that the lung sounds are still heard throughout the lobes. Assess oxygen saturation level. If the tube is dislodged, the oxygen saturation level may change. Assess the chest for symmetric rise and fall during respiration. If the tube is dislodged, the rise and fall of the chest will change. Assess the patient's need for pain medication or sedation. Assess pain. The patient should be calm, free of pain, and relaxed during the retaping so as not to move and cause an accidental **extubation**. Inspect the patient's face, the lips and tongue, and the head in the areas where the securement device and the endotracheal tube sit for alterations in integrity that may result from irritation or pressure from the tube, tape, ties, or endotracheal tube holder.
ACTUAL OR POTENTIAL HEALTH PROBLEMS AND NEEDS	Many actual or potential health problems or issues may require the use of this skill as part of related interventions. An appropriate health problem or issue may include: - Altered skin integrity risk - Impaired oral mucous membrane - Injury risk
OUTCOME IDENTIFICATION AND PLANNING	The expected outcomes to achieve are that the tube remains in place, and the patient maintains bilaterally equal and clear lung sounds. Other outcomes may include that the patient's skin and mucous membranes remain intact; oxygen saturation remains within acceptable parameters, the chest rises symmetrically, the patient's airway remains clear, and the cuff pressure does not exceed 20 to 30 cm H_2O (AACN, 2018; Hess et al., 2021; Hinkle et al., 2022; Turner, Feeney et al., 2020).

IMPLEMENTATION

ACTION	**RATIONALE**
1. Gather equipment.	Assembling equipment provides for an organized approach to the task.
2. Perform hand hygiene and put on PPE, if indicated.	Hand hygiene and PPE prevent the spread of microorganisms. PPE is required based on transmission precautions.
3. Identify the patient.	Identifying the patient ensures the right patient receives the intervention and helps prevent errors.
4. Assemble equipment on the overbed table or other surface within reach.	Arranging items nearby is convenient, saves time, and avoids unnecessary stretching and twisting of muscles on the part of the nurse.
5. Close the curtains around the bed and close the door to the room, if possible.	This ensures the patient's privacy.

(continued on page 914)

Skill 14-11 ▶ Securing an Endotracheal Tube *(continued)*

ACTION	**RATIONALE**
6. Assess the need for endotracheal tube retaping. **Administer pain medication or sedation, as prescribed, before attempting to retape endotracheal tube.** Explain to the patient what you are going to do and why, even if the patient does not appear to be alert.	Retaping the endotracheal tube can stimulate coughing, which may be painful for patients, particularly those with surgical incisions. Explanation alleviates fears, facilitates engagement with care, and provides reassurance for the patient. Any procedure that may compromise respiration is frightening for the patient. Even if the patient appears unconscious, the nurse should explain what is happening.
7. Obtain the assistance of a second person to hold the endotracheal tube in place while the old tape is removed and the new tape is placed.	This prevents accidental extubation.
8. Adjust the bed to a comfortable working position (VHACEOSH, 2016). Lower the side rail closest to you. **Place the patient in an appropriate position based on assessment of individual circumstances.** Move the overbed table close to your work area and raise it to waist height. Place a trash receptacle within easy reach of the work area.	Having the bed at the proper height prevents back and muscle strain. Positioning of the patient is based on the circumstances of the individual patient; health status, health problems, presence of drains and/or monitoring devices, etc., that allows access to the site. The overbed table provides a work surface and maintains the sterility of the objects on the work surface. Placing the trash receptacle within reach allows for an organized approach to care.
9. Put on a face shield or goggles and a mask. Suction the patient as described in Skill 14-9 or 14-10.	PPE prevents exposure to contaminants. Suctioning decreases the likelihood of the patient coughing during the retaping of the endotracheal tube. If the patient coughs, the tube may become dislodged.
10. Measure a piece of tape for the length needed to reach around the patient's head one and a half to two times (Hess et al., 2021). Cut the tape. Lay it adhesive side up on the table.	Extra length is needed so that tape can be wrapped around the endotracheal tube.
11. Cut another piece of tape long enough to reach from one jaw around the back of the neck to the other jaw. Lay this piece on the center of the longer piece on the table, matching the tapes' adhesive sides together.	This prevents the tape from sticking to the patient's hair and the back of the neck (Hess et al., 2021).
12. Take one 3-mL syringe or tongue blade and wrap the sticky tape around the syringe until the nonsticky area is reached. Do this for the other side as well.	This helps the nurse or respiratory therapist to manage the tape without it sticking to the sheets or the patient's hair.
13. Take one of the 3-mL syringes or tongue blades and pass it under the patient's neck so that there is a 3-mL syringe on either side of the patient's head.	This makes the tape easy to access when retaping the tube.
14. Provide oral care, including suctioning the oral cavity. Refer to Skill 14-7 (oral hygiene is covered in Chapter 7).	This helps to decrease secretions in the oral cavity and pharynx region.
15. Take note of the "cm" position markings on the tube. Begin to unwrap the old tape from around the endotracheal tube. After one side is unwrapped, have the assistant hold the endotracheal tube as close to the patient's lips or naris as possible to offer stabilization.	The assistant should hold the tube to prevent accidental extubation. Holding the tube as close to the patient's lips or naris as possible prevents accidental dislodgement of the tube.
16. Carefully remove the remaining tape from the endotracheal tube (Figure 2). **After the tape is removed, have the assistant gently and slowly move the endotracheal tube (if orally intubated) to the other side of the mouth (Figure 3). Assess the mouth for any skin breakdown. Before applying new tape, make sure that the markings on the endotracheal tube are at the same spot as when retaping began.**	The endotracheal tube may cause pressure injuries if left in the same place over time. Repositioning the endotracheal tube may reduce the risk for pressure injury (Gupta et al., 2020; Holdman et al., 2020).
17. Remove the old tape from the patient's cheeks and the side of their face. Use adhesive remover to remove excess adhesive from the tape (Figure 4). Clean the patient's face and neck with a washcloth and cleanser. If the patient has facial hair, consider shaving their cheeks. Pat the cheeks dry with the towel.	To prevent skin breakdown, remove old adhesive. Shaving helps to decrease pain when the tape is removed. The cheeks must be dry before new tape is applied to ensure that it sticks.

ACTION

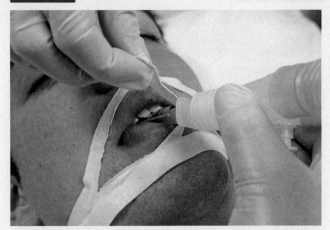

FIGURE 2. Ensuring endotracheal tube is stabilized and removing old tape.

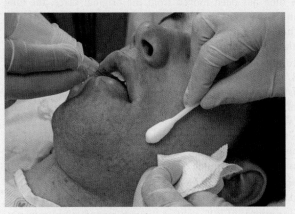

RATIONALE

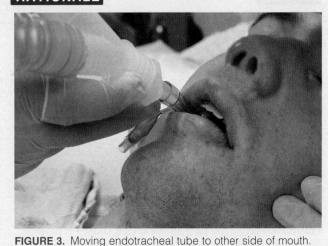

FIGURE 3. Moving endotracheal tube to other side of mouth.

FIGURE 4. Removing excess adhesive on cheeks from tape.

18. Apply the skin barrier to the patient's face (under the nose and on the cheeks and lower lip) where the tape will sit; apply a cushioning/proactive pressure reducing dressing if indicated. Unroll one side of the tape. Ensure that the nonstick part of the tape remains behind the patient's neck while pulling firmly on the tape. Place the adhesive portion of the tape snugly against the patient's cheek. Keep track of the pilot balloon from the endotracheal tube, to avoid taping it to the patient's face. Split the tape in half from the end to the corner of the patient's mouth.

The skin barrier/protectant prevents skin irritation and excoriation from the tape, adhesives, and moisture and helps the tape adhere better to the skin (Fumarola et al., 2020; Kelly-O'Flynn et al., 2020). The use of cushioning/proactive dressings between the skin and the securement device reduce the risk for alterations in skin integrity. The tape should be snug to the side of the patient's face to prevent accidental extubation.

19. Place the top-half piece of tape under the patient's nose (Figure 5). Wrap the lower half around the tube in one direction, such as over and around the tube. Fold over the tab on the end of the tape.

By placing one piece of tape on the lip and the other piece of tape on the tube, the tube remains secure. The tab makes tape removal easier.

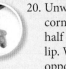

20. Unwrap the second side of the tape. Split to the corner of the patient's mouth. Place the bottom-half piece of tape along the patient's lower lip. Wrap the top half around the tube in the opposite direction, such as below and around the tube. Fold over the tab on the end of the tape. Apply pressure to the tape on the endotracheal tube to ensure the tape is secure (Figure 6). Remove gloves. Perform hand hygiene.

Alternating the placement of the top and bottom pieces of tape provides more anchorage for the tube. Wrapping the tape in an alternating manner ensures that the tape will not accidentally be unwound. Removal of gloves and hand hygiene reduce the risk for pathogen transmission and contamination of other items.

(continued on page 916)

Skill 14-11 ▶ Securing an Endotracheal Tube *(continued)*

ACTION

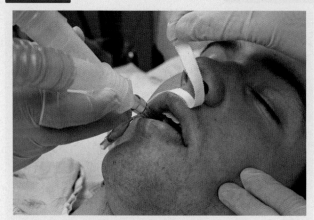

FIGURE 5. Placing the top-half of the tape under the patient's nose.

21. **Auscultate lung sounds. Assess for cyanosis, oxygen saturation, chest symmetry, and endotracheal tube stability. Again check the cm marker on the tube to ensure that the tube is at the correct depth.**

22. **If the endotracheal tube is cuffed, check the pressure of the balloon by attaching a handheld pressure gauge to the pilot balloon of the endotracheal tube.**

23. Assist the patient to a comfortable position. Raise the bed rail and place the bed in the lowest position.

 24. Remove the face shield or goggles and mask. Remove additional PPE, if used. Perform hand hygiene.

RATIONALE

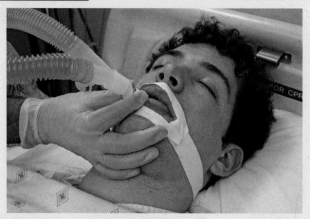

FIGURE 6. Applying pressure to the tape on the endotracheal tube to ensure the tape is secure.

If the tube has been moved from the original place, the lung sounds may change, as well as oxygen saturation and chest symmetry. The tube should be stable and should not move with each respiration cycle.

Careful monitoring of cuff pressure is necessary to decrease the risk for tracheal necrosis, tracheal rupture, laryngeal nerve palsy, tracheal stenosis, microaspiration, and/or inadequate ventilation (Turner, Feeney et al., 2020). The smallest amount of air that results in an airtight seal between the trachea and the tube is desirable and less likely to result in complications; maintain pressure between 20 and 30 cm H_2O (AACN, 2018; Hess et al., 2021; Hinkle et al., 2022; Turner, Feeney et al., 2020).

This ensures patient comfort. Proper positioning with raised side rails and the proper bed height provides for patient comfort and safety.

Proper removal of PPE reduces the risk for infection transmission and contamination of other items. Hand hygiene prevents the spread of microorganisms.

EVALUATION

The expected outcomes have been met when the tube has remained in place and the patient has maintained bilaterally equal and clear lung sounds, the patient's skin and mucous membranes have remained intact, oxygen saturation has remained within acceptable parameters, the chest rises symmetrically, the patient's airway has remained clear, and cuff pressure has not exceeded 20 to 30 cm H_2O (AACN, 2018; Hess et al., 2021; Hinkle et al., 2022; Turner, Feeney et al., 2020).

DOCUMENTATION

Guidelines

Document the procedure, including the depth of the endotracheal tube from the teeth, lips, or naris; the amount, consistency, and color of secretions suctioned; the presence of any skin or mucous membrane changes or pressure injury and associated interventions; and your before and after assessments, including lung sounds, oxygen saturation, cuff pressure, and chest symmetry. Document cuff pressure.

Sample Documentation

9/27/25 1305 Endotracheal tube tape changed; tube remains 12 cm at lips; suctioned for tenacious, yellow secretions, copious in amount; 2-cm pressure injury noted on left side of tongue. Wound care team consult requested. Tube moved to right side of mouth; lung sounds clear and equal after retaping; pulse oximeter remains 98% on 35% FiO_2, cuff pressure 22 cm H_2O; chest rises symmetrically.

—C. Bausler, RN

DEVELOPING CLINICAL REASONING AND CLINICAL JUDGMENT

UNEXPECTED SITUATIONS AND ASSOCIATED INTERVENTIONS

- *Patient is accidentally extubated during tape change:* Remain with the patient. Instruct the assistant to notify the health care team. Assess the patient's vital signs, ability to breathe without assistance, and oxygen saturation. Be ready to deliver assisted breaths with a bag-valve mask (Skill 14-16) or administer oxygen. Anticipate the need for reintubation.
- *Tube depth changes during retaping:* Tube depth should be maintained at the same level unless otherwise prescribed by the health care team. Remove the tape around tube, adjust the tube to prescribed depth, and reapply the tape.
- *Air leak (air escaping around the balloon) is heard on inspiration cycle of ventilator:* Auscultate lung sounds and check the depth of the endotracheal tube to ensure that it has not dislodged. Obtain a handheld pressure gauge and check pressure. Air may need to be added to the balloon to prevent the air leak. If pressure is already 20 to 30 cm H_2O, you may need to contact the health care team before adding more air to balloon. Sometimes, a change in the patient's position will resolve air leaks.
- *Patient is biting on the endotracheal tube:* Obtain a bite block (Hess et al., 2021). With the help of an assistant, place the bite block around the endotracheal tube or in the patient's mouth. If prescribed, consider sedating the patient.
- *Depth of endotracheal tube changes with respiratory cycle:* Remove the old tape. Repeat taping of the endotracheal tube, ensuring that the tape is snug against the patient's face. Consider use of a commercial securement device. There are various types on the market; check with your facility for availability.
- *Patient has trauma to the face that prevents the use of tape when securing the endotracheal tube:* You may need to obtain a commercially prepared endotracheal tube holder. There are various types on the market; check with your facility for availability.
- *Lung sounds are greater on one side:* Check the depth of the endotracheal tube. If the tube has been advanced, the lung sounds will appear greater on the side on which the tube is further down. Remove the tape and move the tube so that it is placed properly. If the depth has not changed, assess the patient's oxygen saturation and respiratory rate. Notify the health care team. Anticipate the need for a chest x-ray.
- *Pressure injury is noted in the mouth or naris (if patient is intubated via naris):* If the ulcer is painful, consider consulting with the health care team regarding the use of a topical numbing medication, such as lidocaine viscous jelly. Apply topically with a cotton-tipped applicator. Consider a consult with the wound care team. Keep the area clean by performing more frequent oral or nasal care. Ensure that the ventilator or oxygen tubing is not pulling on the endotracheal tube, thus applying pressure additional on the patient's skin and mucous membranes.
- *Pilot balloon is accidentally cut while caring for endotracheal tube:* Notify the health care team. Obtain a 22-gauge IV catheter and thread it into the pilot balloon tubing, being careful not to puncture the tubing with the needle, below the cut. Remove the needle from the catheter and apply a stopcock or needleless Luer-Lok to the catheter. Alternatively, a blunt needle can be passed into the pilot balloon tubing and a stopcock or Luer-Lok attached to the needle hub (Hess et al., 2021). If air is needed to reinflate the balloon, a syringe can be attached to the stopcock or Luer-Lok so that air may be added. Anticipate the need for an endotracheal tube change.

SPECIAL CONSIDERATIONS

- Make sure emergency equipment is easily accessible at the bedside. Keep a bag-valve mask, oxygen, an extra endotracheal tube of the same size, and suction equipment at the bedside of a patient with an endotracheal tube at all times.
- Evidence suggests that once adhesive tape is outside of its original packaging, it becomes contaminated with pathogens and presents a risk for transmission of pathogens to the patient and risk for an associated health care–associated infection (Bernatchez & Schommer, 2021; Krug et al., 2014; Krug et al., 2016). Krug et al. suggest contamination of the tape used to secure an endotracheal tube is a significant issue and needs to be considered when choosing equipment, including tape that is clean and individually packaged.

(continued on page 918)

Skill 14-11 ▶ Securing an Endotracheal Tube   *(continued)*

EVIDENCE FOR PRACTICE ▶

ENDOTRACHEAL TUBES AND PATIENT COMMUNICATION
Related Evidence
Karlsen, M. M. W., Ølnes, M. A., & Heyn, L. G. (2019). Communication with patients in intensive care units: A scoping review. *Nursing in Critical Care, 24*(3), 115–131. https://doi.org/10.1111/nicc.12377
    Refer to details in Skill 14-9, Evidence for Practice.

Skill 14-12 ▶ Suctioning a Tracheostomy: Open System

The purpose of suctioning is to maintain a patent airway and remove pulmonary secretions, blood, vomitus, and foreign material from the airway. When suctioning via a tracheostomy tube, the goal is to remove secretions that are not accessible to cilia bypassed by the tube itself. Tracheal suctioning can lead to hypoxemia, cardiac dysrhythmias, airway trauma, atelectasis, hyperinflation, infection, bleeding, and pain. Therefore, it is imperative to be diligent in maintaining aseptic technique and in following best practice and facility guidelines and procedures to prevent potential hazards. Tracheal suctioning should be performed only when clinically indicated based on assessment and not routinely (AARC, 2010; Burns & Delgado, 2019; Hess et al., 2021; Morton & Fontaine, 2018). Indications for the need for suctioning include audible and/or visible secretions, reduced oxygen saturation, presence of coarse crackles over the trachea, deterioration of arterial blood gas values, reduced breath sounds, the patient's inability to generate an effective spontaneous cough, acute respiratory distress, and suspected aspiration of secretions (AARC, 2010; Patton, 2019). In the home setting and other community-based settings, clean technique is used, as the patient is not exposed to disease-causing organisms that may be found in health care settings, such as hospitals (Sterni et al., 2016).

Because suctioning removes secretions not accessible to bypassed cilia, the recommendation is to insert the catheter only as far as the end of the tracheostomy tube. Catheter contact and suction can cause tracheal mucosal damage, loss of cilia, edema, and fibrosis and increase the risk of infection and bleeding. Insertion of the suction catheter to a predetermined distance, no more than the tip of the artificial airway to no more than 1 cm past the length of the endotracheal tube (adults) and 0.5 cm (pediatric patients) (Boroughs & Dougherty, 2015; Hess et al., 2021; Kendrick, 2020), avoids contact with the trachea and carina, reducing the effects of tracheal mucosal damage (Boroughs & Dougherty, 2015; Hahn, 2010; Ireton, 2007; Pasrija & Hall, 2020; Pate & Zapata, 2002). Box 14-2 in Skill 14-9 outlines several methods for determining appropriate suction catheter depth. The suction catheter should be small enough not to occlude the airway being suctioned but large enough to remove secretions; use a suction catheter that occludes less than 50% of the lumen of the endotracheal tube (AARC, 2010; Pasrija & Hall, 2020).

Tracheal suctioning is an uncomfortable procedure at a minimum, and it can be a very painful and/or distressing experience. Individualized pain management must be performed in response to the patient's needs (Arroyo-Novoa et al., 2008; Chaseling et al., 2014; Wrona et al., 2021; Düzkaya & Kuğuoğlu, 2015). Anticipate the administration of pharmacologic (analgesic medication) and use of nonpharmacologic interventions for the patient before suctioning. As mentioned previously, perform suctioning only when clinically necessary because of the many potential risks, including hypoxia, infection, tracheal tissue damage, dysrhythmias, and atelectasis.

Note: In-line, closed suction systems are available to suction mechanically ventilated patients. The use of closed suction catheter systems may avoid some of the infection control issues and other complications associated with open suction techniques. Open- and closed-system suctioning is discussed in the introduction to Skills 14-9 and 14-10. The closed suctioning procedure is the same for patients with tracheostomy tubes and endotracheal tubes connected to mechanical ventilation. Refer to details in Skill 14-10.

DELEGATION CONSIDERATIONS	Suctioning a tracheostomy is not delegated to assistive personnel (AP). Depending on the state's nurse practice act and the organization's policies and procedures, suctioning of a tracheostomy in a stable situation, such as long-term care and other community-based care settings, may be delegated to licensed practical/vocational nurses (LPN/LVNs). The decision to delegate must be based on careful analysis of the patient's needs and circumstances as well as the qualifications of the person to whom the task is being delegated. Refer to the Delegation Guidelines in Appendix A.
EQUIPMENT	• Portable or wall suction unit with tubing • A commercially prepared suction kit with an appropriate-size catheter (see General Considerations) or • Sterile suction catheter with Y-port in the appropriate size • Sterile, disposable container • Sterile gloves • Towel or waterproof pad • Goggles and mask or face shield; N95 mask or equivalent, based on patient's health status • Additional PPE, as indicated • Disposable, clean gloves • Resuscitation bag connected to 100% oxygen
ASSESSMENT	Assess for indications for the need for suctioning: audible and/or visible secretions, reduced oxygen saturation, presence of coarse crackles over the trachea, deterioration of arterial blood gas values, reduced breath sounds, the patient's inability to generate an effective spontaneous cough, acute respiratory distress, and suspected aspiration of secretions (AARC, 2010; Patton, 2019; Sole et al., 2015). Assess lung sounds. Wheezes, crackles, gurgling or diminished breath sounds may indicate the need for suctioning. Assess for the presence of visualized secretions in the artificial airway, audible secretions, and ineffective coughing (Morton & Fontaine, 2018; Sole et al., 2015). Assess the oxygen saturation level. Deterioration in oxygen desaturation may be an indication of the need for suctioning (AARC, 2010). Assess respiratory status, including respiratory rate and depth. Patients may become tachypneic when they need to be suctioned. Assess the patient for signs of respiratory distress, such as nasal flaring, retractions, or grunting. Assess for pain and the potential to cause pain during the intervention. (Arroyo-Novoa et al., 2008; Chaseling et al., 2014; Wrona et al., 2021; Düzkaya & Kuğuoğlu, 2015). Anticipate the administration of pharmacologic (analgesic medication) and use of nonpharmacologic interventions for the patient before suctioning (Arroyo-Novoa et al., 2008; Düzkaya & Kuğuoğlu, 2015). Assess the appropriate suction catheter depth. Refer to Box 14-2 in Skill 14-9. Assess the characteristics and amount of secretions while suctioning.
ACTUAL OR POTENTIAL HEALTH PROBLEMS AND NEEDS	Many actual or potential health problems or issues may require the use of this skill as part of related interventions. An appropriate health problem or issue may include: • Ineffective airway clearance • Altered breathing pattern • Impaired gas exchange
OUTCOME IDENTIFICATION AND PLANNING	The expected outcome to achieve is that the patient will exhibit a clear, patent airway. Other outcomes that may be appropriate include that the patient will exhibit an oxygen saturation level within acceptable parameters, demonstrate a respiratory rate and depth within acceptable parameters, and remain free from any signs of respiratory distress and adverse effect.

IMPLEMENTATION

ACTION	**RATIONALE**
1. Gather equipment.	Assembling equipment provides for an organized approach to the task.
2. Perform hand hygiene and put on PPE, if indicated.	Hand hygiene and PPE prevent the spread of microorganisms. PPE is required based on transmission precautions.

(continued on page 920)

Skill 14-12 ▶ Suctioning a Tracheostomy: Open System *(continued)*

ACTION

3. Identify the patient.

4. Assemble equipment on the overbed table or other surface within reach.

5. Close the curtains around the bed and close the door to the room, if possible.

6. Determine the need for suctioning. Verify the prescribed suctioning intervention in the patient's health record, if necessary. Anticipate the administration of pharmacologic (analgesic medication) and use of nonpharmacologic interventions for the patient before suctioning. **Assess for pain or the potential to cause pain. Administer pain medication, as prescribed, before suctioning.**

7. Explain to the patient what you are going to do and why, even if the patient does not appear to be alert. Reassure the patient that you will interrupt the procedure if they indicate respiratory difficulty.

8. Adjust the bed to a comfortable working position (VHACEOSH, 2016). Lower the side rail closest to you. **If the patient is conscious, place them in a semi-Fowler position (Figure 1). If the patient is unconscious, place them in an appropriate position based on assessment of individual circumstances.** Move the overbed table close to your work area and raise it to waist height.

RATIONALE

Identifying the patient ensures the right patient receives the intervention and helps prevent errors.

Arranging items nearby is convenient, saves time, and avoids unnecessary stretching and twisting of muscles on the part of the nurse.

This ensures the patient's privacy.

Suctioning should be performed only when clinically indicated based on assessment and not routinely (AARC, 2010; Burns & Delgado, 2019; Hess et al., 2021; Morton & Fontaine, 2018). At a minimum, suctioning is an uncomfortable procedure, and it can be a very painful and/or distressing experience. Individualized pain management must be performed in response to the patient's needs (Arroyo-Novoa et al., 2008; Chaseling et al., 2014; Wrona et al., 2021; Düzkaya & Kuğuoğlu, 2015).

Explanation alleviates fears. Even if the patient appears unconscious, the nurse should explain what is happening. Any procedure that compromises respiration is frightening for the patient.

Having the bed at the proper height prevents back and muscle strain. A sitting position helps the patient to cough and makes breathing easier. Gravity also facilitates catheter insertion. Positioning of the unconscious patient is based on the circumstances of the individual patient; health status, health problems, presence of drains and/or monitoring devices, etc. The overbed table provides a work surface and maintains the sterility of the objects on the work surface.

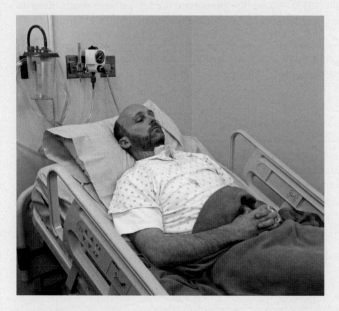

FIGURE 1. Patient in semi-Fowler position.

ACTION

9. Place a towel or waterproof pad across the patient's chest.
10. **Adjust suction to the appropriate pressure** (Hess et al., 2021) (Figure 2).
    - No more than 150 mm Hg for adults and adolescents.
    - No more than 125 mm Hg for children.
    - No more than 100 mm Hg for infants.

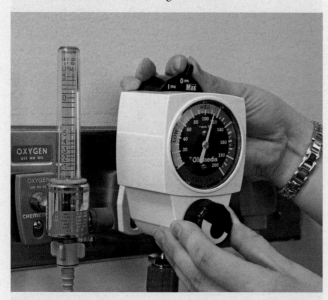

FIGURE 2. Turning suction unit to appropriate pressure.

11. Put on a disposable, clean glove and occlude the end of the connecting tubing to check suction pressure. Place the connecting tubing in a convenient location. If using a resuscitation bag, place it connected to oxygen within convenient reach.
12. Open the sterile suction package using aseptic technique. The open wrapper or container becomes a sterile field to hold other supplies. Carefully remove the sterile container, touching only the outside surface. Set it up on the work surface and pour sterile saline into it.
13. Put on a face shield or goggles and a mask (Figure 3). Put on sterile gloves. Your dominant hand will manipulate the catheter and must remain sterile. The nondominant hand is considered clean rather than sterile and will control the suction valve (Y-port) on the catheter.
14. With your dominant gloved hand, pick up the sterile catheter. Pick up the connecting tubing with your nondominant hand and connect the tubing and suction catheter (Figure 4).

RATIONALE

This protects bed linens and the patient.

Higher pressures can cause excessive trauma, hypoxemia, and atelectasis.
Higher pressures can cause excessive trauma, hypoxemia, and atelectasis.

The glove prevents contact with blood and body fluids. Checking pressure ensures that equipment is working properly. Preparation allows for an organized approach to the procedure.

Sterile normal saline or water is used to lubricate the outside of the catheter, minimizing irritation of the mucosa during introduction. It is also used to clear the catheter between suction attempts.

Handling the sterile catheter using a sterile glove helps prevent introducing organisms into the respiratory tract; the clean glove protects the nurse from microorganisms.

This maintains sterility of the suction catheter.

(continued on page 922)

Skill 14-12 ▶ Suctioning a Tracheostomy: Open System (continued)

ACTION	RATIONALE
15. Moisten the catheter by dipping it into the container of sterile saline, unless it is a silicone catheter (Figure 5). Occlude the Y-tube to check suction (Figure 6).	Lubricating the inside of the catheter with saline helps move secretions in the catheter. Silicone catheters do not require lubrication. Checking ensures that equipment is working properly.

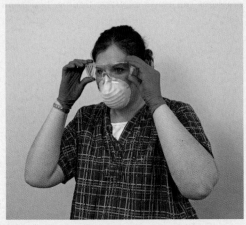

FIGURE 3. Putting on goggles and mask.

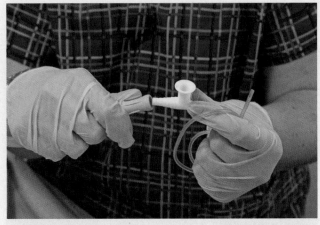

FIGURE 4. Connecting suction catheter to suction tubing.

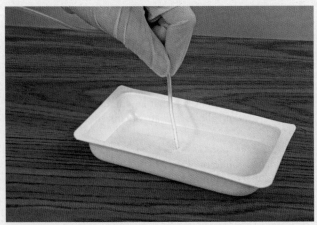

FIGURE 5. Moistening catheter in saline solution.

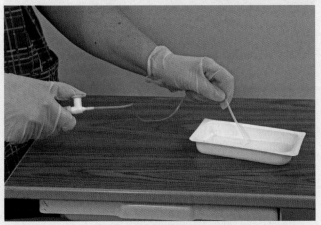

FIGURE 6. Occluding Y-port to check for proper suction.

ACTION	RATIONALE
16. Using your nondominant hand, remove the ventilator tubing or oxygen source (if in use) from the tracheostomy tube and attach the manual resuscitation bag. Hyperoxygenate the patient using your nondominant hand and the manual resuscitation bag for a minimum of 30 seconds (Burns & Delgado, 2019). Alternatively, use the sigh mechanism on a mechanical ventilator.	Hyperoxygenation aids in preventing hypoxemia during suctioning.
17. Using your nondominant hand, remove the manual resuscitation bag from the tracheostomy tube. Alternatively, open the adapter on the mechanical ventilator tubing.	This exposes the tracheostomy tube without contaminating your sterile gloved hand.

ACTION

18. Using your dominant hand, gently and quickly insert the catheter into the tracheostomy tube. **Advance the catheter to the predetermined length. Do not occlude the Y-port when inserting the catheter.**

19. Apply suction by intermittently occluding the Y-port on the catheter with the thumb of your nondominant hand, and gently rotate the catheter as it is being withdrawn (Figure 7). **Do not suction for more than 10 to 15 seconds at a time** (AARC, 2010; Burns & Delgado, 2019; Hess et al., 2021; Pasrija & Hall, 2020).

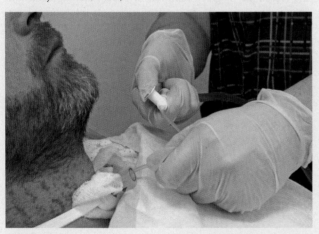

FIGURE 7. Intermittently occluding the Y-port on the catheter to apply suction while withdrawing catheter.

20. Hyperoxygenate the patient using your nondominant hand and a manual resuscitation bag for a minimum of 30 seconds (Burns & Delgado, 2019). Replace the oxygen delivery device, if applicable, using your nondominant hand, and have the patient take several deep breaths. If the patient is mechanically ventilated, close the adapter on the mechanical ventilator tubing and use the sigh mechanism on a mechanical ventilator.

21. Flush the catheter with saline. Assess the effectiveness of suctioning and repeat, as needed, according to the patient's tolerance. Wrap the suction catheter around your dominant hand between attempts.

RATIONALE

Catheter contact and suction cause tracheal mucosal damage, loss of cilia, edema, and fibrosis and increase the risk of infection and bleeding. Insertion of the suction catheter to a predetermined distance, no more than the tip of the artificial airway to no more than 1 cm past the length of the endotracheal tube (adults) and 0.5 cm (pediatric patients) (Boroughs & Dougherty, 2015; Hess et al., 2021; Kendrick, 2020) avoids contact with the trachea and carina, reducing the effects of tracheal mucosal damage (Boroughs & Dougherty, 2015; Hahn, 2010; Ireton, 2007; Pasrija & Hall, 2020; Pate & Zapata, 2002). If resistance is met, the carina or tracheal mucosa has been hit. Withdraw the catheter at least 0.5 inch before applying suction. Occluding the Y-port (i.e., suctioning) when inserting the catheter increases the risk for trauma to the airway mucosa and increases the risk of hypoxemia.

Turning the catheter as it is withdrawn minimizes trauma to the mucosa. Suctioning for longer than 15 seconds robs the respiratory tract of oxygen, which may result in hypoxemia (AARC, 2010; Pasrija & Hall, 2020). Suctioning too quickly may be ineffective at clearing all secretions.

Suctioning removes air from the patient's airway and can cause hypoxemia. Hyperoxygenation can help prevent suction-induced hypoxemia.

Flushing clears the catheter and lubricates it for the next insertion. Reassessment determines the need for additional suctioning. Wrapping the catheter around your hand prevents inadvertent contamination of the catheter.

(continued on page 924)

Skill 14-12 ▶ Suctioning a Tracheostomy: Open System *(continued)*

ACTION	RATIONALE

22. Allow at least a 30-second interval if additional suctioning is needed (Burns & Delgado, 2019). Do not make more than three suction passes per suctioning episode. If the patient is spontaneously breathing, **encourage them to cough and deep breathe between suctioning attempts.** Suction the oropharynx after suctioning the trachea (refer to Skill 14-7). Do not reinsert the tracheostomy tube after suctioning the mouth.

The interval allows for reventilation and reoxygenation of airways. Excessive suction passes contribute to complications. Suctioning the oropharynx clears the mouth of secretions. Routine oral suctioning to aspirate secretions that accumulate above the cuff of the tube is also necessary to reduce the risk of pneumonia and provide patient comfort (AACN, 2018; Hess et al., 2021; Morton & Fontaine, 2018). More microorganisms are usually present in the mouth, so it is suctioned last to prevent transmission of contaminants.

23. Perform oral hygiene after tracheal suctioning. Oral hygiene measures are discussed in Chapter 7.

Respiratory secretions that are allowed to accumulate in the mouth are irritating to mucous membranes, pose a risk for aspiration, are unpleasant for the patient, and contribute to the colonization of the oropharyngeal secretions by respiratory pathogens. Diligent oral hygiene care can improve oral health and limit the growth of pathogens in the oropharyngeal secretions, decreasing the incidence of aspiration pneumonia, community-acquired pneumonia, nonventilator health care–associated pneumonia (NV-HAP), and ventilator-associated pneumonia (VAP) (AACN, 2017; Chick & Wynne, 2020; Jenson et al., 2018; Quinn et al., 2020).

24. When suctioning is completed, coil the catheter in one hand. Remove the glove from the hand over the coiled catheter (the catheter remains inside the glove), pulling the glove off inside out (Figure 8). Remove the glove from the other hand, pulling inside out, and dispose of gloves, catheter, and container with solution in the appropriate receptacle. Perform hand hygiene. Assist the patient to a comfortable position. Raise the bed rail and place the bed in the lowest position.

This technique of glove removal, disposal of equipment, and hand hygiene reduces transmission of microorganisms. Proper positioning with raised side rails and the proper bed height provides for patient comfort and safety.

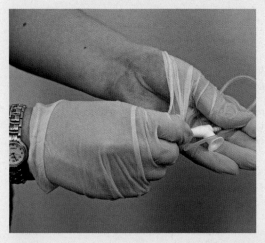

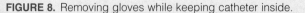
FIGURE 8. Removing gloves while keeping catheter inside.

25. Turn off the suction. Remove the supplemental oxygen placed for suctioning, if appropriate. Remove the face shield or goggles and mask. Perform hand hygiene.

Proper removal of PPE reduces the risk for infection transmission and contamination of other items. Hand hygiene prevents transmission of microorganisms.

26. Reassess the patient's respiratory status, including respiratory rate, effort, oxygen saturation, lung sounds, tracheal sounds, and presence/absence of secretions in artificial airway, and the patient's response to the intervention.

This assesses the effectiveness of suctioning and the presence of complications.

ACTION

27. Remove additional PPE, if used. Perform hand hygiene.

RATIONALE

Proper removal of PPE reduces the risk for infection transmission and contamination of other items. Hand hygiene prevents the spread of microorganisms.

EVALUATION

The expected outcomes have been met when the patient has exhibited a clear, patent airway; an oxygen saturation level within acceptable parameters; and a respiratory rate and depth within acceptable parameters; and the patient has remained free from any signs of respiratory distress and adverse effect.

DOCUMENTATION

Guidelines

Document the time of suctioning, assessments before and after interventions, the reason for suctioning, oxygen saturation levels, and the characteristics and amount of secretions.

Sample Documentation

9/1/25 1515 Yellow secretions noted in opening of tracheostomy tube; coarse crackles noted to auscultation over trachea. Lungs auscultated for wheezes in upper and lower lobes bilaterally. Respirations at 24 breaths/min. Weak, ineffective cough noted. Tracheal suction completed with 12-Fr catheter. Large amount of thick, yellow secretions obtained. Specimen for culture collected and sent. After suctioning, no secretions noted in tracheostomy tube, auscultation over trachea clear, faint wheezing persists, oxygen saturation at 97%, respirations 18 breaths/min.

—C. Bausler, RN

DEVELOPING CLINICAL REASONING AND CLINICAL JUDGMENT

UNEXPECTED SITUATIONS AND ASSOCIATED INTERVENTIONS

• *Patient coughs hard enough to dislodge tracheostomy:* Keep a spare tracheostomy and obturator at the bedside. Insert the obturator into the tracheostomy tube and reinsert the tracheostomy into the stoma. Remove the obturator. Secure the ties and auscultate lung sounds. Palpate the tracheostomy site for any **subcutaneous emphysema**, a result of air or gas collecting under the skin (crepitus).
• *Tracheostomy becomes dislodged and is not easily replaced:* Notify the health care team immediately. This is an emergency situation. Cover the tracheostomy stoma. Assess the patient's respiratory status. Anticipate the possible need for maintaining ventilation using a manual resuscitation device and mask and for possible oro- or nasotracheal intubation.
• *Lung sounds do not improve greatly, and oxygen saturation remains low after three suctioning attempts:* Allow the patient time to recover from previous suctionings. If needed, hyperoxygenate again. Suction the patient again and assess whether the oxygen saturation increases, lung sounds improve, and secretion amount decreases.
• *Patient develops signs of intolerance to suctioning; oxygen saturation level decreases and remains low after hyperoxygenation; patient becomes cyanotic; or patient becomes bradycardic:* Stop suctioning. Auscultate lung sounds. Consider hyperventilating the patient with a manual resuscitation device. Remain with the patient. Alert staff to notify the health care team of the change in the patient's status.

(continued on page 926)

Skill 14-12 ▶ Suctioning a Tracheostomy: Open System *(continued)*

SPECIAL CONSIDERATIONS

General Considerations

- Determine the size of the catheter to use by the size of the tracheostomy tube. The suction catheter should be small enough not to occlude the airway being suctioned but large enough to remove secretions; use a suction catheter that occludes less than 50% of the lumen of the endotracheal tube (AARC, 2010; Pasrija & Hall, 2020). Larger catheters can contribute to trauma and hypoxemia.
- If the patient eats by mouth, it is recommended that the tracheostomy tube be suctioned prior to eating to prevent the need for suctioning during or after meals, which may stimulate excessive coughing and could result in vomiting (Hess et al., 2021, p. 429).
- The practice of instillation of saline solution directly into the airway during tracheal suctioning is not supported by evidence and is not recommended for inclusion as part of evidence-based practice and suctioning (AARC, 2010; Boroughs & Dougherty, 2015; Burns & Delgado, 2019; Leddy & Wilkinson, 2015; Owen et al., 2016; Wang et al., 2017).
- Keep emergency equipment easily accessible at the bedside. Keep a bag-valve mask, oxygen, the obturator from the current tracheostomy, a spare tracheostomy of the same size, a spare tracheostomy one size smaller, and suction equipment at the bedside of a patient with a tracheostomy tube at all times (Dawson, 2014; Patton, 2019). If the patient is currently using a tracheostomy without a cuff, keep a spare tracheostomy of the same size with a cuff at the bedside for emergency use.

Infant and Child Considerations

- Insertion of the suction catheter to a predetermined distance, no more than the tip of the artificial airway to no more than 0.5 cm past the length of the endotracheal tube avoids contact with the trachea and carina, reducing the effects of tracheal mucosal damage (Boroughs & Dougherty, 2015; Kendrick, 2020).
- The maximal time for application of negative pressure (suction) for neonates, children, and adolescents should be less than 5 to 10 seconds (Boroughs & Dougherty, 2015; Dawson et al., 2012, as cited in Edwards, 2018, p. 51; Hockenberry et al., 2019).

EVIDENCE FOR PRACTICE ▶

TRACHEOSTOMY TUBES AND PATIENT COMMUNICATION

Placement of a tracheostomy tube results in the inability to speak, at least initially, for patients; once a patient is stable, the use of certain types of tracheostomy tubes may be appropriate to provide a patient with the ability to talk and communicate verbally. Difficult communication can prevent tracheostomy patients from expressing their needs and emotions, and collaborating in the planning of care, and it may contribute to ineffective responses to patient concerns and needs (Tollotti et al., 2018). What is the experience of patients with a tracheostomy who are unable to communicate verbally?

Related Research

Tolotti, A., Bagnasco, A., Catania, G., Aleo, G., Pagnucci, N., Cadorin, L., Zanini, M., Rocco, G., Stievano, A., Carnevale, F. A., & Sasso, L. (2018). The communication experience of tracheostomy patients with nurses in the intensive care unit: A phenomenological study. *Intensive & Critical Care Nursing, 46*, 24–31. https://doi.org/10.1016/j.iccn.2018.01.001

The purpose of this phenomenologic study was to describe the experience and sources of comfort and discomfort in tracheostomy patients when they communicate with nurses in the intensive care unit (ICU). The study took place in an ICU of a teaching hospital in Northern Italy. Participants included adult patients with a tracheostomy who were intubated for more than 5 days, mechanically ventilated, and not under sedation ($n = 8$) and the nurses ($n = 7$) who the patients remembered best in relation to their communication experiences in the ICU. During the patients' stay in the ICU, observation of the communication interactions between patients and nurses took place. The data collected through the observations were used during the interviews to gain a better understanding of the problems the patients reported in their narrations and during data analysis to gain a clearer and wider view of the context in which the communication events occurred. Within days after discharge from the ICU, semistructured in depth interviews with patients were conducted to explore the difficulties experienced by the patients during their communication experience with the nurses and to identify which elements had facilitated or hindered their communication. Patients were asked which nurses they remembered in particular, and short semistructured interviews were conducted with these nurses to explore the communication events and the context. All interviews were audiorecorded and transcribed verbatim. Transcripts of each patient interview were read and reread and then a line-by-line thematic analysis was conducted. Main themes were identified and grouped into categories. A thematic analysis of the transcripts of the nurses' interviews was completed to identify the similarities and the differences between the patients' and the nurses' transcripts, focusing on the communication difficulties experienced by the patients and comfort and discomfort factors when communicating with the nurses. An analysis of all cases and situations was completed to identify and describe commonalities and differences in the experiences reported by the patients. An examination of which communication comfort and discomfort factors were considered more important by the patients and which by the nurses was also completed. Two main themes were identified in relation to patients' communication experience with the nurses: (1) feeling powerless and frustrated, (2) facing continual misunderstanding, resignation and anger. The main communication discomfort factors identified were struggling with not knowing what was happening, feeling like others had given up on me, living in isolation and feeling invisible. The main comfort factors identified were being with family members, feeling reassured by having a call bell nearby and nurses' presence. The researchers concluded the results highlighted the importance of communication for tracheostomy patients and how communication is intrinsically linked to many aspects of the patient's experience, which cannot be reduced merely to the inability to use their voice.

Relevance for Nursing Practice
Effective communication is a cornerstone of professional nursing care. Communication strategies for patients who are unable to communicate verbally are a critical part of the provision of care. Good communication enables nurses to provide appropriate and person-centered nursing care. Nurses have a responsibility to develop and implement communication strategies to meet the needs of all patients in their care.

Skill 14-13 ▶ Providing Care of a Tracheostomy Tube and Site

Skill Variation: *Cleaning a Nondisposable Tracheostomy Inner Cannula*

Skill Variation: *Using an Alternative Site Dressing if Commercially Prepared Sponge Is Not Available*

Skill Variation: *Securing a Tracheostomy With Ties/Tape*

A tracheostomy is an artificial opening made into the trachea, usually at the level of the second or third cartilaginous ring. A tracheostomy tube is inserted through the opening. A tracheostomy tube consists of an outer cannula or main shaft and an obturator. An obturator, which guides the direction of the outer cannula, is inserted into the tube during placement and removed once the outer cannula of the tube is in place. Many tubes have inner cannulas that may or may not be disposable. The outer cannula remains in place in the trachea, and the inner cannula is removed for cleaning or replaced with a new one (Morton & Fontaine, 2018). Periodic cleaning or replacement of the inner cannula prevents airway obstruction from secretions that have accumulated on the tube's inner surface (Patton, 2019). Replace a disposable inner cannula or clean a nondisposable one at least once every 8 hours; more frequent cleaning may be required based on the patient's

(continued on page 928)

Skill 14-13 ▶ Providing Care of a Tracheostomy Tube and Site *(continued)*

status (Patton, 2019). For example, cleaning or replacement may be necessary every 4 hours or more if thick, viscous, or copious secretions are present (Patton, 2019).

Because soiled tracheostomy dressings place the patient at risk for the development of skin breakdown and infection, regularly change any dressings and tracheostomy collar or ties. If gauze dressings are used at the site, use dressings that are not filled with cotton to prevent aspiration of foreign bodies (e.g., lint or cotton fibers) into the trachea. Clean the skin around a tracheostomy to prevent buildup of dried secretions and skin breakdown. Implement medical device–related pressure injury prevention strategies to reduce the risk for alterations in skin integrity. Interventions may include the use of a hydrocolloid dressing under the tracheostomy flange during the postoperative period, placing a polyurethane foam dressing at the tracheostomy site after suture removal (O'Toole et al., 2017), routine skin and oral assessments, and provision of scheduled skin and oral hygiene interventions (Holdman et al., 2020).

Exercise care when changing the tracheostomy collar or ties to prevent accidental decannulation or expulsion of the tube. Have an assistant hold the tube in place during the changing of a collar. When changing a tracheostomy tie, keep the soiled tie in place until a clean one is securely attached. Patient condition, nursing assessment and judgment, and facility policy determine specific procedures and schedules, but a newly inserted tracheostomy may require attention every 1 to 2 hours.

Patients with tracheostomies frequently have an ineffective cough mechanism and copious secretions, which necessitate tracheal suctioning to remove secretions. Refer to Skill 14-12. Routine oral suctioning to aspirate secretions that accumulate above the cuff of the tube and frequent oral hygiene are also necessary to reduce the risk of pneumonia and provide patient comfort (AACN, 2018; Hess et al., 2021; Morton & Fontaine, 2018). Refer to Skills 14-7 and 7-4.

Because the respiratory tract is sterile and the tracheostomy provides a direct opening, meticulous care is necessary when using aseptic technique. Once the tracheostomy site is healed, in the home and other community-based settings, clean technique is used, as the patient is not exposed to pathogens that may be found in acute health care settings.

DELEGATION CONSIDERATIONS

Care of a tracheostomy tube is not delegated assistive personnel (AP). Depending on the state's nurse practice act and the organization's policies and procedures, care of a tracheostomy tube in a stable situation may be delegated to licensed practical/vocational nurses (LPN/LVNs). The decision to delegate must be based on careful analysis of the patient's needs and circumstances as well as the qualifications of the person to whom the task is being delegated. Refer to the Delegation Guidelines in Appendix A.

EQUIPMENT

- Disposable gloves
- Sterile gloves
- Goggles and mask or face shield; N95 mask or equivalent, based on patient's health status
- Additional PPE, as indicated
- Sterile normal saline
- Sterile cup or basin
- Sterile cotton-tipped applicators
- Sterile gauze sponges

- Disposable inner tracheostomy cannula, appropriate size for the patient
- Sterile suction catheter and glove set
- Commercially prepared tracheostomy or drain dressing
- Commercially prepared tracheostomy holder
- Plastic disposal bag
- Assistant (additional nurse or respiratory therapist)

ASSESSMENT

Assess for the need for tracheostomy care, which may include soiled dressings and holder or ties, secretions in the tracheostomy tube, and diminished airflow through the tracheostomy, or in accordance with facility policy. Assess the patient's respiratory status, including respiratory rate, rhythm, and effort. Assess lung sounds and oxygen saturation levels. Lung sounds should be equal in all lobes, with an oxygen saturation level within acceptable parameters. If the tracheostomy is dislodged, lung sounds and oxygen saturation level will diminish. Assess the patient for pain. If the tracheostomy is new or changes in integrity of the site are present, pain medication may be needed before performing tracheostomy care. Assess the insertion site for any redness or purulent drainage; if present, these may signify an infection. Inspect the insertion site and the patient's neck for any alterations in integrity that may result from irritation or pressure from the tube, ties, or the tracheostomy tube holder.

ACTUAL OR POTENTIAL HEALTH PROBLEMS AND NEEDS	Many actual or potential health problems or issues may require the use of this skill as part of related interventions. An appropriate health problem or issue may include: • Altered skin integrity • Infection risk • Ineffective airway clearance
OUTCOME IDENTIFICATION AND PLANNING	The expected outcomes to achieve when performing tracheostomy care are that the tracheostomy tube remains in place and the patient exhibits a tube and site free from drainage, secretions, and alterations in skin integrity and a patent airway. Other outcomes that may be appropriate include that oxygen saturation levels will be within acceptable parameters, the patient will have no evidence of respiratory distress, and cuff pressure does not exceed 20 to 30 cm H_2O (AACN, 2018; Hess et al., 2021; Hinkle et al., 2022; Patton, 2019).

IMPLEMENTATION

ACTION

1. Gather equipment.

2. Perform hand hygiene and put on PPE, if indicated.

3. Identify the patient.

4. Assemble equipment on the overbed table or other surface within reach.

5. Close the curtains around the bed and close the door to the room, if possible.

6. Determine the need for tracheostomy care. **Assess the patient's pain and administer pain medication, if indicated.**

7. Explain to the patient what you are going to do and why, even if the patient does not appear to be alert. Reassure the patient that you will interrupt the procedure if they indicate respiratory difficulty.

8. Adjust the bed to a comfortable working position (VHACEOSH, 2016). Lower the side rail closest to you. **If the patient is conscious, place them in a semi-Fowler position. Assist the patient to slightly extend their neck, if not contraindicated. If the patient is unconscious, place them in an appropriate position based on assessment of individual circumstances.** Move the overbed table close to your work area and raise it to waist height. Place a trash receptacle within easy reach of the work area.

RATIONALE

Assembling equipment provides for an organized approach to the task.

Hand hygiene and PPE prevent the spread of microorganisms. PPE is required based on transmission precautions.

Identifying the patient ensures the right patient receives the intervention and helps prevent errors.

Arranging items nearby is convenient, saves time, and avoids unnecessary stretching and twisting of muscles on the part of the nurse.

This ensures the patient's privacy.

If the tracheostomy is new or changes in integrity of the site are present, pain medication may be needed before performing tracheostomy care.

Explanation alleviates fears. Even if the patient appears unconscious, the nurse should explain what is happening. Any procedure that compromises respiration is frightening for the patient.

Having the bed at the proper height prevents back and muscle strain. A sitting position helps the patient to cough and makes breathing easier. Gravity also facilitates catheter insertion if suctioning is indicated. Having the neck slightly extended can facilitate easier removal of the inner cannula (Patton, 2019). Positioning of the unconscious patient is based on the circumstances of the individual patient; health status, health problems, presence of drains and/or monitoring devices, etc. The overbed table provides a work surface and maintains sterility of the objects on the work surface. A trash receptacle within reach prevents reaching over the sterile field or turning your back to the field to dispose of trash.

(continued on page 930)

Skill 14-13 ▶ Providing Care of a Tracheostomy Tube and Site *(continued)*

ACTION	RATIONALE
9. Put on a face shield or goggles and a mask. Suction the tracheostomy, if necessary. Refer to Skill 14-12. If the tracheostomy has just been suctioned, remove the soiled site dressing and discard it before removal of the gloves used to perform suctioning.	PPE prevents contact with contaminants. Suctioning removes secretions to prevent occluding the outer cannula while the inner cannula is removed.

Cleaning the Tracheostomy: Disposable Inner Cannula

(See the accompanying Skill Variation for steps for cleaning a nondisposable inner cannula.)

ACTION	RATIONALE
10. Carefully open the package with the new disposable inner cannula, taking care not to contaminate the cannula or the inside of the package (Figure 1). Carefully open the package with the sterile cotton-tipped applicators, taking care not to contaminate them. Open the sterile cup or basin and fill 0.5 inch deep with saline. Open the plastic disposable bag and place it within reach on the work surface.	The inner cannula must remain sterile. Saline and applicators will be used to clean the tracheostomy site. The plastic disposable bag will be used to discard removed inner cannula.

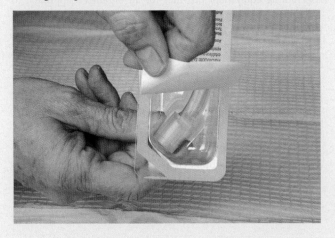

FIGURE 1. Carefully opening package with new disposable inner cannula. (Used with permission from Shutterstock. *Photo by B. Proud.*)

ACTION	RATIONALE
11. Put on disposable gloves.	Gloves protect against exposure to blood and body fluids.
12. Remove the oxygen source if one is present. Stabilize the outer cannula and faceplate of the tracheostomy with your nondominant hand. Grasp the locking mechanism of the inner cannula with your dominant hand. Press the tabs and release the lock (Figure 2). Gently remove the inner cannula and place it in the disposal bag. If not already removed, remove the site dressing and dispose of it in the trash.	Stabilizing the faceplate prevents trauma to, and pain from, the stoma. Releasing the lock permits removal of the inner cannula.
13. Working quickly, discard your current gloves and put on sterile gloves. Pick up the new inner cannula with your dominant hand; stabilize the faceplate with your nondominant hand and gently insert the new inner cannula into the outer cannula. Press the tabs to allow the lock to grab the outer cannula (Figure 3). Reapply the oxygen source, if one is in use.	Sterile gloves are necessary to prevent contamination of the new inner cannula. Locking to the outer cannula secures the inner cannula in place. Reapplying the oxygen source maintains an oxygen supply to the patient.

Applying Clean Dressing and Holder

(See accompanying Skill Variations for steps for an alternative site dressing if a commercially prepared sponge is not available and to secure a tracheostomy with tracheostomy ties/tape instead of a collar.)

ACTION	RATIONALE

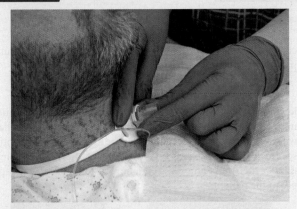

FIGURE 2. Releasing lock on inner cannula.

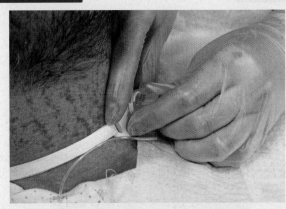

FIGURE 3. Locking new inner cannula in place.

14. Remove the oxygen source, if necessary. Dip the cotton-tipped applicator or gauze sponge in the cup or basin with sterile saline and clean the stoma under the faceplate. Use each applicator or sponge only once, moving from the stoma site outward (Figure 4).

Saline is nonirritating to tissue. Cleansing from the stoma outward and using each applicator only once promotes aseptic technique.

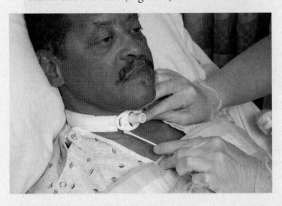

FIGURE 4. Cleaning from stoma site, outward.

15. Pat the skin gently with a dry 4 × 4 gauze sponge.

Gauze removes excess moisture.

16. Slide the commercially prepared tracheostomy dressing or prefolded non–cotton-filled 4 × 4-inches dressing under the faceplate.

Lint or fiber from a cut cotton-filled gauze pad can be aspirated into the trachea, causing respiratory distress, or can embed in the stoma and cause irritation or infection.

17. Alternatively, implement use of a hydrocolloid or polyurethane foam dressing at the tracheostomy site (Dixon et al., 2018; O'Toole et al., 2017). If this type of dressing is already in use, frequency of change is based on the type of dressing in use, assessment of dressing, and facility policy.

Use of a hydrocolloid dressing under the tracheostomy flange during the postoperative period and/or placing a polyurethane foam dressing at the tracheostomy site after suture removal reduces the risk for medical device–related alterations in skin integrity. (Dixon et al., 2018; O'Toole et al., 2017). These types of dressings may remain in place for longer periods of time.

18. Change the tracheostomy tube holder:

    a. **Obtain the assistance of a second person to hold the tracheostomy tube in place while the old collar is removed and the new collar is placed.**

    Holding the tracheostomy tube in place ensures that the tracheostomy will not inadvertently be expelled if the patient coughs or moves. Doing so provides attachment for one side of the faceplate.

    b. Open the package for the new tracheostomy collar.

    This allows access to the new collar.

    c. Both nurses should put on clean gloves.

    Gloves prevent contact with blood, body fluids, and contaminants.

    d. One nurse holds the faceplate while the other pulls up the Velcro tabs. Gently remove the collar.

    Holding the tracheostomy tube in place ensures that the tracheostomy will not inadvertently be expelled if the patient coughs or moves. Pulling up the Velcro tabs loosens the collar.

(continued on page 932)

Skill 14-13 ▶ Providing Care of a Tracheostomy Tube and Site *(continued)*

ACTION	RATIONALE
e. The first nurse continues to hold the tracheostomy faceplate.	This prevents accidental extubation.
f. The other nurse places the collar around the patient's neck and inserts first one tab, then the other, into the openings on the faceplate and secures the Velcro tabs on the tracheostomy holder (Figure 5).	Securing the Velcro tabs holds the tracheostomy in place and prevents accidental expulsion of the tracheostomy tube.
g. Check the fit of the tracheostomy collar. You should be able to fit no more than two fingers between the neck and the collar (Cleveland Clinic, 2021; Morton & Fontaine, 2018). Check to make sure that the patient can flex the neck comfortably. Reapply the oxygen source, if necessary (Figure 6).	Allowing one to two fingerbreadths under the collar permits neck flexion that is comfortable and ensures that the collar will not compromise circulation to the area but is sufficiently secure to prevent excessive movement of the tracheostomy tube in the stoma and decannulation. Maintains oxygen supply to the patient.

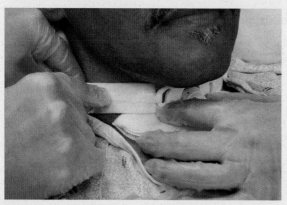

FIGURE 5. Securing tabs on tracheostomy holder.

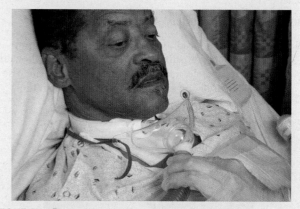

FIGURE 6. Reapplying oxygen source.

19. Remove gloves. Perform hand hygiene. **If the tracheostomy tube is cuffed, check the pressure of the balloon by attaching a handheld pressure gauge to the pilot balloon of the endotracheal tube.**	Removal of gloves and hand hygiene reduce the risk for pathogen transmission and contamination of other items. Careful monitoring of cuff pressure is necessary to decrease the risk for tracheal necrosis, tracheal rupture, laryngeal nerve palsy, tracheal stenosis, microaspiration, and inadequate ventilation (Turner, Feeney et al., 2020). The smallest amount of air that results in an airtight seal between the trachea and the tube is desirable and less likely to result in complications; maintain pressure between 20 and 30 cm H_2O (AACN, 2018; Hess et al., 2021; Hinkle et al., 2022; Patton, 2019).
20. Remove the face shield or goggles and mask. Perform hand hygiene. Assist the patient to a comfortable position. Raise the bed rail and place the bed in the lowest position.	Proper removal of PPE reduces the risk for infection transmission and contamination of other items. Hand hygiene prevents the spread of microorganisms. Proper positioning with raised side rails and the proper bed height provides for patient comfort and safety.
21. Reassess the patient's respiratory status, including respiratory rate, effort, oxygen saturation, and lung sounds.	Assessments determine the effectiveness of interventions and the presence of complications.
22. Remove additional PPE, if used. Perform hand hygiene.	Proper removal of PPE reduces the risk for infection transmission and contamination of other items. Hand hygiene prevents the spread of microorganisms.

EVALUATION

The expected outcomes have been met when the tracheostomy tube has remained in place; the patient has exhibited a tube and site free from drainage, secretions, and alterations in skin integrity and a patent airway; oxygen saturation levels have remained within acceptable parameters; the patient has had no evidence of respiratory distress; and cuff pressure has not exceeded 20 to 30 cm H_2O (AACN, 2018; Hess et al., 2021; Hinkle et al., 2022; Patton, 2019).

DOCUMENTATION

Guidelines

Document your assessments before and after interventions, including site assessment, skin assessment, the presence of pain, lung sounds, and oxygen saturation levels. Document the procedure, including site care, changing of dressing, and tube securement. Document the presence of any alterations in skin integrity and associated interventions. Document cuff pressure.

Sample Documentation

<u>9/26/25</u> 1300 Tracheostomy care completed; lung sounds clear in all lobes; respirations even/unlabored; site without erythema or edema; small amount of thick, yellow secretions noted at site, oxygen saturation 95% on O_2 35% via trach collar, cuff pressure 25 cm H_2O. Site dressing and trach securement collar changed.

—C. Bausler, RN

DEVELOPING CLINICAL REASONING AND CLINICAL JUDGMENT

UNEXPECTED SITUATIONS AND ASSOCIATED INTERVENTIONS

- *Patient coughs hard enough to dislodge tracheostomy:* Keep a spare tracheostomy and obturator at the bedside. Insert the obturator into the new tracheostomy and insert the tracheostomy into the stoma. Remove the obturator. Secure the ties and auscultate lung sounds. Palpate for any subcutaneous emphysema.
- *Tracheostomy becomes dislodged and is not easily replaced:* Notify the health care team immediately. This is an emergency situation. Cover the tracheostomy stoma. Assess the patient's respiratory status. Anticipate the possible need for maintaining ventilation using a manual resuscitation device and mask and for possible oro- or nasotracheal intubation.
- *On palpating around the insertion site, you note a moderate amount of subcutaneous emphysema in tissue:* Assess for dislodgement of the tracheostomy tube. If the tube has become displaced, a buildup of air in the subcutaneous portion of the skin is likely. Notify the health care team if the subcutaneous emphysema is a change in the patient's status.

SPECIAL CONSIDERATIONS

General Considerations

- One nurse working alone should always place new tracheostomy ties before removing old ties to prevent accidental extubation of the tracheostomy. If it is necessary to remove the old ties first, obtain the assistance of a second person to hold the tracheostomy tube in place while the old tie is removed and the new tie is replaced.
- Keep emergency equipment easily accessible at the bedside. Keep a bag-valve mask, oxygen, the obturator from the current tracheostomy, a spare tracheostomy of the same size, a spare tracheostomy one size smaller, and suction equipment at the bedside of a patient with a tracheostomy tube at all times (Dawson, 2014; Patton, 2019).
- If the patient is currently using a tracheostomy without a cuff, keep a spare tracheostomy of the same size with a cuff at the bedside for emergency use.
- Monitoring of the cuff pressure using a handheld cuff pressure manometer should take place at the beginning of each shift or following any procedure during which movement of the tube may have taken place (e.g., dressing/tape/collar change, patient repositioning) (Patton, 2019).
- *Pilot balloon is accidentally cut while caring for a tracheostomy tube with a cuff:* Notify the health care team. Obtain a 22-gauge IV catheter and thread it into the pilot balloon tubing, being careful not to puncture the tubing with the needle, below the cut. Remove the needle from the catheter

(continued on page 934)

Skill 14-13 ▶ Providing Care of a Tracheostomy Tube and Site (continued)

and apply a stopcock or needleless Luer-Lok to the catheter. Alternatively, a blunt needle can be passed into the pilot balloon tubing and a stopcock or Luer-Lok attached to the needle hub (Hess et al., 2021). If air is needed to reinflate the balloon, a syringe can be attached to the stopcock or Luer-Lok so that air may be added. Anticipate the need for a tracheostomy tube change.
- Consider implementation of medical device–related pressure injury prevention strategies to reduce the risk for alterations in skin integrity, including use of a hydrocolloid dressing under the tracheostomy flange during the postoperative period or a polyurethane foam dressing at the tracheostomy site after suture removal instead of a gauze dressing (Dixon et al., 2018; O'Toole et al., 2017).

Community-Based Care Considerations
- Instruct the patient and home caregiver on how to perform tracheostomy care. Observe a return demonstration and provide feedback.
- Clean, rather than sterile, technique can be used in the home setting.
- Sterile saline can be made by mixing 1 teaspoon of table salt in 1 quart of water and boiling for 15 minutes. The solution is cooled and stored in a clean, dry container. Discard the saline at the end of each day to prevent growth of bacteria. In the home, tap water may also be used, but distilled water or homemade saline should be used if the patient has well water (Cleveland Clinic, 2021).
- Instruct the patient who is performing self-care to use a mirror to view the steps in the procedure.

Skill Variation ▶ Cleaning a Nondisposable Tracheostomy Inner Cannula

Some tracheostomies use nondisposable inner cannulas, requiring the nurse to clean the inner cannula. Aseptic technique is maintained during the procedure. Clean, rather than sterile, technique can be used in the home setting. Additional equipment includes a sterile tracheostomy cleaning kit, if available, or three sterile basins; sterile brush/pipe cleaners; and sterile cleaning solutions (hydrogen peroxide and normal saline solution).

1. Follow Steps 1–9 in Skill 14-13.
10. Prepare the supplies: Open the tracheostomy care kit and separate basins, touching only the edges. If a kit is not available, open three sterile basins. Fill one basin 0.5 inch deep with hydrogen peroxide or half hydrogen peroxide and half saline, based on facility policy. Fill the other two basins 0.5 inch with saline. Open the sterile brush or pipe cleaners, cotton-tipped applicators, and gauze pads, if they are not already available in the cleaning kit.
11. Put on disposable gloves.
12. Remove the oxygen source if one is present. If not already removed, remove site dressing and dispose of it in the trash can. Stabilize the outer cannula and faceplate of the tracheostomy with your nondominant hand. Rotate the inner cannula in a counterclockwise motion with your dominant hand to release the lock (Figure A).
13. Continue to hold the faceplate. Gently remove the inner cannula (Figure B) and carefully drop it in the basin with the hydrogen peroxide. Replace the oxygen source over the outer cannula.
14. Discard your current gloves and put on sterile gloves. Remove the inner cannula from the soaking solution. Moisten the brush or pipe cleaner in saline and insert it into tube, using a back-and-forth motion to clean (Figure C).

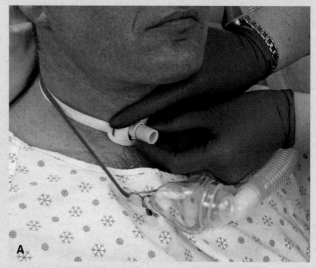

FIGURE A. Rotating inner cannula while stabilizing outer cannula.

15. Agitate the cannula in saline solution. Remove it and tap it against the inner surface of the basin. Place it on the sterile gauze pad. If secretions have accumulated in the outer cannula during cleaning of the inner cannula, suction the outer cannula using sterile technique.
16. Alternatively, hold the inner cannula over an empty basin and pour the peroxide over and into the cannula. Clean the inner cannula with a pipe cleaner or brush. Thoroughly rinse it with saline and tap it to dry. Some sources suggest that the inner cannula should not be soaked due to the increased risk of exposure to pathogens (Cleveland Clinic, 2021; Patton, 2019).

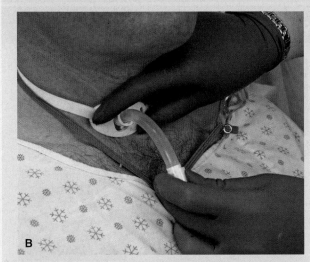

FIGURE B. Removing inner cannula for cleaning.

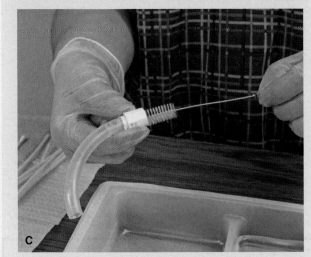

FIGURE C. Using brush to clean inner cannula.

17. Stabilize the outer cannula and faceplate with your non-dominant hand. Replace the inner cannula into the outer cannula with your dominant hand. Turn it clockwise and check that the inner cannula is secure (Figure D). Reapply the oxygen source, if in use.
18. Continue with site care as detailed above in Skill 14-13.

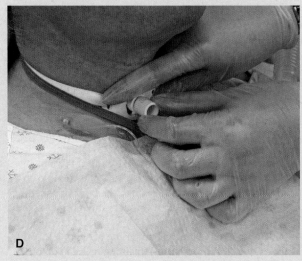

FIGURE D. Replacing inner cannula.

Skill Variation ▶ Using an Alternative Site Dressing if Commercially Prepared Sponge Is Not Available

If a commercially prepared site dressing or drain sponge is not available, do not cut a gauze sponge to use at the tracheostomy site. Cutting the gauze can cause loose fibers, which can become lodged in the stoma, causing irritation or infection. Loose fibers could also be inhaled into the trachea, causing respiratory distress.

1. Clean or replace the inner cannula as described in Skill 14-13 up to Step 15 or in the Skill Variation Cleaning a Nondisposable Inner Cannula.

16. Pat the skin gently with a dry 4 × 4 gauze sponge.
17. Fold two gauze sponges on the diagonal, to form triangles. Slide one triangle under the faceplate on each side of the stoma, with the longest side of the triangle against the tracheostomy tube.

(continued on page 936)

Skill 14-13

Providing Care of a Tracheostomy Tube and Site *(continued)*

Skill Variation ▶ Securing a Tracheostomy With Ties/Tape

A tracheostomy may be secured in place using twill ties or tape. One nurse working alone should always place new tracheostomy ties in place before removing the old ties to prevent accidental extubation of the tracheostomy. If it is necessary to remove the old ties first, obtain the assistance of a second person to hold the tracheostomy tube in place while the old tie is removed and the new tie is replaced.

1. Clean or replace the inner cannula as described in Skill 14-13 up to Step 18 or in the Skill Variation Cleaning a Nondisposable Inner Cannula.
19. Put on clean gloves. If another nurse is assisting, both nurses should put on clean gloves.
20. Cut a piece of the tape twice the length of the neck circumference plus 4 inches. Trim the ends of the tape on the diagonal.
21. Insert one end of the tape through the faceplate opening alongside the old tie. Pull it through until both ends are even length (Figure E).
22. Slide both ends of the tape under the patient's neck and insert one end through the remaining opening on other side of the faceplate. Pull it snugly and tie the ends in a double square knot to the side of the patient's neck. You should be able to fit one finger between the neck and the ties. Avoid tying the knot at the back of patient's neck, as this can cause excess pressure and skin breakdown. In addition, the ties could be confused with the patient's

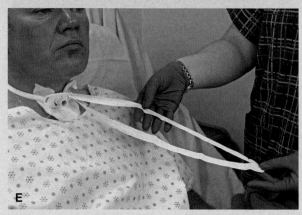

FIGURE E. Pulling tape through faceplate opening alongside old tie until ends are an even length.

gown and mistakenly untied. Reapply the oxygen supply, if in use.
23. Check the fit of the tracheostomy collar. You should be able to fit no more than two fingers between the neck and the collar (Cleveland Clinic, 2021; Morton & Fontaine, 2018). Check to make sure that the patient can flex their neck comfortably.
24. Carefully cut and remove the old ties. Take care to avoid cutting the pilot balloon if the tracheostomy tube has a cuff.

EVIDENCE FOR PRACTICE ▶

TRACHEOSTOMY TUBES AND PATIENT COMMUNICATION
Related Research
Tolotti, A., Bagnasco, A., Catania, G., Aleo, G., Pagnucci, N., Cadorin, L., Zanini, M., Rocco, G., Stievano, A., Carnevale, F. A., & Sasso, L. (2018). The communication experience of tracheostomy patients with nurses in the intensive care unit: A phenomenological study. *Intensive & Critical Care Nursing, 46,* 24–31. https://doi.org/10.1016/j.iccn.2018.01.001
Refer to details in Skill 14-12, Evidence for Practice.

Skill 14-14 ▶ Providing Care of a Chest Drainage System

Skill Variation: *Providing Care of a Chest Drainage System Using Dry Seal or Dry Suction*

A chest tube is indicated when negative pressure in the pleural space is disrupted, as from thoracic surgery (post-thoracotomy) or unanticipated trauma (Muzzy & Butler, 2015). Chest tubes may be inserted to drain fluid (pleural effusion), blood (**hemothorax**), or air (pneumothorax) from the pleural space to restore the negative intrathoracic pressure and allow the compressed lung to reexpand (Hinkle et al., 2022). A chest tube may also be indicated for pleurodesis (pleural sclerosing; installation of anesthetic or sclerosing agent to achieve inflammatory adherence of the visceral and parietal pleural to each other) (Burns & Delgado, 2019; Hinkle et al., 2022). A mediastinal chest tube may be placed after cardiac surgery to drain blood from around the heart (Morton & Fontaine, 2018). A tunneled pleural catheter (tunneled under the skin before entering the pleural space) may be used to improve quality of life in patients with recurrent pleural effusions related to some end-stage diseases, such as malignancy (Miller et al., 2018).

A chest tube is a firm plastic tube with drainage holes in the proximal end that is inserted in the pleural space. Once inserted, the tube is secured with a suture at the insertion site, covered with a dressing, secured with tape a few inches below the insertion site, and attached to a drainage system that may or may not be attached to suction. Other components of the system may include a closed water seal drainage system that prevents air from reentering the chest once it has escaped, and a suction control chamber that prevents excess suction pressure from being applied to the pleural cavity. The suction chamber may be a water-filled or a dry chamber. A water-filled suction chamber is regulated by the amount of water in the chamber, whereas dry suction is controlled by a knob and internal valves to control suction and is automatically regulated to changes in the patient's pleural pressure (Sasa, 2019; Zisis et al., 2015). There are also portable drainage systems that use gravity for drainage. Table 14-2 compares different types of chest drainage systems.

Table 14-2 Comparison of Chest Drainage Systems

TYPE	DESCRIPTION	COMMENTS
Traditional water seal (also referred to as wet-suction) chamber	Has three chambers: a collection chamber, water seal chamber (middle chamber), and wet-suction control chamber. Generally used to provide 20 cm H_2O of suction.	• Requires that sterile fluid be instilled into water seal and suction chambers. • Has positive and negative pressure–release valves. • Intermittent bubbling indicates that system is functioning properly. • Additional suction can be added by connecting system to a suction source.
Dry-suction water seal (also referred to as dry suction)	Has three chambers: a collection chamber, water seal chamber (middle chamber), and dry-suction control chamber. Provides up to 40 cm H_2O of suction.	• Requires that sterile fluid be instilled in water seal chamber at 2-cm level. • No need to fill suction chamber with fluid. • Suction pressure is set with a regulator. • Has positive and negative pressure–release valves. • Has an indicator to signify that the suction pressure is adequate. • Quieter than traditional water seal systems.
Dry-suction (also referred to as one-way valve system)	Has a one-way mechanical valve that allows air to leave the chest and prevents air from moving back into the chest	• No need to fill suction chamber with fluid; can be set up quickly in an emergency. • Works even if knocked over, making it ideal for patients who are ambulatory. • Not able to easily observe air leaks, monitor intrapleural pressures, or use suction

Source: Adapted from Hinkle, J. L., Cheever, K. H., & Overbaugh, K. J. (2022). *Brunner & Suddarth's Textbook of medical-surgical nursing* (15th ed.). Wolters Kluwer; Kane, C. J., York, N. L., & Minton, L. A. (2013). Chest tubes in the critically ill patient. *Dimensions of Critical Care Nursing, 32*(3), 111–117. https://doi.org/1097/DCC.0b013e3182864721; and Sasa, R. I. (2019). Evidence-based update on chest tube management. *American Nurse Today, 14*(4), 10–14.

(continued on page 938)

Skill 14-14 ▶ Providing Care of a Chest Drainage System (continued)

Nursing responsibilities include assisting with insertion, monitoring the patient's status and response to the treatment, monitoring the patency of the chest drainage system, providing patient education, and assisting with removal of the chest tube. Once the tube is in place, monitor the patient's response, including respiratory status and vital signs, check the site and site dressing, and maintain the patency and integrity of the drainage system.

The following procedure is based on the use of a traditional water seal, three-compartment chest drainage system. Figure 1 is an example of this system. The Skill Variation following the procedure describes a technique for caring for a chest drainage system using dry seal or suction.

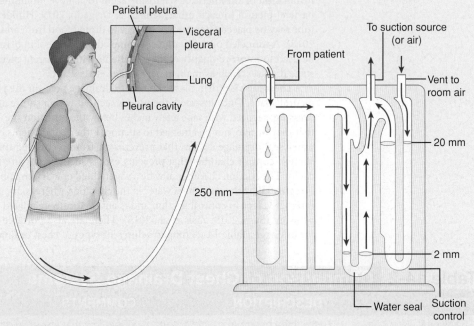

FIGURE 1. Chest drainage system.

DELEGATION CONSIDERATIONS	Care of a chest tube is not delegated to assistive personnel (AP). Depending on the state's nurse practice act and the organization's policies and procedures, care of a chest tube may be delegated to licensed practical/vocational nurses (LPN/LVNs). The decision to delegate must be based on careful analysis of the patient's needs and circumstances as well as the qualifications of the person to whom the task is being delegated. Refer to the Delegation Guidelines in Appendix A.

EQUIPMENT

- Bottle of sterile normal saline or water
- Two pairs of padded or rubber-tipped Kelly clamps (if a clamp is not in place on the drainage system tubing)
- Pair of clean scissors

- Disposable gloves
- Additional PPE, as indicated
- Foam tape
- Prescribed drainage system, if changing is required

ASSESSMENT

Assess the patient's vital signs and mental status. Significant changes from baseline may indicate complications. Assess for restlessness and shortness of breath. Assess the patient's respiratory status, including respiratory rate, rhythm and depth, and oxygen saturation level. If the chest tube is not functioning appropriately, the patient may become tachypneic and hypoxic. Assess the patient's lung sounds. The lung sounds over the chest tube site may be diminished due to the presence of fluid, blood, or air. Also assess the patient for pain. Sudden pressure or increased pain indicates potential complications. In addition, many patients report pain at the chest tube insertion site and request medication for the pain. Assess the patient's knowledge of the chest tube to ensure that they understand the rationale for the chest tube.

ACTUAL OR POTENTIAL HEALTH PROBLEMS AND NEEDS	Many actual or potential health problems or issues may require the use of this skill as part of related interventions. An appropriate health problem or issue may include: • Impaired gas exchange • Knowledge deficiency • Acute pain
OUTCOME IDENTIFICATION AND PLANNING	The expected outcome to achieve is that the patient will not experience complications related to the chest drainage system or experience respiratory distress. Other outcomes that may be appropriate include that the patient will verbalize an understanding of the need for the chest tube, the patient will have adequate pain control at the chest tube insertion site, lung sounds will be clear and equal bilaterally, and the patient will be able to increase activity tolerance gradually.

IMPLEMENTATION

ACTION

1. Gather equipment.

2. Perform hand hygiene and put on PPE, if indicated.

3. Identify the patient.

4. Assemble equipment on the overbed table or other surface within reach.

5. Close the curtains around the bed and close the door to the room, if possible.

6. Explain to the patient what you are going to do and why.

7. **Assess the patient's level of pain. Administer prescribed medication, as needed, and/or implement the use of non-pharmacologic interventions.**

8. Put on gloves.

Assessing the Drainage System

9. Move the patient's gown to expose the chest tube insertion site. Keep the patient covered as much as possible, using a bath blanket to drape the patient, if necessary. Observe the dressing at the chest tube insertion site and confirm that it is dry and intact (Figure 2).

10. Check that all connections are securely taped. Check that the tube is secured with tape to the patient's skin a few inches below the insertion site. Gently palpate around the insertion site, feeling for crepitus, a result of air or gas collecting under the skin (subcutaneous emphysema). This may feel crunchy or spongy, or like "popping" under your fingers.

RATIONALE

Assembling equipment provides for an organized approach to the task.

Hand hygiene and PPE prevent the spread of microorganisms. PPE is required based on transmission precautions.

Identifying the patient ensures the right patient receives the intervention and helps prevent errors.

Arranging items nearby is convenient, saves time, and avoids unnecessary stretching and twisting of muscles on the part of the nurse.

This ensures the patient's privacy.

Explanation relieves anxiety and facilitates engagement.

Regular pain assessments are required to maintain adequate analgesic relief from the discomfort and pain caused by chest drains (Kane et al., 2013; Muzzy & Butler, 2015).

Gloves prevent contact with contaminants and body fluids.

Keeping the patient as covered as possible maintains the patient's privacy and limits unnecessary exposure of the patient. Use of a dressing at the site is supported in the evidence, including petroleum gauze, dry gauze, silicone foam, and transparent film (Gross et al., 2016; Jeffries et al., 2017; Sasa, 2019; Upvall et al., 2019; Wood et al., 2019). Some patients experience significant drainage or bleeding at the insertion site. If this occurs, the dressing needs to be replaced to maintain occlusion of the site.

The chest tube drainage system integrity must be intact to function as intended (Sasa, 2019). Taping secures the tube to help prevent accidental dislodgment and kinking and tension at the insertion site (Sasa, 2019). The body will absorb small amounts of subcutaneous emphysema after the chest tube is removed. Larger or increasing amounts could indicate improper placement of the tube or an air leak and can cause discomfort to the patient.

(continued on page 940)

Skill 14-14 ▶ Providing Care of a Chest Drainage System *(continued)*

ACTION

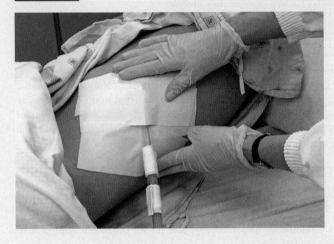

FIGURE 2. Assessing dressing at chest tube insertion site.

11. Check the drainage tubing to ensure that there are no dependent loops or kinks. Position the drainage collection device below the tube insertion site.

12. If the chest tube is prescribed to be connected to suction, note the fluid level in the suction chamber and check it with the amount of prescribed suction. Look for bubbling in the suction chamber. Temporarily disconnect the suction to check the level of water in the chamber. Add sterile water or saline, if necessary, to maintain the correct amount of suction.

13. Observe the water seal chamber for fluctuations of the water level with the patient's inspiration and expiration (tidaling). If suction is used, temporarily disconnect the suction to observe for fluctuation. Assess for the presence of bubbling in the water seal chamber. Add water, if necessary, to maintain the level at the 2-cm mark or the mark recommended by the manufacturer.

14. Assess the amount and type of fluid drainage. Measure drainage output at the end of each shift by marking the level on the container or placing a small piece of tape at the drainage level to indicate date and time (Figure 3). The amount should be a running total because the drainage system is never emptied. If the drainage system fills, remove and replace it (see Guidelines below).

15. Remove gloves. Perform hand hygiene. Assist the patient to a comfortable position. Raise the bed rail and place the bed in the lowest position, as necessary.

16. Remove additional PPE, if used. Perform hand hygiene.

RATIONALE

Dependent loops or kinks in the tubing can prevent the tube from draining properly and result in increased intrathoracic pressure (Sasa, 2019). The drainage collection device must be positioned below the tube insertion site so that drainage can move out of the tubing and into the collection device.

Some fluid is lost due to evaporation. If suction is set too low, the amount needs to be increased to ensure that enough negative pressure is placed in the pleural space to drain the pleural space sufficiently. If suction is set too high, the amount needs to be decreased to prevent any damage to the fragile lung tissue. Gentle bubbling in the suction chamber indicates that suction is being applied to assist drainage.

Fluctuation of the water level in the water seal chamber with inspiration and expiration is an expected and normal finding. Bubbles in the water seal chamber, after the initial insertion of the tube or when air is being removed, are a normal finding. Constant bubbles in the water seal chamber after the initial insertion period indicate an air leak in the system. Leaks can occur within the drainage unit or at the insertion site.

Measurement allows for accurate intake and output measurement and assessment of the effectiveness of therapy, and it contributes to the decision to remove the tube. The drainage system would lose its negative pressure if it were opened.

Proper removal of PPE reduces the risk for infection transmission and contamination of other items. Hand hygiene prevents the spread of microorganisms. Placing the patient in a comfortable position ensures patient comfort. Proper positioning with raised side rails and the proper bed height provides for patient comfort and safety.

Proper removal of PPE reduces the risk for infection transmission and contamination of other items. Hand hygiene prevents the spread of microorganisms.

ACTION

RATIONALE

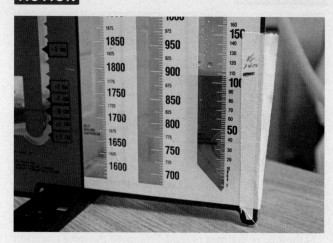

FIGURE 3. Drainage marked on device.

Changing the Drainage System

17. Some drainage systems have a clamp on the drainage tubing. If one is present, there is no need to use other clamps. Otherwise, obtain two-padded Kelly clamps, a new drainage system, and a bottle of sterile water. Add water to the water seal chamber in the new system until it reaches the 2-cm mark or the mark recommended by the manufacturer. Follow the manufacturer's directions to add water to the suction system, if suction is prescribed.

18. Put on clean gloves and additional PPE, as indicated.

19. **Engage the clamp on the drainage tubing.** Alternatively, apply Kelly clamps 1.5 to 2.5 inches from insertion site and 1 inch apart, going in opposite directions (Figure 4).

Gathering equipment provides for an organized approach. An appropriate level of water in the water seal chamber is necessary to prevent air from entering the chest. An appropriate level of water in the suction chamber provides the prescribed amount of suction.

Gloves prevent contact with contaminants and body fluids.

Clamps provide a more complete seal and prevent air from entering the pleural space through the chest tube.

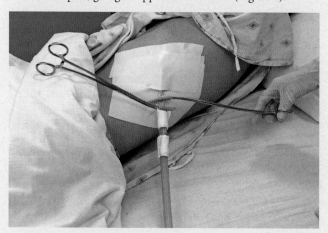

FIGURE 4. Padded clamps on chest tube.

20. Remove the suction from the current drainage system by unrolling (Figure 5) or use scissors to carefully cut away (Figure 6) any foam tape on the connection of the chest tube and drainage system. Using a slight twisting motion, remove the drainage system. **Do not pull on the chest tube.**

Removing suction permits application of the new system. In many facilities, bands or foam tape are placed where the chest tube meets the drainage system to ensure that the chest tube and the drainage system remain connected. Due to the negative pressure, a slight twisting motion may be needed to separate the tubes. The chest tube is sutured in place; do not tug on the chest tube and dislodge it.

(*continued on page 942*)

Skill 14-14 ▶ Providing Care of a Chest Drainage System *(continued)*

ACTION   **RATIONALE**

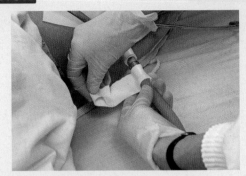

FIGURE 5. Unrolling foam tape.

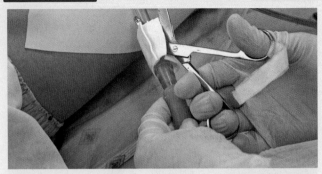

FIGURE 6. Carefully cutting foam tape.

21. Keeping the end of the chest tube sterile, insert the end of the new drainage system into the chest tube (Figure 7). **Unclamp the tubing clamp or remove the Kelly clamps.** Reconnect the suction, if prescribed. Apply foam tape to the chest tube/drainage system connection site.

The chest tube is sterile. The tube must be reconnected to the suction to form a negative pressure and allow for reexpansion of the lung or drainage of fluid. Prolonged clamping can result in a pneumothorax. Bands or foam tape help prevent the separation of the chest tube from the drainage system.

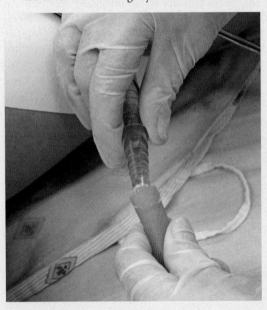

FIGURE 7. Inserting the end of the new drainage system into the chest tube.

22. Assess the patient and the drainage system as outlined (see Steps 9 to 15).

Assess for changes related to the manipulation of the system and placement of a new drainage system.

23. Remove additional PPE, if used. Perform hand hygiene.

Proper removal of PPE reduces the risk for infection transmission and contamination of other items. Hand hygiene prevents the spread of microorganisms.

EVALUATION

The expected outcomes have been met when the chest drainage system has remained patent and functioning. In addition, the patient has remained free of signs and symptoms of respiratory distress and complications related to the chest drainage system, has verbalized adequate pain relief, has gradually increased activity tolerance, and has verbalized an understanding of the need for the chest tube.

DOCUMENTATION

Guidelines

Document the site of the chest tube; the amount and type of drainage; the amount of suction applied; and the presence of any bubbling, tidaling, or subcutaneous emphysema. Document the type of dressing in place and the patient's pain level as well as any measures performed to relieve the patient's pain. Document the changing of the drainage system, if complete.

Sample Documentation

> 9/10/25 1805 Chest tube present in right lower portion of rib cage at the axillary line. Draining moderate amount of serosanguinous fluid. Suction at 20 cm H$_2$O noted; gentle bubbling noted in suction chamber. Tidaling present in water seal chamber, no air leak noted. Small amount of subcutaneous emphysema noted around insertion site, unchanged from previous assessment; patient denies any pain; site dressing intact.
> —C. Bausler, RN

DEVELOPING CLINICAL REASONING AND CLINICAL JUDGMENT

UNEXPECTED SITUATIONS AND ASSOCIATED INTERVENTIONS

- *Chest tube becomes separated from the drainage device:* Put on gloves. Open the normal saline solution or sterile water and submerge the chest tube into the bottle 1 to 2 inches below the surface of the solution, taking care to avoid contaminating the chest tube. This creates a water seal until a new drainage unit can be attached. Assess the patient for any signs of respiratory distress. Notify the health care team. Do not leave the patient. Summon a coworker to obtain a new chest drainage unit and reconnect the drainage system (Sasa, 2019). Alternatively, clamp the chest tube using a rubber-tipped clamp, but only for a few minutes to obtain and reconnect a new chest drainage unit; clamping poses the risk of tension pneumothorax (Sasa, 2019). Anticipate the need for a chest x-ray.
- *Chest tube becomes dislodged:* Put on gloves. Immediately apply an occlusive dressing to the site. There is controversy in the evidence for practice over whether the occlusive dressing should be a sterile petroleum gauze covered with an occlusive tape or a sterile 4 × 4 gauze folded and covered with an occlusive tape. (An example of an occlusive tape would be foam tape or the clear dressing used to cover IV insertion sites.) Assess the patient for any signs of respiratory distress. Notify the health care team of the incident and to determine whether the chest tube should be replaced. Anticipate the need for a chest x-ray.
- *While assessing the chest tube, you notice a lack of drainage when there had been drainage previously:* Check for kinked tubing or a clot in the tubing. Note the amount of suction on which the chest tube is set. Do not "milk" the tubing (i.e., squeezing and releasing small segments of tubing between the fingers) or "strip" the tubing (i.e., squeezing the length of the tube without releasing it) (Makic et al., 2015; Kane et al., 2013; Muzzy & Butler, 2015; Sasa, 2019). Bruising and trauma of lung tissue can occur as a result as well as dangerously increased intrathoracic pressure (Sasa, 2019). If the suction is not set appropriately, adjust it until the prescribed amount is achieved. Keeping the tubing horizontal across the bed or chair before dropping it vertically into the drain device and avoiding dependent loops optimize drainage. Notify the health care team if the lack of drainage persists.
- *Drainage dramatically increases or becomes bright red:* Notify the health care team immediately. This can indicate fresh bleeding.
- *Chest tube drainage suddenly decreases, and the water seal chamber is not tidaling:* Notify the health care team immediately. This could signal that the tube is blocked. Assess the patient's respiratory status.
- *The chest drainage unit is knocked over:* Promptly return it to its upright position and check all connections. Most chest drainage units have mechanisms to contain fluids in their respective chambers, but assess all chambers for any changes (Sasa, 2019). Inspect the water seal chamber to ensure the sterile water is at the 2-cm mark. Check the suction control chamber and add sterile water as needed. Re-mark the drainage chambers if fluid has redistributed between the chambers.

(continued on page 944)

Skill 14-14 ▶ Providing Care of a Chest Drainage System *(continued)*

SPECIAL CONSIDERATIONS

General Considerations

- Ensure that a bottle of sterile water or normal saline is at the bedside at all times. Never clamp chest tubes except to change the drainage system, or when there is a prescribed intervention, such as for a trial before chest tube removal. If the chest tube becomes accidentally disconnected from the drainage system, place the end of the chest tube into the sterile solution (see Unexpected Situations above). This prevents more air from entering the pleural space through the chest tube but allows for any air that does enter the pleural space, through respirations, to escape once pressure builds up.
- Evidence supports the use of a dressing at the chest tube insertion site; historically, petroleum gauze dressings have been the standard of care. Current evidence suggests that the use of petroleum gauze macerates the skin at the site over time and may increase the risk of infection and presents several alternative ways of dressing the chest tube site, including dry gauze, silicone foam, and transparent film (Gross et al., 2016; Jeffries et al., 2017; Morton & Fontaine, 2018; Sasa, 2019; Upvall et al., 2019; Wood et al., 2019).
- Keep two rubber-tipped clamps and additional dressing material at the bedside for quick access, if needed.
- **Do not** "milk" the tubing (i.e., squeezing and releasing small segments of tubing between the fingers) or "strip" the tubing (i.e., squeezing the length of the tube without releasing it) to promote drainage. This creates excessive negative pressure that can damage delicate lung tissue. Stripping and milking are not necessary to maintain chest tube patency and probably do more harm than good (Makic et al., 2015, p. 44; Sasa, 2019).
- If the patient has a small pneumothorax with little or no drainage and suction is not used, the tube may be connected to a Heimlich valve. A Heimlich valve is a small one-way valve chamber that allows air or drainage to exit from, but not enter, the chest tube (Burns & Delgado, 2019) (Figure 8). The valve drains into a plastic bag that can be held at any level, allowing the patient to be ambulatory simply by carrying the bag (Gogakos et al., 2015). Check to assure that the valve is pointing in the correct direction. The arrow on the casing points away from the patient.
- Maintain the chest drainage system in an upright position and lower than the level of the tube insertion site. This is necessary for proper functioning of the system and to aid drainage.
- Encourage the use of an incentive spirometer, if prescribed, and/or frequent deep breathing and coughing by the patient. This helps drain the lungs, promotes lung expansion, and prevents atelectasis.

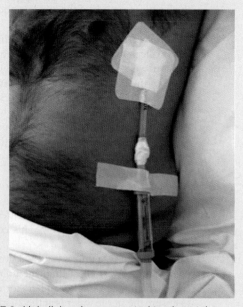

FIGURE 8. Heimlich valve connected to chest tube.

Skill Variation ▶ Providing Care of a Chest Drainage System Using Dry Seal or Dry Suction

1. Perform hand hygiene and put on PPE, if indicated.

2. Identify the patient.

3. Assemble equipment on the bedside stand or overbed table or other surface within reach.
4. Close the curtains around the bed and close the door to the room, if possible.
5. Explain to the patient what you are going to do and why.
6. **Assess the patient's level of pain. Administer prescribed medication, as needed.**
7. Put on gloves. Move the patient's gown to expose the chest tube insertion site. Keep the patient covered as much as possible, using a bath blanket to drape the patient, if necessary. Observe the dressing around the chest tube insertion site and confirm that it is dry and intact.
8. Check that all connections are taped securely. Check that the tube is secured with tape to the patient's skin a few inches below the insertion site. Gently palpate around the insertion site, feeling for subcutaneous emphysema, a collection of air or gas under the skin. This may feel crunchy or spongy, or like "popping" under your fingers.
9. Check the drainage tubing to ensure that there are no dependent loops or kinks. The drainage collection device must be positioned below the tube insertion site.

10. If the chest tube is to be connected to suction, assess the amount of suction set on the chest tube against the amount of suction prescribed. Assess for the presence of the suction control indicator, which is a bellows or float device, when adjusting the regulator to the desired level of suction, if prescribed.
11. Assess for fluctuations in the diagnostic indicator with the patient's inspiration and expiration.
12. Check the air-leak indicator for leaks in dry systems with a one-way valve.
13. Assess the amount and type of fluid drainage. Measure the drainage output at the end of each shift by marking the level on the container or placing a small piece of tape at the drainage level to indicate date and time. The amount should be a running total because the drainage system is never emptied. If the drainage system fills, it is removed and replaced.
14. Some portable chest drainage systems require manual emptying of the collection chamber. Follow the manufacturer's recommendations for timing of emptying. Typically, the unit should not be allowed to fill completely because drainage could spill out. Wear gloves, clean the syringe port with an alcohol wipe, use a 60-mL Luer-Lok syringe, screw the syringe into the port, and aspirate to withdraw fluid. Repeat, as necessary, to empty the chamber. Dispose of the fluid according to facility policy.
15. Remove gloves and additional PPE, if used. Perform hand hygiene.

Skill 14-15 ▶ Assisting With Removal of a Chest Tube

Chest tubes are removed after the lung is reexpanded, the patient's overall respiratory function improves, drainage is minimal, and no air has leaked (Morton & Fontaine, 2018; Sasa, 2019). An advanced practice professional usually performs chest tube removal. The practitioner will determine when the chest tube is ready for removal by evaluating the chest x-ray and assessing the patient and the amount of drainage from the tube.

DELEGATION CONSIDERATIONS

Assisting with the removal of a chest tube is not delegated to assistive personnel (AP). Depending on the state's nurse practice act and the organization's policies and procedures, assisting with the removal of a chest tube may be delegated to licensed practical/vocational nurses (LPN/LVNs). The decision to delegate must be based on careful analysis of the patient's needs and circumstances as well as the qualifications of the person to whom the task is being delegated. Refer to the Delegation Guidelines in Appendix A.

(continued on page 946)

Skill 14-15 ▶ Assisting With Removal of a Chest Tube   *(continued)*

EQUIPMENT
- Disposable gloves
- Additional PPE, as indicated
- Suture removal kit (tweezers and scissors)
- Sterile petroleum jelly-impregnated gauze and 4 × 4 gauze dressings or other occlusive dressings, based on facility policy
- Occlusive tape, such as foam tape

ASSESSMENT

Assess the patient's respiratory status, including respiratory rate and oxygen saturation level. This provides a baseline for comparison after the tube is removed. If the patient begins to have respiratory distress, they will usually become tachypneic and hypoxic. Assess the patient's lung sounds. The lung sounds over the chest tube site may be diminished due to the tube. Assess the patient for pain. Many patients report pain at the chest tube insertion site and request medication for the pain. If the patient has not recently received pain medication, give it before the chest tube removal to decrease the pain felt with the procedure and ease anxiety (Hood et al., 2014; Morton & Fontaine, 2018; Muzzy & Butler, 2015; Sasa, 2019; Yarahmadi et al., 2018).

ACTUAL OR POTENTIAL HEALTH PROBLEMS AND NEEDS

Many actual or potential health problems or issues may require the use of this skill as part of related interventions. An appropriate health problem or issue may include:
- Knowledge deficiency
- Acute pain
- Injury risk

OUTCOME IDENTIFICATION AND PLANNING

The expected outcomes to achieve when caring for a patient after removal of a chest tube are that the tube is removed without patient injury, and the patient remains free from respiratory distress. Other outcomes that may be appropriate include that the insertion site will remain clean and dry without evidence of infection, the patient will experience adequate pain control during the chest tube removal, and lung sounds will be clear and equal bilaterally.

IMPLEMENTATION

ACTION	RATIONALE
1. Gather equipment.	Assembling equipment provides for an organized approach to the task.
2. **Perform hand hygiene and put on PPE, if indicated.**	Hand hygiene and PPE prevent the spread of microorganisms. PPE is required based on transmission precautions.
3. Identify the patient.	Identifying the patient ensures the right patient receives the intervention and helps prevent errors.
4. Assemble equipment on the overbed table or other surface within reach.	Arranging items nearby is convenient, saves time, and avoids unnecessary stretching and twisting of muscles on the part of the nurse.
5. Administer pain medication, as prescribed. **Premedicate the patient before the chest tube removal, at a sufficient interval to allow for the medication to take effect, based on the medication prescribed.** In addition, consider the use of nonpharmacologic measures to reduce pain upon removal of tube (Muzzy & Butler, 2015; Yarahmadi et al., 2018).	Most patients report discomfort during chest tube removal (Hood et al., 2014; Morton & Fontaine, 2018; Muzzy & Butler, 2015; Sasa, 2019; Yarahmadi et al., 2018).
6. Close the curtains around the bed and close the door to the room, if possible.	This ensures the patient's privacy.
7. Explain to the patient what you are going to do and why. Explain any nonpharmacologic pain interventions the patient may use to decrease discomfort during tube removal.	Explanation relieves anxiety and facilitates engagement with care. Nonpharmacologic pain management interventions, such as relaxation exercises and the application of cold, have been shown to help decrease pain during chest tube removal (Ertuğ & Ülker, 2012; Yarahmadi et al., 2018).

ACTION

8. Explain to the patient that they will be required to take and hold a deep breath or exhale during chest tube removal. Instruct the patient to practice taking deep breaths and holding them. Alternatively, the patient may be asked to take a deep breath and hum during removal of the tube (Muzzy & Butler, 2015).

9. Put on clean gloves.

10. Assist the patient to a position with the head of the bed elevated 45 to 90 degrees (Morton & Fontaine, 2018; Sasa, 2019). Provide reassurance to the patient while the practitioner removes the dressing and then the tube.

11. **After the practitioner has removed the chest tube and secured the occlusive dressing, assess patient's respiratory status, lung sounds, vital signs, oxygen saturation, and pain level.**

12. Anticipate a prescribed intervention for a chest x-ray.

13. Dispose of equipment appropriately.

14. Remove gloves and additional PPE, if used. Perform hand hygiene.

15. Continue to monitor the patient's cardiopulmonary status and comfort level. Monitor the site and dressing.

RATIONALE

The chest tube must be removed during breath holding or expiration to prevent air from reentering the pleural space (Hood et al., 2014; Muzzy & Butler, 2015; Morton & Fontaine, 2018).

Gloves prevent contact with contaminants and body fluids.

The removal of the dressing and the tube can increase the patient's anxiety level. Offering reassurance will help the patient feel more secure and help decrease anxiety.

In most facilities, advanced practice professionals remove chest tubes, but some facilities have developed programs to train and support nurses to remove chest tubes (Hood et al., 2014; Muzzy & Butler, 2015). An occlusive dressing is placed to prevent leakage of air into the site. Once the tube is removed, the patient's status will need to be assessed for signs of adverse effects or complications.

A chest x-ray is performed to evaluate the status of the lungs after chest tube removal to ensure that the lung is still fully inflated.

This reduces the risk for transmission of microorganisms and contamination of other items.

Proper removal of PPE reduces the risk for infection transmission and contamination of other items. Hand hygiene prevents the spread of microorganisms.

Continued monitoring allows for assessment of possible respiratory distress if the lung does not remain inflated. Checking the dressing ensures the assessment of changes in the patient's condition and enables timely intervention to prevent complications.

EVALUATION

The expected outcomes have been met when the tube has been removed without patient injury and the patient has remained free from respiratory distress, the insertion site has remained clean and dry without evidence of infection, the patient has verbalized adequate pain control, and lung sounds have remained clear and equal bilaterally.

DOCUMENTATION

Guidelines

Document the respiratory assessment, oxygen saturation, lung sounds, total chest tube output, pain assessment, and status of the insertion site and dressing.

Sample Documentation

9/16/25 1950 Procedure explained to patient. Morphine sulfate 2 mg IV given. Patient used earbuds to listen to music choice during procedure. Dr. Reynolds at bedside, and right mid-axillary lower lobe chest tube removed. Vaseline gauze and gauze dressings applied over insertion site covered by foam tape. Lung sounds clear, slightly diminished over right lower lobe. Respirations unlabored at 16 breaths/min, pulse 88, blood pressure 118/64. Oxygen saturation 97% on room air; 322 mL of serosanguinous drainage noted in drainage device at time of removal. Patient denies pain or respiratory distress.

—C. Bausler, RN

(*continued on page 948*)

Skill 14-15 ▶ Assisting With Removal of a Chest Tube *(continued)*

DEVELOPING CLINICAL REASONING AND CLINICAL JUDGMENT

UNEXPECTED SITUATIONS AND ASSOCIATED INTERVENTIONS

- *Patient experiences respiratory distress after chest tube removal:* Assess respiratory status, vital signs, and oxygen saturation. Auscultate lung sounds. Diminished or absent lung sounds could be a sign that the lung has not fully reinflated or that the fluid has returned. Notify the health care team immediately. Anticipate a prescribed intervention for a chest x-ray and possible reinsertion of a chest tube.
- *Chest tube dressing becomes loosened:* Change the chest tube dressing per facility policy in order to assess the site for erythema and drainage. Replace the dressing using sterile technique. The dressing should remain occlusive for at least 3 days.

SPECIAL CONSIDERATIONS

Infant and Child Considerations

- It may be difficult to gain the cooperation of the child to hold their breath during tube removal. Distraction may be helpful. Ask the child to blow up a balloon or blow bubbles (Crawford, 2011).

EVIDENCE FOR PRACTICE ▶

PAIN AND CHEST TUBE REMOVAL

Chest tube removal is a painful procedure for many, if not most, patients. Pharmacologic and nonpharmacologic interventions have been used to decrease patients' discomfort during this procedure.

Related Research

Yarahmadi, S., Mohammadi, N., Ardalan, A., Najafizadeh, H., & Gholami, M. (2018). The combined effects of cold therapy and music therapy on pain following chest tube removal among patients with cardiac bypass surgery. *Complementary Therapies in Clinical Practice, 31,* 71–75. https://doi.org/10.1016/j.ctcp.2018.01.006

The purpose of this randomized controlled trial was to examine the effect of cold and music therapy individually and in combination on reducing pain related to chest tube removal. Patients who had cardiac bypass surgery ($n = 180$) and had a chest tube placed were randomized into four groups. Group A ($n = 45$) used ice packs for 20 minutes prior to chest tube removal. Participants in group B ($n = 45$) listened to music for a total of 30 minutes, beginning 15 minutes prior to removal of the chest tube. Group C ($n = 45$) used an ice pack for 20 minutes prior to removal of the chest tube and listened to music for a total of 30 minutes, beginning 15 minutes prior to removal of the tube. Participants in group D ($n = 45$) received no intervention in relation to removal of the chest There was a statistically significant difference in pain intensity scores at the time of chest tube removal between the cold therapy group (group A) and the combination cold and music therapy group (group C) compared to the control group (group D) ($p < .00001$). There were no statistically significant differences in pain intensity scores between any groups at 15 minutes following chest tube removal. The researchers concluded the application of either cold therapy or a combination of cold and music therapy as a nonpharmacologic intervention can potentially control the pain caused by chest tube removal.

Relevance to Nursing Practice

Nursing interventions related to decreasing pain and increasing patient comfort are an important nursing responsibility. Interventions should include the use of nonpharmacologic interventions, in addition to the administration of analgesics. The application of cold to the chest wall and listening to music can be implemented to manage pain and discomfort experienced by a patient during removal of a chest tube. Nurses could easily incorporate these simple interventions as part of nursing care for these patients.

Skill 14-16 ▶ Using a Manual Resuscitation Bag and Mask

If the patient is not breathing with an adequate rate and depth, or if the patient has lost the respiratory drive, a bag and mask may be used to deliver oxygen and assist with ventilation until the patient is resuscitated or can be intubated with an endotracheal tube. Bag and mask devices may be referred to as Ambu bags (air mask bag units) or BVMs (bag-valve masks). The bags come in infant, pediatric, and adult sizes. The bag consists of an oxygen reservoir, oxygen tubing, the bag itself, a one-way valve to prevent secretions from entering the bag, an exhalation port, an elbow so that the bag can lie across the patient's chest, and a mask. When the bag is compressed, the nonrebreathing valve directs gas from the bag through the mask and to the patient; when the bag is released, the exhaled gas exits through the exhalation port, and the bag simultaneously reinflates (Hess et al., 2021). The mask is removed to fit onto an endotracheal or tracheostomy tube.

DELEGATION CONSIDERATIONS

The use of a BVM may be delegated to assistive personnel (AP) in an emergency situation. The use of a BVM may be delegated to licensed practical/vocational nurses (LPN/LVNs). The decision to delegate must be based on careful analysis of the patient's needs and circumstances as well as the qualifications of the person to whom the task is being delegated. Refer to the Delegation Guidelines in Appendix A.

EQUIPMENT

- Handheld resuscitation device with a mask
- Oxygen source
- Disposable gloves
- Face shield or goggles and mask
- Additional PPE, as indicated

ASSESSMENT

Assess the patient's respiratory effort and drive. If the patient is breathing less than 10 breaths/min, is breathing too shallowly, or is not breathing at all, assistance with a BVM may be needed. Assess the oxygen saturation level. Patients who have decreased respiratory effort and drive may also have a decreased oxygen saturation level. Assess the heart rate and rhythm. Bradycardia may occur with a decreased oxygen saturation level, leading to a cardiac dysrhythmia. Many times, a BVM is used in a crisis situation. Manual ventilation may also be used during airway suctioning.

ACTUAL OR POTENTIAL HEALTH PROBLEMS AND NEEDS

Many actual or potential health problems or issues may require the use of this skill as part of related interventions. An appropriate health problem or issue may include:
- Altered breathing pattern
- Impaired gas exchange

OUTCOME IDENTIFICATION AND PLANNING

The expected outcome to achieve is that the patient will exhibit signs and symptoms of adequate respirations and oxygenation. Other outcomes that may be appropriate include that the patient will receive adequate volume of respirations with the BVM, and the patient will maintain oxygen saturation within acceptable parameters.

IMPLEMENTATION

ACTION	RATIONALE
1. If this is not a crisis situation, perform hand hygiene.	Hand hygiene prevents the spread of microorganisms.
2. Put on PPE, as indicated.	PPE prevents the spread of microorganisms. PPE is required based on transmission precautions.

(continued on page 950)

Skill 14-16 ▶ Using a Manual Resuscitation Bag and Mask *(continued)*

ACTION	**RATIONALE**
3. If this is not a crisis situation, identify the patient.	Identifying the patient ensures the right patient receives the intervention and helps prevent errors.
4. Explain to the patient what you are going to do and why, even if the patient does not appear to be alert.	Explanation alleviates fears. Even if the patient appears unconscious, the nurse should explain what is happening.
5. Put on disposable gloves. Put on a face shield or goggles and a mask.	Using gloves deters the spread of microorganisms. PPE protects the nurse from pathogens.
6. **Connect the mask to the bag device (Figure 1) and connect the oxygen tubing to the oxygen source (Figure 2). Turn on the oxygen to a flow rate of 10 to 15 L/min** (Hess et al., 2021). This may be done by visualizing or by listening to the open end of the reservoir or tail: if air is heard flowing, the oxygen tubing is attached and on.	The expected results might not be accomplished if the oxygen tubing is not attached and on.

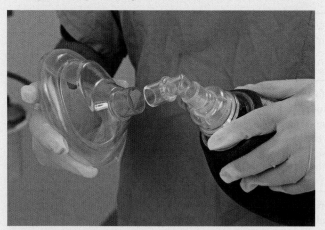

FIGURE 1. Connecting mask to bag-valve device.

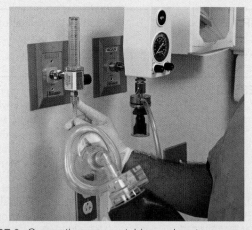

FIGURE 2. Connecting oxygen tubing on bag to oxygen source.

7. Initiate cardiopulmonary resuscitation (CPR), if indicated. Refer to Skill 15-1.	Start CPR in any situation in which either breathing alone or breathing and a heartbeat are absent. The brain is sensitive to hypoxia and will sustain irreversible damage after 4 to 6 minutes of no oxygen. The faster CPR is initiated, the greater the chance of survival.
8. Position yourself at the patient's head. If possible, get behind the head of the bed and remove the headboard. **Tilt the patient's head back and lift their jaw forward.**	Standing at the head of the bed makes positioning easier when obtaining a seal of the mask to the face. Hyperextending the neck opens the airway.
9. Place the mask over the patient's face with the opening over their oral cavity. If the mask is teardrop shaped, the narrow portion should be placed over the bridge of the patient's nose.	This helps ensure an adequate seal so that oxygen can be forced into the lungs.
10. **Use the thumb and index finger of one of your hands to make a "C" on the side of the mask, pressing the edges of the mask to the patient's face to form a seal. Use the remaining three fingers on the same hand to lift the angles of the patient's jaw to open the airway and press the mask to the face** (Hess et al., 2021).	This helps ensure that an adequate seal is formed so that oxygen can be forced into the lungs.
11. Using your other hand, squeeze the bag to give a breath over 1 second (Figure 3), watching the chest for symmetric rise.	The volume of air needed is based on patient's size. Enough has been delivered if their chest is rising. If air is introduced rapidly, it may enter the stomach.

ACTION

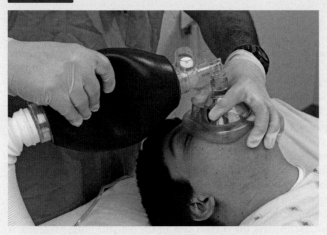

FIGURE 3. Squeezing the resuscitation bag with mask sealed on face.

12. Deliver the breaths with the patient's own inspiratory effort, if present. Avoid delivering breaths when the patient exhales. Deliver one breath every 6 seconds (about 10 breaths/min, adults) (American Heart Association [AHA], 2020b), if the patient's own respiratory drive is absent. Continue delivering breaths until the patient's drive returns or until the patient is intubated and attached to mechanical ventilation.

13. When use of the manual resuscitation bag and mask is no longer required, dispose of equipment appropriately.

 14. Remove the face shield or goggles and mask. Remove gloves and additional PPE, if used. Perform hand hygiene.

RATIONALE

If a patient has spontaneous inspiratory effort, breaths delivered to them must be timed to coincide with the spontaneous breaths to avoid the discomfort of dyssynchronous breathing, anxiety, and resistance to ventilation (Morton & Fontaine, 2018).

Once the patient's airway has been stabilized or the patient is breathing on their own, bag-mask delivery can be stopped.

This reduces the risk for transmission of microorganisms and contamination of other items.

Proper removal of PPE reduces the risk for infection transmission and contamination of other items. Hand hygiene prevents the spread of microorganisms.

EVALUATION   The expected outcomes have been met when the patient has exhibited signs and symptoms of adequate respirations and oxygenation, has received an adequate volume of respirations with the BVM, and has maintained oxygen saturation within acceptable parameters.

DOCUMENTATION

Guidelines   Document the incident, including the patient's respiratory effort before initiation of bag-mask breaths, lung sounds, oxygen saturation, chest symmetry, and resolution of the incident (e.g., intubation or patient's respiratory drive returns).

Sample Documentation

> 9/1/25 2015 Patient arrived to emergency department with respiratory rate of 4 breaths/min; respirations shallow; pulse 58; manual breaths delivered using adult bag with mask and 100% oxygen, oxygen saturation increased from 78% to 100% after eight breaths delivered; Dr. Alsup at bedside; patient sedated with 5 mg midazolam before intubation with 7.5-mm oral endotracheal tube, taped 10 cm at lips; lung sounds clear and equal in all lobes; see graphics for ventilator settings. Nasogastric tube placed via R naris to low intermittent suction, small amount of dark green drainage noted, chest x-ray obtained.
>
> —C. Bausler, RN

(continued on page 952)

Skill 14-16 ▶ Using a Manual Resuscitation Bag and Mask *(continued)*

DEVELOPING CLINICAL REASONING AND CLINICAL JUDGMENT

UNEXPECTED SITUATIONS AND ASSOCIATED INTERVENTIONS

- *Chest is not rising when breaths are delivered, and resistance is felt:* Reposition the head or perform the jaw-thrust maneuver. If the chest is not rising at all and resistance is being met, the tongue or another object may be obstructing the airway. If repositioning does not resolve the effort, consider performing the Heimlich maneuver.
- *Chest is rising asymmetrically:* Instruct the assistant to listen to lung sounds bilaterally. The patient may need a chest tube placed due to pneumothorax. Anticipate the need for chest tube placement.
- *Oxygen saturation decreases from 100% to 80%:* Assess whether the chest is rising. If the chest is rising asymmetrically, the patient may have a pneumothorax. Anticipate the need for a chest tube. Check the oxygen tubing. Someone may have stepped on the tubing, either kinking the tubing or pulling the tubing from the oxygen device.
- *Seal cannot be formed around the patient's face, and a large amount of air is escaping around mask:* Assess the patient's face and mask. Is the mask the correct size for the patient? If the mask size is correct, reposition your fingers, or have a second person hold the mask while you compress the bag.

SPECIAL CONSIDERATIONS

General Considerations

- If a patient has spontaneous inspiratory effort, breaths delivered to the patient must be timed to coincide with their spontaneous breaths to avoid the discomfort of dyssynchronous breathing, anxiety, and resistance to ventilation (Morton & Fontaine, 2018).
- If three or more rescuers are present, two rescuers can provide more effective bag-mask ventilation than one rescuer (AHA, 2020b; Hess et al., 2021). One rescuer maintains a seal on the mask and an open airway with two hands using the technique described above, while the other squeezes the bag to deliver the ventilation and oxygenation.
- Have equipment to suction airway readily available when using a BVM. Air can be forced into the stomach during manual ventilation with a mask, causing abdominal distention. This distention can cause vomiting and possible aspiration. Be alert for vomiting; watch through the mask. If the patient starts to vomit, stop ventilating immediately, remove the mask, wipe and suction vomitus as needed, then resume ventilation.

Infant and Child Considerations

- Deliver breaths at a rate of 20 to 30 breaths/min for infants and children who have a pulse but absent or inadequate respiratory effort (AHA, 2020b).

EVIDENCE FOR PRACTICE ▶

CARDIOPULMONARY RESUSCITATION AND EMERGENCY CARDIAC CARE
Related Guideline

The American Heart Association provides guidelines for cardiopulmonary resuscitation and emergency cardiac care and has incorporated these guidelines into the Basic Life Support and Advanced Life Support education for health care providers who respond to respiratory and cardiovascular emergencies.

American Heart Association (AHA). (2020). 2020 American Heart Association guidelines for cardiopulmonary resuscitation and emergency cardiovascular care. Parts 1–7. *Circulation,* *142*(16 Suppl 2). https://www.ahajournals.org/toc/circ/142/16_suppl_2

Enhance Your Understanding

Focusing on Patient Care: Developing Clinical Reasoning and Clinical Judgment

Consider the case scenarios at the beginning of the chapter as you answer the following questions to enhance your understanding and apply what you have learned.

QUESTIONS

1. Scott Mingus has a chest drain in place after thoracic surgery. The chest tube has been draining 20 to 30 mL of serosanguinous fluid every hour. Suddenly, the chest tube output is 110 mL/hr and the drainage is bright red. What should the nurse do?

2. Saranam Srivastava has a history of smoking and is scheduled for abdominal surgery. They need to learn how to use an incentive spirometer. What should the nurse include in patient education regarding the use of an incentive spirometer?

3. The nurse caring for Paula Cunningham determines that Ms. Cunningham needs to be suctioned via her endotracheal tube. What assessment findings might lead to this conclusion? How would the nurse determine if the suctioning of Ms. Cunningham's airway was effective?

You can find suggested answers after the Bibliography at the end of this chapter.

Integrated Case Study Connection

The case studies in the back of the book focus on integrating concepts. Refer to the following case studies to enhance your understanding of the concepts and skills in this chapter.

- Basic Case Studies: Kate Townsend, page 1205.
- Intermediate Case Studies: Olivia Greenbaum, page 1209; George Patel, page 1223.
- Advanced Case Studies: Cole McKean, page 1225; Damian Wallace, page 1227; George Patel, Gwen Galloway, Claudia Tran, and James White, page 1232.

Bibliography

Adams, D. (2018). Is there any incentive? A review on the use of incentive spirometry in postoperative abdominal surgery patients. *Canadian Journal of Respiratory Therapy, 54*(2), 50.

Al-Kindi, S. G., Brook, R. D., Biswal, S., & Rajagopalan, S. (2020). Environmental determinants of cardiovascular disease: Lessons learned from air pollution. *Nature Reviews Cardiology, 17*(10), 656–672. https://doi.org/10.1038/s41569-020-0371-2

Al-lede, M., Kumaran, R., & Waters, K. (2018). Home continuous positive airway pressure for cardiopulmonary indications in infants and children. *Sleep Medicine, 48*, 86–92. https://doi.org/10.1016/j.sleep.2018.04.004

Alqahtani, J. S., Worsley, P., & Voegeli, D. (2018). Effect of humidified noninvasive ventilation on the development of facial skin breakdown. *Respiratory Care, 63*(9), 1102–1110. https://doi.org/10.4187/respcare.06087

Amalakanti, S., & Pentakota, M. R. (2016). Pulse oximetry overestimates oxygen saturation in COPD. *Respiratory Care, 61*(4), 423–427. https://doi.org/10.4187/respcare.04435

American Association for Respiratory Care (AARC) Clinical Practice Guidelines. (2010). Endotracheal suctioning of mechanically ventilated patients with artificial airways 2010. *Respiratory Care, 55*(6), 758–764. https://www.aarc.org/wp-content/uploads/2014/08/06.10.0758.pdf

American Association of Critical-Care Nurses (AACN). (2017). AACN practice alert: Oral care for acutely and critically ill patients. *Critical Care Nurse, 37*(3), e19–e21. https://doi.org/10.4037/ccn2017179

American Association of Critical-Care Nurses (AACN). (2018). *AACN Practice alert. Prevention of aspiration in adults.* https://www.aacn.org/clinical-resources/practice-alerts/prevention-of-aspiration

American Heart Association (AHA). (2020a, October 20). 2020 American Heart Association guidelines for cardiopulmonary resuscitation and emergency cardiovascular care. Parts 1–7. *Circulation, 142*(16 Suppl 2). https://www.ahajournals.org/toc/circ/142/16_suppl_2

American Heart Association (AHA). (2020b). *2020 CPR & ECC guidelines. BLS provider manual.* AHA product number: 20–1102. https://shopcpr.heart.org/bls-provider-manual

American Lung Association. (2020a, May 27). Managing asthma. Measuring your peak flow rate. https://www.lung.org/lung-health-diseases/lung-disease-lookup/asthma/living-with-asthma/managing-asthma/measuring-your-peak-flow-rate

American Lung Association. (2020b, July 21). *Oxygen delivery devices and accessories.* https://www.lung.org/lung-health-diseases/lung-procedures-and-tests/oxygen-therapy/oxygen-delivery-devices

American Sleep Association (ASA). (2021). *CPAP user guide.* https://www.sleepassociation.org/sleep-apnea/cpap-treatment/cpap-user-guide/

American Thoracic Society (ATS). (2021). *Patient education/Information series. Pulse oximetry.* https://www.thoracic.org/patients/patient-resources/resources/pulse-oximetry.pdf

Andrews, M., Boyle, J. S., & Collins, J. (2020). *Transcultural concepts in nursing care* (8th ed.). Wolters Kluwer.

Arroyo-Novoa, C., Figueroa-Ramos, M., Puntillo, K., Stanik-Hutt, J., Thompson, C. L., White, C., & Wild, L. R. (2008). Pain related to tracheal suctioning in awake acutely and critically ill adults: A descriptive study. *Intensive & Critical Care Nursing, 24*(1), 20–27. https://doi.org/10.1016/j.iccn.2007.05.002

Asthma and Allergy Foundation of America (AAFA). (2017, December). Asthma. Peak flow meters. https://www.aafa.org/asthma/asthma-diagnosis/lung-function-tests/peak-flow-meters.aspx

Asthma Initiative of Michigan (AIM). (n.d.). *Spacers and valved-holding chambers.* https://getasthmahelp.org/spacer-holding.aspx

Baranoski, S., & Ayello, E. A. (2020). *Wound care essentials. Practice principles* (5th ed.). Wolters Kluwer.

Bauldoff, G., Gubrud, P., & Carno, M. A. (2020). *LeMone and Burke's Medical-surgical nursing: Clinical reasoning in patient care* (7th ed.). Pearson.

Bernatchez, S. F., & Schommer, K. (2021). Infection prevention practices and the use of medical tapes. *American Journal of Infection Control, 49*(9), 1177–1182. https://doi.org/10.1016/j.ajic.2021.03.007

Boroughs, D. S., & Dougherty, J. M. (2015). Pediatric tracheostomy care: What home care nurses need to know. *American Nurse Today, 10*(3), 8–10. https://www.myamericannurse.com/wp-content/uploads/2015/03/ant3-Pediatric-Home-Trach-225.pdf

Burns, S. M., & Delgado, S. A. (2019). *AACN essentials of critical care nursing* (4th ed.). McGraw Hill Education.

Camacho-Del Rio, G. (2018). Evidence-based practice: Medical device-related pressure injury prevention. *American Nurse Today, 13*(10), 50–52.

Centers for Disease Control and Prevention (CDC). (2021, January 19). *Heart disease.* https://www.cdc.gov/heartdisease/

Chaseling, W., Bayliss, S. L., Rose, K., Armstrong, L., Boyle, M., Caldwel, J., Chung, C., Girffiths, K., Johnson, K., Rolls, K., & Davidson, P. (2014). Suctioning an adult ICU patient with an artificial airway. Agency for Clinical Innovation NSW Government. Version 2. NSW, Australia. https://www.aci.health.nsw.gov.au/__data/assets/pdf_file/0010/239554/ACI14_Suction_2-2.pdf

Chick, A., & Wynne, A. (2020). Introducing an oral care assessment tool with advanced cleaning products into a high-risk clinical setting. *British Journal of Nursing, 29*(5), 290–296. doi: 10.12968/bjon.2020.29.5.290

Cleveland Clinic. (2020, December 15). *Peak flow meter.* https://my.clevelandclinic.org/health/articles/4298-peak-flow-meter

Cleveland Clinic. (2021). *Tracheostomy care.* https://my.clevelandclinic.org/health/treatments/17568-tracheostomy-care

Crawford, D. (2011). Care and nursing management of a child with a chest drain. *Nursing Children and Young People, 23*(10), 27–33. https://doi.org/10.7748/ncyp2011.12.23.10.27.c8836

Dawson, D. (2014). Essential principles: Tracheostomy care in the adult patient. *British Association of Critical Care Nurses, 19*(2), 63–72. https://doi.org/10.1111/nicc.12076

Dix, A. (2018). Respiratory rate: The benefits of continuous monitoring. *Nursing Times, 114*(11), 36–37. https://www.nursingtimes.net/clinical-archive/respiratory-clinical-archive/respiratory-rate-6-the-benefits-of-continuous-monitoring-29-10-2018/

Dixon, L. M., Mascioli, S., Mixell, J. H., Gillin, T., Upchurch, C. N., & Bradley, K. M. (2018). Reducing tracheostomy-related pressure injuries. *AACN Advanced Critical Care, 29*(4), 426–431. https://dx.doi.org/10.4037/aacnacc2018426

Düzkaya, D. S., & Kuğuoğlu, S. (2015). Assessment of pain during endotracheal suction in the pediatric intensive care unit. *Pain Management Nursing, 16*(1), 11–19. https://doi.org/10.1016/j.pmn.2014.02.003

Edwards, E. (2018). Principles of suctioning in infants, children and young people. *Nursing Children & Young People, 30*(4), 46–54. https://doi.org/10.7748/ncyp.2018.e846

Eliopoulos, C. (2018). *Gerontological nursing* (9th ed.). Wolters Kluwer.

Elliott, M., & Baird, J. (2019). Pulse oximetry and the enduring neglect of respiratory rate assessment: A commentary on patient surveillance. *British Journal of Nursing, 28*(19) 1156–1159. https://doi.org/10.12968/bjon.2019.28.19.1256

Eltorai, A. E. M., Martin, T. J., Patel, S. A., Tran, M., Eltorai, A. S., Daniels, A. H., & Baird, G. L. (2019). Visual obstruction of flow of indicator increases inspiratory volumes in incentive spirometry. *Respiratory Care, 64*(5), 590–594. https://doi.org/10.4187/respcare.06331

Eltorai, A. E. M., Szabo, A. L., Antoci Jr., V., Ventetuolo, C. E., Elias, J. A., Daniels, A. H., & Hess, D. R. (2018). Clinical effectiveness of incentive spirometry for the prevention of postoperative pulmonary complications. *Respiratory Care, 63*(3), 347–352. https://doi.org/10.4187/respcare.05679

Ertuğ, N., & Ülker, S. (2012). The effect of cold application on pain due to chest tube removal. *Journal of Clinical Nursing, 21*(5–6), 784–790. https://doi.org/10.1111/j.1365-2702.2011.03955.x

European Pressure Ulcer Advisory Panel (EPUAP), National Pressure Injury Advisory Panel (NPIAP), and Pan Pacific Pressure Injury Alliance (PPPIA). Haesler, E. (Ed). (2019). *Prevention and treatment of pressure ulcers/injuries: Clinical Practice guideline. The international guideline.* http://www.internationalguideline.com/

Fischbach, F. T., & Fischbach, M. A. (2018). *A manual of laboratory and diagnostic tests* (10th ed.). Wolters Kluwer.

Fisk, A. C. (2018). The effects of endotracheal suctioning in the pediatric population. An integrative review. *Dimension of Critical Care Nursing, 37*(1), 44–56. https://doi.org/10.1097/DCC.0000000000000275

Ford, C., & Roberson, M. (2021). Oxygen therapy in a hospital setting. *British Journal of Nursing, 30*(2), 96–100. https://doi.org/10.12968/bjon.2021.30.2.96

Fountain, L. (2021a, January 22). CPAP vs BiPAP. Sleep Foundation. https://www.sleepfoundation.org/cpap/cpap-vs-bipap

Fountain, L. (2021b, January 28). How to clean a CPAP machine. Sleep Foundation. https://www.sleepfoundation.org/cpap/how-to-clean-a-cpap-machine

Franklin, D., Fraser, J. F., & Schibler, A. (2019). Respiratory support for infants with bronchiolitis, a narrative review of the literature. *Paediatric Respiratory Reviews, 30*, 16–24. https://doi.org/10.1016/j.prrv.2018.10.001

Fumarola, S., Allaway, R., Callaghan, R., Collier, M., Downie, F., Geraghty, J., Kiernan, S., & Spratt, F. (2020). Overlooked and underestimated: Medical adhesive-related skin injuries. Best practice consensus document on prevention. *Journal of Wound Care, 29*(Suppl 3c), S1–S24. https://doi.org/10.12968/jowc.2020.29.Sup3c.S1

Gilder, E., McGuinness, S. P., Cavadino, A., Jull, A., & Parke, R. L. (2020). Avoidance of routine endotracheal suction in subjects ventilated for ≤ 12 hours following elective cardiac surgery. *Respiratory Care, 65*(12), 1838–1846. https://doi.org/10.4187/respcare.07821

Gogakos, A., Barbetakis, N., Lazaridis, G., Papaiwannou, A., Karavergou, A., Lampaki, S., Baka, S., Mpoukovinas, I., Karavasilis, V., Kioumis, I., Pitsiou, G., Katsikogiannis, N., Tsakiridis, K., Rapti, A., Trakada, G., Iissimopoulos, A., Tsirgogianni, K., Zarogoulidis, K., & Zarogoulidis, P. (2015). Heimlich valve and pneumothorax. *Annals of Translational Medicine, 3*(4), 54. https://doi.org/10.3978/j.issn.2305-5839.2015.03.25

Gross, S. L., Jennings, C. D., & Clark, R. C. (2016). Comparison of three practices for dressing chest tube insertion sites: A randomized controlled trial. *MedSurg Nursing, 25*(4), 229–250.

Gupta, P., Shiju, S., Chacko, G., Thomas, M., Abas, A., Savarimuthu, I., Omari, E., Al-Balushi, S., Jessymol, P., Mathew, S., Quinto, J., McDonald, I., & Andrews, W. (2020). A quality improvement programme to reduce hospital-acquired pressure injuries. *BMJ Open Quality, 9*, e000905. https://doi.org/10.1136/bmjoq-2019-000905

Hahn, M. (2010). 10 considerations for endotracheal suctioning. *The Journal for Respiratory Care Practitioners, 23*(7), 32–33. https://rtmagazine.com/department-management/clinical/10-considerations-for-endotracheal-suctioning/

Hayes, D. Jr, Wilson, K. C., Krivchenia, K., Hawkins, S. M., Balfour-Lynn, I. M., Gozal, D., Panitch, H. B., Splaingard, M. L., Rhein, L. M., Kurland, G., Abman, S. H., Hoffman, T. M., Carroll, C. L., Cataletto, M. E., Tumin, D., Oren, E., Martin, R. J., Baker, J., Porta, G. R., … on behalf of the American Thoracic Society Assembly on Pediatrics. (2019). Home oxygen therapy for children. An official American Thoracic Society Clinical Practice Guideline. *American Journal of Respiratory and Critical Care Medicine, 199*(3), e5–e23. https://doi.org/10.1164/rccm.201812-2276ST

Hernández, G., Roca, O., & Colinas, L. (2017). High-flow nasal cannula support therapy: New insights and improving performance. *Critical Care, 21*, 1–11. https://doi.org/10.1186/s13054-017-1640-2

Hess, D. R., MacIntyre, N. R., Galvin, W. F., & Mishoe, S. C. (2021). *Respiratory care: Principles and practice* (4th ed.). Jones & Bartlett Learning.

Higginson, R., Parry, A., & Williams, M. (2016). Airway management in the hospital environment. *British Journal of Nursing, 25*(2), 94–100. https://doi.org/10.12968/bjon.2016.25.2.94

Hinkle, J. L., Cheever, K. H., & Overbaugh, K. J. (2022). *Brunner & Suddarth's textbook of medical-surgical nursing* (15th ed.). Wolters Kluwer.

Hockenberry, M. J., Wilson, D., & Rodgers, C. C. (2019). *Wong's nursing care of infants and children* (11th ed.). Elsevier.

Holdman, J., Rozansky, C., & Baldwyn, T. (2020, January 10). *Reduction of respiratory device-related pressure injuries.* Respiratory Therapy Magazine. [Online]. https://rtmagazine.com/department-management/clinical/reduction-of-respiratory-device-related-pressure-injuries/

Hood, B. S., Henderson, W., & Pasero, C. (2014). Chest tube removal: An expanded role for the bedside nurse. *Journal of PeriAnesthesia Nursing, 29*(1), 53–59. https://doi.org/http://dx.doi.org/10.1016/j.jopan.2013.11.001

Imbriaco, G., & Monesi, A. (2021). Closed tracheal suctioning systems in the era of COVID-19: Is it time to consider them as a gold standard? *Journal of Infection Prevention, 22*(1), 44–45. https://doi.org/10.1177/1757177420963775

International Council of Nurses (ICN). (2019). *Nursing diagnosis and outcome statements.* https://www.icn.ch/sites/default/files/inline-files/ICNP2019-DC.pdf

Ireton, J. (2007). Tracheostomy suction: A protocol for practice. *Paediatric Nursing, 19*(10), 14–18.

Jacobs, S. S., Krishnan, J. A., Lederer, D. J., Ghazipura, M., Hossain, T., Tan, A. Y. M., Carlin, B., Drummond, M. B., Ekström, M., Garvey, C., Graney, B. A., Jackson, B., Kallstrom, T., Knight, S. L., Lindell, K., Prieto-Centurion, V., Renzoni, E. A., Ryerson, C. J., Schneidman, A., … on behalf of the American Thoracic Society Assembly on Nursing. (2020). Home oxygen therapy for adults with chronic lung disease. An official American Thoracic Society Clinical Practice Guideline. *American Journal of Respiratory and Critical Care Medicine, 202*(10), e121–e141. https://doi.org/10.1164/rccm.202009-3608ST

Jarvis, C., & Echkardt, A. (2020). *Physical examination & health assessment* (8th ed.). Elsevier.

Jeffries, M., Flanagan, J., Daviews, D., & Knoll, S. (2017). Evidence3 to support the use of occlusive dry sterile dressings for chest tubes. *MedSurg Nursing, 26*(3), 171–174.

Jensen, S. (2019). *Nursing health assessment. A best practice approach* (3rd ed.). Wolters Kluwer.

Jenson, H., Maddux, S., & Waldo, M. (2018). Improving oral care in hospitalized non-ventilated patients: Standardizing products and protocol. *MEDSURG Nursing, 27*(1), 38–45.

Johns Hopkins Medicine. (n.d.). *Tracheostomy service. Cleaning and caring for tracheostomy equipment.* https://www.hopkinsmedicine.org/tracheostomy/living/equipment_cleaning.html#trach

Johns Hopkins Medicine. (2021). *Occupational lung diseases.* https://www.hopkinsmedicine.org/health/conditions-and-diseases/occupational-lung-diseases

Joint Commission. (2018, July 23). Quick safety 43: Managing medical device-related pressure injuries. https://www.jointcommission.org/resources/news-and-multimedia/newsletters/newsletters/quick-safety/quick-safety-43-managing-medical-devicerelated-pressure-injuries/

Kane, C. J., York, N. L., & Minton, L. A. (2013). Chest tubes in the critically ill patient. *Dimensions of Critical Care Nursing, 32*(3), 111–117. https://doi.org/10.1097/DCC.0b013e3182864721

Karch, A. M. (2020). *Focus on nursing pharmacology* (8th ed.). Wolters Kluwer.

Karlsen, M. M. W., Ølnes, M. A., & Heyn, L. G. (2019). Communication with patients in intensive care units: A scoping review. *Nursing in Critical Care, 24*(3), 115–131. https://doi.org/10.1111/nicc.12377

Kelly-O'Flynn, S., Mohamud, L., & Copson, D. (2020). Medical adhesive-related skin injury. *British Journal of Nursing, 29*(6), S20–S26. https://doi.org/10.12968/bjon.2020.29.6.S20

Kendrick, A. (2020). Clinical guidelines (nursing). *Endotracheal tube suction of ventilated neonates.* The Royal Children's Hospital Melbourne. https://www.rch.org.au/rchcpg/hospital_clinical_guideline_index/Endotracheal_tube_suction_of_ventilated_neonates/

Kotta, P. A., & Ali, J. M. (2021). Incentive spirometry for prevention of postoperative pulmonary complications after thoracic surgery. *Respiratory Care, 66*(2), 327–333. https://doi.org/10.4187/respcare.07972

Krug, L., Machan, M., & Villalba, J. (2014). Securing the endotracheal tube with adhesive tape: An integrative literature review. *AANA Journal, 82*(6), 457–464.

Krug, L., Machan, M. D., & Villalba, J. (2016). Changing endotracheal tube taping practice: An evidence-based practice project. *AANA Journal, 84*(4), 261–270.

Kurt, O. K., Zhang, J., & Pinkerton, K. E. (2016). Pulmonary health effects of air pollution. *Current Opinion in Pulmonary Medicine, 22*(2), 138–143. https://doi.org/10.1097/MCP.0000000000000248

Kyle, T., & Carman, S. (2021). *Essentials of pediatric nursing* (4th ed.). Wolters Kluwer.

Leddy, R., & Wilkinson, J. M. (2015). Endotracheal suctioning practices of nurses and respiratory therapists: How well do they align with clinical practice guidelines? *Canadian Journal of Respiratory Therapy, 51*(3), 60–64. https://www.ncbi.nlm.nih.gov/pmc/articles/PMC4530836/

Liu, F., Shao, Q., Jiang, R., Zeng, Z., Liu, Y., LI, Y., Liu, Q., Ding, C., Zhao, N., Peng, Z., & Qian, K. (2019). High-flow oxygen therapy to speed weaning from mechanical ventilation: A prospective randomized study. *American Journal of Critical Care, 28*(5), 370–376. https://doi.org/10.4037/ajcc2019130

López-López, L., Torres-Sánchez, I., Cabrera-Martos, I., Ortíz-Rubio, A., Granados-Santiago, M., & Valenza, M. C. (2020). Nursing interventions improve continuous positive airway pressure adherence in obstructive sleep apnea with excessive daytime sleepiness: A systematic review. *Rehabilitation Nursing, 45*(3), 140–146. https://doi.org/10.1097/rnj.0000000000000190

Makic, M. B., Rauen, C., Jones, K., & Fisk, A. C. (2015). Continuing to challenge practice to be evidence based. *Critical Care Nurse, 35*(2), 39–50. https://doi.org/http://dx.doi.org/10.4037/ccn2015693

Maraş, G. B., Eşer, I., Şenoğlu, N., Yilmaz, N. Ö., & Derici, Y. K. (2020). Increasing suction pressure during endotracheal suctioning increases the volume of suctioned secretions, but not the procedure-related complications: A comparative study in open system endotracheal suctioning. *Intensive & Critical Care Nursing, 61*, 102928. https://doi.org/10.1016/j.iccn.2020.102928

Martin, T. J. (2020, August 19). *Treatment and prognosis of the obesity hypoventilation syndrome.* UpToDate. https://www.uptodate.com/contents/treatment-and-prognosis-of-the-obesity-hypoventilation-syndrome

Mayfield, S., Jauncey-Cooke, J., Hough, J. L., Schibler, A., Gibbons, K., & Bogossian, F. (2014). High-glow nasal cannula therapy for respiratory support in children. *Cochrane Database of Systematic Reviews, 2014*(3), CD009850. https://doi.org/10.1002/14651858.CD009850.pub2.

Mayo Foundation for Medical Education and Research (MFMER). (2018a, May 17). CPAP machines: Tips for avoiding 10 common problems. https://www.mayoclinic.org/diseases-conditions/sleep-apnea/in-depth/cpap/art-20044164

Mayo Foundation for Medical Education and Research (MFMER). (2018b, December 1). Hypoxemia. https://www.mayoclinic.org/symptoms/hypoxemia/basics/definition/sym-20050930

Mayo Foundation for Medical Education and Research (MFMER). (2020, April 9). Peak flow meter. https://www.mayoclinic.org/tests-procedures/peak-flow-meter/about/pac-20394858

MedlinePlus. (2020, January 12). *Oxygen safety.* https://medlineplus.gov/ency/patientinstructions/000049.htm

MedlinePlus. (2021, June 9). *Positive airway pressure treatment.* https://medlineplus.gov/ency/article/001916.htm

Mirza, S., Clay, R. D., Koslow, M. A., & Scanlon, P. D. (2018). COPD guidelines: A review of the 2018 GOLD report. *Mayo Clinic Proceedings, 93*(10), 1488–1502. https://doi.org/10.1016/j.mayocp.2018.05.026

Mitchell, J. (2015). Pathophysiology of COPD: Part 2. *Practice Nursing, 26*(9), 444–449. https://doi.org/10.12968/pnur.2015.26.9.444

Moore, Y., Shotton, E., Brown, R., Gremmel, J., Lindsey, S., & Pankey, J. (2018). Effects of incentive spirometry on perceived dyspnea in patients hospitalized with pneumonia. *MEDSURG Nursing, 27*(1), 19–37.

Morton, P. G., & Fontaine, D. K. (2018). *Critical care nursing. A holistic approach* (11th ed.). Wolters Kluwer.

Mussa, C. C., Gomaa, D., Rowley, D. D., Schmidt, U., Ginier, E., & Strickland, S. L. (2021). AARC clinical practice guideline: Management of adult patients with tracheostomy in the acute care setting. *Respiratory Care, 66*(1), 156–169. https://doi.org/https://doi.org/10.4187/respcare.08206

Mussa, C. C., Meksraityte, E., Li, J., Gulczynski, B., Liu, J., & Kuruc, A. (2018). Factors associated with endotracheal tube related pressure injury. *SM Journal of Nursing, 4*(1), 1018. https://jsmcentral.org/sm-nursing/smjn-v4-1018.pdf

Muzzy, A. C., & Butler, A. K. (2015). Managing chest tubes: Air leaks and unplanned tube removal. *American Nurse Today, 10*(5), 10–13. https://www.myamericannurse.com/managing-chest-tubes-air-leaks-unplanned-tube-removal/

National Fire Protection Association. (2016). *NFPA safety tip sheet: Medical oxygen.* https://www.nfpa.org/-/media/Files/Public-Education/Resources/Safety-tip-sheets/OxygenSafety.ashx

National Heart Lung and Blood Institute (NHLBI). (n.d.a). *CPAP. Also known as continuous positive airway pressure.* https://www.nhlbi.nih.gov/health-topics/cpap

National Heart, Lung, and Blood Institute (NHLBI). (2013). *COPD.* http://www.nhlbi.nih.gov/health/health-topics/topics/copd/atrisk

National Heart Lung and Blood Institute (NHLBI). (2019). COPD. Also known as chronic obstructive pulmonary disease, emphysema. https://www.nhlbi.nih.gov/health-topics/copd

Nishimura, M. (2016). High-flow nasal cannula oxygen therapy in adults: Physiological benefits, indication, clinical benefits, and adverse effects. *Respiratory Care, 61*(4), 529–541. https://doi.org/10.4187/respcare.04577

Norris, T. L. (2020). *Porth's essentials of pathophysiology* (5th ed.). Wolters Kluwer.

O'Driscoll, B. R., Howard, L. S., Earis, J., Mak, V., & British Thoracic Society Emergency Oxygen Guideline Group; on behalf of the British Thoracic Society Emergency Oxygen Guideline Group. (2017). BTS guideline for oxygen use in adults in healthcare and emergency settings. *Thorax, 72*(Supp 1), ii1–ii90. https://doi.org/10.1136/thoraxjnl-2016-209729

O'Toole, T. R., Jacobs, N., Hondorp, B., Crawford, L., Boudrereau, L. R., Jeffe, J., Stein, B., & LoSavio, P. (2017). Prevention of tracheostomy-related hospital-acquired pressure ulcers. *Otolaryngology—Head and Neck Surgery, 156*(4), 642–651. doi: 10.1177/0194599816689584

Owen, E. B., Woods, C. R., O'Flynn, J. A., Boone, M. C., Calhoun, A. W., & Montgomery V. L. (2016). A bedside decision tree for use of saline with endotracheal tube suctioning in children. *Critical Care Nurse, 36*(1), e1–e10. https://doi.org/http://dx.doi.org/10.4037/ccn2016358

Pacheco, D. (2021, July 8). *Continuous positive airway pressure (CPAP).* Sleep Foundation. https://www.sleepfoundation.org/cpap

Pasrija, D., & Hall, C. A. (2020, June 2). *Airway suctioning.* StatPearls. https://www.ncbi.nlm.nih.gov/books/NBK557386/

Pate, M., & Zapata, T. (2002). Ask the experts: How deeply should I go when I suction an endotracheal or tracheostomy tube? *Critical Care Nurse, 22*(2), 130–131.

Patton, J. (2019). Tracheostomy care. *British Journal of Nursing, 28*(16), 1060–1062. https://doi.org/10.12968/bjon.2019.28.16.1060

Pinto, V. L., & Sharma, S. (2021, May 7). *Continuous positive airway pressure.* StatPearls. https://www.ncbi.nlm.nih.gov/books/NBK482178/

Pittman, J., & Gillespie, C. (2020). Medical device-related pressure injuries. *Critical Care Nursing Clinics of North America, 32*(4), 533–542. https://doi.org/10.1016/j.cnc.2020.08.004

Quinn, B., Giuliano, K. K., & Baker, D. (2020). Non-ventilator health care-associated pneumonia (NV-HAP): Best practices for prevention of NV-HAP. *American Journal of Infection Control, 48*(5), A23–A27. https://doi.org/10.1016/j.ajic.2020.03.006

Raimundo, R. D., Sato, M. A., da Silva, T. D., de Abreu, L. C., Valenti, B. E., Riggs, D. W., & Carll, A. P. (2021). Open and closed endotracheal suction systems divergently affect pulmonary function in mechanically ventilated subjects. *Respiratory Care, 66*(5), 785–792. https://doi.org/10.4187/respcare.08511

Rolfe, S., & Paul, F. (2018). Oxygen therapy in adult patients. Part 2: Promoting safe and effective practice in patients' care and management. *British Journal of Nursing, 27*(17), 988–995. https://doi.org/10.12968/bjon.2018.27.17.988

Ruan, Q., Khasanah, I. H., Kongkeaw, O., & Maneewat, K. (2017). Pain management during endotracheal tube suctioning: An evidence-based approach for nurses. *Nursing & Primary Care, 1*(4), 1–3. https://www.scivisionpub.com/pdfs/pain-management-during-endotracheal-tube-suctioning-an-evidencebased-approach-for-nurses-168.pdf

Sasa, R. I. (2019). Evidence-based update on chest tube management. *American Nurse Today, 14*(4), 4. XXX

Schreiber, M. L. (2015). Tracheostomy: Site care, suctioning, and readiness. *MEDSURG Nursing, 24*(2), 121–124.

Silbert-Flagg, J., & Pillitteri, A. (2018). *Maternal and child health nursing* (8th ed.). Wolters Kluwer.

Sjoding, M. W., Dickson, R. P., Iwashyna, T. J., Gay, S. E., & Valley, T. S. (2020). Racial bias in pulse oximetry measurement. *New England Journal of Medicine, 383*(25), 2477–2478. https://doi.org/10.1056/NEJMc2029240

Sole, M. L., Bennet, M. B., & Ashworth, S. (2015). Clinical indicators for endotracheal suctioning in adult patients receiving mechanical ventilation. *American Journal of Critical Care, 24*(4), 318–324. https://doi.org/10.4037/ajcc2015794

Stanford Children's Health. (2021). *Respiratory distress syndrome (RDS) in premature babies.* https://www.stanfordchildrens.org/en/topic/default?id=respiratory-distress-syndrome-90-P02371

Sterni, L. M., Collaco, J. M., Baker, C. D., Carroll, J. L., Sharma, G. D., Brozek, J. L., Finder, J. D., Ackerman, V. L., Arens, R., Boroughs, D. S., Carter, J., Daigle, K. L., Dougherty, J., Gozal, D., Kevill, K., Kravitz, R. M., Kriseman, T., MacLusky, I., Rivera-Spoljaric, K., … ATS Pediatric Chronic Home Ventilation Workgroup. (2016). An official American Thoracic Society Clinical Practice Guideline: Pediatric chronic home invasive ventilation. *American Journal of Respiratory and Critical Care Medicine, 193*(8), e16–e35. https://doi.org/10.1164/rccm.201602-0276ST

Suni, E. (2020, September 11). *How to use a CPAP machine for better sleep.* Sleep Foundation. https://www.sleepfoundation.org/cpap/how-to-use-cpap-machine

Taylor, C., Lynn, P., & Bartlett, J. (2023). *Fundamentals of nursing: The art and science of person-centered care* (10th ed.). Wolters Kluwer.

Tolotti, A., Bagnasco, A., Catania, G., Aleo, G., Pagnucci, N., Cadorin, L., Zanini, M., Rocco, G., Stievano, A., Carnevale, F. A., & Sasso, L. (2018). The communication experience of tracheostomy patients with nurses in the intensive care unit: A phenomenological study. *Intensive & Critical Care Nursing, 46*, 24–31. https://doi.org/10.1016/j.iccn.2018.01.001

Turner, M. A., Feeney, M., & Deeds, J. L. (2020). Improving endotracheal cuff inflation pressures: An evidence-based project in a military medical center. *AANA Journal, 88*(3), 203–208.

Turner, M. C., Andersen, Z. J., Baccarelli, A., Diver, W. R., Gapstur, S. M., Pope, C. A. III, Prada, D., Samet, J., Thurston, G., & Cohen, A. (2020). Outdoor air pollution and cancer: An overview of the current evidence and public health recommendations. *CA: A Cancer Journal for Clinicians, 70*, 460–479. https://doi.org/org/10.3322/caac.21632

Upvall, M. J., Bourgault, A. M., Pigon, C., & Swartzman, C. A. (2019). Exemplars illustrating de-implementation of tradition-based practices. *Critical Care Nurse, 39*(6), 64–69. https://doi.org/10.4037/ccn2019534

U.S. Food and Drug Administration (USFDA). (2021, February 19). *Pulse oximeter accuracy and limitations: FDA safety communication.* https://www.fda.gov/medical-devices/safety-communications/pulse-oximeter-accuracy-and-limitations-fda-safety-communication

VHA Center for Engineering & Occupational Safety and Health (CEOSH). (2016). Safe patient handling and mobility guidebook. http://www.tnpatientsafety.com/pubfiles/Initiatives/workplace-violence/sphm-pdf.pdf

Walters, H. R., Young, H. E., & Young, P. J. (2018). A modified tie technique for securing endotracheal tubes. *Respiratory Care, 63*(4), 424–429. doi: 10.4187/respcare.05655

Wang, C. H., Tsai, J. C., Chen, S. F., Su, C. L., Chen, L., Lin, C. C., & Tam, K. W. (2017). Normal saline installation before suctioning: A meta-analysis of randomized controlled trials. *Australian Critical Care, 30*(5), 260–265. https://doi.org/10.1016/j.aucc.2016.11.001

Wolters Kluwer. (2022). Problem-based care plans. In *Lippincott Advisor.* Wolters Kluwer.

Wood, M. D., Powers, J., & Rechter, J. L. (2019). Comparative evaluation of chest tube insertion site dressings: A randomized controlled trial. *American Journal of Critical Care, 28*(6), 415–423. https://doi.org/10.4037/ajcc2019645

World Health Organization (WHO). (2011). Patient safety. Using the pulse oximeter. http://www.who.int/patientsafety/safesurgery/pulse_oximetry/who_ps_pulse_oxymetry_tutorial2_advanced_en.pdf

Wrona, S. K., Quinlan-Colwell, A., Brown, L., & Jannuzzi, R. G. E. (2021, December 27). Procedural pain management: Clinical practice recommendations American Society for Pain Management Nursing. *Pain Management Nursing*, S1524-9042(21)00245-9. Advance online publication. https://doi.org/10.1016/j.pmn.2021.11.008

Yarahmadi, S., Mohammadi, N., Ardalan, A., Najafizadeh, H., & Gholami, M. (2018). The combined effects of cold therapy and music therapy on pain following chest tube removal among patients with cardiac bypass surgery. *Complementary Therapies in Clinical Practice, 31,* 71–75. https://doi.org/10.1016/j.ctcp.2018.01.006

Yazdannik, A., Saghaei, M., Haghighat, S., & Eghbali-Babadi, M. (2019). Efficacy of closed endotracheal suctioning in critically ill patients: A clinical trial of comparing two levels of negative suctioning pressure. *Journal of Nursing Practice Today, 6*(2), 60–67.

Yönt, G. H., Korhan, E. A., & Dizer, B. (2014). The effect of nail polish on pulse oximetry readings. *Intensive and Critical Care Nursing, 30*(2), 111–115. https://doi.org/10.1016/j.iccn.2013.08.003

Zemach, S., Helviz, Y., Shitrit, M., Friedman, R., & Levin, P. D. (2019). The use of high-flow nasal cannula oxygen outside the ICU. *Respiratory Care, 64*(11), 1333–1342. https://doi.org/10.4187/respcare.06611

Zisis, C., Tsirgogianni, K., Lazaridis, G., Lampaki, S., Baka, S., Mpoukovinas, I., Karavasilis, V., Kioumis, I., Pitsiou, G., Katsikogiannis, N., Tsakiridis, K., Rapti, A., Trakada, G., Karapantzos, I., Karapantzou, C., Zissimopoulos, A., Zarogoulidis, K., & Zarogoulidis, P. (2015). Chest drainage systems in use. *Annals of Translational Medicine, 3*(3), 43. https://doi.org/10.3978/j.issn.2305-5839.2015.02.09

SUGGESTED ANSWERS FOR FOCUSING ON PATIENT CARE: DEVELOPING CLINICAL REASONING AND CLINICAL JUDGMENT

1. Notify the health care team immediately. This can indicate fresh bleeding. Assess the patient's vital signs and level of consciousness. Significant changes from baseline may indicate complications. Assess the patient's respiratory status, including oxygen saturation level. The patient may become tachypneic and hypoxic. Assess the patient's lung sounds. The lung sounds over the chest tube site may be diminished due to the presence of increased blood. Also assess the patient for pain. Sudden pressure or increased pain indicates potential complications. Reassure the patient, as necessary, to decrease anxiety. Maintain the patient on bed rest and monitor closely. Anticipate the need for additional IV fluids or blood transfusions, as well as the potential for surgery to control the bleeding.

2. Assess the patient's level of knowledge regarding the use of an incentive spirometer. Assess the patient's level of pain. Administer pain medication, as prescribed, if needed. Wait the appropriate amount of time for the medication to take effect. Explain the rationale for use of an incentive spirometer and the goal of the activity. If the patient has recently undergone abdominal or chest surgery, place a pillow or folded blanket over a chest or abdominal incision for splinting. Demonstrate how to steady the device with one hand and hold the mouthpiece with the other hand. If the patient cannot use hands, assist the patient with the incentive spirometer. Instruct the patient to exhale normally and then place lips securely around the mouthpiece. Instruct the patient to inhale slowly and as deeply as possible through the mouthpiece without using the nose (if necessary, a nose clip may be used). When the patient cannot inhale anymore, the patient should hold their breath and count to three. Check the position of gauge to determine progress and level attained. If the patient begins to cough, splint an abdominal or chest incision. Instruct the patient to remove lips from mouthpiece and exhale normally. If the patient becomes lightheaded during the process, tell their to stop and take a few normal breaths before resuming incentive spirometry. Encourage the patient to perform incentive spirometry 5 to 10 times every 1 to 2 hours, if possible. Clean the mouthpiece with water and shake to dry. Patient should verbalize an understanding of the rationale, procedure, and cleaning of equipment and be able to give a return demonstration of the use of the incentive spirometer.

3. Assess lung sounds. Patients who need to be suctioned may have crackles or gurgling present. Assess oxygen saturation level. Oxygen saturation usually decreases when a patient needs to be suctioned. Assess respiratory status, including respiratory rate and depth. Patients may become tachypneic when they need to be suctioned. Assess patient for signs of respiratory distress, such as nasal flaring, retractions, or grunting. Additional indications for suctioning via an endotracheal tube include secretions in the tube, acute respiratory distress, and frequent or sustained coughing. Also assess for pain and the potential to cause pain during the intervention. Individualized pain management must be performed in response to the patient's needs (Arroyo-Novoa et al., 2008; Chaseling et al., 2014; Wrona et al., 2021; Düzkaya & Kuğuoğlu, 2015). If the patient has had abdominal surgery or other procedures, administer pain medication before suctioning. Assess appropriate suction catheter depth (refer to Box 14-2 in Skill 14-9). Determine if suctioning the patient's airway was effective by reassessing the patient. The symptoms that indicated the need for airway suctioning should be absent or greatly diminished. The patient should not exhibit signs of respiratory distress and should have an oxygen saturation level within normal limits.

15

Perfusion and Cardiovascular Care

Focusing on Patient Care

This chapter will help you develop some of the skills related to perfusion and cardiovascular care necessary to care for the following patients:

Coby Pruder, age 40, is to undergo an electrocardiogram as part of a physical examination. Although they report feeling healthy, they are also nervous.

Harry Stebbings, age 67, is admitted to the emergency department for chest pain and cardiac monitoring.

Ann Kribell, age 54, is a patient in the cardiac care unit. Ann has been diagnosed with heart failure and is receiving cardiac monitoring. The cardiac monitoring alarms are alarming very frequently, multiple times an hour.

Refer to Focusing on Patient Care: Developing Clinical Reasoning and Clinical Judgment at the end of the chapter to apply what you learn.

Learning Outcomes

After completing the chapter, you will be able to accomplish the following:

1. Perform cardiopulmonary resuscitation.
2. Perform emergency automated external defibrillation.
3. Perform emergency manual external defibrillation (asynchronous).
4. Obtain a 12-lead electrocardiogram.
5. Apply a cardiac monitor.
6. Apply and monitor a transcutaneous (external) pacemaker.
7. Remove a peripheral arterial catheter.

Nursing Concepts

- Assessment
- Clinical Decision Making/Clinical Judgment
- Perfusion
- Safety
- Tissue Integrity

Life depends on a constant supply of oxygen. This demand for oxygen is met by the function of the respiratory and cardiovascular systems, together known as the cardiopulmonary system. Gas exchange, the intake of oxygen and the release of carbon dioxide, is made possible by the respiratory system (refer to Chapter 14). The cardiovascular system (Fig. 14-2 in Chapter 14) delivers oxygen to the cells. Perfusion of body tissues depends on essentially three factors:

- Integrity of the airway system to transport air to and from the lungs
- A properly functioning alveolar system in the lungs to oxygenate venous blood and to remove carbon dioxide from the blood
- A properly functioning cardiovascular system and blood supply to carry nutrients and wastes to and from body cells

The cardiovascular system is composed of the heart and the blood vessels. The heart is the main organ of **circulation**, which is the continuous one-way circuit of blood through the blood vessels (Norris, 2020). The heart is the circulatory pump, squeezing through the heart and out into the body. This is accomplished by contractions starting in the atria, followed by contraction of the ventricles, with a subsequent resting of the heart. Figure 15-1 provides an overview of cardiac anatomy. Deoxygenated blood (low in oxygen; high in carbon dioxide) is carried from the right side of the heart to the lungs, where oxygen is picked up and carbon dioxide is released, and then returned to the left side of the heart. This oxygenated blood (high in oxygen; low in carbon dioxide) is pumped out to all other parts of the body and back again (refer to Fig. 14-2 in Chapter 14). The contraction of the muscles of the heart is controlled by electrical impulses produced in and carried over specialized tissue within the heart. These tissues make up the heart's conduction system. Figure 15-2 provides a review of the cardiac conduction system.

Assessment of cardiovascular function commonly involves noninvasive techniques such as inspection, auscultation, and palpation. Additional basic and important indicators of the heart's effectiveness are pulse rate, strength, and rhythm; blood pressure; skin color and temperature; and level of consciousness. Refer to Chapters 2 and 3 for additional information related to these assessments. Chapter 14 provides additional information related to oxygenation and cardiopulmonary function.

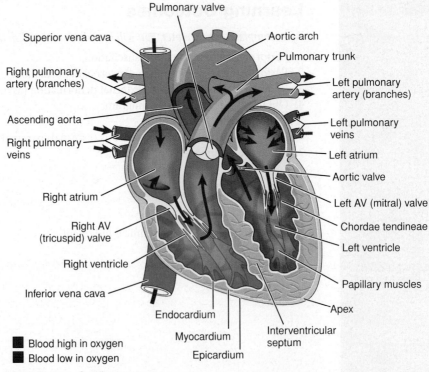

FIGURE 15-1. Cardiac anatomy.

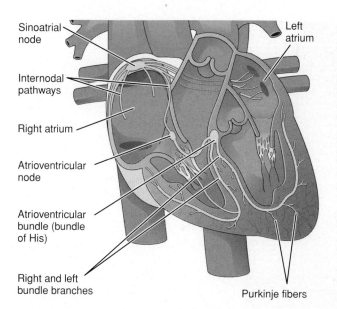

Sinoatrial node

Left atrium

Internodal pathways

Right atrium

Atrioventricular node

Atrioventricular bundle (bundle of His)

Right and left bundle branches

Purkinje fibers

FIGURE 15-2. Cardiac conduction system.

   This chapter covers select skills necessary for the nurse to promote perfusion and provide cardiovascular care. While performing skills related to perfusion, keep in mind factors that affect cardiopulmonary function, leading to impaired perfusion, and how these factors might affect a particular patient (see Fundamentals Review 14-1 in Chapter 14). Chapter 14 presents skills related to oxygenation, which assist nurses in providing cardiovascular care. Should the heart stop pumping, it can be manually pumped via **cardiopulmonary resuscitation (CPR)** until electrical **defibrillation** and additional health care support arrives. Noninvasive heart monitoring involves **electrocardiography** and **cardiac monitoring**. Figure 15-3 highlights cardiac landmark reference lines that are used in assessment and for placing devices related to perfusion and cardiovascular care, such as a transcutaneous (external) pacemaker. Other electrical therapy devices are discussed in Fundamentals Review 15-1.

   Invasive techniques, such as pulmonary artery pressure monitoring, Swan-Ganz catheterization, cardiac output determination, and cardiac support via an intra-aortic balloon pump (IABP) typically are used by trained critical care personnel to provide additional monitoring and support. These techniques are beyond the scope of this text.

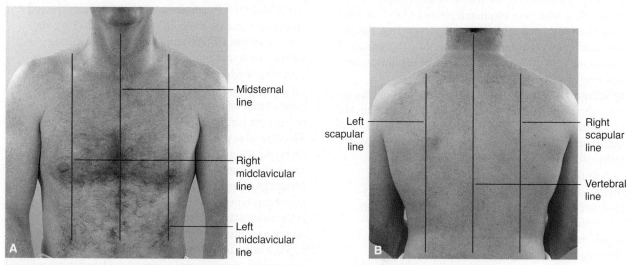

Midsternal line

Right midclavicular line

Left midclavicular line

Left scapular line

Right scapular line

Vertebral line

A

B

FIGURE 15-3. Cardiac landmarks: Reference lines. **A.** Anterior chest. **B.** Posterior chest. (*continued*)

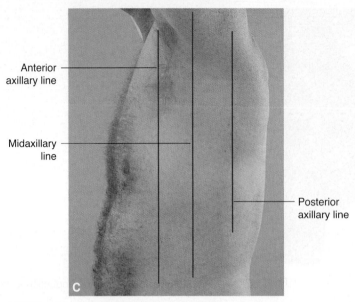

Anterior
axillary line

Midaxillary
line

Posterior
axillary line

C

FIGURE 15-3. (*Continued*) **C.** Lateral chest.

Fundamentals Review 15-1

ELECTRICAL THERAPY DEVICES

In addition to defibrillation, electrical therapy may be delivered via the following devices:

- **Implantable cardioverter–defibrillator (ICD)** is a sophisticated device that automatically discharges an electric current to provide bradycardia and antitachycardia pacing, synchronized cardioversion, and defibrillation (convert abnormal cardiac rhythms to normal sinus rhythm) when it senses ventricular bradycardia and tachyarrhythmias. Patients with a history of ventricular fibrillation or ventricular tachycardia, with poor ejection fraction (<35%), or with nonischemic dilated cardiomyopathy (New York Heart Association [NYHA] functional class II or III), as well as patients with other conditions may be candidates for this type of device (Morton & Fontaine, 2018).
- **Synchronized cardioversion** is the treatment of choice for arrhythmias that do not respond to vagal maneuvers or to drug therapy, such as atrial tachycardia, atrial flutter, atrial fibrillation, and symptomatic ventricular tachycardia. Cardioversion is performed similarly to defibrillation but is synchronized with the heart rhythm and uses fewer joules. Cardioversion works by delivering an electrical charge to the myocardium at the peak of the R wave. This causes immediate depolarization, interrupting reentry circuits, and allowing the sinoatrial node to resume control. Synchronizing the electrical charge with the R wave ensures that the current will not be delivered on the vulnerable T wave and thus disrupting repolarization.

It is usually performed in a critical care area, in the presence of a physician, an anesthesiologist, and emergency equipment. The patient is sedated as the procedure is painful (Burns & Delgado, 2019).
- **Pacemakers** are electronic devices that can be used to initiate the heartbeat when the heart's intrinsic electrical system cannot effectively generate a rate adequate to support cardiac output. Pacemakers are used to treat some arrhythmias and may be used for patients with heart failure to improve cardiac output (NHLBI, 2021). Pacemakers can be temporary: placed on the skin (transcutaneous) (refer to Skill 15-6); via temporary epicardial pacing wires inserted during surgery; or transvenous via a pacing electrode wire passed through a vein (the brachial, internal, or external jugular, subclavian, or femoral) and into the right atrium or right ventricle. Pacemakers can also be permanent surgically implanted devices.
- **Biventricular pacemakers** (cardiac resynchronization therapy pacing device) use electrical current to improve synchronization of left ventricular contraction. Biventricular pacemakers are used in patients with heart failure (NYHA class III or IV), with an intraventricular conduction delay (QRS >120 ms), and in patients with left ventricular ejection fraction <35%. These devices improve right and left ventricle contraction, resulting in improved cardiac function, with improved ejection fraction (Cleveland Clinic, 2019).

Skill 15-1 ▶ Performing Cardiopulmonary Resuscitation

The American Heart Association (AHA, 2020b) identifies interventions to provide emergency cardiovascular care, using the metaphor "Chain of Survival." Elements of this emergency care include cardiopulmonary resuscitation (CPR), the combination of chest compressions (to circulate blood), mouth-to-mouth breathing (to supply oxygen to the lungs), and defibrillation (to interrupt or stop an abnormal heart rhythm using controlled electrical shocks). The elements and order of actions in the Chain of Survival differ based on the situation, whether the patient has the cardiac arrest outside the hospital or inside the hospital and whether the patient is an adult, child, or infant (AHA, 2020b). The brain is very sensitive to hypoxia, and damage to the brain begins to occur within minutes without oxygen; after 5 minutes, permanent anoxic brain injury can occur (Headway, 2021; Lacerte et al., 2020). The faster emergency cardiovascular care (CPR) is initiated, the greater the chance of survival (AHA, 2020b).

After making sure the environment is safe for rescuers and the patient and checking the patient for responsiveness, health care providers in the hospital activate the emergency response system, get an automated external defibrillator (AED) or defibrillator and emergency equipment, and begin CPR. In the health care setting, it is imperative that personnel be aware of the patient's stated instructions regarding any wish not to be resuscitated. This should be clearly expressed and documented in the patient's health record.

The AHA provides guidelines related to emergency interventions outside of health care facilities. Learning conventional CPR is still recommended, and trained lay rescuers should provide rescue breaths in addition to chest compressions (AHA, 2020a). However, the AHA guidelines recommend that when a teen or adult suddenly collapses, untrained lay bystanders should call 911 (activate the emergency response system) and push hard and fast in the center of the patient's chest (AHA, 2020a). These two steps, called Hands-Only CPR, can be as effective as conventional CPR (AHA, 2021). Providing Hands-Only CPR to a teen or adult who has collapsed from a sudden **cardiac arrest** can more than double or triple that person's chance of survival (AHA, 2021).

DELEGATION CONSIDERATIONS	The initiation and provision of cardiopulmonary resuscitation is appropriate for all health care providers.
EQUIPMENT	• PPE, such as a face shield or one-way valve mask and gloves, if available • Bag-valve-mask device and oxygen, if available • Automated external defibrillator (Skill 15-2 details use) or • Manual external defibrillator (Skill 15-3 details use)
ASSESSMENT	Assess the patient's vital parameters and determine the patient's level of responsiveness. Check for partial or complete airway obstruction. Assess for the absence or ineffectiveness of respirations. Assess for the absence of signs of circulation and pulses.
ACTUAL OR POTENTIAL HEALTH PROBLEMS AND NEEDS	Many actual or potential health problems or issues may require the use of this skill as part of related interventions. An appropriate health problem or issue may include: • Impaired cardiac output • Impaired gas exchange • Altered breathing pattern
OUTCOME IDENTIFICATION AND PLANNING	The expected outcome to achieve when performing CPR is that CPR is performed effectively without adverse effect to the patient. Additional outcomes include that the patient regains a pulse and respirations; the patient's heart and lungs maintain adequate function to sustain life; advanced cardiac life support (ACLS) is initiated, if indicated; and the patient does not experience serious injury.

(continued on page 962)

Skill 15-1 ▶ Performing Cardiopulmonary Resuscitation *(continued)*

IMPLEMENTATION

ACTION	RATIONALE

1. Verify scene safety. Check for responsiveness in the patient. Call for help, pull the call bell, and call the facility emergency response number. Call for emergency equipment and the AED or defibrillator, if available.

   Verification of scene safety makes sure the environment is safe for rescuers and the patient. Assessing responsiveness prevents starting CPR on a conscious patient. Activating the emergency response system initiates a rapid response, and accessing equipment supports appropriate interventions.

2. Put on gloves, if available. Position the patient supine on their back on a firm, flat surface, with their arms alongside their body. If the patient is in bed, place a backboard or other rigid surface under them (often the footboard of the patient's bed). Position yourself at the patient's side.

   Gloves prevent contact with blood and body fluids. The supine position is required for resuscitative efforts and evaluation to be effective. A firm surface allows compression of the chest and heart to create adequate blood flow (AHA, 2020b). A backboard provides a firm surface on which to apply compressions.

3. **Provide defibrillation (if indicated) at the earliest possible moment, as soon as an AED becomes available.** Refer to Skills 15-2 and 15-3.

   Early defibrillation (along with high-quality CPR and all components of the Chain of Survival) is necessary to improve chances of survival from pulseless ventricular tachycardia and ventricular **fibrillation** (AHA, 2020b). The AED quickly delivers a shock (defibrillation) to the heart muscle to interrupt shockable rhythms and resets the heart's electrical system so a normal (organized) heart rhythm can return (AHA, 2020b).

4. Simultaneously look for no breathing or only gasping and check for a pulse, palpating the carotid pulse, for no more than 10 seconds. If the patient has no breathing or is only gasping and no pulse is felt, begin CPR using the compression/ventilation ratio of 30 compressions to two breaths, starting with chest compressions (**CAB sequence**) (Step 5). Alternatively, if there is no normal breathing but the patient has a pulse, see Step 14. Alternatively, if the patient is breathing normally and has a pulse, monitor until advanced care providers take over.

   Pulse assessment evaluates cardiac function. Gasping is not normal breathing and is a sign of cardiac arrest (AHA, 2020b). Delays in chest compressions should be minimized, so the health care provider should take no more than 10 seconds to check for a pulse. If it is not felt within that time period, chest compressions should be started (AHA, 2020b).

   Rescue breathing should be provided to maintain effective oxygenation and ventilation (AHA, 2020b).

5. **Chest compressions (C):** Position the heel of one of your hands in the center of the patient's chest between the nipples, directly over the lower half of the sternum. Place the heel of your other hand directly on top of your first hand. Extend or interlace your fingers to keep them above the chest. Straighten your arms and position your shoulders directly over your hands (Figure 1). Alternatively, put one hand on the patient's sternum to push on the chest and grasp the wrist of that hand with your other hand to support the first hand as you push down on the chest (Figure 2) (AHA, 2020b).

   Proper hand positioning ensures that the force of compressions is on the sternum, ensuring that the chest compressions are as effective as possible.

6. Push hard and fast. Chest compressions should depress the sternum to a depth of at least 2 inches (adult). Push straight down on the patient's sternum. Perform 30 chest compressions at a rate of 100–120/min, counting "1, 2, etc." up to 30, keeping your elbows locked, arms straight, and shoulders directly over your hands (refer to Figure 1). Allow full chest recoil (reexpansion) after each compression. **Do not lean on chest wall between compressions.** Chest compression and chest recoil/relaxation times should be approximately equal (AHA, 2020b).

   Direct cardiac compression and manipulation of intrathoracic pressure supply blood flow during CPR. Compressing the chest at least 2 inches ensures that compressions are not too shallow and provides adequate blood flow. Full chest recoil allows adequate venous return to the heart. Avoid leaning on the chest wall between compressions to ensure complete chest recoil (AHA, 2020b).

7. Ventilate using a barrier device (face mask or bag-valve-mask device, if available, or face shield) (refer to Skill 14-16 in Chapter 14). Give two breaths (as described below) after each set of 30 compressions. Cycles of 30 compressions and 2 ventilations are recommended (AHA, 2020b).

   Breathing and compressions simulate lung and heart function, providing oxygen and circulation.

ACTION

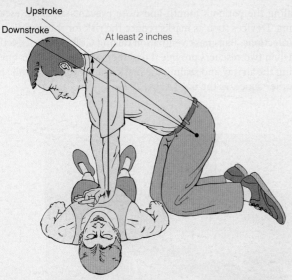

FIGURE 1. Using correct body alignment for chest compressions. Depress the sternum 2 inches.

8. **Airway (A):** Use the head tilt–chin lift maneuver to open the patient's airway (Figure 3). Place one hand on the patient's forehead and apply firm, backward pressure with your palm to tilt the head back. Place the fingers of your other hand under the bony part of the lower jaw near the chin and lift the jaw upward to bring the chin forward.

9. **If trauma to the head or neck is present or suspected,** use the jaw-thrust maneuver to open the airway (Figure 4). Position yourself at the patient's head. Place one hand on each side of the patient's head. Rest your elbows on the flat surface under the patient, grasp the angle of the patient's lower jaw, and lift with both hands, displacing the jaw forward. If the jaw thrust does not open the airway, use the head tilt–chin lift maneuver (AHA, 2020b).

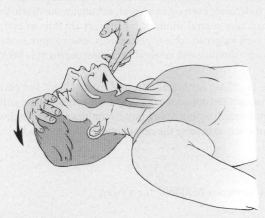

FIGURE 3. Using the head tilt–chin lift method to open the airway.

RATIONALE

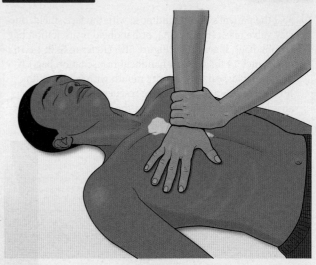

FIGURE 2. Alternate hand position for chest compressions.

The head tilt–chin lift maneuver lifts the tongue, relieving airway obstruction by the tongue in an unresponsive person (AHA, 2020b).

The jaw-thrust maneuver may reduce neck and spine movement.

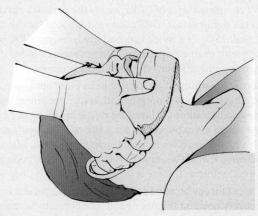

FIGURE 4. Using the jaw-thrust maneuver to open the airway.

(continued on page 964)

Skill 15-1 ▶ Performing Cardiopulmonary Resuscitation *(continued)*

ACTION

10. Seal the patient's mouth and nose with the face shield, one-way valve mask (Figure 5A), or handheld resuscitation bag (Ambu bag), if available (Figure 5B). (Refer to Skill 14-16 in Chapter 14 for use of a handheld resuscitation bag.) If not available, seal the patient's mouth with your mouth. If two rescuers are present, one rescuer should open the airway and seal the mask against the face, while the other rescuer squeezes the bag (AHA, 2020b).

RATIONALE

Sealing the patient's mouth and nose prevents air from escaping. Devices such as masks reduce the risk for transmission of infections. Bag-mask ventilation during CPR is more effective when two rescuers provide it together, with one rescuer opening the airway and sealing the mask against the face, while the other squeezes the bag (AHA, 2020b).

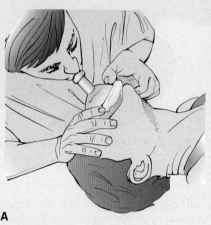
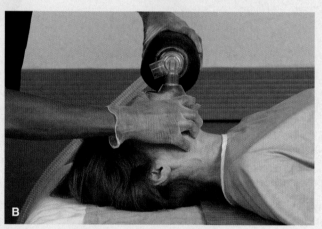

A   **B**

FIGURE 5. A. Using a one-way valve mask. **B.** Using a handheld resuscitation bag. (*Source:* Used with permission from Shutterstock. *Photo by B. Proud.*)

11. **Breathing (B):** Instill two breaths, each lasting 1 second, making the chest rise.

Breathing into the patient provides oxygen to the patient's lungs. Noting the rise of the chest affirms adequate ventilation.

12. If you are unable to ventilate or the chest does not rise during ventilation, reposition the patient's head and reattempt to ventilate. If still unable to ventilate, resume CPR. Each subsequent time the airway is opened to administer breaths, look for an object. If an object is visible in the mouth, remove it. If no object is visible, continue with CPR.

Inability to ventilate indicates that the airway may be obstructed. Repositioning maneuvers may be sufficient to open the airway and promote spontaneous respirations. It is critical to minimize interruptions in chest compressions to maintain circulatory perfusion.

13. After about 2 minutes (until prompted by AED or about five complete cycles of CPR), **assess the patient's rhythm on the defibrillator**. Defibrillate as indicated (see Skill 15-2 or Skill 15-3). If a shock is not advised, resume CPR, beginning with chest compressions. Do not recheck to see if there is a pulse. Follow the AED voice prompts.

This evaluates cardiac function. Resuming CPR provides optimal treatment. Even when a shock eliminates the dysrhythmia it may take several minutes for a heart rhythm to establish and even longer to achieve perfusion. Chest compressions can provide coronary and cerebral perfusion during this period.

14. **Rescue breathing:** If the patient has a pulse but is not breathing normally, continue with rescue breathing, without chest compressions. Administer rescue breathing at a rate of one breath every 6 seconds, for a rate of 10 breaths/min. If the situation involves a possible opioid overdose, administer naloxone if available, as per protocol. Check the pulse about every 2 minutes. If there is no pulse, begin CPR (Step 5).

Rescue breathing maintains adequate oxygenation. For patients with suspected opioid overdose who are unresponsive with no normal breathing but have a pulse, administration of naloxone is indicated to reverse the opioid effects (AHA, 2020b).

15. If spontaneous breathing resumes, place the patient in the recovery position (Figure 6) and monitor until advance care providers take over.

This prevents obstruction of the airway.

16. Otherwise, continue CPR and use of the AED until advanced care providers take over, the patient starts to breathe or move or otherwise react, you are too exhausted to continue, or an advanced health care provider discontinues CPR.

Once started, CPR must continue until one of these conditions is met. In an acute care setting, help should arrive within a few minutes.

ACTION	**RATIONALE**

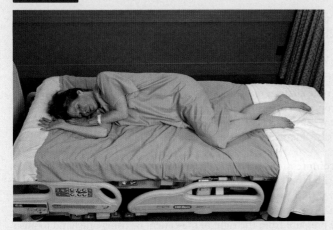

FIGURE 6. Recovery position. (*Source:* Used with permission from Shutterstock. *Photo by B. Proud.*)

 17. Remove gloves, if used. Perform hand hygiene.

Proper removal of PPE reduces the risk for infection transmission and contamination of other items. Hand hygiene prevents transmission of microorganisms.

EVALUATION

The expected outcomes have been met when CPR has been performed effectively without adverse effect to the patient, the patient has regained a pulse and respirations, the patient's heart and lungs have maintained adequate function to sustain life, ACLS has been initiated, and the patient has not experienced serious injury.

DOCUMENTATION

Guidelines

Document the time the patient was discovered unresponsive and CPR was initiated. Continued intervention, such as by the code team, is typically documented on a code form, which identifies the actions and drugs provided during the code. Provide a summary of these events in the patient's health record.

Sample Documentation

07/06/25 2230 Called to patient's room by wife. Patient noted to be without evidence of respirations or circulation. Emergency response system activated, CPR initiated. See code sheet.

—B. Clapp, RN

DEVELOPING CLINICAL REASONING AND CLINICAL JUDGMENT

UNEXPECTED SITUATIONS AND ASSOCIATED INTERVENTIONS

- *When performing chest compression, there is an audible crack:* Be aware that this sound most commonly indicates cracking of the ribs. Recheck your hand position. Then continue compressions.
- *You find a patient lying on the floor:* Determine the patient's level of responsiveness. If the patient is unresponsive, quickly clear an area, call for assistance and AED, and begin CPR as indicated.

(continued on page 966)

Skill 15-1 ▶ Performing Cardiopulmonary Resuscitation *(continued)*

SPECIAL CONSIDERATIONS

General Considerations

- Every effort should be taken to minimize interruptions in chest compressions. A shorter duration of interruptions in chest compressions is associated with better outcomes (AHA, 2020b).
- Do not move the patient while CPR is in progress unless the patient is in a dangerous environment (such as a burning building), or you believe you cannot perform CPR effectively under the current circumstances; the resuscitation team may choose to continue CPR at the scene or transport the patient to an appropriate environment (AHA, 2020b).
- Perform CPR in the same manner if the patient is obese. Techniques may need to be adjusted in the presence of morbid obesity, due to the physical attributes of individual patients (AHA, 2020b).
- Do not delay providing chest compressions for a pregnant woman in cardiac arrest. Perform CPR for pregnant patients using the same guidelines. Perform continuous manual lateral uterine displacement (LUD) for visibly pregnant women (approximately 20 weeks'; uterus at or above the umbilicus) if additional rescuers are present (AHA, 2020b). Manually move the uterus to the patient's left to relieve the pressure from the right of the patient by using one hand to push upward and leftward off the maternal vessels, or from the left of the patient, using two hands to cup and lift up and leftward off the maternal vessels; LUD relieves the pressure of the uterus on the large blood vessels in the abdomen, to improve blood flow to the heart (AHA, 2020b).
- If it is not possible to seal the patient's mouth completely for reasons such as oral trauma, perform mouth-to-nose breathing. If the patient has a tracheostomy, provide ventilation through the tracheostomy instead of the mouth.
- A nonconventional CPR approach has been suggested for patients with an advanced airway in the prone position if turning the patient supine would lead to delays or risk to providers or patients (Bhatnager et al., 2018). Compressions in the prone position are delivered on the thoracic spine (T7/T10), 0 to 2 vertebral segments below the scapulae (reversed precordial compressions) (Bhatnager et al., 2018; Douma et al., 2020; Edelson et al., 2020). Evidence on the provision of CPR in the prone position is ongoing and further research is needed (Moscarelli et al., 2020).
- The AHA provides guidelines related to emergency interventions outside of health care facilities. Learning conventional CPR is recommended, and trained lay rescuers should provide rescue breaths in addition to chest compressions (AHA, 2020b). However, when a teen or adult suddenly collapses, untrained lay bystanders should call 911 (to activate the emergency response system), and push hard and fast in the center of the patient's chest (AHA, 2021). These two steps, called Hands-Only CPR, can be as effective as conventional CPR (AHA, 2021). Providing Hands-Only CPR to a teen or adult who has collapsed from a sudden cardiac arrest can more than double or triple that person's chance of survival (AHA, 2021). The AHA (2021) still recommends CPR with compressions and breaths for infants and children, victims of drowning or drug overdose, and for people who have collapsed due to breathing problems.
- Be familiar with facility guidelines and/or standards of care related to family presence during resuscitation (FPDR), and advocate for the presence of a family facilitator and support for family needs. The presence of people who are relatives or significant others with whom the patient shares an established relationship during resuscitation or invasive procedures is controversial. Evidence in the literature suggests family members desire FPDR and identifies multiple associated benefits (AACN, 2016; McAlvin & Carew-Lyons, 2014; Pankop et al., 2013; Soleimanpur et al., 2017; Toronto & LaRocco, 2018; Vanhoy et al., 2019). The AACN (2016) and the Emergency Nurses Association (Vanhoy et al., 2019) recommend family members of all patients undergoing resuscitation and invasive procedures should be given the option of presence at the bedside (AACN, 2016; Vanhoy et al., 2019). The development of related policies or standards of practice in all patient care areas to address the needs of family members when they are present during invasive procedures and resuscitative events is recommended (AACN, 2016; Toronto & LaRoco, 2018; Vanhoy et al., 2019).

Infant and Child Considerations

- Once a child reaches puberty (breast development and/or underarm hair), use adult CPR guidelines for resuscitation (AHA, 2020b).
- As soon as it is determined that the scene is safe and an infant or child is unresponsive, shout for help to activate the emergency response system. Assess for breathing and a pulse (brachial artery in an infant and carotid or femoral artery in a child); this should take no more than 10 seconds.

If a pulse is not detected or not detected for certain, begin chest compressions. The only difference in chest compressions is for infants. A lone health care provider can use either the 2-finger or 2-thumb–encircling hands technique (AHA, 2020b). The two-thumb–encircling hands technique is recommended when CPR is provided by two rescuers. If it is not possible to encircle the patient's chest, compress the chest with the two fingers (AHA, 2020b).

- Perform the head tilt–chin lift and give two breaths after 30 compressions (15 compressions if two rescuers) (AHA, 2020b).
- Children with unwitnessed collapse: Give 2 minutes of CPR, then leave the patient to activate the emergency response system and get the AED. Return and resume CPR; use the AED as soon as it is available (AHA, 2020b).
- Most AED models are designed for both pediatric and adult resuscitation attempts; use the pediatric AED pads for children younger than age 8 years (AHA, 2020b).
- Many AEDs are equipped with a pediatric attenuator to decrease (attenuate) the delivered energy to make them suitable for infants and children younger than age 8 years; a pediatric attenuator is often attached to the pediatric AED pads (AHA, 2020b).
- Check the AED for a key or switch that will deliver a child shock dose; turn the key or switch before activating the AED (AHA, 2020b).

Older Adult Considerations

- Nurses can help promote informed, shared decision making about CPR to older adults and their families. Educate, support, and advocate for patients as they face this critical choice (Einav et al., 2021). Provide evidence-based information, supportive listening, and a willingness to respect their choices (Sharma et al., 2016).

EVIDENCE FOR PRACTICE ▶

CARDIOPULMONARY RESUSCITATION AND EMERGENCY CARDIAC CARE

The AHA provides guidelines for cardiopulmonary resuscitation and emergency cardiac care and has incorporated these guidelines into the Basic Life Support and Advanced Life Support education for health care providers who respond to cardiovascular and respiratory emergencies.

- American Heart Association (AHA). (2020a, October 20). 2020 American Heart Association guidelines for cardiopulmonary resuscitation and emergency cardiovascular care. Parts 1–7. *Circulation, 142*(16 Suppl 2). https://www.ahajournals.org/toc/circ/142/16_suppl_2/
- American Heart Association (AHA). (2020b). *2020 CPR & ECC guidelines. BLS provider manual.* AHA product number: 20–1102.
- American Heart Association (AHA). (2020c). *2020 ACLS for experienced providers. Manual and resource text.* AHA product number: 15–3134.

EVIDENCE FOR PRACTICE ▶

CARDIOPULMONARY RESUSCITATION AND FAMILY PRESENCE

The option for family presence during resuscitation (FPDR) or invasive procedures is recommended by multiple professional organizations (AACN, 2016; Toronto & LaRoco, 2018; Vanhoy et al., 2019) but remains controversial among nurses (Powers & Reeve, 2020). What interventions might improve nurses' support for and implementation of FPDR?

Related Research

Powers, K., & Reeve, C. L. (2020). Family presence during resuscitation: Medical-surgical nurses' perceptions, self-confidence, and use of invitations. *American Journal of Nursing, 120*(11), 28–38. https://doi.org/10.1097/01.naj.0000721244.16344.ee

The purpose of this study was to examine the personal, professional, and workplace factors associated with medical-surgical nurses' perceptions, self-confidence, and use of invitations regarding family presence during resuscitation (FPDR). Potential barriers to FPDR were also

(continued)

Skill 15-1 ▶ Performing Cardiopulmonary Resuscitation   *(continued)*

explored to inform the design of interventions that might improve FPDR implementation in the medical-surgical practice setting. A cross-sectional survey design was used to investigate which factors are predictors of medical-surgical nurses' FPDR perceptions, self-confidence, and use of invitations regarding FPDR; nurses' perceptions of barriers to FPDR; and nurses' educational preferences related to FPDR. A convenience sample of medical-surgical nurses ($n = 51$) was obtained through a study advertisement in a professional journal for medical-surgical nurses and through an email sent to members of the organization. Participants completed the study survey tools via an online survey site platform. Participants reported overall neutral perceptions of FPDR; 63% had never invited family members to experience resuscitation. The most significant predictor of more favorable perceptions, higher self-confidence, and greater use of invitations was having prior experience with FPDR. Analysis of perceived barriers indicated that these can be addressed through providing nurses with supportive FPDR policies and education. Only 14% of participants reported that their facility or unit had a written FPDR policy and only 16% had ever received any FPDR education. The authors concluded that FPDR is not commonly practiced on medical-surgical units. The authors recommended that medical-surgical nurses should be provided with experience, policies, and education related to FPDR to improve FPDR implementation rates in this setting. The authors suggest opportunities to implement FPDR in medical-surgical settings are abundant and should be utilized to support the patient–family unit and promote positive outcomes.

Relevance for Nursing Practice

Nurses are important patient advocates. Evidence supports the development, implementation, and evaluation of family presence protocols to ensure that patient- and family-centered care is provided. Nurses should be active participants in the development of educational interventions to address options for FPDR. Nurse educators should consider implementing educational interventions to improve nurses' support for FPDR and prepare them to implement FPDR in clinical practice.

Skill 15-2 ▶ Performing Emergency Automated External Defibrillation

Rapid defibrillation for shockable rhythms (ventricular fibrillation [VF] and pulseless ventricular tachycardia [VT]) is a critical part of Basic Life Support and administration of cardiopulmonary resuscitation (CPR) (see Skill 15-1) (AHA, 2020a). Early defibrillation is critical to increase patient survival (AHA, 2020a). Electrical therapy can be administered by defibrillation, **cardioversion**, or a pacemaker (see Fundamentals Review 15-1 at the beginning of the chapter).

Defibrillation delivers large amounts of electric current to a patient over brief periods of time. It is the standard treatment for VF and is also used to treat pulseless VT. The goal is to depolarize the irregularly beating heart temporarily and allow more coordinated contractile activity to resume. It does so by completely depolarizing the myocardium, producing a momentary asystole. This provides an opportunity for the natural pacemaker centers of the heart to resume normal activity.

The automated external defibrillator (AED) is a portable, computer-based external defibrillator that automatically detects and interprets the heart's rhythm and informs the operator if a shock is indicated (Figure 1). The defibrillator responds to the patient information by advising "shock" or "no shock." Fully automatic models automatically perform rhythm analysis and shock, if indicated. These are usually found in out-of-hospital settings. Semiautomatic models require the operator to press an "Analyze" button to initiate rhythm analysis and then press a "Shock" button to deliver the shock, if indicated. Semiautomatic models are usually found in acute care and other health care settings. An AED will not deliver a shock unless the electrode pads are correctly attached, and a shockable rhythm is detected. Some AEDs have motion-detection devices that ensure the defibrillator will not discharge if there is motion, such as motion from personnel in contact with

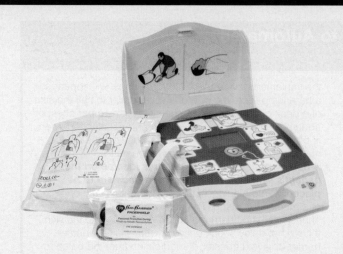

FIGURE 1. Automated external defibrillator (AED).

the patient. The strength of the charge is preset. Once the pads are in place and the device is turned on, follow the prompts given by the device. The following guidelines are based on the AHA (2020b) guidelines. AHA guidelines state that these recommendations may be modified for the in-hospital setting, where continuous electrocardiographic or hemodynamic monitoring may be in place. CPR should be immediately initiated (see Skill 15-1), and the AED/defibrillator should be used as soon as it is available.

The application of the AED as soon as it is available allows for analysis of cardiac status and delivery of an initial shock, if indicated, for adults and children. After an initial shock, resume CPR immediately for about 2 minutes (until prompted by AED to allow rhythm check). Provide sets of one shock alternating with 2 minutes of CPR until the AED indicates a "no shock indicated" message; the patient starts to move, breathe, or otherwise react; or until advanced cardiac life support (ACLS) is available (AHA, 2020b).

In the health care setting, including community-based care settings, it is imperative that personnel be aware of the patient's stated instructions regarding a wish not to be resuscitated. This should be clearly expressed and documented in the patient's health record.

DELEGATION CONSIDERATIONS	The initiation and provision of CPR, including use of an AED, is appropriate for all health care providers.
EQUIPMENT	• AED (some models have the pads, cables, and AED preconnected) • Self-adhesive, pregelled electrode monitor–defibrillator pads (6) • Cables to connect the pads and AED • Razor • Towel
ASSESSMENT	Assess the patient for unresponsiveness, effective breathing, and signs of circulation. Assess the patient's vital parameters and determine the patient's level of responsiveness. Check for partial or complete airway obstruction. Assess for the absence or ineffectiveness of respirations. Assess for the absence of signs of circulation and pulses. An AED should be used only when a patient is unresponsive, not breathing, or not breathing normally and lacks signs of circulation (pulseless, lack of effective respirations, coughing, movement). Determine the age of the patient; some AED systems are designed to deliver both adult and child shock doses. Choose the correct electrode pad for the size/age of the patient. If available, use child pads or a child system for children younger than age 8 years (refer to Special Considerations at the end of this Skill). Determine whether special situations exist that require additional actions before the AED is used or that contraindicate its use (refer to Box 15-1 for details of these situations and appropriate actions).

(continued on page 970)

Skill 15-2 ▶ Performing Emergency Automated External Defibrillation *(continued)*

Box 15-1   Special Situations Related to Automated External Defibrillation

- ***The patient is in water.*** Water is a good conductor of electricity. **Do not use an automated external defibrillator (AED) in water.** Defibrillation administered to a patient in water could result in shocking the AED operator and bystanders. Another possible effect is that water on the patient's skin will provide a direct path for the electrical current from one electrode to the other. The arcing of the electrical current between the electrodes bypasses the heart, resulting in the delivery of inadequate current to the heart. If the patient is in water, pull the patient out of the water. If water is covering the patient's chest, quickly dry the chest before attaching the AED pads. If the patient is lying on snow or in a small puddle, the AED may be used after quickly wiping the chest (AHA, 2020b).

- ***The patient has an implanted pacemaker or defibrillator.*** If possible, avoid placing the AED pad directly over the implanted device (AHA, 2020b), which will appear as a hard lump (from the size of a silver dollar to half the size of a deck of cards) beneath the skin of the upper chest or abdomen with an overlying scar. If an AED electrode pad is placed directly over an implanted device, the device may block delivery of the shock to the heart.

- ***A transdermal medication patch is located on the patient's skin where the electrode pads are to be placed.*** Avoid placing AED pads in contact with or on top of a medication patch. The patch may block the delivery of energy to the heart and cause small burns to the skin. If it will not delay shock delivery, wear gloves or other barrier (to avoid transfer of medication from the patch to you) to quickly remove the patch and wipe the area before attaching the AED pad (AHA, 2020b).

ACTUAL OR POTENTIAL HEALTH PROBLEMS AND NEEDS

Many actual or potential health problems or issues may require the use of this skill as part of related interventions. An appropriate health problem or issue may include:
- Impaired cardiac output
- Altered tissue perfusion
- Altered breathing pattern

OUTCOME IDENTIFICATION AND PLANNING

The expected outcomes to achieve when performing AED are that it is performed correctly without adverse effect to the patient, and the patient regains signs of circulation, with organized electrical rhythm and pulse. Additional outcomes include that the patient regains respirations; the patient's heart and lungs maintain adequate function to sustain life; the patient does not experience serious injury; and ACLS is initiated, as indicated.

IMPLEMENTATION

ACTION	RATIONALE
1. Verify scene safety. Check for patient responsiveness. Look for no breathing or only gasping. Call for help, pull the call bell, and call the facility emergency response number. Call for emergency equipment and the AED or defibrillator, if available. Put on gloves, if available. Begin CPR (see Skill 15-1).	Verification of scene safety makes sure the environment is safe for rescuers and the patient. Assessing responsiveness prevents starting CPR on a conscious patient. Activating the emergency response system initiates a rapid response. Accessing equipment supports appropriate interventions. Gloves prevent contact with blood and body fluids. Initiating CPR preserves the patient's heart and brain function while awaiting defibrillation.
2. **Provide defibrillation (if indicated) at the earliest possible moment, as soon as the AED becomes available.**	Early defibrillation (along with high-quality CPR and all components of the Chain of Survival) is necessary to improve chances of survival from pulseless VT and VF (AHA, 2020b). The AED quickly delivers a shock (defibrillation) to the heart muscle to interrupt shockable rhythms and resets the heart's electrical system so a normal (organized) heart rhythm can return (AHA, 2020b).
3. Prepare the AED. Power on the AED by pushing the power button. Some devices will turn on automatically when the lid or case is opened.	Proper setup ensures proper functioning.

ACTION

4. Attach the AED cables to the adhesive electrode pads (may be preconnected).

5. Stop chest compressions. Peel away the covering from the electrode pads to expose the adhesive surface. Attach the electrode pads to the patient's chest. Place one pad on the upper right sternal border, directly below the clavicle. Place the second pad lateral to the left nipple, with the top margin of the pad a few inches below the axilla (anterolateral positioning) (Figure 2). Alternatively, if two or more rescuers are present, one rescuer should continue chest compressions while another rescuer attaches the AED pads. Attach the AED connecting cables to the AED box, if not preconnected.

6. Once the pads are in place and the device is turned on, follow the prompts given by the device. Clear the patient and analyze the rhythm. Ensure no one is touching the patient. Loudly state a "Clear the patient" message. Press the "Analyze" button to initiate analysis, if necessary. Some devices automatically begin analysis when the pads are attached. Avoid all movement affecting the patient during analysis.

7. If a shockable rhythm is present, the device will announce that a shock is indicated and begin charging. Once the AED is charged, a message will be delivered to shock the patient.

8. **Before pressing the "Shock" button, loudly state a "Clear the patient" message. Visually check that no one is in contact with the patient or the bed** (Figure 3). Press the "Shock" button. If the AED is fully automatic, a shock will be delivered automatically.

RATIONALE

Proper setup ensures proper functioning.

Proper setup ensures proper functioning. The most common placement of the electrode pads is the anterior-lateral position (Morton & Fontaine, 2018). This placement puts the heart directly in the current pathway (Morton & Fontaine, 2018). Application by a second rescuer minimizes interruptions in chest compressions.

Movement and electrical impulses cause artifacts during analysis. Avoidance of artifacts ensures accurate rhythm analysis.

The shock message is delivered through a written or visual message on the AED screen, an auditory alarm, or a voice-synthesized statement.

Ensuring a clear patient avoids accidental shocking of personnel. Avoidance of contact with the patient avoids accidental shock to personnel.

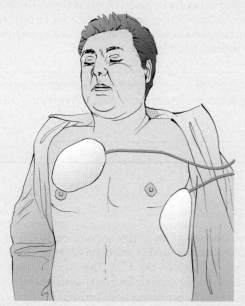

FIGURE 2. AED electrode pad placement.

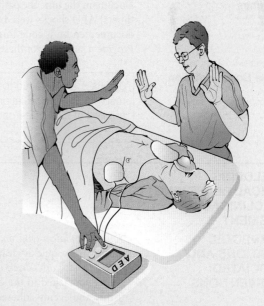

FIGURE 3. Stating a "Clear the patient" message.

(continued on page 972)

Skill 15-2 ▶ Performing Emergency Automated External Defibrillation *(continued)*

ACTION	**RATIONALE**
9. Immediately resume CPR, beginning with chest compressions. After about 2 minutes (until prompted by AED or about five complete cycles of CPR), allow the AED to analyze the heart rhythm. If a shock is not advised, resume CPR, beginning with chest compressions. Do not recheck to see if there is a pulse. Follow the AED voice prompts.	Resuming CPR provides optimal treatment. Even when a shock eliminates the **dysrhythmia**, it may take several minutes for a heart rhythm to establish and even longer to achieve perfusion. Chest compressions can provide coronary and cerebral perfusion during this period. Some AEDs in the community for use by untrained lay rescuers are automatically programmed to cycle through three analysis/shock cycles in one set. This would necessitate turning off the AED after the first shock and turning it back on for future analysis and defibrillation. Be familiar with the type of AED available for use.
10. Continue CPR and use of the AED until advanced care providers take over, the patient starts to breathe or move or otherwise react, you are too exhausted to continue, or an advanced health care provider discontinues CPR.	Once started, CPR must continue until one of these conditions is met. In an acute care setting, help should arrive within a few minutes.
11. Remove gloves and other PPE, if used. Perform hand hygiene.	Proper removal of PPE reduces the risk for infection transmission and contamination of other items. Hand hygiene prevents transmission of microorganisms.

EVALUATION

The expected outcomes have been met when defibrillation has been performed correctly without adverse effect to the patient; the patient has regained signs of circulation, with organized electrical rhythm and pulse; the patient has regained respirations; the patient's heart and lungs have maintained adequate function to sustain life; the patient has not experienced serious injury; and ACLS has been initiated, as indicated.

DOCUMENTATION

Guidelines

Document the time the patient was discovered unresponsive and CPR was initiated. Document the time(s) AED shocks were initiated. Continued intervention, such as by the code team, is typically documented on a code form, which identifies the actions and drugs provided during the code. Provide a summary of these events in the patient's health record.

Sample Documentation

> 07/06/25 2230 Called to patient's room by wife. Patient noted to be without evidence of respirations or circulation. Emergency response system activated, CPR initiated. AED applied at 2232. See code sheet.
>
> —B. Clapp, RN

DEVELOPING CLINICAL REASONING AND CLINICAL JUDGMENT

UNEXPECTED SITUATIONS AND ASSOCIATED INTERVENTIONS

- *You find a patient lying on the floor:* Determine the patient's level of responsiveness. If the patient is unresponsive, quickly clear an area, call for assistance and AED, and begin CPR (refer to Skill 15-1).
- *"Check pads" or "Check electrodes" message appears on the AED:* The electrode pads are not securely attached to the chest, or the cables are not securely fastened. Check that the pads are firmly and evenly adhered to the patient's skin. Verify connections between the cables and the AED and the cables and electrode pads. Check that the patient is not wet or diaphoretic or has excessive chest hair. See actions below for appropriate interventions in these situations.
- *Patient has a hairy chest:* The adhesive electrode pads may stick to the chest hair instead of to the skin, preventing adequate contact with the skin. Note whether the patient has a hairy chest before the AED pads are applied; if needed, use a razor to shave the area where the AED pads will be placed (AHA, 2020b). If AED pads are already in place and there is insufficient contact

or seal due to excess hair, press firmly on the current pads to attempt to provide sufficient adhesion. If unsuccessful, briskly remove the current pads to remove a good portion of the chest hair. If a significant amount of hair remains, quickly shave the area with the razor in the AED case, minimizing delay in shock delivery (Olasveengen et al., 2020). Apply a second set of electrode pads over the same sites. Continue with the procedure.
- *Patient is noticeably diaphoretic, or the skin is wet:* The electrode pads will not attach firmly to wet or diaphoretic skin. Quickly wipe the chest with a cloth or towel before attaching the electrode pads (AHA, 2020b).

SPECIAL CONSIDERATIONS

General Considerations

- **Every effort should be taken to minimize interruptions in chest compressions. A shorter duration of interruptions in chest compressions is associated with better outcomes** (AHA, 2020b).
- Most defibrillators use multifunctional electrode patches to both monitor and administer electrical therapy. Although paddles are still available, they are seldom used, as positioning requires additional "hands off" time, which depletes myocardial oxygen and energy stores (Morton & Fontaine, 2018, p. 330).
- Nurses should know the distinction between automatic and automated AEDs. *Automatic* AEDs charge and independently deliver a shock when indicated. *Automated* AEDs require action on the part of the user to deliver the shock. Familiarity with the device is important to its safe and effective use (Morton & Fontaine, 2018, p. 331).
- Appropriate maintenance of the AED is critical for proper operation. Check the AED for any visible signs of damage. Check the "ready for use" indicator on the AED daily. Perform maintenance according to the manufacturer's recommendations and facility policy.

Infant and Child Considerations

- Most AED models are designed for both pediatric and adult resuscitation attempts; use the pediatric AED pads for children younger than age 8 years (AHA, 2020b). Follow the AED manufacturer's instructions for placement of pediatric AED pads; some require placing pediatric pads in a front and back (anteroposterior) position, while others require right–left (anterolateral) placement. Anteroposterior placement is common for infants (AHA, 2020b).
- If pediatric pads are not available, use adult pads. Make sure the pads do not touch each other or overlap (AHA, 2020b). Adult pads deliver a higher shock dose, but a higher shock dose is better than no shock (AHA, 2020b).
- Many AEDs are equipped with a pediatric attenuator to decrease (attenuate) the delivered energy to make them suitable for infants and children younger than age 8 years; a pediatric attenuator is often attached to the pediatric AED pads (AHA, 2020b).

Older Adult Considerations

- Nurses can help promote informed, shared decision making about CPR to older adults and their families. Educate, support, and advocate for patients as they face this critical choice (Einav et al., 2021). Provide evidence-based information, supportive listening, and a willingness to respect their choices (Sharma et al., 2016).

EVIDENCE FOR PRACTICE ▶

CARDIOPULMONARY RESUSCITATION AND EMERGENCY CARDIAC CARE
The AHA provides guidelines for cardiopulmonary resuscitation and emergency cardiac care and has incorporated these guidelines into the Basic Life Support and Advanced Life Support education for health care providers who respond to cardiovascular and respiratory emergencies. Refer to the Evidence for Practice in Skill 15-1 for details.

Skill 15-3 ▶ Performing Emergency Manual External Defibrillation (Asynchronous)

Rapid defibrillation for shockable rhythms (ventricular fibrillation [VF] and pulseless ventricular tachycardia [VT]) is a critical part of Basic Life Support and administration of cardiopulmonary resuscitation (CPR) (see Skill 15-1) (AHA, 2020a). Early defibrillation is critical to increase patient survival (AHA, 2020a). Electrical therapy can be administered by defibrillation, cardioversion, or a pacemaker (see Fundamentals Review 15-1 at the beginning of the chapter).

Defibrillation delivers large amounts of electric current to a patient over brief periods of time. It is the standard treatment for VF and is also used to treat pulseless VT. The goal is to depolarize the irregularly beating heart temporarily and allow more coordinated contractile activity to resume. It does so by completely depolarizing the myocardium, producing a momentary asystole. This provides an opportunity for the natural pacemaker centers of the heart to resume normal activity. The self-adhering electrode pads delivering the current are placed on the patient's chest; during cardiac surgery, electrode paddles are placed directly on the myocardium.

Manual defibrillation is accomplished with an external defibrillator (Figure 1) and depends on the operator for analysis of rhythm, charging, proper application of the self-adhering electrode pads to the patient's thorax, and delivery of the shock. It requires the user to have immediate and accurate dysrhythmia recognition skills. The following guidelines are based on the AHA (2020b) guidelines.

In the health care setting, including community-based care settings, it is imperative that personnel be aware of the patient's stated instructions regarding a wish not to be resuscitated. This should be clearly expressed and documented in the patient's health record.

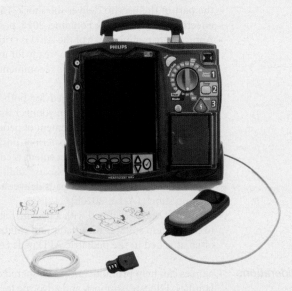

FIGURE 1. External defibrillator. (*Source:* Image from https://www.usa.philips.com/healthcare/product/HCM3535A/heartstart-mrx#galleryTab=PI Courtesy of Royal Philips ©.)

DELEGATION CONSIDERATIONS	The initiation and provision of manual external defibrillation should be performed by health care providers who are certified in advanced cardiac life support (ACLS) measures.

EQUIPMENT	• Defibrillator (biphasic*) • External self-adhering electrode pads (or internal paddles sterilized for cardiac surgery) • Electrocardiogram (ECG) monitor with recorder, depending on equipment available (usually part of the defibrillator) • Oxygen therapy equipment • Bag-valve-mask • Airway equipment • Emergency pacing equipment • Emergency cardiac medications • Razor *Biphasic defibrillators have replaced monophasic shock defibrillators, which are no longer manufactured. Biphasic defibrillators are safer and more effective (AHA, 2020a).

ASSESSMENT	Assess the patient for unresponsiveness, effective breathing, and signs of circulation. Assess the patient's vital parameters and determine the patient's level of responsiveness. Check for partial or complete airway obstruction. Assess for the absence or ineffectiveness of respirations. Assess for the absence of signs of circulation and pulses.
ACTUAL OR POTENTIAL HEALTH PROBLEMS AND NEEDS	Many actual or potential health problems or issues may require the use of this skill as part of related interventions. An appropriate health problem or issue may include: • Impaired cardiac output • Altered breathing pattern • Injury risk
OUTCOME IDENTIFICATION AND PLANNING	The expected outcomes to achieve when performing manual external defibrillation are that it is performed correctly without adverse effect to the patient, and the patient regains signs of circulation with organized electrical rhythm and pulse. Additional outcomes may include that the patient regains respirations; the patient's heart and lungs maintain adequate function to sustain life; the patient does not experience serious injury; and ACLS is initiated, as indicated.

IMPLEMENTATION

ACTION

1. Verify scene safety. Check for responsiveness. Look for no breathing or only gasping. Call for help, pull the call bell, and call the facility emergency response number. Call for emergency equipment and the automated external defibrillator (AED) or defibrillator, if available. Put on gloves, if available. Begin CPR, as indicated (see Skill 15-1).

2. **Provide defibrillation (if indicated) at the earliest possible moment, as soon as the AED becomes available.**

3. Turn on the defibrillator.

4. Expose the patient's chest and apply electrode pads to the chest. Place one pad on the upper right sternal border, directly below the clavicle. Place the second pad lateral to the left nipple, with the top margin of the pad a few inches below the axilla (anterolateral positioning) (Figure 2). Alternatively, if two or more rescuers are present, one rescuer should continue chest compressions, while another rescuer attaches the electrode pads. Assess the cardiac rhythm.

5. Set the energy level for a clinically appropriate energy level for the defibrillator, beginning with 120 to 200 J (joules) (depending on the specific biphasic defibrillator in use) (AHA, 2020a).

6. If the patient remains in VF or pulseless VT, **loudly state a "Clear the patient" message. Visually check that no one is in contact with the patient or the bed.** Press the button to deliver the shock.

RATIONALE

Verification of scene safety makes sure the environment is safe for rescuers and the patient. Assessing responsiveness prevents starting CPR on a conscious patient. Activating the emergency response system initiates a rapid response. Accessing equipment supports appropriate interventions. Gloves prevent contact with blood and body fluids. Initiating CPR preserves heart and brain function while awaiting defibrillation.

Early defibrillation (along with high-quality CPR and all components of the Chain of Survival) is necessary to improve chances of survival from pulseless VT and VF (AHA, 2020b). The AED quickly delivers a shock (defibrillation) to the heart muscle to interrupt shockable rhythms and resets the heart's electrical system so a normal (organized) heart rhythm can return (AHA, 2020b).

Charging prepares for defibrillation.

Proper setup ensures proper functioning. This placement puts the heart directly in the current pathway (Morton & Fontaine, 2018). Application by a second rescuer minimizes interruptions in chest compressions. Connecting the monitor leads to the patient allows for assessment of the cardiac rhythm and determination of the need for defibrillation.

Proper setup ensures proper functioning and appropriate intervention.

Standing clear of the bed and patient avoids accidental shocking of personnel. Pressing the shock button discharges the electric current for defibrillation.

(continued on page 976)

Skill 15-3 ▶ Performing Emergency Manual External Defibrillation (Asynchronous) *(continued)*

| ACTION | RATIONALE |

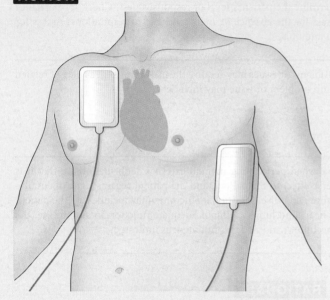

FIGURE 2. Anterolateral placement of self-adhering electrode pads.

7. After the shock, immediately resume CPR, beginning with chest compressions. After five cycles (about 2 minutes), reassess the cardiac rhythm. Continue until advanced care providers take over; the patient starts to breathe, move, or otherwise react; you are too exhausted to continue; or an advanced health care provider discontinues CPR.

Resuming CPR provides optimal treatment. Even when a shock eliminates the dysrhythmia, it may take several minutes for a heart rhythm to establish and even longer to achieve perfusion. Chest compressions can provide coronary and cerebral perfusion during this period. Once started, CPR must continue until one of these conditions is met. In an acute care setting, help should arrive within a few minutes.

8. If necessary, prepare to defibrillate subsequent shocks per ACLS protocol; if initial cardioversion is unsuccessful, energy is increased in subsequent attempts, depending on the defibrillator in use (AHA, 2020a).

Additional shocking may be needed to stimulate the heart. Commercially available defibrillators will either provide fixed energy settings or allow for escalating energy settings (AHA, 2020a).

9. Announce that you are preparing to defibrillate and follow the procedure described above.

Additional shocking may be needed to stimulate the heart.

10. If defibrillation restores a normal rhythm:

a. Check for signs of circulation; check the central and peripheral pulses, and obtain a blood pressure reading, heart rate, and respiratory rate.

The patient will need continuous monitoring to prevent further problems. Continuous monitoring helps provide for early detection and prompt intervention should additional problems arise.

b. If signs of circulation are present, check breathing. If breathing is inadequate, assist with breathing. Administer rescue breathing at a rate of one breath every 6 seconds, for a rate of 10 breaths/min (refer to Skill 15-1).

Rescue breathing maintains adequate oxygenation.

c. If breathing is adequate, place the patient in the recovery position. Continue to assess the patient.

d. Assess the patient's level of consciousness, cardiac rhythm, blood pressure, breath sounds, skin color, and temperature.

Reassessment determines the need for continued intervention and provides optimal treatment.

e. Obtain baseline ABG levels (Skill 18-11) and a 12-lead ECG (Skill 15-4), if prescribed.

These assessments provide data to help inform continued intervention and optimal treatment.

f. Provide supplemental oxygen, ventilation, and medications, as needed.

This provides optimal treatment.

g. Anticipate the possible use of targeted temperature management, including therapeutic hypothermia.

Lowering of a patient's core temperature after cardiac arrest may improve survival and functional recovery (AHA, 2020a; Morton & Fontaine, 2018).

ACTION

11. Keep the electrode pads on the patient in case of recurrent VT or VF.

12. Remove gloves and other PPE, if used. Perform hand hygiene.

13. Prepare the defibrillator for immediate reuse.

RATIONALE

Keeping the pads in place provides preparation for future use.

Proper removal of PPE reduces the risk for infection transmission and contamination of other items. Hand hygiene prevents transmission of microorganisms.

The patient may remain unstable and could require further intervention.

EVALUATION

The expected outcomes have been met when defibrillation has been performed correctly without adverse effect to the patient; the patient has regained signs of circulation, with organized electrical rhythm and pulse; the patient has regained respirations; the patient's heart and lungs have maintained adequate function to sustain life; the patient has not experienced serious injury; and ACLS has been initiated, as indicated.

DOCUMENTATION

Guidelines

Document the time you discovered the patient unresponsive and started CPR. Document the procedure, including the patient's ECG rhythms both before and after defibrillation; the number of times defibrillation was performed; the voltage used during each attempt; whether a pulse returned; the dosage, route, and time of drug administration; whether CPR was used; how the airway was maintained; and the patient's outcome. Continued intervention, such as by the code team, is typically documented on a code form, which identifies the actions and drugs provided during the code. Provide a summary of these events in the patient's health record.

Sample Documentation

07/06/25 2230 Called to patient's room by wife. Patient noted to be without evidence of respirations or circulation. Emergency response system activated, CPR initiated. Manual defibrillation initiated at 2232. See code sheet.

—B. Clapp, RN

DEVELOPING CLINICAL REASONING AND CLINICAL JUDGMENT

UNEXPECTED SITUATIONS AND ASSOCIATED INTERVENTIONS

- *Defibrillator fails to fire:* Check that the power is turned on. If the defibrillator is battery operated, check if the battery is low. Check that it is fully charged.
- *You find a patient lying on the floor:* Determine the patient's level of responsiveness. If the patient is unresponsive, quickly clear an area, call for assistance and AED, and begin CPR (refer to Skill 15-1).
- *Patient has a hairy chest:* The adhesive electrode pads may stick to the chest hair instead of to the skin, preventing adequate contact with the skin. Press firmly on the current pads to attempt to provide sufficient adhesion. If unsuccessful, briskly remove the current pads to remove a good portion of the chest hair. If a significant amount of hair remains, quickly shave the area with the razor in the AED case, minimizing delay in shock delivery (Olasveengen et al., 2020). Apply a second set of electrode pads over the same sites. Continue with the procedure.
- *Patient is noticeably diaphoretic, or the skin is wet:* The electrode pads will not attach firmly to wet or diaphoretic skin. Dry the chest with a cloth or towel before attaching the electrode pads.

(continued on page 978)

Skill 15-3 ▶ Performing Emergency Manual External Defibrillation (Asynchronous) *(continued)*

SPECIAL CONSIDERATIONS

General Considerations

- Every effort should be taken to minimize interruptions in chest compressions. A shorter duration of interruptions in chest compressions is associated with better outcomes (AHA, 2020b).
- Alternative placement of self-adhering electrode pads: Anterior–posterior placement. Place one pad anteriorly at the precordium to the left of the lower sternal border and the other pad posteriorly under the patient's body beneath the heart and immediately below the scapula (Figure 3).
- Most defibrillators use multifunctional electrode patches to both monitor and administer electrical therapy. Although paddles are still available, they are seldom used, as positioning requires additional "hands off" time, which depletes myocardial oxygen and energy stores (Morton & Fontaine, 2018, p. 330).
- Defibrillation can cause accidental electric shock to those providing care.
- Defibrillators vary from one manufacturer to another, so familiarize yourself with your facility's equipment. Perform maintenance according to the manufacturer's recommendations and facility policy.

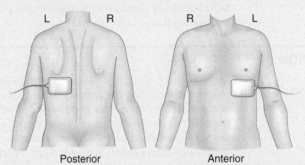

FIGURE 3. Anteroposterior placement of self-adhering electrode pads.

Infant and Child Considerations

- If pediatric defibrillator pads are not available, use adult pads. Make sure the pads do not touch each other or overlap (AHA, 2020b).

Older Adult Considerations

- Nurses can help promote informed decision making about CPR to older adults and their families. Educate, support, and advocate for patients as they face this critical choice (Einav et al., 2021). Provide evidence-based information, supportive listening, and a willingness to respect their choices (Sharma et al., 2016).

EVIDENCE FOR PRACTICE ▶

CARDIOPULMONARY RESUSCITATION AND EMERGENCY CARDIAC CARE

The AHA provides guidelines for CPR and emergency cardiac care and has incorporated these guidelines into the Basic Life Support and Advanced Life Support education for health care providers who respond to cardiovascular and respiratory emergencies.

Refer to the Evidence for Practice in Skill 15-1 for details.

Skill 15-4 ▶ Obtaining an Electrocardiogram

Electrocardiography measures the heart's electrical activity and is one of the most valuable and frequently used diagnostic tools. Impulses moving through the heart's conduction system create electric currents that can be monitored on the body's surface. Electrodes attached to the skin can detect these electric currents and transmit them to an instrument that produces a record of cardiac activity, the **electrocardiogram (ECG)**. The data are graphed as waveforms (Figure 1). ECGs can be used to

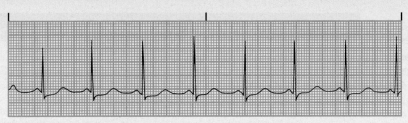

FIGURE 1. Electrocardiogram (waveform) strip.

assess and diagnose patients with suspected arrhythmias, hypertension, coronary heart disease, and heart failure (Menzies-Gow, 2018) and to identify myocardial ischemia and infarction, rhythm and conduction disturbances, chamber enlargement, electrolyte imbalances, and drug toxicity.

The standard 12-lead ECG uses a series of electrodes placed on the extremities and the chest wall to assess the heart from 12 different viewpoints (leads) by attaching 10 cables with electrodes to the patient's limbs and chest: 4 limb electrodes and 6 chest electrodes (Figure 2). Each lead provides an electrographic snapshot of electrochemical activity of the myocardial cell membrane. The ECG device measures and averages the differences between the electrical potential of the electrode sites for each lead and graphs them over time, creating the standard ECG complex, called PQRST (Box 15-2). These electrodes provide views of the heart from the frontal plane as well as the horizontal plane. It is essential that connection or placement of the ECG electrodes/leads is accurate to prevent misdiagnosis (Bickerton & Pooler, 2019; Pearce, 2019). The ECG tracing needs to be clear to enable accurate and reliable interpretation.

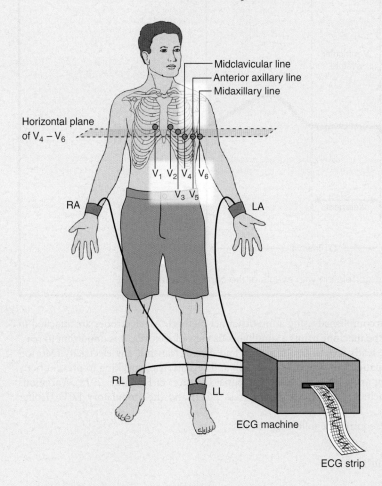

FIGURE 2. 12-lead ECG lead placement. (*Source:* From Morton, P. G., & Fontaine, D. K. [2018]. *Essentials of critical care nursing. A holistic approach* [11th ed.]. Wolters Kluwer, with permission.)

(*continued on page 980*)

Skill 15-4 ▶ Obtaining an Electrocardiogram *(continued)*

Box 15-2 | Electrocardiograph Complex

The electrocardiograph (ECG) complex consists of five waveforms labeled with the letters P, Q, R, S, and T. In addition, sometimes a U wave appears.

- **P wave:** Represents atrial depolarization (conduction of the electrical impulse through the atria); the first component of ECG waveform.
- **PR interval:** Tracks the atrial impulse from the atria through the AV node, from the SA node to the AV node. Measures from the beginning of the P wave to the beginning of the QRS complex. Normal PR is 0.12 to 0.2 seconds.
- **QRS complex:** Follows the PR interval and represents depolarization of the ventricles (the time it takes for the impulse to travel through the bundle branches to the Purkinje fibers) or impulse conduction and contraction of the myocardial cells (ventricular systole). The Q wave appears as the first negative deflection in the QRS complex, the R wave as the first positive deflection. The

S wave appears as the second negative deflection or the first negative deflection after the R wave. Normal QRS is 0.06 to 0.1 seconds.

- **ST segment:** Represents the end of ventricular conduction or depolarization and the beginning of ventricular recovery or repolarization; the J point marks the end of the QRS complex and the beginning of the ST segment.
- **T wave:** Represents ventricular recovery or repolarization.
- **QT interval:** Measures ventricular depolarization and repolarization; varies with the heart rate (i.e., the faster the heart rate, the shorter the QT interval); extends from the beginning of the QRS complex to the end of the T wave. Normal QT is <0.4 seconds but can vary with heart rate.
- **U wave:** Represents the recovery period of the Purkinje fibers or ventricular conduction fibers; not present on every rhythm strip.

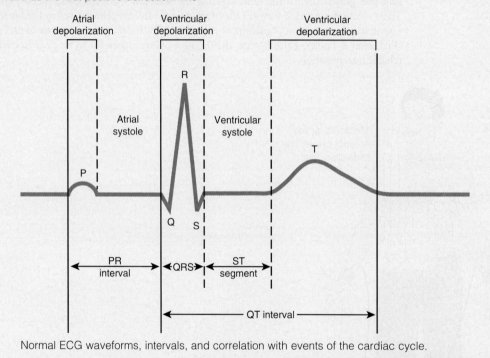

Normal ECG waveforms, intervals, and correlation with events of the cardiac cycle.

An ECG is typically accomplished using a multichannel method. All electrodes are attached to the patient at once, and the machine prints a simultaneous view of all leads. It is important to reassure the patient that the leads just sense and record and do not transmit any electricity (Morton & Fontaine, 2018). The patient must be able to lie still and refrain from speaking to prevent body movement from creating artifacts in the electrical signal (Morton & Fontaine, 2018). Variations of the standard ECG include the exercise ECG (stress ECG) and the ambulatory ECG (Holter monitoring).

Interpreting the ECG requires the following actions:

- Determining the rate
- Determining the rhythm
- Evaluating the P wave
- Determining the duration of the PR interval
- Determining the duration of the QRS complex

- Evaluating the T wave
- Determining the duration of the QT interval
- Evaluating the ST segment
- Evaluating any other components

DELEGATION CONSIDERATIONS	Obtaining an ECG is not delegated to assistive personnel (AP); in some facilities, technicians are trained to obtain an ECG. Depending on the state's nurse practice act and the organization's policies and procedures, this procedure may be delegated to licensed practical/vocational nurses (LPN/LVNs). The decision to delegate must be based on careful analysis of the patient's needs and circumstances as well as the qualifications of the person to whom the task is being delegated. Refer to the Delegation Guidelines in Appendix A.
EQUIPMENT	• ECG machine • Recording paper • Disposable pregelled electrodes • Adhesive remover swabs • 4 × 4 gauze pads • Skin cleanser and water, if necessary • PPE, as indicated • Bath blanket
ASSESSMENT	Review the patient's health record and care plan for information about the patient's need for an ECG. Assess the patient's cardiac status, including heart rate, blood pressure, and auscultation of heart sounds. If the patient is already connected to a cardiac monitor, remove the electrodes to accommodate the precordial leads and minimize electrical interference on the ECG tracing. Keep the patient away from objects that might cause electrical interference, such as equipment, fixtures, and power cords. Inspect the patient's chest for areas of irritation, skin breakdown, or excessive hair that might interfere with electrode placement.
ACTUAL OR POTENTIAL HEALTH PROBLEMS AND NEEDS	Many actual or potential health problems or issues may require the use of this skill as part of related interventions. An appropriate health problem or issue may include: • Impaired cardiac output • Acute pain • Activity intolerance
OUTCOME IDENTIFICATION AND PLANNING	The expected outcomes to achieve are that an ECG is obtained without any complications, and the patient demonstrates an understanding of the need for and about the ECG.

IMPLEMENTATION

ACTION	**RATIONALE**
1. Verify the prescribed intervention for the ECG in the patient's health record.	Verifying the prescribed intervention ensures that the correct intervention is administered to the right patient.
2. Gather all equipment.	Assembling equipment provides for an organized approach to the task.
3. Perform hand hygiene and put on PPE, if indicated.	Hand hygiene and PPE prevent the spread of microorganisms. PPE is required based on transmission precautions.
4. Identify the patient.	Identifying the patient ensures the right patient receives the intervention and helps prevent errors.

(continued on page 982)

Skill 15-4 ▶ Obtaining an Electrocardiogram *(continued)*

ACTION	RATIONALE
5. Close the curtains around the bed and close the door to the room, if possible. As you set up the machine to record a 12-lead ECG, explain to the patient what you are going to do and why. Tell the patient that the test records their heart's electrical activity, and it may be repeated at certain intervals. Emphasize that no electrical current will enter their body. Tell the patient the test typically takes about 5 minutes. Ask the patient about allergies to adhesive, as appropriate.	This ensures the patient's privacy. Explanation relieves anxiety and facilitates engagement. Possible allergies may exist related to the adhesive on ECG leads.
6. Place the ECG machine close to the patient's bed and plug the power cord into the wall outlet.	Having equipment available saves time and facilitates accomplishment of the task.
7. If the bed is adjustable, raise it to a comfortable working height (VHACEOSH, 2016).	Having the bed at the proper height prevents back and muscle strain on the part of the nurse.
8. Position the patient in a semi-recumbent position (head of the bed at approximately 45 degrees) or supine position in the center of the bed with their arms at their sides (Campbell et al., 2017). Expose the patient's arms and legs, and drape appropriately. Encourage the patient to relax their arms and legs. Ensure their wrists do not touch their waist. Make sure their feet do not touch the bed's footboard.	Proper positioning helps promote patient comfort and will produce a better tracing. Proper positioning, supporting the patient's limbs on the bed, and relaxing their arms and legs minimizes muscle tension and trembling and resulting electrical interference (Campbell et al., 2017). The ECG appearance can be affected by the angle of incline of the torso at the time of the recording (Campbell et al., 2017). Document the patient's position so that subsequent tracings are performed with the patient in the same position (Campbell et al., 2017; Garcia, 2015; Morton & Fontaine, 2018).
9. If necessary, prepare the skin for electrode placement (AACN, 2018). If an area is excessively hairy, clip the hair (AACN, 2018; Oster, n.d.) or shave the hair with a single-use razor (Campbell et al., 2017), according to facility policy. Clean excess oil or other substances from the skin with a skin cleanser and water. Use a gauze pad to vigorously rub and dry the skin.	Shaving may cause microabrasions on the skin, possibly resulting in portals of entry for microorganisms. Oils and excess hair interfere with electrode contact and function. Rubbing with gauze abrades and dries the skin. Proper skin preparation is essential to reduce artifacts in and increase quality of the ECG tracing (AACN, 2018; Campbell et al., 2017; Garcia, 2015; Oster, n.d.).
10. Apply the limb electrodes (Figure 3). Peel the contact paper off the self-sticking disposable electrode and apply directly to the prepared site, as recommended by the manufacturer. Connect the limb lead wires to the electrodes. The tip of each lead wire is lettered and color coded for easy identification. The white, or RA, lead goes to the right arm, just above the wrist bone; the green, or RL, lead to the right leg, just above the ankle bone; the red, or LL, lead to the left leg, just above the ankle bone; and the black, or LA, lead to the left arm, just above the wrist bone. Refer to Figure 2 for electrode placement.	Use of recommended standard sites for limb electrodes is essential to obtain an accurate recording (Campbell et al., 2017; Garcia, 2015; Morton & Fontaine, 2018).

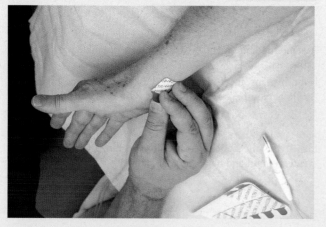

FIGURE 3. Applying limb electrode.

ACTION

11. Expose the patient's chest. Apply the chest electrodes (Figure 4A). Peel the contact paper off the self-sticking, disposable electrode and apply them directly to the prepared site, as recommended by the manufacturer. Connect the chest lead wires to the electrodes (Figure 4B). The tip of each lead wire is lettered and color coded for easy identification. The V_1 to V_6 leads are applied to the chest. Position chest electrodes as follows (refer to Figure 2):
    - V_1 (red): Fourth intercostal space at right sternal border
    - V_2 (yellow): Fourth intercostal space at left sternal border
    - V_3 (green): Exactly midway between V_2 and V_4
    - V_4 (blue): Fifth intercostal space at the left midclavicular line
    - V_5 (orange): Left anterior axillary line, same horizontal plane as V_4 and V_6
    - V_6 (purple): Left midaxillary line, same horizontal plane as V_4 and V_5

RATIONALE

Proper lead placement is necessary for accurate test results (AACN, 2018; Campbell et al., 2017; Garcia, 2015; Morton & Fontaine, 2018).

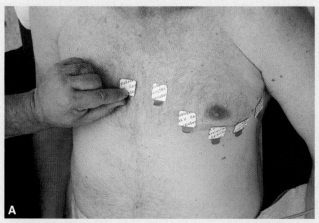
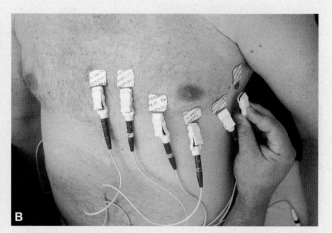

FIGURE 4. **A.** Applying chest electrode. **B.** Applying chest lead.

12. After the application of all the leads (Figure 5), ensure that the cables are not pulling on the electrodes or lying over each other. Make sure the paper-speed selector is set to the standard 25 mm/sec and that the machine is set to full voltage (10 mm/mV) (Menzies-Gow, 2018).

Lack of pulling and tension minimizes electrical artifacts and improves quality and accuracy of the ECG. The correct paper speed affects the timing of the ECG with respect to measurement of rate and duration of intervals (Garcia, 2015). The machine will record a normal standardization mark—a square that is the height of 2 large squares or 10 small squares on the recording paper.

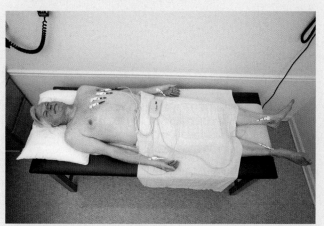

FIGURE 5. Completed application of 12-lead ECG.

(continued on page 984)

Skill 15-4 ▶ Obtaining an Electrocardiogram *(continued)*

ACTION	RATIONALE
13. Enter the appropriate patient identification data into the machine. Depending on facility policy, enter the patient's name, health record number, and age and biologic sex.	This allows for proper identification of the ECG strip. The ECG device requires minimum data input of age and biologic sex to correctly analyze the data (Garcia, 2015).
14. Ask the patient to relax and breathe normally. **Instruct the patient to lie still and not to talk while the ECG is being recorded.**	Lying still and not talking avoids resulting artifacts in the electrical signal, producing a better tracing (Campbell et al., 2017; Morton & Fontaine, 2018).
15. Press the AUTO or START button. Observe the tracing quality (Figure 6). The machine will record all 12 leads automatically, recording 3 consecutive leads simultaneously. Some machines have a display screen so you can preview waveforms before the machine records them on paper. Adjust the waveform, if necessary. If any part of the waveform extends beyond the paper when you record the ECG, adjust the normal standardization to half-standardization and repeat. Note this adjustment on the ECG strip, because this will need to be considered in interpreting the results.	Observation of tracing quality allows for adjustments to be made, if necessary. Notation of adjustments ensures accurate interpretation of results.

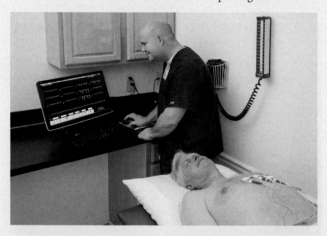

FIGURE 6. Observing tracing quality.

ACTION	RATIONALE
16. When the machine finishes recording the 12-lead ECG (Figure 7), remove the electrodes and clean the patient's skin, if necessary, with adhesive remover for sticky residue.	Removal and cleaning promote patient comfort.

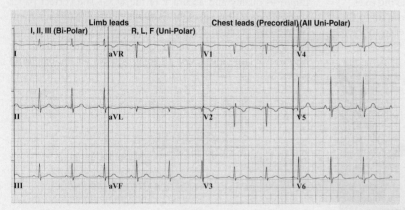

FIGURE 7. 12-Lead ECG configuration. (*Source:* From Diepenbrock, N. [2021]. *Quick reference to critical care* [6th ed.]; Fig. 2-33. Wolters Kluwer, with permission.)

ACTION	RATIONALE
17. After disconnecting the lead wires from the electrodes, dispose of the electrodes. Return the patient to a comfortable position. Lower the bed height and adjust the head of the bed to a comfortable position.	Proper disposal deters the spread of microorganisms. Positioning with head adjustment promotes patient comfort. Lowering the bed height promotes patient safety.

ACTION	RATIONALE
18. If not done electronically from data entered into the machine, label the ECG with the patient's name, date of birth, location, date and time of recording, and other relevant information (such as symptoms that occurred during the recording). Note any deviations to the standard approach to the recording, such as alternative placement of leads (see Special Considerations below).	Accurate labeling ensures the ECG is recorded for the correct patient as well as accurate and reliable interpretation.
19. Clean the ECG machine per facility policy. Clean reusable ECG cables and clips, according to facility policy; dispose of single-use ECG cables and clips.	Cleaning equipment between each patient use decreases the risk for transmission of microorganisms. Use non–bleach-based cleaning wipes to avoid deterioration of the wires (Bloe, 2021). Even after cleaning, the presence of microorganisms on reusable ECG lead wires increases the risk of transmission between patients, increasing the risk of health care–associated infections (Bloe, 2021). The use of single-use ECG leads reduces the risk of infection (Bloe, 2021).
20. Remove additional PPE, if used. Perform hand hygiene.	Proper removal of PPE reduces the risk for infection transmission and contamination of other items. Hand hygiene prevents transmission of microorganisms.

EVALUATION

The expected outcomes have been met when an ECG has been obtained without any complications, and the patient has demonstrated an understanding of the need for and about the ECG.

DOCUMENTATION

Guidelines

Document significant assessment findings, the date and time that the ECG was obtained, and the patient's response to the procedure. Label the ECG recording with the patient's name; room number; and facility identification number, if this was not done by the machine. Also record the date, time, and the patient's position as well as any appropriate clinical information on the ECG, such as blood pressure measurement, if the patient was experiencing chest pain. Record any deviations to the standard approach to the recording, such as alternative placement of leads (see Special Considerations below).

Sample Documentation

> 11/10/25 1745 Patient admitted to room 663. Denies pain, nausea, and shortness of breath. Apical heart rate 82 and regular. Blood pressure 146/88. ECG obtained. Copy faxed to Dr. Martin.
>
> —B. Clapp, RN

DEVELOPING CLINICAL REASONING AND CLINICAL JUDGMENT

UNEXPECTED SITUATIONS AND ASSOCIATED INTERVENTIONS

- *Artifact appears on the tracing:* An artifact may be due to loose electrodes or patient movement. Reassess the electrode connections. Ensure the ECG electrodes have not expired and are not dry; change the electrodes, if necessary. Ask the patient to lie extremely still. Consider additional skin preparation; refer to Step 9 in the Skill. Redo the ECG, if necessary.
- *Minimal complexes are seen:* This may be due to extreme bradycardia. Run longer strips.

(continued on page 986)

Skill 15-4 ▶ Obtaining an Electrocardiogram *(continued)*

SPECIAL CONSIDERATIONS

- Nurses must be familiar with the particular equipment in use; accuracy of the information is dependent on following the specifications of the manufacturer (Garcia, 2015). Some manufacturers may use different color combinations for the precordial leads; refer to the instructions for the particular equipment in use (Menzies-Gow, 2018).
- The standard limb electrode locations are slightly proximal (just above) to the wrist and ankle bones (Campbell et al., 2017). Limb electrodes may be placed on the inside or outside aspects of the patient's wrist and ankle. Allow patients to position themselves comfortably, and then use the most accessible aspect for electrode placement. Do not obtain recordings from any other limb position unless there is a clinical reason, such as an amputation, surgical wounds, or burns. In patients with amputations, it is important to place the electrodes in the same position bilaterally (Garcia, 2015). Upper arms and upper legs may be used as alternative sites in these situations. ECGs recorded using any other limb position or precordial positions must be labeled to account for changes that might affect the interpretation and clinical decisions made (Campbell et al., 2017; Garcia, 2015).
- Limb electrodes must not be placed on the torso to avoid significant alteration to the recorded information (Campbell et al., 2017).
- To position the chest leads (V_1 to V_6) correctly, it is important to be able to accurately locate the relevant intercostal spaces (Campbell et al., 2017).
- For female patients, place the V_4 electrode, as well as V_5 and V_6 as necessary, under the breast tissue as close to the chest wall as possible (Campbell et al., 2017; Garcia, 2015). In a large-breasted patient, you may need to displace the breast tissue laterally and/or superiorly.
- Skin preparation is essential to ensure optimal electrode contact; a significant amount of dry or dead skin cells, grease, sweat, or hair can negatively affect the quality of the ECG recording (Menzies-Gow, 2018).
- If it is necessary to adapt the recording techniques for an individual patient's circumstances, clearly describe the adaptations on the hard copy of the recording and in the electronically stored ECG (Campbell et al., 2017).

Skill 15-5 ▶ Applying a Cardiac Monitor

Continuous cardiac (electrocardiographic) monitoring provides constant observation of the heart's electrical activity. It is used to monitor a patient's heart rate and rhythm or the effects of a therapy (Morton & Fontaine, 2018). Cardiac monitoring is used for patients with conduction disturbances, for those at risk for life-threatening arrhythmias; such as postoperative patients and patients who are sedated; to diagnose myocardial ischemia; and in whom the administration of certain medications could result in dysrhythmias (Burns & Delgado, 2019; Sampson, 2018a). As with other forms of electrocardiography, cardiac monitoring uses electrodes placed on the patient's chest to transmit electrical signals that are converted into a tracing of cardiac rhythm on an oscilloscope. Either 3- or 5-lead systems may be used (Figure 1). The 3-lead–wire monitoring system facilitates monitoring of the patient in limb leads I, II, and III (Morton & Fontaine, 2018). The 5-lead–wire monitoring system facilitates monitoring of the patient in any one of the standard 12 leads.

Two types of monitoring may be performed: hardwire or telemetry. In hardwire monitoring, the patient is connected to a monitor at the bedside. The rhythm display appears at the bedside but may also be transmitted to a console at a remote location. Telemetry uses a small transmitter (connected to a patient) to send electrical signals to another location, where the electrical signals are displayed on a monitor screen, providing remote viewing of the heart's electrical activity. Battery-powered and portable, telemetry frees patients from cumbersome wires and cables and lets them be comfortably mobile. Telemetry is especially useful for monitoring arrhythmias that occur during sleep, rest, exercise, and stressful situations.

Regardless of the type, cardiac monitors can display the patient's heart rate and rhythm, produce a printed record of cardiac rhythm, and sound an alarm if the heart rate exceeds or falls below specified limits. Monitors also recognize and count abnormal heartbeats as well as changes. Cardiac monitoring systems may incorporate computer systems that store, analyze, and trend monitored data; automatic chart documentation; and wireless communication devices that provide data and alarms that can be carried by the nurse (Morton & Fontaine, 2018).

Gel foam electrodes are commonly used. Electrodes should be changed every 24 hours to prevent skin irritation and maintain quality of data (AACN, 2018; McGuffin & Ortiz, 2019). Hypoallergenic electrodes are available for patients with hypersensitivity to tape or adhesive. Any loose or nonadhering electrode should be replaced immediately to prevent inaccurate or missing data.

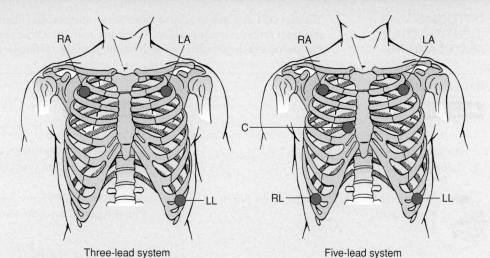

FIGURE 1. Electrode positions for 3- (*left*) and 5-lead (*right*) systems.
Positions for the 3-lead system:
RA (white electrode) below right clavicle, second ICS, right midclavicular line
LA (black electrode) below left clavicle, second ICS, left midclavicular line
LL (red electrode) left lower rib cage, eighth ICS, left midclavicular line
Positions for the 5-lead system:
RA (white electrode) below right clavicle, second ICS, right midclavicular line
RL (green electrode) right lower rib cage, eighth ICS, right midclavicular line
LA (black electrode) below left clavicle, second ICS, left midclavicular line
LL (red electrode) left lower rib cage, eighth ICS, left midclavicular line
Chest (brown electrode) any V lead position, usually V_1 (fourth ICS, right sternal border)

DELEGATION CONSIDERATIONS	The application of a cardiac monitor is not delegated to assistive personnel (AP); in some facilities, technicians are trained to apply the leads. Depending on the state's nurse practice act and the organization's policies and procedures, application of a cardiac monitor may be delegated to licensed practical/vocational nurses (LPN/LVNs). The decision to delegate must be based on careful analysis of the patient's needs and circumstances as well as the qualifications of the person to whom the task is being delegated. Refer to the Delegation Guidelines in Appendix A.

EQUIPMENT

- Lead wires
- Pregelled (gel foam) electrodes (number varies from 3 to 5)
- Gauze pads
- Skin cleanser

- Patient cable for hardwire cardiac monitoring
- Transmitter, transmitter pouch, and telemetry battery pack for telemetry
- PPE, as indicated

ASSESSMENT	Review the patient's health record and care plan for information about their need for cardiac monitoring. Assess the patient's cardiac status, including heart rate, blood pressure, and auscultation of heart sounds. Inspect the patient's chest for areas of irritation, skin breakdown, or excessive hair that might interfere with electrode placement. Electrode sites must be dry, with minimal hair. The patient may be sitting or supine, in a bed or a chair.

ACTUAL OR POTENTIAL HEALTH PROBLEMS AND NEEDS	Many actual or potential health problems or issues may require the use of this skill as part of related interventions. An appropriate health problem or issue may include: • Impaired cardiac output • Acute pain • Knowledge deficiency

(continued on page 988)

Skill 15-5 ▶ Applying a Cardiac Monitor *(continued)*

OUTCOME IDENTIFICATION AND PLANNING

The expected outcome to achieve when performing cardiac monitoring is that a clear waveform, free from artifacts, is displayed on the cardiac monitor. Other appropriate outcomes may include that the patient demonstrates an understanding of the reason for monitoring.

IMPLEMENTATION

ACTION	RATIONALE
1. Verify the prescribed intervention for cardiac monitoring in the patient's health record.	Verifying the prescribed intervention ensures that the correct intervention is administered to the right patient.
2. Gather equipment.	Assembling equipment provides for an organized approach to the task.
3. Perform hand hygiene and put on PPE, if indicated.	Hand hygiene and PPE prevent the spread of microorganisms. PPE is required based on transmission precautions.
4. Identify the patient.	Identifying the patient ensures the right patient receives the intervention and helps prevent errors.
5. Close the curtains around the bed and close the door to the room, if possible. Explain to the patient what you are going to do and why. Tell the patient that the monitoring records their heart's electrical activity. Emphasize that no electrical current will enter their body. Ask the patient about allergies to adhesive, as appropriate.	This ensures the patient's privacy. Explanation relieves anxiety and facilitates engagement. Possible allergies may exist related to the adhesive on ECG leads.
6. For hardwire monitoring, plug the cardiac monitor into an electrical outlet and turn it on to warm up the unit while preparing the equipment and the patient. For telemetry monitoring, insert a new battery into the transmitter. Match the poles on the battery with the polar markings on the transmitter case. Press the button at the top of the unit, test the battery's charge, and test the unit to ensure that the battery is operational.	Proper setup ensures proper functioning. Not all models have a test button. Test according to the manufacturer's directions.
7. Insert the cable into the appropriate socket in the monitor.	Proper setup ensures proper functioning.
8. Connect the lead wires to the cable. In some systems, the lead wires are permanently secured to the cable. For telemetry, if the lead wires are not permanently affixed to the telemetry unit, attach them securely. If they must be attached individually, connect each one to the correct outlet.	Proper setup ensures proper functioning.
9. Connect an electrode to each of the lead wires, carefully checking that each lead wire is in its correct outlet.	Proper setup ensures proper functioning.
10. If the bed is adjustable, raise it to a comfortable working height (VHACEOSH, 2016).	Having the bed at the proper height prevents back and muscle strain on the part of the nurse.
11. Expose the patient's chest and determine electrode positions, based on which system and leads are being used (refer to Figure 1). If necessary, prepare the skin for electrode placement (AACN, 2018). If an area is excessively hairy, clip the hair (AACN, 2018; Oster, n.d.) or shave the hair with a single-use razor (Campbell et al., 2017), according to facility policy. Clean excess oil or other substances from the skin with a skin cleanser and water. Use a gauze pad to vigorously rub and dry the skin.	Shaving may cause microabrasions on the skin, possibly resulting in portals of entry for microorganisms. Oils and excess hair interfere with electrode contact and function. Rubbing with gauze abrades and dries the skin. Proper skin preparation is essential to reduce artifacts in and increase quality of the ECG tracing (AACN, 2018; Campbell et al., 2017; Garcia, 2015; Oster, n.d.). Proper skin preparation and application of electrodes are imperative for good ECG monitoring (Morton & Fontaine, 2018, p. 215).

ACTION

RATIONALE

12. Remove the backing from the pregelled electrode. Check the gel for moistness. If the gel is dry, discard it and replace it with a fresh electrode. **Apply the electrode to the site and press it firmly to ensure a tight seal.** Repeat with the remaining electrodes to complete the 3- or 5-lead system (Figure 2).

Gel acts as a conduit and must be moist and secured tightly.

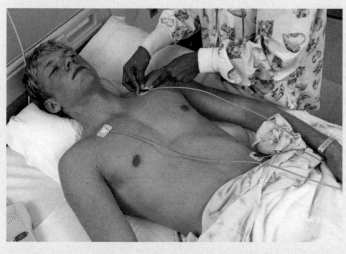

FIGURE 2. Applying the electrodes.

13. When all the electrodes are in place, connect the appropriate lead wire to each electrode. Select the appropriate monitoring lead based on the patient's clinical situation (AACN, 2018; Burns & Delgado, 2019; Sampson, 2018b). Check the waveform for clarity, position, and size. **To verify that the monitor is detecting each beat, compare the digital heart rate display with an auscultated count of the patient's heart rate.** If necessary, use the gain control to adjust the size of the rhythm tracing, and use the position control to adjust the waveform position on the monitor.

This ensures accuracy of the reading and relevant information for the individual patient.

14. Set the upper and lower limits of the heart rate alarm and other alarm settings, based on the patient's condition and the goals of patient care (AACN, 2018).

Setting alarms allows for audible notification if the heart rate or other variables are beyond limits. The default setting for the monitor automatically turns on all alarms; limits should be set for each patient.

15. For telemetry, place the transmitter in the pouch in the patient's gown. If no pouch is available in the gown, use a portable pouch. Tie the pouch strings around the patient's neck and waist, making sure that the pouch fits snugly without causing discomfort. If no pouch is available, place the transmitter in the patient's bathrobe pocket.

This prevents tension on the lead wires and promotes patient comfort.

16. Return the patient to a comfortable position. Lower the bed height and adjust the head of the bed to a comfortable position.

Repositioning promotes patient comfort. Lowering the bed promotes patient safety.

17. To obtain a rhythm strip, press the RECORD key, either at the bedside for monitoring or at the central station for telemetry. Analyze the strip, as appropriate. If the rhythm strip is a printed copy, label the strip with the patient's name and room number, date, time, and rhythm identification. Place the rhythm strip in the appropriate location in the patient's health record, based on facility policy.

A rhythm strip provides a baseline for future comparison. Accurate labeling ensures the ECG is recorded for the correct patient and accurate and reliable interpretation.

18. Remove additional PPE, if used. Perform hand hygiene.

Proper removal of PPE reduces the risk for infection transmission and contamination of other items. Hand hygiene prevents transmission of microorganisms.

(continued on page 990)

Skill 15-5 ▶ Applying a Cardiac Monitor *(continued)*

EVALUATION

The expected outcomes have been met when a clear waveform, free from artifacts, has been displayed on the cardiac monitor and the patient has demonstrated an understanding of the reason for monitoring.

DOCUMENTATION

Guidelines

Document significant assessment findings, the date and time that monitoring began, the monitoring lead used, and the patient's response to the procedure. Document a rhythm strip at least every 8 hours and with any changes in the patient's condition (or as stated by facility policy). Label the rhythm strip with the patient's name, room number, and facility identification number, if this was not done by the machine. Also record the date, time, and the patient's position as well as any appropriate clinical information. Record any deviations to the standard approach to the recording, such as alternative placement of leads.

Sample Documentation

> 12/16/25 1615 Patient admitted to room. Cardiac telemetry monitor in place; monitoring in lead II. See EHR for assessment data and initial rhythm strip.
>
> —T. Shah, RN

DEVELOPING CLINICAL REASONING AND CLINICAL JUDGMENT

UNEXPECTED SITUATIONS AND ASSOCIATED INTERVENTIONS

- *Low amplitude:* Assess if the size control is adjusted properly. Assess for poor contact between skin and electrodes, dried gel, broken or loose lead wires, a poor connection between the patient and the monitor, or a malfunctioning monitor. Check connections on all lead wires and the monitoring cable. Replace electrodes, as necessary. Reapply electrodes, if required.
- *Wandering baseline:* Assess for poor position, poor contact between electrodes and the patient's skin, or thoracic movement with respirations. Reposition or replace electrodes.
- *Artifact (waveform interference):* Assess for patient movement, improperly applied electrodes, or static electricity. Check the plugs to make sure the prongs are not loose.
- *Skin excoriation under electrodes:* Assess for an allergic reaction to electrode adhesive or electrodes being left on the skin too long. Change the electrodes daily. Remove the electrodes and apply hypoallergenic electrodes and hypoallergenic tape, or remove the electrode, clean the site, and reapply the electrode at the new site.

SPECIAL CONSIDERATIONS

General Considerations

- Make sure all electrical equipment and outlets are grounded to avoid electric shock and interference (artifacts).
- Change electrodes daily to prevent skin irritation and maintain quality of data (AACN, 2018; McGuffin & Ortiz, 2019).
- Avoid opening the electrode package until just before using to prevent the gel from drying out.
- Avoid placing the electrodes on bony prominences, hairy locations, areas where defibrillator pads will be placed, and areas for chest compression.
- Assess skin integrity and examine the leads every 8 hours. Replace and reposition the electrodes, as necessary, and at least daily.
- If the patient is being monitored by telemetry, show them how the transmitter works. If applicable, identify the button that will produce a recording of the ECG at the central station. Instruct the patient to push the button whenever symptoms occur; this causes the central console to print a rhythm strip. Also, advise the patient to notify the nurse immediately if symptoms occur.
- If the prescribed intervention is in place, tell the patient to remove the transmitter during showering or bathing, if appropriate, but stress that they should let the nurse know the unit is being removed.

Infant and Child Considerations

- Having the infant or child wear a snug undershirt over the leads helps to keep the leads in place (Kyle & Carman, 2021).

Community-Based Care Considerations

- Holter monitoring involves the use of continuous ECG monitoring to quantify cardiac activity that occurs during a patient's usual activities (Morton & Fontaine, 2018). Electrodes are place on the chest and connected to a portable recording device, which is worn for 24 hours up to 14 days (McLaughlin, 2020). Holder monitoring may be used to assess and diagnose the patient with syncope, near syncope, dizziness, or palpitations (Morton & Fontaine, 2018). Instruct patients to keep a diary to record medications, activities, and symptoms during the monitoring period; patients should maintain normal activities and record an entry in the diary at least every 2 hours (Morton & Fontaine, 2018).

EVIDENCE FOR PRACTICE ▶

CARDIAC MONITORING

Many patients admitted to acute care settings with cardiac, respiratory, and other acute health problems are placed on electrocardiographic monitoring. Frequent monitor alarms are distracting, interfere with the ability to perform critical tasks and contribute to alarm fatigue. The Joint Commission identifies improvement in the safety of clinical alarm systems, including the contribution of alarm signals to unnecessary alarm noise and alarm fatigue, as part of the National Patient Safety Goals (The Joint Commission, 2021). How can nurses reduce false alarms to promote safe patient care?

Related Evidence

McGuffin, K. S., & Ortiz, S. (2019). Daily electrocardiogram electrode change and the effect on frequency of nuisance alarms. *Dimensions of Critical Care Nursing, 38*(4), 187–191. https://doi.org/10.1097/DCC.0000000000000362

The purpose of the quality improvement project was to determine if changing electrocardiogram (ECG) electrodes daily would decrease the frequency of telemetry alarms. The project was implemented on an adult inpatient cardiac telemetry unit over a 28-day period, with a patient census during this period of 33 to 36 patients. Data were collected about the total number of telemetry alarms for 14 days prior to implementation, during which time the usual care was provided for changing of cardiac monitoring electrodes; cardiac monitoring electrodes were changed every 72 hours at inconsistent times during the day. During this preimplementation period, education on proper skin preparation (cleansing the skin with soap and water before electrode placement) and correct placement of ECG electrodes was provided to the day and night shift nurses three times per week. Data were then collected for 14 days during the intervention, in which staff changed electrodes daily on all patients receiving telemetry monitoring. Staff organized electrode changes by shift. For the first 7 days, the night shift changed electrodes; in the final 7 days, the day shift changed electrodes, between the hours of 6 am and 9 am. Staff recorded the date and time of each electrode change. Data were collected about the total number of telemetry alarms for 14 days during implementation. Comparison analysis determined if the frequency of alarms decreased after the intervention with daily electrode change. Prior to the intervention, there were 14,179 alarms in the 14-day period. There were 3,664 alarms during the 14-day intervention period (difference of 10, 515 alarms). There was a 74.15% reduction in telemetry alarms on the unit following implementation of a daily electrode change. The authors concluded daily ECG electrode changes may be an effective strategy for reducing nuisance alarms on telemetry units.

Relevance for Nursing Practice

Nurses have the responsibility to include interventions to provide for the best patient care outcomes possible. Ensuring proper skin preparation before applying monitor electrodes and daily changing of electrodes are simple interventions that can be implemented by nurses. These interventions can lead to fewer cardiac monitor alarms, contributing to reduced alarm fatigue and increased patient safety.

Skill 15-6 ▶ Using a Transcutaneous (External) Pacemaker

Temporary cardiac pacing is used to electrically stimulate the myocardium to correct life-threatening cardiac dysrhythmias such as bradycardia (Burns & Delgado, 2019). A temporary pacemaker consists of an external, battery-powered pulse generator and a lead or electrode system to electrically stimulate heartbeat. Most manual defibrillators and some AEDs are equipped to perform transcutaneous pacing (Hinkle et al., 2022). Transcutaneous pacing can temporarily supply an electrical current in the heart when electrical conduction is abnormal. This device works by sending an electrical impulse from the pulse generator to the patient's heart by way of two large-surface electrodes, which are placed on the front and back of the patient's chest. This stimulates the contraction of cardiac muscle fibers through electrical stimulation (depolarization) of the myocardium. Transcutaneous pacing is quick and effective but is usually used as short-term therapy until the situation resolves or transvenous or permanent pacing can be initiated (Burns & Delgado, 2019; Morton & Fontaine, 2018).

Transcutaneous pacing can cause significant discomfort (burning sensation and involuntary muscle contraction) (Hinkle et al., 2022). The patient should be informed, adequately sedated, and provided analgesia whenever possible (Burns & Delgado, 2019; Morton & Fontaine, 2018, p. 312; Stout, 2017).

DELEGATION CONSIDERATIONS	The use of a transcutaneous pacemaker is not delegated to assistive personnel (AP). Depending on the state's nurse practice act and the organization's policies and procedures, this procedure may be delegated to licensed practical/vocational nurses (LPN/LVNs). The decision to delegate must be based on careful analysis of the patient's needs and circumstances as well as the qualifications of the person to whom the task is being delegated. Refer to the Delegation Guidelines in Appendix A.
EQUIPMENT	• Transcutaneous noninvasive pacemaker • Transcutaneous pacing electrodes and cables • ECG electrodes and cables • Cardiac monitor • Medication for analgesia and/or sedation, as prescribed
ASSESSMENT	Review the patient's health record and care plan for information about the patient's need for pacing and as a prescribed intervention. Transcutaneous pacing is generally an emergency measure. Assess the patient's initial cardiac rhythm, including a rhythm strip and 12-lead ECG. Monitor heart rate, respiratory status, level of consciousness, and skin color. If the patient is pulseless, initiate CPR.
ACTUAL OR POTENTIAL HEALTH PROBLEMS AND NEEDS	Many actual or potential health problems or issues may require the use of this skill as part of related interventions. An appropriate health problem or issue may include: • Impaired cardiac output • Altered tissue perfusion • Injury Risk
OUTCOME IDENTIFICATION AND PLANNING	The expected outcomes to achieve when using an external transcutaneous pacemaker are that it is applied correctly without adverse effect; the patient regains and/or maintains signs of adequate circulation, including the capture of at least the minimal set heart rate; and the patient does not experience injury.

IMPLEMENTATION

ACTION	RATIONALE
1. Verify the prescribed intervention for a transcutaneous pacemaker in the patient's health record.	Verifying the prescribed intervention ensures that the correct intervention is administered to the right patient.
2. Gather all equipment.	Assembling equipment provides for an organized approach to the task.

ACTION	RATIONALE
3. Perform hand hygiene and put on PPE, if indicated.	Hand hygiene and PPE prevent the transmission of microorganisms. PPE is required based on transmission precautions.
4. Identify the patient.	Verifying the patient's identity validates that the correct procedure is being done on the correct patient.
5. If the patient is responsive, explain the procedure to them. Explain that it involves some discomfort and that you will administer medication to keep them comfortable and help them to relax. **Administer analgesia and sedation, as prescribed, if it is not an emergency situation.**	Most alert patients cannot tolerate the uncomfortable sensations produced by the high energy levels needed to pace externally (Zagkli et al., 2020). If responsive, the patient will most likely be sedated and given analgesia (Burns & Delgado, 2019; Hinkle et al., 2022; Morton & Fontaine, 2018; Stout, 2017).
6. Close the curtains around the bed and close the door to the room, if possible. Obtain vital signs.	This provides for patient privacy. Vital signs provide a baseline for assessing pacing effectiveness.
7. If necessary, prepare the skin for electrode placement (AACN, 2018). If an area is excessively hairy, clip the hair (AACN, 2018; Oster, n.d.), or shave the hair with a single-use razor (Campbell et al., 2017), according to facility policy. Clean excess oil or other substances from the skin with a skin cleanser and water. Use a gauze pad to vigorously rub and dry the skin.	Shaving may cause microabrasions on the skin, possibly resulting in portals of entry for microorganisms. Oils and excess hair interfere with electrode contact and function. Rubbing with gauze abrades and dries the skin. Proper skin preparation is essential to reduce artifacts in and increase quality of the pacing (AACN, 2018; Campbell et al., 2017; Garcia, 2015; Oster, n.d.).
8. Attach the cardiac monitoring electrodes to the patient in the lead I, II, and III positions (refer to Skill 15-5). Do this even if the patient is already on telemetry monitoring. If you select the lead II position, adjust the left leg (LL) electrode placement to accommodate the anterior pacing electrode and the patient's anatomy.	Cardiac monitoring electrodes must be placed in addition to the pacing electrodes in order for the pacemaker to read the patient's cardiac rhythm while the pacing electrodes deliver the energy needed to pace the heart (Stout, 2017). Connecting the telemetry electrodes to the pacemaker is required.
9. Attach the patient monitoring electrodes to the ECG cable and into the ECG input connection on the front of the pacing generator. Set the selector switch to the "Monitor on" position.	These actions ensure that the equipment is functioning properly.
10. Note the ECG waveform on the monitor. Adjust the R-wave beeper volume to a suitable level and activate the alarm by pressing the "Alarm on" button. Set the alarm for 10 to 20 beats lower and 20 to 30 beats higher than the patient's target pacing rate.	These actions ensure that the equipment is functioning properly. Alarms alert the nurse to potential concerns regarding the patient's status.
11. Press the "Start/Stop" button for a printout of the waveform.	A printout provides objective data.
12. Apply the two pacing electrodes, starting with the posterior electrode. Pull the protective strip from the posterior electrode (marked "Back") and apply the electrode on the left side of the thoracic spinal column, just below the scapula (Figure 1).	This placement ensures that the electrical stimulus will travel only a short distance to the heart.
13. Apply the anterior pacing electrode (marked "Front"), which has two protective strips—one covering the gelled area and one covering the outer rim. Expose the gelled area and apply it to the skin in the anterior position, to the left of the precordium in the V_2 to the V_5 position (see Figure 1). Move this electrode around to get the best waveform. Then expose the electrode's outer rim and firmly press it to the skin.	This placement ensures that the electrical stimulus will travel only a short distance to the heart.
14. Prepare to pace the heart. After making sure the energy output in milliamperes (mA) is on 0, connect the electrode cable to the monitor output cable.	This sets the pacing threshold.

(continued on page 994)

Skill 15-6 ▶ Using a Transcutaneous (External) Pacemaker *(continued)*

ACTION

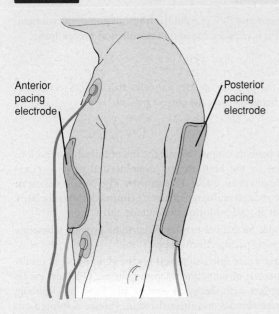

Anterior pacing electrode

Posterior pacing electrode

FIGURE 1. Transcutaneous pacemaker pads in place.

15. Check the waveform, looking for a tall QRS complex in lead II.

16. Check the selector switch to "Pacer on." Select synchronous (demand) or asynchronous (fixed-rate or nondemand) mode, as prescribed. **Tell the patient they may feel a thumping or twitching sensation. Reassure the patient you will provide analgesic medication if the discomfort is intolerable.**

17. Set the pacing rate dial to a target pacing rate of 60 to 70 beats/min. Look for pacer artifact or spikes, which will appear as you increase the rate.

18. Set the pacing current output (in mA), if not automatically done by the pacemaker. For patients with bradycardia, start with the minimal setting and **slowly increase the amount of energy delivered to the heart by adjusting the "Output" mA dial. Do this until electrical capture is achieved: you will see a pacer spike followed by a widened QRS complex and a tall broad T wave that resembles a premature ventricular contraction.**

19. Increase output by 2 mA or 10% to ensure capture. **Do not go higher (unless prescribed or indicated) because of the increased risk of discomfort to the patient.** Print a strip and place it in the patient's health record.

RATIONALE

Asynchronous pacing delivers a stimulus at a set (fixed) rate regardless of the occurrence of spontaneous myocardial depolarizations (the patient's own underlying heart rate). Synchronous pacing delivers a stimulus only when the heart's intrinsic pacemaker fails to function at a predetermined rate (if the patient's own heart rate drops below the demand rate set on the pacemaker). Analgesia and/or sedation may be administered, as prescribed and indicated, for discomfort associated with pacing (Burns & Delgado, 2019; Hinkle et al., 2022; Morton & Fontaine, 2018; Stout, 2017).

Setting the pacing rate dial higher than the intrinsic rhythm ensures adequate cardiac output.

Setting the pacing current output ensures adequate cardiac output.

Increasing the output ensures consistent capture. With full capture, the patient's heart rate should be the same as the pacemaker rate shown on the machine. The usual pacing threshold is between 40 and 80 mA. Thresholds may vary due to recent cardiothoracic surgery, pericardial effusions, cardiac tamponade, acidosis, and hypoxia. These conditions may require higher thresholds. Printing a strip documents the patient's paced rhythm.

ACTION	RATIONALE
20. Assess for effectiveness of pacing and mechanical capture: observe for a pacemaker spike with subsequent capture; assess heart rate and rhythm (using the right carotid, brachial, or femoral artery), assess blood pressure, and assess for signs of improved cardiac output (increased blood pressure, improved level of consciousness, improved body temperature).	Both electrical and mechanical capture must occur to benefit the patient (Stout, 2017). Transcutaneous pacing spikes are usually very large and may distort the QRS complex in electrocardiography (Burns & Delgado, 2019). The presence of a pulse with every pacing spike confirms ventricular capture (Burns & Delgado, 2019). Use of the patient's right side for pulse assessment avoids inaccuracy related to strong contractions from the pacemaker.
21. Secure the pacing leads and cable to the patient's body.	This prevents accidental displacement of the electrode, resulting in failure to pace or sense.
22. Remove PPE, if used. Perform hand hygiene.	Proper removal of PPE reduces the risk for infection transmission and contamination of other items. Hand hygiene and proper disposal of equipment reduce the transmission of microorganisms.
23. Continue to monitor the patient's heart rate and rhythm to assess ventricular response to pacing. Assess the patient's vital signs, skin color, level of consciousness, and peripheral pulses. Take blood pressure in both arms.	Assessment helps determine the effectiveness of the paced rhythm. If the blood pressure reading is significantly higher in one arm, use that arm for measurements.
24. Continue to assess the patient's pain and administer analgesia/sedation, as prescribed, to ease the discomfort of chest wall muscle contractions.	Analgesia and sedation promote patient comfort.
25. Perform a 12-lead ECG and additional ECGs daily or with clinical changes.	ECG monitoring provides a baseline for further evaluation.
26. Continually monitor the ECG readings, noting capture, sensing, rate, intrinsic beats, and competition of paced and intrinsic rhythms. If the pacemaker is sensing correctly, the sense indicator on the pulse generator should flash with each beat.	Continuous monitoring helps evaluate the patient's condition and determine the effectiveness of therapy.

EVALUATION

The expected outcomes have been met when the external transcutaneous pacemaker has been applied correctly without adverse effect; the patient has regained and/or maintained signs of adequate circulation, including the capture of at least the minimal set heart rate; and the patient has not experienced injury.

DOCUMENTATION

Guidelines

Document the reason for pacemaker use, time that pacing began, electrode locations, pacemaker settings, the patient's response to the procedure and to temporary pacing, complications, and nursing actions taken. Document the patient's pain intensity rating, analgesia or sedation administered, and the patient's response. If possible, obtain a rhythm strip before, during, and after pacemaker placement; anytime the pacemaker settings are changed; and whenever the patient receives treatment because of a complication due to the pacemaker.

Sample Documentation

1/2/25 1218 Baseline rhythm strip obtained, sinus bradycardia at 43 beats/min; see flow sheet. External temporary pacemaker placed by Dr. Goodman. Cardiac monitoring electrodes placed in the lead I, II, and III positions. Pacer set in synchronous mode at rate of 80 beats/min; pacing current output 72 mA. Patient with strong femoral pulses; see flow sheet for vital signs. Patient reports chest discomfort of 4/10. Medicated with morphine 2 mg IV. Pacer alarms set at 50 and 90 beats/min.

—R. Robinson, RN

1/2/25 1250 Patient reports decreased pain, 1/10.

—R. Robinson, RN

(continued on page 996)

Skill 15-6 ▶ Using a Transcutaneous (External) Pacemaker *(continued)*

DEVELOPING CLINICAL REASONING AND CLINICAL JUDGMENT

UNEXPECTED SITUATIONS AND ASSOCIATED INTERVENTIONS

- *Failure to pace:* This happens when the pacemaker either does not fire or fires too often. The pulse generator may not be working properly, or it may not be conducting the impulse to the patient. If the pacing or sensing indicator flashes, check the connections to the cable and the position/contact of the pacing electrodes on the patient. The cable may have come loose, or the electrode may not be making contact. If the pulse generator is turned on, but the indicators still are not flashing, change the battery. If that does not help, use a different pulse generator. Check the settings if the pacemaker is firing too rapidly. If they are correct, or if altering them (according to your facility's policy or the prescribed intervention) does not help, change the pulse generator.
- *Failure to capture:* Pacemaker spikes are seen, but the heart is not responding. The most common reason is failure to increase the current sufficiently. It may also be caused by changes in the pacing threshold from ischemia, an electrolyte imbalance (high or low potassium or magnesium levels), acidosis, an adverse reaction to a medication, or fibrosis. If the patient's condition has changed, notify the health care provider, and ask for new settings. Carefully check all connections, making sure they are placed properly and securely. Increase the milliamperes slowly (according to facility policy or the prescribed intervention).
- *Failure to sense intrinsic beats:* This could cause ventricular tachycardia or ventricular fibrillation if the pacemaker fires on the vulnerable T wave. This could be caused by the pacemaker sensing an external stimulus as a QRS complex, which could lead to asystole, or by the pacemaker not being sufficiently sensitive, which means it could fire anywhere within the cardiac cycle. If the pacing is undersensing, turn the sensitivity dial toward lower millivolt value. If it is oversensing, reduce the sensitivity; the value in millivolts should be larger to make the pacer less sensitive (Morton & Fontaine, 2018). If the pacemaker is not functioning correctly, change the battery or the pulse generator.

SPECIAL CONSIDERATIONS

- Transcutaneous pacing spikes are usually very large, often distorting the QRS complex in electrocardiography (Burns & Delgado, 2019). The presence of a pulse with every pacing spike confirms ventricular capture (Burns & Delgado, 2019).
- Do not leave patients unattended during noninvasive pacing. It is safe to touch the patient and perform procedures during pacing (e.g., CPR). Gloves should be worn. Do not touch the conductive surface of the electrodes.
- Check the skin where the electrodes are placed for skin burns or tissue damage (Hinkle et al., 2022). Reposition, as needed.

Skill 15-7 ▶ Removing a Peripheral Arterial Catheter

Arterial catheters may be used for intensive and continuous cardiac monitoring and intra-arterial access. The most common sites in adults are the radial (Burns & Delgado, 2019) and brachial arteries to reduce the risk of infection (O'Grady et al., 2017), although the femoral site can be used as well (Morton & Fontaine, 2018). Alternative and less frequent sites include the axillary and pedal arteries in adults (Burn & Delgado, 2019) and temporal and umbilical arteries in neonates (Gorski et al., 2021; Morton & Fontaine, 2018). As soon as the arterial catheter is no longer needed or has become ineffective, it should be removed (Burns & Delgado, 2019; Gorski et al., 2021; O'Grady et al., 2017). Consult facility policy to determine whether nurses are permitted to perform this procedure. Two nurses should be at the bedside until bleeding is controlled and to be available to give emergency medications or assistance, if necessary.

| DELEGATION CONSIDERATIONS | Removal of an arterial catheter is not delegated to assistive personnel (AP) or licensed practical/vocational nurses (LPN/LVNs). |

EQUIPMENT

- Sterile gloves
- Clean gloves
- Goggles and mask or face shield
- Waterproof, disposable gown
- Sterile gauze pads
- Waterproof protective pad
- Sterile suture removal set

- Transparent dressing
- Hypoallergenic tape
- Emergency medications (e.g., atropine, for a vasovagal response with femoral catheter removal) for emergency response, per facility policy and guidelines

ASSESSMENT

Review the patient's health record and care plan for information and prescribed intervention about discontinuation of the arterial catheter. Assess the patient's coagulation status, including laboratory studies, to reduce the risk of complications secondary to impaired clotting ability. Assess the patient's understanding of the procedure. Inspect the site for leakage, bleeding, or hematoma. Assess skin color and temperature and assess distal pulses for strength and quality. Mark distal pulses with an "X" for easy identification after the procedure.

ACTUAL OR POTENTIAL HEALTH PROBLEMS AND NEEDS

Many actual or potential health problems or issues may require the use of this skill as part of related interventions. An appropriate health problem or issue may include:

- Injury risk
- Altered skin integrity
- Infection risk

OUTCOME IDENTIFICATION AND PLANNING

The expected outcomes to achieve when removing an arterial catheter are that the catheter is removed intact and without injury to the patient. Additional outcomes include that the patient maintains intact peripheral circulation, and the site remains clean and dry, without evidence of infection, bleeding, or hematoma.

IMPLEMENTATION

ACTION	**RATIONALE**
1. Verify the prescribed intervention for removal of the arterial catheter in the patient's health record.	Verifying the prescribed intervention ensures that the correct intervention is administered to the right patient.
2. Gather all equipment.	Assembling equipment provides for an organized approach to the task.
3. Perform hand hygiene and put on PPE, if indicated.	Hand hygiene and PPE prevent the spread of microorganisms. PPE is required based on transmission precautions.
4. Identify the patient.	Identifying the patient ensures the right patient receives the intervention and helps prevent errors.
5. Close the curtains around the bed and close the door to the room, if possible. Explain the procedure to the patient.	This ensures the patient's privacy. Explanation relieves anxiety and facilitates engagement in care.
6. Maintain an IV infusion of normal saline via another venous access during the procedure, as prescribed or per facility guidelines.	IV access may be needed in case of hypotension or bradycardia.
7. If the bed is adjustable, raise it to a comfortable working height (VHACEOSH, 2016).	Having the bed at the proper height prevents back and muscle strain on the part of the nurse.

(continued on page 998)

Skill 15-7 ▶ Removing a Peripheral Arterial Catheter *(continued)*

ACTION	**RATIONALE**
8. Put on clean gloves, goggles and a mask or face shield, and a gown.	These prevent contact with blood and body fluids.
9. Turn off the monitor alarms and then turn off the flow clamp to the flush solution. Carefully remove the stabilization device and/or dressing over the insertion site. Remove any sutures using the suture removal kit; make sure all sutures have been removed.	These measures help prepare for withdrawal of the catheter.
10. **Withdraw the catheter using a gentle, steady motion. Keep the catheter parallel to the blood vessel during withdrawal.** Watch for hematoma formation during catheter removal by gently palpating surrounding tissue. If a hematoma starts to form, reposition your hands until optimal pressure is obtained to prevent further leakage of blood.	Using a gentle, steady motion parallel to the blood vessel helps reduce the risk for traumatic injury.
11. **Immediately after withdrawing the catheter, apply pressure at and just above the cannula site with a sterile 4 × 4 gauze pad. Maintain pressure over the site for at least 5 minutes** (Burns & Delgado, 2019), **or until hemostasis is achieved** (Burns & Delgado, 2019; Gorski et al., 2021). Apply additional pressure (10 minutes or longer) (Burns & Delgado, 2019) to a femoral site, or if the patient has a coagulation abnormality or is receiving anticoagulants (Burns & Delgado, 2019; Crumlett & Johnson, 2016).	This prevents bleeding and hematoma formation.
12. Cover the site with a sterile dressing once hemostasis is achieved (Gorski et al., 2021). Once hemostasis is achieved, a pressure dressing may be used but is generally not needed (Burns & Delgado, 2019).	This prevents introduction of microorganisms and reduces the risk of infection.
13. Remove gloves and perform hand hygiene. Lower the bed height and assist the patient to a position of comfort.	Proper removal of PPE and hand hygiene reduce the risk for infection transmission and contamination of other items. Positioning promotes patient safety and comfort.
14. Remove additional PPE. Perform hand hygiene.	Proper removal of PPE reduces the risk for infection transmission and contamination of other items. Hand hygiene prevents transmission of microorganisms.
15. Observe the site for bleeding and thrombosis of the artery frequently after catheter removal (Burns & Delgado, 2019), according to facility policy. Assess and document the circulatory status distal to the site frequently for the first few hours after catheter removal (Burns & Delgado, 2019), according to facility policy.	Continued assessment allows for early detection and prompt intervention, should problems arise.

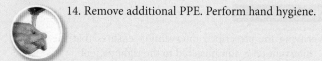

EVALUATION

The expected outcomes have been met when the patient has exhibited a clean and dry arterial catheter site without evidence of injury, infection, bleeding, or hematoma, and the patient demonstrated intact peripheral circulation.

DOCUMENTATION

Guidelines

Document the time the catheter was removed and how long pressure was applied. Document assessment of peripheral circulation, appearance of the site, the type of dressing applied, the timed assessments, the patient's response, and any medications administered.

Sample Documentation

12/20/25 1830 Right radial arterial catheter removed. Pressure applied to site for 10 minutes. Site intact without signs of hematoma; radial pulse present, +2 and regular. Hand warm and dry; hand skin tone consistent with left hand. Sterile transparent dressing applied to site. Patient denies pain, nausea, shortness of breath. Vital signs stable before, during, and after procedure. See vital signs tab.

—B. Clapp, RN

DEVELOPING CLINICAL REASONING AND CLINICAL JUDGMENT

UNEXPECTED SITUATIONS AND ASSOCIATED INTERVENTIONS

- *Assessment reveals fresh blood on the site dressing:* Apply pressure. If bleeding continues, notify the health care team.
- *Affected extremity is cold and/or pulseless:* Immediately notify the health care team.
- *Patient reports severe back pain or is noted to be hypotensive:* Symptoms may be due to retroperitoneal bleeding. Notify the health care team immediately.

SPECIAL CONSIDERATIONS

- Culture of the catheter tip may be indicated upon removal if the patient has a suspected catheter-associated blood stream infection (CABSI) (Gorski et al., 2021). If prescribed, place the catheter tip on a 4 × 4 sterile gauze pad. After the bleeding is under control and the dressing is secure, hold the catheter over the sterile container. Cut the tip of the catheter with sterile scissors and allow it to fall into the sterile container. Label the specimen and send it to the laboratory.

Enhance Your Understanding

Focusing on Patient Care: Developing Clinical Reasoning and Clinical Judgment

Consider the case scenarios at the beginning of the chapter as you answer the following questions to enhance your understanding and apply what you have learned.

QUESTIONS

1. Coby Pruder becomes visibly anxious when you bring in the ECG machine and begin to open the supplies. What could you do to help alleviate their anxiety?

2. You go in to assess Harry Stebbings and find them unresponsive. How should you respond?

3. You go in to respond to the alarm on the cardiac monitor. Ann Kribell is asymptomatic, and their vital signs are stable, but the monitor tracing has a lot of artifacts. Ann reports being tired and irritable as a result of being unable to rest or sleep because of the alarms. Discuss the appropriate actions to problem solve this unexpected situation.

You can find suggested answers after the Bibliography at the end of this chapter.

Integrated Case Study Connection

The case studies in the back of the book focus on integrating concepts. Refer to the following case studies to enhance your understanding of the concepts and skills in this chapter.

- Advanced Case Studies: Cole McKean, page 1225.

Bibliography

American Association of Critical-Care Nurses (AACN). (2016). *AACN practice alert. Family presence during resuscitation and invasive procedures. Critical Care Nurse*, 36(1), e11–e14. http://dx.doi.org/10.4037/ccn2016980

American Association of Critical-Care Nurses (AACN). (2018). *AACN practice alert. Accurate dysrhythmia monitoring in adults. Critical Care Nurse*, 36(6), e26–e34. http://dx.doi.org/10.4037/ccn2016767

American Heart Association (AHA). (2016, September 30). *Implantable cardioverter defibrillator (ICD).* https://www.heart.org/en/health-topics/arrhythmia/prevention–treatment-of-arrhythmia/implantable-cardioverter-defibrillator-icd#.WN6CIfnyuUk

American Heart Association (AHA). (2020a, October 20). 2020 American Heart Association guidelines for cardiopulmonary resuscitation and emergency cardiovascular care. Parts 1-7. *Circulation, 142*(16 Suppl 2). https://www.ahajournals.org/toc/circ/142/16_suppl_2

American Heart Association (AHA). (2020b). *2020 CPR & ECC guidelines. BLS provider manual.* AHA product number: 20–1102.

American Heart Association (AHA). (2021). *Hands-only CPR. Fact sheet.* https://cpr.heart.org/-/media/cpr-files/courses-and-kits/hands-only-cpr/2021hocpr-documents/ds17758_cprweek_fact-sheeteng.pdf?la=en

Andrews, M., Boyle, J. S., & Collins, J. (2020). *Transcultural concepts in nursing care* (8th ed.). Wolters Kluwer.

Bauldoff, G., Gubrud, P., & Carno, M. A. (2020). *LeMone and Burke's Medical-surgical nursing: Clinical reasoning in patient care* (7th ed.). Pearson.

Bhatnager, V., Jinjil, K., Dwivedi, D., Verma, R., & Tandon, U. (2018). Cardiopulmonary resuscitation: Unusual techniques for unusual situations. *Journal of Emergencies, Trauma, and Shock, 11*(1), 31–37. https://doi.org/10.4103/JETS.JETS_58_17

Bickerton, M., & Pooler, A. (2019). Misplaced ECG electrodes and the need for continuing training. *British Journal of Cardiac Nursing, 14*(3), 123–132. https://doi.org/10.12968/bjca.2019.14.3.123

Bloe, C. (2021). The role of single-use ECG leads in reducing healthcare-associated infections. *British Journal of Nursing, 30*(11), 628–633. https://doi.org/10.12968/bjon.2021.30.11.628

Burns, S. M, & Delgado, S. A. (2019). *AACN essentials of critical care nursing* (4th ed.). McGraw Hill Education.

Campbell, B., Richley, D., Ross, C., & Eggett, C. J. (2017). *Clinical guidelines by consensus: Recording a standard 12-lead electrocardiogram. An approved method by the Society for Cardiological Science and Technology (SCST).* https://scst.org.uk/wp-content/uploads/2020/02/SCST_ECG_Recording_Guidelines_2017am.pdf

Cleveland Clinic. (2019, April 25). *Biventricular pacemaker.* https://my.clevelandclinic.org/health/treatments/16784-biventricular-pacemaker

Crumlett, H., & Johnson, A. (2016). Procedure 59. Arterial catheter insertion (assist), care, and removal. In D. L. Wiegand (Ed.), *AACN Procedure manual for high acuity, progressive, and critical care* (7th ed., pp. 508–522). Elsevier.

Di Biase, M., Casani, A., & Orfeo, L. (2015). Invasive arterial blood pressure in the neonatal intensive care: A valuable tool to manage very ill preterm and term neonates. *Italian Journal of Pediatrics, 41*(Suppl 1), A9. https://doi.org/10.1186/1824-7288-41-S1-A9

Douma, M. J., MacKenzie, E., Loch, T., Tan, M. C., Anderson, D., Picard, C., Milovanovic, L., O'Dochartaigh, D., & Brindley, P. G. (2020). Prone cardiopulmonary resuscitation:? A scoping and expanded grey literature review for the COVID-19 pandemic. *Resuscitation, 155,* 103–111. https://doi.org/10.1016/j.resuscitation.2020.07.010

Edelson, D. P., Sasson, C., Chan, P. S., Atkins, D. L., Aziz, K., Becker, L. B., Berg, R. A., Bradley, S. M., Brooks, S. C., Cheng, A., Escobedo, M., Flores, G. E., Girotra, S., Hsu, A., Kamath-Rayne, B. D., Lee, H. C., Lehotsky, R. E., Mancini, M. E., Merchant, R. M., … Topjian, A. A. (2020). Interim guidance for basic and advanced life support in adults, children, and neonates with suspected or confirmed COVID-19. *Circulation, 141*(25), e933–e943. https://doi.org/10.1161/CIRCULATIONAHA.120.047463

Einav, S., Cortegiani, A., & Marcus, E. L. (2021). Cardiac arrest in older patients. *Current Opinion in Anesthesiology, 34*(1), 40–47. https://doi.org/10.1097/ACO.0000000000000942

Eliopoulos, C. (2018). *Gerontological nursing* (9th ed.). Wolters Kluwer.

Fischbach, F. T., & Fischbach, M. A. (2018). *A manual of laboratory and diagnostic tests* (10th ed.). Wolters Kluwer.

Garcia, T. (2015). Acquiring the 12-lead electrocardiogram: Doing it right every time. *Journal of Emergency Nursing, 41*(6), 474–478. https://doi.org/10.1016/j.jen.2015.04.014

Gorski, L. A., Hadaway, L., Hagle, M. E., Broadhurst, D., Clare, S., Kleidon, T., Meyer, B. M., Nickel, B., Rowley, S., Sharpe, E., & Alexander, M.; Infusion Nurses Society (INS). (2021). Infusion therapy. Standards of practice. *Journal of Infusion Nursing, 44*(Suppl 1), S1–S224. https://doi.org/10.1097/NAN.0000000000000396

Headway. (2021). *Hypoxic and anoxic brain injury.* https://www.headway.org.uk/about-brain-injury/individuals/types-of-brain-injury/hypoxic-and-anoxic-brain-injury/

Hinkle, J. L., Cheever, K. H., & Overbaugh, K. (2022). *Brunner & Suddarth's Textbook of medical-surgical nursing* (15th ed.). Wolters Kluwer.

International Council of Nurses (ICN). (2019). *Nursing diagnosis and outcome statements.* https://www.icn.ch/sites/default/files/inline-files/ICNP2019-DC.pdf

Jarvis, C., & Echkardt, A. (2020). *Physical examination & health assessment* (8th ed.). Elsevier.

Jensen, S. (2019). *Nursing health assessment. A best practice approach* (3rd ed.). Wolters Kluwer.

Jevon, P. (2010). Procedure for recording a standard 12-lead electrocardiogram. *British Journal of Nursing (Mark Allen Publishing), 19*(10), 649–651.

The Joint Commission. (2021, January 1). *Hospital: 2021 National Patient Safety Goals.* https://www.jointcommission.org/standards/national-patient-safety-goals/hospital-national-patient-safety-goals/

Karch, A. M. (2020). *Focus on nursing pharmacology* (8th ed.). Wolters Kluwer.

Kyle, T., & Carman, S. (2021). *Essentials of pediatric nursing* (4th ed.). Wolters Kluwer.

Lacerte, M., Shapshak, A. H., & Mesfin, F. B. (2020, November 19). *Hypoxic brain injury.* StatPearls. https://www.ncbi.nlm.nih.gov/books/NBK537310/

McAlvin, S. S., & Carew-Lyons, A. (2014). Family presence during resuscitation and invasive procedures in pediatric critical care: A systematic review. *American Journal of Critical Care, 23*(6), 477–484. https://doi.org/10.4037/ajcc2014922

McGuffin, K. S., & Ortiz, S. (2019). Daily electrocardiogram electrode change and the effect on frequency of nuisance alarms. *Dimensions of Critical Care Nursing, 38*(4), 187–191. https://doi.org/10.1097/DCC.0000000000000362

McLaughlin, M. A. (Ed.). (2020). *Cardiovascular care made incredibly easy* (4th ed.). Wolters Kluwer.

Menzies-Gow, E. (2018). How to record a 12-lead electrocardiogram. *Nursing Standard, 33*(2), 38–42. https://doi.org/10.7748/ns.2018.e11066

Miller, S. K. (2019). 12-lead electrocardiographic interpretation for nurse practitioners. *The Journal for Nurse Practitioners, 15*(1), 110–117. https://doi.org/10.1016/j.nurpra.2018.10.014

Morton, P. G., & Fontaine, D. K. (2018). *Essentials of critical care nursing: A holistic approach* (11th ed.). Wolters Kluwer.

Moscarelli, A., Iozzo, P., Ippolito, M., Catalisano, G., Gregoretti, C., Giarratano, A., Baldi, E., & Cortegiani, A. (2020). Cardiopulmonary resuscitation in prone position: A scoping review. *American Journal of Emergency Medicine, 38*(11), 2416–2424. https://doi.org/10.1016/j.ajem.2020.08.097

National Heart, Lung, and Blood Institute (NHLBI). (2021, January 8). *Pacemakers.* https://www.nhlbi.nih.gov/health-topics/pacemakers

Norris, T. L. (2020). *Porth's essentials of pathophysiology* (5th ed.). Wolters Kluwer.

O'Grady, N. P., Alexander, M., Burns, L. A., Dellinger, E. P., Garland, J., Heard, S. O., Lipsett, P. A., Masur, H., Mermel, L. A., Pearson, M. L., Raad, I. I., Randolph, A. G., Rupp, M. E., Saint, S., & Healthcare Infection

Control Practices Advisory Committee (HICPAC). (2017, July). *Guidelines for the prevention of intravascular catheter-related infections.* Centers for Disease Control and Prevention. *Clinical Infectious Diseases, 52*(9), e162–193. https://www.cdc.gov/infectioncontrol/pdf/guidelines/bsi-guidelines-H.pdf

Olasveengen, T. M., Mancinie, M. E., Perkins, G. D., Avis, S., Brooks, S., Castrén, M., Chung, S. P., Considine, J., Couper, K., Escalante, R., Hatanaka, T., Hung, K. K. C., Kudenchuk, P., Lim, S. H., Nishiyama, C., Ristagno, G., Semeraro, F., Smith, C. M., Smyth, M. A., … Morley, P. T. (2020). Adult basic life support: 2020 international consensus on cardiopulmonary resuscitation and emergency cardiovascular care science with treatment recommendations. *Circulation, 142*(16 Supp 1), S41–S91. https://doi.org/10.1161/CIR.0000000000000892

Oster, C. D. (n.d.). *Proper skin prep helps ensure ECG trace quality.* 3M Medical. https://multimedia.3m.com/mws/media/358372O/proper-skin-prep-ecg-trace-quality-white-paper.pdf

Pankop, R., Chang, K., Thorlton, J., & Spitzer, T. (2013). Implemented family presence protocols: An integrative review. *Journal of Nursing Care Quality, 28*(3), 281–288. https://doi.org/10.1097/NCQ.0b013e31827a472a

Pearce, A. (2019). Examining the causes and effects of electrode misplacement during electrocardiography: A literature review. *British Journal of Cardiac Nursing* [online], *14*(7), 1–15. https://doi.org/10.12968/bjca.2019.0010

Powers, K., & Reeve, C. L. (2020). Family presence during resuscitation: Medical-surgical nurses' perceptions, self-confidence, and use of invitations. *American Journal of Nursing, 120*(11), 28–38. https://doi.org/10.1097/01.naj.0000721244.16344.ee

Sampson, M. (2018a). Continuous ECG monitoring in hospital: Part 1, indications. *British Journal of Cardiac Nursing, 13*(2), 80–85. https://doi.org/10.12968/bjca.2018.13.2.80

Sampson, M. (2018b). Continuous ECG monitoring in hospital: Part 2, practical issues. *British Journal of Cardiac Nursing, 13*(3), 128–134. https://doi.org/10.12968/bjca.2018.13.3.128

Sharma, R., Jayathissa, S., & Weatherall, M. (2016). Cardiopulmonary resuscitation knowledge and opinions on end of life decision making of older adults admitted to an acute medical service. *New Zealand Medical Journal, 129*(1428), 26–36.

Silbert-Flagg, J., & Pillitteri, A. (2018). *Maternal and child health nursing* (8th ed.). Wolters Kluwer.

Soleimanpour, H., Tabrizi, J. S., Rouhi, A. J., Golzari, S. E. J., Mahmoodpoor, A., Esfanjani, R. M., & Soleimanpour, M. (2017). Psychological effects on patient's relatives regarding their presence during resuscitation. *Journal of Cardiovascular and Thoracic Research, 9*(2), 113–117. https://doi.org/10.15171/jcvtr.2017.19

Stout, K. (Ed.). (2017). *ACLS review made incredibly easy* (3rd ed.). Wolters Kluwer.

Taylor, C., Lynn, P., & Bartlett, J. (2023). *Fundamentals of nursing: The art and science of person-centered care* (10th ed.). Wolters Kluwer.

Toronto, C. E., & LaRocco, S. A. (2018). Family perception of and experience with family presence during cardiopulmonary resuscitation: An integrative review. *Journal of Clinical Nursing, 28*(1–2), 32–46. https://doi.org/10.1111/jocn.14649

Vanhoy, M. A., Horigan, A., Stapleton, S. J., Valdez, A. M., Bradford, J. Y., Killian, M., Reeve, N. E., Slivinski, A., Zaleski, M. E., Proehl, J., Wolf, L., Delao, A., Gates, L. Sr., & 2017 ENA Clinical Practice Guideline Committee. (2019). Clinical Practice Guideline: Family presence. *Journal of Emergency Nursing, 45*(1), e1–e76. e29. https://doi.org/10.1016/j.jen.2018.11.012

VHA Center for Engineering & Occupational Safety and Health (CEOSH). (2016). *Safe patient handling and mobility guidebook.* http://www.tnpatientsafety.com/pubfiles/Initiatives/workplace-violence/sphm-pdf.pdf

Wolters Kluwer. (2022). Problem-based care plans. In *Lippincott Advisor.* Wolters Kluwer.

Zagkli, F., Georgakopoulou, A., & Chilandakis, J. (2020). Effects of transcutaneous cardiac pacing on ventricular repolarization and comparison with transvenous pacing. *Pacing and Clinical Electrophysiology, 43*(9), 1004–1011. https://doi.org/10.1111/pace.14000

SUGGESTED ANSWERS FOR FOCUSING ON PATIENT CARE: DEVELOPING CLINICAL REASONING AND CLINICAL JUDGMENT

1. Explain the steps involved in obtaining an ECG. Tell Mr. Pruder that the test records the heart's electrical activity, and it may be repeated at certain intervals. Emphasize that no electrical current will enter their body and that the ECG will provide important information to help guide their health care. Tell them the test typically takes about 5 minutes.

2. Call for help, pull call bell, and call the facility emergency response number. Call for emergency equipment and the automated external defibrillator (AED) or defibrillator. Put on gloves, if available. Position Mr. Stebbings supine on their back on a firm, flat surface, with arms alongside the body. If they are in bed, place a backboard or other rigid surface under them (often the footboard of the patient's bed). Initiate CPR. Provide defibrillation as soon as an AED becomes available.

3. Check the cardiac monitor alarm settings to ensure the upper and lower limits of the heart rate alarm and other alarm settings are based on the patient's condition and goals of patient care. If the alarms are set for parameters that are not relevant to this patient, the alarms may be triggering at inappropriate times. Check that the electrodes are securely adhered to the patient's skin. Change the electrodes; clean excess oil or other substances from the skin. Use a gauze pad to vigorously rub and dry the skin. Oils and excess hair interfere with electrode contact and function. Rubbing with gauze abrades and dries the skin. Poor contact with the skin may result in an inaccurate signal. Proper skin preparation is essential to reduce artifacts in and increase the quality of the ECG tracing. When you open the electrode package, check the gel for moistness before applying the new electrode. Dried electrodes do not conduct the signal well or accurately. Apply the electrode to the skin by pressing firmly to ensure a tight seal. Poor contact with the skin may result in an inaccurate signal.

16

Fluid, Electrolyte, and Acid–Base Balance

Focusing on Patient Care

This chapter will help you develop some of the skills related to fluid, electrolyte, and acid–base balance necessary to care for the following patients:

Simon Lawrence, age 3 years, has been admitted to the pediatric floor with fluid volume deficit after vomiting for 2 days. They will be treated with intravenous fluids to assist in rehydration.

Melissa Cohen, age 32, was just involved in a motor vehicle crash. They have lost a large amount of blood and need a blood transfusion.

Jack Tracy, age 67, is undergoing chemotherapy at the outpatient chemotherapy center. Their recently implanted port will be deaccessed prior to leaving the center.

Refer to Focusing on Patient Care: Developing Clinical Reasoning and Clinical Judgment at the end of the chapter to apply what you learn.

Learning Outcomes

After completing the chapter, you will be able to accomplish the following:

1. Initiate a peripheral intravenous catheter access and intravenous infusion.
2. Monitor an IV site and infusion.
3. Change an IV solution container and administration set.
4. Change a peripheral venous access device site dressing.
5. Cap for intermittent use and flush a peripheral venous access device.
6. Administer a blood transfusion.
7. Change the site dressing and flush a central venous access device.
8. Access an implanted port.
9. Deaccess an implanted port.
10. Remove a peripherally inserted central catheter.

Nursing Concepts

- Assessment
- Clinical Decision Making/Clinical Judgment
- Fluids and Electrolytes
- Safety

T his chapter discusses skills needed to care for patients with fluid, electrolyte, and acid–base balance needs. The total amount of body water makes up approximately 50% to 60% of body weight in a healthy person (Brinkman et al., 2021). The balance, or homeo-stasis, of fluid, electrolytes, and acid–base is interrelated and maintained through the func-tions of almost every organ of the body. In a healthy person, fluid intake and fluid losses are about equal. Fundamentals Review 16-1 lists the average adult daily fluid sources and losses. Abnormalities in fluid, electrolyte, and acid–base balance are also interrelated and may occur together.

The use of infused intravenous (IV) solutions may be prescribed as part of patient care related to fluid, electrolyte, and acid–base disturbances. The nurse is responsible for critically evaluating all patient orders prior to administration, as well as for initiating, monitoring, and discontinuing the therapy. If the prescribed intervention is unclear in any way or does not seem appropriate based on the patient's condition and/or status, it is the nurse's responsibility to ask the prescribing practitioner for clarification prior to be-ginning administration. The contents of selected IV solutions and comments about their use are listed in Fundamentals Review 16-2. As with other therapeutic agents, the nurse must understand the rationale for the use of IV therapy for the individual patient, the type of solution being used, its desired effect, and potential complications (Fundamen-tals Review 16-3). Blood product transfusions are other infusions that may be adminis-tered through IV access devices and include red blood cells, platelets, and coagulation factors.

Fundamentals Review 16-1

AVERAGE ADULT DAILY FLUID SOURCES AND LOSSES

Fluid Intake (mL)		Fluid Output (mL)	
Ingested water	1,500	Kidneys	1,500
Ingested food	800	Skin	600
Metabolic oxidation	300	Lungs	400
		Gastrointestinal	100
Total	*2,600*	*Total*	*2,600*

Source: Data from Willis, L. M. (Ed.). (2020). *Fluids & electrolytes made incredibly easy!* (7th ed.). Wolters Kluwer.

Fundamentals Review 16-2

SELECTED IV SOLUTIONS

Solution	Comments
Isotonic Solutions	
Total osmolality close to that of the ECF; replace the ECF	
0.9% NaCl (normal saline)	Not desirable as routine maintenance solution because it provides only Na^+ and Cl^-, which are provided in excessive amounts
	May be used to expand temporarily the extracellular compartment if circulatory insufficiency is a problem; also used to treat hypovolemia, metabolic alkalosis, mild hyponatremia, hypercalcemia
	Used with administration of blood transfusions
Lactated Ringer solution	Contains multiple electrolytes in about the same concentrations as found in plasma (note that this solution is lacking in Mg^{2+})
	Used in the treatment of hypovolemia, burns, and fluid lost from GI sources
Hypotonic Solutions	
Hypotonic to plasma; replace ICF	
0.33% NaCl (1/3-strength normal saline)	Provides Na^+, Cl^-, and free water
	Na^+ and Cl^- allows kidneys to select and retain needed amounts
	Free water desirable as aid to kidneys in elimination of solutes
	Used in treating hypernatremia
0.45% NaCl (½-strength normal saline)	A hypotonic solution that provides Na^+, Cl^-, and free water
	Used as a basic fluid for maintenance needs
	Often used to treat hypernatremia (because this solution contains a small amount of Na^+, it dilutes the plasma sodium while not allowing it to drop too rapidly)
Hypertonic Solutions	
Hypertonic to plasma	
5% dextrose in Lactated Ringer solution	Supplies fluid and calories to the body
	Replaces electrolytes; shifts fluid from the intracellular compartment into the intravascular space, expanding vascular volume
5% dextrose in 0.9% NaCl	Used to treat SIADH
	Can temporarily be used to treat hypovolemia if plasma expander is not available

Source: Adapted from Hale, A., & Hovey, M. J. (2014). *Fluid, electrolyte, and acid-base imbalances.* F.A. Davis Company; Hinkle, J. L., Cheever, K. H., & Overbaugh, K. (2022). *Brunner & Suddarth's Textbook of medical-surgical nursing* (15th ed.). Wolters Kluwer; and Willis, L. M. (Ed.). (2020). *Fluids & electrolytes made incredibly easy!* (7th ed.). Wolters Kluwer.

Fundamentals Review 16-3

COMPLICATIONS ASSOCIATED WITH INTRAVENOUS INFUSIONS

Complication/Cause	Signs and Symptoms	Nursing Considerations
Infiltration: the escape of fluid into the subcutaneous tissue Dislodged needle Penetrated vessel wall	Swelling, pallor, coldness, or pain around the infusion site; significant decrease in the flow rate	Check the infusion site every hour for signs/symptoms. Discontinue the infusion if symptoms occur. Restart the infusion at a different site. Use site-stabilization device.
Venous access device–related infection: Improper hand decontamination/hand hygiene Frequent disconnection of tubing, access ports, and/or access caps Poor insertion technique, multiple insertion attempts Multilumen catheters Long-term catheter insertion Frequent dressing changes Inadequate/improper decontamination of hub prior to use An IV solution that becomes contaminated when solutions are changed, a medication is added, or the solution is allowed to infuse for too long a period Inappropriate administration set changes	Erythema, edema, induration, drainage at the insertion site Fever, malaise, chills, other vital sign changes	Perform hand hygiene before and after palpating catheter insertion sites; before and after inserting, replacing, accessing, and dressing a VAD. Assess catheter site routinely. Notify health care team immediately if any signs of infection. Use scrupulous aseptic technique when starting an infusion. Follow best-practice guidelines for site care, changing of administration tubing sets, connectors, caps, and other administration equipment. Follow facility protocol for culture of drainage. Consider use of 2% chlorhexidine wash for daily skin cleansing.
Phlebitis: an inflammation of a vein Mechanical trauma from needle or catheter Chemical trauma from solution	Local, acute tenderness; redness, warmth, and slight edema of the vein above the insertion site	Use a phlebitis scale to assess and document phlebitis. Discontinue the infusion immediately. Apply warm compresses to the affected site. Avoid further use of the vein. Restart the infusion in another vein.
Thrombus: a blood clot Tissue trauma from needle or catheter	Symptoms similar to phlebitis IV fluid flow may cease if clot obstructs needle.	Stop the infusion immediately. Apply warm compresses as prescribed or according to facility policy. Restart the IV at another site. *Do not rub or massage the affected area.*
Speed shock: the body's reaction to a substance that is injected into the circulatory system too rapidly Too rapid a rate of fluid infusion into circulation	Pounding headache, fainting, rapid pulse rate, apprehension, chills, back pains, and dyspnea	Use the proper IV tubing. Carefully monitor the rate of fluid flow. Check the rate frequently for accuracy. A time tape is useful for this purpose.
Fluid overload: the condition caused when too large a volume of fluid infuses into the circulatory system Too large a volume of fluid infused into circulation	Engorged neck veins, increased blood pressure, and difficulty in breathing (dyspnea)	If symptoms develop, slow the rate of infusion. Notify the health care team immediately. Monitor vital signs. Carefully monitor the rate of fluid flow. Check the rate frequently for accuracy.
Air embolus: air in the circulatory system Break in the IV system above the heart level, allowing air in the circulatory system as a bolus	Respiratory distress Increased heart rate Cyanosis Decreased blood pressure Change in level of consciousness	Pinch off catheter or secure system to prevent entry of air. Place patient on left side in Trendelenburg position. Call for immediate assistance. Monitor vital signs and pulse oximetry.

Skill 16-1 ▶ Initiating a Peripheral Intravenous Catheter Access and Intravenous Infusion

The infusion of intravenous (IV) solutions may be prescribed to address fluid and/or electrolyte disturbances. The health care provider with prescriptive privileges is responsible for prescribing the type and amount of solution to be infused in a specified period of time. The nurse determines the infusion rate based on the amount of solution to be infused over 1 hour to achieve the prescribed infusion volume over the prescribed period of time. For IV fluid and other therapies to be administered, an IV access must be established. The nurse initiating a peripheral intravenous catheter (PIVC) needs to assess for the safest, most appropriate site for each particular patient. The accessibility and condition of the vein and the type of fluid to be infused should be considered when determining the location for intravenous access via a PIVC. Refer to the Assessment section of this skill. Figure 1 illustrates potential infusion sites for peripheral venous catheters. Consider the use of methods to reduce pain and discomfort of catheter insertion, such as local anesthetic agents and nonpharmacologic interventions (cognitive, behavioral, and complementary therapies) (Basak et al., 2020; Gorski et al., 2021).

Verify the amount and type of solution to be administered as well as the prescribed infusion rate. Critically evaluating all prescribed infusions prior to administration. Any concerns regarding the type or amount of therapy prescribed should be immediately and clearly communicated to the prescribing practitioner for clarification prior to beginning administration. Evaluate the patient's need for IV therapy, the type of solution being used, its desired effect, and potential adverse reactions

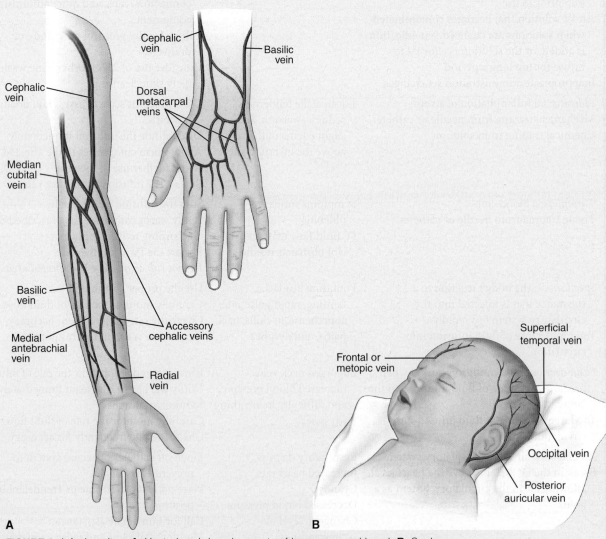

FIGURE 1. Infusion sites. **A.** Ventral and dorsal aspects of lower arm and hand. **B.** Scalp.

and effects. Follow the facility's policies and guidelines to determine if the infusion should be administered by electronic infusion device or by gravity/free flow. Refer to Box 16-1 for guidelines to calculate the flow rate for gravity/free-flow infusion.

Box 16-1 Regulating Intravenous Flow Rate

Follow facility guidelines to determine if infusion should be administered by electronic infusion device or by gravity/free flow.

- Verify prescribed IV solution.
- Check patency of IV access.

If the infusion is to be administered by gravity/free-flow infusion:

- Verify drop factor (number of drops in 1 mL) of the equipment in use.
- Calculate the flow rate:
  EXAMPLE—Administer 1,000 mL D$_5$W over 10 hours (set delivers 60 drops/1 mL).

a. Standard formula

$$\text{gtt (drops)/min} = \frac{\text{volume (mL)} \times \text{drop factor (gtt (drops)/mL)}}{\text{time (in minutes)}}$$

$$\text{gtt (drops)/min} = \frac{1{,}000 \text{ mL} \times 60}{600 \text{ (60 min} \times 10 \text{ h)}}$$

$$= \frac{60{,}000}{600}$$

$$= 100 \text{ gtt (drops)/min}$$

b. Short formula using milliliters per hour

$$\text{gtt (drops)/min} = \frac{\text{milliliters per hour} \times \text{drop factor (gtt (drops)/mL)}}{\text{time (60 min)}}$$

Find milliliters per hour by dividing 1,000 mL by 10 hours:

$$\frac{1{,}000}{10} = 100 \text{ mL/60}$$

$$\text{gtt (drops)/min} = \frac{100 \text{ mL} \times 60}{60 \text{ min}}$$

$$= \frac{6{,}000}{60}$$

$$= 100 \text{ drops/min}$$

DELEGATION GUIDELINES	The initiation of a PIVC and IV infusion is not delegated to assistive personnel (AP). Depending on the state's nurse practice act and the organization's policies and procedures, initiation of a PIVC and IV infusion may be delegated to licensed practical/vocational nurses (LPN/LVNs). The decision to delegate must be based on careful analysis of the patient's needs and circumstances as well as the qualifications of the person to whom the task is being delegated. Refer to the Delegation Guidelines in Appendix A.
EQUIPMENT	• IV solution, as prescribed • Electronic MAR (eMAR) or medication administration record (MAR) • Towel or disposable pad • Nonallergenic tape • IV administration set • Label for infusion set (for next change date) • Transparent semipermeable membrane (TSM) dressing • Electronic infusion device (if appropriate) • Tourniquet • Time tape and/or label (for IV container) • Cleansing swabs >0.5% chlorhexidine in alcohol solution is preferred; tincture of iodine, an iodophor ([povidone-iodine], or 70% alcohol may also be used) (Gorski et al., 2021; Mimoz et al., 2015; O'Grady et al., 2017) • IV securement/stabilization device, as appropriate • Clean gloves • Additional PPE, as indicated • IV pole • Local anesthetic (based on facility policy and/or if prescribed) • PIVC

(continued on page 1008)

Skill 16-1 ▶ Initiating a Peripheral Intravenous Catheter Access and Intravenous Infusion *(continued)*

- Short extension tubing, if not permanently attached to the PIVC
- Needleless connector or end cap for extension tubing
- Antimicrobial wipes
- Passive disinfection caps (based on facility policy)
- Skin barrier protectant wipe (e.g., Skin-Prep®)
- Single-use clippers or scissors for hair removal (as indicated)
- Single-use, commercially prepared, prefilled syringe with sterile normal saline for injection, minimum volume equal to twice the internal volume of the catheter system (Gorski et al., 2021), according to facility policy.

ASSESSMENT

Review the patient's record for baseline data, such as vital signs; intake and output balance; and pertinent laboratory values, such as serum electrolytes. Assess the appropriateness of the solution for the patient. Inspect the IV infusion solution for any particulates and check the IV label. Confirm it is the solution prescribed. Review assessment and laboratory data that may influence solution administration. Evaluate the patient's history for any allergies or sensitivity to skin antiseptics (Gorski et al., 2021). The suitability of particular veins for peripheral IV infusions varies with individual circumstances. Determine site selection after considering the accessibility of a vein, the condition of a vein, and the type of fluid to be infused. Assess the patient's arms for potential sites for initiating the PIVC and IV infusion. Keep in mind the following guidelines related to PIVCs and access sites:

- Determine the most desirable accessible vein. For a short PIVC, use the forearm to prolong dwell time, increase the likelihood of the PIVC lasting the full length of the prescribed therapy, decrease pain during dwell time, promote self-care, and prevent accidental removal and occlusions (Gorski et al., 2021). The dorsal and ventral surfaces of the upper extremities, including the metacarpal, cephalic, basilic, and median veins, are appropriate sites for infusion (Gorski et al., 2021). Avoid the cephalic vein at the radial wrist, inner aspect of the wrist, and sites at/above the antecubital fossa because of the potential risk for nerve damage (Gorski et al., 2021). For a long PIVC, use the veins on the dorsal and ventral surfaces of the upper extremities, including the cephalic, basilic, and median veins; insertion should be in the forearm without crossing into the antecubital fossa (Gorski et al., 2021). Consider use of the basilic, cephalic, or brachial veins when inserting a midline catheter (Gorski et al., 2021). Figure 1A illustrates infusion sites on the arm and hand for adult patients.
- In adults, hand veins may be considered for short-term therapy (>24 hours); catheter insertion in areas of flexion such as the hand is associated with higher failure rates over time (Gorski et al., 2021).
- In general, either arm may be used for IV therapy. Use of the nondominant arm is preferred for patient comfort and to limit movement in the impacted extremity (Gorski et al., 2021). For example, if the patient is right-handed, the IV is preferably placed on the left extremity to improve the patient's ability to complete activities of daily living. This is particularly important if the duration of infusion is expected to be prolonged.
- Determine accessibility based on the patient's condition. The use of an extremity for IV therapy may be contraindicated in some circumstances. For example, patients with a history of breast cancer with same-side surgical axillary lymph node removal; patients with burns, infections, or traumatic injury to the extremity; and patients with an upper extremity arteriovenous fistula or graft or other catheters for dialysis treatment will not be able to have an IV catheter placed on the impacted extremity.
- Avoid PIVC insertion in areas of flexion, if there is pain on palpation, in compromised skin and sites distal to these areas (such as open wounds), in extremities with infection, and in extremities with planned procedures (Gorski et al., 2021).
- Do not use the antecubital veins if another vein is available. They are not a good choice for infusion because flexion of the patient's arm can displace the IV catheter over time. By avoiding the antecubital veins for peripheral venous catheters, a PICC line may be inserted later, if needed.
- Do not use veins in the leg of an adult, unless needed for an emergent insertion; if used, remove as soon as possible, as use of the lower extremities is associated with risk of tissue damage, thrombophlebitis, and ulceration (Gorski et al., 2021). Some facilities require a prescribed intervention to insert an IV catheter in an adult patient's lower extremity.

ACTUAL OR POTENTIAL HEALTH PROBLEMS AND NEEDS	Many actual or potential health problems or issues may require the use of this skill as part of related interventions. An appropriate health problem or issue may include: • Fluid imbalance • Electrolyte imbalance • Fluid overload risk
OUTCOME IDENTIFICATION AND PLANNING	The expected outcome to achieve when initiating a PIVC and IV infusion is that the PIVC is inserted using sterile technique on the first attempt. Other outcomes include that the patient experiences minimal discomfort, and the IV solution infuses without difficulty.

IMPLEMENTATION

ACTION	**RATIONALE**
1. Verify the prescribed IV solution on the eMAR/MAR. Consider the appropriateness of the prescribed therapy in relation to the patient. Clarify any inconsistencies. Check the patient's health record for allergies. Know techniques for IV insertion, precautions, and the purpose of the IV solution administration, if prescribed. Check the solution for color and the container for leaking and expiration date, if prescribed. Gather the necessary supplies.	This ensures that the correct IV solution and rate of infusion and/or medication will be administered. The nurse is responsible for critically evaluating all patient orders prior to administration. Any concerns regarding the type or amount of therapy prescribed should be immediately and clearly communicated to the prescribing health care provider. This knowledge and skill are essential for safe and accurate IV and medication administration. Preparation promotes efficient time management and an organized approach to the task.
2. Perform hand hygiene and put on PPE, if indicated.	Hand hygiene and PPE prevent the spread of microorganisms. PPE is required based on transmission precautions.
3. Identify the patient.	Identifying the patient ensures the right patient receives the intervention and helps prevent errors.
4. Assemble equipment on the bedside stand or overbed table or other surface within reach.	Bringing everything to the bedside conserves time and energy. Arranging items nearby is convenient, saves time, and avoids unnecessary stretching and twisting of muscles on the part of the nurse.
5. Close the curtains around the bed and close the door to the room, if possible. Explain to the patient what you are going to do and why. Ask the patient about allergies to medications, tape, or skin antiseptics, as appropriate. If considering using a local anesthetic, inquire about allergies for these substances as well. Consider use of nonpharmacologic interventions to reduce pain associated with PIVC insertion.	This ensures the patient's privacy. Explanation relieves anxiety and facilitates engagement. Possible allergies may exist related to medications, tape, or local anesthetic. Injectable anesthetic can result in allergic reactions and tissue damage. Nonpharmacologic interventions suggested for use to reduce PIVC insertion–related pain and discomfort include distraction, relaxation, breathing exercises, and virtual reality (VR) (Basak et al., 2020; Gorski et al., 2021). The choices of interventions for pediatric patients include swaddling, breastfeeding, pacifiers, rocking, blowing bubbles, reading books, use of VR, and local vibrating cold devices and should be made with consideration of growth and development level (Gorski et al., 2021).

(continued on page 1010)

Skill 16-1 ▶ Initiating a Peripheral Intravenous Catheter Access and Intravenous Infusion *(continued)*

ACTION	RATIONALE
6. If using a local anesthetic, explain the rationale and procedure to the patient. Apply the anesthetic to a few potential insertion sites. Allow sufficient time for the anesthetic to take effect.	Explanations provide reassurance and facilitate engagement. Local anesthetic agents should be used to reduce pain in all adult and pediatric populations (Gorski et al., 2021). Local anesthetic agents to reduce pain associated with PIVC insertion include vapocoolant sprays, topical transdermal agents, jet injection of pressure-accelerated lidocaine (needle-free), application of hot or cold to the site, and intradermal injection of lidocaine or bacteriostatic 0.9% sodium chloride (Gorski et al., 2021; Korkut et al., 2020; Welyczko, 2020). Some anesthetics take up to an hour to become effective.

Prepare the IV Solution and Administration Set

ACTION	RATIONALE
7. Compare the IV container label with the eMAR/MAR. Remove the IV bag from the outer wrapper, if indicated. Check expiration dates. Scan the bar code on container, if necessary. Compare the patient identification band with the eMAR/MAR. Alternatively, label the solution container with the patient's name, solution type, additives, date, and time. Complete a time strip for the infusion and apply to the IV container.	Checking the label with eMAR/MAR ensures the correct IV solution will be administered. Identifying the patient ensures the right patient receives the medications and helps prevent errors. The time strip allows for quick visual reference by the nurse to monitor infusion accuracy.
8. Maintain aseptic technique when opening sterile packages and the IV solution. Remove the administration set from the package (Figure 2). Apply the label to the tubing reflecting the day/date for the next set change, per facility guidelines.	Asepsis is essential for preventing the spread of microorganisms. Labeling the tubing ensures adherence to facility policy regarding administration set changes and reduces the risk of the spread of microorganisms. Refer to Box 16-3 in Skill 16-3 for recommended administration set change guidelines.

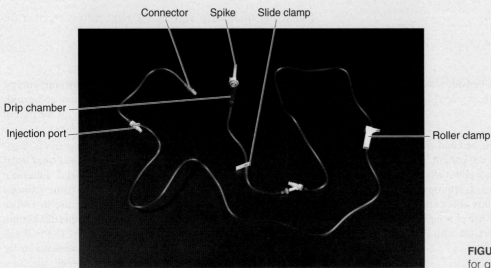

FIGURE 2. Basic administration set for gravity/free-flow infusion.

ACTION	RATIONALE
9. Close the roller clamp or slide the clamp on the IV administration set (Figure 3). Invert the IV solution container and remove the cap on the entry site, taking care not to touch the exposed entry site. Remove the cap from the spike on the administration set. Using a twisting and pushing motion, insert the administration set spike into the entry site of the IV container (Figure 4). Alternatively, follow the manufacturer's directions for insertion.	Clamping the IV tubing prevents air and fluid from entering the IV tubing. Inverting the container allows easy access to the entry site. Touching the opened entry site on the IV container and/or the spike on the administration set results in contamination, resulting in the need to discard the container/administration set. Inserting the spike punctures the seal in the IV container and allows access to the contents.

ACTION

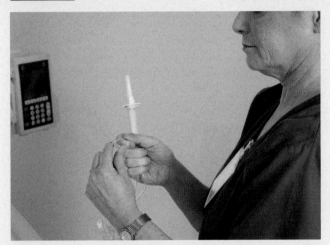

FIGURE 3. Closing clamp on administration set.

10. Hang the IV container on the IV pole. Squeeze the drip chamber and fill it at least halfway (Figure 5).

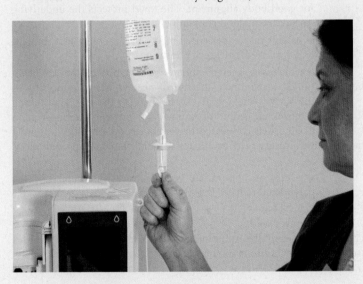

11. Open the IV tubing clamp and allow fluid to move through the tubing. Follow the additional manufacturer's instructions for the specific electronic infusion pump, as indicated. **Allow fluid to flow until all air bubbles have disappeared, and the entire length of the tubing is primed (filled) with IV solution (Figure 6).** Close the clamp. Alternatively, some brands of tubing may require removal of the cap at the end of the IV tubing to allow the fluid to flow. Maintain its sterility. After the fluid has filled the tubing, recap the end of the tubing.

12. If an electronic device is to be used, follow the manufacturer's instructions for inserting the tubing into the device (Figure 7).

RATIONALE

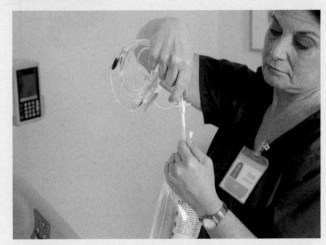

FIGURE 4. Inserting administration set spike into entry site of IV fluid container.

Suction causes fluid to move into the drip chamber. Fluid prevents air from moving down the tubing.

FIGURE 5. Squeezing drip chamber to fill at least halfway.

This technique prepares for IV fluid administration and removes air from the tubing. Air should be purged from all administration sets to prevent air embolism (Gorski et al., 2021). Touching the open end of the tubing results in contamination, resulting in the need to discard the administration set.

This ensures proper use of equipment.

(continued on page 1012)

Skill 16-1 ▶ Initiating a Peripheral Intravenous Catheter Access and Intravenous Infusion *(continued)*

ACTION

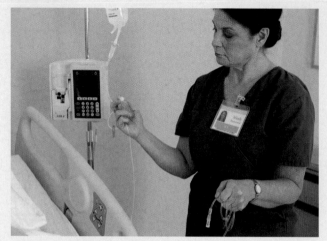

FIGURE 6. Priming administration set.

RATIONALE

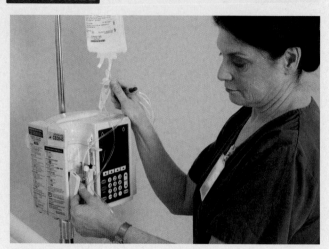

FIGURE 7. Inserting administration set into electronic infusion device.

Initiate Peripheral Venous Access

13. Place the patient in the low-Fowler position in bed. Place a protective towel or pad under the patient's arm.

The supine position permits either arm to be used and allows for good body alignment. The towel protects the underlying surface from blood contamination.

14. Provide emotional support, as needed.

The patient may experience anxiety because they may, in general, fear needlestick or IV infusion.

15. Open the short extension tubing package. Attach the needleless connector or end cap, if not in place. Clean the needleless connector or end cap with an alcohol wipe. Insert a syringe with normal saline into the extension tubing. Fill the extension tubing with normal saline and place the extension tubing and syringe back on the package, within easy reach.

A needleless connector should be attached to the extension tubing to eliminate the use of needles when connecting to the VAD (Gorski et al., 2021). Priming the extension tubing removes air from the tubing and prevents administration of air when connected to venous access. Having the tubing within easy reach facilitates accomplishment of procedure.

16. Select and palpate for an appropriate vein. Refer to the guidelines in the previous Assessment section. If the intended insertion site is visibly soiled, clean the area with soap and water (Gorski et al., 2021).

The use of an appropriate vein decreases discomfort for the patient and reduces the risk for damage to body tissues.

17. Remove excess hair at the insertion site, if needed, to facilitate application of the site dressing. Use single-patient-use scissors or disposable-head surgical clippers to remove hair at the insertion site and dressing area.

Hair can inhibit adhesion of the site dressing. Shaving causes microabrasions and may increase the risk for infection (Gorski et al., 2021).

18. Put on gloves.

Gloves prevent contact with blood and body fluids.

19. Apply a single-patient-use tourniquet (Gorski et al., 2021) 3 to 4 inches above the venipuncture site to obstruct venous blood flow and distend the vein (Figure 8). Direct the ends of the tourniquet away from the entry site. Make sure the radial pulse is still present.

A single-patient-use tourniquet prevents transmission of microorganisms. Impeding venous blood flow causes the vein to distend while maintaining arterial circulation. Distended veins are easy to see, palpate, and enter. The end of the tourniquet could contaminate the area of injection if directed toward the entry site. The tourniquet may be applied too tightly, so assessment for the radial pulse is important. Checking radial pulse ensures arterial supply is not compromised.

20. Instruct the patient to hold their arm lower than their heart.

Lowering the arm below the heart level helps distend the veins by filling them.

ACTION

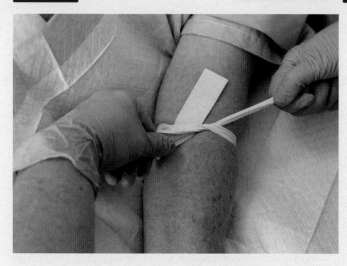

FIGURE 8. Applying tourniquet.

RATIONALE

21. Ask the patient to open and close their fist. Observe and palpate for a suitable vein. If a vein cannot be felt, consider the use of vascular visualization technology or ultrasound to assist with identification of peripheral veins (Gorski et al., 2021).

Contracting the muscles of the forearm forces blood into the veins, thereby distending them further. Vascular visualization technology can be used to assist with identification of peripheral veins, with resulting increased insertion success; reduced insertion-related complications; and minimization of the need to escalate to unnecessary, more invasive VADs (Gorski et al., 2021). Ultrasound-guided PIVC insertion is a safe, efficient intervention and should be used for placement of a short PIVC in difficult-to-access adult patients (Gorski et al., 2021; Houston, 2013), the insertion of long PIVCs (Gorski et al., 2021), and after failed venipuncture attempts (Edwards & Jones, 2018; Egan et al., 2013).

22. Use a single-use sterile applicator containing sterile antiseptic solution to **cleanse the site with >5% chlorhexidine in alcohol solution or the solution identified by facility policy. Follow the manufacturer's directions for use to determine the product application process and dry times (Gorski et al., 2021). Allow the antiseptic to dry naturally; do not wipe, fan, or blow on the skin** (Gorski et al., 2021).

Cleansing is necessary because organisms on the skin can be introduced into the tissues or the bloodstream with the needle. Use of >0.5% chlorhexidine in alcohol solution is preferred for skin antisepsis (Gorski et al., 2021; Sarani et al., 2018). If there is a contraindication to alcoholic chlorhexidine solution, tincture of iodine, an iodophor (povidone-iodine), or 70% alcohol may instead be used (Gorski et al., 2021; Mimoz et al., 2015; O'Grady et al., 2017).

23. **Do not touch/palpate the insertion site after skin antisepsis. Use sterile gloves if repalpation of the vein is necessary after skin antisepsis.**

Touching the site after skin antisepsis recontaminates the insertion site. Use of sterile gloves for palpation prevents contamination of the insertion site.

24. Using your nondominant hand placed about 1 or 2 inches below the entry site, hold the patient's skin taut against the vein. **Avoid touching the prepared site.** Ask the patient to remain still while performing the venipuncture.

Pressure on the vein and surrounding tissues stabilizes the vein and helps prevent movement of the vein as the needle or catheter is being inserted. The planned IV insertion site is not palpated after skin cleansing unless sterile gloves are worn to prevent contamination (Gorski et al., 2021). Patient movement may prevent proper technique for IV insertion.

25. Align the IV catheter on top of the vein; enter the skin gently, holding the catheter by the hub in your dominant hand, bevel side up, at a 10- to 15-degree angle (Figure 9). Insert the catheter from directly over the vein or from the side of the vein. While following the course of the vein, advance the needle or catheter into the vein. A sensation of "give" can be felt when the needle enters the vein.

This allows the needle or catheter to enter the vein with minimal trauma and deters passage of the needle through the vein.

(*continued on page 1014*)

Skill 16-1 ▶ Initiating a Peripheral Intravenous Catheter Access and Intravenous Infusion *(continued)*

ACTION	RATIONALE
26. Continue to hold the skin taut. When blood returns through the catheter and/or the flashback chamber of the catheter, use the push-off tab to separate the catheter from the needle stylet and advance the catheter into the vein until the hub is at the venipuncture site. The exact technique depends on the type of device used.	The tourniquet causes increased venous pressure, resulting in automatic backflow. Placing the access device well into the vein helps to prevent dislodgement.
27. Release the tourniquet. Activate the safety mechanism on the needle stylet. Compress the skin well above the catheter tip to stop the flow of blood. Quickly remove the protective cap from the extension tubing, attach it to the catheter hub, and tighten the Luer lock. Stabilize the catheter or needle with your nondominant hand.	Bleeding is minimized and the patency of the vein is maintained if the connection is made smoothly between the catheter and extension tubing.
28. Continue to stabilize the catheter or needle and pull back on the syringe to assess for blood return, then flush gently with the saline, observing the site for infiltration and leaking. Remove the syringe from the end cap.	Presence of a blood return upon aspiration and lack of resistance when flushing indicate patency of the VAD (Gorski et al., 2021). Infiltration and/or leaking and the patient reports of pain and/or discomfort indicate that the insertion into the vein is not successful and should be discontinued. The syringe is no longer needed once flushing is complete.
29. Open the skin protectant wipe. Apply the skin protectant to the site, making sure to apply—at a minimum—the area to be covered with the dressing. Place a sterile transparent dressing and/or catheter securing/stabilization device over the venipuncture site. Loop the tubing near the entry site, and anchor it with tape (nonallergenic) close to the site.	The skin protectant aids in adhesion of the dressing and decreases the risk for skin trauma when the dressing is removed. A transparent dressing allows easy visualization and protects the site. Stabilization/securing devices preserve the integrity of the access device, minimize catheter movement at the hub, and prevent catheter dislodgement and loss of access (Gorski et al., 2021). Some stabilization devices also act as a site dressing. The weight of the tubing is sufficient to pull it out of the vein if it is not well anchored. Nonallergenic tape is less likely to tear fragile skin.
30. Label the IV dressing with the date, time, site, and type and size of the catheter placed (Figure 10).	Other personnel working with the infusion will know the site, type of device being used, and when it was inserted.

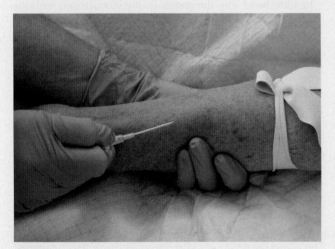

FIGURE 9. Stretching skin taut and inserting needle.

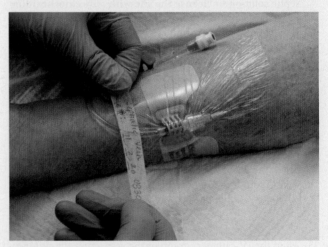

FIGURE 10. Venous access site with labeled dressing.

ACTION

31. Using an antimicrobial swab, vigorously disinfect the connection surface and sides of the needleless connector or end cap on the extension tubing and allow it to dry. Remove the end cap from the administration set. Insert the end of the administration set into the needleless connector or end cap (Figure 11). Loop the administration set tubing near the entry site, and anchor it with tape (nonallergenic) close to the site. Remove your gloves. Perform hand hygiene.

RATIONALE

Venous access device (VAD) administration set entry points, end caps, and needleless connectors must be disinfected prior to each access to reduce the risk for introduction of microorganisms and prevent VAD-related infection (Frimpong et al., 2015; Gorski et al., 2021; Harper, 2014; Loveday et al., 2014). Friction is needed to physically remove microorganisms from the top, sides, and threads of the needleless connector or end cap. Allow the antiseptic to dry completely following the manufacturer's directions for use (Gorski et al., 2021). Inserting the administration set allows initiation of the fluid infusion. The weight of the tubing is sufficient to pull it out of the vein if it is not well anchored. Nonallergenic tape is less likely to tear fragile skin. Removing gloves properly reduces the risk for infection transmission and contamination of other items. Hand hygiene prevents transmission of microorganisms.

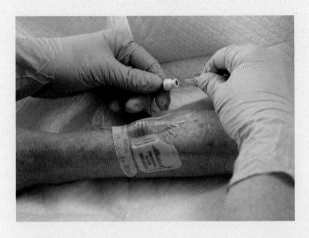

FIGURE 11. Inserting administration set into the end cap of venous access device.

32. Open the clamp on the administration set. Set the flow rate and begin the fluid infusion (Figure 12). Alternatively, start the flow of solution by releasing the clamp on the tubing and counting the drops. Adjust until the correct drop rate is achieved. Assess the flow of the solution and function of the infusion device. Inspect the insertion site for signs of infiltration (Figure 13).

Verifying the rate and device settings ensures the patient receives the correct volume of solution. If the catheter slips out of the vein, the solution will accumulate (infiltrate) into the surrounding tissue.

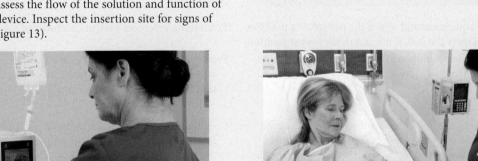

FIGURE 12. Initiating IV fluid infusion.

FIGURE 13. Inspecting insertion site.

(continued on page 1016)

Skill 16-1 ▶ Initiating a Peripheral Intravenous Catheter Access and Intravenous Infusion *(continued)*

ACTION	RATIONALE
33. Apply an IV securement/stabilization device if not already in place as part of the dressing, as indicated, based on facility policy. Explain to the patient the purpose of the device and the importance of safeguarding the site when using the extremity.	These systems are recommended for use on all venous access sites, particularly central venous access sites, to preserve the integrity of the access device, minimize catheter movement at the hub, and prevent catheter dislodgement and loss of access (Gorski et al., 2021). Some devices also act as a site dressing and may already have been applied.
34. Apply a passive disinfection cap to each access site on the administration set; use an antimicrobial swab to vigorously disinfect the connection surface and sides of each access site and allow it to dry. Attach a passive disinfection cap to each site (Figure 14).	Passive disinfection caps contain an antiseptic-impregnated sponge that dispenses the antiseptic over the connector's top and threads and protects the hub from contamination by touch or airborne sources (Gorski et al., 2021; Stango et al., 2014). VAD administration set entry points, end caps, and needleless connectors must be vigorously scrubbed and disinfected prior to each access to reduce the risk for introduction of microorganisms and prevent VAD-related infection (Frimpong et al., 2015; Gorski et al., 2021; Harper, 2014; Loveday et al., 2014). Friction is needed to physically remove microorganisms from the top, sides, and threads of the needleless connector or end cap. Allow the antiseptic to dry completely to ensure complete effectiveness.

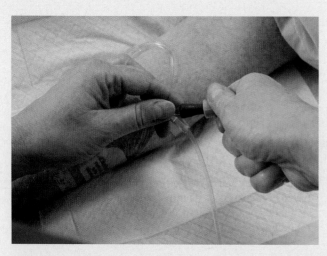

FIGURE 14. Attaching a passive disinfection cap to each access site.

35. Remove the equipment and return the patient to a position of comfort. Lower the bed, if it is not in the lowest position.	Positioning promotes patient comfort and safety.
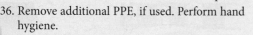 36. Remove additional PPE, if used. Perform hand hygiene.	Proper removal of PPE reduces the risk for infection transmission and contamination of other items. Hand hygiene prevents transmission of microorganisms.
37. Return to check the flow rate and observe the IV site for infiltration and/or other complications 30 minutes after starting the infusion and at least hourly thereafter. Ask the patient if they are experiencing any pain or discomfort related to the IV infusion.	Continued monitoring is important to maintain the correct flow rate. Early detection of problems ensures prompt intervention.

EVALUATION

The expected outcomes have been met when the IV access has been initiated on the first attempt, fluid has flown easily into the vein without any sign of infiltration, and the patient has verbalized minimal discomfort related to insertion and has demonstrated an understanding of the reasons for the IV.

DOCUMENTATION

Guidelines

Document the date and time of insertion, number of attempts, and location (anatomical descriptors, laterality, landmarks) where the IV access was placed as well as the type, length and gauge/size of the PIVC inserted, type of anesthetic (if used), type of IV solution, rate of the IV infusion (often done in the eMAR/MAR), and the use of a securing or stabilization device. Document the use of visualization technology (if used). Document the condition of the site. Record the patient's reaction to the procedure and pertinent patient teaching, such as alerting the nurse if the patient experiences any pain from the IV or notices any swelling at the site. Document the IV fluid solution on the intake and output record.

Sample Documentation

Lippincott DocuCare

Practice documenting peripheral venous access infusion in *Lippincott DocuCare*.

> <u>11/02/25</u> 0830 20-gauge IV started in dorsal surface of the L forearm via the cephalic vein; positive blood return, lack of resistance when flushed. Transparent dressing and peripheral stabilization device applied. Site without redness, drainage, or edema; patient denies discomfort. $D_5$1/2 NS with 20 mEq KCl begun at 110 mL/hr. Patient instructed to call with any pain, discomfort, or swelling and verbalizes an understanding of instructions.
>
> —*S. Barnes, RN*

DEVELOPING CLINICAL REASONING AND CLINICAL JUDGMENT

UNEXPECTED SITUATIONS AND ASSOCIATED INTERVENTIONS

- *An artery is inadvertently accessed or the patient reports paresthesias, numbness, or tingling upon insertion:* Immediately remove the catheter, apply pressure to the insertion site, and notify the health care team (Gorski et al., 2021).
- *Fluid does not easily flow into the vein:* Reposition the extremity because certain positions that the patient may assume may prevent the IV from infusing properly. If the IV is a free-flowing IV, raise the height of the IV pole. This may promote an increase in IV flow. Attempt to flush the PIVC with saline. Check the IV connector to ensure that the clamp is fully open. If fluid still does not flow easily, or if resistance is met while flushing, the IV may be against a valve and may need to be restarted in a different location.
- *Fluid does not flow easily into the vein and the skin around the insertion site is edematous and cool to the touch:* The IV has infiltrated. Put on gloves and remove the catheter. Use a skin marker to outline the area with visible signs of infiltration to allow for assessment of changes (Gorski et al., 2021). Secure the gauze with tape over the insertion site without applying pressure. Assess the area distal to the VAD for capillary refill, sensation, and motor function Gorski et al., 2021). Restart the IV in a new location. Estimate the volume of fluid that escaped into the tissue based on the rate of infusion and length of time since the last assessment. Notify the health care team and use an appropriate method for clinical management of the infiltrate site, based on the infused solution and facility guidelines (Gorski et al., 2021). Record the site assessment and interventions as well as the site for new venous access.
- *A small hematoma is forming at the site while you are inserting the catheter:* The vein is "blowing," which means a small hole has been made in the vein, and blood is leaking out into the tissues. Remove and discard the catheter and choose an alternative insertion site.
- *Fluids are leaking around the insertion site:* Check connections. Change the dressing on the site. If the site continues to leak, remove the IV and restart it in a new location.
- *IV infusion set becomes disconnected from IV:* Discard the administration set to prevent infection. Assess patency and attempt to flush the PIVC. If the PIVC is still patent, the site may still be used as long as the catheter hub has not been contaminated.
- *IV catheter is partially pulled out of the insertion site (migrates externally):* Do not readvance the catheter. Whether the access is salvageable depends on how much of the catheter remains in the vein. Assess for proper placement in the vein before further use and consider the infusion therapy and circumstances to determine viability and secure at the current location (Gorski et al., 2021). Removal and reinsertion at a new site might be the most appropriate intervention if the PIVC is no longer in an appropriate position for the prescribed infusion (Gorski et al., 2021). If the PIVC is not removed, monitor it closely for signs of infiltration and infection.

(*continued on page 1018*)

Skill 16-1 ▶ Initiating a Peripheral Intravenous Catheter Access and Intravenous Infusion *(continued)*

SPECIAL CONSIDERATIONS

General Considerations

- The smallest-gauge PIVC that will accommodate the prescribed therapy and patient need should be selected (Gorski et al., 2021). A 20- to 24-gauge catheter is recommended for most infusions to decrease the risk of phlebitis (Gorski et al., 2021).
- A 22- to 26-gauge catheter is recommended for patients with limited venous options to minimize insertion-related trauma (Gorski et al., 2021).
- An individual nurse should not make more than two attempts at vascular access placement when initiating venous access for a patient (Gorski et al., 2021). If unsuccessful after two attempts, a colleague with advanced skills, such as a member of the nurse IV team, should attempt to initiate the venous access (Gorski et al., 2021). Multiple unsuccessful attempts cause pain to the patient and result in delayed treatment, limited future vascular access, increased costs, and increased risk for complications (Gorski et al., 2021).
- Factors that may interfere with successful evaluation of the condition of the patient's veins and subsequent placement of a peripheral catheter include obesity, diabetes, hypertension, variations in skin between patient populations (e.g., darker skin tones, excessive hair, presence of scars or tattoos), increased patient age, neonates, fluid volume deficit, injection drug use, the presence of multiple chronic health conditions (e.g., diabetes, renal disease), vascular disease, chemotherapy, and/or frequent hospitalizations (Dougherty, 2013; Dychter et al., 2012; Fields et al., 2014; Gorski et al, 2021; Morata & Bowers, 2020; Partovi-Deilami et al., 2016). These factors interfere with use of traditional techniques of direct visualization, anatomic landmarks, and palpation and make placement of the PIVC difficult (Gorski et al., 2021; Houston, 2013).
- Ultrasound-guided PIVC insertion is a safe, efficient intervention and should be used for placement of a short PIVC in difficult-to-access adult patients (Gorski et al., 2021; Houston, 2013), the insertion of long PIVCs (Gorski et al., 2021), and after failed venipuncture attempts (Edwards & Jones, 2018; Egan et al., 2013).
- Closed-system peripheral intravenous catheters are available. These systems integrate the catheter and extension tubing as one piece (Galang et al., 2020), eliminating the need for the addition of separate extension tubing, reducing potential contamination.
- Drying time with 70% isopropyl alcohol is 5 seconds; alcohol-based chlorhexidine requires 20 seconds. Povidone iodine requires longer than 6 minutes to be thoroughly dry, making it less favorable to clinical practice (Gorski et al., 2021).
- Transparent semipermeable membrane (TSM) dressings are commonly used to protect the insertion site. A gauze dressing is recommended if the patient is diaphoretic, the site is bleeding or oozing, or there is drainage from the exit site; replace it with a TSM once this is resolved (Gorski et al., 2021; O'Grady et al., 2017).
- Avoid blood pressure measurement or placement of a tourniquet over the site/upper extremity with a peripheral VAD during periods of infusion (Gorski et al., 2021).
- When the patient is showering or bathing, protect the peripheral VAD with clear plastic wrap or a device designed for this purpose. Cover the connections and protect the hub connections from water contamination (Gorski et al., 2021).

Infant and Child Considerations

- Potential sites for short PIVCs for neonates and pediatric patients include veins in the hand; forearm; and, if not walking, the foot. Avoid the antecubital fossa, which has a higher failure rate (Gorski et al., 2021). Consider veins in the forearm and the saphenous vein for long PIVCs (Gorski et al., 2021). Select an upper arm site using the basilic, cephalic, or brachial veins; veins in the leg (saphenous, popliteal, femoral) with the tip below the inguinal crease; and in the scalp with the tip in the neck, above the thorax for placement of a midline catheter (Gorski et al., 2021).
- When no alternative site is available, veins of the scalp may be used as a last resort; avoid the use of the hands, thumbs, or fingers (Gorski et al., 2021).
- A 22- to 26-gauge catheter is recommended for neonates and pediatric patients to minimize insertion-related trauma (Gorski et al., 2021).
- Use chlorhexidine with caution in infants up to age 14 days, premature infants, and low-birth-weight infants due to the risk of skin irritation and chemical burns (Gorski et al., 2021).

Older Adult Considerations
- A 22- to 26-gauge catheter is recommended for older adults to minimize insertion-related trauma (Gorski et al., 2021).
- Insert the PIVC using a 5- to 15-degree angle for older adults (Gorski et al., 2021).

EVIDENCE FOR PRACTICE ▶

INTRAVENOUS ACCESS AND INFUSION
Related Guideline Infusion Nurses Society (INS) Standards of Practice

Gorski, L. A., Hadaway, L., Hagle, M. E., Broadhurst, D., Clare, S., Kleidon, T., Meyer, B. M., Nickel, B., Rowley, S., Sharpe, E., & Alexander, M.; Infusion Nurses Society. (2021). Infusion therapy. Standards of practice, 8th edition. *Journal of Infusion Nursing, 44*(Suppl 1), S1–S224. https://doi.org/10.1097/NAN.0000000000000396

The Infusion Nurses Society is recognized as the global authority in infusion therapy. The *Infusion Nursing Standards of Practice* is an evidence-based document, providing guidelines for nurses related to infusion therapy for use in all patient settings and addressing all patient populations.

EVIDENCE FOR PRACTICE ▶

PERIPHERAL INTRAVENOUS CATHETER INSERTION AND PAIN MANAGEMENT

Insertion of a peripheral intravenous catheter (PIVC) is associated with potentially significant risks and complications, which can cause pain for patients (Welyczko, 2020). Nurses' awareness and ability to mitigate pain when inserting a PIVC has the potential to reduce complications and pain and improve quality of care and patient satisfaction.

Related Research

Korkut, S., Karadağ, S., & Doğan, Z. (2020). The effectiveness of local hot and cold applications on peripheral intravenous catheterization: A randomized controlled trial. *Journal of PeriAnesthesia Nursing, 35*(6), 597–602. https://doi.org/10.1016/j.jopan.2020.04.011

The purpose of this randomized-controlled trial was to examine the effect of local hot and cold applications before peripheral intravenous catheter (PIVC) insertion on pain, anxiety, insertion time, and vein evaluation. Patients who were hospitalized in the cardiology department of a university hospital ($n = 90$) participated in the study. Participants were randomly assigned to an intervention I group (hot application) ($n = 30$), intervention II (cold application) group ($n = 30$), and a control group (no application; standard practice of the clinic) ($n = 30$). Participants completed a patient information form that included questions about demographic data, chronic disease, history of peripheral vascular disease, status of satisfaction with hot or cold application, and whether they would choose the same application in the future. Vein assessment was performed before and after the hot and cold application (intervention groups) and immediately before PIVC insertion (all groups). A numeric rating scale was used to measure pain and anxiety before and during PIVC insertion. A hot or cold pack was applied for 1 minute to participants in the respective intervention groups before insertion of the PIVC. A stopwatch was set up to determine how long it took to place the catheters; in all three groups the stopwatch was started in the beginning of the insertion procedure and was stopped at the end of the insertion procedure. Pain level was found to be significantly lower in the hot and cold application groups than the control group ($p < .05$); no difference was determined between the hot and cold application groups. Anxiety levels of the patients were significantly lower in the hot application group than in the cold application and control groups ($p < .05$). Insertion duration was significantly lower in the hot application group than the other two groups ($p < .05$). Researchers had no difficulty inserting the catheter into 73% of the hot application group and had various degrees of difficulty in inserting the catheter into 87% of the cold application group and 70% of the patients in the control group. Ninety-three percent of the participants in the hot application group reported being satisfied with the application, and 80% reported they wanted the application again. Fifty percent of those in the cold application group reported being not satisfied with the application, and 57% reported that they did not want the application again. Vein visibility was increased after the

(continued)

Skill 16-1 ▶ Initiating a Peripheral Intravenous Catheter Access and Intravenous Infusion *(continued)*

hot application. The researchers concluded applying local hot and cold application before inserting a PIVC reduced pain and anxiety levels. Application of hot increased vein visibility and patient satisfaction and shortened insertion time; cold application decreased vein visibility/prolonged the insertion time and decreased patient satisfaction. The researchers recommended the use of hot application to reduce pain and anxiety levels associated with PIVC insertion and nurse-perceived difficulty in inserting peripheral venous catheters.

Relevance for Nursing Practice

Nurses play a large role in designing interventions to positively impact patient outcomes. Nurses should include pain management strategies to improve patient experience of PIVC insertion. The application of heat is a simple, readily available intervention and may be considered to support positive patient outcomes.

Skill 16-2 ▶ Monitoring an Intravenous Site and Infusion

The nurse is responsible for maintaining the proper intravenous infusion flow rate and monitoring the intravenous (IV) site. This is routinely done as part of the initial patient assessment and at regular intervals, based on patient condition and facility policy. In addition, IV sites are checked at specific intervals and each time an IV medication is given, as dictated by the facility's policies. It is common to check the IV infusion and site every hour, but it is important to be familiar with the requirements of your facility. Monitoring the infusion rate is a very important part of the patient's overall management. If the patient does not receive the prescribed rate, they may experience a fluid volume deficit. In contrast, if the patient is administered too much fluid over a period of time, they may experience fluid volume overload. Other responsibilities involve checking the IV site for possible complications and assessing for both the desired effects of an IV infusion as well as potential adverse reactions to the IV therapy.

DELEGATION CONSIDERATIONS

The monitoring of an IV site and infusion is not delegated to assistive personnel (AP). Depending on the state's nurse practice act and the organization's policies and procedures, these procedures may be delegated to licensed practical/vocational nurses (LPN/LVNs). The decision to delegate must be based on careful analysis of the patient's needs and circumstances as well as the qualifications of the person to whom the task is being delegated. Refer to the Delegation Guidelines in Appendix A.

EQUIPMENT

- PPE, as indicated
- Standardized scale for assessing and documenting phlebitis (Box 16-2 provides an example of one scale)

ASSESSMENT

Assess the continued appropriateness of the solution for the patient. Inspect the IV infusion solution for any particulates and check the IV label. Confirm it is the solution prescribed. Review assessment and laboratory data that may influence solution administration. Assess the current rate of flow by verifying the settings on the electronic infusion device or timing the drops if it is a gravity/free-flow infusion. Check the tubing for kinks or anything that might clamp or interfere with the flow of the solution. Inspect the IV site. The dressing should be intact, adhering to the skin on all edges. Check for any leaks or fluid under or around the dressing. Inspect the tissue around the IV entry site for swelling, coolness, or pallor. These are signs of fluid infiltration into the tissue around the IV catheter. Also inspect the site for redness, swelling, and warmth. These signs might

Box 16-2 | Phlebitis Scale

Grade and document phlebitis according to the most severe presenting indicator.

Grade	Clinical Criteria	Grade	Clinical Criteria
0	No symptoms	4	Pain at access site with erythema and/or edema
1	Erythema at access site with or without pain		Streak formation
2	Pain at access site with erythema and/or edema		Palpable venous cord >1 inch in length
3	Pain at access site with erythema and/or edema Streak formation Palpable venous cord		Purulent drainage

Source: Gorski, L. A., Hadaway, L., Hagle, M. E., Broadhurst, D., Clare, S., Kleidon, T., Meyer, B. M., Nickel, B., Rowley, S., Sharpe, E., & Alexander, M.; Infusion Nurses Society. (2021). Infusion therapy. Standards of practice, 8th edition. *Journal of Infusion Nursing, 44*(Suppl 1), S139. https://doi.org/10.1097/NAN.0000000000000396

indicate the development of phlebitis or an inflammation of the blood vessel at the site. Grade phlebitis, if present. Refer to Box 16-2. Ask the patient if they are experiencing any pain or discomfort related to the IV line. Pain or discomfort can be a sign of infiltration, extravasation, phlebitis, thrombophlebitis, and infection related to IV therapy; refer to Fundamentals Review 16-3. Assess the patient's fluid intake and output. Assess the patient's knowledge of IV therapy.

ACTUAL OR POTENTIAL HEALTH PROBLEMS AND NEEDS

Many actual or potential health problems or issues may require the use of this skill as part of related interventions. An appropriate health problem or issue may include:
• Fluid imbalance
• Infection risk
• Altered skin integrity risk

OUTCOME IDENTIFICATION AND PLANNING

The expected outcomes to be achieved when monitoring the IV infusion and site are that the patient remains free of complications related to IV therapy and exhibits a patent IV site, and the IV solution infuses at the prescribed flow rate.

IMPLEMENTATION

ACTION

RATIONALE

1. Verify the IV prescribed solution on the eMAR/MAR with the health record. Consider the appropriateness of the prescribed therapy in relation to the patient. Clarify any inconsistencies. Check the patient's health record for allergies. Check solution for color and the container for leaking and expiration date. Know the purpose of the IV administration.

This ensures that the correct IV solution and rate of infusion and/or medication will be administered. The nurse is responsible for critically evaluating all patient orders. Any concerns regarding the type or amount of therapy prescribed should be immediately and clearly communicated to the prescribing health care provider. This knowledge and skill are essential for safe and accurate IV and medication administration.

2. **Monitor the IV infusion every hour or per facility policy. More frequent checks may be necessary if medication is being infused.**

This promotes safe administration of IV fluids and medication.

3. Perform hand hygiene and put on PPE, if indicated.

Hand hygiene and PPE prevent the spread of microorganisms. PPE is required based on transmission precautions.

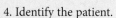

4. Identify the patient.

Identifying the patient ensures the right patient receives the intervention and helps prevent errors.

(continued on page 1022)

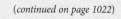

Skill 16-2 ▶ Monitoring an Intravenous Site and Infusion *(continued)*

ACTION

5. Close the curtains around the bed and close the door to the room, if possible. Explain to the patient what you are going to do and why.

6. If an electronic infusion device is being used, check settings, alarm, and indicator lights. Check the set infusion rate (Figure 1). Note the position of fluid in the IV container in relation to the time tape. Teach the patient about the alarm features on the electronic infusion device.

7. If the IV is infusing via gravity/free flow, check the drip chamber and time the drops (Figure 2). Refer to Box 16-1 in Skill 16-1 to review calculation of IV flow rates for gravity/free-flow infusion.

RATIONALE

This ensures the patient's privacy. Explanation relieves anxiety and facilitates engagement.

Observation ensures that the infusion control device and the alarm are functioning. Lack of knowledge about "alarms" may create anxiety for the patient.

This ensures that the flow rate is correct. Use a watch with a second hand for counting the drops in regulating a gravity/free-flow drip IV infusion.

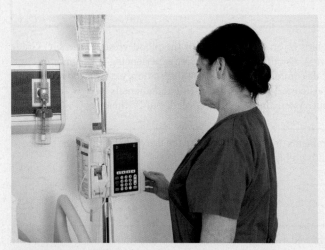

FIGURE 1. Checking infusion device settings.

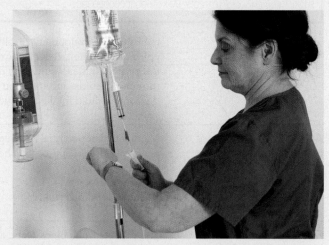

FIGURE 2. Checking drip chamber and timing drops.

8. Check the tubing for anything that might interfere with the flow (Figure 3). Be sure the clamps are in the open position.

9. Observe the dressing for leakage of the IV solution.

10. Inspect the site for swelling, leakage at the site, coolness, or pallor, which may indicate infiltration (Figure 4). Ask if the patient is experiencing any pain or discomfort. If any of these symptoms are present, the IV will need to be removed and restarted at another site. Check facility policy for treating infiltration. See Fundamentals Review 16-3.

11. Inspect the site for redness, swelling, and heat. Palpate for induration. Ask if the patient is experiencing pain. These findings may indicate phlebitis, making it necessary to discontinue and restart the IV at another site. Grade phlebitis (refer to Box 16-2 and Fundamentals Review 16-3). Check facility policy for treatment of phlebitis.

Any kink or pressure on the tubing may interfere with the flow.

Leakage may occur at the connection of the tubing with the hub of the catheter and allow for loss of the IV solution.

The catheter may become dislodged from the vein, and IV solution may flow into the subcutaneous tissue.

Chemical irritation, mechanical trauma, and microorganisms may cause injury to the vein and can lead to phlebitis.

ACTION

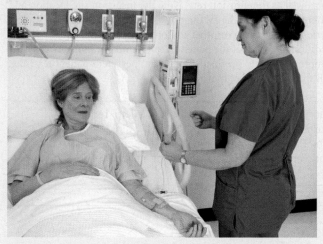

FIGURE 3. Checking tubing for anything that might interfere with flow rate.

RATIONALE

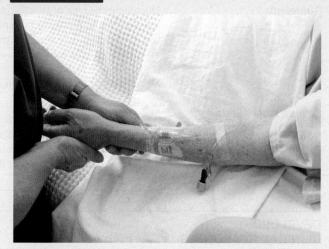

FIGURE 4. Inspecting IV site.

12. Check for local manifestations (redness, pus, warmth, induration, and pain) that may indicate an infection is present at the site. Also check for systemic manifestations (chills, fever, tachycardia, hypotension) that may accompany local infection at the site. If signs of infection are present, discontinue the IV and notify the health care team. Be careful not to disconnect the IV tubing when putting on the patient's hospital gown or assisting the patient with movement to avoid contamination.

Poor aseptic technique may allow bacteria to enter the catheter insertion site or the tubing connection and may occur with manipulation of equipment.

13. Be alert for additional complications of IV therapy, such as fluid overload or bleeding. Refer to Fundamentals Review 16-3.

   a. Fluid overload can result in signs of cardiac and/or respiratory failure. Monitor intake and output and vital signs. Assess for edema and auscultate lung sounds. Ask if the patient is experiencing any shortness of breath.

   b. Check for bleeding at the site.

Infusing too much IV solution results in an increase of circulating fluid volume.

Older adults are most at risk for this complication due to possible decrease in cardiac and/or renal functions.

Bleeding may be caused by anticoagulant medication. Bleeding at the site is most likely to occur when the IV is discontinued.

14. If appropriate, instruct the patient to call for assistance if any discomfort is noted at the site, the solution container is nearly empty, the flow has changed in any way, or if the electronic pump alarm sounds.

This facilitates patient engagement and safe administration of IV solution.

15. Remove PPE, if used. Perform hand hygiene.

Proper removal of PPE reduces the risk for infection transmission and contamination of other items. Hand hygiene prevents transmission of microorganisms.

EVALUATION

The expected outcomes have been met when the patient has remained free of complications related to IV therapy and has exhibited a patent IV site, and the IV solution has infused at the prescribed flow rate.

(continued on page 1024)

Skill 16-2 ▶ Monitoring an Intravenous Site and Infusion (continued)

DOCUMENTATION

Guidelines

Document the type of IV solution as well as the infusion rate. Note the insertion site location and site assessment. Document the patient's reaction to the IV therapy as well as the absence of subjective reports that they are not experiencing any pain or other discomfort, such as coolness or heat associated with the infusion. In addition, record that the patient is not demonstrating any other IV complications, such as signs or symptoms of fluid overload. Document pertinent patient teaching. Document the IV fluid solution on the intake and output record.

Sample Documentation

> 11/6/25 1020 IV site right forearm/cephalic vein intact without swelling, redness, or drainage; dressing and stabilization device intact. D_5 0.9% NS with 20 mEq KCl continues to infuse at 110 mL/hr. Patient and partner instructed to call nurse with any swelling, discomfort or pain and verbalize an understanding of instructions.
> —S. Barnes, RN

DEVELOPING CLINICAL REASONING AND CLINICAL JUDGMENT

UNEXPECTED SITUATIONS AND ASSOCIATED INTERVENTIONS

- *Patient's lung sounds were previously clear, but now some crackles in the bases are auscultated, and the patient reports some shortness of breath:* Notify the health care team immediately. The patient may be exhibiting signs of fluid overload. Be prepared to tell the health care provider what the past intake and output totals were as well as the patient's vital signs and pulse oximetry assessment findings.
- *IV is not flowing as easily as it previously had been:* Check all clamps on the tubing, and check the tubing for any kinking. Check that the patient is not lying on the tubing. If the IV is over a joint, reposition the extremity and see if this helps the flow. Attempt to flush the PIVC with normal saline. If the IV is painful, you meet resistance when attempting to flush, or fluid still does not flow easily, discontinue the IV and restart it in another place.

EVIDENCE FOR PRACTICE ▶

INTRAVENOUS ACCESS AND INFUSION
Related Guideline Infusion Nurses Society (INS) Standards of Practice
Gorski, L. A., Hadaway, L., Hagle, M. E., Broadhurst, D., Clare, S., Kleidon, T., Meyer, B. M., Nickel, B., Rowley, S., Sharpe, E., & Alexander, M.; Infusion Nurses Society. (2021). Infusion therapy. Standards of practice, 8th edition. *Journal of Infusion Nursing, 44*(Suppl 1), S1–S224. https://doi.org/10.1097/NAN.0000000000000396
    Refer to details in Skill 16-1, Evidence for Practice.

EVIDENCE FOR PRACTICE ▶

SHORT PERIPHERAL INTRAVENOUS CATHETERS AND PHLEBITIS
Phlebitis (inflammation of the wall of a vein) is one venous access device–related infection that causes pain, interrupts infusion therapy, necessitates insertion of a new intravenous catheter, may compromise subsequent vascular access, and is a potentially serious complication related to IV therapy (Gorski et al., 2021; Gunasegaran et al., 2018). What can nurses do to decrease the risk of this potential complication of IV therapy?

Related Research
Gunasegaran, N., See, M. T. A., Leong, S. T., Yuan, L. X., & Ang, S. Y. (2018). A randomized controlled study to evaluate the effectiveness of two treatment methods in reducing incidence of short peripheral catheter-related phlebitis. *Journal of Infusion Nursing, 41*(2), 131–137. https://doi.org/10.1097/NAN.0000000000000271

The purpose of this randomized-controlled trial was to evaluate the effectiveness of two treatment methods in reducing the incidence of short-peripheral catheter (SPC)-related phlebitis. Patients from a medical ward of an acute tertiary hospital in Singapore ($n = 969$) who had an SPC in an upper limb and were between ages 21 and 99 years participated in the study. Patients were excluded who were critically ill, allergic to alcohol and/or chlorhexidine, admitted for upper limb phlebitis and/or cellulitis, or known to have dermatologic issues. Participants were randomly assigned a treatment method by week of admission; all patients admitted to the unit in any one particular week received the same preinsertion SPC skin antisepsis treatment method and post removal dressing material. Treatment method 1 consisted of preinsertion skin antisepsis with 70% isopropyl alcohol applied in a circular motion that was allowed to dry, and post removal dressing of sterile gauze and application of an adhesive bandage after hemostasis was achieved. Treatment method 2 consisted of preinsertion skin antisepsis with 2% chlorhexidine in 70% isopropyl alcohol applied in a circular motion that was allowed to dry, and post removal dressing of sterile gauze and application of film dressing (spray-on) after hemostasis was achieved. Participants in both treatment groups received the same care while the catheter was in place: use of aseptic technique when manipulating the SPC; flushing before and after drug administration; and routine removal after 72 to 96 hours. The primary outcome was signs of phlebitis during the course of infusion therapy or within 48 hours after removal. Participants were evaluated for signs of phlebitis daily, once every shift, using the visual infusion phlebitis (VIP) score tool to determine the presence and severity of phlebitis. Participants who were discharged before the 48 hours following the removal of the catheter were educated on the signs and symptoms of phlebitis before discharge and were contacted by phone to inquire about the presence of signs and symptoms of phlebitis. There was no significant difference in the incidence of phlebitis between participants in the two treatment methods. The researchers concluded that the type of cleansing solution and post removal dressing material used may not be the most important factor in reducing the incidence of phlebitis. The researchers suggested strict adherence to aseptic techniques and prompt removal of the SPC remain the cornerstone in the prevention of phlebitis.

Relevance for Nursing Practice

Nurses are responsible for identifying clinical practice concerns and possible solutions, working to improve patient care. Nurses should consider interventions to provide the best care for patients. Safe clinical practice including strict adherence to aseptic technique and compliance with best practice related to skin antisepsis and management of intravenous access sites are important to improve patient outcomes.

Skill 16-3 ▶ Changing an Intravenous Solution Container and Administration Set

Intravenous (IV) fluid administration frequently involves multiple containers of fluid for infusion. Verify the amount and type of solution to be administered as well as the prescribed volume and/ or infusion rate. Critically evaluate all prescribed infusions prior to administration. Any concerns regarding the type or amount of therapy prescribed should be immediately and clearly communicated to the prescribing practitioner. Evaluate the patient's need for IV therapy, the type of solution being used, its desired effect, and potential adverse reactions and effects. Follow the facility's policies and guidelines to determine if the infusion should be administered by electronic infusion device or by gravity/free flow. Refer to Box 16-1 in Skill 16-1 for guidelines to calculate the flow

(*continued on page 1026*)

Skill 16-3 ▶ Changing an Intravenous Solution Container and Administration Set *(continued)*

rate for gravity/free-flow infusion. Monitor these fluid infusions and replace the fluid containers, as needed. Focus on the following points:

- If more than one IV solution or medication is ordered, check facility policy and the appropriate literature to make sure that the additional IV solution can be attached to the existing tubing.
- As one bag is infusing, prepare the next bag so it is ready for a change when less than 50 mL of fluid remains in the original container.
- Ongoing assessments related to the desired outcomes of the IV therapy, as well as assessing for both local and systemic IV infusion complications, are required. Refer to Fundamentals Review 16-3.
- Before switching the IV solution containers, check the date and time of the infusion administration set to ensure it does not also need to be replaced. Check facility policy for guidelines for changing IV administration sets. Refer to Box 16-3 for recommended administration set change guidelines based on the type of infusion and device, as suggested by Infusion Nurses Society Standards (Gorski et al., 2021).
- Infusion administration sets should be changed immediately upon suspected contamination, or when the integrity of the administration product or system has been compromised (Gorski et al., 2021, p. S123). Infusion administration sets should also be changed when a new VAD is placed (Gorski et al., 2021, p. S124).

Box 16-3 | Recommended Administration Set Change Schedule

Type of Infusion/Type of Device	Recommended Frequency
• Primary and secondary continuous administration sets used to administer fluids other than lipid, blood, or blood products	• Change no more frequently than every 96 hours. • Change at least every 7 days. • Change if VAD is changed Change if the integrity of the product or system has been compromised • If the first unit of blood requires 4 hours for transfusion, do not reuse toe administration set or filter. Most standard filters have a 4-unit maximum capacity for reuse.
Intermittent administration sets	Every 24 hours
Administration sets with inline or add-on filters used to administer PN	Change every 24 hours or with each new PN container.
Administration sets used to administer IV lipid emulsions (ILE)	Change every 12 hours and/or with each new ILE container.
Administration sets used to administer blood and blood components	If the first unit of blood requires 4 hours for transfusion, do not reuse toe administration set or filter. Most standard filters have a 4-unit maximum capacity for reuse.
• Primary and secondary continuous administration sets used to administer fluids other than lipid, blood, or blood products	• Change no more frequently than every 96 hours. • Change at least every 7 days. • Change if VAD is changed Change if the integrity of the product or system has been compromised • If the first unit of blood requires 4 hours for transfusion, do not reuse toe administration set or filter. Most standard filters have a 4-unit maximum capacity for reuse.
Intermittent administration sets	Every 24 hours

Source: Adapted from Gorski, L. A., Hadaway, L., Hagle, M. E., Broadhurst, D., Clare, S., Kleidon, T., Meyer, B. M., Nickel, B., Rowley, S., Sharpe, E., & Alexander, M.; Infusion Nurses Society. (2021). Infusion therapy. Standards of practice, 8th edition. *Journal of Infusion Nursing, 44*(Suppl 1), S1–S224. https://doi.org/10.1097/NAN.0000000000000396

DELEGATION CONSIDERATIONS

The changing of an IV solution container and administration set is not delegated to assistive personnel (AP). Depending on the state's nurse practice act and the organization's policies and procedures, these procedures may be delegated to licensed practical/vocational nurses (LPN/LVNs). The decision to delegate must be based on careful analysis of the patient's needs and circumstances as well as the qualifications of the person to whom the task is being delegated. Refer to the Delegation Guidelines in Appendix A.

EQUIPMENT	**For solution container change:** • IV solution, as prescribed • eMAR/MAR • Time tape and/or label (for IV container) • PPE, as indicated **For tubing change:** • IV administration set • Label for administration set (for next change date)	• Transparent semipermeable membrane (TSM) dressing • Nonallergenic tape • IV securement/stabilization device, as appropriate • Passive disinfection caps (based on facility policy) • Gloves • Additional PPE, as indicated • Antimicrobial wipes

---

ASSESSMENT

Review the patient's record for baseline data, such as vital signs and intake and output balance, and pertinent laboratory values, such as serum electrolytes. Assess the appropriateness of the solution for the patient. Inspect the IV infusion solution for any particulates and check the IV label. Confirm it is the solution prescribed. Review assessment and laboratory data that may influence solution administration.

Inspect the IV site. The dressing should be intact, adhering to the skin on all edges. Check for any leaks or fluid under or around the dressing. Inspect the tissue around the IV entry site for swelling, coolness, or pallor. These are signs of fluid infiltration into the tissue around the IV catheter. Also inspect the site for redness, swelling, and warmth. These signs might indicate the development of phlebitis or an inflammation of the blood vessel at the site. Ask the patient if they are experiencing any pain or discomfort related to the IV line. Pain or discomfort can be a sign of infiltration, extravasation, phlebitis, thrombophlebitis, and infection related to IV therapy. Refer to Fundamentals Review 16-3. Skill 16-4 provides additional detail related to monitoring an IV site.

ACTUAL OR POTENTIAL HEALTH PROBLEMS AND NEEDS

Many actual or potential health problems or issues may require the use of this skill as part of related interventions. An appropriate health problem or issue may include:
• Fluid imbalance
• Infection risk
• Altered skin integrity risk

OUTCOME IDENTIFICATION AND PLANNING

The expected outcomes to achieve when changing an IV solution container and tubing are that the prescribed IV infusion continues without interruption, and no infusion complications are identified.

IMPLEMENTATION

ACTION	**RATIONALE**
1. Verify the prescribed IV solution order on the eMAR/MAR. Consider the appropriateness of the prescribed therapy in relation to the patient. Clarify any inconsistencies. Check the patient's health record for allergies. Check the solution for color and the container for leaking and expiration date. Know the purpose of the IV solution administration. Gather the necessary supplies.	This ensures that the correct IV solution and rate of infusion and/or medication will be administered. The nurse is responsible for critically evaluating all patient orders prior to administration. Any concerns regarding the type or amount of therapy prescribed should be immediately and clearly communicated to the prescribing health care provider. This knowledge and skill are essential for safe and accurate IV and medication administration. Preparation promotes efficient time management and an organized approach to the task.
2. Perform hand hygiene and put on PPE, if indicated.	Hand hygiene and PPE prevent the spread of microorganisms. PPE is required based on transmission precautions.
3. Identify the patient.	Identifying the patient ensures the right patient receives the intervention and helps prevent errors.

(continued on page 1028)

Skill 16-3 ▶ Changing an Intravenous Solution Container and Administration Set *(continued)*

ACTION	RATIONALE
4. Assemble equipment on the bedside stand or overbed table or other surface within reach.	Bringing everything to the bedside conserves time and energy. Arranging items nearby is convenient, saves time, and avoids unnecessary stretching and twisting of muscles on the part of the nurse.
5. Close the curtains around the bed and close the door to the room, if possible. Explain to the patient what you are going to do and why. Ask the patient about allergies to medications or tape, as appropriate.	This ensures the patient's privacy. Explanation relieves anxiety and facilitates engagement. Possible allergies may exist related to the IV solution additive or tape.
6. Compare the IV container label with the eMAR/MAR. Remove the IV bag from the outer wrapper, if indicated. Check expiration dates. Scan the bar code on the container, if necessary (Figure 1). Compare the patient identification band with the eMAR/MAR. Alternatively, label the solution container with the patient's name, solution type, additives, date, and time. Complete a time strip for the infusion and apply it to the IV container.	Checking the label with the eMAR/MAR ensures the correct IV solution will be administered. Identifying the patient ensures the right patient receives the medications and helps prevent errors. Time strip allows for quick visual reference by the nurse to monitor infusion accuracy.

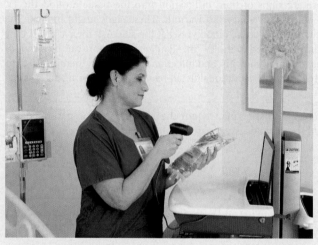

FIGURE 1. Scanning the bar code on container.

7. Maintain aseptic technique when opening sterile packages and the IV solution. Remove the administration set from the package. Apply the label to the tubing reflecting the day/date for the next set change, per facility guidelines.	Asepsis is essential for preventing the spread of microorganisms. Labeling the tubing ensures adherence to facility policy regarding administration set changes and reduces the risk of the spread of microorganisms. Refer to Box 16-3 for recommended administration set change guidelines.

To Change IV Solution Container

8. If using an electronic infusion device, pause the device or put on "hold." Close the slide clamp on the administration set closest to the drip chamber. If using a gravity/free-flow infusion, close the roller clamp on the administration set.	The action of the infusion device needs to be paused while the solution container is changed. Closing the clamp prevents the fluid in the drip chamber from emptying and air from entering the tubing during the procedure.
9. Carefully remove the cap on the entry site of the new IV solution container and expose the entry site, **taking care not to touch the exposed entry site.**	Touching the opened entry site on the IV container results in contamination, resulting in the need to discard the container.
10. Lift the completed container off the IV pole and invert it. Quickly remove the spike from the old IV container, **taking care to not contaminate the spike.** Discard the old IV container.	Touching the spike on the administration set results in contamination, resulting in the need to discard the tubing.
11. Using a twisting and pushing motion, insert the administration set spike into the entry site of the IV container. Alternatively, follow the manufacturer's directions for insertion. Hang the container on the IV pole.	Inserting the spike punctures the seal in the IV container and allows access to the contents.

ACTION

12. Alternatively, hang the new IV fluid container on an open hook on the IV pole. Carefully remove the cap on the entry site of the new IV solution container and expose the entry site, **taking care not to touch the exposed entry site.** Lift the completed container off the IV pole and invert it. Quickly remove the spike from the old IV container, **taking care to not contaminate the spike** (Figure 2). Discard the old IV container. Using a twisting and pushing motion, insert the administration set spike into the entry port of the new IV container as it hangs on the IV pole (Figure 3).

RATIONALE

Touching the opened entry site on the IV container or the administration set spike results in contamination, resulting in the need to discard both. Inserting the spike punctures the seal in the IV container and allows access to the contents.

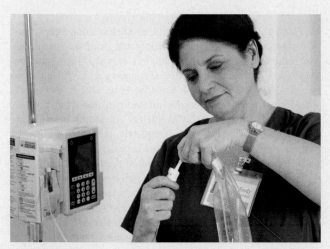

FIGURE 2. Removing administration spike from old IV fluid container.

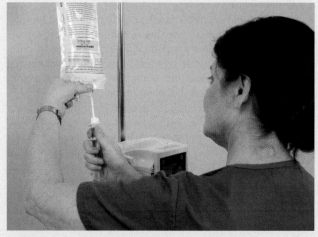

FIGURE 3. Inserting administration set spike into entry port of new IV fluid container.

13. If using an electronic infusion device, open the slide clamp, check the drip chamber of the administration set, verify the flow rate programmed in the infusion device, and turn the device to "run" or "infuse."

Verifying the rate and device settings ensures the patient receives the correct volume of the solution.

14. If using a gravity/free-flow infusion, slowly open the roller clamp on the administration set and count the drops. Adjust until the correct drop rate is achieved (Figure 4).

Opening the clamp regulates the flow rate into the drip chamber. Verifying the rate ensures that the patient receives the correct volume of solution.

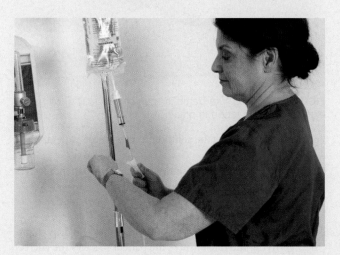

FIGURE 4. Reopening clamp and adjusting flow rate.

(*continued on page 1030*)

Skill 16-3 ▶ Changing an Intravenous Solution Container and Administration Set *(continued)*

ACTION	RATIONALE

To Change IV Solution Container and Administration Set

15. Prepare the IV solution and administration set. Refer to Skill 16-1, Steps 7–11.

16. Hang the new IV container on an open hook on the IV pole. Close the clamp on the existing IV administration set. Also, close the clamp on the short extension tubing connected to the IV catheter in the patient's arm.

Clamping the existing IV tubing prevents leakage of fluid from the administration set after it is disconnected. Clamping the tubing on the extension set prevents introduction of air into the extension tubing.

17. If using an electronic infusion device, remove the current administration set from the device. Following the manufacturer's directions, insert a new administration set into the infusion device.

The administration set must be removed in order to insert a new tubing into the device.

18. Put on gloves. Remove the current infusion tubing from the needleless connector or end cap on the short extension IV tubing. Using an antimicrobial swab, vigorously disinfect the connection surface and sides of the needleless connector or end cap on the extension tubing and allow them to dry. Remove the end cap from the new administration set. Insert the end of the administration set into the needleless connector or end cap (Figure 5). Loop the administration set tubing near the entry site, and anchor it with tape (nonallergenic) close to the site (Figure 6). Remove your gloves. Perform hand hygiene.

VAD entry points, end caps, and needleless connectors must be vigorously scrubbed and disinfected prior to each access to reduce the risk for introduction of microorganisms and prevent VAD-related infection (Frimpong et al., 2015; Gorski et al., 2021; Harper, 2014; Loveday et al., 2014). Friction is needed to physically remove microorganisms from the top, sides, and threads of the needleless connector or end cap. Allow the antiseptic to dry completely, following the manufacturer's directions for use (Gorski et al., 2021). Inserting the administration set allows initiation of the fluid infusion. The weight of the tubing is sufficient to pull it out of the vein if it is not well anchored. Nonallergenic tape is less likely to tear fragile skin. Proper removal of PPE reduces the risk for infection transmission and contamination of other items. Hand hygiene prevents transmission of microorganisms.

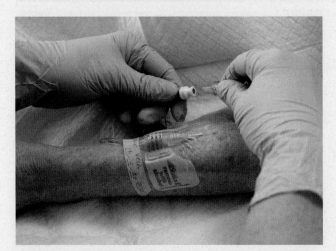

FIGURE 5. Inserting the end of the administration set into the needleless connector or end cap.

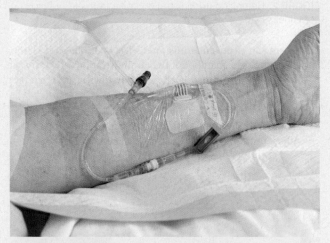

FIGURE 6. Making sure clamp is open on new tubing, with short extension tubing taped in place.

19. Open the clamp on the extension tubing. Open the clamp on the administration set.

Opening clamps allows the solution to flow to the patient.

20. If using an electronic infusion device, check the drip chamber of the administration set, verify the flow rate programmed in the infusion device, and turn the device to "run" or "infuse."

Verifying the rate and device settings ensures the patient receives the correct volume of solution.

21. If using a gravity/free-flow infusion, slowly open the roller clamp on the administration set and count the drops. Adjust until the correct drop rate is achieved.

Opening the clamp regulates the flow rate into the drip chamber. Verifying the rate ensures the patient receives the correct volume of solution.

ACTION

22. Apply a passive disinfection cap to each access site on the administration set; use an antimicrobial swab to vigorously disinfect the connection surface and sides of each access site and allow them to dry. Attach a passive disinfection cap to each site.

23. Remove equipment. Ensure the patient's comfort. Lower the bed, if it is not in the lowest position.

24. Remove additional PPE, if used. Perform hand hygiene.

25. Return to check the flow rate and observe the IV site for infiltration and/or other complications 30 minutes after starting the infusion and at least hourly thereafter. Ask the patient if they are experiencing any pain or discomfort related to the IV infusion.

RATIONALE

Passive disinfection caps contain an antiseptic-impregnated sponge that dispenses the antiseptic over the connector's top and threads and protects the hub from contamination by touch or airborne sources (Gorski et al., 2021; Stango et al., 2014). VAD administration set entry points, end caps, and needleless connectors must be vigorously scrubbed and disinfected prior to each access to reduce the risk for introduction of microorganisms and prevent VAD-related infection (Frimpong et al., 2015; Gorski et al., 2021; Harper, 2014; Loveday et al., 2014). Friction is needed to physically remove microorganisms from the top, sides, and threads of the needleless connector or end cap. Allow the antiseptic to dry completely to ensure complete effectiveness.

This promotes patient comfort and safety.

Proper removal of PPE reduces the risk for infection transmission and contamination of other items. Hand hygiene prevents transmission of microorganisms.

Continued monitoring is important to maintain the correct flow rate. Early detection of problems ensures prompt intervention.

EVALUATION

The expected outcomes have been met when the IV solution container and administration set have been changed, the IV infusion has continued without interruption, and no infusion complications have been identified.

DOCUMENTATION

Guidelines

Document the type of IV solution and the rate of infusion (often done in the eMAR/MAR) and the assessment of the access site. Record the patient's reaction to the procedure and pertinent patient teaching, such as alerting the nurse if the patient experiences any pain from the IV or notices any swelling at the site. Document the IV fluid solution on the intake and output record.

Sample Documentation

11/3/25 1015 IV fluid changed from $D_5$1/2 NS with 20 mEq KCl/L at 125 mL/hr to D_5 0.9% NS with 20 mEq KCl/L at 80 mL/hr via infusion pump. IV site and dressing/stabilization device intact; no swelling, redness, or drainage noted.

—S. Barnes, RN

DEVELOPING CLINICAL REASONING AND CLINICAL JUDGMENT

UNEXPECTED SITUATIONS AND ASSOCIATED INTERVENTIONS

- *Infusion does not flow or flow rate changes after bag and tubing are changed (gravity/free flow):* Make sure that the flow clamp is open, and the drip chamber is approximately half full. Check the electronic device for proper functioning. Check the IV site for possible problems with the catheter, such as bending of the catheter or the position of the patient's extremity and inspect the IV site for signs and symptoms of complications. Readjust the flow rate as necessary (gravity/free flow).
- *After attaching new IV tubing, you note air bubbles in the tubing:* If the bubbles are above the roller clamp, you can easily remove them by closing the roller clamp, stretching the tubing downward,

(continued on page 1032)

Skill 16-3 ▶ Changing an Intravenous Solution Container and Administration Set *(continued)*

and tapping the tubing with your finger so the bubbles rise to the drip chamber. If there is a larger amount of air in the tubing, swab the medication port on the tubing below the air with an antimicrobial solution and attach a syringe to the port below the air. Clamp the tubing below the access port. Aspirate the air from the tubing via the syringe. Remember that air bubbles in the tubing can be reduced if the tubing is primed slowly with fluid instead of allowing a wide-open flow of the solution.

EVIDENCE FOR PRACTICE ▶	**INTRAVENOUS ACCESS AND INFUSION** **Related Guideline Infusion Nurses Society (INS) Standards of Practice** Gorski, L. A., Hadaway, L., Hagle, M. E., Broadhurst, D., Clare, S., Kleidon, T., Meyer, B. M., Nickel, B., Rowley, S., Sharpe, E., & Alexander, M.; Infusion Nurses Society. (2021). Infusion therapy. Standards of practice, 8th edition. *Journal of Infusion Nursing, 44*(Suppl 1), S1–S224. https://doi.org/10.1097/NAN.0000000000000396 Refer to details in Skill 16-1, Evidence for Practice.

Skill 16-4 ▶ Changing a Peripheral Venous Access Device Site Dressing

The intravenous (IV) site is a potential entry point for microorganisms into the bloodstream. Maintenance of an intact and patent dressing at the insertion site is an important means of preventing infection and other complications. Transparent semipermeable membrane (TSM) dressings are commonly used to protect the insertion site. TSM dressings (e.g., Tegaderm™ or OpSite IV™) allow easy inspection of the IV site and permit evaporation of moisture that accumulates under the dressing. Sterile gauze may also be used to cover the catheter site. A gauze dressing is recommended if the patient is diaphoretic, the site is bleeding or oozing, or there is drainage from the exit site; replace it with a TSM once this is resolved (Gorski, 2020; O'Grady et al., 2017).

Facility policy generally determines the type of dressing used and the intervals for dressing change. Perform site care and replace TSM dressings at least every 7 days (except neonatal patients) or immediately if the dressing becomes damp, loosened, visibly soiled, or has a lifted/detached border; blood or drainage is present; or there is compromised skin integrity under the dressing (Gorski et al., 2021). Change sterile gauze dressings at least every 2 days, or if the integrity of the dressing is disrupted (damp, loosened, visibly soiled) (Gorski et al., 2021). Consider the use of sterile adhesive removers and skin barrier film to prevent medical adhesive–related skin injury (MARSI) (Fumarola et al., 2020; Gorski et al., 2021; Zhao et al., 2018). However, dressing changes might be required more often, based on nursing assessment and judgment. Site care and dressing changes are performed using aseptic nontouch technique to minimize the possibility of contamination when changing these dressings (ANTT) (Gorski et al., 2021). In the nontouch technique, the practitioner touches a site or equipment only as absolutely necessary, even when wearing sterile gloves (Taylor et al., 2023).

DELEGATION CONSIDERATIONS

The changing of a peripheral venous access dressing is not delegated to assistive personnel (AP). Depending on the state's nurse practice act and the organization's policies and procedures, the changing of a peripheral venous access dressing may be delegated to licensed practical/vocational nurses (LPN/LVNs). The decision to delegate must be based on careful analysis of the patient's needs and circumstances as well as the qualifications of the person to whom the task is being delegated. Refer to the Delegation Guidelines in Appendix A.

EQUIPMENT

- Transparent semipermeable membrane (TSM) dressing
- Cleansing swabs (>0.5% chlorhexidine in alcohol solution preferred [Gorski et al., 2021; Sarani et al., 2018]); if there is a contra-indication to alcoholic chlorhexidine solution, tincture of iodine, an iodophor (povidone-iodine), or 70% alcohol may also be used (Gorski et al., 2021; Mimoz et al., 2015; O'Grady et al., 2017). Use chlorhexidine with caution in infants up to age 14 days, premature infants, and low-birth-weight infants due to the risk of skin irritation and chemical burns (Gorski et al., 2021).

- Adhesive remover
- Antimicrobial wipes
- Skin protectant wipes (e.g., Skin-Prep™)
- IV securement/stabilization device, as appropriate
- Nonallergenic tape
- Standardized scale for assessing and documenting phlebitis (Box 16-3 in Skill 16-3 provides an example of one scale)
- Gloves
- Towel or disposable pad
- Additional PPE, as indicated

ASSESSMENT

Assess the PIVC site. The dressing should be intact, adhering to the skin on all edges. Check for any leaks or fluid under or around the dressing or other indications that the dressing needs to be changed. Inspect the tissue around the IV entry site for swelling, coolness, or pallor. These are signs of fluid infiltration into the tissue around the IV catheter. Also inspect the site for redness, swelling, and warmth. These signs might indicate the development of phlebitis or an inflammation of the blood vessel at the site. Ask the patient if they are experiencing any pain or discomfort related to the IV line. Pain or discomfort can be a sign of infiltration, extravasation, phlebitis, thrombophlebitis, and infection related to IV therapy. Grade phlebitis, if present. Refer to Box 16-2. Refer also to Fundamentals Review 16-3. Note the insertion date and date of last dressing change, if different from the insertion date. Assess the patient's need to maintain venous access. If the patient does not need the access, discuss the possibility of discontinuation with the health care team. Evaluate the patient's history for any allergies or sensitivity to skin antiseptics (Gorski et al., 2021). Assess the patient's knowledge of PIVC therapy.

ACTUAL OR POTENTIAL HEALTH PROBLEMS AND NEEDS

Many actual or potential health problems or issues may require the use of this skill as part of related interventions. An appropriate health problem or issue may include:
- Infection risk
- Injury risk
- Altered skin integrity risk

OUTCOME IDENTIFICATION AND PLANNING

The expected outcomes to achieve when changing a peripheral venous access dressing are that the dressing is changed without adverse effect, and the patient exhibits an access site that is clean, dry, and without evidence of any signs and symptoms of infection, infiltration, or phlebitis.

IMPLEMENTATION

ACTION	RATIONALE
1. Assess and discuss with the health care team the need for continued peripheral venous access. Determine the need for a dressing change. Check facility policy. Gather equipment.	The clinical need for the IV catheter should be assessed on a daily basis in acute inpatient settings and during regular assessment visits in community-based care settings (Gorski et al., 2021). The particular facility's policies determine the type of dressing used and when these dressings are changed. Dressing changes might be required more often, based on nursing assessment and judgment. Immediately change any dressing that is damp, loosened, visibly soiled, or has a lifted/detached border; if blood or drainage is present; or if there is compromised skin integrity under the dressing (Gorski et al., 2021). Preparation promotes efficient time management and an organized approach to the task.

(continued on page 1034)

Skill 16-4 ▶ Changing a Peripheral Venous Access Device Site Dressing *(continued)*

ACTION	RATIONALE
2. Perform hand hygiene and put on PPE, if indicated.	Hand hygiene and PPE prevent the spread of microorganisms. PPE is required based on transmission precautions.
3. Identify the patient.	Identifying the patient ensures the right patient receives the intervention and helps prevent errors.
4. Assemble equipment on the bedside stand or overbed table or other surface within reach.	Bringing everything to the bedside conserves time and energy. Arranging items nearby is convenient, saves time, and avoids unnecessary stretching and twisting of muscles on the part of the nurse.
5. Close the curtains around the bed and close the door to the room, if possible. Explain to the patient what you are going to do and why. Ask the patient about allergies to tape and skin antiseptics.	This ensures the patient's privacy. Explanation relieves anxiety and facilitates engagement. Possible allergies may exist related to the tape or antiseptics.
6. Put on gloves. Place a towel or disposable pad under the patient's arm with the venous access. If the solution is currently infusing, temporarily stop the infusion.	Gloves prevent contact with blood and body fluids. The pad protects the underlying surface.
7. **Hold the catheter in place with your nondominant hand and support the patient's skin.** Beginning at the device hub, **gently lift the edge of the dressing away from the skin, then gently push the skin down and away from the dressing/adhesive** (Fumarola et al., 2020). **Lift the dressing perpendicular to the skin toward the insertion site, carefully removing the old dressing and/or stabilization/securing device** (Figure 1). If the patient is at increased risk for medical adhesive–related skin injury (MARSI), or there is resistance, use an adhesive remover (Barton, 2020; Fumarola et al., 2020; Kelly-O'Flynn et al., 2020). Avoid inadvertently dislodging the catheter, as it may be adhered to the dressing/stabilization device (Gorski et al., 2021). Discard the dressing.	Pushing the skin down and away from the adhesive reduces the risk for medical adhesive–related skin injury (MARSI) (Fumarola et al., 2020). The use of adhesive remover allows for easy, rapid, and painless removal without the associated problems of skin stripping and helps reduce patient discomfort (Barton, 2020; Fumarola et al., 2020; Kelly-O'Flynn et al., 2020). Proper disposal of the dressing prevents transmission of microorganisms.
8. Inspect the IV site for the presence of phlebitis (inflammation), infection, or infiltration. If noted, grade phlebitis and discontinue and relocate PIVC. Refer to Fundamentals Review 16-3 and Box 16-2 (in Skill 16-2). Assess the integrity of the stabilization device if it is separate from the dressing; change the stabilization device according to the manufacturer's directions and/or facility policy.	Inflammation (phlebitis), infection, or infiltration causes trauma to tissues and necessitates removal of the VAD. A standardized scale should be used to assess and document phlebitis (Gorski et al., 2021). The integrity of the stabilization device should be assessed with each dressing change, and the device itself should be changed according to the manufacturer's directions (Gorski et al., 2021).
9. Use a single-use sterile applicator containing sterile antiseptic solution to **cleanse the site with >5% chlorhexidine in alcohol solution or the solution identified by facility policy (Figure 2). Follow the manufacturer's directions for use to determine product application process and dry times (Gorski et al., 2021). Allow the antiseptic to dry naturally; do not wipe, fan, or blow on the skin** (Gorski et al., 2021).	Cleansing is necessary because organisms on the skin can be introduced into the tissues or the bloodstream with the needle. Use of >0.5% chlorhexidine in an alcohol solution is preferred for skin antisepsis (Gorski et al., 2021; Sarani et al., 2018). If there is a contraindication to alcoholic chlorhexidine solution, tincture of iodine, an iodophor (povidone-iodine), or 70% alcohol may also be used (Gorski et al., 2021; Mimoz et al., 2015; O'Grady et al., 2017).

ACTION

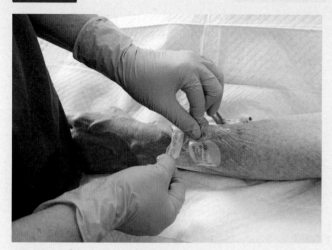

FIGURE 1. Carefully removing old dressing.

10. Open the skin protectant wipe. Apply it to the site, making sure to cover, at minimum, the area to be covered with the dressing (Figure 3). Allow it to dry. Place the sterile transparent dressing and/or catheter securing/stabilization device over the venipuncture site (Figure 4).

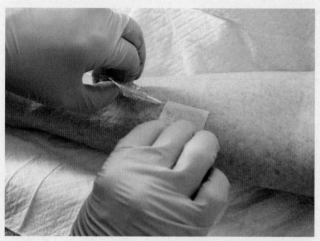

FIGURE 3. Applying skin protectant to site.

11. Label the dressing with the date, time of change, and your initials. Loop the tubing near the entry site, and anchor it with tape (nonallergenic) close to the site (Figure 5). Resume fluid infusion, if indicated. Check that the IV flow is accurate and the system is patent. Refer to Skill 16-2.

12. Apply an IV securement/stabilization device if not already in place as part of the dressing, as indicated, based on facility policy. Explain to the patient the purpose of the device and the importance of safeguarding the site when using the extremity.

RATIONALE

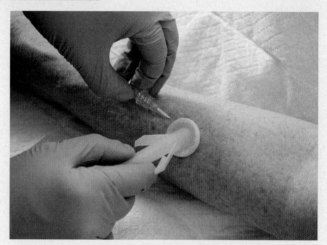

FIGURE 2. Cleansing the site with an antiseptic solution.

The skin protectant aids in adhesion of the dressing and decreases the risk for skin trauma when the dressing is removed. A transparent dressing allows easy visualization and protects the site. Stabilization/securing devices preserve the integrity of the access device, minimize catheter movement at the hub, and prevent catheter dislodgement and loss of access (Gorski et al., 2021). Some stabilization devices also act as a site dressing.

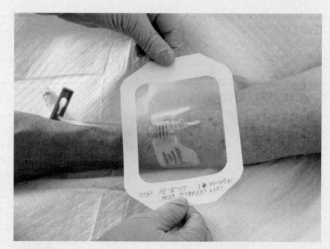

FIGURE 4. Applying transparent dressing to site.

Other personnel working with the infusion will know what type of device is being used, the site, and when it was inserted. The weight of the tubing is sufficient to pull it out of the vein if it is not well anchored. Nonallergenic tape is less likely to tear fragile skin.

These systems are recommended for use on all venous access sites, and particularly central venous access sites, to preserve the integrity of the access device, minimize catheter movement at the hub, and prevent catheter dislodgement and loss of access (Gorski et al., 2021). Some devices also act as a site dressing and may already have been applied.

(*continued on page 1036*)

Skill 16-4 ▶ **Changing a Peripheral Venous Access Device Site Dressing** *(continued)*

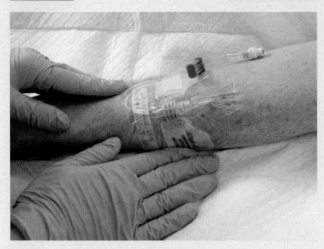

ACTION	RATIONALE

FIGURE 5. Site dressing with label and anchored tubing.

13. Remove equipment. Remove gloves and perform hand hygiene. Ensure the patient's comfort. Lower the bed, if it is not in the lowest position.

Removing PPE properly and performing hand hygiene reduce the risk for infection transmission and contamination of other items. Positioning promotes patient comfort and safety.

14. Remove additional PPE, if used. Perform hand hygiene.

Removing PPE properly reduces the risk for infection transmission and contamination of other items. Hand hygiene prevents transmission of microorganisms.

EVALUATION

The expected outcomes have been met when the dressing has been changed without adverse effect, and the patient has exhibited an access site that is clean, dry, and without evidence of any signs and symptoms of infection, infiltration, or phlebitis.

DOCUMENTATION

Guidelines

Document the location of the venous access as well as the condition of the site. Include the presence or absence of signs of erythema, redness, swelling, or drainage. Document the clinical criteria for site complications. Refer to Fundamentals Review 16-3 and Box 16-2 (in Skill 16-2). Record the patient's subjective comments regarding the absence or presence of pain at the site. Record the patient's reaction to the procedure and pertinent patient teaching, such as alerting the nurse if the patient experiences any pain from or swelling at the site.

Sample Documentation

11/15/25 1120 Dressing change to IV site in L hand (dorsal metacarpal) complete. Transparent dressing and peripheral stabilization device applied. Site without erythema, redness, edema, or drainage. D$_5$ NS infusing at 75 mL/hr. Patient instructed to call nurse with any pain, discomfort, swelling, or questions.

—S. Barnes, RN

DEVELOPING CLINICAL REASONING AND CLINICAL JUDGMENT

UNEXPECTED SITUATIONS AND ASSOCIATED INTERVENTIONS

• *Patient reports that IV site feels "funny" and hurts:* Observe the venous access site for redness, edema, and warmth, and/or swelling, pallor, and coolness. If present, clamp the tubing to stop the IV solution flow, put on gloves, and remove the catheter. Use a skin marker to outline the area with visible signs of infiltration to allow for assessment of changes (Gorski et al., 2021). Secure the gauze with tape over the insertion site without applying pressure. Assess the area distal to the VAD for capillary refill, sensation, and motor function (Gorski et al., 2021). Restart the IV in a new location. Estimate the volume of fluid that escaped into the tissue based on the rate of infusion and length of time since the last assessment. Notify the health care team and use an appropriate method for clinical management of the infiltrate site, based on the infused solution and facility guidelines (Gorski et al., 2021). Record the site assessment and interventions as well as the site for new venous access.

- *IV catheter is partially pulled out of insertion site (migrates externally):* Do not readvance the catheter. Whether the access is salvageable depends on how much of the catheter remains in the vein. Assess for proper placement in the vein before further use and consider the infusion therapy and circumstances to determine viability and secure at the current location (Gorski et al., 2021). Removal and reinsertion at a new site might be the most appropriate intervention if the PIVC is no longer in an appropriate position for the prescribed infusion (Gorski et al., 2021). If the PIVC is not removed, monitor it closely for signs of infiltration and infection.

SPECIAL CONSIDERATIONS

General Considerations

- Use of >0.5% chlorhexidine in alcohol solution is preferred for skin antisepsis (Gorski et al., 2021; Sarani et al., 2018). If there is a contraindication to alcoholic chlorhexidine solution, tincture of iodine, an iodophor (povidone-iodine), or 70% alcohol may instead be used (Gorski et al., 2021; Mimoz et al., 2015; O'Grady et al., 2017).
- Drying time with 70% isopropyl alcohol is 5 seconds; alcohol-based chlorhexidine requires 20 seconds. Povidone iodine requires longer than 6 minutes to be thoroughly dry, making it less favorable to clinical practice (Gorski et al., 2021).
- Use of topical antibiotic ointments or creams on insertion sites as part of routine site care is not recommended because of their potential to promote fungal infections and antimicrobial resistance (Gorski et al., 2021; O'Grady et al., 2017).
- Do not submerge venous catheters and catheter sites in water (O'Grady et al., 2017). When the patient is showering or bathing, protect the peripheral VAD with clear plastic wrap or a device designed for this purpose. Cover the connections and protect the hub connections from water contamination (Gorski et al., 2021).

Infant and Child Considerations

- Use chlorhexidine with caution in infants up to age 14 days, premature infants, and low-birth-weight infants due to the risk of skin irritation and chemical burns (Gorski et al., 2021).

Older Adult Considerations

- Avoid using vigorous friction at the insertion site, which can traumatize fragile skin and veins in older adults.

EVIDENCE FOR PRACTICE ▶

INTRAVENOUS ACCESS AND INFUSION
Related Guideline Infusion Nurses Society (INS) Standards of Practice
Gorski, L. A., Hadaway, L., Hagle, M. E., Broadhurst, D., Clare, S., Kleidon, T., Meyer, B. M., Nickel, B., Rowley, S., Sharpe, E., & Alexander, M.; Infusion Nurses Society. (2021). Infusion therapy. Standards of practice, 8th edition. *Journal of Infusion Nursing, 44*(Suppl 1), S1–S224. https://doi.org/10.1097/NAN.0000000000000396
　　Refer to details in Skill 16-1, Evidence for Practice.

Skill 16-5 ▶ Capping for Intermittent Use and Flushing a Peripheral Venous Access Device

When a continuous intravenous (IV) is no longer necessary, the primary IV line (PIVC or CVAD) can be capped and converted to an intermittent infusion device. A capped line consists of the IV catheter connected to a short length of extension tubing sealed with a cap. Capping of a short peripheral venous catheter is commonly referred to as a medication or saline lock. Capping of a vascular access device provides venous access for intermittent infusions or emergency medications. Capping of a VAD can be accomplished in different ways. Refer to facility policy for the procedure to convert an access for intermittent use.

VADs used for intermittent infusions should be flushed with preservative-free 0.9% sodium chloride solution and aspirated for a blood return prior to each infusion to assess catheter function (Gorski et al., 2021). Flushing of the device is also required after each infusion to clear the infused medication or other solution from the catheter lumen. Vascular access devices are "locked" after completion of the flush solution at each use to decrease the risk of occlusion (Gorski et al., 2021). According to the guidelines from the INS, PIVCs are locked with preservative-free 0.9% sodium chloride (Gorski et al., 2021). If the device is not in use, periodic flushing according to facility policy is required to keep the catheter patent.

It is important to follow the manufacturer's directions for use when flushing, clamping, and disconnecting syringes and IV administration tubing or any other device from needleless connectors. In the absence of manufacturer directions, identify the internal mechanism for fluid displacement reported by the manufacturer for the type of needleless connector being used and use the appropriate sequence for flushing, clamping, and disconnecting based on the type of needleless connector to prevent connection/disconnection reflux (Box 16-4) (Gorski et al, 2021).

Box 16-4 ▌ Needleless Connectors

Sequence for Flushing, Clamping, and Disconnecting
- Follow the manufacturers' directions for use if available.
- In the absence of manufacturer directions, identify the internal mechanism for fluid displacement reported by the manufacturer for the type of needleless connector being used and use the following sequence (Gorski et al., 2021):

Internal Mechanism for Fluid Displacement	Sequence for Flushing, Clamping, and Disconnecting
Negative displacement	Flush, clamp, disconnect
Positive displacement	Flush, disconnect, clamp
Neutral and antireflux	No specific sequence required

Source: Adapted from Gorski, L. A., Hadaway, L., Hagle, M. E., Broadhurst, D., Clare, S., Kleidon, T., Meyer, B. M., Nickel, B., Rowley, S., Sharpe, E., & Alexander, M.; Infusion Nurses Society. (2021). Infusion therapy. Standards of practice, 8th edition. *Journal of Infusion Nursing, 44*(Suppl 1), S1–S224. https://doi.org/10.1097/NAN.0000000000000396

DELEGATION CONSIDERATIONS	Capping and flushing of a peripheral VAC is not delegated to assistive personnel (AP). Depending on the state's nurse practice act and the organization's policies and procedures, these procedures may be delegated to licensed practical/vocational nurses (LPN/LVNs). The decision to delegate must be based on careful analysis of the patient's needs and circumstances as well as the qualifications of the person to whom the task is being delegated. Refer to the Delegation Guidelines in Appendix A.
EQUIPMENT	• End cap device, according to facility policy • Gloves • Additional PPE, as indicated • 4 × 4 gauze pad • Single-use, commercially prepared, pre-filled syringe with sterile normal saline for injection, minimum volume equal to twice the internal volume of the catheter system (Gorski et al., 2021), according to facility policy • Passive disinfection caps (based on facility policy) • Antimicrobial wipes • Nonallergenic tape

ASSESSMENT	Assess the insertion site for signs of any complications. Refer to Fundamentals Review 16-3 and Box 16-2 (in Skill 16-2). Assess the appropriateness of discontinuation of the fluid infusion for the patient. Verify the prescribed intervention for discontinuation of IV fluid infusion. Evaluate the patient's history for any allergies or sensitivity to skin antiseptics (Gorski et al., 2021).
ACTUAL OR POTENTIAL HEALTH PROBLEMS AND NEEDS	Many actual or potential health problems or issues may require the use of this skill as part of related interventions. An appropriate health problem or issue may include: • Infection risk • Injury risk
OUTCOME IDENTIFICATION AND PLANNING	The expected outcome to achieve when capping a peripheral intravenous infusion is that the peripheral VAD is converted for intermittent use and the patient remains free from injury and signs and symptoms of complications. In addition, the capped VAD remains patent.

IMPLEMENTATION

ACTION	**RATIONALE**
1. Determine the need for conversion to an intermittent access. Verify the prescribed intervention for discontinuation of IV fluid infusion. Check facility policy. Gather the necessary supplies.	This ensures the correct intervention for the correct patient. Preparation promotes efficient time management and an organized approach to the task.
2. Perform hand hygiene and put on PPE, if indicated.	Hand hygiene and PPE prevent the spread of microorganisms. PPE is required based on transmission precautions.
3. Identify the patient.	Identifying the patient ensures the right patient receives the intervention and helps prevent errors.
4. Assemble equipment on the bedside stand or overbed table or other surface within reach.	Bringing everything to the bedside conserves time and energy. Arranging items nearby is convenient, saves time, and avoids unnecessary stretching and twisting of muscles on the part of the nurse.
5. Close the curtains around the bed and close the door to the room, if possible. Explain to the patient what you are going to do and why. Ask the patient about allergies to tape and skin antiseptics.	This ensures the patient's privacy. Explanation relieves anxiety and facilitates engagement. Possible allergies may exist related to the tape or antiseptics.
6. Assess the peripheral VAD site. Refer to Skill 16-2.	Complications, such as infiltration, phlebitis, or infection, necessitate discontinuation of the IV infusion at that site.
7. If using an electronic infusion device, stop the device. Close the roller clamp on the administration set. If using a gravity/free-flow infusion, close the roller clamp on the administration set.	The action of the infusion device needs to be stopped and the clamp closed to prevent leaking of fluid when the tubing is disconnected.
8. Put on gloves. Close the clamp on the short extension tubing connected to the IV catheter in the patient's arm.	Clamping the tubing on the extension set prevents introduction of air into the extension tubing.

(continued on page 1040)

Skill 16-5 ▶ Capping for Intermittent Use and Flushing a Peripheral Venous Access Device *(continued)*

ACTION

9. Remove the administration set tubing from the needleless connector or end cap on the extension set. Using an antimicrobial swab, disinfect the connection surface and sides of the needleless connector or end cap on the extension tubing and allow them to dry (Figure 1).

10. Insert the saline flush syringe into the needleless connector or end cap on the extension tubing. Pull back on the syringe to aspirate the catheter for positive blood return. If positive, instill the solution over 1 minute or flush the line according to facility policy (Figure 2). Prevent connection/disconnection reflux by using the appropriate sequence for flushing, clamping, and disconnecting determined by the type of needleless connector being used (Box 16-4) (Gorski et al., 2021).

RATIONALE

Removing the infusion tubing discontinues the infusion. VAD administration set entry points, end caps, and needleless connectors must be disinfected prior to each access to reduce the risk for introduction of microorganisms and prevent VAD-related infection (Frimpong et al., 2015; Gorski et al., 2021; Harper, 2014; Loveday et al., 2014). Friction is needed to physically remove microorganisms from the top, sides, and threads of the needleless connector or end cap. Allow the antiseptic to dry completely, following the manufacturer's directions for use (Gorski et al., 2021).

The presence of a blood return upon aspiration and lack of resistance when flushing indicate patency of the VAD (Gorski et al., 2021). Flushing maintains patency of the IV line. The action of the positive pressure end cap is maintained with the appropriate sequence for flushing, clamping, and disconnecting determined by the type of needleless connector in use (Gorski et al., 2021). Clamping prevents air from entering the extension set.

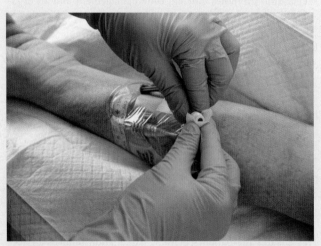

FIGURE 1. Using an antimicrobial swab to disinfect the connection surface and sides of the needleless connector or end cap on the extension tubing.

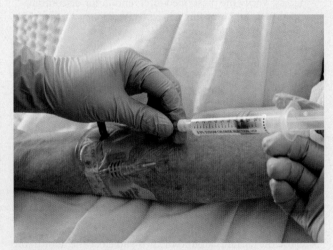

FIGURE 2. Flushing venous access device.

11. If necessary, loop the extension tubing near the entry site and anchor it with tape (nonallergenic) close to the site.

12. Using an antimicrobial swab, vigorously disinfect the needleless connector or end cap on the extension tubing and allow it to dry. Attach a passive disinfection cap.

The weight of the tubing is sufficient to pull it out of the vein if it is not well anchored. Nonallergenic tape is less likely to tear fragile skin.

VAD administration set entry points, end caps, and needleless connectors must be vigorously scrubbed and disinfected prior to each access to reduce the risk of introducing microorganisms and to prevent VAD-related infection (Frimpong et al., 2015; Gorski et al., 2021; Harper, 2014; Loveday et al., 2014). Friction is needed to physically remove microorganisms from the top, sides, and threads of the needleless connector or end cap. Allow the antiseptic to dry completely to ensure complete effectiveness. Passive disinfection caps contain an antiseptic-impregnated sponge that dispenses the antiseptic over the connector's top and threads and protects the hub from contamination by touch or airborne sources (Gorski et al., 2021; Stango et al., 2014).

ACTION	RATIONALE

 13. Remove equipment. Remove gloves and perform hand hygiene. Ensure the patient's comfort. Lower the bed, if it is not in the lowest position.

Removing gloves properly and hand hygiene reduce the risk for infection transmission and contamination of other items. Positioning promotes patient comfort and safety.

 14. Remove additional PPE, if used. Perform hand hygiene.

Proper removal of PPE reduces the risk for infection transmission and contamination of other items. Hand hygiene prevents transmission of microorganisms.

EVALUATION

The expected outcomes have been met when the peripheral VAD has been converted for intermittent use, the patient has remained free from injury and signs and symptoms of complications, and the capped VAD has remained patent.

DOCUMENTATION

Guidelines

Document discontinuation of the IV fluid infusion. Record the condition of the venous access site. Document the flushing of the VAD. This is often done in the eMAR/MAR. Record the patient's reaction to the procedure and any patient teaching that occurred.

Sample Documentation

12/13/25 1/20 IV infusion capped per order. Peripheral site in right forearm (cephalic) flushed without resistance using 3 mL of saline. Dressing remains intact. Site without redness, swelling, drainage, or heat. Patient denies discomfort. Patient verbalized an understanding of the need to maintain IV access.

—A. Lynn, RN

DEVELOPING CLINICAL REASONING AND CLINICAL JUDGMENT

UNEXPECTED SITUATIONS AND ASSOCIATED INTERVENTIONS

- *Peripheral venous access site leaks fluid when flushed:* Check connections. If the site continues to leak, remove it from the site to prevent infection and other complications. Evaluate the need for continued access; if a clinical need is present, restart it in another location.
- *IV does not flush easily:* Assess the insertion site. Infiltration and/or phlebitis may be present. If present, remove the IV. Use a skin marker to outline the area with visible signs of infiltration to allow for assessment of changes (Gorski et al., 2021). Secure the gauze with tape over the insertion site without applying pressure. Assess the area distal to the VAD for capillary refill, sensation, and motor function (Gorski et al., 2021). Assess the need for continued venous access. If a clinical need is present, restart the IV in a new location. Estimate the volume of fluid that escaped into the tissue based on the rate of infusion and length of time since the last assessment. Notify the health care team and use an appropriate method for clinical management of the infiltrate site, based on infused solution and facility guidelines (Gorski et al., 2021). Record the site assessment and interventions as well as the site for new venous access.
- *IV does not flush easily:* The catheter may be blocked or clotted due to a kinked catheter at the insertion site. Aspirate and attempt to flush again. If resistance remains, do not force. Forceful flushing can dislodge a clot at the end of the catheter. Remove the IV. Assess the need for continued venous access. If a clinical need is present, restart the IV in a new location.
- *IV catheter is partially pulled out of insertion site (migrates externally):* Do not readvance the catheter. Whether the access is salvageable depends on how much of the catheter remains in the vein. Assess for proper placement in the vein before further use and consider the infusion therapy and circumstances to determine viability and secure at the current location (Gorski et al., 2021). Removal and reinsertion at a new site might be the most appropriate intervention if the PIVC is no longer in an appropriate position for the prescribed infusion (Gorski et al., 2021). If the PIVC is not removed, monitor it closely for signs of infiltration and infection.

(continued on page 1042)

| Skill 16-5 ▶ | **Capping for Intermittent Use and Flushing a Peripheral Venous Access Device** *(continued)* |

SPECIAL CONSIDERATIONS

- Some facilities may use end caps for VADs that are not positive pressure devices. In this case, flush with the recommended volume of saline, ending with 0.5 mL of solution remaining in the syringe. While maintaining pressure on the syringe, clamp the extension tubing. This provides positive pressure, preventing backflow of blood into the catheter, decreasing risk for occlusion.
- If the administration tubing was connected directly to the hub of the IV catheter when the access was initiated, short extension tubing should be added when the line is capped.

EVIDENCE FOR PRACTICE ▶

INTRAVENOUS ACCESS AND INFUSION
Related Guideline Infusion Nurses Society (INS) Standards of Practice
Gorski, L. A., Hadaway, L., Hagle, M. E., Broadhurst, D., Clare, S., Kleidon, T., Meyer, B. M., Nickel, B., Rowley, S., Sharpe, E., & Alexander, M.; Infusion Nurses Society. (2021). Infusion therapy. Standards of practice, 8th edition. *Journal of Infusion Nursing, 44*(Suppl 1), S1–S224. https://doi.org/10.1097/NAN.0000000000000396
    Refer to details in Skill 16-1, Evidence for Practice.

| Skill 16-6 ▶ | **Administering a Blood Transfusion** |

A blood transfusion is the infusion of whole blood or a blood component, such as plasma, red blood cells (RBCs), cryoprecipitate, or platelets, into the patient's venous circulation (Table 16-1). A blood product transfusion is given when a patient's RBCs, platelets, or coagulation factors decrease to levels that compromise a patient's health. Blood transfusions are not without risk, however. Potentially life-threatening complications include allergic reaction and anaphylactic reaction, hemolytic reaction, transfusion-related acute lung injury, circulatory volume overload, immunosuppression, and transmission of infectious diseases (Carman et al., 2018). It is important that the potential benefits of the transfusion be considered against the potential risks (American Red Cross, 2021; Carman et al., 2018). Before a patient can receive a blood product, their blood must be typed to ensure that they receive compatible blood (**blood typing** and **crossmatching**). If incompatible, clumping and hemolysis of the recipient's blood cells result and death can occur (Table 16-2). Alternatively, a patient may receive an **autologous transfusion**, in which case, the potential for transfusion reaction is significantly decreased (Silvergleid, 2022). The nurse must also verify the infusion rate, based on facility policy or prescribed intervention. Follow the facility's policies and guidelines to determine if the transfusion should be administered by an electronic infusion device or by gravity/free flow. Refer to Box 16-1 in Skill 16-1 for guidelines to calculate the flow rate for gravity/free-flow infusion. Identification of patients at risk for complications and patient monitoring during and after transfusion of blood products is essential because of ongoing risk for transfusion reaction (Carman et al., 2018; DeLisle, 2018).

DELEGATION CONSIDERATIONS

The administration of a blood transfusion is not delegated to assistive personnel (AP). Depending on the state's nurse practice act and the organization's policies and procedures, the initiation and monitoring of a blood transfusion may be delegated in certain circumstances to licensed practical/vocational nurses (LPN/LVNs) who have received appropriate training. The decision to delegate must be based on careful analysis of the patient's needs and circumstances as well as the qualifications of the person to whom the task is being delegated. Refer to the Delegation Guidelines in Appendix A.

Table 16-1 Blood Products

BLOOD PRODUCT	FILTER	RATE OF ADMINISTRATION	ABO COMPATIBILITY	DOUBLE-CHECKED BY TWO LICENSED PRACTITIONERS/ ADULTS (e.g., registered nurse, physician/adult caregiver)
Packed red blood cells	Yes	1 unit over 2–3 hours; no longer than 4 hours	Yes	Yes
Platelets	Yes	Over 1–2 hours; no longer than 4 hours	No	Yes
Cryoprecipitate	Yes	As quickly as tolerated by the patient; no longer than 4 hours	Recommended	Yes
Fresh-frozen plasma	Yes	As quickly as tolerated by the patient or over 15–60 minutes; no longer than 4 hours	Yes	Yes
Albumin	Yes	5% solution: 1–2 mL/min (5%) to start up to 4 mL/min 25% solution no more than 1 mL/min	No	No

Source: Adapted from Global RPH. (2018, April 21). Albumin. https://globalrph.com/dilution/albumin/; Gorski, L. A., Hadaway, L., Hagle, M. E., Broadhurst, D., Clare, S., Kleidon, T., Meyer, B. M., Nickel, B., Rowley, S., Sharpe, E., & Alexander, M.; Infusion Nurses Society. (2021). Infusion therapy. Standards of practice, 8th edition. *Journal of Infusion Nursing*, *44*(Suppl 1), S1–S224. https://doi.org/10.1097/NAN.0000000000000396.

Table 16-2 Transfusion Reactions

REACTION	SIGNS AND SYMPTOMS	NURSING ACTIVITY
Allergic reaction: allergy to transfused blood	Hives, itching Anaphylaxis	• Stop transfusion immediately and keep vein open with normal saline. • Notify health care team immediately. • Administer antihistamine parenterally as necessary.
Febrile reaction: fever develops during infusion	Fever and chills Headache Malaise	• Stop transfusion immediately and keep vein open with normal saline. • Notify health care team. • Treat symptoms.
Hemolytic transfusion reaction: incompatibility of blood product	Immediate onset Facial flushing Fever, chills Headache Low back pain Shock	• Stop infusion immediately and keep vein open with normal saline. • Notify health care team immediately. • Obtain blood samples from site. • Obtain first voided urine. • Treat shock if present. • Send unit, tubing, and filter to lab. • Draw blood sample for serologic testing and send urine specimen to lab.
Circulatory overload: too much blood administered	Dyspnea Dry cough Pulmonary edema	• Slow or stop infusion. • Monitor vital signs. • Notify health care team. • Place in upright position with feet dependent.
Bacterial reaction: bacteria present in blood	Fever Hypertension Dry, flushed skin Abdominal pain	• Stop infusion immediately. • Obtain culture of patient's blood and return blood bag to lab. • Monitor vital signs. • Notify health care team. • Administer antibiotics as ordered.

(continued on page 1044)

Skill 16-6 ▶ Administering a Blood Transfusion *(continued)*

EQUIPMENT	• Blood product • Blood administration set (tubing with in-line filter, or add-on filter, and Y for saline administration) • 0.9% normal saline for IV infusion • Electronic infusion pump labeled for blood transfusion • Venous access; if peripheral site, initiated with a 20- to 24-gauge catheter based on vein size (adults) (Gorski et al., 2021) • Antimicrobial wipes • Gloves • Additional PPE, as indicated • Nonallergenic tape • Second adult trained in the identification of the recipient and blood components (i.e., registered nurse, other licensed practitioner [hospital/outpatient setting]); responsible adult (home setting) to verify blood product and patient information (Gorski et al., 2021)
ASSESSMENT	Review the most recent laboratory values, in particular, the complete blood count (CBC). Ask the patient about any previous transfusions, including the number they have had and any reactions experienced during a transfusion. Inspect the VAD insertion site, noting the gauge of the IV catheter. Blood or blood components may be transfused via a 20- to 24-gauge peripheral VAD (adult) (Gorski et al., 2021). Central venous access devices (CVADs) may also be used to administer a transfusion. Baseline assessment prior to obtaining blood for transfusion should include measurement of vital signs, lung assessment, identification of conditions that may increase the risk of transfusion-related adverse reactions (e.g., current fever, heart failure, renal disease, risk of fluid volume excess), the presence of an appropriate and patent VAD, and current laboratory values (Gorski et al., 2021). Institution policies vary on the frequency of assessment. The Infusion Nurses Society Standards of Practice recommend checking the patient's vital signs within 30 minutes prior to transfusion, 15 minutes after initiating the transfusion, after the transfusion is completed, 1 hour after the transfusion has been completed, and as needed based on clinical observation of the patient's condition (Gorski et al., 2021).
ACTUAL OR POTENTIAL HEALTH PROBLEMS AND NEEDS	Many actual or potential health problems or issues may require the use of this skill as part of related interventions. An appropriate health problem or issue may include: • Infection risk • Fluid imbalance • Impaired cardiac output
OUTCOME IDENTIFICATION AND PLANNING	The expected outcomes to achieve when administering a blood transfusion are that the patient receives the blood transfusion without any evidence of a transfusion reaction or complications, and the patient exhibits signs and symptoms of fluid balance, improved cardiac output, and enhanced tissue perfusion.

IMPLEMENTATION

ACTION	**RATIONALE**
1. Verify the prescribed intervention for transfusion of a blood product. Verify the completion of informed consent documentation in the health record.	Verification of the prescribed intervention ensures the right patient receives the correct intervention.
2. Gather all equipment.	Preparation promotes efficient time management and an organized approach to the task.
3. Perform hand hygiene and put on PPE, if indicated.	Hand hygiene and PPE prevent the spread of microorganisms. PPE is required based on transmission precautions.

ACTION	**RATIONALE**
4. Identify the patient.	Identifying the patient ensures the right patient receives the intervention and helps prevent errors.
5. Assemble equipment on the bedside stand or overbed table or other surface within reach.	Bringing everything to the bedside conserves time and energy. Arranging items nearby is convenient, saves time, and avoids unnecessary stretching and twisting of muscles on the part of the nurse.
6. Close the curtains around the bed, and close the door to the room, if possible. Explain to the patient what you are going to do and why. Ask the patient about previous experience with a transfusion and any reactions. Advise the patient to report any signs/symptoms associated with complications of transfusion therapy (e.g., uneasy feeling, pain, dizziness, rash, chills, itching, rash, or other unusual symptoms).	This ensures the patient's privacy. Explanation relieves anxiety and facilitates engagement. Previous reactions may increase the risk for reaction to this transfusion. Any reaction to the transfusion necessitates stopping the transfusion immediately and evaluating the situation.
7. Prime the blood administration set with the normal saline IV fluid. Refer to Skill 6-1.	Normal saline (0.9% sodium chloride) is the solution of choice for blood product administration (Gorski et al., 2021).
8. Put on gloves. If the patient does not have a VAD in place, initiate peripheral venous access. (Refer to Skill 16-1.) Connect the administration set to the VAD via the extension tubing. (Refer to Skill 16-1.) Infuse the normal saline per facility policy.	Gloves prevent contact with blood and body fluids. Infusion of fluid via venous access maintains patency until the blood product is administered. Start an IV before obtaining the blood product in case the initiation takes longer than 30 minutes. Blood must be stored at a carefully controlled temperature (Hill & Derbyshire, 2021), and transfusion must begin within the length of time blood or a blood product must be returned after it is obtained from the blood bank/source, as identified by facility policy.
9. Obtain the blood product from blood bank/transfusion service according to facility policy. Verify the patient information and blood product information; inspect the blood component for abnormalities. Scan the bar codes/biometric scanning on the blood products if in use and required.	Confirmation of patient and blood component information is necessary at the time the blood component is released from the transfusion service to ensure the right patient receives the correct intervention (Gorski et al., 2021). Computerized checking systems using bar codes/radio frequency identification devices/biometric scanning on blood products are being implemented to identify, track, and assign data to transfusions as an additional safety measure (Gorski et al., 2021; Hill & Derbyshire, 2021).
10. Two registered nurses (or other practitioners trained in the identification of the recipient and blood components [i.e., licensed practitioner in the hospital/outpatient setting; responsible adult in the home setting]) compare and validate the following information in the presence of the patient with the health record, the patient identification band (hospital/outpatient setting), and the label of the blood product (Gorski et al., 2021): • Prescribed intervention for transfusion of blood product • Informed consent • Two independent patient identifiers (e.g., patient name, patient identification number) • Blood group and type • Blood product donation identification number, expiration date/time, date/time of issue • Inspection of the blood component: intact container, abnormal color, presence of clots, clumping, excessive air/bubbles	Verification of this information reduces the risk for error in administration. If appearance is not normal (e.g., abnormal color, clots, excessive air/bubbles, unusual odor), the product may be contaminated; return the blood to the blood bank/transfusion service (Gorski et al., 2021).

(continued on page 1046)

Skill 16-6 ▶ Administering a Blood Transfusion *(continued)*

ACTION

11. **Obtain a baseline assessment (refer to the previous Assessment section) including a set of vital signs before beginning the transfusion.**

12. Put on gloves. Put the electronic infusion pump on "hold." Close the roller clamp closest to the drip chamber on the saline side of the administration set. Close the roller clamp on the administration set below the infusion device. Alternatively, if infusing via gravity/free flow, close the roller clamp on the administration set.

13. Close the roller clamp closest to the drip chamber on the blood product side of the administration set. Remove the protective cap from the access port on the blood container. Remove the cap from the access spike on the administration set. Using a pushing and twisting motion, insert the spike into the access port on the blood container, taking care not to contaminate the spike. Hang the blood container on the IV pole. Open the roller clamp on the blood side of the administration set. Squeeze the drip chamber until the in-line filter is saturated (Figure 1). Remove your gloves. Perform hand hygiene.

14. **Start administration slowly (approximately 2–3 mL/min for the first 15 minutes** (Gorski et al., 2021). **Stay with the patient for the first 15 minutes of transfusion.** Open the roller clamp on the administration set below the infusion device. Set the flow rate and begin the transfusion. Alternatively (if infusing by gravity/free flow), start the flow of solution by releasing the clamp on the tubing and counting the drops. Adjust until the correct drop rate is achieved. Assess the flow of the blood and function of the infusion device. Inspect the insertion site for signs of infiltration.

15. Observe the patient for signs/symptoms associated with complications of transfusion therapy (e.g., uneasy feeling, pain, dizziness, rash, chills, itching, rash, or other unusual symptoms) or any unusual comments.

16. Reassess vital signs after 15 minutes (Figure 2). Obtain vital signs thereafter according to facility policy and nursing assessment.

RATIONALE

Assessment helps identify conditions that may increase the risk of transfusion-related adverse reactions and establishes a baseline for future comparison (Carman et al., 2018; Gorski et al., 2021). The presence of fever may be a cause for delay in the administration of the blood component (Gorski et al., 2021). Any change in vital signs during the transfusion may indicate a reaction.

Gloves prevent contact with blood and body fluids. Stopping the infusion prevents blood from infusing to the patient before completion of preparations. Closing the clamp to saline allows the blood product to be infused via the electronic infusion pump. Electronic infusion pumps (labeled for blood transfusion) can be used to deliver blood or blood components without significant risk of hemolysis of RBCs or platelet damage (Gorski et al., 2021).

Filling the drip chamber prevents air from entering the administration set. The filter in the blood administration set removes particulate material formed during storage of the blood. If the administration set becomes contaminated, the entire set must be discarded and replaced.

Major transfusion reactions usually appear before the first 50 mL have been transfused, and a slow rate will minimize the volume of RBCs infused (Gorski et al., 2021). Increasing the rate after 15 minutes when there are no signs of reaction helps to ensure the completion of the transfusion within 4 hours of leaving the controlled temperature storage of the blood bank/transfusion service (Gorski et al., 2021; Hill & Derbyshire, 2021).

Verifying the rate and device settings ensures the patient receives the correct volume of solution. If the catheter slips out of the vein, the blood will accumulate (infiltrate) into the surrounding tissue.

These signs and symptoms may be an early indication of a transfusion reaction.

Vital signs must be assessed as part of monitoring for possible adverse reaction. Facility policy and nursing judgment will dictate frequency. Guidelines suggest vital signs should be checked within 30 minutes prior to transfusion, 15 minutes after initiating the transfusion (Hill & Derbyshire, 2021), after the transfusion is completed, 1 hour after the transfusion has been completed, and as needed based on clinical observation of the patient's condition (Gorski et al., 2021).

ACTION

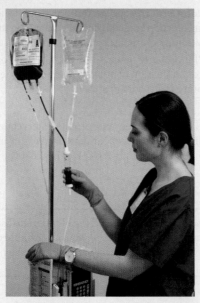

FIGURE 1. Squeezing the drip chamber to saturate the filter.

17. After the observation period (15 minutes), increase the infusion rate to the calculated rate to complete the infusion within the prescribed time frame, no more than 4 hours.

18. Maintain the prescribed flow rate as ordered or as deemed appropriate based on the patient's overall condition, keeping in mind the outer limits for safe administration. Ongoing monitoring is crucial throughout the entire duration of the blood transfusion for early identification of any adverse reactions.

19. **During transfusion, assess the patient at least every 30 minutes for adverse reactions. Stop the blood transfusion if you suspect a reaction. Quickly replace the blood tubing with a new administration set primed with normal saline for IV infusion. Initiate an infusion of normal saline for IV at a keep open rate, usually 40 mL/hr. Obtain vital signs. Notify the health care team and the blood bank/transfusion service** (Gorski et al., 2021).

20. When the transfusion is complete, close the roller clamp on the blood side of the administration set and open the roller clamp on the normal saline side of the administration set. Initiate infusion of normal saline. When all of the blood has infused into the patient, clamp the administration set. Obtain vital signs. Put on gloves. Cap the access site or resume the previous IV infusion (refer to Skills 16-1 and 16-5). Alternatively, disconnect the transfusion when complete without flushing the remainder of the blood in the line and flush the VAD with 0.9% sodium chloride according to facility policy. Dispose of blood-transfusion equipment or return it to the blood bank, according to facility policy.

RATIONALE

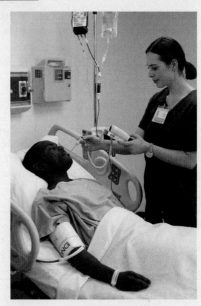

FIGURE 2. Assessing vital signs after 15 minutes.

If no adverse effects occurred during this time, the infusion rate is increased. Increasing the rate after 15 minutes when there are no signs of reaction helps to ensure the completion of the transfusion within 4 hours (Gorski et al., 2021). If complications occur, they can be observed, and the transfusion can be stopped immediately. Verifying the rate and device settings ensures the patient receives the correct volume of solution. Transfusion must be completed within 4 hours (Gorski et al., 2021) due to the potential for bacterial growth in a blood product at room temperature.

The rate must be carefully controlled, and the patient's reaction must be monitored frequently.

If a transfusion reaction is suspected, the blood must be stopped. Do not infuse the normal saline through the blood tubing because you would be allowing more of the blood into the patient's body, which could complicate a reaction. Besides a serious life-threatening blood transfusion reaction, the potential for fluid–volume overload exists in older adults and patients with decreased cardiac function.

Saline prevents hemolysis of RBCs and clears the remainder of blood in the IV line.

Proper disposal of equipment reduces transmission of microorganisms and potential contact with blood and body fluids. Some guidelines suggest that flushing through the remainder of the blood in the line with 0.9% sodium chloride is unnecessary and is not recommended because it may result in particles being flushed through the filter (JPAC, 2014).

(continued on page 1048)

Skill 16-6 ▶ Administering a Blood Transfusion *(continued)*

ACTION	RATIONALE
21. Remove equipment. Remove your gloves and perform hand hygiene. Ensure the patient's comfort. Lower the bed, if it is not in the lowest position.	Removing gloves properly and performing hand hygiene reduces the risk for infection transmission and contamination of other items. Positioning promotes patient comfort and safety.
22. Remove additional PPE, if used. Perform hand hygiene.	Removing PPE properly reduces the risk for infection transmission and contamination of other items. Hand hygiene prevents transmission of microorganisms.
23. Monitor the patient to detect febrile or pulmonary transfusion reactions for at least 4 to 6 hours; educate patients who are not under direct observation after their transfusion about signs and symptoms of delayed transfusion reaction and the importance of reporting.	This ensures early detection and prompt intervention. Delayed transfusion reactions can occur days to weeks or months after transfusion (Carman et al., 2018; DeLIsle, 2018).

EVALUATION

The expected outcomes have been met when the patient has received the blood transfusion without any evidence of a transfusion reaction or complication, and the patient has exhibited signs and symptoms of fluid balance, improved cardiac output, and enhanced peripheral tissue perfusion.

DOCUMENTATION

Guidelines

Document that the patient received the blood transfusion; include the type of blood product. Record the patient's condition throughout the transfusion, including pertinent data, such as vital signs, lung sounds, and the patient's subjective response to the transfusion. Document any complications or reactions and whether the patient had received the transfusion without any complications or reactions. Document the assessment of the IV site and any other fluids infused during the procedure. Document the transfusion volume and other IV fluid intake on the patient's intake and output record.

Sample Documentation

> 11/2/25 1100 T 97.6°F P 82 R 14 B/P 116/74. 1 unit of packed blood red cells initiated via left forearm (basilic) 20-gauge venous access without difficulty using infusion pump. Patient states "no discomfort." IV site intact, no swelling, redness, or pain. See transfusion record.
>
> —S. Barnes, RN

> 11/2/25 1115 T 97.6°F P 78 R 16 B/P 118/68. 1 unit of packed blood red cells infusing via left forearm (basilic) 20-gauge venous access without difficulty, infusion rate 65 mL/hr. Patient states "no discomfort." IV site intact, no swelling, redness, or pain. See transfusion record.
>
> —S. Barnes, RN

> 11/2/25 1445 T 97.6°F P 82 R 14 B/P 120/74. 1 unit of packed blood red cells completed via left forearm (basilic) 20-gauge venous access without difficulty. Patient denies symptoms of complications. IV site intact, no swelling, redness, or pain.
>
> —S. Barnes, RN

DEVELOPING CLINICAL REASONING AND CLINICAL JUDGMENT

UNEXPECTED SITUATIONS AND ASSOCIATED INTERVENTIONS

- *Patient experiences slight increase in temperature but is exhibiting no other signs of a transfusion reaction:* Notify the health care team. Document and continue to monitor. A temperature increase of 1.8°F (1°C) or higher can be the first sign of a serious transfusion reaction, and the transfusion should be stopped (Suddock & Crookston, 2021).
- *Patient reports shortness of breath; on auscultation, you note crackles bilaterally in the bases:* Compare vital signs and lung sounds with previous vital signs and lung sounds for this patient. Obtain a pulse oximetry reading. Notify the health care team. Anticipate a possible prescribed intervention for a dose of a diuretic or decrease in the rate of the transfusion. Document and continue to assess and monitor the patient for signs and symptoms of fluid overload.
- *Patient is febrile (temperature increase of 1.8°F [1°C] or higher), tachycardic, and reporting a headache and/or back pain or other sign/symptom of adverse reaction:* Stop the transfusion immediately (Gorski et al., 2021; Hill & Derbyshire, 2021). Disconnect the infusion and administer an infusion of 0.9% sodium chloride using a new administration set at a keep-open rate. Notify the health care team and the blood bank/transfusion service. Administer medications as prescribed. Send the blood unit, administration set, and filter to the laboratory. Obtain additional diagnostic tests, such as blood and urine tests, based on facility policy and prescribed interventions. Document and continue to monitor.

SPECIAL CONSIDERATIONS

General Considerations

- Do not add or infuse any other solutions or medications through the same administration set with blood or blood components and do not piggyback blood administration sets into other infusion administration sets (Gorski et al., 2021).
- When rapid transfusion is required, a larger-sized catheter gauge is recommended (18 to 20 gauge) (Gorski et al., 2021).
- CVADs are acceptable for blood administration (Gorski et al., 2021).
- Computerized checking systems using bar codes/radio frequency identification devices/biometric scanning on blood products are being implemented to identify, track, and assign data to transfusions as an additional safety measure (Gorski et al., 2021; Hill & Derbyshire, 2021).
- Transfusions of platelets should be administered over 1 to 2 hours (Gorski et al., 2021).
- Transfusions of plasma should be administered as quickly as tolerated by the patient or over 15 to 60 minutes (Gorski et al., 2021).
- Never warm blood in a microwave. Use a blood-warming device that is indicated for this purpose, following the manufacturer's directions for use (Gorski et al., 2021). A blood warmer should be used when indicated by patient history, clinical condition, and/or prescribed therapy/intervention. Blood warmers should also be used for large-volume transfusions (Suddock & Crookston, 2021), therapeutic apheresis exchange transfusions in patients known to have significant cold agglutinins, patients with clinically significant conditions, and for neonate exchange transfusions (Gorski et al., 2021).
- External compression devices, if used for rapid transfusions, should be equipped with a pressure gauge, should totally encase the blood bag, and should apply uniform pressure against all parts of the blood container. Pressure should not exceed 300 mm Hg (Gorski et al., 2021). A large-gauge catheter (PIVC) may be more effective than a pressure device to achieve rapid infusion (Gorski et al., 2021).

Infant and Child Considerations

- Use an appropriate and patent VAD for transfusion for infants and children; options include the umbilical vein (neonates) or a vein large enough to accommodate a 22- to 24-gauge catheter (Gorski et al., 2021).

Community-Based Care Considerations

- Transfusion of blood products in a community-based setting may be appropriate for medically stable patients with chronic conditions (Garciá et al., 2018; Sharp et al., 2021) and have been associated with low rates of individual and system adverse events (Sharp et al., 2021).

(continued on page 1050)

Skill 16-6 ▶ Administering a Blood Transfusion *(continued)*

EVIDENCE FOR PRACTICE ▶

INTRAVENOUS ACCESS AND INFUSION
Related Guideline Infusion Nurses Society (INS) Standards of Practice
Gorski, L. A., Hadaway, L., Hagle, M. E., Broadhurst, D., Clare, S., Kleidon, T., Meyer, B. M., Nickel, B., Rowley, S., Sharpe, E., & Alexander, M.; Infusion Nurses Society. (2021). Infusion therapy. Standards of practice, 8th edition. *Journal of Infusion Nursing, 44*(Suppl 1), S1–S224. https://doi.org/10.1097/NAN.0000000000000396
   Refer to details in Skill 16-1, Evidence for Practice.

Skill 16-7 ▶ Changing the Dressing and Flushing Central Venous Access Devices

Central venous access devices (CVADs) are venous access devices in which the tip of the catheter terminates in the central venous circulation, usually in the lower one third of the superior vena cava near its junction with the right atrium (Gorski et al., 2021). Types of CVADs include peripherally inserted central catheters (PICCs) (Figure 1), nontunneled percutaneous central venous catheters (Figure 2), tunneled percutaneous central venous catheters (Figure 3), and implanted ports. (Refer to Skill 16-8, Figure 1.) CVADs provide access for a variety of IV fluids, medications, blood products, and PN solutions and provide a means for hemodynamic monitoring and blood sampling. The use of a CVAD should be considered when the anticipated duration of infusion therapy is >15 days (Gorski et al., 2021). The type and duration of infusion therapy, patient preference, the patient's physiologic condition (age, health problems, comorbidities), and the patient's vascular condition (history of vascular access attempts, vessel, and skin health at potential insertion sites) determines the type of CVAD used (Gorski et al., 2021).

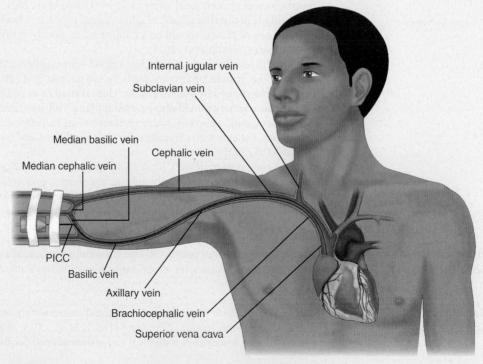

FIGURE 1. Placement of peripherally inserted central catheter (PICC).

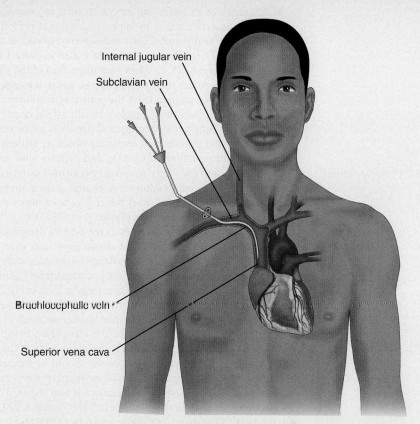

FIGURE 2. Placement of triple-lumen, nontunneled percutaneous central venous catheter.

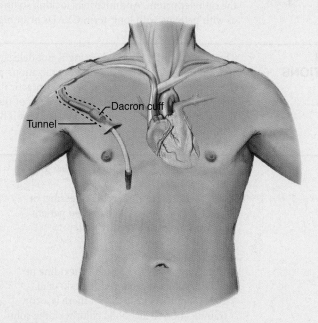

FIGURE 3. Tunneled percutaneous central venous catheter.

(*continued on page 1052*)

Skill 16-7 ▶ Changing the Dressing and Flushing Central Venous Access Devices *(continued)*

Maintenance of an intact and patent dressing in combination or integrated with a securement device at the insertion site is an important means of preventing infection, protecting the site, and promoting skin health and CVAD securement (Gorski et al., 2021). Transparent semipermeable membrane (TSM) dressings are commonly used to protect the insertion site. TSM dressings (e.g., Tegaderm™ or OpSite IV™) allow easy inspection of the site and permit evaporation of moisture that accumulates under the dressing. Sterile gauze may also be used to cover the catheter site. A gauze dressing is recommended if the patient is diaphoretic, or if the site is bleeding or oozing or has drainage from the exit site; replace it with a TSM once this is resolved (Gorski, 2020; O'Grady et al., 2017). Chlorhexidine-impregnated dressings are recommended for use as VAD site dressings for certain patient populations, including oncology patients with implanted ports, adult patients with short-term nontunneled CVADs, and patients with an epidural access device (Gorski et al., 2021). Site care and dressing changes are performed using aseptic nontouch technique to minimize the possibility of contamination when changing these dressings (ANTT) (Gorski et al., 2021). In the nontouch technique, the practitioner touches a site or equipment only as absolutely necessary, even when wearing sterile gloves (Taylor et al., 2023).

Facility policy generally determines the type of dressing and the intervals for dressing change. Perform site care and replace TSM dressings at least every 7 days (except neonatal patients) or immediately if the dressing becomes damp, loosened, visibly soiled, or has a lifted/detached border; blood or drainage is present; or there is compromised skin integrity under the dressing (Gorski et al., 2021). Change sterile gauze dressings at least every 2 days, or if the integrity of the dressing is disrupted (damp, loosened, visibly soiled) (Gorski et al., 2021). Consider the use of sterile adhesive removers and skin barrier film to prevent medical adhesive–related skin injury (MARSI) (Fumarola et al., 2020; Gorski et al., 2021; Zhao et al., 2018). Tunneled, cuffed CVADs may require a site dressing when the subcutaneous tunnel is healed (Gorski et al., 2021).

CVADs used for intermittent infusions should be flushed with preservative-free 0.9% sodium chloride solution and aspirated for a blood return prior to each infusion to assess catheter function (Gorski et al., 2021). Flushing of the device is also required after each infusion to clear the infused medication or other solution from the catheter lumen. CVADs should be locked with either a heparin solution (10 units/mL) or preservative-free 0.9% sodium chloride after each intermittent use, according to the directions for use for the specific CVAD and needleless connector (Gorski et al., 2021). If the device is not in use, periodic flushing according to facility policy is required to keep the catheter patent. Antimicrobial locking solutions are sometimes used in specific situations, such as with patients with long-term CVADs or in high-risk patient populations (Gorski et al., 2021).

DELEGATION CONSIDERATIONS

The changing of a CVAD dressing is not delegated to assistive personnel (AP). Depending on the state's nurse practice act and the organization's policies and procedures, the changing of a CVAD dressing may be delegated to licensed practical/vocational nurses (LPN/LVNs). The decision to delegate must be based on careful analysis of the patient's needs and circumstances as well as the qualifications of the person to whom the task is being delegated. Refer to the Delegation Guidelines in Appendix A.

EQUIPMENT

- Sterile tape or sterile adhesive skin closure strips (i.e., Steri-Strips™)
- TSM dressing; antimicrobial dressing; or gauze pad for dressing, based on patient circumstances and facility policy
- Several 2 × 2 gauzes
- Sterile towel or drape
- Cleansing swabs (>0.5% chlorhexidine in alcohol solution preferred [Gorski et al., 2021; Sarani et al., 2018]); if there is a contraindication to alcoholic chlorhexidine solution, tincture of iodine, an iodophor (povidone-iodine), or 70% alcohol may also be used (Gorski et al., 2021; Mimoz et al., 2015;

O'Grady et al., 2017). Use chlorhexidine with caution in infants up to age 14 days, premature infants, and low-birth-weight infants due to the risk of skin irritation and chemical burns (Gorski et al., 2021)
- Prefilled commercially prepared syringes with 10-mL sterile normal saline for injection (minimum volume equal to twice the internal volume of the catheter system) (Gorski et al., 2021); one for each lumen of the CVAD
- Prefilled commercially prepared syringes with heparin 10 units/mL in 10-mL; one for each lumen of the CVAD (based on the manufacturer's directions for the use of the

CVAD and needleless connector, and facility policy)
- Masks (2), depending on facility policy
- Gloves
- Sterile gloves
- Additional PPE, as indicated
- Adhesive remover
- Skin protectant/barrier wipe (e.g., Skin-Prep™)
- Antimicrobial wipes

- Needleless connector or positive pressure end caps; one for each lumen of the CVAD
- Passive disinfection caps (based on facility policy)
- IV securement/stabilization device, as appropriate
- Sterile measuring tape
- Bath blanket
- Additional PPE, as indicated

ASSESSMENT

Assess the CVAD site. The CVAD site should be assessed with each infusion and at least daily in patients being treated in inpatient and nursing facility settings (Gorski et al., 2021). In community-care settings, the CVAD should be assess at every visit, and the patient or caregiver should be taught to check the CVAD site with each infusion or at least once per day (Gorski et al., 2021). The dressing should be intact, adhering to the skin on all edges. Check for any leaks or fluid under or around the dressing or other indications that the dressing needs to be changed. Inspect the tissue around the entry site for redness, swelling, tenderness, and warmth. These signs might indicate the development of localized infection. Ask the patient if they are experiencing any pain or discomfort related to the VAD, paresthesias, numbness, or tingling. Pain or discomfort can be a sign of infiltration, extravasation, phlebitis, thrombophlebitis, deep vein thrombosis, and/or infection. Refer to Fundamentals Review 16-3. Note the insertion date/access date and the date of the last dressing change. Assess the patient's need to maintain the CVAD. If the patient does not need the access, discuss the possibility of discontinuation with the health care team. Evaluate the patient's history for any allergies or sensitivity to skin antiseptics (Gorski et al., 2021). Assess the patient's knowledge of CVAD therapy. Assess the CVAD condition. Verify if the current locking solution dwelling in the CVAD needs to be aspirated and discarded or may be infused as part of the flushing procedure; all antimicrobial lock solutions must be aspirated and discarded (Gorski et al., 2021).

ACTUAL OR POTENTIAL HEALTH PROBLEMS AND NEEDS

Many actual or potential health problems or issues may require the use of this skill as part of related interventions. An appropriate health problem or issue may include:
- Infection risk
- Knowledge deficiency
- Altered skin integrity risk

OUTCOME IDENTIFICATION AND PLANNING

The expected outcomes to achieve when changing a dressing and flushing a CVAD are that site care is provided, and the dressing is changed and the device is flushed without adverse effect. In addition, the patient exhibits an access site that is clean, dry, and without evidence of any signs and symptoms of infection or other adverse effect, and the CVAD remains patent.

IMPLEMENTATION

ACTION

1. Assess and discuss with the health care team the need for continued CVAD access. Determine the need for a dressing change. Check facility policy. Often, the procedure for CVAD flushing and dressing changes will be a standing protocol. Gather equipment.

RATIONALE

The clinical need for the CVAD should be assessed on a daily basis in acute inpatient settings and during regular assessment visits in community-based care settings (Gorski et al., 2021). The particular facility's policies determine the type of dressing used and when these dressings are changed. Dressing changes might be required more often, based on nursing assessment and judgment. Immediately change any dressing that is damp, loosened, visibly soiled, or has a lifted/detached border; blood or drainage is present; or if there is compromised skin integrity under the dressing (Gorski et al., 2021). Preparation promotes efficient time management and an organized approach to the task.

(continued on page 1054)

Skill 16-7 ▶ Changing the Dressing and Flushing Central Venous Access Devices *(continued)*

ACTION	**RATIONALE**

2. Perform hand hygiene and put on PPE, if indicated.

Hand hygiene and PPE prevent the spread of microorganisms. Unclean hands and improper technique are potential sources for infecting a CVAD. PPE is required based on transmission precautions.

3. Identify the patient.

Identifying the patient ensures the right patient receives the intervention and helps prevent errors.

4. Assemble equipment on the bedside stand or overbed table or other surface within reach.

Bringing everything to the bedside conserves time and energy. Arranging items nearby is convenient, saves time, and avoids unnecessary stretching and twisting of muscles on the part of the nurse.

5. Close the curtains around the bed and close the door to the room, if possible. Explain to the patient what you are going to do and why. Ask the patient about allergies to tape and skin antiseptics.

This ensures the patient's privacy. Explanation relieves anxiety and facilitates engagement. Possible allergies may exist related to the tape or antiseptics.

6. Place a waste receptacle or bag at a convenient location for use during the procedure.

Having a waste container handy means the soiled dressing can be discarded easily, without the spread of microorganisms.

7. Adjust the bed to a comfortable working height (VHACEOSH, 2016).

Having the bed at the proper height prevents back and muscle strain.

8. Assist the patient to a comfortable position that provides easy access to the CVAD insertion site and dressing. If the patient has a PICC, position the patient with their arm extended from the body below heart level. Use the bath blanket to cover any exposed area other than the site.

Patient positioning and use of a bath blanket provide for comfort and warmth. This position is recommended to reduce the risk of air embolism.

9. Apply a mask. Ask the patient to turn their head away from the access site. Alternatively, have the patient put on a mask, depending on facility policy. Move the overbed table to a convenient location within easy reach. Set up a sterile field on the table. Open the dressing supplies and add them to the sterile field. If IV solution is infusing via CVAD, interrupt it and place it on hold during dressing change. Apply the slide clamp on each lumen of the CVAD.

Masks help to deter the spread of microorganisms. The patient should wear a mask if they are unable to turn their head away from the site or based on facility policy. Many facilities have all sterile dressing supplies gathered in a single package. Stopping infusion and clamping each lumen prevents air from entering CVAD.

10. Put on clean gloves. Alternatively, use sterile gloves if there is a need to touch the insertion site (Gorski et al., 2021). Assess the CVAD insertion site through the old dressing (Figure 4). (Refer to previous Assessment discussion.) Palpate the site, noting pain, tenderness, or discomfort. **Stabilize the catheter by holding it in place with your nondominant hand and support the skin.** Beginning at the device hub, **gently lift the edge of the dressing away from the skin, then gently push the skin down and away from the dressing/adhesive** (Fumarola et al., 2020). **Lift the dressing perpendicular to the skin toward the insertion site, carefully removing the old dressing and/or stabilization/securing device.** If the patient is at increased risk for medical adhesive–related skin injury (MARSI), or there is resistance, use an adhesive remover (Barton, 2020; Fumarola et al., 2020; Kelly-O'Flynn et al., 2020). Avoid inadvertently dislodging the CVAD, as it may be adhered to the dressing/stabilization device (Gorski et al., 2021). Discard the dressing.

Gloves prevent contact with blood and body fluids. Pain, tenderness, or discomfort on palpation may be a sign of infection. The catheter/needle may be adhered to the dressing, increasing the risk of accidental dislodgment. Pushing the skin down and away from the adhesive reduces the risk for medical adhesive–related skin injury (MARSI) (Fumarola et al., 2020). Rapid and/or vertical pulling or insufficient support of skin when removing the dressing should be avoided (Gorski et al., 2021). The use of adhesive remover allows for the easy, rapid, and painless removal without the associated problems of skin stripping and helps reduce patient discomfort (Barton, 2020; Fumarola et al., 2020; Kelly-O'Flynn et al., 2020). Proper disposal of dressing prevents transmission of microorganisms.

ACTION

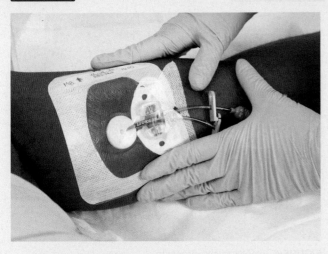

FIGURE 4. Inspecting CVAD insertion site.

11. Based on the device in use, remove the stabilization device according to the manufacturer's directions. Securement devices designed to remain in place for the life of the CVAD (e.g., a subcutaneous anchor securement system) does not need to be removed and replaced regularly with each dressing change but should be assessed during site care to ensure its integrity (Gorski et al., 2021). Remove your gloves and discard them.

12. Perform hand hygiene. Put on sterile gloves. Starting at the insertion site and continuing in a circle, wipe off any old blood or drainage with a sterile antimicrobial wipe. Use a single-use sterile applicator containing sterile antiseptic solution to **cleanse the site with >5% chlorhexidine in alcohol solution or the solution identified in facility policy, making sure to cover, at minimum, the area to be covered with the dressing. Follow the manufacturer's directions for use to determine product application process and dry times (Gorski et al., 2021). Allow the antiseptic to dry naturally; do not wipe, fan, or blow on the skin** (Gorski et al., 2021).

13. Apply antimicrobial dressing (chlorhexidine-impregnated) at the insertion site, based on facility policy (Figure 5). Apply the skin protectant to the same area, avoiding direct application to the antimicrobial dressing or the insertion site, and allow it to dry. Apply the securement/stabilization device, if used, and/or the TSM dressing, centering it over the insertion site (Figure 6). Measure the external CVAD length and compare it to the external CVAD length documented at insertion.

RATIONALE

The stabilization device is changed with the dressing change, based on the manufacturer's directions (Gorski et al., 2021). Removing gloves properly reduces the risk for infection transmission and contamination of other items.

Hand hygiene prevents transmission of microorganisms. Site care and replacement of the dressing are accomplished using sterile ANTT technique. Cleansing is necessary because organisms on the skin can be introduced into the tissues or the bloodstream with the needle. Use of >0.5% chlorhexidine in alcohol solution is preferred for skin antisepsis (Gorski et al., 2021; Sarani et al., 2018). If there is a contraindication to alcoholic chlorhexidine solution, tincture of iodine, an iodophor (povidone-iodine), or 70% alcohol may instead be used (Gorski et al., 2021; Mimoz et al., 2015; O'Grady et al., 2017).

Use chlorhexidine-impregnated dressing for all patients ages 18 years and older with short-term nontunneled CVADs (Gorski et al., 2021). Skin protectant under the antimicrobial dressing interferes with the action of the dressing. Skin protectant improves adhesion of the dressing and protects the skin from damage and irritation when the dressing is removed. The TSM dressing allows easy visualization and protects the site. Stabilization/securing devices preserve the integrity of the access device, minimize catheter movement at the hub, and prevent catheter dislodgement and loss of access (Gorski et al., 2021). Some stabilization devices also act as a site dressing. Measurement of the extending catheter can be compared with the documented length at the time of insertion to assess if the catheter has migrated inward or moved outward (Gorski et al., 2021).

(continued on page 1056)

Skill 16-7 ▶ Changing the Dressing and Flushing Central Venous Access Devices *(continued)*

ACTION	RATIONALE

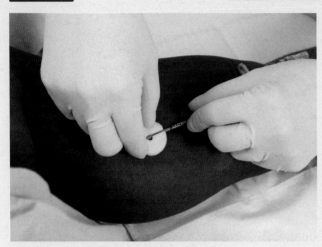

FIGURE 5. Applying antimicrobial dressing.

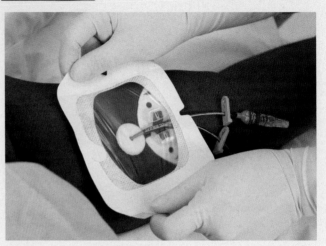

FIGURE 6. Applying site dressing.

14. Based on facility policy, replace the end caps/needless connection devices, as indicated. Working with one lumen at a time, remove the needleless connector or end cap. Using an antimicrobial swab, vigorously disinfect the connection surface and sides of each access site and allow it to dry. Attach a new needleless connector or end cap. Repeat for each lumen.

Change the needleless connectors no more frequently than at 96-hour intervals or according to the manufacturer's directions for use; changing more frequently adds no benefit and has been shown to increase the risk of catheter-associated blood stream infections (Gorski et al., 2021). VAD administration set entry points, end caps, and needleless connectors must be vigorously scrubbed and disinfected prior to each access to reduce the risk for introduction of microorganisms and prevent VAD-related infection (Frimpong et al., 2015; Gorski et al., 2021; Harper, 2014; Loveday et al., 2014). Friction is needed to physically remove microorganisms from the top, sides, and threads of the needleless connector or end cap. Allow the antiseptic to dry completely to ensure complete effectiveness. Passive disinfection caps contain an antiseptic-impregnated sponge that dispenses the antiseptic over the connector's top and threads and protects the hub from contamination by touch or airborne sources (Gorski et al., 2021; Stango et al., 2014).

15. If required, flush each lumen of the CVAD. The amount of saline and heparin flushes varies depending on the specific CVAD and on facility policy.

Flushing maintains patency of the CVAD.

ACTION

To Flush the Lumen(s)

16. Using an antimicrobial swab, vigorously scrub the needleless connector or end cap on one of the lumens and allow it to dry. Prevent connection/disconnection reflux by using the appropriate sequence for flushing, clamping, and disconnecting determined by the type of needleless connector being used (Box 16-4 in Skill 16-5) (Gorski et al., 2021). Insert the saline flush syringe into the needleless connector. Open the clamp on the lumen. Slowly inject the saline flush, noting any resistance or sluggishness, and slowly pull back on the syringe to aspirate for positive blood return. If positive, instill the remaining solution over 1 minute or by using a pulsatile flushing technique of 10 short boluses of 1 mL interrupted by brief pauses; flush the line according to facility policy. Remove the syringe. Insert the locking solution syringe and instill the volume of solution designated by facility policy over 1 minute or according to facility policy. Remove your gloves. Perform hand hygiene.

17. Using an antimicrobial swab, vigorously disinfect the connection surface and sides of each access site and allow them to dry. Attach a passive disinfection cap to each access site (Figure 7).

RATIONALE

VAD administration set entry points, end caps, and needleless connectors must be disinfected prior to each access to reduce the risk for introduction of microorganisms and prevent VAD-related infection (Frimpong et al., 2015; Gorski et al., 2021; Harper, 2014; Loveday et al., 2014). Friction is needed to physically remove microorganisms from the top, sides, and threads of the needleless connector or end cap. Allow the antiseptic to dry completely following the manufacturer's directions for use (Gorski et al., 2021). The action of the positive pressure end cap is maintained with the appropriate sequence for flushing, clamping, and disconnecting determined by the type of needleless connector in use (Gorski et al., 2021). The presence of a blood return upon aspiration and lack of resistance when flushing indicate patency of the VAD (Gorski et al., 2021). Flushing maintains patency of the IV line. A pulsatile flushing technique of 10 short boluses of 1 mL interrupted by brief pauses may be more effective in removing solid deposits (e.g., fibrin, drug precipitate, intraluminal bacteria) (Gorski et al., 2021). Clamping prevents air from entering the CVAD. Vascular access devices are locked after completion of the flush solution at each use to decrease the risk of occlusion (Gorski et al., 2021). CVADs should be locked with either a heparin solution (10 units/mL) or preservative-free 0.9% sodium chloride after each intermittent use, according to the directions for use for the specific CVAD and needleless connector (Gorski et al., 2021). Removing gloves properly and hand hygiene reduce the risk for infection transmission and contamination of other items.

Passive disinfection caps contain an antiseptic-impregnated sponge that dispenses the antiseptic over the connector's top and threads and protects the hub from contamination by touch or airborne sources (Gorski et al., 2021; Stango et al., 2014). VAD administration set entry points, end caps, and needleless connectors must be vigorously scrubbed and disinfected prior to each access to reduce the risk for introduction of microorganisms and prevent VAD-related infection (Frimpong et al., 2015; Gorski et al., 2021; Harper, 2014; Loveday et al., 2014). Friction is needed to physically remove microorganisms from the top, sides, and threads of the needleless connector or end cap. Allow the antiseptic to dry completely to ensure complete effectiveness.

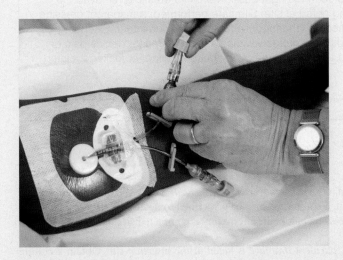

FIGURE 7. Attaching a passive disinfection cap to each access site.

(continued on page 1058)

Skill 16-7 ▶ Changing the Dressing and Flushing Central Venous Access Devices *(continued)*

ACTION	**RATIONALE**
18. Label the dressing with the date, time of change, and your initials. Resume fluid infusion, if indicated. Check that the IV flow is accurate and the system is patent. (Refer to Skill 16-2.)	Other personnel working with the infusion will know what type of device is being used, the site, and when the dressing was last changed.
19. Apply an IV securement/stabilization device if not already in place as part of the dressing, as indicated, based on facility policy. Explain to the patient the purpose of the device and the importance of safeguarding the site when using the extremity.	The weight of the tubing and/or tugging on the tubing could cause catheter dislodgement. These systems are recommended for use on all venous access sites, and particularly central venous access sites, to preserve the integrity of the access device, minimize catheter movement at the hub, and prevent catheter dislodgement and loss of access (Gorski et al., 2021). Some devices also act as a site dressing and may already have been applied.
20. Remove equipment. Ensure the patient's comfort. Lower the bed, if it is not in the lowest position.	Positioning promotes patient comfort and safety.
21. Remove additional PPE, if used. Perform hand hygiene.	Proper removal of PPE reduces the risk for infection transmission and contamination of other items. Hand hygiene prevents transmission of microorganisms.

EVALUATION

The expected outcomes have been met when site care has been provided and the dressing has been changed and the device flushed without adverse effect. In addition, the patient has exhibited an access site that is clan, dry, and without evidence of any signs and symptoms of infection or other adverse effect, and the CVAD remains patent.

DOCUMENTATION

Guidelines

Document the location, appearance, and condition of the CVAD site. Include the presence or absence of signs of erythema, redness, swelling, or drainage and the external CVAD length. Record whether the patient is experiencing any pain or discomfort related to the CVAD. Document the clinical criteria for site complications. Refer to Fundamentals Review 16-3 and Box 16-2 (in Skill 16-2). Record the patient's subjective comments regarding the absence or presence of pain at the site. Record the patient's reaction to the procedure and pertinent patient teaching, such as alerting the nurse if the patient experiences any pain from the site or notices any swelling at the site. The CVAD lumens should flush without difficulty. Communicate any abnormal findings, such as dislodgement of the CVAD, abnormal insertion assessment findings, or inability to flush the CVAD, to the health care team.

Sample Documentation

> 11/12/25 0400 PICC line located in the right basilic vein. Old dressing removed, no drainage, redness, or swelling noted at site. Site care performed; transparent dressing applied and needleless connectors changed; securement device intact. Extending catheter length 5 cm. NSS flush per protocol without difficulty. Patient denies pain or discomfort. Patient instructed to inform nurse of any pain, swelling, or leakage related to PICC line.
>
> —S. Barnes, RN

DEVELOPING CLINICAL REASONING AND CLINICAL JUDGMENT

UNEXPECTED SITUATIONS AND ASSOCIATED INTERVENTIONS

- *While dressing is being changed, CVAD is inadvertently dislodged:* Notify the health care team. If the CVAD is not all the way out, a chest x-ray may be prescribed to determine the location of the end of the CVAD. Reapply a dressing before the chest x-ray is completed so that the CVAD is not further dislodged.
- *When the dressing is removed, purulent drainage is noted at the insertion site:* Obtain a culture of the site, clean the area, reapply a dressing, and notify the health care team. This prevents the

CVAD from being open to air and unprotected while you are notifying the health care team. In addition, the culture is obtained without having to remove the dressing a second time. If a culture of the site is not prescribed, discard it in the appropriate receptacle.

- *When flushing the catheter, you are unable to withdraw blood, there is a sluggish flow, and/or you are unable to flush or infuse through the CVAD:* These signs may indicate CVAD occlusion. Consult with the nurse IV team and the health care team for appropriate catheter clearance/repair procedures to preserve the function of the CVAD (Gorski et al., 2021).

SPECIAL CONSIDERATIONS	• Use a 10-mL syringe or a syringe specifically designed to generate lower injection pressure to assess CVAD patency (Gorski et al., 2021). • The use of single-use, commercially prepared, prefilled syringes of appropriate solution to flush and lock VADs reduces the risk of catheter-associated bloodstream infection and saves time for syringe preparation (Gorski et al., 2021). • The minimum volume for 0.9% sodium chloride flush solution is the volume equal to twice the internal volume of the catheter system, the catheter plus add-on devices (Gorski et al., 2021). • If edema is present and/or upper extremity venous thrombosis is suspected in a patient with a PICC, measure the arm 10 cm above the antecubital fossa and compare the measurement with the documented measurement from the time of PICC insertion to confirm the presence of edema (Cicolini et al., as cited in Kline & Katrancha, 2019). • The continued need for *PICCs* and *nontunneled* CVADs should be assess on a daily basis and removed when there is a change in the patient's infusion needs, or it is no longer needed for the plan of care (Gorski et al., 2021). • The continued need for *tunneled* and *implanted* CVADs should be assessed on a regular basis; removal may be indicated when infusion therapy is completed, in the presence of an unresolved complication, or when it is no longer needed for the plan of care; consideration should be given to the possibility for infusion therapy to resume in the future (Gorski et al., 2021). • Use of >0.5% chlorhexidine in alcohol solution is preferred for skin antisepsis (Gorski et al., 2021; Sarani et al., 2018). If there is a contraindication to alcoholic chlorhexidine solution, tincture of iodine, an iodophor (povidone-iodine), or 70% alcohol may instead be used (Gorski et al., 2021; Mimoz et al., 2015; O'Grady et al., 2017). • Drying time with 70% isopropyl alcohol is 5 seconds; alcohol-based chlorhexidine requires 20 seconds. Povidone-iodine requires longer than 6 minutes to be thoroughly dry, making it less favorable to clinical practice (Gorski et al., 2021). • Chlorhexidine-impregnated dressings are recommended for use as VAD site dressings for certain patient populations, including oncology patients with implanted ports, adult patients with short-term nontunneled CVADs, and patients with an epidural access device (Gorski et al., 2021). • Heparin-induced thrombocytopenia (HIT) has been reported with the use of heparin flush solutions. Monitor all patients closely for signs and symptoms of HIT. If present or suspected, discontinue heparin (Gorski et al., 2021). • Use of topical antibiotic ointments or creams on insertion sites as part of routine site care is not recommended because of their potential to promote fungal infections and antimicrobial resistance (Gorski et al., 2021; O'Grady et al., 2017). • Do not submerge venous catheters and catheter sites in water; showering is permitted with the use of impermeable coverings (clear plastic wrap or a device designed for this purpose) to protect the catheter and connections (Gorski et al., 2021; O'Grady et al., 2017; York et al., 2020).
Infant and Child Considerations	• Use chlorhexidine with caution in infants up to age 14 days, premature infants, and low-birth-weight infants due to the risk of skin irritation and chemical burns (Gorski et al., 2021).
Older Adult Considerations	• Avoid using vigorous friction at the insertion site, which can traumatize fragile skin and veins in older adults.

(continued on page 1060)

Skill 16-7 ▶ Changing the Dressing and Flushing Central Venous Access Devices *(continued)*

Community-Based Care Considerations

- In community-based settings, the CVAD should be assessed at every visit, and the patient or caregiver should be taught to check the CVAD site with each infusion or at least once per day (Gorski et al., 2021).
- Patient and family/caregiver education should include managing activities of daily living (bathing, clothing, seatbelts) to prevent needle dislodgement, reporting any signs or symptoms of complications (pain, burning, stinging, or soreness), and follow-up actions (Gorski et al., 2021).

EVIDENCE FOR PRACTICE ▶

INTRAVENOUS ACCESS AND INFUSION
Related Guideline Infusion Nurses Society (INS) Standards of Practice
Gorski, L. A., Hadaway, L., Hagle, M. E., Broadhurst, D., Clare, S., Kleidon, T., Meyer, B. M., Nickel, B., Rowley, S., Sharpe, E., & Alexander, M.; Infusion Nurses Society. (2021). Infusion therapy. Standards of practice, 8th edition. *Journal of Infusion Nursing, 44*(Suppl 1), S1–S224. https://doi.org/10.1097/NAN.0000000000000396
  Refer to details in Skill 16-1, Evidence for Practice.

Skill 16-8 ▶ Accessing an Implanted Port

An implanted port consists of a subcutaneous injection port attached to a catheter. The distal catheter tip dwells in the lower segment of the superior vena cava at or near the cavoatrial junction (CAJ) (the point at which the superior vena cava meets and melds into the superior wall of the right atrium), and the proximal end or port is usually implanted in a subcutaneous pocket of the upper chest (typical) or abdominal wall (Figure 1). Implanted ports placed in the upper arm (or less commonly,

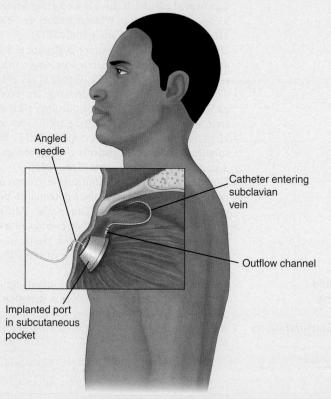

Angled needle

Catheter entering subclavian vein

Outflow channel

Implanted port in subcutaneous pocket

FIGURE 1. An implanted port with catheter inserted in subclavian vein and noncoring needle inserted into port.

lower extremity) are referred to as *peripheral access system ports.* Confirmation of tip location either by postprocedure chest radiograph or by technology used during the placement procedure is required prior to use and should be documented in the patient's health record (Gorski et al., 2021).

When not in use, no external parts of the system are visible. When venous access is desired, the location of the injection port must be palpated. A special angled, noncoring needle is inserted through the skin and septum and into the port reservoir to access the system. Once accessed, patency is maintained by periodic flushing. The length and gauge of the needle used to access the port should be selected based on the patient's anatomy, amount of subcutaneous tissue at the site, and anticipated infusion requirements. Access the port with the smallest-gauge noncoring needle to accommodate the prescribed therapy (Gorski et al., 2021). The length of the noncoring needle should be such that it allows the external components to sit level with the skin and securely within the port (needle touches bottom of port upon insertion) (Gorski et al., 2021). Transparent semipermeable membrane (TSM) dressings that cover the needle and access site are maintained and changed as outlined in Skill 16-7.

Consider the use of methods to reduce pain and discomfort during port access, such as local anesthetic agents and nonpharmacologic interventions (cognitive, behavioral, and complementary therapies) (Gorski et al., 2021).

CVADs used for intermittent infusions should be flushed with preservative-free 0.9% sodium chloride solution and aspirated for a blood return prior to each infusion to assess catheter function (Gorski et al., 2021). Flushing of the device is also required after each infusion to clear the infused medication or other solution from the catheter lumen. CVADs should be locked with either a heparin solution (10 units/mL) or preservative-free 0.9% sodium chloride after each intermittent use, according to the directions for use for the specific CVAD and needleless connector (Gorski et al., 2021). If the device is not in use, periodic flushing according to facility policy is required to keep the catheter patent. Antimicrobial locking solutions are sometimes used in specific situations, such as with patients with long-term CVADs or in high-risk patient populations (Gorski et al., 2021).

Facility policy generally determines the type of dressing and the intervals for dressing change. Perform site care and replace TSM dressings at least every 7 days (except neonatal patients) or immediately if the dressing becomes damp, loosened, visibly soiled, or has a lifted/detached border; blood or drainage is present; or there is compromised skin integrity under the dressing (Gorski et al., 2021). Change sterile gauze dressings at least every 2 days, or if the integrity of the dressing is disrupted (damp, loosened, visibly soiled) (Gorski et al., 2021). Consider the use of sterile adhesive removers and skin barrier film to prevent medical adhesive–related skin injury (MARSI) (Fumarola et al., 2020; Gorski et al., 2021; Zhao et al., 2018).

DELEGATION CONSIDERATIONS	Accessing an implanted port is not delegated to assistive personnel (AP) or to licensed practical/vocational nurses (LPN/LVNs).
EQUIPMENT	• Sterile tape or sterile adhesive skin closure strips (i.e., Steri-Strips™) • Transparent semipermeable membrane (TSM) dressing; antimicrobial dressing; or gauze pad for dressing, based on facility policy • Several 2 × 2 gauzes • Sterile towel or drape • Cleansing swabs (>0.5% chlorhexidine in alcohol solution preferred [Gorski et al., 2021; Sarani et al., 2018]); if there is a contraindication to alcoholic chlorhexidine solution, tincture of iodine, an iodophor (povidone-iodine), or 70% alcohol may also be used (Gorski et al., 2021; Mimoz et al., 2015; O'Grady et al., 2017). Use chlorhexidine with caution in infants up to age 14 days, premature infants, and low-birth-weight infants due to the risk of skin irritation and chemical burns (Gorski et al., 2021) • Prefilled commercially prepared syringe with sterile 0.9% sodium chloride for injection, at least 10 mL for implanted ports (Gorski et al., 2021) • Noncoring safety needle of appropriate length and gauge • Local anesthetic (based on facility policy and/or if prescribed) • Masks (2), depending on facility policy • Gloves • Sterile gloves • Additional PPE, as indicated

(continued on page 1062)

Skill 16-8 ▶ Accessing an Implanted Port *(continued)*

- Skin barrier protectant wipe (e.g., Skin-Prep®)
- Antimicrobial wipes
- Needleless connector or positive pressure end cap
- Passive disinfection caps (based on facility policy)
- IV securement/stabilization device
- Sterile measuring tape
- Bath blanket

ASSESSMENT

Assess the port site. Inspect the skin over the port, looking for any swelling, redness, or drainage. Assess the site over the port for any pain or tenderness, erythema, and drainage. These signs might indicate the development of localized infection. Ask the patient if they are experiencing any pain or discomfort related to the VAD, paresthesias, numbness, or tingling. Pain or discomfort can be a sign of infiltration, extravasation, phlebitis, thrombophlebitis, deep vein thrombosis, and/or infection. Refer to Fundamentals Review 16-3. Review the patient's history for the length of time the port has been in place. If the port has been placed recently, assess the surgical incision. Note the presence of adhesive skin closure strips, approximation, ecchymosis, redness, edema, and/or drainage. Evaluate the patient's history for any allergies or sensitivity to skin antiseptics (Gorski et al., 2021). Assess the patient's knowledge of CVAD therapy. Verify if the current locking solution dwelling in the CVAD needs to be aspirated and discarded or may be infused as part of the flushing procedure; all antimicrobial lock solutions, for example, must be aspirated and discarded (Gorski et al., 2021).

ACTUAL OR POTENTIAL HEALTH PROBLEMS AND NEEDS

Many actual or potential health problems or issues may require the use of this skill as part of related interventions. An appropriate health problem or issue may include:
- Infection risk
- Knowledge deficiency
- Altered skin integrity risk

OUTCOME IDENTIFICATION AND PLANNING

The expected outcomes to achieve when accessing an implanted port are that the port is accessed with minimal discomfort to the patient, the patient experiences no trauma to the site or infection, and the patient verbalizes an understanding of care associated with the port.

IMPLEMENTATION

ACTION	RATIONALE
1. Verify the prescribed intervention requiring port access and facility policy and/or procedure. Often, the procedure for accessing an implanted port and dressing changes will be a standing protocol. Gather equipment.	Checking the prescribed intervention and policy ensures that the proper procedure is initiated. Preparation promotes efficient time management and an organized approach to the task.
2. Perform hand hygiene and put on PPE, if indicated.	Hand hygiene and PPE prevent the spread of microorganisms. Unclean hands and improper technique are potential sources for infecting a CVAD. PPE is required based on transmission precautions.
3. Identify the patient.	Identifying the patient ensures the right patient receives the intervention and helps prevent errors.
4. Assemble equipment on the bedside stand or overbed table or other surface within reach.	Bringing everything to the bedside conserves time and energy. Arranging items nearby is convenient, saves time, and avoids unnecessary stretching and twisting of muscles on the part of the nurse.

ACTION

5. Close the curtains around the bed and close the door to the room, if possible. Explain to the patient what you are going to do and why. Ask the patient about allergies to tape and skin antiseptics. If considering using a local anesthetic, inquire about allergies for these substances as well. Consider use of nonpharmacologic interventions to reduce pain associated with PIVC insertion.

6. If using a local anesthetic, explain the rationale and procedure to the patient. Apply the anesthetic as indicated to the port site. Allow sufficient time for the anesthetic to take effect.

7. Place a waste receptacle or bag at a convenient location for use during the procedure.

8. Adjust the bed to a comfortable working height (VHACEOSH, 2016).

9. Assist the patient to a comfortable position that provides easy access to the port site. Use the bath blanket to cover any exposed area other than the site.

10. Apply a mask. Ask the patient to turn their head away from the access site. Alternatively, have the patient put on a mask, depending on facility policy. Move the overbed table to a convenient location within easy reach. Set up a sterile field on the table. Open the dressing supplies and add them to the sterile field.

11. Put on gloves. Palpate the location of the port; palpate and note the location of the outflow channel where the catheter is attached to the port body (refer to Figure 1). Assess the site. Note the status of any surgical incisions that may be present. Remove your gloves and discard them. Perform hand hygiene.

12. Put on sterile gloves. Connect the needleless connector or end cap to the extension tubing on the noncoring needle. Using an antimicrobial swab, vigorously disinfect the connection surface and sides of each access site and allow them to dry. Insert a syringe with 10-mL normal saline into the needleless connector or end cap. Fill the extension tubing with normal saline and apply the clamp. Remove the syringe. Place it on the sterile field.

RATIONALE

This ensures the patient's privacy. Explanation relieves anxiety and facilitates engagement. Possible allergies may exist related to the tape or antiseptics. Injectable anesthetic can result in allergic reactions and tissue damage. Nonpharmacologic interventions suggested for use to reduce PIVC insertion-related pain and discomfort include distraction, relaxation, breathing exercises, and virtual reality (VR) (Basak et al., 2020; Gorski et al., 2021). The choices of interventions for pediatric patients include swaddling, breastfeeding, pacifiers, rocking, blowing bubbles, reading books, use of VR, and local vibrating cold devices and should be made with consideration of growth and development level (Gorski et al., 2021).

Explanations provide reassurance and facilitate engagement. Local anesthetic agents should be used to reduce pain in all adult and pediatric populations (Gorski et al., 2021). Local anesthetic agents to reduce pain associated with needle insertion include vapocoolant sprays, topical transdermal agents, jet injection of pressure-accelerated lidocaine (needle-free), application of hot or cold to the site, and intradermal injection of lidocaine or bacteriostatic 0.9% sodium chloride (Gorski et al., 2021; Korkut et al., 2020; Welyczko, 2020). Some anesthetics take up to an hour to become effective.

Having a waste container handy means the soiled dressing can be discarded easily, without the spread of microorganisms.

Having the bed at the proper height prevents back and muscle strain.

Patient positioning and use of a bath blanket provide for comfort and warmth.

Masks are recommended to reduce the risk of droplet transmission of oropharyngeal flora (Gorski et al., 2021). The patient should wear a mask if they are unable to turn their head away from the site or based on facility policy. Many facilities have all sterile dressing supplies gathered in a single package.

Knowledge of location and boundaries of the port are necessary to access the site safely. Orientation of the needle bevel in the opposite direction from the outflow channel is associated with a greater amount of protein removal during flushing of the port (Gorski et al., 2021).

Port access is accomplished using sterile technique. Organisms on the skin can be introduced into the tissues or the bloodstream with the needle. VAD administration set entry points, end caps, and needleless connectors must be vigorously scrubbed and disinfected prior to each access to reduce the risk for introduction of microorganisms and prevent VAD-related infection (Frimpong et al., 2015; Gorski et al., 2021; Harper, 2014; Loveday et al., 2014). Friction is needed to physically remove microorganisms from the top, sides, and threads of the needleless connector or end cap. Allow the antiseptic to dry completely to ensure complete effectiveness. Priming the extension tubing removes air from the tubing and prevents administration of air when connected to the port.

(continued on page 1064)

Skill 16-8 ▶ Accessing an Implanted Port *(continued)*

ACTION	**RATIONALE**

ACTION

13. Use a single-use sterile applicator containing sterile antiseptic solution to **cleanse the site with >5% chlorhexidine in alcohol solution or the solution identified in facility policy, making sure to cover at minimum the area to be covered with the dressing. Follow the manufacturer's directions for use to determine product application process and dry times** (Gorski et al., 2021). **Allow the antiseptic to dry naturally; do not wipe, fan, or blow on the skin** (Gorski et al., 2021).

14. Pick up the noncoring needle and extension tubing. Coil the extension tubing into the palm of your hand. Using your nondominant hand, locate the port by palpating the edges through the patient's skin. Hold the port stable, keeping the skin taut (Figure 2).

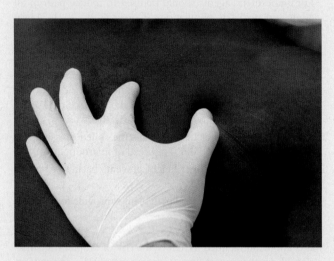

FIGURE 2. Stabilizing port with nondominant hand.

15. Visualize the center of the port. Insert the needle with the needle bevel oriented in the opposite direction from the outflow channel where the catheter is attached to the port body. Holding the needle at a 90-degree angle to the skin, insert the needle **through the skin into the port septum (Figure 3) until the needle hits the back of the port (Figure 4).**

16. Using an antimicrobial swab, vigorously disinfect the connection surface and sides of each access site and allow them to dry. **Alert: if an antimicrobial locking solution was used when the port was last locked, withdraw the solution from the port prior to flushing and discard** (Gorski et al., 2021). Insert the syringe with normal saline. **Open the clamp on the extension tubing and flush with 3 to 5 mL of saline, while observing the site for fluid leak or infiltration. It should flush easily, without resistance.**

RATIONALE

Cleansing is necessary because organisms on the skin can be introduced into the tissues or the bloodstream with the needle. Use of >0.5% chlorhexidine in alcohol solution is preferred for skin antisepsis (Gorski et al., 2021; Sarani et al., 2018). If there is a contraindication to alcoholic chlorhexidine solution, tincture of iodine, an iodophor (povidone-iodine), or 70% alcohol may instead be used (Gorski et al., 2021; Mimoz et al., 2015; O'Grady et al., 2017).

Keeping the equipment contained in your hand prevents accidental contact with nonsterile surfaces and resulting contamination. The edges of the port must be palpated so that the needle can be inserted into the center of the port. Hold the port with your nondominant hand so that the needle is inserted into the port with your dominant hand.

To function properly, the needle must be located in the middle of the port and inserted to the back internal wall of the port. Orientation of the needle bevel in the opposite direction from the outflow channel is associated with a greater amount of protein removal during flushing of the port (Gorski et al., 2021). Use of a noncoring needle of a length that allows the external components (e.g., wings) to sit level with the skin and securely within the port (needle touches bottom of port upon insertion) reduces the risk of needle dislodgement after access (Gorski et al., 2021).

VAD administration set entry points, end caps, and needleless connectors must be vigorously scrubbed and disinfected prior to each access to reduce the risk for introduction of microorganisms and prevent VAD-related infection (Frimpong et al., 2015; Gorski et al., 2021; Harper, 2014; Loveday et al., 2014). Friction is needed to physically remove microorganisms from the top, sides, and threads of the needleless connector or end cap. Allow the antiseptic to dry completely to ensure complete effectiveness.

Flushing an antibiotic solution into the patient's blood stream could increase development of antibiotic resistance and other adverse effects (Gorski et al., 2021).

If the needle is not inserted onto the port correctly, fluid will leak into the tissue, causing the tissue to swell and producing signs of infiltration. Flushing without resistance is also a sign that the needle is inserted correctly.

ACTION

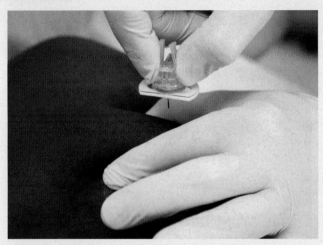

FIGURE 3. Inserting needle through skin into port.

RATIONALE

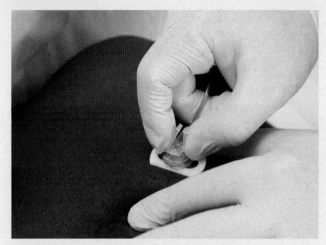

FIGURE 4. Noncoring (Huber) needle in place.

17. Slowly pull back on the syringe plunger to aspirate for blood return (Figure 5). Do not allow blood to enter the syringe. If positive, instill the solution over 1 minute or by using a pulsatile flushing technique of 10 short boluses of 1 mL interrupted by brief pauses; flush the line according to facility policy. Remove the syringe. Using an antimicrobial swab, vigorously scrub the needleless connector or end cap on the extension tubing and allow them to dry. Insert the locking solution syringe and instill the volume of solution designated by facility policy over 1 minute or according to facility policy. Prevent connection/disconnection reflux by using the appropriate sequence for flushing, clamping, and disconnecting determined by the type of needleless connector being used (refer to Box 16-4 in Skill 16-5) (Gorski et al., 2021). Alternatively, if IV fluid infusion is to be initiated, do not flush with heparin.

The presence of a blood return upon aspiration and lack of resistance when flushing indicate patency of the VAD (Gorski et al., 2021). Not allowing blood to enter the syringe ensures that the needle will be flushed with pure saline. A pulsatile flushing technique of 10 short boluses of 1 mL interrupted by brief pauses may be more effective in removing solid deposits (e.g., fibrin, drug precipitate, intraluminal bacteria) (Gorski et al., 2021).

VAD administration set entry points, end caps, and needleless connectors must be vigorously scrubbed and disinfected prior to each access to reduce the risk for introduction of microorganisms and prevent VAD-related infection (Frimpong et al., 2015; Gorski et al., 2021; Harper, 2014; Loveday et al., 2014). Friction is needed to physically remove microorganisms from the top, sides, and threads of the needleless connector or end cap. Allow the antiseptic to dry completely to ensure complete effectiveness.

The action of the positive pressure end cap is maintained with the appropriate sequence for flushing, clamping, and disconnecting determined by the type of needleless connector in use (Gorski et al., 2021). Clamping prevents air from entering the CVAD. Vascular access devices are locked after completion of the flush solution at each use to decrease the risk of occlusion (Gorski et al., 2021). CVADs should be locked with either a heparin solution (10 units/mL) or preservative-free 0.9% sodium chloride after each intermittent use, according to the directions for use for the specific CVAD and needleless connector (Gorski et al., 2021).

18. If using a "gripper" needle, remove the gripper portion from the needle by squeezing the sides together and lifting off the needle while holding the needle securely to the port with your other hand (Figure 6).

A gripper facilitates needle insertion and needs to be removed before application of the dressing.

(continued on page 1066)

Skill 16-8 ▶ Accessing an Implanted Port *(continued)*

ACTION

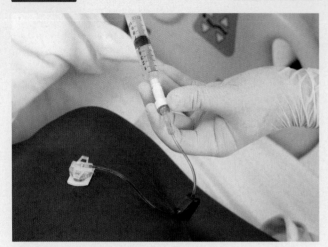

FIGURE 5. Aspirating for blood return.

19. Apply antimicrobial dressing (chlorhexidine-impregnated) at the insertion site, based on facility policy. Apply the skin protectant to the same area, avoiding direct application to the antimicrobial dressing or the insertion site, and allow it to dry. Apply the securement/stabilization device, if used, and/or the TSM dressing, centering it over the insertion site. Refer to Skill 16-7.

20. Apply a passive disinfection cap to the needleless connector or end cap on the extension tubing (Figure 7). Remove your gloves and perform hand hygiene.

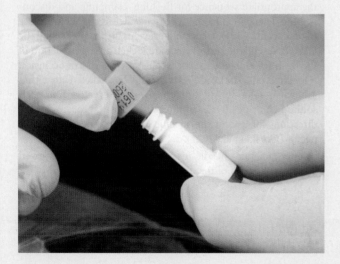

RATIONALE

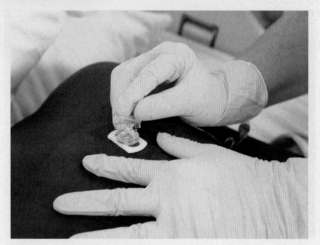

FIGURE 6. Removing gripper from needle.

Use chlorhexidine-impregnated dressing for all patients ages 18 years and older with short-term nontunneled CVADs (Gorski et al., 2021). Skin protectant under the antimicrobial dressing interferes with the action of the dressing. Skin protectant improves adhesion of the dressing and protects the skin from damage and irritation when the dressing is removed. The TSM dressing allows easy visualization and protects the site. Stabilization/securing devices preserve the integrity of the access device, minimize catheter movement at the hub, and prevent catheter dislodgement and loss of access (Gorski et al., 2021). Some stabilization devices also act as a site dressing.

Passive disinfection caps contain an antiseptic-impregnated sponge that dispenses the antiseptic over the connector's top and threads and protects the hub from contamination by touch or airborne sources (Gorski et al., 2021; Stango et al., 2014). Removal of gloves reduces the risk for infection transmission and contamination of other items. Hand hygiene prevents transmission of microorganisms.

FIGURE 7. Attaching a passive disinfection cap.

ACTION

21. Label the dressing with the date, time of change, and your initials. Apply an IV securement/stabilization device if not already in place as part of the dressing, as indicated, based on facility policy. Explain to the patient the purpose of the device and the importance of safeguarding the site when using the extremity.

22. Remove equipment. Ensure the patient's comfort. Lower the bed, if it is not in the lowest position.

 23. Remove additional PPE, if used. Perform hand hygiene.

RATIONALE

Other personnel working with the infusion will know what type of device is being used, the site, and when the dressing was last changed.

The weight of the tubing and/or tugging on the tubing could cause catheter dislodgement. These systems are recommended for use on all venous access sites, and particularly central venous access sites, to preserve the integrity of the access device, minimize catheter movement at the hub, and prevent catheter dislodgement and loss of access (Gorski et al., 2021). Some devices also act as a site dressing and may already have been applied.

Positioning promotes patient comfort and safety.

Proper removal of PPE reduces the risk for infection transmission and contamination of other items. Hand hygiene prevents transmission of microorganisms.

EVALUATION

The expected outcomes have been met when the port has been accessed with minimal discomfort to the patient, the patient has not experienced trauma to the site or infection, and the patient has verbalized an understanding of care associated with the port.

DOCUMENTATION

Guidelines

Document the location of the port, site appearance and condition, and the size of needle used to access the port. Document the presence of a blood return and the ease of ability to flush the port. Record if the patient is experiencing any pain or discomfort related to the CVAD. Document the clinical criteria for site complications. Refer to Fundamentals Review 16-3 and Box 16-2 (in Skill 16-2). Record the patient's subjective comments regarding the absence or presence of pain at the site. Record the patient's reaction to the procedure and pertinent patient teaching, such as alerting the nurse if the patient experiences any pain from the site or notices any swelling at the site.

Sample Documentation

> 11/22/25 1245 Implanted port R chest wall. Site without drainage, swelling, or redness. 20-gauge 0.75-inch Huber needle used to access port. Flushes easily with good blood return. Transparent dressing and external stabilization device applied. Patient denies pain or discomfort. Patient instructed to call nurse with any swelling, pain, or leaking.
> —S. Barnes, RN

DEVELOPING CLINICAL REASONING AND CLINICAL JUDGMENT

UNEXPECTED SITUATIONS AND ASSOCIATED INTERVENTIONS

- *Port insertion site begins to swell when flushing with saline:* Stop flushing. Verify that the needle is in place and has not become dislodged. Attempt to flush. If swelling persists, do not continue to flush. Remove the needle. Obtain additional supplies and reaccess the port with a new needle. Check blood return and flush. If swelling persists, stop flushing. Depending on facility policy, leave the access needle in place. Cover it with a transparent dressing. Notify the health care team. Anticipate diagnostic tests to determine the patency of the port.

- *Port does not flush:* Check the clamp to make sure it is open. Gently push down on the needle and again try to flush. Ask the patient to perform a Valsalva maneuver. Try having the patient change position or place the affected arm over their head, or try raising or lowering the head of the bed. If the port still does not flush, remove the needle. Obtain additional supplies and reaccess with a new needle. Check blood return and flush. If still unable to flush, notify the health care team. Depending on facility policy, leave the access needle in place. Cover it with a transparent dressing. Anticipate diagnostic tests to determine the patency of the port.

(continued on page 1068)

Skill 16-8 ▶ Accessing an Implanted Port *(continued)*

- *Port flushes but does not have a blood return:* Ask the patient to perform a Valsalva maneuver. Try having the patient change position or place the affected arm over their head, or try raising or lowering the head of the bed. If the port still does not have a blood return, remove the needle. Obtain additional supplies and reaccess with the new needle. Check blood return and flush. If it still does not have a blood return, notify the health care team. Depending on facility policy, leave the access needle in place. Cover it with a transparent dressing. Anticipate diagnostic tests to determine the patency of the port and/or instillation of thrombolytic.

SPECIAL CONSIDERATIONS

General Considerations

- The needle should be inserted with the needle bevel oriented in the opposite direction from the outflow channel where the catheter is attached to the port body. Orientation of the needle bevel in the opposite direction from the outflow channel is associated with a greater amount of protein removal during flushing of the port (Gorski et al., 2021).
- The CVAD site should be assessed with each infusion and at least daily in patients being treated in inpatient and nursing facility settings (Gorski et al., 2021).
- Confirm that a port is indicated for power injection before using it for this purpose.
- The use of single-use, commercially prepared, prefilled syringes of appropriate solution to flush and lock VADs reduces the risk of catheter-associated bloodstream infection and saves time for syringe preparation (Gorski et al., 2021).
- Flush accessed but noninfusing implanted vascular access ports daily (Gorski et al., 2021).
- A sterile, single-use product that sits on the skin over the implanted port insertion site is available to enable successful insertion of the access needle into the center of the port (Barton et al., 2018).
- For vascular access ports that are not actively accessed for infusion therapy, there is insufficient evidence to recommend the optimal frequency for flushing and locking: use at least 10 mL of 0.9% sodium chloride; use of 0.9% sodium chloride alone may be as effective as heparin in maintaining patency; extending maintenance flushing to every 3 months with 10 mL of 0.9% sodium chloride and 3 or 5 mL of heparin (100 units/mL) was found to be safe and effective in maintaining patency (Gorski et al., 2021).
- There is insufficient evidence to recommend the frequency of replacement of the noncoring needle when the port is used for a continuous infusion. Replace the noncoring needle according to the manufacturer's directions for use or in accordance with organizational procedures (Gorski et al., 2021).
- Implanted ports require larger flush volumes due to the volume required to fill the device.
- The continued need for *tunneled* and *implanted* CVADs should be assessed on a regular basis; removal may be indicated when infusion therapy is completed, in the presence of an unresolved complication, or when it is no longer needed for the plan of care; consideration should be given to the possibility for infusion therapy to resume in the future (Gorski et al., 2021).
- Drying time with 70% isopropyl alcohol is 5 seconds; alcohol-based chlorhexidine requires 20 seconds. Povidone-iodine requires longer than 6 minutes to be thoroughly dry, making it less favorable to clinical practice (Gorski et al., 2021).
- Chlorhexidine-impregnated dressings are recommended for use as VAD site dressings for certain patient populations, including oncology patients with implanted ports, adult patients with short-term nontunneled CVADs, and patients with an epidural access device (Gorski et al., 2021).
- Heparin-induced thrombocytopenia (HIT) has been reported with the use of heparin flush solutions. Monitor all patients closely for signs and symptoms of HIT. If present or suspected, discontinue heparin (Gorski et al., 2021).
- Use of topical antibiotic ointments or creams on insertion sites as part of routine site care is not recommended because of their potential to promote fungal infections and antimicrobial resistance (Gorski et al., 2021; O'Grady et al., 2017).
- Do not submerge accessed port sites in water; showering is permitted with the use of impermeable coverings (clear plastic wrap or a device designed for this purpose) to protect the catheter and connections (Gorski et al., 2021; O'Grady et al., 2017; York et al., 2020).

Infant and Child Considerations

- Use chlorhexidine with caution in infants up to age 14 days, premature infants, and low-birth-weight infants due to the risk of skin irritation and chemical burns (Gorski et al., 2021).

Older Adult Considerations
- Avoid using vigorous friction at the insertion site, which can traumatize fragile skin and veins in older adults.

Community-Based Care Considerations
- Patients often are discharged with a CVAD. The patient and family/caregiver require teaching to care for CVAD in the home.
- In community-care settings, the CVAD should be assess at every visit, and the patient or caregiver should be taught to check the CVAD site with each infusion or at least once per day (Gorski et al., 2021).
- Patient and family/caregiver education should include managing activities of daily living (bathing, clothing, seatbelts) to prevent needle dislodgement; reporting any signs or symptoms of complications (pain, burning, stinging, or soreness); and follow-up actions (Gorski et al., 2021).

EVIDENCE FOR PRACTICE ▶

INTRAVENOUS ACCESS AND INFUSION
Related Guideline Infusion Nurses Society (INS) Standards of Practice
Gorski, L. A., Hadaway, L., Hagle, M. E., Broadhurst, D., Clare, S., Kleidon, T., Meyer, B. M., Nickel, B., Rowley, S., Sharpe, E., & Alexander, M.; Infusion Nurses Society. (2021). Infusion therapy. Standards of practice, 8th edition. *Journal of Infusion Nursing, 44*(Suppl 1), S1–S224. https://doi.org/10.1097/NAN.0000000000000396
Refer to details in Skill 16-1, Evidence for Practice.

Skill 16-9 ▶ Deaccessing an Implanted Port

When an implanted port will not be used for a period of time, the port is deaccessed. Deaccessing a port involves flushing and locking the port and removing the needle.

DELEGATION CONSIDERATIONS

Deaccessing an implanted port is not delegated to assistive personnel (AP) or to licensed practical/vocational nurses (LPN/LVNs).

EQUIPMENT
- Gloves
- Additional PPE, as indicated
- Prefilled commercially prepared syringe with 10-mL sterile normal saline for injection (minimum volume equal to twice the internal volume of the catheter system) (Gorski et al., 2021)
- Prefilled commercially prepared syringe with heparin 10 units/mL in 10-mL
- Sterile gauze sponge
- Antimicrobial wipes
- Small adhesive bandage

ASSESSMENT

Assess the port site. Inspect the skin over the port, looking for any swelling, redness, or drainage. Assess the site over the port for any pain or tenderness, erythema, and drainage. These signs might indicate the development of localized infection. Ask the patient if they are experiencing any pain or discomfort related to the VAD, paresthesias, numbness, or tingling. Pain or discomfort can be a sign of infiltration, extravasation, phlebitis, thrombophlebitis, deep vein thrombosis, and/or infection. Refer to Fundamentals Review 16-3. Review the patient's history for the length of time the port has been in place. If the port has been placed recently, assess the surgical incision. Note the presence of adhesive skin closure strips, approximation, ecchymosis, redness, edema, and/or drainage. Evaluate the patient's history for any allergies or sensitivity to skin antiseptics (Gorski et al., 2021). Assess the patient's knowledge of CVAD therapy. Verify if the current locking solution dwelling in the CVAD needs to be aspirated and discarded or may be infused as part of the flushing procedure; all antimicrobial lock solutions, for example, must be aspirated and discarded (Gorski et al., 2021).

(continued on page 1070)

Skill 16-9 ▶ Deaccessing an Implanted Port *(continued)*

ACTUAL OR POTENTIAL HEALTH PROBLEMS AND NEEDS	Many actual or potential health problems or issues may require the use of this skill as part of related interventions. An appropriate health problem or issue may include: • Infection risk • Knowledge deficiency • Altered skin integrity risk
OUTCOME IDENTIFICATION AND PLANNING	The expected outcomes to achieve when deaccessing an implanted port are that the port is flushed and locked without adverse effect, and the needle is removed with minimal to no discomfort to the patient; the patient experiences no trauma or infection; and the patient verbalizes an understanding of port care.

IMPLEMENTATION

ACTION	**RATIONALE**
1. Verify the prescribed intervention requiring port access and facility policy and/or procedure. Often, the procedure for deaccessing an implanted port and dressing changes will be a standing protocol. Gather equipment.	Checking the prescribed intervention and/or policy ensures that the proper procedure is initiated. Preparation promotes efficient time management and an organized approach to the task.
2. Perform hand hygiene and put on PPE, if indicated.	Hand hygiene and PPE prevent the spread of microorganisms. Unclean hands and improper technique are potential sources for infecting a CVAD. PPE is required based on transmission precautions.
3. Identify the patient.	Identifying the patient ensures the right patient receives the intervention and helps prevent errors.
4. Assemble equipment on the bedside stand or overbed table or other surface within reach.	Bringing everything to the bedside conserves time and energy. Arranging items nearby is convenient, saves time, and avoids unnecessary stretching and twisting of muscles on the part of the nurse.
5. Close the curtains around the bed, and close the door to the room, if possible. Explain to the patient what you are going to do and why.	This ensures the patient's privacy. Explanation relieves anxiety and facilitates engagement.
6. Adjust the bed to a comfortable working height (VHACEOSH, 2016).	Having the bed at the proper height prevents back and muscle strain.
7. Assist the patient to a comfortable position that provides easy access to the port site. Use the bath blanket to cover any exposed area other than the site.	Patient positioning and use of a bath blanket provide for comfort and warmth.
8. Put on gloves. Using an antimicrobial swab, vigorously disinfect the connection surface and sides of each access site and allow them to dry. **Alert: if an antimicrobial locking solution was used when the port was last locked, withdraw the solution from the port prior to flushing and discard** (Gorski et al., 2021). Insert the syringe with normal saline. Unclamp the extension tubing and check for a blood return as indicated in Skill 16-8. Do not allow blood to enter the syringe. If positive, instill the solution over 1 minute or by using a pulsatile flushing technique of 10 short boluses of 1 mL interrupted by brief pauses; flush the line according to facility policy (Figure 1).	Gloves prevent contact with blood and body fluids. VAD administration set entry points, end caps, and needleless connectors must be vigorously scrubbed and disinfected prior to each access to reduce the risk for introduction of microorganisms and prevent VAD-related infection (Frimpong et al., 2015; Gorski et al., 2021; Harper, 2014; Loveday et al., 2014). Friction is needed to physically remove microorganisms from the top, sides, and threads of the needleless connector or end cap. Allow the antiseptic to dry completely to ensure complete effectiveness. Flushing an antibiotic solution into the patient's blood stream could increase development of antibiotic resistance and other adverse effects (Gorski et al., 2021).

ACTION

RATIONALE

It is important to flush all substances out of the well of the implanted port, because it may be inactive for an extended period of time. Presence of a blood return upon aspiration and lack of resistance when flushing indicate patency of the VAD (Gorski et al., 2021). Not allowing blood to enter the syringe ensures that the needle will be flushed with pure saline. A pulsatile flushing technique of 10 short boluses of 1 mL interrupted by brief pauses may be more effective in removing solid deposits (e.g., fibrin, drug precipitate, intraluminal bacteria) (Gorski et al., 2021).

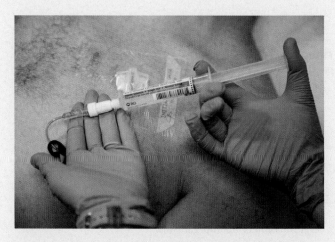

FIGURE 1. Flushing port with saline.

9. Remove the syringe. Using an antimicrobial swab, vigorously disinfect the connection surface and sides of each access site and allow them to dry. Insert the locking solution syringe and instill the volume of solution designated by facility policy over 1 minute or according to facility policy. Prevent connection/disconnection reflux by using the appropriate sequence for flushing, clamping, and disconnecting determined by the type of needleless connector being used (Box 16-4 in Skill 16-5) (Gorski et al, 2021).

VAD administration set entry points, end caps, and needleless connectors must be vigorously scrubbed and disinfected prior to each access to reduce the risk for introduction of microorganisms and prevent VAD-related infection (Frimpong et al., 2015; Gorski et al., 2021; Harper, 2014; Loveday et al., 2014). Friction is needed to physically remove microorganisms from the top, sides, and threads of the needleless connector or end cap. Allow the antiseptic to dry completely to ensure complete effectiveness.

CVADs should be locked with either a heparin solution (10 units/mL) or preservative-free 0.9% sodium chloride after each intermittent use, according to the directions for use for the specific CVAD and needleless connector (Gorski et al., 2021).

The action of the positive pressure end cap is maintained with the appropriate sequence for flushing, clamping, and disconnecting determined by the type of needleless connector in use (Gorski et al., 2021). Clamping prevents air from entering the CVAD.

10. Remove the dressing and/or stabilization device, noting any drainage and discard (refer to Skill 16-7).

Removal of the stabilization device and dressing is necessary to remove the access needle.

11. Stabilize the port on either side with the thumb and forefinger of your nondominant hand. Grasp the needle/wings with the fingers of the dominant hand. Firmly and smoothly, pull the needle straight up at a 90-degree angle from the skin to remove it from the port septum (Figure 2). Engage the needle guard, if this is not automatic on removal. Dispose of the needle with the extension tubing in the sharps container.

The port is held in place while the needle is removed. Proper disposal of the needle prevents accidental injury.

(*continued on page 1072*)

Skill 16-9 ▶ Deaccessing an Implanted Port *(continued)*

ACTION

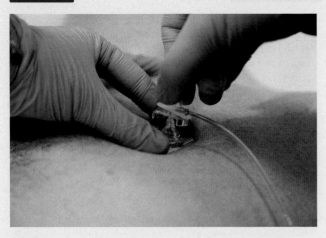

RATIONALE

FIGURE 2. Pulling needle from port with autoengagement of needle guard.

12. Apply gentle pressure with the gauze to the insertion site. Apply a small adhesive bandage over the port if any oozing occurs. Otherwise, a dressing is not necessary. Remove your gloves. Perform hand hygiene.

A small amount of blood may form from the needlestick. Intact skin provides a barrier to infection. Proper removal of PPE reduces the risk for infection transmission and contamination of other items. Hand hygiene prevents transmission of microorganisms.

13. Ensure the patient's comfort. Lower the bed, if it is not in the lowest position.

Positioning promotes patient comfort and safety.

14. Remove additional PPE, if used. Perform hand hygiene.

Removing PPE properly reduces the risk for infection transmission and contamination of other items. Hand hygiene prevents transmission of microorganisms.

EVALUATION

The expected outcomes have been met when the port has been flushed easily; the needle has been removed without difficulty; the site has remained clean, dry, and without evidence of redness, irritation, or warmth; and the patient has verbalized an understanding of port care.

DOCUMENTATION

Guidelines

Document the location of the port, assessment of site, and the ease or difficulty of flushing the port. Record the locking of the port. This may be done on the eMAR/MAR. Document removal of the access needle. Record the appearance of the site, including if there is any drainage, swelling, or redness. Record any appropriate patient teaching.

Sample Documentation

11/13/25 1020 Implanted port L chest wall flushed without resistance using 10 mL of saline and 5 mL of heparin/10 U/mL. No hematoma noted. Access needle removed without difficulty. Site without redness, swelling, drainage, or heat. Patient denies discomfort. Patient verbalized an understanding of site care.

—S. Barnes, RN

DEVELOPING CLINICAL REASONING AND CLINICAL JUDGMENT

UNEXPECTED SITUATIONS AND ASSOCIATED INTERVENTIONS

• *Port does not flush:* Check the clamp to make sure the tubing is open. Gently push down on the needle and again try to flush. Ask the patient to perform a Valsalva maneuver. Have the patient change position or place the affected arm over their head and raise or lower the head of the bed. If the port still does not flush, notify the health care team. Leave the access needle in place. Cover it with a transparent dressing. Anticipate diagnostic tests to determine patency of port.

• *Site does not stop bleeding:* Continue to hold pressure. If the patient has some clotting disturbances, pressure may need to be applied for a longer duration.

SPECIAL CONSIDERATIONS

General Considerations

- For vascular access ports that are not actively accessed for infusion therapy, there is insufficient evidence to recommend the optimal frequency for flushing and locking: use at least 10 mL of 0.9% sodium chloride; use of 0.9% sodium chloride alone may be as effective as heparin in maintaining patency; extending maintenance flushing to every 3 months with 10 mL of 0.9% sodium chloride and 3 or 5 mL of heparin (100 units/mL) was found to be safe and effective in maintaining patency (Gorski et al., 2021).
- The continued need for *tunneled* and *implanted* CVADs should be assessed on a regular basis; removal may be indicated when infusion therapy is completed, in the presence of an unresolved complication, or when it is no longer needed for the plan of care; consideration should be given to the possibility for infusion therapy to resume in the future (Gorski et al., 2021).
- The use of single-use, commercially prepared, prefilled syringes of appropriate solution to flush and lock VADs reduces the risk of catheter-associated bloodstream infection and saves time for syringe preparation (Gorski et al., 2021).
- Implanted ports require larger flush volumes due to the volume required to fill the device.
- Antimicrobial locking solutions are sometimes used in specific situations, such as with patients with long-term CVADs or in high-risk patient populations (Gorski et al., 2021).

Community-Based Care Considerations

- Patient and family/caregiver education should include managing activities of daily living (bathing, clothing, seatbelts) to prevent needle dislodgement; reporting any signs or symptoms of complications (pain, burning, stinging, or soreness); and follow-up actions (Gorski et al., 2021).

EVIDENCE FOR PRACTICE ▶

INTRAVENOUS ACCESS AND INFUSION
Related Guideline Infusion Nurses Society (INS) Standards of Practice
Gorski, L. A., Hadaway, L., Hagle, M. E., Broadhurst, D., Clare, S., Kleidon, T., Meyer, B. M., Nickel, B., Rowley, S., Sharpe, E., & Alexander, M.; Infusion Nurses Society. (2021). Infusion therapy. Standards of practice, 8th edition. *Journal of Infusion Nursing, 44*(Suppl 1), S1–S224. https://doi.org/10.1097/NAN.0000000000000396
Refer to details in Skill 16-1, Evidence for Practice.

Skill 16-10 ▶ Removing a Peripherally Inserted Central Catheter

When a peripherally inserted central catheter (PICC) is no longer required, or when the patient has developed complications, it will be discontinued. Nurses or specialized IV team nurses may be responsible for removing a PICC line. Specific protocols must be followed to prevent breakage or fracture of the catheter.

DELEGATION CONSIDERATIONS

The removal of a PICC is not delegated to assistive personnel (AP) or to licensed practical/vocational nurses (LPN/LVNs).

EQUIPMENT

- Gloves
- Additional PPE, as indicated
- Sterile gauze sponges
- Suture removal set, as needed
- Transparent semipermeable membrane dressing
- Disposable measuring tape

ASSESSMENT

Assess the insertion site, looking for any swelling, redness, or drainage. Assess the site for any pain, tenderness, discomfort, and paresthesias. Check pertinent laboratory values, particularly coagulation times and platelet counts. Patients with alterations in coagulation require that pressure be applied for a longer period of time after catheter removal. Measure the length of the PICC after removal.

Skill 16-10 ▶ Removing a Peripherally Inserted Central Catheter *(continued)*

ACTUAL OR POTENTIAL HEALTH PROBLEMS AND NEEDS

Many actual or potential health problems or issues may require the use of this skill as part of related interventions. An appropriate health problem or issue may include:
- Infection risk
- Injury risk
- Knowledge deficiency

OUTCOME IDENTIFICATION AND PLANNING

The expected outcomes to achieve when removing a PICC are that the PICC is removed intact with minimal to no discomfort to the patient, and the patient experiences no adverse effect or infection.

IMPLEMENTATION

ACTION	RATIONALE
1. Verify the prescribed intervention for PICC removal and facility policy and procedure. Gather equipment.	Checking the prescribed intervention and/or policy ensures that the proper procedure is initiated. Preparation promotes efficient time management and an organized approach to the task.
2. Perform hand hygiene and put on PPE, if indicated.	Hand hygiene and PPE prevent the spread of microorganisms. Unclean hands and improper technique are potential sources for infecting a CVAD. PPE is required based on transmission precautions.
3. Identify the patient.	Identifying the patient ensures the right patient receives the intervention and helps prevent errors.
4. Close the curtains around the bed and close the door to the room, if possible. Explain to the patient what you are going to do and why.	This ensures the patient's privacy. Explanation relieves anxiety and facilitates engagement.
5. Adjust the bed to a comfortable working height (VHACEOSH, 2016).	Having the bed at the proper height prevents back and muscle strain.
6. Assist the patient to a supine flat or Trendelenburg position with their arm straight and the catheter insertion site at or below heart level. Use the bath blanket to cover any exposed area other than the site.	This position is recommended to reduce the risk of air embolism during removal (Gorski et al., 2021). Use of a bath blanket provides for comfort and warmth.
7. Put on gloves. Stabilize the catheter hub with your nondominant hand. Remove the dressing and/or stabilization device, noting any drainage and discard (refer to Skill 16-7).	Gloves prevent contact with blood and body fluids. Removal of the stabilization device and dressing is necessary to remove PICC.
8. Instruct the patient to hold their breath and perform a Valsalva maneuver as the last portion of the catheter is removed. If the Valsalva maneuver is contraindicated or the patient is unable to perform it, use a Trendelenburg or left lateral decubitus position, have the patient hold their breath, or time the removal to their exhalation (Gorski et al., 2021).	Use of the recommended interventions reduces the risk for air embolism (Gorski et al., 2021).
9. Using your dominant hand, remove the catheter slowly. Grasp the catheter close to the insertion site and slowly ease it out, keeping it parallel to the skin. Continue removing in small increments, using a smooth and constant motion (Figure 1).	Gentle pressure reduces the risk of breakage. The catheter should come out easily.
10. After removal, apply pressure to the site with the sterile gauze at and just above the insertion site until hemostasis is achieved by manual compression (Gorski et al., 2021). Apply an air-occlusive dressing.	Adequate pressure prevents hematoma formation. Use of an air-occlusive dressing occludes the skin-to-vein tract and decreases the risk of retrograde air emboli (Gorski et al., 2021).

ACTION	RATIONALE

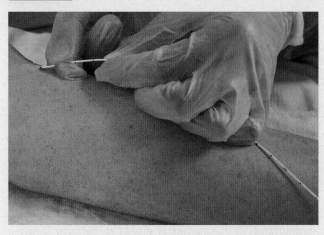

FIGURE 1. Removing PICC in small increments, using a smooth and constant motion. (*Source:* Used with permission from Shutterstock. *Photo by B. Proud.*)

11. Measure the catheter and compare it with the length listed in the chart when it was inserted. Inspect the catheter for patency to ensure it is fully intact. Dispose of the PICC according to facility policy.

Measurement and inspection ensure that the entire catheter was removed. Proper disposal reduces transmission of microorganisms and prevents contact with blood and body fluids.

12. Remove your gloves. Perform hand hygiene. Ensure the patient's comfort. Lower the bed, if it is not in the lowest position.

Removal of PPE and performance of hand hygiene reduce the risk for transmission of microorganisms. Positioning promotes patient comfort and safety.

13. Encourage the patient to remain in a flat or reclining position, if able, for 30 minutes post removal.

Remaining in a flat or reclining position decreases the risk of air entering through an intact skin-to-vein tract (Gorski et al., 2021).

14. Remove additional PPE, if used. Perform hand hygiene.

Proper removal of PPE reduces the risk for infection transmission and contamination of other items. Hand hygiene prevents transmission of microorganisms.

15. Leave the occlusive dressing in place for at least 24 hours (Gorski et al., 2021).

Use of an air-occlusive dressing at the site for at least 24 hours occludes the skin-to-vein tract and decreases the risk of retrograde air emboli (Gorski et al., 2021).

EVALUATION

The expected outcomes have been met when the PICC has been removed with minimal to no discomfort to the patient and without adverse event or infection.

DOCUMENTATION

Guidelines

Document the location of the PICC and its removal. Record the catheter length and patency. Record the appearance of the site, including drainage, swelling, or redness, and the placement of the occlusive dressing. Record any appropriate patient teaching.

Sample Documentation

4/1/25 1230 PICC removed from L brachial. Length of catheter 37.5 cm; entire length intact. Pressure applied to insertion site for 2 minutes; site without bleeding, ecchymosis, redness, drainage. Dry occlusive dressing applied. Patient instructed to notify nurse if pain, discomfort or bleeding noted.

—S. Stone, RN

(*continued on page 1076*)

Skill 16-10 ▶ Removing a Peripherally Inserted Central Catheter (continued)

DEVELOPING CLINICAL REASONING AND CLINICAL JUDGMENT

UNEXPECTED SITUATIONS AND ASSOCIATED INTERVENTIONS

- *You encounter resistance while attempting to remove the PICC:* If resistance is felt when removing a catheter, stop removal. Resistance may be caused by a smooth muscle spasm inside the vein wall. Encourage the patient to relax and take deep breaths. Wait a few minutes and then try again (Hadaway, 2009). Do not forcibly remove the catheter (Gorski et al., 2021). Replace the sterile dressing and collaborate with the health care team to discuss appropriate interventions for successful removal (Gorski et al., 2021).
- *You measure the catheter after removal, and it is shorter than the documented length at insertion:* Notify the health care team. Monitor the patient for signs of distress. The piece of catheter could be lodged in the venous system or have migrated to the right atrium. Anticipate the need for radiology studies to locate the piece of catheter and possible endovascular techniques to retrieve the catheter piece(s).

SPECIAL CONSIDERATIONS

- If the Valsalva maneuver is contraindicated, or the patient is unable to perform it, use a Trendelenburg or left lateral decubitus position, have the patient hold their breath, or time the removal to their exhalation (Gorski et al., 2021).

EVIDENCE FOR PRACTICE ▶

INTRAVENOUS ACCESS AND INFUSION
Related Guideline Infusion Nurses Society (INS) Standards of Practice
Gorski, L. A., Hadaway, L., Hagle, M. E., Broadhurst, D., Clare, S., Kleidon, T., Meyer, B. M., Nickel, B., Rowley, S., Sharpe, E., & Alexander, M.; Infusion Nurses Society. (2021). Infusion therapy. Standards of practice, 8th edition. *Journal of Infusion Nursing*, 44(Suppl 1), S1–S224. https://doi.org/10.1097/NAN.0000000000000396
Refer to details in Skill 16-1, Evidence for Practice.

Enhance Your Understanding

Focusing on Patient Care: Developing Clinical Reasoning and Clinical Judgment

Consider the case scenarios at the beginning of the chapter as you answer the following questions to enhance your understanding and apply what you have learned.

QUESTIONS

1. Simon Lawrence's mother is asking about the risks associated with IV placement. What would you tell her about the risks associated with IV placement and rehydration?

2. During the first 5 minutes of Melissa Cohen's transfusion of packed red blood cells, she reports a headache and low back pain. When you assess her, you find that she has a temperature of 101°F (up from 98.9°F earlier) and she is shivering. What actions would be most appropriate at this time?

3. Mr. Tracy asks about care of his recently implanted port. What are some patient education topics you should discuss with him while he is at the outpatient chemotherapy center?

You can find suggested answers after the Bibliography at the end of this chapter.

Enhance Your Understanding (Continued)

Integrated Case Study Connection

The case studies in the back of the book focus on integrating concepts. Refer to the following case studies to enhance your understanding of the concepts and skills in this chapter.

- Intermediate Case Studies: Olivia Greenbaum, page 1209; Jason Brown, page 1215; Kent Clark, page 1217; Janice Romero, page 1220; Gwen Galloway, page 1221.
- Advanced Case Studies: Robert Espinoza, page 1230.

Bibliography

AABB. (n.d.). *Clinical resources. Clinical guidelines and guidance.* Retrieved August 4, 2021, https://www.aabb.org/news-resources/resources/clinical-resources

Adams, M. P., Holland, N., & Urban, C. Q. (2020). *Pharmacology for nurses. A pathophysiologic approach* (6th ed.). Pearson.

American Red Cross. (n.d.a). *Requirements by donation type.* Retrieved August 4, 2021, from https://www.redcrossblood.org/donate-blood/how-to-donate/eligibility-requirements.html

American Red Cross. (n.d.b). *Why give blood.* Retrieved August 4, 2021, from https://www.redcrossblood.org/donate-blood/how-to-donate/common-concerns/first-time-donors.html

American Red Cross. (n.d.c). *Blood donation process. Frequently asked questions.* Retrieved August 4, 2021, from https://www.redcrossblood.org/faq.html

American Red Cross. (n.d.d). *Autologous and directed donations.* https://www.redcrossblood.org/donate-blood/how-to-donate/types-of-blood-donations/autologous-and-directed-donations.html

American Red Cross. (2021, January). *A Compendium of transfusion practice guidelines* (4th ed.). https://www.redcrossblood.org/content/dam/redcross-blood/hospital-page-documents/334401_compendium_v04jan2021_bookmarkedworking_rwv01.pdf

Andrews, M., Boyle, J. S., & Collins, J. (2020). *Transcultural concepts in nursing care* (8th ed.). Wolters Kluwer.

Barton, A. (2020). Medical adhesive-related skin injuries associated with vascular access: Minimising risk with Appeel sterile. *British Journal of Nursing, 29*(8), S20–S27. https://doi.org/10.12968/bjon.2020.29.8.S20

Barton, A., Pamment, K., & Fizpatrick, D. (2018). Evaluation of a device to improve non-coring needle insertion into implanted intravenous ports. *British Journal of Nursing, 27*(19), S20–S24. https://doi.org/10.12968/bjon.2018.27.19.S20

Basak, T., Duman, S., & Demirtas, A. (2020). Distraction-based relief of pain associated with peripheral intravenous catheterisation in adults: A randomised controlled trial. *Journal of Clinical Nursing, 29*(5–6), 770–777. https://doi.org/10.1111/jocn.15131

Bauldoff, G., Gubrud, P., & Carno, M. (2020). *LeMone and Burke's Medical-surgical nursing: Clinical reasoning in patient care* (7th ed.). Pearson.

Berndt, D., & Steinheiser, M. (2019). Central vascular access device complications. *American Nurse, 14*(10), 6–13.

Brinkman, J. E., Dorius, B., & Sharma, S. (2021, May 9). *Physiology, body fluids.* StatPearls. https://www.ncbi.nlm.nih.gov/books/NBK482447/

Carman, M., Uhlenbrock, J. S., & McClintock, S. M. (2018). A review of current practice in transfusion therapy. *American Journal of Nursing, 118*(5), 36–44. https://doi.org/10.1097/01.NAJ.0000532808.81713.fc

Centers for Disease Control and Prevention (CDC). (2020, March 18). *Blood safety basics.* https://www.cdc.gov/bloodsafety/basics.html

Corley, A., Ullman, A. J., Mihala, G., Ray-Barruel, G., Alexandrou, E., & Rickard, C. M. (2019). Peripheral intravenous catheter dressing and securement practice is associated with site complications and suboptimal dressing integrity: A secondary analysis of 40,637 catheters. *International Journal of Nursing Studies, 100,* 103409. https://doi.org/10.1016/j.ijnurstu.2019.103409

DeLisle, J. (2018). Is this a blood transfusion reaction? Don't hesitate; check it out. *Journal of Infusion Nursing, 41*(1), 43–51. https://doi.org/10.1097/NAN.0000000000000261

Dougherty, L. (2013). Intravenous therapy in older patients. *Nursing Standard, 28*(6), 50–58. https://doi.org/10.7748/ns2013.10.28.6.50.e7333

Dudek, S. (2022). *Nutrition essentials for nursing practice* (9th ed.). Wolters Kluwer.

Dychter, S., Gold, D., Carson, D., & Haller, M. (2012). Intravenous therapy: A review of complications and economic considerations of peripheral access. *Journal of Infusion Nursing, 35*(2), 84–91. https://doi.org/10.1097/NAN.0b013e31824237ce

Edwards, C., & Jones, J. (2018). Development and implementation of an ultrasound-guided peripheral intravenous catheter program for emergency nurses. *Journal of Emergency Nursing, 44*(1), 33–36. http://dx.doi.org/10.1016/j.jen.2017.07.009

Egan, G., Healy, D., O'Neill, H., Clarke-Maloney, M., Grace, P. A., & Walsh, S. R. (2013). Ultrasound guidance for difficult peripheral venous access: A systematic review and meta-analysis. *Emergency Medicine Journal, 30*(7), 521–526. https://doi.org/10.1136/emermed-2012-201652

Eliopoulos, C. (2018). *Gerontological nursing* (9th ed.). Wolters Kluwer.

Fields, B. E., Whitney, R. L., & Bell, J. F. (2020). Managing home infusion therapy. *American Journal of Nursing, 120*(12), 53–59. https://doi.org/10.1097/01.naj.0000724252.22812.a2

Fields, J. M., Piela, N. E., Au, A. K., & Ku, B. S. (2014). Risk factors associated with difficult venous access in adult ED patients. *American Journal of Emergency Medicine, 32*(10), 1179–1182. https://doi.org/10.1016/j.ajem.2014.07.008

Fischbach, F. T., & Fischbach, M. A. (2018). *A manual of laboratory and diagnostic tests* (10th ed.). Wolters Kluwer.

Flynn, J. M., Larsen, E. N., Keogh, S., Ullman, A. J., & Rickard, C. M. (2019). Methods for microbial needleless connector decontamination: A systematic review and meta-analysis. *American Journal of Infection Control, 47*(8), 956–962. https://doi.org/10.1016/j.ajic.2019.01.002

Fowler, S. B., Penoyer, D. A., & Bourgault, A. M. (2018). Insertion and removal of PIVCs: Exploring best practices. *Nursing, 48*(7), 65–67. https://doi.org/10.1097/01.NURSE.0000534108.88895.e2

Frimpong, A., Caguioa, J., & Octavo, G. (2015). Promoting safe IV management in practice using H.A.N.D.S. *British Journal of Nursing, 24*(2), S18–S23. https://doi.org/10.12968/bjon.2015.24.Sup2.S18

Fumarola, S., Allaway, R., Callaghan, R., Collier, M., Downie, F., Geraghty, J., Kiernan, S., Spratt, F., Bianchi, J., Bethell, E., Downe, A., Griffin, J., Hughes, M., King, B., LeBlanc, K., Savine, L., Stubbs, N., & Voegeli, D. (2020). Overlooked and underestimated: Medical adhesive-related skin injuries. Best practice consensus document on prevention. *Journal of Wound Care, 29*(Suppl 3c), S1–S24. https://doi.org/10.12968/jowc.2020.29.Sup3c.S1

Galang, H., Hubbard-Wright, C., Hahn, D. S., Yost, G., Yoder, L., Maduro, R. S., Morgan, M. K., & Zimbro, K. S. (2020). A randomized trial comparing outcomes of 3 types of peripheral intravenous catheters. *Journal of Nursing Care Quality, 35*(1), 6–12. https://doi.org/10.1097/NCQ.0000000000000421

Garciá, D., Aguilera, A., Antolin, F., Arroyo, J. L. Lozano, M., Sanroma, P., & Romón, I. (2018). Home transfusion: Three decades of practice at a tertiary care hospital. *Transfusion, 58*(10), 2309–2319. https://doi.org/10.1111/trf.14816

Global RPH. (2018, April 21). *Albumin.* https://globalrph.com/dilution/albumin/

Gorski, L. A. (2020). Infusion therapy: A model for safe practice in the home setting. *American Nurse Today, 15*(6), 12.

Gorski, L. A., Hadaway, L., Hagle, M. E., Broadhurst, D., Clare, S., Kleidon, T., Meyer, B. M., Nickel, B., Rowley, S., Sharpe, E., & Alexander, M.; Infusion Nurses Society. (2021). Infusion therapy. Standards of practice, 8th edition. *Journal of Infusion Nursing, 44*(Suppl 1), S1–S224. https://doi.org/10.1097/NAN.0000000000000396

Gunasegaran, N., See, M. T. A., Leong, S. T., Yuan, L. X., & Ang, S. Y. (2018). A randomized controlled study to evaluate the effectiveness of 2 treatment methods in reducing incidence of short peripheral catheter-related phlebitis. *Journal of Infusion Nursing, 41*(2), 131–137. https://doi.org/10.1097/NAN.0000000000000271

Hadaway, L. C. (2009). Central venous access devices. *Nursing 2009 Critical Care, 3*(5), 26–33.

Hale, A., & Hovey, M. J. (2014). *Fluid, electrolyte, and acid–base imbalances.* F.A. Davis Company.

Harper, D. (2014). I.V. Rounds. Infusion therapy: Much more than a simple task. *Nursing, 44*(7), 66–67. https://doi.org/10.1097/01.NURSE.0000446643.87747.1f

Harrold, K. (2019, July 26). Guide to the safe use of needle free connectors. *British Journal of Nursing, 28*(Sup14b). [Online]. https://www.magonlinelibrary.com/doi/abs/10.12968/bjon.2019.28.Sup14b.1

Hill, B., & Derbyshire, J. (2021). Blood transfusions: Ensuring patient safety. *British Journal of Nursing, 30*(9), 520–524. https://doi.org/10.12968/bjon.2021.30.9.520

Hinkle, J. L., Cheever, K. H., & Overbaugh, K. (2022). *Brunner & Suddarth's Textbook of medical-surgical nursing* (15th ed.). Wolters Kluwer.

Houston, P. A. (2013). Obtaining vascular access in the obese patient population. *Journal of Infusion Nursing, 36*(1), 52–56. https://doi.org/10.1097/NAN.0b013e31827989d8

Institute for Safe Medication Practices (ISMP). (2020). *Guidelines for optimizing safe implementation and use of smart infusion pumps.* https://www.ismp.org/guidelines/safe-implementation-and-use-smart-pumps

Jarvis, C., & Echkardt, A. (2020). *Physical examination & health assessment* (8th ed.). Elsevier.

Jensen, S. (2019). *Nursing health assessment. A best practice approach* (3rd ed.). Wolters Kluwer.

The Joint Commission. (2021). *National patient safety goals.* https://www.jointcommission.org/standards/national-patient-safety-goals

Joint United Kingdom (UK) Blood Transfusion and Tissue Transplantation Services Professional Advisory Committee (JPAC). (2014, September 1). *4.12: Technical aspects of transfusion.* https://www.transfusionguidelines.org/transfusion-handbook/4-safe-transfusion-right-blood-right-patient-right-time-and-right-place/4-12-technical-aspects-of-transfusion

Karch, A. M. (2020). *Focus on nursing pharmacology* (8th ed.). Wolters Kluwer.

Kelly, L., & Snowden, A. (2021). 'Pinholes in my arms': The vicious cycle of vascular access. *British*

Journal of Nursing, 30(14), S4–S13. https://doi.org/
10.12968/bjon.2021.30.14.S4

Kelly-O'Flynn, S., Mohamud, L., & Copson, D.
(2020). Medical adhesive-related skin injury. *British
Journal of Nursing, 29*(6), S20–S26. https://doi.org/
10.12968/bjon.2020.29.6.S20

Kline, M., & Katrancha, E. D. (2019). Central venous
access devices: An overview for nursing students.
Nursing, 49(7), 63–64. https://doi.org/10.1097/01.
NURSE.0000559922.99814.f8

Korkut, S., Karadağ, S., & Doğan, Z. (2020). The
effectiveness of local hot and cold applications on
peripheral intravenous catheterization: A randomized
controlled trial. *Journal of PeriAnesthesia Nursing, 35*(6),
597–602. https://doi.org/10.1016/j.jopan.2020.04.011

Krein, S. L., Kuhn, L., Ratz, D., & Chopra, V. (2019).
Use of designated nurse PICC teams and CLABSI prevention practices among U.S. hospitals: A survey-based
study. *Journal of Patient Safety, 15*(4), 293–295. https://
doi.org/10.1097/PTS.0000000000000246

Kyle, T., & Carman, S. (2021). *Essentials of pediatric
nursing* (4th ed.). Wolters Kluwer.

Loveday, H. P., Wilson, J. A., & Pratt, R. J. (2014).
Epic3: National evidence-based guidelines for preventing healthcare-associated infections in NHS hospitals
in England. *Journal of Hospital Infection, 86*(1), S1–S70.
https://doi.org/10.1016/S0195-6701(13)60012-2

McArthur, B. (2018). Peripherally inserted central
catheters (PICCs): A review of complications and innovative solutions. *Vascular Access, 12*(1), 32–37.

Memorial Sloan Kettering Cancer Center. (2021,
March 29). *About your peripherally inserted central
catheter (PICC).* https://www.mskcc.org/cancer-care/
patient-education/about-your-peripherally-inserted-
central-catheter-picc

Mimoz, O., Lucet, J. C., & Kerforne, T. (2015). Skin
antisepsis with chlorhexidine-alcohol versus povidone
iodine-alcohol, with and without skin scrubbing, for
prevention of intravascular-catheter-related infection (CLEAN): An open-label, multicenter, randomized, controlled, two-by-two factorial trial. *Lancet,
386*(10008), 2069–2077. https://doi.org/10.1016/S0140-
6736(15)00244-5

Morata, L., & Bowers, M. (2020). Ultrasound-guided
peripheral intravenous catheter insertion: The nurse's
manual. *CriticalCareNurse, 40*(5), 38–46. https://doi.org/
10.4037/ccn2020240

Morrell, E. (2020). Reducing risks and improv-
ing vascular access outcomes. *Journal of Infusion
Nursing, 43*(4), 222–228. https://doi.org/10.1097/
NAN.0000000000000377

Morton, P. G., & Fontaine, D. K. (2018). *Critical care
nursing. A holistic approach* (11th ed.). Wolters Kluwer.

Nailon, R. E., Rupp, M. E., & Lynden, E. (2019).
A day in the life of a CVAD. *Journal of Infusion
Nursing, 42*(3), 125–131. https://doi.org/10.1097/
NAN.0000000000000321

Norris, T. L. (2020). *Porth's essentials of pathophysiology* (5th ed.). Wolters Kluwer.

O'Grady, N. P., Alexander, M., & Burns, L. A.;
The Healthcare Infection Control Practices Advisory
Committee (HICPAC). (2011). Guidelines for the preven-
tion of intravascular catheter-related infections. *American
Journal of Infection Control, 39*(4 Suppl), S1–S34. https://
www.cdc.gov/infectioncontrol/guidelines/bsi/index.html

O'Grady, N. P., Alexander, M., & Burns, L. A.;
The Healthcare Infection Control Practices Advisory
Committee (HICPAC). (2017). *Guidelines for the prevention of intravascular catheter-related infections.* https://
www.cdc.gov/infectioncontrol/guidelines/bsi/index.html

Pan, M., Meng, A., Yin, R., Zhi, X., Du, S., Shi, R.,
Zhu, P., Cheng, F., Sun, M., Li, C., & Fang, H. (2019).
Nursing interventions to reduce peripherally inserted
central catheter occlusion for cancer patients. *Cancer
Nursing, 42*(6), E49–E58. https://doi.org/10.1097/
NCC.0000000000000664

Partovi-Deilami, K., Nielsen, J. K., Møller, A. M.,
Nesheim, S. S., & Jørgensen, V. L. (2016). Effect of
ultrasound-guided placement of difficult-to-place
peripheral venous catheters: A prospective study of a
training program for nurse anesthetists. *AANA Journal,
84*(2), 86–92.

Sarani, H., Moulaei, N., Tabas, E. E., Safarzai, E., &
Jahani, S. (2018). Comparison of the effects of alcohol,
chlorhexidine, and alcohol-chlorhexidine on local
catheter-related infections rate: A double-blind clinical trial study. *Medical-Surgical Nursing Journal, 7*(2),
e85962. https://doi.org/10.5812/msnj.85962

Sharp, R., Turner, L., Altschwager, J., Corsini, N., &
Esterman, A. (2021). Adverse events associated with
home blood transfusion: A retrospective cohort study.
Journal of Clinical Nursing, 30(11–12), 1751–1759.
https://doi.org/10.1111/jocn.15734

Silbert-Flagg, J., & Pillitteri, A. (2018). *Maternal and
child health nursing* (8th ed.). Wolters Kluwer.

Silvergleid, A. J. (2022, February 18). *Surgical blood
conservation: Preoperative autologous blood donation.*
UpToDate. https://www.uptodate.com/contents/
surgical-blood-conservation-preoperative-autologous-
blood-donation

Slater, K., Cooke, M., Fullerton, F., Whitby, M., Hay,
J., Lingard, S., Douglas, J., & Rickard, C. M. (2020).
Peripheral intravenous catheter needleless connector
decontamination study—Randomized controlled trial.
American Journal of Infection Control, 48(9), 1013–1018.
https://doi.org/10.1016/j.ajic.2019.11.030

Slater, K., Fullerton, F., Cooke, M., Snell, S., &
Rickard, C. M. (2018). Needleless connector drying
tome—how long does it take? *American Journal of
Infection Control, 46*(9), 1080–1081. https://doi.org/
10.1016/j.ajic.2018.05.007

Stango, C., Runyan, D., Stern, J., Macri, I., &
Vacca, M. (2014). A successful approach to reducing
bloodstream infections based on a disinfection
device for intravenous needleless connector hubs.
Journal of Infusion Nursing, 37(6), 462–465.
https://doi.org/10.1097/NAN.0000000000000075

Suddock, J. T., & Crookston, K. P. (2021, August 11).
Transfusion reactions. In *StatPearls [Internet]* StatPearls
Publishing. https://www.ncbi.nlm.nih.gov/books/
NBK482202/#article-30465.s10

Taylor, C., Lynn, P., & Bartlett, J. (2023). *Fundamentals
of nursing: The art and science of person-centered care*
(10th ed.). Wolters Kluwer.

Toughy, T. A., & Jett, K. (2018). *Ebersol and Hess'
gerontological nursing & healthy aging* (5th ed.).
Elsevier.

VHA Center for Engineering & Occupational
Safety and Health (CEOSH). (2016). *Safe patient
handling and mobility guidebook.* http://www.
tnpatientsafety.com/pubfiles/Initiatives/workplace-
violence/sphm-pdf.pdf

Walters, B., & Price, C. (2019). Quality improvement initiative reduces the occurrence of complications
in peripherally inserted central catheters. *Journal of
Infusion Nursing, 42*(1), 29–36. https://doi.org/10.1097/
NAN.0000000000000310

Welyczko, N. (2020). Peripheral intravenous can-
nulation: Reducing pain and local complications. *British
Journal of Nursing, 29*(8), S12–S19. https://doi.org/
10.12968/bjon.2020.29.8.S12

Willis, L. M. (Ed.). (2020). *Fluids & electrolytes made
incredibly easy!* (7th ed.). Wolters Kluwer.

WoltersKluwer. (2022). Problem-based care plans. In
Lippincott Advisor. Wolters Kluwer.

Wortley, V., & Almerol, L. A. (2020). Misplacement
of PICCs following power-injected CT contrast media.
British Journal of Nursing, 29(19), S4–S10. https://doi.org/
10.12968/bjon.2020.29.19.S4

York, N., Angell-Barrick, N., Carter, J., & Aquino-
Guerrero, M. (2020). Avoiding contamination of
CVADs when bathing and showering. *Journal of
Kidney Care, 5*(2), 71–78. https://doi.org/10.12968/
jokc.2020.5.2.71

Zhao, H., He, Y., Wei, Q., & Ying, Y. (2018). Medical
adhesive-related skin injury prevalence at the peripherally inserted central catheter insertion site. *Journal of
Wound, Ostomy, and Continence Nursing, 45*(1), 22–25.
https://doi.org/10.1097/WON.0000000000000394

SUGGESTED ANSWERS FOR FOCUSING ON PATIENT CARE: DEVELOPING CLINICAL REASONING AND CLINICAL JUDGMENT

1. Explain the reason the IV access is necessary and the rationale for IV fluid replacement. Discuss the potential complications related to peripheral venous access and IV fluid infusion, including infiltration, phlebitis, and infection. Explain the steps the nurses will take to prevent these complications; discuss the steps Ms. Lawrence can take to help prevent complications, as well as the signs and symptoms of which she should be aware. Encourage her to continue to ask questions and report any signs or symptoms she feels her son exhibits. Discuss the advantages related to using a topical anesthetic before peripheral venous access insertion. Explain any securement/stabilization devices that will be used with Simon to prevent accidental dislodgement or removal of the venous access device.

2. Ms. Cohen is exhibiting signs and symptoms consistent with a hemolytic transfusion reaction. This type of reaction typically occurs immediately and is the result of incompatibility of the donor blood with the recipient's blood. Stop the blood immediately. Disconnect the blood and begin infusing normal saline via a different, new administration set. Notify the health care team immediately. Monitor vital signs and symptoms. Anticipate the administration of medications to treat the reaction, including hypotension. Prepare to obtain required blood samples for serologic testing and a urine specimen. Return blood product and administration tubing to laboratory.

3. Provide Mr. Tracy with information regarding skin care and assessment related to his port site. Inform him about how to care for his port if it is accessed. It is important that he is aware of signs and symptoms that he should report to his health care provider. He also needs to be aware of the time interval for surgical follow-up and the interval for appointments to flush and lock the port, if not in use.

17

Neurologic Care

Focusing on Patient Care

This chapter will help you develop some of the skills related to neurologic care necessary for the following patients:

Aleta Jackson, age 68, was involved in a head-on collision. She has been prescribed and will be discharged with a cervical collar to stabilize her neck.

Yuka Chong, age 7, was recently diagnosed with epilepsy, and has arrived at the clinic for a follow-up visit. Her mothers have a lot of questions and concerns about how to react when Yuka has a seizure.

Nikki Gladstone, age 19, is in your intensive care unit following surgery related to a cranial malignancy. She has an external ventriculostomy device in place to monitor intracranial pressure.

Refer to Focusing on Patient Care: Developing Clinical Reasoning and Clinical Judgment at the end of the chapter to apply what you learn.

Learning Outcomes

After completing the chapter, you will be able to accomplish the following:

1. Apply a two-piece cervical collar.
2. Implement seizure precautions and seizure management.
3. Care for patient with a halo external fixation device (halo traction).
4. Care for a patient with an external ventriculostomy device.
5. Care for a patient with a fiberoptic intracranial catheter.

Nursing Concepts

- Assessment
- Clinical Decision Making/Clinical Judgment
- Intracranial Regulation
- Safety
- Sensory Perception

Many patients experience injury to the head, neck, or spinal column. In addition, numerous disorders, such as infections and tumors, can affect the brain and spinal cord, interfering with neurologic function. Specialized devices may be used to monitor and control intracranial pressure (ICP). Meticulous care is needed after injury or trauma to ensure that further injury does not occur. This chapter covers skills to assist the nurse in providing neurologic care.

Behavioral scales are used to standardize observations for the objective and accurate assessment of **level of consciousness (LOC)** (degree of wakefulness or ability to be aroused) and monitor changes related to neurologic injury and **coma** (Hickey & Strayer, 2020). Fundamentals Review 17-1 provides descriptions of terms used to describe levels of consciousness. The Glasgow Coma Scale (GCS) and the Full Outline of UnResponsiveness (FOUR) score are examples of two tools used to assess LOC. The GCS is used as a rapid evaluation of the status of acutely ill patients at risk of acute brain damage (Derbyshire & Hill, 2018). The FOUR score coma scale is an assessment tool for adult and pediatric patients with severe neurologic impairment (Hickey & Strayer, 2020). It includes information not assessed by the GCS, including measurement of brainstem reflexes; determination of eye opening, blinking, and tracking; a broad spectrum of motor responses; and the presence of abnormal breath rhythms and a respiratory drive, providing a more comprehensive neurologic assessment (Jalali & Rezaei, 2014; Zappa et al., 2020). The FOUR score tool does not include an assessment of verbal response and may be more useful for assessing critically ill patients with depressed level of consciousness or those who have undergone intubation (Almojuela et al., 2018; Iyer et al., 2009; Sadaka et al., 2012). Fundamentals Review 17-2 reviews a brief neurologic exam. Refer to Fundamentals Review 17-3 and Fundamentals Review 17-4 for the GCS and the FOUR Score assessment tools. Refer to Chapter 3 for a review of other components of a neurologic assessment.

Fundamentals Review 17-1

Full consciousness	Awake, alert; oriented to person, place, and time; comprehends spoken and written word; able to express ideas verbally or in writing; responds to all stimuli, including verbal commands
Confusion	Disoriented to person, place and/or time; shortened attention span; memory difficulty; difficulty following commands; may be agitated, restless
Lethargy	Appears oriented to time, place and person; drowsy but makes spontaneous movements; can be aroused with verbal stimuli; slowed and sluggish speech, thought and actions; delayed responses
Obtunded	Responds verbally with a word; arousable with loud verbal or light tactile stimuli; drifts off when not stimulated; appears very drowsy, able to follow simple commands
Stupor	Generally unresponsive; minimal spontaneous movement; must be shaken or shouted at to arouse; incomprehensible verbalization, may open eyes; responds appropriately to painful stimuli
Coma	Appears to be sleeping; cannot be aroused, even with use of painful stimuli; no verbal response; may have some reflex activity (such as gag reflex) depending on the level of coma

Source: Adapted from Hickey, J. V., & Strayer, A. L. (Eds.). (2020). *The clinical practice of neurological and neurosurgical nursing* (8th ed.). Wolters Kluwer and Hinkle, J. L., Cheever, K. H., & Overbaugh, K. (2022). *Brunner & Suddarth's Textbook of medical-surgical nursing* (15th ed.). Wolters Kluwer.

Fundamentals Review 17-2

BRIEF NEUROLOGIC EXAM

By assessing the patient's appearance and verbal and physical responses, you can obtain important information about the patient's neurologic status, including:

- Is it unchanged/changed from baseline?
- Has the patient developed changes that may indicate a problem with the nervous system?
- Are there symptoms that need further investigation?

This basic examination can be used during every patient encounter. Refer to Chapter 3 for details related to other components of a neurologic assessment.

What?	How?	Why?
<ul><li>Assess level of consciousness, cognition, position, posture, facial symmetry, respiratory pattern.</li><li>Assess ability to speak at normal conversational volume.</li><li>Identify external forces (e.g., medications, other injuries, or altered laboratory values) that may affect the patient's responses during the assessment.</li><li>Identify abnormalities that existed before the patient's current health problem.</li></ul>	Does the patient: <ul><li>Wake up easily?</li><li>Hear introduction and question?</li><li>Open both eyes and keep them open?</li><li>Pay attention to you and remain awake and alert?</li><li>Demonstrate behavior appropriate for situation?</li><li>Track you with head and eye movements as you move around room?</li><li>Speak clearly?</li><li>Provide appropriate responses?</li><li>Demonstrate symmetry of movement in extremities?</li></ul>	<ul><li>Alertness, attention, arousal: Assesses reticular activating system, hypothalamus, and thalamus</li><li>Interpretation of what is heard and responds appropriately: Assesses cerebral cortex</li><li>Motor function: Assesses corticospinal motor pathway and basal ganglia system</li><li>Clear, organized, and appropriate speech: Assesses motor speech and language centers in left cerebral hemisphere</li></ul>

Source: Adapted from Henley Haugh, K. (2015). Head-to-toe: Organizing your baseline patient physical assessment. *Nursing, 45*(12), 58–61; Hickey, J. V., & Strayer, A. L. (Eds.). (2020). *The clinical practice of neurological and neurosurgical nursing* (8th ed.). Wolters Kluwer; McCallum, C., & Leonard, M. (2013). The connection between neurosciences and dialysis: A quick neurological assessment for hemodialysis nurses. *CANNT Journal, 23*(3), 20–26.

Fundamentals Review 17-3

GLASGOW COMA SCALE

The Glasgow Coma Scale (GCS) evaluates three key categories of behavior that most closely reflect activity in the higher centers of the brain: eye opening, verbal response, and motor response. Within each category, each level of response is given a numerical value. The maximal score is 15, indicating a fully awake, alert, and oriented patient; the lowest score is 3, indicating deep coma (Hickey & Strayer, 2020). The GCS is used in conjunction with other neurologic assessments, including pupillary reaction and vital sign measurement, to evaluate a patient's status.

Component	Score	Response
Eye opening	4	Opens eyes spontaneously when someone approaches
	3	Opens eyes in response to speech (normal tone or shouting)
	2	Opens eyes only to painful stimuli (apply pressure with a pen to the lateral outer aspect of the second or third finger, up to 10 seconds, then release)
	1	No response to painful stimuli
Best motor response	6	Accurately responds to instructions; obeys a simple command, such as "Lift your left hand off the bed"
	5	Localizes (moves hand to point of stimulation) to painful stimuli and attempts to remove source
	4	Flexion reflex action, but unable to locate the source of pain; purposeless movement in response to pain
	3	Flexes elbows and wrists while extending lower legs to pain; **decorticate** posturing
	2	Extends upper and lower extremities to pain; **decerebrate** posturing
	1	No motor response to pain on any limb
Best verbal response	5	Converses; oriented to time, place, and person
	4	Converses; disoriented to time, place, or person; any one or all indicators
	3	Converses only in words or phrases that make little sense in the context of the questions
	2	Responds with incomprehensible sounds; no understandable words and/or moaning, groaning, or crying in response to painful stimuli
	1	No response

Source: Adapted from Hickey, J. V., & Strayer, A. L. (Eds.). (2020). *The clinical practice of neurological and neurosurgical nursing* (8th ed.). Wolters Kluwer; Okamura, K. (2014). Glasgow Coma Scale flow chart: A beginner's guide. *British Journal of Nursing, 23*(20), 1068–1073; and Teasdale, G., & Jennett, B. (1974). Assessment of coma and impaired consciousness. A practical scale. *Lancet, 2*(7872), 81–84.

Fundamentals Review 17-4

THE FULL OUTLINE OF UNRESPONSIVENESS (FOUR)

Researchers at the Mayo Clinic designed the FOUR score coma scale, which has been proposed as an alternative to the Glasgow Coma Scale (GCS). The FOUR score assigns a value of 0 to 4 to each of the four functional categories: eye response, motor response, brainstem reflexes, and respiration. In each of these categories, a score of 0 indicates nonfunctioning status, and a score of 4 represents normal functioning. The FOUR score may provide greater neurologic detail than the GCS due to its ability to evaluate brainstem reflexes and to recognize changes in breathing patterns and stages of brain herniation (Hickey & Strayer, 2020; Kocak et al., 2012). The FOUR score is used in conjunction with other neurologic assessments and vital sign measurement to evaluate a patient's status.

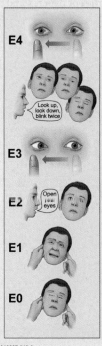 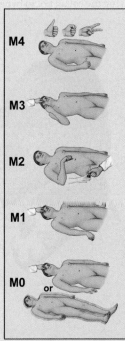 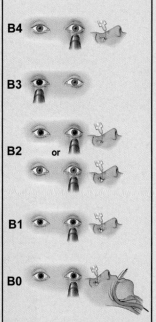 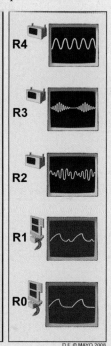

Ec1316227-013-0

D.F. © MAYO 2008

Eye response (E):
E4 = eyelids open or opened, tracking or blinking to command
E3 = eyelids open, but not tracking
E2 = eyelids closed, but open to loud voice
E1 = eyelids closed, but open to pain

Motor response (M):
M4 = demonstrated thumbs-up, fist, or peach sign to command
M3 = localizing to pain
M2 = flexion response to pain
M1 = extensor posturing
M0 = no response to pain or generalized myoclonus status epilepticus (prolonged repetitive epileptic myoclonic [involuntary twitching of a muscle] activity)

Brainstem reflexes (B):
B4 = pupil and corneal reflexes present
B3 = one pupil wide and fixed
B2 = pupil or corneal reflexes absent
B1 = pupil and corneal reflexes absent
B0 = absent pupil, corneal, and cough reflex

Respiration (R):
R4 = not intubated, regular breathing
R3 = not intubated, Cheyne–Stokes breathing pattern
R2 = not intubated, irregular breathing pattern
R1 = breathes above ventilator rate
R0 = breathes at ventilator rate or apnea

Skill 17-1 ▶ Applying a Two-Piece Cervical Collar

Patients suspected of having injuries to the cervical spine may be immobilized with a cervical collar to stabilize the neck and prevent further damage to the spinal cord (Hickey & Strayer, 2020; Morton & Fontaine, 2018). A cervical collar may be used as external immobilization for simple cervical compression fractures or other cervical vertebral injuries (Hickey & Strayer, 2020). A cervical collar maintains the neck in a straight line, with the chin slightly elevated and tucked inward. The collar is removed as soon as is feasible after radiologic clearance (Montgomery & Goode, 2014). Cervical collars may also be used to support the weight of the head and limit cervical motion as part of nonpharmacologic management of pain associated with degeneration in rheumatic disorders (Figure 1) (Hinkle et al., 2022). Care must be taken, when applying the collar, not to hyperflex or hyperextend the patient's neck.

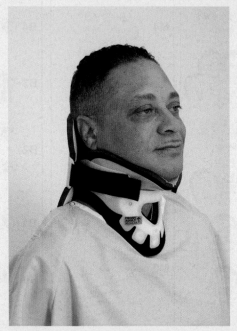

FIGURE 1. Cervical collar in place.

DELEGATION CONSIDERATIONS	Application of a cervical collar is not delegated to assistive personnel (AP). Depending on the state's nurse practice act and the organization's policies and procedures, application of a cervical collar may be delegated to licensed practical/vocational nurses (LPN/LVNs). The decision to delegate must be based on careful analysis of the patient's needs and circumstances as well as the qualifications of the person to whom the task is being delegated. Refer to the Delegation Guidelines in Appendix A.
EQUIPMENT	• Nonsterile gloves • Additional PPE, as indicated • Tape measure • Cervical collar of appropriate size • Disposable skin cleansing wipes or washcloth, skin cleanser and water • Towel
ASSESSMENT	Perform a neurologic assessment (see Fundamentals Review 17-2 and Chapter 3). Assess the patient's level of consciousness and ability to follow commands to determine any neurologic dysfunction. If application of the cervical collar is in response to trauma or injury, assess for a patent airway. If the airway is occluded, try repositioning using the jaw-thrust–chin lift method, which helps open the airway without moving the patient's neck. Inspect and palpate the cervical spine area for tenderness, swelling, deformities, or crepitus. Do not ask the patient to move their neck if a cervical spinal cord injury is suspected. If the patient is able to follow commands, instruct them not to move the head or neck. Have a second person stabilize the cervical spine by holding the patient's head firmly on either side directly above their ears.

ACTUAL OR POTENTIAL HEALTH PROBLEMS AND NEEDS	Many actual or potential health problems or issues may require the use of this skill as part of related interventions. An appropriate health problem or issue may include: • Injury risk • Acute pain • Altered skin integrity risk
OUTCOME IDENTIFICATION AND PLANNING	The expected outcome to achieve is that the patient's cervical spine is immobilized. Other outcomes that may be appropriate include prevention of further injury to the spinal cord, and the patient does not experience alterations in skin integrity, experiences minimal to no pain, and demonstrates an understanding about the need for immobilization and use of the device.

IMPLEMENTATION

ACTION	**RATIONALE**
1. Review the health record and plan of care to determine the need for placement of a cervical collar. Identify any movement limitations. Gather the necessary supplies.	Reviewing the record and plan of care validates the correct patient and correct procedure. Identification of limitations prevents injury. Assembling equipment provides for an organized approach to the task.
2. Perform hand hygiene and put on PPE, if indicated.	Hand hygiene and PPE prevent the spread of microorganisms. PPE is required based on transmission precautions.
3. Identify the patient.	Identifying the patient ensures the right patient receives the intervention and helps prevent errors.
4. Assemble equipment on the bedside stand, overbed table, or other surface within reach.	Arranging items nearby is convenient, saves time, and avoids unnecessary stretching and twisting of muscles on the part of the nurse.
5. Close the curtains around the bed and close the door to the room, if possible. Explain to the patient what you are going to do and why.	This ensures the patient's privacy. Explanation relieves anxiety and facilitates engagement with care.
6. Assess the patient for any changes in neurologic status (see Fundamentals Review 17-2 and Chapter 3 for assessment details).	Patients with cervical spine injuries are at risk for problems with the neurologic system.
7. Place the bed at an appropriate and comfortable working height (VHACEOSH, 2016). Lower the side rails as necessary.	Having the bed at the proper height and lowering the rails prevents back and muscle strain.
8. Put on gloves. Gently clean the patient's face and neck with a skin cleanser and water. If the patient has experienced trauma, inspect the area for broken glass or other material that could cut them or you. Pat the area dry. Remove your gloves and perform hand hygiene.	Gloves prevent contact with blood and body fluids. Blood, glass, leaves, and twigs may be present on the patient's neck. The area should be clean before applying the cervical collar to help prevent skin breakdown. Removal of gloves and performing hand hygiene prevents transmission of microorganisms.
9. If the patient has experienced trauma or injury, have a second caregiver in position to hold the patient's head firmly on either side above their ears. Measure from the bottom of the chin to the top of the sternum, and measure around the neck. Match these height and circumference measurements to the manufacturer's recommended size chart.	This action stabilizes the cervical spine by holding the head firmly on either side above the ears. To immobilize the cervical spine and to prevent skin breakdown under the collar, the correct collar size must be used (Cooper, 2013).
10. Slide the flattened back portion of the collar under the patient's head (Figure 2). The center of the collar should line up with the center of the patient's neck. **Do not allow the patient's head to move when passing the collar under the head.** Align the top section (occipital pad) with the middle of the patient's ear (Haertel, 2019).	Stabilizing the cervical spine is crucial to prevent the head from moving, which could cause further damage to the cervical spine. Placing the collar in the center ensures that the neck is aligned properly.

(continued on page 1086)

Skill 17-1 ▶ Applying a Two-Piece Cervical Collar *(continued)*

ACTION

RATIONALE

11. Place the front of the collar centered over the chin, while ensuring that the chin area fits snugly in the recess. Be sure that the front half of the collar overlaps the back half. Secure Velcro straps on both sides (Figure 3). Check to see that at least one finger can be inserted between the collar and the patient's neck.

The collar should fit snugly to prevent the patient from moving their neck and causing further damage to the cervical spine. Velcro will help hold the collar securely in place. The collar should not be too tight to cause discomfort.

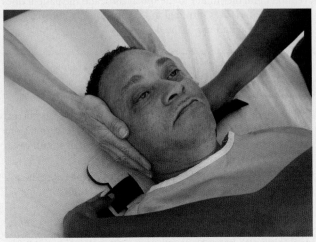

FIGURE 2. Sliding the flattened back portion of the collar under the patient's head.

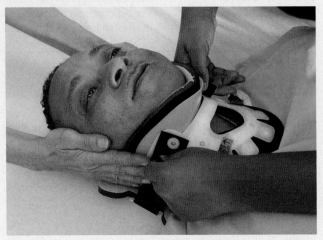

FIGURE 3. Securing the front and back halves of the cervical collar.

12. Raise the side rails. Place the bed in the lowest position. Make sure the call bell is in reach.

The bed in the lowest position and access to the call bell contribute to patient safety.

13. Reassess the patient's neurologic status and comfort level.

Reassessment helps to evaluate the effects of movement on the patient.

14. Remove additional PPE, if used. Perform hand hygiene.

Proper removal of PPE reduces the risk for infection transmission and contamination of other items. Hand hygiene prevents transmission of microorganisms.

15. Assess the skin under the cervical collar and at contact points on the chin, shoulder, and ear at least every 4 hours for any signs of skin breakdown (Morton & Fontaine, 2018). Consider use of a silicone border or hydrocolloid dressings over bony prominences or other areas that come in contact with the device and between the device and the skin (Camacho-Del Rio, 2018). Remove the collar per facility policy and inspect and cleanse the skin under the collar, drying well before replacement. When the collar is removed, if the patient has experienced trauma or injury, have a second person immobilize the cervical spine.

Alterations in skin integrity/medical device–related pressure injuries may occur under the cervical collar and at contact points (Baranoski & Ayello, 2020; EPUAP, NPIAP, & PPPIAa, 2019; Lacey et al., 2019; Morton & Fontaine, 2020). The neck is particularly prone to sweating, necessitating cleansing of the skin and thorough drying to prevent increased risk of skin breakdown (Cooper, 2013).

EVALUATION

The expected outcomes have been met when the cervical collar has been placed without adverse effect; the patient's cervical spine has been immobilized without further injury; and the patient has not experienced alterations in skin integrity, has experienced minimal to no pain or discomfort, and has demonstrated an understanding of the use of the device and the need for immobilization.

DOCUMENTATION

Guidelines

Document the application of the collar, including size and any skin care necessary before the application, condition of the skin under the cervical collar and at pressure points, the patient's pain level, and neurologic and any other assessment findings.

Sample Documentation

<u>11/22/25</u> 0900 Patient arrived on unit; cervical spine immobilized; medium-sized cervical collar applied. Patient awake, alert, and oriented. Admits to right neck pain; denies other pain. See flow sheet for neurologic assessment. Skin pink, warm, and dry. A 3-cm laceration noted on R anterior side of neck. Wound cleansed and antibiotic ointment applied. Patient instructed to refrain from moving without assistance; call bell placed in right hand.

—*B. Clapp, RN*

DEVELOPING CLINICAL REASONING AND CLINICAL JUDGMENT

UNEXPECTED SITUATIONS AND ASSOCIATED INTERVENTIONS

- *Height and neck circumference measurements are between two sizes:* Start with the smaller size. If the collar is too large, the neck may not be immobilized.
- *Skin breakdown is noted on the shoulder, neck, or ear:* Apply a protective dressing over the area and continue to assess for further skin breakdown. Assess for continued need for the application of the collar (Cooper, 2013; Wang et al., 2020).
- *Patient reports that the collar is "choking" them:* If not contraindicated, place the patient in the reverse Trendelenburg position to see if this helps. Elevation of the upper body lessens pressure on the head and neck from the collar. Assess the tightness of the cervical collar; at least one finger should slide under the collar.
- *Patient is able to move their head from side to side with the cervical collar on:* Tighten the cervical collar, if possible. If the collar is as tight as possible, apply a collar one size smaller and evaluate for a better fit.

SPECIAL CONSIDERATIONS

- Cervical collar–related pressure injuries may develop on the occiput, chin, ears, mandible, supra-scapular area, and over the larynx. Implement medical device–related pressure injury prevention strategies to reduce the risk for alterations in skin integrity. Interventions may include the use of a prophylactic cushioning/proactive dressings between the skin and the device, routine skin assessments, and provision of scheduled skin hygiene interventions (Baranoski & Ayello, 2020; EPUAP, NPIAP, & PPPIAa, 2019; Lacey et al., 2019; Morton & Fontaine, 2020).
- Most rigid collars have removable inner pads; obtain an extra set of pads to remove and replace pads to allow for cleansing and complete drying of soiled pads (Cooper, 2013). Recommendations for frequency of pad changing vary (Cooper, 2013; Lacey et al., 2019). Use of a washcloth and a mild skin cleanser and water to wipe the collar has been suggested as another strategy that results in quicker drying time (Haertel, 2019).
- Nurses should collaborate with the health care team regarding the care and management of patients wearing cervical collars, including assessment of the continued need for use of the device (Lacey et al., 2019).

EVIDENCE FOR PRACTICE ▶

PRESSURE INJURY AND CERVICAL COLLARS

Patients in intensive care units may have experienced trauma and/or serious injury to the head or neck and require the application of a cervical collar. These critically ill patients have multiple factors that increase the risk of the development of pressure injuries. What are the risk factors associated with the development of pressure injuries related to the use of cervical collars?

Related Research

Wang, H. R. N., Campbell, J., Doubrovsky, A., Singh, V., Collins, J., & Coyer, F. (2020). Pressure injury development in critically ill patients with a cervical collar in situ: A retrospective longitudinal study. *International Wound Journal, 17*(4), 944–956. https://doi.org/10.1111/iwj.13363

The purpose of this retrospective longitudinal cohort study was to determine the incidence and risk factors associated with the development of cervical collar–related pressure injuries in an intensive care unit (ICU) in Australia. The health care records of all patients ages 18 years

(continued)

Skill 17-1 ▶ Applying a Two-Piece Cervical Collar *(continued)*

and older admitted to the ICU with a cervical collar over a 9-year period ($n = 906$) were examined. Data were retrieved from the clinical databases regarding length of time the patient was in the ICU, the time the patient had the cervical collar in place; frequency of repositioning of the patient, lowest Glasgow Coma Scale score every day, and the time to direct and indirect development of a cervical collar–related pressure injury and other pressure injury. Chi square and t-tests were used to identify variables associated with cervical collar–related pressure injury development, and a logistic regression model was used to analyze the risk factors. Incidence of pressure injury over the 9 years was 16.9% ($n = 154/906$). Development of pressure injury directly associated with a cervical collar increased by 33% with each repositioning event ($p = .033$). Time in the cervical collar ($p = .002$) and length of stay in the ICU ($p < .001$) were associated with pressure injury development. The researchers concluded that patients with cervical collars are a vulnerable group at risk for pressure injury development. The authors suggested education programs and interdisciplinary collaboration focused on the removal of cervical collars as soon as possible and development of evidence-based practice guidelines to standardize nursing practice and improve care of patients in cervical collars are necessary.

Relevance to Nursing Practice
Nurses play a large role in designing interventions to positively impact patient outcomes. Nurses should advocate for patients and work to develop nursing care guidelines to provide interventions to reduce patient risk for development of pressure injuries related to cervical collars and other medical devices.

Skill 17-2 ▶ Employing Seizure Precautions and Seizure Management

Seizures occur when the electrical system of the brain malfunctions. Sudden uncontrolled electrical disturbance in the brain from abnormal and excessive discharge from cerebral neurons results in episodes of abnormal motor, sensory, autonomic, or psychic activity or a combination of these (Hickey & Strayer, 2020; Mayo Foundation for Medical Education and Research [MFMER], 2021b). A **seizure** manifests as an alteration in sensation (vision, hearing, taste), behavior, movement, perception, mood, cognitive abilities, or consciousness that may be barely noticeable to abnormal, involuntary contractions and rapid shaking (convulsion) with loss of consciousness (Centers for Disease Control and Prevention [CDC], 2020a; Hinkle et al., 2022; World Health Organization [WHO], 2017).

During a seizure, patients are at risk for hypoxia, vomiting, and pulmonary aspiration. Patients who are at risk for seizures and those who have had a seizure(s) are often placed under seizure precautions to minimize the risk of physical injury. Most seizures last from 30 seconds to 2 minutes; a seizure that lasts longer than 5 minutes is a medical emergency (MFMER, 2021b). Causes of seizures include cerebrovascular disease, hypoxemia, head injury, hypertension, central nervous system infections, metabolic and toxic conditions, brain tumor, drug and alcohol withdrawal, allergies, coronavirus infection, and a history of epilepsy (seizure disorder) (Hinkle et al., 2022; MFMER, 2021b). Seizure management includes interventions by the nurse to prevent aspiration, protect the patient from injury, provide care after the seizure, and observe and document the details of the event (Hickey & Strayer, 2020; Hinkle et al., 2022). Figure 1 illustrates nursing measures to protect the patient from injury.

DELEGATION CONSIDERATIONS

The implementation of seizure precautions may be delegated to assistive personnel (AP). The implementation of seizure management may not be delegated to AP. Implementation of seizure precautions as well as seizure management may be delegated to licensed practical/vocational nurses (LPN/LVNs). The decision to delegate must be based on careful analysis of the patient's needs and circumstances as well as the qualifications of the person to whom the task is being delegated. Refer to the Delegation Guidelines in Appendix A.

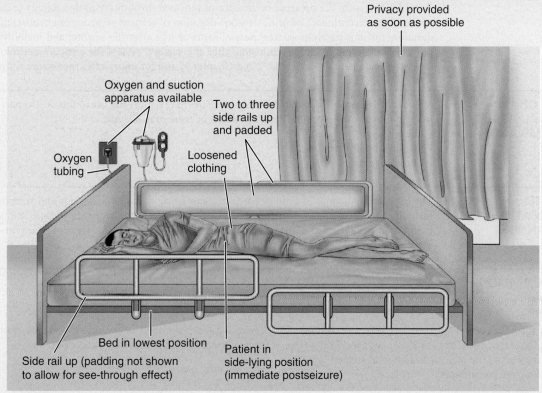

FIGURE 1. Protecting patient from injury. (*Source:* Hinkle, J. L., Cheever, K. H., & Overbaugh, K. (2022). *Brunner & Suddarth's Textbook of medical-surgical nursing* (15th ed.). Wolters Kluwer; and adapted from American Association of Neuroscience Nurses [AANN]. [2016]. *Care of adults and children with seizures and epilepsy: AANN clinical practice guideline series.* https://apps.aann.org/store/product-details?productId=192053329)

EQUIPMENT	
	• PPE, as indicated
	• Portable or wall suction unit with tubing
	• A commercially prepared suction kit with an appropriate size catheter or:
	• Sterile suction catheter with Y-port of the appropriate size (adult: 10 to 16 Fr)
	• Sterile disposable container
	• Sterile gloves
	• Oral airway
	• Bed rail padding
	• Oxygen apparatus
	• Nasal cannula or mask to deliver oxygen
	• Handheld bag valve/resuscitation bag

ASSESSMENT

Assess for preexisting conditions that increase the patient's risk for seizure activity. For example, assess for a history of seizure disorder or epilepsy, cerebrovascular disease, hypoxemia, head injury, hypertension, central nervous system infections, metabolic conditions (e.g., renal failure, hypocalcemia, hypoglycemia), brain tumor, drug/alcohol withdrawal, and allergies. Assess circumstances before the seizure, such as visual, auditory, olfactory, or tactile stimuli; emotional or psychological disturbances; sleep or hyperventilation. Assess for the occurrence of an **aura**. Note where the movements or stiffness and the gaze position and position of the head when the seizure begins. Assess the body part(s) and the type of movement(s) involved in the seizure. Assess pupil sizes, whether the eyes remained open during the seizure, and whether the eyes or head turned to

(continued on page 1090)

Skill 17-2 ▶ Employing Seizure Precautions and Seizure Management *(continued)*

one side. Assess for the presence or absence of repeated involuntary motor activity (e.g., repeated swallowing); incontinence of urine or stool; duration of seizure; presence of unconsciousness and duration; obvious paralysis or weakness of arms or legs after the seizure; and inability to speak, movements, sleeping, and/or confusion after the seizure. Assess the patient's neurologic status (refer to Fundamentals Review 17-2 and Chapter 3) and for injury after the seizure is over.

ACTUAL OR POTENTIAL HEALTH PROBLEMS AND NEEDS	Many actual or potential health problems or issues may require the use of this skill as part of related interventions. An appropriate health problem or issue may include: • Injury risk • Aspiration risk • Knowledge deficiency
OUTCOME IDENTIFICATION AND PLANNING	The expected outcomes to achieve when implementing seizure precautions and seizure management are that the patient remains free from injury and that the sequence of signs and symptoms is observed and recorded. Other specific outcomes will be formulated depending on the identified actual or potential health problem(s) or need(s).

IMPLEMENTATION

ACTION	**RATIONALE**
1. Review the health record and plan of care for conditions that would place the patient at risk for seizures. Review the health record and the plan of care for a prescribed intervention for seizure precautions.	Reviewing the prescribed interventions and care plan validates the correct patient and correct procedure.
Seizure Precautions	
2. Gather the necessary supplies.	Preparation promotes efficient time management and an organized approach to the task.
3. Perform hand hygiene and put on PPE, if indicated.	Hand hygiene and PPE prevent the spread of microorganisms. PPE is required based on transmission precautions.
4. Identify the patient.	Identifying the patient ensures the right patient receives the intervention and helps prevent errors.
5. Assemble equipment on the bedside stand, overbed table, or other surface within reach.	Arranging items nearby is convenient, saves time, and avoids unnecessary stretching and twisting of muscles on the part of the nurse.
6. Close the curtains around the bed and close the door to the room, if possible. Explain to the patient what you are going to do and why.	This ensures the patient's privacy. Explanation relieves anxiety and facilitates engagement.
7. Place the bed in the lowest position with two to three side rails elevated. Apply padding to the side rails.	The bed in the lowest position promotes safety and decreases risk of injury. Rail padding decreases the risk of injury (Kyle & Carman, 2021).
8. Attach the oxygen apparatus to the oxygen access in the wall at the head of the bed. Place the nasal cannula or mask equipment in a location where it can be easily reached, if needed.	During a seizure, patients are at risk for hypoxia, vomiting, and pulmonary aspiration. Ready access ensures availability of oxygen in the event of a seizure.
9. Attach the suction apparatus to the vacuum access in the wall at the head of the bed. Place the suction catheter, oral airway, and resuscitation bag in a location where they are easily reached, if needed.	During a seizure, patients are at risk for hypoxia, vomiting, and pulmonary aspiration. Ready access ensures availability of suction in the event of a seizure. The oral airway and resuscitation bag ensure availability of emergency ventilation in the event of respiratory arrest.

ACTION

10. Remove PPE, if used. Perform hand hygiene.

Seizure Management

11. For patients with known seizures, be alert for the occurrence of an aura, if known. If the patient reports experiencing an aura, have them lie down. If possible, provide a safe, private place, away from curious onlookers (Lawal et al., 2018).

12. Once a seizure begins, if in a health care facility, close the curtains around the bed and close the door to the room, if possible.

13. If the patient is seated, ease them to the floor.

14. Remove the patient's eyeglasses. Loosen any constricting clothing (Lawal et al., 2018). Place something flat and soft, such as a folded blanket, under their head. Push aside furniture or other objects in area.

15. If the patient is in bed, remove the pillow, place the bed in the lowest position, and raise the side rails (Lawal et al., 2018).

16. Do not restrain the patient. Guide their movements, if necessary. Do not try to insert anything in the patient's mouth or open their jaws (Lawal et al., 2018).

17. If possible, place the patient on their side with their head flexed forward and the head of the bed elevated 30 degrees. Begin administration of oxygen, based on facility policy. Clear the airway using suction, as appropriate (refer to Skill 14-7 in Chapter 14).

18. Provide supervision throughout the seizure and time the length of the seizure.

19. Establish/maintain intravenous access, as necessary. Administer medications, as appropriate, based on the prescribed intervention and facility policy.

20. After the seizure, place the patient in a side-lying position. Clear their airway using suction, as appropriate.

21. Monitor vital signs, oxygen saturation, response to medications administered, and capillary glucose, as appropriate.

22. Place the bed in the lowest position. Make sure the call bell is in reach.

23. Reassess the patient's neurologic status and comfort level.

24. Allow the patient to sleep after the seizure. On awakening, orient and reassure the patient. Reassess, as indicated.

25. Remove PPE, if used. Perform hand hygiene.

RATIONALE

Proper removal of PPE reduces the risk for infection transmission and contamination of other items. Hand hygiene prevents the spread of microorganisms.

Some patients report a warning or premonition before seizures occur; an aura can be a visual, auditory, or olfactory sensation that indicates a seizure is going to occur. Lying down prevents injury that might occur if the patient falls to the floor. Providing a private place ensures patient privacy.

Closing the door or curtain provides for patient privacy.

Getting the patient to the floor prevents injury that might occur if the patient were to fall.

Removing objects and loosening clothing prevent possible injury. The blanket prevents injury from striking a hard surface (floor).

These precautions prevent injury.

Restraint can injure the patient. Guiding movements prevents injury. Attempting to open their mouth and/or insert anything into their mouth can result in broken teeth and injury to their mouth, lips, or tongue.

During a seizure, patients are at risk for hypoxia, vomiting, and pulmonary aspiration. This position allows the tongue to fall forward, facilitates drainage of saliva and mucus, and minimizes risk for aspiration. Oxygen supports the increased metabolism associated with neurologic and muscular hyperactivity. A patent airway is necessary to support ventilation.

Supervision of the patient ensures safety. Timing of the event contributes to accurate information and documentation.

Pharmacologic therapy may be appropriate, based on patient history and health status. Intravenous access is necessary to administer emergency medications.

The side-lying position facilitates drainage of secretions. A patent airway is necessary to support ventilation.

Monitoring of parameters provides information for accurate assessment of patient status.

The bed in the lowest position and access to the call bell contribute to patient safety.

Reassessment helps to evaluate the effects of the event on the patient.

The patient will probably experience an inability to recall the seizure; patients may also experience confusion, anxiety, embarrassment, and/or fatigue after a seizure. Reassessment helps to evaluate the effects of the event on the patient.

Proper removal of PPE reduces the risk for infection transmission and contamination of other items. Hand hygiene prevents the spread of microorganisms.

(continued on page 1092)

Skill 17-2 ▶ Employing Seizure Precautions and Seizure Management *(continued)*

EVALUATION

The expected outcomes have been met when the patient has remained free from injury, and the sequence of signs and symptoms has been observed and recorded. Other specific outcomes should be evaluated depending on the identified actual or potential health problem(s) or need(s).

DOCUMENTATION

Guidelines

Document initiation of seizure precautions, including specific interventions put in place. Document if the beginning of the seizure was witnessed. If so, record noted circumstances before the seizure, such as visual, auditory, or olfactory stimuli, tactile stimuli, emotional or psychological disturbances, sleep, or hyperventilation. Note the occurrence of an aura and where the movements or stiffness, gaze position, and position of the head were when the seizure began. Record the body part(s) and the type of movement(s) involved in the seizure. Document pupil sizes; whether the eyes remained open during the seizure; whether the eyes or head turned to one side; the presence or absence of repeated involuntary motor activity (e.g., repeated swallowing); incontinence of urine or stool; duration of the seizure; the presence of unconsciousness and duration; obvious paralysis or weakness of arms or legs after seizure; and the inability to speak, movements, sleeping, and/or confusion after the seizure. Document oxygen administration, airway suction, safety measures, and medication administration, if used. If the patient was injured during the seizure, document assessment of injury. Document follow-up interventions.

Sample Documentation

> <u>1/22/25</u> 0745 Patient bathing with assistance. Stated "I don't feel right." Patient suddenly verbally unresponsive, stiff contractions of legs and arms, with arms extended, lasting approximately 15 seconds; 5-second period of apnea; and bladder incontinence. Continued with approximately 30 seconds of muscle contraction of extremities; eyes closed, facial grimacing. Patient then appeared to sleep; BP 102/68; P 88; R 16; oxygen saturation 94%. Patient awakened after 20 minutes, reporting headache and fatigue and returned to sleep. Dr. Mason notified of events and assessment. Seizure precautions implemented.
>
> *—D. Tyne, RN*

DEVELOPING CLINICAL REASONING AND CLINICAL JUDGMENT

UNEXPECTED SITUATIONS AND ASSOCIATED INTERVENTIONS

- *You enter room and find patient in the midst of a seizure:* Initiate seizure management interventions outlined above. Note in documentation that the seizure onset was not initially witnessed.

SPECIAL CONSIDERATIONS

General Considerations

- The average seizure stops within 2 minutes without requiring medication (Burns & Delgado, 2019). First-line treatment for patients with prolonged seizures or status epilepticus (seizure lasts longer than 5 minutes or seizures occurring close together without recovery by the patient between seizures) is administration of a benzodiazepine (Burns & Delgado, 2019).

Infant and Child Considerations

- Most seizures in children are caused by disorders that originate outside of the brain, such as high fever, infection, head trauma, toxins, or cardiac arrhythmias (Kyle & Carman, 2021). Febrile seizures are the most common type of seizure in children younger than age 5 years (Kavanagh et al., 2018; Millichap, 2018).
- Seizures in newborns are associated with underlying conditions, such as hypoxic ischemic encephalopathy, hypoglycemia, hypocalcemia, meningitis, encephalitis, cerebral infarction, and intracranial hemorrhage (Kyle & Carman, 2021). The prognosis depends on the underlying cause and severity of the seizure (Kyle & Carman, 2021).

- Children with recurrent seizures should wear a medical alert bracelet (Kyle & Carmen, 2021).
- Provide education regarding prescribed medications, including administration, potential side effects, and the importance of not running out of medication (El-Radhi, 2015).
- Encourage patients and their families/caregivers to keep a seizure diary (El-Radhi, 2015). The Epilepsy Foundation (2016) provides an online self-management tool and companion app for seizures and epilepsy with a focus on self-monitoring, tracking seizures and other symptoms, managing medication and other therapies, recognizing triggers, and communicating with their health care providers.
- Encourage supervision during bathing, swimming, ambulation, and other potentially hazardous activities (Kyle & Carman, 2021).
- Encourage regular sleep and avoidance of fatigue (El-Radhi, 2015; Kyle & Carman, 2021; Smith et al., 2015).
- Emergency assistance should be obtained for multiple or prolonged (>5 minutes in duration) seizures (CDC, 2020b).
- Provide information about support groups for children, parents, and families adjusting to a diagnosis of epilepsy.
- Suggest that families have a seizure action/response plan and periodic "seizure drills" to practice what every family member/caregiver should do if the child has a seizure (Epilepsy Foundation, 2014b; Epilepsy Foundation, 2020; Smith et al., 2015).

Community-Based Care Considerations

- Include patient and family/caregiver teaching for patients with documented seizures as well as those at risk for seizures. Teaching should include basic first aid management and the following tips (CDC, 2020b):
  - Help the person to lie down.
  - Remove eyeglasses and loosen constrictive clothing.
  - Clear the area around the person of anything hard or sharp.
  - Place something flat and soft (e.g., a folded jacket) under their head. Turn the person gently on their side, if possible.
  - Do not try to force anything into the patient's mouth.
  - Stay with the person during the seizure.
  - Remain calm.
  - Time the seizure.
  - After the seizure, place the person on their side and stay with them until consciousness is regained; reorient as necessary.
- Encourage patients and their families/caregivers to keep a seizure diary. The Epilepsy Foundation (2016) provides an online self-management tool and companion app for seizures and epilepsy with a focus on self-monitoring, tracking seizures and other symptoms, managing medication and other therapies, recognizing triggers, and communicating with their health care providers.
- Suggest that families have a seizure action/response plan and periodic "seizure drills" to practice what every family member/caregiver should do in the event of a seizure (Epilepsy Foundation, 2014b; Epilepsy Foundation, 2020).
- Teach the patient and family/caregiver guidelines about when to call 911 or otherwise seek emergency medical assistance (CDC, 2020b):
  - If the seizure lasts longer than 5 minutes
  - If the person has never had a seizure before
  - If the person has difficulty breathing or waking after the seizure
  - If the person has another seizure soon after the first; the person is hurt during the seizure; if the seizure happens in water; or if the person has another health condition such as diabetes, heart disease, or is pregnant
- Patients with recurrent seizures should wear a medical alert bracelet.

(continued on page 1094)

Skill 17-2 ▶ Employing Seizure Precautions and Seizure Management *(continued)*

EVIDENCE FOR PRACTICE ▶

STUDENTS WITH SEIZURES AND EPILEPSY
Related Guideline
Lepkowski, A. M., & Maughan, E. D. (2019). School nursing evidence-based clinical practice guideline: Students with Seizures and Epilepsy. https://www.pathlms.com/nasn/courses/8992

The National Association of School Nurses' (NASN). *School Nursing Evidence-Based Practice Clinical Guideline: Students with Seizures and Epilepsy* provides recommendations based on the available evidence and expert consensus for provision of high-quality care of students with seizure disorders to improve the health and safety of students. The Guideline is a decision-making tool to be implemented in conjunction with the use of nursing judgment.

EVIDENCE FOR PRACTICE ▶

PARENTS' KNOWLEDGE AND FEARS
Providing children and their parents/family/caregiver support and education are important aspects of nursing care related to seizures (Kyle & Carman, 2021). Parents of children with seizures and seizure disorders face uncertainty and need knowledge and skills to care for their children and deal with fears related to helping their child live with this health issue (Fowler et al., 2021). Assessment of parents' knowledge and concerns/fears provides important information to assist nurses in planning and providing person- and family/caregiver-centered care.

Related Research
Fowler, S. B., Hauck, M. J., Allport, S., & Dailidonis, R. (2021). Knowledge and fears of parents of children diagnosed with epilepsy. *Journal of Pediatric Nursing, 60,* 311–313. https://doi.org/10.1016/j.pedn.2021.08.008

The purpose of this descriptive comparative study was to describe and compare the knowledge and fears of parents of children diagnosed with epilepsy in the hospital and clinic settings. The convenience sample consisted of parents of children receiving health care at the neuro/ortho unit of a pediatric hospital or pediatric neurology clinic for children diagnosed with epilepsy. Parents completed two surveys. The Epilepsy Knowledge Scale (Chronbach alpha 0.755) was used to measure knowledge levels about epilepsy. The Epilepsy-related fears in Parents Questionnaire (EEPQ) (Chronbach alpha 0.92) were used to measure fears related to epilepsy. Forty parents completed the two surveys; 80% identified as mothers. The percentage of correct responses to the Epilepsy Knowledge Scale questions ranged from 31% to 100% (mean = 75%). Responses to the EEPQ indicated parents had many fears, including short-term and future long-term fears. Parents indicated they were afraid when their child was in the care of others, and they had fears of negative outcomes that included death if their child would have a seizure while being cared for others. There was no statistically significant difference in responses between hospital or clinic parents. The researchers concluded that participating parents had knowledge of seizures and epilepsy but were fearful with immediate and long-term concerns. The authors suggested nurses need to provide verbal and written educational materials, talk to parents about their fears related to epilepsy, and validate parents' skills in responding to a seizure.

Relevance to Nursing Practice
Nurses play a key role in providing patient and family/caregiver support. Nurses must include patient/family/caregiver education and support; allow parents to share their thoughts and feelings; and integrate collaboration with support services, such as support groups, psychologists, and/or social workers, as necessary. Nurses should speak with families about their concerns and fears in order to assist them to achieve the best outcomes possible.

Skill 17-3 ▶ Caring for a Patient With a Halo External Fixation Device (Halo Traction)

A halo external fixation device (halo traction) may be used to provide stabilization of the cervical spine for patients with spinal cord injury (Bauldoff et al., 2020; Hickey & Strayer, 2020). Halo traction consists of a metal ring that fits over the patient's head, connected with skull pins into the skull, and metal bars that connect the ring to a vest that distributes the weight of the device around the chest. This type of traction immobilizes the head and neck after traumatic injury to the cervical vertebrae and allows early mobility (Hinkle et al., 2022).

Nursing responsibilities include reassuring the patient, maintaining the device, monitoring neurovascular status, monitoring respiratory status, promoting exercise, preventing complications from the therapy, preventing infection by providing pin-site care, and providing teaching to ensure compliance and self-care. A growing evidence base supports effective management of pin sites but with no clear consensus (Cam & Korkmaz, 2014; Ktistakis et al., 2015; Lagerquist et al., 2012; Lethaby et al., 2013). There remains considerable diversity of practice in caring for pin sites (Abbariao, 2018; Kazmers et al., 2016; Lethaby et al., 2013; Walker et al., 2018). Pin-site care varies based on prescribed interventions and facility policy. Dressings may be applied for the first 48 to 72 hours, and then sites may be left open to air (Abbariao, 2018). Pin-site care may be performed frequently in the first 48 to 72 hours after application, when drainage may be heavy; other evidence suggests pin care should begin after the first 48 to 72 hours (Abbariao, 2018). Pin-site care may be done daily or weekly or not at all (Georgiades, 2018; Lagerquist et al., 2012; Timms & Pugh, 2012). Pin-site care is completed using aseptic technique in the immediate postoperative period. Refer to specific prescribed interventions and facility guidelines.

DELEGATION CONSIDERATIONS	The care of a patient with a halo external fixation device may not be delegated to assistive personnel (AP). Depending on the state's nurse practice act and the organization's policies and procedures, care for these patients may be delegated to licensed practical/vocational nurses (LPN/LVNs). The decision to delegate must be based on careful analysis of the patient's needs and circumstances as well as the qualifications of the person to whom the task is being delegated. Refer to the Delegation Guidelines in Appendix A.
EQUIPMENT	• Basin of warm water, bath towels and skin cleanser, based on facility policy • Antimicrobial ointment, per prescribed intervention or facility policy • Sterile applicators • Sterile container • Cleansing agent for pin care, sterile normal saline for initial cleaning, but may be an antimicrobial such as chlorhexidine or povidone-iodine (Hickey & Strayer, 2020; Sáenz-Jalón et al., 2020; Walker et al., 2018), per prescribed intervention or facility policy • Sterile gauze or dressing prescribed intervention or facility policy • Analgesic, as prescribed • Gloves • Sterile or nonsterile gloves for performing pin care, depending on prescribed intervention or facility policy • Additional PPE, as indicated
ASSESSMENT	Review the patient's health record, prescribed interventions, and plan of care to determine the type of device being used and the prescribed care. Assess the halo external fixation device to ensure proper function and position. Perform respiratory, neurologic, and skin assessments. Inspect the pin-insertion sites for inflammation and infection, including swelling, cloudy or offensive drainage, pain, or redness. Assess the patient's knowledge regarding the device, self-care activities and responsibilities, and their feelings related to treatment.
ACTUAL OR POTENTIAL HEALTH PROBLEMS AND NEEDS	Many actual or potential health problems or issues may require the use of this skill as part of related interventions. An appropriate health problem or issue may include: • Altered body image perception • Bathing/hygiene ADL deficit • Infection risk

(continued on page 1096)

Skill 17-3 ▶ Caring for a Patient With a Halo External Fixation Device (Halo Traction) *(continued)*

OUTCOME IDENTIFICATION AND PLANNING	The expected outcome to achieve when caring for a patient with a halo external fixation device is that the patient maintains cervical alignment. Additional outcomes that may be appropriate include that the patient shows no evidence of infection, and the patient is free from injury.

IMPLEMENTATION

ACTION	RATIONALE
1. Review the health record and the plan of care to determine the type of device being used and prescribed care.	Reviewing the health record and care plan validates the correct patient and correct procedure.
2. Gather the necessary equipment.	Preparation promotes efficient time management and an organized approach to the task.
3. Perform hand hygiene and put on PPE, if indicated.	Hand hygiene and PPE prevent the spread of microorganisms. PPE is required based on transmission precautions.
4. Identify the patient.	Identifying the patient ensures the right patient receives the intervention and helps prevent errors.
5. Assemble equipment on the bedside stand, overbed table, or other surface within reach.	Arranging items nearby is convenient, saves time, and avoids unnecessary stretching and twisting of muscles on the part of the nurse.
6. Close the curtains around the bed and close the door to the room, if possible. Explain to the patient what you are going to do and why.	This ensures the patient's privacy. Explanation relieves anxiety and facilitates engagement.
7. Assess the patient for the possible need for nonpharmacologic, pain-reducing interventions or analgesic medication before beginning. Administer the appropriate prescribed analgesic. Allow sufficient time for the analgesic to achieve its effectiveness before beginning the procedure.	Pain is a subjective experience influenced by past experience. Pin care may cause pain for some patients. Assessing for pain and administering analgesics promotes patient comfort.
8. Place a waste receptacle at a convenient location for use during the procedure.	Having a waste container handy means that the soiled dressing may be discarded easily, without the spread of microorganisms.
9. Adjust the bed to a comfortable working height, if the patient will remain in bed (VHACEOSH, 2016). Alternatively, have the patient sit up, if appropriate.	Having the bed at the proper height prevents back and muscle strain.
10. Assist the patient to a comfortable position that provides easy access to their head. Place a waterproof pad under their head if they are lying down.	Patient positioning provides for comfort. A waterproof pad protects underlying surfaces.
11. Monitor vital signs and perform a neurologic assessment, including level of consciousness, motor function, and sensation, per facility policy (see Fundamentals Review 17-2 and Chapter 3). This is usually done at least every 2 hours for 24 hours or possibly every hour for 48 hours.	Changes in the neurologic assessment could indicate spinal cord trauma, which would require immediate intervention.
12. Examine the halo vest unit every 8 hours for stability, secure connections, and positioning (Figure 1). Make sure the patient's head is centered in the halo without neck flexion or extension. Check each bolt for loosening.	Assessment ensures correct function of the device and patient safety. Loose bolts require attention from an appropriate advanced practice professional to maintain correct positioning, proper alignment, and unit stability.
13. Check the fit of the vest. With the patient in a supine position, you should be able to insert one or two fingers under the jacket at the shoulder and chest.	Checking the fit prevents compression on the chest, which could interfere with respiratory status.

ACTION

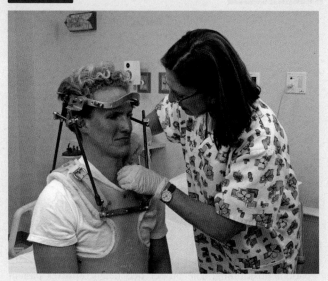

FIGURE 1. Examining halo vest for stability, secure connections, and positioning.

14. Put on gloves, if appropriate. Remove the patient's shirt or gown. Wash the patient's chest and back daily; avoid putting stress on the halo vest or crown while bathing. Loosen the bottom Velcro straps based on the prescribed intervention or facility policy. Protect the vest liner with a waterproof pad.

15. Wring out a bath towel soaked in warm water (and skin cleanser, depending on facility policy). Pull the towel back and forth in a drying motion beneath the front.

16. Thoroughly dry the skin in the same manner with a dry towel. Inspect the skin for tender, reddened areas or pressure spots. Do not use powder or lotion under the vest.

17. Turn the patient on their side, less than 45 degrees if lying supine, and repeat the process on their back. Remove the waterproof pad from the vest liner. Close the Velcro straps.

18. Implement medical device–related pressure injury prevention strategies, including use of a prophylactic cushioning/proactive dressing between the skin and vest (Pittman & Gillespie, 2020). Assist the patient with putting on a new shirt, if desired.

19. Perform a respiratory assessment. Check for respiratory impairment, such as absence of breath sounds, the presence of adventitious sounds, reduced inspiratory effort, or shortness of breath.

20. Assess the site at and around the pins for redness, edema, and odor. Assess for skin tenting, prolonged or purulent drainage, elevated body temperature, elevated pin-site temperature, and bowing or bending of the pins.

21. Perform pin-site care (Figure 2) (see Skills 9-18 and 9-19 in Chapter 9).

RATIONALE

Gloves prevent contact with blood and body fluids. Removal of clothing from the torso allows visualization of, and access to, appropriate areas. Daily cleaning prevents skin breakdown and allows assessment. Loosening the straps allows access to the chest and back. The waterproof pad keeps the vest liner dry and prevents skin irritation and breakdown.

Using an overly wet towel could lead to skin maceration and breakdown.

Drying prevents skin irritation and breakdown. Powders and lotions can cause skin irritation.

This prevents skin breakdown. Cleansers and lotions can cause skin irritation.

Pressure injuries may be related to a medical device or other object (EPUAP, NPIAP, & PPPIA, 2019). Any tube, electrode, sensor, or other rigid or stiff device element under pressure can create pressure damage (Baranoski & Ayello, 2020; EPUAP, NPIAP, & PPPIA, 2019). A cotton undershirt may be worn to absorb moisture (Neurosurgery Education and Outreach Network [NEON], 2018).

The halo vest limits chest expansion, which could lead to alterations in respiratory function. Pulmonary embolus is a common complication associated with spinal cord injury.

Pin sites provide an entry for microorganisms. Assessment allows for early detection and prompt intervention should problems arise.

Pin-site care reduces the risk of infection and subsequent osteomyelitis.

(continued on page 1098)

Skill 17-3 ▶ Caring for a Patient With a Halo External Fixation Device (Halo Traction) *(continued)*

ACTION   **RATIONALE**

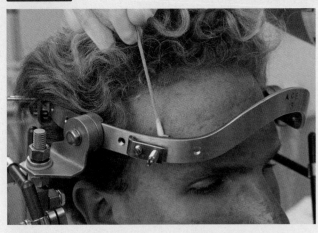

FIGURE 2. Cleansing pin sites.

22. Remove gloves and perform hand hygiene. Raise the rails, as appropriate, and place the bed in the lowest position. Assist the patient to a comfortable position.

23. Remove additional PPE, if used. Perform hand hygiene.

Disposing of gloves and performing hand hygiene reduce the risk of microorganism transmission. The rails assist with patient positioning. The proper bed height ensures patient safety.

Proper removal of PPE reduces the risk for infection transmission and contamination of other items. Hand hygiene prevents the spread of microorganisms.

EVALUATION

The expected outcomes have been met when the patient has maintained cervical alignment, has exhibited no evidence of infection, and has remained free from injury.

DOCUMENTATION

Guidelines

Document the time, date, and type of device in place. Include the skin assessment, pin-site assessment, personal hygiene, and pin-site care. Document the patient's response to the device and the neurologic assessment and respiratory assessment.

Sample Documentation

11/10/25 2030 Halo traction in place. Skin care provided under jacket; two fingers fit at shoulders and chest. Skin intact without redness or irritation. Pin-site care performed. Pin sites cleaned with normal saline and open to the air. Sites without redness, swelling, and drainage. Neurovascular status intact. Patient reports pain at pin sites 4/10. Medicated with ibuprofen 600 mg per order. Will reevaluate pain in 1 hour.
—M. Leroux, RN

DEVELOPING CLINICAL REASONING AND CLINICAL JUDGMENT

UNEXPECTED SITUATIONS AND ASSOCIATED INTERVENTIONS

- *Patient being treated with halo traction reports headache after tightening of the skull pins:* pin sites may be associated with pain for the first few days (Hinkle et al., 2022; NEON, 2018); administer a prescribed analgesic. However, if the pain is associated with jaw movement (chewing and or swallowing), notify the health care team immediately (NEON, 2018); the pins may have slipped onto the temporal plate.
- *Patient reports one pin-site hurting more than the others:* the pin is probably loose; notify the health care team (NEON, 2018).

SPECIAL CONSIDERATIONS

General Considerations

- Always keep the wrench/Allen key specific for the vest attached to the front of the vest for emergency removal of the anterior portion of the vest should it be necessary to perform cardiopulmonary resuscitation (NEON, 2018).
- Patient teaching to prevent injury is very important. Patients need to learn to turn slowly and refrain from bending forward to avoid falls.
- Stress to the frame could cause misalignment of the spine and straining or tearing of the skin. Do not use the frame as handles to transfer or position the patient.
- Notify the health care team about the following signs/symptoms (Hickey & Strayer, 2020): If a pin site becomes unusually painful or tender, if there is any fluid discharge (may be a signal that the pin has loosened or become infected); or if the patient reports that the halo feels loose, imbalanced, or that it is shifting. Pin loosening may also be indicated by a "tight" feeling or a "clicking" sound (Lagerquist et al., 2012).
- The patient's hair should be washed regularly; protect the vest lining from getting wet with a moisture-proof pad (Hickey & Strayer, 2020; NEON, 2018).

Community-Based Care Considerations

- Patients and families require information and guidance about the care of their halo in the community. Written information, as well as specific discharge teaching, is important in helping to prevent complications. Teaching should include the importance of vigilant skin care and signs and symptoms of pin-site infection.
- Encourage exercise by walking; teach the patient to avoid other exercise activities.
- Keeping the hair clean is important. Hair should be shampooed regularly. This can be accomplished by having the patient lie supine in bed, with their head out over foot of the mattress so it is suspended beyond the mattress; their shoulders should remain on the mattress with a towel or plastic bag along the back and shoulders of the vest to keep it from getting wet. A garbage can under the patient's head can be used to catch the water. Alternatively, the patient could rest their elbows on the edge of a bathtub, with a towel on the edge of the tub for padding, and lean over the tub. Use a spray attachment or pitcher of water to wash hair. Protect the vest lining from getting wet with a moisture-proof pad (Hickey & Strayer, 2020; NEON, 2018).

EVIDENCE FOR PRACTICE ▶

EXTERNAL FIXATOR PIN-SITE CARE

Different methods of cleansing external fixator percutaneous pin sites have been suggested to prevent pin-site infections, with no clear consensus on a cleansing regimen or other aspects of pin-site care (Kazmers et al., 2016; Lathaby et al., 2013). Chlorhexidine-alcohol solution and povidone-iodine solution are commonly used to provide pin-site care. Is there a significant difference between the number and severity of infections in fixators among those who are cared for using one or the other of these solutions?

Related Evidence

Sáenz-Jalón, M., Sarabia-Cobo, C. M., Bartolome, E. R., Fernández, M. S., Vélez, B., Escudero, M., Miguel, M. E., Artabe, P., Cabañas, I., Fernández, A., Garcés, C., & Couceiro, J. (2020). A randomized clinical trial on the use of antiseptic solutions for the pin-site care of external fixators: Chlorhexidine-alcohol versus povidone-iodine. *Journal of Trauma Nursing, 27*(3), 146–150. https://doi.org/10.1097/JTN.0000000000000503

This randomized clinical trial investigated the superiority of chlorhexidine-alcohol solution versus povidone-iodine solution for external fixator pin-site care in pin-site infection. The study took place in one hospital in Spain with 128 patients who underwent placement of an external fixator. Participants were randomly assigned to receive pin-site care using either a 2% chlorhexidine-alcohol solution or a 10% povidone-iodine solution. The average number of pins per patient was 4.3 with a total of 568 pins initially available for analysis. Ultimately, 489 pins were analyzed for the development of a pin-site infection, with 79 pins not analyzed for various reasons, including improper collection of the sample or inappropriate condition of the sample

(continued)

Skill 17-3 ► **Caring for a Patient With a Halo External Fixation Device (Halo Traction)** *(continued)*

upon arrival to the laboratory. The majority of patients (82%) remained free of pin-site infection. Results indicated no significant differences of rate of infection between groups. Statistically significant differences were found regarding time and infection variables. The longer the person had the fixator, the higher the risk of infection ($p = .002$). The researchers concluded both chlorhexidine-alcohol and povidone-iodine solutions are equally effective for preventing infection in external fixator pin sites. The researchers suggested other factors should also be taken into consideration when developing pin-site care guidelines, including cost and simplicity of use to optimal care.

Relevance for Nursing Practice
The results of this study suggest that implementing pin-site care with either antimicrobial solution is effective in preventing pin-site infections and that other factors should also be considered to ensure consistent implementation of pin-site care. Nurses should consider adoption of evidence-based pin-site care guidelines to support quality patient care and improve patient outcomes.

EVIDENCE FOR PRACTICE ►

EXTERNAL FIXATOR PIN-SITE CARE
The goal of pin-site care is to reduce the risk for or, when possible, to prevent pin-site infection. Removal of crusts from pin sites is controversial; some evidence suggests removal of crusts prevents excessive pressure at the site and allows for drainage and prevents infection (Abbariao, 2018; Cam & Korkmaz, 2014; Walker et al., 2018). Other evidence suggests crusts should be left in place to act as a biologic barrier to prevent introduction of microorganisms and decrease the risk of pin-site infection (Abbariao, 2018; Georgiades, 2018; Walker et al., 2018).

Related Evidence
Georgiades, D. S. (2018). A systematic integrative review of pin site crusts. *Orthopaedic Nursing*, *37*(1), 36–42. https://doi.org/10.1097/NOR.0000000000000416

   The aim of this systematic review was to explore the effectiveness of pin-site crusts as a biologic dressing versus the removal of pin-site crusts in pin-site care and prevention of pin-site infection. A systematic search was conducted using CINAHL, Cochrane Library, and ProQuest, resulting in 29 initial studies. Five studies that met the inclusion criteria were appraised using the Mixed Method Appraisal Tool. Findings of a narrative synthesis revealed that pin-site crusts have similar properties to that of a dressing, as the crusts are able to act as a barrier between the insertion site of the pin and the external environment, which can reduce infection. The authors concluded pin-site crusts could reduce risk of pin-site infection and could be maintained in place.

Relevance for Nursing Practice
The results of this study suggest that pin-site crusts could be left in place as a biologic dressing, decreasing patients' risk of pin-site infection and improving patient outcomes. Nurses should consider adoption of evidence-based pin-site care guidelines to support quality patient care and improve patient outcomes.

Skill 17-4 ▶ Caring for a Patient With an External Ventriculostomy (Intraventricular Catheter–Closed Fluid-Filled System)

Intracranial pressure (ICP) is the pressure inside the cranium. The components that occupy the intracranial space, blood, tissue, and cerebrospinal fluid (CSF) circulating in the ventricles and subarachnoid space, contribute to the ICP (Hickey & Strayer, 2020). ICP monitoring is used to assess cerebral perfusion. When ICP increases, as a result of conditions such as a mass (e.g., a tumor), bleeding into the brain or fluid around the brain, or swelling within the brain matter itself, neurologic consequences may range from minor to severe, including death. Normal ICP is less than 15 mm Hg. Elevated ICP, intracranial hypertension, is a sustained ICP of 20 to 25 mm Hg or higher for greater than 5 minutes (Hickey & Strayer, 2020). Box 17-1 identifies signs and symptoms of increased ICP in adults.

An external **ventriculostomy** is one method used to rapidly reduce ICP and monitor ICP (Hickey & Strayer, 2020; Hinkle et al., 2022). It is part of a system that includes an external drainage system and an external transducer. This device is inserted into a ventricle of the brain, most commonly the nondominant lateral ventricle, through a hole drilled into the skull. The catheter is connected by a fluid-filled system to a transducer, which records the pressure in the form of an electrical impulse (Hinkle et al., 2022). The ventriculostomy can be used to measure the ICP; to drain CSF, such as removing excess fluid associated with hydrocephalus; or to decrease the volume in the cranial vault, thereby decreasing the ICP, and to instill medications. ICP and blood pressure measurements are used to calculate **cerebral perfusion pressure (CPP)**, the blood pressure gradient across the brain and the pressure necessary to maintain an adequate force for blood throughout the brain, to prevent cerebral ischemia (Hickey & Strayer, 2020). ICP monitoring also provides information about **intracranial compliance**, the ability of the brain to change volume related to a change in pressure; to tolerate stimulation or increase in intracranial volume without an increase in pressure through waveform assessment (Box 17-2) (Hickey & Strayer, 2020; Morton & Fontaine, 2018).

Ventricular drainage is associated with an increased risk of infection. Strict sterile technique should be observed when manipulating the ventricular drain (American Association of Critical-Care Nurses [AACN], 2017; Hickey & Strayer, 2020).

DELEGATION CONSIDERATIONS	The care of a patient with an external ventriculostomy may not be delegated to assistive personnel (AP). Depending on the state's nurse practice act and the organization's policies and procedures, care for these patients may be delegated to licensed practical/vocational nurses (LPN/LVNs). The decision to delegate must be based on careful analysis of the patient's needs and circumstances as well as the qualifications of the person to whom the task is being delegated. Refer to the Delegation Guidelines in Appendix A.
EQUIPMENT	• Ventriculostomy setup • Carpenter level, bubble-line level, or laser level, according to facility policy • PPE, as indicated

Box 17-1 Signs and Symptoms of Increased Intracranial Pressure in Adults

- Decreased level of consciousness
- Changes in mental status
- Lethargy
- Coma
- Headache
- Confusion
- Restlessness, agitation
- Irritability
- Hypoactive reflexes
- Slowed response time
- Ataxia

- Aphasia
- Slowed speech
- Progressively severe headache
- Nausea and vomiting (usually projectile vomiting)
- Seizures
- Changes in pupil size; unequal pupils
- Slowed or lack of pupillary response to light
- Widening of pulse pressure
- Respiratory pattern changes
- Leakage of clear yellow or pinkish fluid from ear or nose

(continued on page 1102)

Skill 17-4 ▶ Caring for a Patient With an External Ventriculostomy (Intraventricular Catheter–Closed Fluid-Filled System) *(continued)*

Box 17-2 | Interpreting ICP Waveforms

Sustained periods (>5 minutes) of ICPs greater than 20 to 25 mm Hg are considered significant and can be extremely dangerous. Sustained periods of ICPs greater than 60 mm Hg are usually fatal (Morton & Fontaine, 2018). A normal waveform correlates with hemodynamic changes. Plotting extended periods of increased ICP measurements over time provides patterns known as A, B, and C waves (waveform trends).

Normal Intracranial Waveform

A normal ICP waveform typically shows a steep upward slope followed by a downward slope with three descending peaks that correlate with hemodynamic changes (forces related to the circulation of blood). P1 correlates with systole; P2 most directly reflects the state of intracranial compliance, so as ICP rises, P2 elevates; P3 tapers down to correlate with diastole (Morton & Fontaine, 2018). In normal circumstances, this waveform occurs continuously and indicates an ICP between 0 and 15 mm Hg—normal pressure. The amplitude of P2 may exceed P1 with increased ICP or decreased intracranial compliance (Morton & Fontaine, 2018).

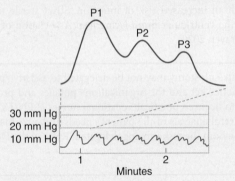

A Waves

A waves are produced by spontaneous, transient, rapid increases of pressure over a period of time (ICP values of 50 to 200 mm Hg, lasting 5 to 20 minutes) and are associated with compromised cerebral perfusion and deteriorating neurologic status.

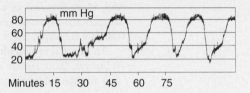

B Waves

B waves, which appear sharp and rhythmic with a sawtooth pattern, are shorter (30 seconds to 2 minutes) with ICP values of 20 to 50 mm Hg. They are seen in patients with intracranial hypertension and decreased intracranial compliance. B waves are an early indication of deteriorating neurologic status and may precede A waves.

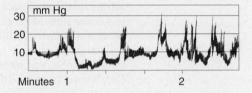

C Waves

C waves are rapid and rhythmic, but they are not as sharp as B waves. C waves are associated with ICPs as high as 20 mm Hg that persist for less than 5 minutes. They may fluctuate with respirations or systemic blood pressure changes and are without clinical significance (AACN, 2017; Burns & Delgado, 2019).

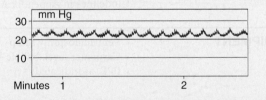

Source: Adapted from American Association of Critical-Care Nurses (AACN). (2017). In D. L. Wiegand (Ed.). *AACN procedure manual for high acuity, progressive, and critical care* (7th ed.). Elsevier; Burns, S. M., & Delgado, S. A. (2019). *AACN Essentials of critical care nursing* (4th ed.). McGraw Hill Education; Hinkle, J. L., Cheever, K. H., & Overbaugh, K. (2022). *Brunner & Suddarth's Textbook of medical-surgical nursing* (15th ed.). Wolters Kluwer; and Morton, P. G., & Fontaine, D. K. (2018). *Critical care nursing. A holistic approach* (11th ed.). Wolters Kluwer.

ASSESSMENT

Assess the color of the fluid draining from the ventriculostomy. Normal CSF is clear or straw colored. Cloudy CSF may suggest an infection. Red or pink CSF may indicate bleeding. Assess vital signs, because changes in vital signs can reflect a neurologic problem. Assess the patient's pain level. The patient may be experiencing pain at the ventriculostomy insertion site. Assess the insertion site.

Perform a neurologic assessment (see Fundamentals Review 17-2 and Chapter 3). Assess the patient's level of consciousness (LOC). If the patient is awake, assess for their orientation to person, place, and time. If the patient's LOC is decreased, note their ability to respond and to be aroused. Inspect pupil size and response to light. Pupils should be equal and round and should react to light bilaterally. Any changes in LOC or pupillary response may suggest a neurologic problem. If the patient can move their extremities, assess the strength of their hands and feet (see Chapter 3 for detailed instructions on assessing muscle strength). A change in strength or a difference in strength on one side compared with the other may indicate a neurologic problem.

ACTUAL OR POTENTIAL HEALTH PROBLEMS AND NEEDS	Many actual or potential health problems or issues may require the use of this skill as part of related interventions. An appropriate health problem or issue may include: • Injury risk • Increased intracranial pressure • Infection risk
OUTCOME IDENTIFICATION AND PLANNING	The expected outcomes to achieve are that the patient maintains ICP at less than 15 mm Hg and CPP of 50 to 70 mm Hg (adults) (Burns & Delgado, 2019; Hickey & Strayer, 2020; Hinkle et al., 2022; Morton & Fontaine, 2018). Other outcomes that may be appropriate include that the patient is free from infection, and the patient/family/caregivers understand the need for the ventriculostomy.

IMPLEMENTATION

ACTION	**RATIONALE**
1. Review the prescribed interventions and patient health record for specific information about ventriculostomy parameters.	The nurse needs to know the most recent prescribed intervention for the height of the ventriculostomy. For example, if the health care practitioner has ordered that the ventriculostomy is to be at 10 cm, this means the patient's ICP must rise above 10 cm before the ventriculostomy will drain CSF.
2. Gather the necessary supplies.	Preparation promotes efficient time management and an organized approach to the task.
3. Perform hand hygiene and put on PPE, if indicated.	Hand hygiene and PPE prevent the spread of microorganisms. PPE is required based on transmission precautions.
4. Identify the patient.	Identifying the patient ensures the right patient receives the intervention and helps prevent errors.
5. Assemble equipment on the bedside stand, overbed table, or other surface within reach.	Arranging items nearby is convenient, saves time, and avoids unnecessary stretching and twisting of muscles on the part of the nurse.
6. Close the curtains around the bed and close the door to the room, if possible. Explain to the patient what you are going to do and why.	This ensures the patient's privacy. Explanation relieves anxiety and facilitates engagement.
7. Assess the patient for any changes in neurologic status (see Fundamentals Review 17-2 and Chapter 3 for details of assessment).	Patients with ventriculostomies are at risk for problems with the neurologic system.
8. Set the zero reference level. **Assess the height of the ventriculostomy system to ensure that the stopcock is at the appropriate reference point: the tragus of the ear (Figure 1), the outer canthus of the patient's eye, or the patient's external auditory canal** (Hickey & Strayer, 2020; Munakomi & Das, 2021) using a carpenter level, bubble-line level, or laser level, according to facility policy. Adjust the height of the system, if needed.	For measurements to be accurate, the stopcock must be at a reference point to approximate the catheter tip at the level of the foramen of Monro. Use of the same reference point for all readings is critical to ensure accuracy. Use of a carpenter level, bubble-line level, or laser level, ensures accuracy (Hickey & Strayer, 2020). If the ventriculostomy is used just to measure the ICP and not to drain the CSF, the stopcock will be turned off to the drip chamber.

(continued on page 1104)

Skill 17-4 ▸ Caring for a Patient With an External Ventriculostomy (Intraventricular Catheter–Closed Fluid-Filled System) *(continued)*

| ACTION | RATIONALE |

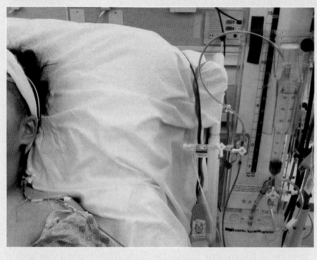

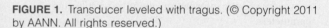

FIGURE 1. Transducer leveled with tragus. (© Copyright 2011 by AANN. All rights reserved.)

9. Set the pressure level based on the prescribed pressure. Move the drip chamber to the ordered height. Assess the amount of CSF in the drip chamber if the ventriculostomy is draining.

When the ICP is higher than the prescribed pressure level, CSF will drain into the drip chamber. If the ventriculostomy is to drain CSF, the nurse must turn the stopcock off to the drip chamber to obtain a measurement of ICP. After the ICP value is obtained, remember to turn the stopcock back off to the transducer so that CSF is allowed to drain.

10. **Zero the transducer.** Turn the stopcock off to the patient. Remove the cap from the transducer, being careful not to touch the end of the cap. Press and hold the calibration button on the monitor until the monitor beeps. Return the cap to the transducer. **Turn the stopcock off to the drip chamber to obtain an ICP reading and waveform tracing. After obtaining a reading, turn the stopcock off to the transducer.**

The readings would not be considered accurate if the transducer had not been recently zeroed. If the stopcock is not turned off to the patient, when opened to room air, CSF will flow out of the stopcock. The end of the cap must remain sterile to prevent an infection. The stopcock must be off to the drip chamber (open to the transducer) to obtain an ICP. If the ventriculostomy is to drain CSF, the nurse must turn the stopcock off to the drip chamber. After the ICP value is obtained, remember to turn the stopcock back off to the transducer so that CSF is allowed to drain into the drip chamber.

11. **Adjust the ventriculostomy height to prevent too much drainage, too little drainage, or inaccurate ICP readings.**

If the patient's head is lower than the ventriculostomy, the drainage of CSF will slow or stop. If the patient's head is higher than the ventriculostomy, the drainage of CSF will increase. Any ICP readings taken when the ventriculostomy is not level with the outer canthus of the eye would be inaccurate.

12. Care for the insertion site according to the facility's policy. Maintain the system using strict sterile technique. Assess the site for any signs of infection, such as purulent drainage, redness, or warmth. Ensure the catheter is secured at the site per facility policy. If the catheter is sutured to the scalp, assess integrity of the sutures (Figure 2).

Site care varies, possibly ranging from leaving the site open to air to applying antibiotic ointment and gauze. Sterile technique helps to prevent infection (AACN, 2017; Hickey & Strayer, 2020; Munakomi & Das, 2021). Securing the catheters after insertion prevents dislodgement and breakage of the device.

13. Calculate the CPP, if necessary. Calculate the difference between the systemic MAP and the ICP.

CPP is an estimate of the adequacy of the blood supply to the brain.

14. Remove PPE, if used. Perform hand hygiene.

Proper removal of PPE reduces the risk for infection transmission and contamination of other items. Hand hygiene prevents the spread of microorganisms.

ACTION

RATIONALE

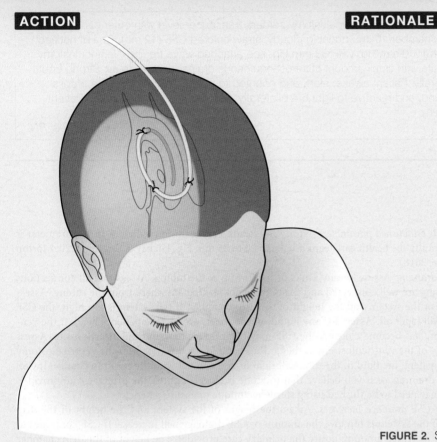

FIGURE 2. Sutured external ventriculostomy catheter.

15. Assess ICP, MAP, and CPP continuously or intermittently as prescribed (AACN, 2017). Note drainage amount, color, and clarity.

Frequent assessment provides valuable indicators for identifying subtle trends that may suggest developing problems.

16. Assess ICP drainage system at least every 4 hours, checking the insertion site, all drainage system tubing and parts, for cracks in the system, and for leakage from the insertion site or system. Label the external ventriculostomy tubing and access ports clearly.

Frequent monitoring allows for early identification of problems and prompt intervention. Clear labeling prevents accidental use as an intravenous access.

EVALUATION

The expected outcomes have been met when the patient has maintained ICP at less than 15 mm Hg and CPP of 50 to 70 mm Hg (adults) (Burns & Delgado, 2019; Hickey & Strayer, 2020), the patient has remained free from infection, and the patient/family/caregivers have verbalized an understanding of the need for the ventriculostomy.

DOCUMENTATION

Guidelines

Document the following information: amount and color of CSF, ICP, and CPP; pupil status; motor strength bilaterally; orientation to time, person, and place; LOC; vital signs; pain; assessment of insertion site; and height of the ventriculostomy.

(continued on page 1106)

Skill 17-4 Caring for a Patient With an External Ventriculostomy (Intraventricular Catheter–Closed Fluid-Filled System) *(continued)*

Sample Documentation

> <u>11/2/25</u> 1410 External ventriculostomy zeroed; transducer level with outer canthus of eye, drip chamber 10 cm; draining cloudy, straw-colored CSF (12 mL), Dr. Hill notified of clarity. ICP 10 mm Hg; CPP 83 mm Hg, see attached wave tracing. Ventriculostomy insertion site with small amount of serosanguineous drainage; open to air. Strong equal grip bilaterally. Patient awake, alert, and oriented to person, place, and time. Pupils equal, round, and reactive to light 6/4 bilaterally. See graphics for vital signs. Patient denies pain.
>
> —B. Traudes, RN

DEVELOPING CLINICAL REASONING AND CLINICAL JUDGMENT

UNEXPECTED SITUATIONS AND ASSOCIATED INTERVENTIONS

- *ICP exceeds established parameters:* Notify the health care team immediately. If no parameter is specified, notify the health care team if ICP is >20 to 25 mm Hg (Hickey & Strayer, 2020; Morton & Fontaine, 2018).
- *CSF stops draining:* Assess for any kinks or narrowing of the tubing. Assess that all connections on the tubing are well connected and that CSF is not leaking anywhere from the tubing. Assess the height of the system and the height of the drip chamber. If the system is too high, the CSF drainage will taper off. Assess for any liquid on the sheets around the patient's head. If the ventriculostomy has become clogged, the CSF may begin to leak around the insertion site. Assess the patency of the ventriculostomy catheter. Raise and lower the system. If the ventriculostomy catheter is patent, the fluid in the tube will tidal or rise and fall with the position change. If CSF still is not draining, or if you believe that the tube is clogged, notify the primary care provider. The tube may need to be flushed using sterile technique to ensure patency.
- *Amount of CSF drainage increases:* Assess the height of the system and the height of the drip chamber. If the system is too low, the amount of CSF drainage will increase. If CSF continues to drain at an increased amount, notify the primary care provider. The height of the drip chamber may need to be increased.
- *CSF has changed from clear to cloudy:* Notify the health care team immediately. This can signify an infection, and antibiotics may need to be started.
- *CSF has changed from straw-colored to pink tinged or serosanguineous:* Notify the health care team immediately. This can signify bleeding in the ventricles of the brain.
- *Catheter is accidentally dislodged:* Notify the health care team immediately. Put on sterile gloves and cover the insertion site with sterile gauze. Monitor for color and amount of CSF if draining from the site.

SPECIAL CONSIDERATIONS

- Secure and label the catheters according to facility policy after insertion, and use care when moving patients to prevent dislodgement and breakage of these devices.
- Repositioning is important to prevent skin alterations and to decrease the risks associated with immobility. During position changes, clamp the ventriculostomy; after repositioning, maintain the reference level and ensure the system is patent (AACN, 2017). Modest, initial increases in ICP experienced with repositioning quickly return to baseline after repositioning is complete (McNett & Olson, 2013). Turn and position the patient in proper body alignment, avoiding angulation of body parts. Extreme hip flexion or flexion of the upper legs can increase intraabdominal pressure, leading to increased ICP. Maintain the neck in the neutral position at all times to avoid neck vein compression, which can interfere with venous return (Hickey & Strayer, 2020).
- Maintain the head of the bed elevated 30 degrees to promote venous return from the brain, depending on prescribed interventions and facility procedure (AACN, 2017; Hickey & Strayer, 2020).
- Endotracheal suctioning episodes should be limited to one to two passes of the catheter (Hickey & Strayer, 2020). The ICP increases associated with suctioning, tracheal stimulation, and coughing are modest and transient (McNett & Olson, 2013).

- Oral care is a safe intervention; ICP increases experienced with oral care are modest, transient, and resolve quickly when oral care is complete (McNett & Olson, 2013).
- Auditory stimulation for critically ill neurologically impaired patients does not increase ICP and is considered a safe intervention (McNett & Olson, 2013).
- Drainage should be turned off at the collection chamber before any intervention involving patient movement, such as suctioning, walking, physiotherapy, and repositioning (Humphrey, 2018).
- Plan care to avoid grouping activities and procedures known to increase ICP. Bathing, turning, and other routine care often have a cumulative effect to increase ICP when performed in succession. Allow rest periods between procedures and carefully assess the patient's response to interventions (Hickey & Strayer, 2020).

EVIDENCE FOR PRACTICE ▶	**CLINICAL PRACTICE GUIDELINE: UNIVERSAL STANDARD FOR EXTERNAL VENTRICULAR DRAIN CARE** Hepburn-Smith, M., Dynkevich, I., Spektor, M., Lord, A., Czeisler, B., & Lewis, A. (2016). Establishment of an external ventricular drain best practice guideline: The quest for a comprehensive, universal standard for external ventricular drain care. *Journal of Neuroscience Nursing, 48*(1), 54–65. An interdisciplinary team of nurses, advanced practice nurses, and neurointensivists reviewed medical and nursing literature as well as research-based institutional protocols on external ventricular drain (EVD) insertion and maintenance to determine global best practices. The resulting guideline addresses preinsertion hair removal and skin preparation, aseptic technique, catheter selection, monitoring of EVD insertion technique using a bundle approach, postinsertion dressing type and frequency of dressing changes, techniques for maintenance and CSF sampling, duration of catheter placement, and staff education/competence, and surveillance.

Skill 17-5 ▶ Caring for a Patient With a Fiberoptic Intracranial Catheter

Intracranial pressure (ICP) is the pressure inside the cranium. The components that occupy the intracranial space, blood, tissue, and cerebrospinal fluid circulating in the ventricles and subarachnoid space, contribute to the ICP (Hickey & Strayer, 2020). ICP monitoring is used to assess cerebral perfusion. When ICP increases, as a result of conditions such as a mass (e.g., a tumor), bleeding into the brain or fluid around the brain, or swelling within the brain matter itself, neurologic consequences may range from minor to severe, including death. Normal ICP is less than 15 mm Hg. Elevated ICP, intracranial hypertension, is a sustained ICP of 20 to 25 mm Hg or higher for greater than 5 minutes (Hickey & Strayer, 2020). Refer to Box 17-1 in Skill 17-4 for signs and symptoms of increased ICP in adults.

Fiberoptic catheters are one method used to monitor ICP. Fiberoptic catheters directly monitor ICP using an intracranial transducer located in the tip of the catheter. A miniature transducer in the catheter tip is coupled by a long, continuous wire or fiberoptic cable to an external electronic module. This device can be inserted into the lateral ventricle, subarachnoid space, subdural space, brain parenchyma, or under a bone flap (Figure 1). These devices are not fluid-filled systems, eliminating the problems associated with an external transducer and pressure tubing, such as an external ventriculostomy (see Skill 17-4). Fiberoptic catheters can be used to monitor the ICP and cerebral perfusion pressure (CPP). These devices are calibrated by the manufacturer and zero-balanced only once at the time of insertion.

ICP and blood pressure measurements are used to calculate CPP, the blood pressure gradient across the brain and the pressure necessary to maintain an adequate force for blood throughout

Skill 17-5 ▶ Caring for a Patient With a Fiberoptic Intracranial Catheter *(continued)*

the brain, to prevent cerebral ischemia (Hickey & Strayer, 2020). ICP monitoring also provides information about intracranial compliance, the ability of the brain to change volume related to a change in pressure, to tolerate stimulation or increase in intracranial volume without an increase in pressure through waveform assessment (Hickey & Strayer, 2020; Morton & Fontaine, 2018). Box 17-2 in Skill 17-4 reviews ICP waveforms.

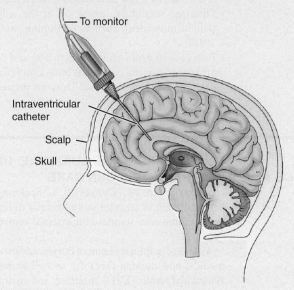

To monitor

Intraventricular catheter

Scalp

Skull

FIGURE 1. Fiberoptic catheter in ventricle. (*Source:* Adapted from Hinkle, J. L., Cheever, K. H., & Overbaugh, K. (2022). *Brunner & Suddarth's Textbook of medical-surgical nursing* (15th ed.). Wolters Kluwer, p. 2002.)

DELEGATION CONSIDERATIONS	The care of a patient with a fiberoptic intracranial catheter may not be delegated to assistive personnel (AP). Depending on the state's nurse practice act and the organization's policies and procedures, care for these patients may be delegated to licensed practical/vocational nurses (LPN/LVNs). The decision to delegate must be based on careful analysis of the patient's needs and circumstances as well as the qualifications of the person to whom the task is being delegated. Refer to the Delegation Guidelines in Appendix A.
EQUIPMENT	• PPE, as indicated
ASSESSMENT	Perform a neurologic assessment (see Fundamentals Review 17-2 and Chapter 3). Assess the patient's level of consciousness (LOC). If the patient is awake, assess their orientation to person, place, and time. If the patient's LOC is decreased, note their ability to respond and to be aroused. Inspect pupil size and response to light. Pupils should be equal and round and should react to light bilaterally. Any changes in LOC or pupillary response may suggest a neurologic problem. If the patient can move their extremities, assess the strength of their hands and feet (see Chapter 3 for detailed instructions on assessing muscle strength). A change in strength or a difference in strength on one side compared with the other may indicate a neurologic problem. Assess vital signs, because changes in vital signs can reflect a neurologic problem. Assess the patient's pain level. The patient may be experiencing pain at the fiberoptic catheter insertion site. Assess the insertion site.
ACTUAL OR POTENTIAL HEALTH PROBLEMS AND NEEDS	Many actual or potential health problems or issues may require the use of this skill as part of related interventions. An appropriate health problem or issue may include: • Injury risk • Increased intracranial pressure • Infection risk

| OUTCOME IDENTIFICATION AND PLANNING | The expected outcomes to achieve are that the patient maintains ICP at less than 15 mm Hg and CPP of 50 to 70 mm Hg (adults) (Burns & Delgado, 2019; Hickey & Strayer, 2020). Other outcomes that may be appropriate include that the patient is free from infection, and the patient/family/caregivers understand the need for the intracranial catheter. |

IMPLEMENTATION

ACTION	**RATIONALE**
1. Review the prescribed interventions and health record for specific information about monitoring parameters.	The nurse needs to know the most recent order for acceptable ICP and CPP values.
2. Perform hand hygiene and put on PPE, if indicated.	Hand hygiene and PPE prevent the spread of microorganisms. PPE is required based on transmission precautions.
 3. Identify the patient.	Identifying the patient ensures the right patient receives the intervention and helps prevent errors.
4. Close the curtains around the bed and close the door to the room, if possible. Explain to the patient what you are going to do and why.	This ensures the patient's privacy. Explanation relieves anxiety and facilitates engagement.
5. Assess the patient for any changes in neurologic status (see Fundamentals Review 17-2 and Chapter 3 for details of assessment).	Patients with ventriculostomies are at risk for problems with the neurologic system.
6. Assess ICP, MAP, and CPP continuously or intermittently as prescribed (AACN, 2017). Note ICP value and waveforms as shown on the monitor.	Frequent assessment provides valuable indicators for identifying subtle trends that may suggest developing problems.
7. Care for the insertion site according to the facility's policy. Maintain the system using strict sterile technique. Assess the site for any signs of infection, such as drainage, redness, or warmth. Ensure the catheter is secured at the site per facility policy.	Site care varies, possibly ranging from leaving the site open to air to applying antibiotic ointment and gauze. Site care aids in reducing the risk for infection. Sterile technique helps to prevent infection (AACN, 2017; Hickey & Strayer, 2020; Munakomi & Das, 2021). Securing the catheters after insertion prevents dislodgement and breakage of the device.
8. Calculate the CPP, if necessary. Calculate the difference between the systemic MAP and the ICP.	CPP is an estimate of the adequacy of the blood supply to the brain.
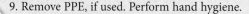 9. Remove PPE, if used. Perform hand hygiene.	Proper removal of PPE reduces the risk for infection transmission and contamination of other items. Hand hygiene prevents the spread of microorganisms.

| EVALUATION | The expected outcomes have been met when the patient has maintained ICP at less than 15 mm Hg and CPP of 50 to 70 mm Hg (adults), the patient has remained free from infection, and the patient/family/caregivers have verbalized an understanding of the need for the intraventricular catheter. |

DOCUMENTATION

| **General Guidelines** | Document the neurologic assessment, ICP and CPP, vital signs, pain, and assessment of the insertion site. |

(continued on page 1110)

Skill 17-5   ▶ Caring for a Patient With a Fiberoptic Intracranial Catheter   *(continued)*

Sample Documentation

<u>11/2/25</u> 1710 Patient sedated; disoriented and combative when awake. Pupils equal round and reactive to light 6/4 bilaterally. See graphics for vital signs. ICP 22 mm Hg; CPP 61 mm Hg; primary care provider notified. Dopamine drip increased to 8 μg/kg/min. Insertion site with small amount of serosanguineous drainage.

—B. Traudes, RN

DEVELOPING CLINICAL REASONING AND CLINICAL JUDGMENT

UNEXPECTED SITUATIONS AND ASSOCIATED INTERVENTIONS

- *ICP exceeds established parameters:* Notify the health care team immediately. If no parameter is specified, notify the health care team if ICP is >20 to 25 mm Hg (Hickey & Strayer, 2020; Morton & Fontaine, 2018).
- *Fiberoptic catheter is accidentally dislodged:* Notify the health care team immediately. Put on sterile gloves and cover the site with sterile gauze. Observe for any CSF leakage from the site.
- *Waveforms are not changing with procedures known to cause an increase in the ICP (e.g., suctioning):* The fiberoptic catheter may be damaged. Check the manufacturer's instructions for troubleshooting. Notify the health care team.
- *CSF is leaking from insertion site:* Notify the health care team. CSF is a prime medium for bacteria, and leakage can lead to an infection. Follow the facility's policy. Some facilities may have the nurse apply a sterile dressing around the insertion site; others may require more frequent cleansing of the area.

SPECIAL CONSIDERATIONS

- Label and secure the catheters according to facility policy after insertion and use care when moving patients to prevent dislodgement and breakage.
- Repositioning is important to prevent skin alterations and to decrease the risks associated with immobility. Modest, initial increases in ICP experienced with repositioning quickly return to baseline after repositioning is complete (McNett & Olson, 2013). Turn and position the patient in proper body alignment, avoiding angulation of body parts. Extreme hip flexion or flexion of the upper legs can increase intraabdominal pressure, leading to increased ICP. Maintain the neck in the neutral position at all times to avoid neck vein compression, which can interfere with venous return (Hickey & Strayer, 2020).
- Maintain the head of the bed elevated 30 degrees to promote venous return from the brain, depending on the prescribed intervention and facility procedure (AACN, 2017; Hickey & Strayer, 2020).
- Limit endotracheal suctioning episodes to one to two passes of the catheter (Hickey & Strayer, 2020). The ICP increases associated with suctioning, tracheal stimulation, and coughing are modest and transient (McNett & Olson, 2013).
- Oral care is a safe intervention; ICP increases experienced with oral care are modest, transient, and resolve quickly when oral care is complete (McNett & Olson, 2013).
- Auditory stimulation for critically ill neurologically impaired patients does not increase ICP and is considered a safe intervention (McNett & Olson, 2013).
- Plan care to avoid grouping activities and procedures known to increase ICP. Bathing, turning, and other routine care often have a cumulative effect to increase ICP when performed in succession. Allow rest periods between procedures and carefully assess the patient's response to interventions (Hickey & Strayer, 2020).

Enhance Your Understanding

Focusing on Patient Care: Developing Clinical Reasoning and Clinical Judgment

Consider the case scenarios at the beginning of the chapter as you answer the following questions to enhance your understanding and apply what you have learned.

QUESTIONS

1. Alcta Jackson, age 68, was involved in a head-on collision. She has begun to report that the cervical collar is hurting her neck. How should you address this issue?

2. Yuka Chong has not had a seizure since being diagnosed with epilepsy. Her mothers seem anxious and fearful and have a lot of questions and concerns about what to do if Yuka has a seizure. What information should be included in teaching for Yuka's mothers?

What safety interventions are appropriate to prevent potential injury during a seizure? How will the mothers know when it is necessary to call for emergency assistance related to a seizure?

3. Mr. and Mrs. Gladstone ask about "the tube coming out of Nikki's head," referring to her ventriculostomy. What should you tell them regarding the ventriculostomy? What should be included in the teaching for her parents? What guidelines regarding positioning and turning Nikki should you keep in mind when caring for her?

You can find suggested answers after the Bibliography at the end of this chapter.

Integrated Case Study Connection

The case studies in the back of the book focus on integrating concepts. Refer to the following case studies to enhance your understanding of the concepts and skills in this chapter.

- Intermediate Case Studies: Kent Clark, page 1217.

Bibliography

Abbariao, M. (2018). Can pin-site infection be prevented? *KaiTiaki Nursing New Zealand, 24*(9), 27–29.

Almojuela, A., Hasen, M., & Zeiler, F. A. (2018). The full outline of UnResponsiveness (FOUR) score and its use in outcome prediction: A scoping systematic review of the adult literature. *Neurocritical Care, 31*(1), 162–175. https://doi.org/10.1007/s12028-018-0630-9

American Association of Neuroscience Nurses (AANN). (2016). Care of adults and children with seizures and epilepsy: AANN clinical practice guideline series. https://apps.aann.org/store/product-details?productId=192053329

American Association of Critical-Care Nurses (AACN). (2017). In D. L. Wiegand (Ed.), *AACN procedure manual for high acuity, progressive, and critical care* (7th ed.). Elsevier.

Andrews, M., Boyle, J. S., & Collins, J. (2020). *Transcultural concepts in nursing care* (8th ed.). Wolters Kluwer.

Baranoski, S., & Ayello, E. A. (2020). *Wound care essentials. Practice principles* (5th ed.). Wolters Kluwer.

Buelow, J., Miller, W., & Fishman, F. (2018). Development of an epilepsy nursing communication tool: Improving the quality of interactions between nurses and patients with seizures. *Journal of Neuroscience Nursing, 50*(2), 74–80. https://doi.org/10.1097/JNN.0000000000000353

Burns, S. M., & Delgado, S. A. (2019). *AACN Essentials of critical care nursing* (4th ed.). McGraw Hill Education.

Cam, R., & Korkmaz, F. D. (2014). The effect of long-term care and follow-up on complications in patients with external fixators. *International Journal of Nursing Practice, 20*(1), 89–96. https://doi.org/10.1111/ijn.12126

Camacho-Del Rio, G. (2018). Evidence-based practice: Medical device-related pressure injury prevention. *American Nurse Today, 13*(10), 50–52.

Centers for Disease Control and Prevention (CDC). (2020a, September 30). *Epilepsy. About epilepsy. Types of seizures.* https://www.cdc.gov/epilepsy/about/types-of-seizures.htm?CDC_AA_refVal=https%3A%2F%2Fwww.cdc.gov%2Fepilepsy%2Fbasics%2Ftypes-of-seizures.htm

Centers for Disease Control and Prevention (CDC). (2020b, September 30). *Epilepsy. About epilepsy.Seizure first aid.* https://www.cdc.gov/epilepsy/about/first-aid.htm

Cooper, K. L. (2013). Evidence-based prevention of pressure ulcers in the intensive care unit. *Critical Care Nurse, 33*(6), 57–66. https://doi.org/10.4037/ccn2013985

Derbyshire, J., & Hill, B. (2018). Performing neurological observations. *British Journal of Nursing, 27*(19), 1110–1114.

Elia, C., Huynh, K., Dong, F., & Miulli, D. (2018). Proper education on spinal orthotics: A way to minimize associated complications. *Journal of Trauma Nursing, 25*(1), 45–48. https://doi.org/10.1097/JTN.0000000000000341

Eliopoulos, C. (2018). *Gerontological nursing* (9th ed.). Wolters Kluwer.

El-Radhi, A. S. (2015). Management of seizures in children. *British Journal of Nursing, 24*(3), 152–155. https://doi.org/10.12968/bjon.2015.24.3.152

Epilepsy Foundation. (2014a). *What is a seizure.* https://www.epilepsy.com/learn/about-epilepsy-basics/what-seizure

Epilepsy Foundation. (2014b). *Seizure drills.* https://www.epilepsy.com/learn/managing-your-epilepsy/seizure-drills

Epilepsy Foundation. (2016). *Epilepsy Foundation My Seizure Diary.* https://www.epilepsy.com/living-epilepsy/epilepsy-foundation-my-seizure-diary

Epilepsy Foundation. (2020, June 10). *First aid for seizures—Stay, safe, side.* https://www.epilepsy.com/living-epilepsy/seizure-first-aid-and-safety/first-aid-seizures-stay-safe-side

European Pressure Ulcer Advisory Panel (EPUAP), National Pressure Injury Advisory Panel (NPIAP), and Pan Pacific Pressure Injury Alliance (PPPIA). Haesler, E. (Ed.). (2019). Prevention and treatment of pressure ulcers/injuries: Clinical Practice guideline. The international guideline. http://www.internationalguideline.com

Fowler, S. B., Hauck, M. J., Allport, S., & Dailidonis, R. (2021). Knowledge and fears of parents of children diagnosed with epilepsy. *Journal of Pediatric Nursing, 60*, 311–313. https://doi.org/10.1016/j.pedn.2021.08.008

Fumarola, S., Allaway, R., Callaghan, R., Collier, M., Downie, F., Geraghty, J., Kiernan, S., & Spratt, F. (2020). Overlooked and underestimated: Medical adhesive-related skin injuries. Best practice consensus document on prevention. *Journal of Wound Care, 29*(Suppl 3c), S1–S24. https://doi.org/10.12968/jowc.2020.29.Sup3c.S1

Georgiades, D. S. (2018). A systematic integrative review of pin site crusts. *Orthopaedic Nursing, 37*(1), 36–42. https://doi.org/10.1097/NOR.0000000000000416

Greenshields, S. (2019). An introduction to nursing children and young people with epilepsy. *British Journal of Nursing, 28*(17), 1115–1117. https://doi.org/10.12968/bjon.2019.28.17.1115

Haertel, S. R. (2019). Cervical spine collars. *Orthopaedic Nursing, 38*(6), 403–405. https://doi.org/10.1097/NOR.0000000000000612

Hepburn-Smith, M., Dynkevich, I., Spektor, M., Lord, A., Czeisler, B., & Lewis, A. (2016). Establishment of an external ventricular drain best practice guideline: The quest for a comprehensive, universal standard for external ventricular drain care. *Journal of Neuroscience Nursing, 48*(1), 54–65. https://doi.org/10.1097/JNN.0000000000000174

Hickey, J. V., & Strayer, A. L. (Eds.). (2020). *The clinical practice of neurological and neurosurgical nursing* (8th ed.). Wolters Kluwer.

Hinkle, J. L., Cheever, K. H., & Overbaugh, K. (2022). *Brunner & Suddarth's Textbook of medical-surgical nursing* (15th ed.). Wolters Kluwer.

Hockenberry, M. J., & Wilson, D, & Rodgers, C. C. (2019). *Wong's nursing care of infants and children* (11th ed.). Elsevier.

Humphrey, E. (2018). Caring for neurosurgical patients with external ventricular drains. *Nursing Times* [online], *114*(4), 52–56. https://www.nursingtimes.net/clinical-archive/neurology/caring-for-neurosurgical-patients-with-external-ventricular-drains-26-03-2018/

International Council of Nurses (ICN). (2019). *Nursing diagnosis and outcome statements.* https://www.icn.ch/sites/default/files/inline-files/ICNP2019-DC.pdf

Iyer, V. N., Mandrekar, J. N., Danielson, R. D., Zubkov, A. Y., Elmer, J. L., & Wijdicks, E. F. (2009). Validity of the FOUR score coma scale in the medical intensive care unit. *Mayo Clinic Proceedings, 84*(8), 694–701.

Jalali, R., & Rezaei, M. (2014). A comparison of the Glasgow coma scale score with full outline of unresponsiveness scale to predict patients' traumatic brain injury outcomes in intensive care units. *Critical Care Research and Practice. 2014*, 289803. https://doi.org/10.1155/2014/289803

Jarvis, C., & Echkardt, A. (2020). *Physical examination & health assessment* (8th ed.). Elsevier.

Jensen, S. (2019). *Nursing health assessment: A best practice approach* (3rd ed.). Wolters Kluwer.

Kavanagh, F. A., Heaton, P. S., Cannon, A., & Paul, S. P. (2018). Recognition and management of febrile convulsions in children. *British Journal of Nursing, 27*(20), 1156–1162. https://doi.org/10.12968/bjon.2018.27.20.1156

Kazmers, N. H., Fragomen, A. T., & Rozbruch, S. R. (2016). Prevention of pin site infection in external fixation: A review of the literature. *Strategies in Trauma and Limb Reconstruction, 11*, 75–85. https://doi.org/10.1007/s11751-016-0256-4

Kocak, Y., Ozturk, S., Ege, F., & Ekmekci, H. (2012). A useful new coma scale in acute stroke patients: FOUR score. *Anaesthesia and Intensive Care, 40*(1), 131–136. https://doi.org/10.1177/0310057X1204000115

Ktistakis, I., Guerado, E., & Giannoudis, P. V. (2015). Pin-site care: Can we reduce the incidence of infections? *Injury, 46*(Suppl 3), S35–S39. https://doi.org/10.1016/S0020-1383(15)30009-7

Kyle, T., & Carman, S. (2021). *Essentials of pediatric nursing* (4th ed.). Wolters Kluwer.

Lacey, L., Palokas, M., & Walker, J. (2019). Preventative interventions, protocols or guidelines for trauma patients at risk of cervical collar-related pressure ulcers: A scoping review. *JBI Database of Systematic Reviews & Implementation Reports, 17*(12), 2452–2475. https://doi.org/10.11124/JBISRIR-2017-003872

Lagerquist, D., Dabrowski, M., Dock, C., Fox, A., Daymond, M., Sandau, K. E., & Halm, M. (2012). Care of external fixator pin sites. *American Journal of Critical Care, 21*(4), 288–292. https://doi.org/10.4037/ajcc2012600

Lawal, M., Omobayo, H., & Lawal., K. (2018). Epilepsy: Pathophysiology, clinical manifestations and treatment options. *British Journal of Neuroscience Nursing, 14*(2), 58–72. https://doi.org/10.12968/bjnn.2018.14.2.58

Lepkowski, A. M., & Maughan, E. D. (2018). Introducing NASN's new evidence-based clinical guideline. Students with Seizures and Epilepsy. *NASN School Nurse, 33*(6), 345–350. https://doi.org/10.1177/1942602X18806824

Lepkowski, A. M., & Maughan, E. D. (2019). School nursing evidence-based clinical practice guideline: Students with Seizures and Epilepsy. https://www.pathlms.com/nasn/courses/8992

Lethaby, A., Temple, J., & Santy Tomlinson, J. (2013). Pin site care for preventing infections associated with external bone fixators and pins. *The Cochrane Database of Systematic Reviews, 3*(12), CD004551. https://doi.org/10.1002/14651858.CD004551.pub3

Mayo Foundation for Medical Education and Research (MFMER). (2021a, May 25). Spinal injury: First aid. https://www.mayoclinic.org/first-aid/first-aid-spinal-injury/basics/art-20056677

Mayo Foundation for Medical Education and Research (MFMER). (2021b, February 24). *Seizures.* https://www.mayoclinic.org/diseases-conditions/seizure/symptoms-causes/syc-20365711

McCallum, C., & Leonard, M. (2013). The connection between neurosciences and dialysis: A quick neurological assessment for hemodialysis nurses. *CANNT Journal, 23*(3), 20–26.

McNett, M. M., & Olson, D. M. (2013). Evidence to guide nursing interventions for critically ill neurologically impaired patients with ICP monitoring. *Journal of Neuroscience Nursing, 45*(3), 120–123. https://doi.org/10.1097/JNN.0b013e3182901f0a

Millichap, J. J. (2018). *Treatment and prognosis of febrile seizures.* UpToDate. https://www.uptodate.com/contents/treatment-and-prognosis-of-febrile-seizures?search=febrile%20seizure&topicRef=6183&source=see_link

Montgomery, N., & Goode, D. (2014). Managing patients with cervical spine injury. *Emergency Nurse, 22*(2), 18–22. https://doi.org/10.7748/en2014.04.22.2.18.e1216

Morton, P. G., & Fontaine, D. K. (2018). *Critical care nursing: A holistic approach* (11th ed.). Wolters Kluwer.

Munakomi, S., & Das, J. M. (2021, August 9). *Ventriculostomy.* StatPearls. https://www.ncbi.nlm.nih.gov/books/NBK545317

Neurosurgery Education and Outreach Network (NEON). (2018). *Nursing care and management of a patient with a halo device.* https://criticalcareontario.ca/wp-content/uploads/2020/10/NEON_Halo_Device_-Booklet_Dec.28_-2018_FINAL.pdf

Norris, T. L. (2020). *Porth's essentials of pathophysiology* (5th ed.). Wolters Kluwer.

Okamura, K. (2014). Glasgow Coma Scale flow chart: A beginner's guide. *British Journal of Nursing, 23*(20), 1068–1073. https://doi.org/10.12968/bjon.2014.23.20.1068

Pittman, J., & Gillespie, C. (2020). Medical device-related pressure injuries. *Critical Care Nursing Clinics of North America, 32*(4), 533–542. https://doi.org/10.1016/j.cnc.2020.08.004

Problem-based care plans. (2022). In *Lippincott Advisor.* Wolters Kluwer. https://advisor.lww.com/lna/home.do

Sadaka, F., Patel, D., & Lakshmanan, R. (2012). The FOUR score predicts outcome in patients after traumatic brain injury. *Neurocritical Care, 16*(1), 95–101.

Sáenz-Jalón, M., Sarabia-Cobo, C. M., Bartolome, E. R., Fernández, M. S., Vélez, B., Escudero, M., Miguel, M. E., Artabe, P., Cabañas, I., Fernández, A., Garcés, C., & Couceiro, J. (2020). A randomized clinical trial on the use of antiseptic solutions for the pin-site care of external fixators: Chlorhexidine-alcohol versus povidone-iodine. *Journal of Trauma Nursing, 27*(3), 146–150. https://doi.org/10.1097/JTN.0000000000000503

Silbert-Flagg, J., & Pillitteri, A. (2018). *Maternal and child health nursing* (8th ed.). Wolters Kluwer.

Smith, G., Wagner, J. L., & Edwards, J. C. (2015). Epilepsy update, part 2: Nursing care and evidence-based treatment. *American Journal of Nursing, 115*(6), 34–44. https://doi.org/10.1097/01.NAJ.0000466314.46508.00

Taylor, C., Lynn, P., & Bartlett, J. (2023). *Fundamentals of nursing: The art and science of person-centered care* (10th ed.). Wolters Kluwer.

Timms, A., & Pugh, H. (2012). Pin site care: Guidance and key recommendations. *Nursing Standard, 27*(1), 50–55. https://doi.org/10.7748/ns2012.09.27.1.50.c9271

VHA Center for Engineering & Occupational Safety and Health (CEOSH). (2016). Safe patient handling and mobility guidebook. http://www.tnpatientsafety.com/pubfiles/Initiatives/workplace-violence/sphm-pdf.pdf

Walker, J. A., Scammell, B. E., & Bayston, R. (2018). A web-based survey to identify current practice in skeletal pin site management. *International Wound Journal, 15*(2), 250–257. https://doi.org/10.1111/iwj.12858

Wang, H. R. N., Campbell, J., Doubrovsky, A., Singh, V., Collins, J., & Coyer, F. (2020). Pressure injury development in critically ill patients with a cervical collar in situ: A retrospective longitudinal study. *International Wound Journal, 17*(4), 944–956. https://doi.org/10.1111/iwj.13363

Wijdicks, E. F., Bamlet, W. R., Maramattom, B. V., Manno, E. M., & McClelland, R. L. (2005) Validation of a new coma scale: The FOUR score. *Annals of Neurology, 58*(4), 585–593. https://doi.org/10.1002/ana.20611

World Health Organization (WHO). (2017). *Fact sheets. Epilepsy.* https://www.who.int/news-room/fact-sheets/detail/epilepsy

Zappa, S., Fagoni, N., Bertoni, M., Selleri, C., Venturini, M. A., Finazzi, P., Metelli, M., Rasulo, F., Piva, S., & Latronico, N. (2020). Determination of imminent brain death using the full outline of unresponsiveness score and the Glasgow Coma Scale: A prospective, multicenter, pilot feasibility study. *Journal of Intensive Care medicine, 35*(2), 203–207. https://doi.org/10.1177/0885066617738714

SUGGESTED ANSWERS FOR FOCUSING ON PATIENT CARE: DEVELOPING CLINICAL REASONING AND CLINICAL JUDGMENT

1. Check the fit and placement of the collar. The center of the collar should line up with the center of the patient's neck. Center the front of the collar over the patient's chin, ensuring that the chin area fits snugly in the recess of the collar. Be sure that the front half of the collar overlaps the back half. Check to see that at least one finger can be inserted between collar and patient's neck. Check the skin under the cervical collar for any signs of skin breakdown. Have a second person immobilize the cervical spine. Remove the top half of the collar and cleanse the skin under the collar. Assess the skin for signs of irritation and/or breakdown. If not contraindicated, place the patient in the reverse Trendelenburg position to see if this helps. After replacing the collar, assess the tightness of the cervical collar; at least one finger should slide under the collar.

2. Patient and family/caregiver education should include not only important information related to epilepsy and patient care, but encouragement and support for the patient and family/caregiver as well. Provide the following in discussions with Yuka and her mothers: Provide education regarding prescribed medications, including administration, potential side effects, and the importance of not running out of medication (El-Radhi, 2015). Yuka and her mothers should be encouraged to keep a seizure diary (El-Radhi, 2015). Suggest that Yuka and her mothers have periodic "seizure drills" to practice what every family member/caregiver should do if Yuka has a seizure (Epilepsy Foundation, 2014b, 2020). Provide information regarding the actions to take if Yuka has a seizure. Encourage supervision during bathing, swimming, ambulation, or other potentially hazardous activities

(Kyle & Carman, 2021). Encourage regular sleep and avoidance of fatigue (El-Radhi, 2015; Kyle & Carman, 2021; Smith et al., 2015). Emergency assistance should be obtained for multiple or prolonged (>5 minutes in duration) seizures; if Yuka has trouble breathing or waking after a seizure; if Yuka has one seizure soon after the first one; or if Yuka is injured during the seizure (CDC, 2020b). Provide information about support groups for Yuka, her mothers and families dealing with a diagnosis of epilepsy. Inform Yuka and her mothers that Yuka should wear a medical alert bracelet.

3. Include the following in discussions with the patient and her family/caregiver: Explain what a ventriculostomy is, the rationale for placing it, and how it helps with the patient's care. Answer any questions they may have regarding the equipment. When positioning and turning the patient, be aware of the location of the ventriculostomy and attached tubing. Ensure that the tubing is not kinked or obstructed by the activity.

After positioning the patient, reassess the height of the system to ensure that the location of the stopcock remains at the appropriate reference point: the tragus of the ear, the outer canthus of the patient's eye, or the patient's external auditory canal (AACN, 2017). Turn and position the patient in proper body alignment, avoiding angulation of body parts. Avoid extreme hip flexion or flexion of the upper legs, which can increase intraabdominal pressure, leading to increased ICP. Maintain the neck in a neutral position at all times to avoid neck vein compression, which can interfere with venous return (Hickey & Strayer, 2020). Keep the head of the bed elevated at 30 degrees to promote venous return from the brain, depending on prescribed interventions and facility procedure (AACN, 2017; Hickey & Strayer, 2020). Bathing, turning, and other routine care often have a cumulative effect to increase ICP when performed in succession. Allow rest periods between procedures and carefully assess the patient's response to interventions (Hickey & Strayer, 2020).

18

Laboratory Specimen Collection

Focusing on Patient Care

This chapter will help you develop some of the skills related to collecting specimens of body fluids when caring for the following patients:

Joseph Conklin, age 90, has been admitted to the hospital due to confusion related to a suspected urinary tract infection. You are to obtain a urine specimen for urinalysis and culture.

Huana Yon, age 67, has made an appointment to see her health care provider for a yearly examination. She is to collect a stool specimen for occult blood testing.

Catherine Yeletsky, age 54, is a patient in the telemetry unit. She has been diagnosed with heart failure and is receiving cardiac monitoring. Ms. Yeletsky also has diabetes and requires peripheral capillary (fingerstick) blood sampling to monitor her blood glucose levels.

Refer to Focusing on Patient Care: Developing Clinical Reasoning and Clinical Judgment at the end of the chapter to apply what you learn.

Learning Outcomes

After completing the chapter, you will be able to accomplish the following:

1. Obtain a nasal swab.
2. Obtain a nasopharyngeal swab.
3. Collect a sputum specimen (expectorated) for culture.
4. Obtain a urine specimen (clean catch, midstream).
5. Obtain a urine specimen from an indwelling urinary catheter.
6. Test a stool specimen for occult blood.
7. Collect a stool specimen.
8. Obtain a capillary blood sample for glucose testing.
9. Collect a venous blood specimen by venipuncture for routine laboratory testing.
10. Obtain a venous blood specimen for culture and sensitivity.
11. Obtain an arterial blood specimen for blood gas analysis.
12. Obtain a blood specimen from a central venous access device
13. Obtain a blood specimen from an arterial catheter.

Nursing Concepts

- Assessment
- Clinical Decision Making/Clinical Judgment
- Safety

Laboratory specimens are collected to aid in the screening and diagnosing of patient health problems, in directing treatment, and in monitoring the treatment effectiveness. Blood, urine, and stool samples are commonly collected types of specimens. Follow facility **protocol** to collect, handle, and transport specimens. Always observe **Standard Precautions** (refer to Fundamentals Review 1-3 in Chapter 1) and **Transmission-Based Precautions** (as indicated) (refer to Fundamentals Review 1-4 in Chapter 1) and use **sterile technique** where appropriate. It is very important to adhere to protocols, best practice guidelines and standards, collect the appropriate amount, use appropriate containers and media, and store and transfer the specimen within specified timelines. It is also extremely important to ensure accurate labeling of any specimen collected, according to facility policy. These measures prevent invalid and inaccurate test results.

Patient teaching is an important part of specimen collection. Explain the rationale for the sample collection and the process for obtaining the specimen. Evaluate the patient's ability to follow the specific procedure for collecting the specimen.

When collecting a specimen, take care to prevent the outside of the container from becoming contaminated with any secretions or body fluids. Place all laboratory specimens in plastic bags marked "Biohazard" and seal the bags to prevent leakage during transportation.

This chapter reviews methods to obtain specimens for common laboratory and diagnostic tests. Nurses must also be knowledgeable about normal and abnormal findings associated with these laboratory tests. Fundamentals Review 18-1 and 18-2 highlight the normal findings associated with urine and stool specimens. Refer to Appendix C for identification of normal adult values for common laboratory tests.

Fundamentals Review 18-1

CHARACTERISTICS OF URINE

Characteristic	Normal Findings	Special Considerations
Color	A freshly voided specimen is pale yellow, straw-colored, or amber, depending on its concentration.	Urine is darker than normal when it is scanty and concentrated. Urine is lighter than normal when it is excessive and diluted. Certain drugs, such as cascara, L-dopa, and sulfonamides, alter the color of urine. Some foods can alter the color; for example, beets can cause urine to appear red in color.
Odor	Normal urine smell is aromatic. As urine stands, it often develops an ammonia odor because of bacterial action.	Some foods cause urine to have a characteristic odor; for example, asparagus causes urine to have a strong, musty odor. Urine high in glucose content has a sweet odor. Urine that is heavily infected has a fetid odor.
Turbidity	Fresh urine should be clear or translucent; as urine stands and cools, it becomes cloudy.	Cloudiness observed in freshly voided urine is abnormal and may be due to the presence of red blood cells, white blood cells, bacteria, vaginal discharge, sperm, or prostatic fluid.
pH	The normal pH is about 6.0, with a range of 4.6 to 8. (Urine alkalinity or acidity may be promoted through diet to inhibit bacterial growth or urinary stone development or to facilitate the therapeutic activity of certain medications.) Urine becomes alkaline on standing when carbon dioxide diffuses into the air.	A high-protein diet causes urine to become excessively acidic. Certain foods tend to produce alkaline urine, such as citrus fruits, dairy products, and vegetables, especially legumes. Certain foods, such as meats, tend to produce acidic urine. Certain drugs influence the acidity or alkalinity of urine; for example, ammonium chloride produces acidic urine, and potassium citrate and sodium bicarbonate produce alkaline urine.

(continued)

Fundamentals Review 18-1 continued

CHARACTERISTICS OF URINE

Characteristic	Normal Findings	Special Considerations
Specific gravity	This is a measure of the concentration of dissolved solids in the urine. The normal range is 1.015 to 1.025.	Concentrated urine will have a higher-than-normal specific gravity, and diluted urine will have a lower-than-normal specific gravity. In the absence of kidney disease, a high specific gravity usually indicates dehydration, and a low specific gravity indicates overhydration.
Constituents	*Organic* constituents of urine include urea, uric acid, creatinine, hippuric acid, indican, urine pigments, and undetermined nitrogen. *Inorganic* constituents are ammonia, sodium, chloride, traces of iron, phosphorus, sulfur, potassium, and calcium.	*Abnormal constituents* of urine include blood, pus, albumin, glucose, ketone bodies, casts, gross bacteria, and bile.

Fundamentals Review 18-2

CHARACTERISTICS OF STOOL

Characteristic	Normal Findings	Special Considerations for Observation
Volume	Variable	Volume of the stool depends on the amount the person eats and the nature of the diet. For example, a diet high in roughage produces more feces than a soft, bland diet. Consistently large diarrheal stools suggest a disorder in the small bowel or proximal colon; small, frequent stools with urgency to pass them suggest a disorder of the left colon or rectum.
Color	Infant: Yellow to brown Adult: Brown	The brown color of the stool is due to stercobilin, a bile pigment derivative. The rapid rate of peristalsis in the breastfed infant causes the stool to be yellow. Stool color is influenced by diet. For example, the stool will be almost black if the person eats red meat and dark green vegetables, such as spinach. The stool will be light brown if the diet is high in milk and milk products and low in meat. The absence of bile may cause the stool to appear white or clay colored. Certain drugs influence the color of the stool. For example, iron salts cause the stool to be black. Antacids cause it to be whitish. Bleeding high in the intestinal tract causes a stool to be black due to the digestion of the blood. Bleeding low in the intestinal tract results in fresh blood in the stool. The stool darkens with standing.
Odor	Pungent; may be affected by foods ingested.	The characteristic odor of the stool is due to **indole** and **skatole**, caused by putrefaction and fermentation in the lower intestinal tract. Stool odor is influenced by its pH value, which normally is neutral or slightly alkaline. Excessive putrefaction causes a strong odor. The presence of blood in the stool causes a unique odor.

Fundamentals Review 18-2 continued

CHARACTERISTICS OF STOOL

Characteristic	Normal Findings	Special Considerations for Observation
Consistency	Soft, semisolid, and formed	Stool consistency is influenced by fluid and food intake and gastric motility. The less time stool spends in the intestine (or the shorter the intestine), the more liquid the stool. Many pathologic conditions influence consistency.
Shape	Formed stool is usually about 1 inch (2.5 cm) in diameter and has the tubular shape of the colon, but may be larger or smaller, depending on the condition of the colon.	A gastrointestinal obstruction may result in a narrow, pencil-shaped stool. Rapid peristalsis thins the stool. Increased time spent in the large intestine may result in a hard, marble-like fecal mass.
Constituents	Waste residues of digestion: bile, intestinal secretions, shed epithelial cells, bacteria, and inorganic material (chiefly calcium and phosphates); seeds, meat fibers, and fat may be present in small amounts.	Internal bleeding, infection, inflammation, and other pathologic conditions may result in abnormal constituents. These include blood, pus, excessive fat, parasites, ova, and mucus. Foreign bodies also may be found in the stool.

Skill 18-1 ▶ Obtaining a Nasal Swab

A nasal swab provides a sample of cells from the nostril that can be cultured, which can aid in the detection of viruses and bacteria that cause respiratory infections, such as influenza, COVID-19, and respiratory syncytial virus (RSV) (MedlinePlus, 2021a). A nasal swab can be part of the screening process to detect infection with drug-resistant microorganisms, such as methicillin-resistant *Staphylococcus aureus* (MRSA) (MedlinePlus, 2021a), and coronavirus testing (CDC, 2019c).

DELEGATION CONSIDERATIONS

Obtaining a nasal swab is not delegated to assistive personnel (AP). Depending on the state's nurse practice act and the organization's policies and procedures, this procedure may be delegated to licensed practical/vocational nurses (LPN/LVNs). The decision to delegate must be based on careful analysis of the patient's needs and circumstances as well as the qualifications of the person to whom the task is being delegated. Refer to the Delegation Guidelines in Appendix A.

EQUIPMENT

- Nasal swab
- Sterile water (optional)
- Nonsterile gloves
- Goggles and face mask, or face shield
- Additional PPE, as indicated
- Biohazard bag
- Appropriate label for specimen, based on facility policy and procedure

ASSESSMENT

Assess the patient's understanding of the collection procedure, the reason for testing, and their ability to engage in care. Inspect the patient's **nares** and for the presence of nasal symptoms, such as discharge, erythema, or congestion. Assess for conditions that would contraindicate obtaining a nasal swab, such as injury to the nares or nose, and surgery of the nose.

ACTUAL OR POTENTIAL HEALTH PROBLEMS AND NEEDS

Many actual or potential health problems or issues may require the use of this skill as part of related interventions. An appropriate health problem or issue may include:
- Infection risk
- Acute pain
- Knowledge deficiency

(continued on page 1118)

Skill 18-1 ▶ Obtaining a Nasal Swab *(continued)*

OUTCOME IDENTIFICATION AND PLANNING

The expected outcomes to achieve are that an uncontaminated specimen is obtained without injury to the patient and sent to the laboratory promptly. Additional outcomes that may be appropriate include that the patient verbalizes an understanding of the rationale for and the steps of the procedure.

IMPLEMENTATION

ACTION	RATIONALE
1. Verify the prescribed intervention for a nasal swab in the patient's health record. Gather equipment. Check the expiration date on the swab package.	Verifying the prescribed intervention is crucial for ensuring that the proper procedure is administered to the right patient. Assembling equipment provides for an organized approach to the task. The swab package is sterile and should not be used past the expiration date.
2. Perform hand hygiene and put on PPE, if indicated.	Hand hygiene and PPE prevent the transmission of microorganisms. PPE is required based on transmission precautions.
3. Identify the patient.	Identifying the patient ensures the right patient receives the intervention and helps prevent errors.
4. Explain the procedure to the patient. Discuss with the patient the need for a nasal swab. Explain to the patient the process by which the specimen will be collected.	Discussion and explanation help to allay some of the patient's anxiety and prepare the patient for what to expect.
5. Check the specimen label with the patient identification bracelet. The label should include the patient's name and identification number, the time the specimen was collected, the route of collection, identification of the person obtaining the sample, and any other information required by facility policy.	Confirmation of patient identification information ensures the specimen is labeled correctly for the right patient.
6. Assemble equipment on the overbed table or other surface within reach.	Arranging items nearby is convenient, saves time, and avoids unnecessary stretching and twisting of muscles on the part of the nurse.
7. Close the curtains around the bed or close the door to the room, if possible.	Closing the door or curtain provides for patient privacy.
8. Put on goggles, a face mask or face shield, and nonsterile gloves.	Goggles, a face mask or face shield, and gloves protect the nurse from exposure to blood or body fluids and prevent the transmission of microorganisms. Irritation to the nose during collection with the nasal swab may cause the patient to sneeze or cough.
9. Place the bed at an appropriate and comfortable working height (VHACEOSH, 2016). Ask the patient to tip their head back slightly. Assist, as necessary.	Having the bed at the proper height prevents back and muscle strain. Tilting the head allows optimal access to the nares, which is where the swab will be inserted.
10. Peel open the swab kit packaging to expose the swab and collection tube. Remove the white plug from the collection tube and discard. Remove the swab from the packaging by grasping the exposed end. Take care not to contaminate the swab by touching it to any other surface. Moisten with sterile water, depending on facility policy.	The swab must remain sterile to ensure the specimen is not contaminated. Moistening the end of the swab minimizes discomfort to the patient.
11. Insert the swab 1.5 cm into one **naris** (Figure 1) and rotate it against the anterior nasal mucosa at least four times for a total of 15 seconds (CDC, 2019; MedlinePlus, 2021a).	Contact with the mucosa is necessary to obtain potential pathogens.

ACTION

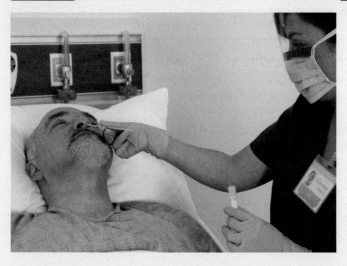

FIGURE 1. Inserting nasal swab into naris.

12. Remove the swab and repeat in the second naris, using the same swab.

13. Insert the swab fully into the collection tube, taking care not to touch any other surface. The handle end of the swab should fit snugly into the collection tube, and the end of the swab should be in the culture medium at the distal end of the collection tube. Lightly squeeze the bottom of the collection tube as necessary, depending on the type of tube in use in the facility, to break the seal on the culture medium.

14. Dispose of used equipment per facility policy. Remove gloves. Perform hand hygiene.

15. Place a label on the collection tube per facility policy. Place the container in a plastic, sealable biohazard bag.

16. Remove the face shield and other PPE, if used. Perform hand hygiene.

17. Transport specimen to the laboratory immediately. If immediate transport is not possible, check with laboratory personnel or the policy manual to see whether refrigeration is contraindicated.

RATIONALE

Repeating in the second naris ensures accurate specimen.

The swab must remain uncontaminated to ensure accurate results. Full insertion of the swab ensures it will remain in the collection tube. Placement of the swab end in culture medium and releasing the liquid transport medium are necessary to ensure accurate specimen processing.

Proper disposal of equipment reduces the transmission of microorganisms. Removing gloves properly reduces the risk for infection transmission and contamination of other items. Hand hygiene reduces the transmission of microorganisms.

This ensures the specimen is labeled correctly for the right patient and ensures proper processing of the specimen. Packaging the specimen in a biohazard bag prevents the person transporting the container from coming in contact with the specimen.

Proper removal of PPE reduces the risk for infection transmission and contamination of other items. Hand hygiene reduces the transmission of microorganisms.

Timely transport ensures accurate results.

EVALUATION

The expected outcomes have been met when an uncontaminated specimen has been obtained without injury to the patient and sent to the laboratory promptly, and the patient has verbalized an understanding of the rationale for and the steps of the procedure.

DOCUMENTATION

Guidelines

Record the time the specimen was collected and sent to the laboratory. Document any pertinent assessments of the patient's nares and the presence of nasal symptoms, such as discharge, erythema, or congestion.

(continued on page 1120)

Skill 18-1 ▶ Obtaining a Nasal Swab *(continued)*

Sample Documentation

> <u>8/21/25</u> 1545 Nasal swab collected and sent to the laboratory. Patient's nares noted to be patent without drainage, congestion, and erythema.
>
> —*S. Turner, RN*

DEVELOPING CLINICAL REASONING AND CLINICAL JUDGMENT

UNEXPECTED SITUATIONS AND ASSOCIATED INTERVENTIONS

- *Swab touches surface other than inner aspect of nares on entry or exit:* Discard the swab, obtain a new culture swab, and recollect the specimen.

SPECIAL CONSIDERATIONS

- If the patient has injury to the nares or nose or has had nose surgery, the nurse should contact the health care team to discuss collection of the specimen. These conditions may prohibit collection.

Skill 18-2 ▶ Obtaining a Nasopharyngeal Swab

A nasopharyngeal swab provides a sample that can be cultured to aid in the diagnosis of infection and to detect the carrier state for certain organisms. A swab on a flexible wire collects a specimen from the posterior **nasopharynx**. It can be used to detect viral and bacterial infections, including *Bordetella pertussis,* respiratory syncytial virus (RSV), *Neisseria meningitidis*, methicillin-resistant *Staphylococcus aureus*, influenza, and coronavirus (Higgins et al., 2020; MedlinePlus, 2021b).

DELEGATION CONSIDERATIONS

Obtaining a nasopharyngeal swab is not delegated to assistive personnel (AP). Depending on the state's nurse practice act and the organization's policies and procedures, this procedure may be delegated to licensed practical/vocational nurses (LPN/LVNs). The decision to delegate must be based on careful analysis of the patient's needs and circumstances as well as the qualifications of the person to whom the task is being delegated. Refer to the Delegation Guidelines in Appendix A.

EQUIPMENT

- Nasopharyngeal swab (flexible wire)
- Penlight
- Tongue depressor
- Facial tissue
- Nonsterile gloves
- Additional PPE, as indicated
- Biohazard bag
- Appropriate label for specimen, based on facility policy and procedure

ASSESSMENT

Assess the patient's understanding of the collection procedure, the reason for testing, and their ability to engage in care. Assess the patient's nares and for the presence of nasal symptoms, such as discharge, erythema, or congestion. Inspect the patient's nasopharynx. Assess for conditions that would contraindicate obtaining a nasopharyngeal swab, such as injury to the nares or nose, and surgery of the nose or throat.

ACTUAL OR POTENTIAL HEALTH PROBLEMS AND NEEDS

Many actual or potential health problems or issues may require the use of this skill as part of related interventions. An appropriate health problem or issue may include:
- Infection risk
- Acute pain
- Knowledge deficiency

OUTCOME IDENTIFICATION AND PLANNING	The expected outcomes to achieve are that an uncontaminated specimen is obtained without injury to the patient and sent to the laboratory promptly. Additional outcomes that may be appropriate include that the patient verbalizes an understanding of the rationale for and the steps of the procedure.

IMPLEMENTATION

ACTION	**RATIONALE**
1. Verify the prescribed intervention for a nasopharyngeal swab in the patient's health record. Gather equipment. Check the expiration date on the swab package.	Verifying the prescribed intervention is crucial for ensuring that the proper procedure is administered to the right patient. Assembling equipment provides for an organized approach to task. The swab package is sterile and should not be used past the expiration date.
2. Perform hand hygiene and put on PPE, if indicated.	Hand hygiene and PPE prevent the transmission of microorganisms. PPE is required based on transmission precautions.
3. Identify the patient.	Identifying the patient ensures the right patient receives the intervention and helps prevent errors.
4. Discuss with the patient the need for a nasopharyngeal swab. Explain the process by which the specimen will be collected. Inform the patient that they may experience discomfort and may gag but should not experience severe pain (Higgins et al., 2020).	Discussion and explanation help to allay some of the patient's anxiety and prepare the patient for what to expect.
5. Check the specimen label with the patient's identification bracelet. The label should include the patient's name and identification number, the time the specimen was collected, the route of collection, identification of person obtaining the sample, and any other information required by facility policy.	Confirmation of patient identification information ensures the specimen is labeled correctly for the right patient.
6. Assemble equipment on the overbed table or other surface within reach.	Arranging items nearby is convenient, saves time, and avoids unnecessary stretching and twisting of muscles on the part of the nurse.
7. Close the curtains around the bed or close the door to the room, if possible.	Closing the door or curtain provides for patient privacy.
8. Put on goggles, a face mask or face shield, and nonsterile gloves.	Goggles, a face mask or face shield, and gloves protect the nurse from exposure to blood or body fluids and prevent the transmission of microorganisms. Irritation to the nose and pharynx during collection with the nasal swab may cause the patient to sneeze or cough.
9. Place the bed at an appropriate and comfortable working height (VHACEOSH, 2016). Ask the patient to blow their nose into facial tissue. Ask the patient to cough into facial tissue, and then to tip back their head. Assist, as necessary.	Having the bed at the proper height prevents back and muscle strain. Blowing the nose clears nasal passages of excess mucus (CDC, 2019b), and coughing clears the nasopharynx of material that may interfere with accurate sampling. Tilting the head allows optimal access to the nares, where the swab will be inserted.
10. Peel open the swab packaging to expose the swab and collection tube. Remove the cap from the collection tube and discard. Remove the swab from packaging by grasping the exposed end. Take care not to contaminate the swab by touching it to any other surface.	The swab must remain sterile to ensure specimen is not contaminated.
11. Ask the patient to open their mouth. Inspect the back of the patient's throat using the tongue depressor.	The swab must make contact with the mucosa to ensure collection of potential pathogens.

(continued on page 1122)

Skill 18-2 ▶ Obtaining a Nasopharyngeal Swab *(continued)*

ACTION

12. Continue to observe the nasopharynx and gently insert the swab straight back into the nostril (parallel to the palate, not upward), aiming posteriorly along the floor of the nasal cavity (CDC, 2019e) (Figure 1A). Insert it approximately 9 to 10 cm (adult) (approximately the distance from the nose to the ear) to the posterior wall of the nasopharynx (CDC, 2019e; Higgins et al., 2020) (Figure 1B). **Do not insert the swab upward. Do not force the swab.** Rotate the swab. Leave the swab in the nasopharynx for several to 30 seconds and remove (CDC, 2019e; MedlinePlus, 2021b). Take care not to touch the swab to the sides of the nostrils.

RATIONALE

Observation of the nasopharynx during collection ensures an accurate specimen is collected. The swab must remain uncontaminated to ensure accurate results.

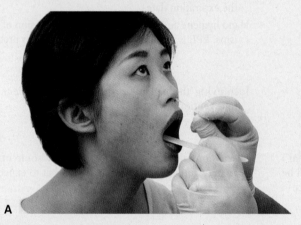
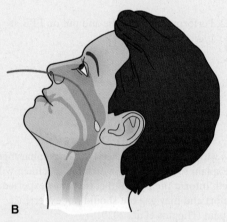

FIGURE 1. A. Observing the nasopharynx and inserting swab. **B.** Nasopharyngeal swab inserted to the posterior wall of the nasopharynx.

13. Insert the swab fully into the collection tube, taking care not to touch any other surface. The handle end of the swab should fit snugly into the collection tube, and the end of the swab should be in the culture medium at the distal end of the collection tube. Lightly squeeze the bottom of the collection tube as necessary, depending on the type of tube in use in the facility, to break the seal on the culture medium.

The swab must remain uncontaminated to ensure accurate results. Full insertion of the swab ensures it will remain in the collection tube. Placement of the swab end in culture medium and releasing of liquid transport medium is necessary to ensure accurate specimen processing.

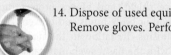 14. Dispose of used equipment per facility policy. Remove gloves. Perform hand hygiene.

Proper disposal of equipment reduces the transmission of microorganisms. Removing gloves properly reduces the risk for infection transmission and contamination of other items. Hand hygiene reduces the transmission of microorganisms.

15. Place a label on the collection tube per facility policy. Place the container in a plastic, sealable biohazard bag.

This ensures the specimen is labeled correctly for the right patient as well as proper processing of the specimen. Packaging the specimen in a biohazard bag prevents the person transporting the container from coming in contact with the specimen.

 16. Remove other PPE, if used. Perform hand hygiene.

Proper removal of PPE reduces the risk for infection transmission and contamination of other items. Hand hygiene reduces the transmission of microorganisms.

17. Transport the specimen to the laboratory immediately. If immediate transport is not possible, check with laboratory personnel or the policy manual to see whether refrigeration is contraindicated.

Timely transport ensures accurate results.

EVALUATION

The expected outcomes have been met when an uncontaminated specimen has been obtained without injury to the patient and sent to the laboratory promptly, and the patient has verbalized an understanding of the rationale for and the steps of the procedure.

DOCUMENTATION

Guidelines

Record the time the specimen was collected and sent to the laboratory. Document any pertinent assessments of the patient's nares and the presence of nasal symptoms, such as discharge, erythema, or congestion. Record significant assessments of the patient's oral cavity and throat.

Sample Documentation

> 8/21/25 1545 Nasopharyngeal swab specimen collected and sent to laboratory. Patient's nares noted to be patent without drainage, congestion, and erythema; nasopharynx bright red with tan discharge.
> —S. Turner, RN

DEVELOPING CLINICAL REASONING AND CLINICAL JUDGMENT

UNEXPECTED SITUATIONS AND ASSOCIATED INTERVENTIONS

- *Patient gags as soon as the tongue depressor is placed in their mouth:* Depress the tongue with the tongue depressor by pushing down halfway back on the tongue. Press slightly off center to avoid eliciting the gag reflex (Jarvis & Eckhardt, 2020).

SPECIAL CONSIDERATIONS

General Considerations

- Warn the patient that the procedure may cause slight discomfort.
- Caution the patient that the procedure may cause gagging.
- Do not force the swab. Forcing could cause injury. If an obstruction is encountered, try the other nostril (CDC, 2019b).
- If the patient has a deviated septum or nasal obstruction, contact the health care team to discuss collection of the specimen (CDC, 2019a). These conditions may prohibit collection.

Infant and Child Considerations

- A young child will require restraint so the nurse can depress the tongue and visualize the back of the mouth without injuring the child (Kyle & Carman, 2021).

Skill 18-3 ▶ Collecting a Sputum Specimen for Culture

Skill Variation: *Collecting a Sputum Specimen via Endotracheal Suctioning*

Sputum production is the result of the reaction of the lungs to any constant recurring irritant (Hinkle et al., 2022). A sputum specimen comes from deep within the bronchi, not from the post-nasal region. Sputum analysis is used to diagnose disease, test for drug sensitivity, and guide patient treatment. Sputum may be obtained to identify pathogenic organisms, determine if malignant cells are present, and assess for hypersensitivity states. A sputum specimen may be prescribed if a bacterial, viral, or fungal infection of the pulmonary system is suspected.

A sputum specimen can be collected by having the patient cough into a sterile container, by endotracheal suctioning, during bronchoscopy, and via transtracheal aspiration. Because secretions have accumulated during the night, it is desirable to collect an expectorated sputum specimen first thing in the morning when the patient rises, which aids in the collection process (Fischbach et al.,

(continued on page 1124)

Skill 18-3 ▶ Collecting a Sputum Specimen for Culture *(continued)*

2022; Hess et al., 2021). Characteristics of sputum and potential causes are outlined in Box 18-1. The following procedure describes collecting an expectorated sample. Collecting a sputum specimen by suctioning via an endotracheal tube is discussed in the Skill Variation at the end of this skill.

Box 18-1 Characteristics of Sputum and Potential Causes

Sputum Characteristic	Potential Cause
• Thick and yellow or green (purulent)	Bacterial infection
• Thin, white, or clear, mucoid (mucous)	Colds, viral infections, bronchitis
• Rust colored	Tuberculosis, pneumococcal pneumonia
• Gradual increase of sputum over time	Chronic bronchitis
• Pink-tinged, mucoid (mucous) sputum	Lung tumor, tuberculosis
• Profuse, frothy, pink sputum	Pulmonary edema
• Foul-smelling sputum and bad breath	Lung abscess, bronchiectasis, anaerobic infection

Source: Adapted from Hinkle, J. L., Cheever, K. H., & Overbaugh, K. (2022). *Brunner & Suddarth's Textbook of medical-surgical nursing* (15th ed.). Wolters Kluwer; Jarvis, C. (2020). *Physical examination and health assessment* (8th ed.). Elsevier; and Jensen, S. (2019). *Nursing health assessment: A best practice approach* (3rd ed.). Wolters Kluwer.

DELEGATION CONSIDERATIONS	Obtaining a sputum specimen is not delegated to assistive personnel (AP). Obtaining a sputum specimen may be delegated to licensed practical/vocational nurses (LPN/LVNs). The decision to delegate must be based on careful analysis of the patient's needs and circumstances as well as the qualifications of the person to whom the task is being delegated. Refer to the Delegation Guidelines in Appendix A.
EQUIPMENT	• Sterile sputum specimen container • Nonsterile gloves • Goggles or safety glasses or face shield • Additional PPE, as indicated • Biohazard bag • Appropriate label for specimen, based on facility policy and procedure
ASSESSMENT	Assess the patient's respiratory rate; rhythm and depth; and lung sounds. Patients with a productive cough may have increased respiratory effort and crackles, rhonchi, wheezing, or diminished lung sounds. Monitor oxygen saturation levels, as patients with excessive pulmonary secretions may have decreased oxygen saturation. Assess the patient's level of pain. Consider administering pain medication before obtaining the sample, because the patient will have to cough. Assess the characteristics of the sputum: color, quantity, presence of blood, and viscosity.
ACTUAL OR POTENTIAL HEALTH PROBLEMS AND NEEDS	Many actual or potential health problems or issues may require the use of this skill as part of related interventions. An appropriate health problem or issue may include: • Acute pain • Ineffective airway clearance • Impaired gas exchange
OUTCOME IDENTIFICATION AND PLANNING	The expected outcome to achieve when collecting a sputum specimen is that the patient produces an adequate sample (based on facility policy) from the lower respiratory tract. Other outcomes that may be appropriate include that airway patency is maintained, and the patient demonstrates an understanding about the need and process for specimen collection.

IMPLEMENTATION

ACTION

1. Verify the prescribed intervention for a sputum specimen collection in the patient's health record. Gather equipment.

2. Perform hand hygiene and put on PPE, if indicated.

3. Identify the patient.

4. Explain the procedure to the patient. Administer pain medication (if prescribed) if the patient might have pain with coughing. If the patient can perform the task without assistance after instruction, leave the container at the bedside with instructions to call the nurse as soon as a specimen is produced.

5. Check the specimen label with the patient's identification bracelet. The label should include the patient's name and identification number, the time the specimen was collected, the route of collection, identification of the person obtaining the sample, and any other information required by facility policy.

6. Assemble equipment on the overbed table or other surface within reach.

7. Close the curtains around the bed and close the door to the room, if possible.

8. Put on disposable gloves, goggles, and safety glasses or a face shield, as indicated.

9. Place the bed at an appropriate and comfortable working height (VHACEOSH, 2016). Lower the side rail closest to you. Place patient in the semi-Fowler position. **Have the patient clear their nose and throat and rinse their mouth with water before beginning the procedure.**

10. Caution the patient to avoid spitting saliva into the sterile container. Explain the importance of obtaining sputum from the lower respiratory tract. If the patient has had abdominal or thoracic surgery, assist the patient to splint the surgical site. **Instruct the patient to inhale deeply two or three times and forcefully cough with exhalation.**

11. If the patient produces sputum, open the lid to the container and have the patient **expectorate** the specimen into the container (Figure 1). Caution the patient to avoid touching the edge or the inside of the collection container.

RATIONALE

Verifying the prescribed intervention is crucial for ensuring that the proper procedure is administered to the right patient. Assembling equipment provides for an organized approach to the task.

Hand hygiene and PPE prevent the transmission of microorganisms. PPE is required based on transmission precautions.

Identifying the patient ensures the right patient receives the intervention and helps prevent errors.

Explanation provides reassurance and promotes engagement. Pain relief facilitates engagement in care.

Confirmation of patient identification information ensures the specimen is labeled correctly for the right patient.

Arranging items nearby is convenient, saves time, and avoids unnecessary stretching and twisting of muscles on the part of the nurse.

Closing the curtain or door provides for patient privacy.

Gloves and eye protection prevent contact with blood and body fluids. Eye protection may be indicated based on the patient's underlying health concerns and risk for contact with body fluids.

Having the bed at the proper height prevents back and muscle strain. The semi-Fowler position will help the patient to cough and expectorate the sputum specimen. Water will rinse the oral cavity of saliva and any food particles.

Saliva can contaminate the sputum specimen. The specimen will need to come from the lungs; saliva is not acceptable. Splinting helps to reduce the pain in the incision and surgical area.

The specimen needs to come from the lungs; saliva is not acceptable. Touching the edge or inside of the sterile collection container contaminates the specimen.

(continued on page 1126)

Skill 18-3 ▶ Collecting a Sputum Specimen for Culture *(continued)*

ACTION

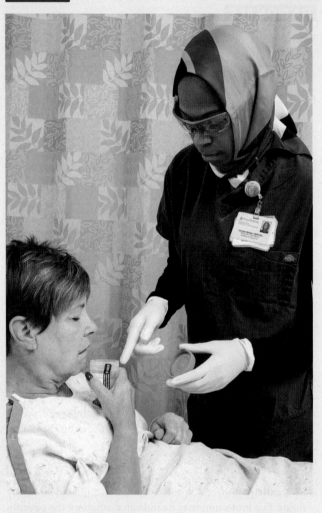

FIGURE 1. Instructing patient to expectorate into the collection container.

12. If the patient believes they can produce more sputum for the specimen, have them repeat the procedure. Collect a volume of sputum based on facility policy.

13. Close the container lid. Offer oral hygiene to the patient. Remove your gloves and goggles. Perform hand hygiene.

14. Remove equipment and return the patient to a position of comfort. Raise the side rails and lower the bed.

15. Place a label on the container per facility policy (Figure 2). Place the container in a plastic, sealable biohazard bag (Figure 3).

16. Remove other PPE, if used. Perform hand hygiene.

RATIONALE

This ensures an adequate amount of sputum specimen is obtained for analysis; 1 to 3 mL is sufficient for most examinations (Fischbach et al., 2022).

Closing the container prevents contamination of the specimen and possible infection transmission. Oral hygiene helps to remove pathogens from the oral cavity. Removing gloves and goggles properly reduces the risk for infection transmission and contamination of other items. Hand hygiene reduces the transmission of microorganisms.

Repositioning promotes patient comfort. Raising the rails promotes safety.

Proper labeling of the specimen ensures the specimen is for the right patient. Packaging the specimen in a biohazard bag prevents the person transporting the container from coming in contact with the specimen.

Proper removal of PPE reduces the risk for infection transmission and contamination of other items. Hand hygiene reduces the transmission of microorganisms.

ACTION	RATIONALE

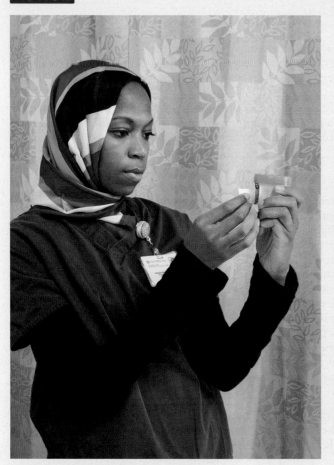

FIGURE 2. Labeling specimen container.

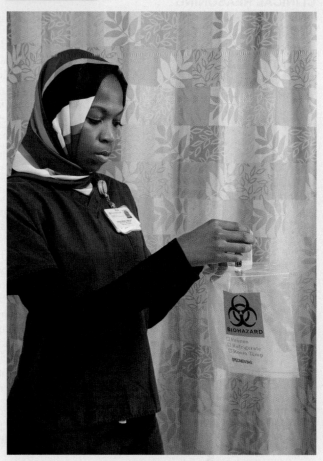

FIGURE 3. Placing specimen container in biohazard bag.

17. Transport the specimen to the laboratory immediately. If immediate transport is not possible, do not refrigerate the specimens (Fischbach et al., 2022).	Timely transport ensures accurate results.

EVALUATION

The expected outcomes have been met when the patient has produced an adequate sample (based on facility policy) from the lower respiratory tract, airway patency has been maintained, and the patient has demonstrated an understanding about the need and process for specimen collection.

DOCUMENTATION

Guidelines

Record the time the sputum specimen was collected and sent to the laboratory, and the characteristics and amount of secretions. Document the tests for which the specimen was collected. Note the respiratory assessment pre- and postcollection. Note antibiotics administered in the past 24 hours on the laboratory request form, if required by the facility.

Sample Documentation

> 9/13/25 0615 Respirations unlabored; lungs with decreased breath sounds at posterior bases. Sputum specimen obtained; patient has moderate amount of thick, yellow sputum; specimen sent to laboratory for culture and sensitivity.
>
> —C. Bausler, RN

(continued on page 1128)

Skill 18-3 ▶ Collecting a Sputum Specimen for Culture *(continued)*

DEVELOPING CLINICAL REASONING AND CLINICAL JUDGMENT

UNEXPECTED SITUATIONS AND ASSOCIATED INTERVENTIONS

- *Patient produced a specimen but did not tell you, so you do not know how long the specimen has been sitting at the bedside:* Unless the patient is able to tell you when the specimen was produced, discard the sample and recollect. Specimens should be sent to the laboratory as soon as possible to ensure valid results.
- *Patient spits saliva into container, without specimen from lungs:* Instruct the patient that the specimen needs to come from the lungs. Review the procedure for collection. Discard the contaminated container, obtain a new container, and recollect a sample.

SPECIAL CONSIDERATIONS

General Considerations

- If possible, collect the sputum sample when the patient arises in the morning, to improve chances of obtaining an adequate amount of sputum. Specimens from deep in the lungs are obtained in the early morning after secretions have accumulated overnight (Hess et al., 2021; Hinkle et al., 2022).
- Instruct the patient to not use mouthwash before collecting a sputum sample because it may contain antibacterial agents (Hess et al., 2021).
- At least three consecutive sputum specimens are needed for diagnostic purposes for patients suspected of having tuberculosis (CDC, 2021a). Sputum specimens for acid-fast bacilli (AFB; to test for tuberculosis) should be collected at least 8 to 24 hours apart, with at least one specimen produced in the early morning (CDC, 2021a).
- If the patient understands directions and is able to engage in their care, the specimen collection container may be left at the bedside for the patient to collect sputum when available. The container lid should remain in place until the patient is ready to expectorate sputum. Instruct the patient to call to inform staff as soon as sputum is produced, so it can be transported to the laboratory in a timely manner.

Community-Based Care Considerations

- If the patient is to collect specimen at home, ensure that they have a clear understanding of the collection procedure and that the specimen needs to be transported immediately to the laboratory. Reinforce to the patient that it is important not to touch the inside of the collection container.

Skill Variation ▶ Collecting a Sputum Specimen via Endotracheal Suctioning

1. Sputum specimens can be collected by suctioning an endotracheal tube or tracheostomy tube. A sterile collection receptacle is attached between the suction catheter and the suction tubing to trap sputum as it is removed from the patient's airway, before reaching the suction collection canister.
2. Refer to Skills 14-7, 14-9, and 14-10 for the procedure for endotracheal suctioning.
3. After checking suction pressure (Step 10, Skill 14-7; Step 10, Skill 14-9; Step 9, Skill 14-10), attach a sterile specimen trap to the suction tubing, taking care to avoid contaminating the open ends (Figure A).
4. Check the specimen label with the patient's identification bracelet. The label should include the patient's name and identification number, the time the specimen was collected, the route of collection, identification of person obtaining the sample, and any other information required by facility policy.
5. Continue with Step 11, Skill 14-7; Step 11, Skill 14-9; Step 10, Skill 14-10, taking care to handle the suction

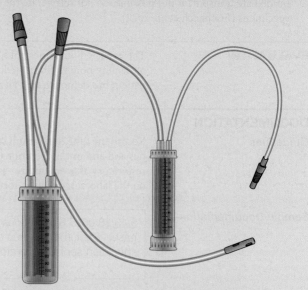

FIGURE A. Suction trap for sputum collection.

tubing and sputum trap with your nondominant hand. Proceed with suction procedure.

6. After the first suction pass, if 1 to 3 mL of sputum has been obtained, disconnect the specimen container, and set it aside (Fischbach et al., 2022). If less than this amount has been collected, resuction the patient after waiting the appropriate amount of time for them to recover.

7. If secretions are extremely thick or tenacious, flush the catheter with a small amount (1 to 2 mL) of sterile normal saline to aid in moving the secretions into the trap.

8. Once the sputum trap is removed, connect the suction tubing to the suction catheter. The catheter may then be flushed with normal saline before suctioning again. Continue with the suctioning procedure, if necessary, based on remaining steps in Skill 14-7, Skill 14-9, or Skill 14-10.

9. When suctioning is completed, place a label on the container per facility policy. Place the container in a plastic, sealable biohazard bag and send it to the laboratory immediately.

Skill 18-4 ▶ Collecting a Urine Specimen (Clean Catch, Midstream)

Skill Variation: *Obtaining a Urine Specimen From a Urinary Diversion*

Obtaining a urine specimen for random collection, urinalysis, and culture is an assessment measure to determine the characteristics of a patient's urine. A voided urine specimen for culture is collected during midstream voiding to minimize bacterial contamination from adjacent anatomical areas (Fischbach et al., 2022; MedlinePlus, 2021c) and to provide a specimen that most closely reflects the characteristics of the urine being produced by the body. If the patient is able to understand and follow the procedure, they may collect the sample on their own, after explanation and instruction.

DELEGATION CONSIDERATIONS	Obtaining a urine specimen by midstream collection may be delegated to assistive personnel (AP) as well as to licensed practical/vocational nurses (LPN/LVNs). The decision to delegate must be based on careful analysis of the patient's needs and circumstances as well as the qualifications of the person to whom the task is being delegated. Refer to the Delegation Guidelines in Appendix A.
EQUIPMENT	• Moist cleansing towelettes or skin cleanser, water, and washcloth • Gloves • Additional PPE, as indicated • Sterile specimen container; urine collection tubes, based on facility policy • Biohazard bag • Appropriate label for specimen, based on facility policy and procedure
ASSESSMENT	Ask the patient about any medications they are taking; medications may affect the results of the test. Assess for any signs and symptoms of a urinary tract infection, such as burning and/or pain with urination (dysuria), or urinary frequency. Assess the patient's ability to engage with the collection process. Determine the patient's need for assistance to obtain specimen correctly.
ACTUAL OR POTENTIAL HEALTH PROBLEMS AND NEEDS	Many actual or potential health problems or issues may require the use of this skill as part of related interventions. An appropriate health problem or issue may include: • Impaired urination • Knowledge deficiency • Urinary frequency

(continued on page 1130)

Skill 18-4 ▶ Collecting a Urine Specimen (Clean Catch, Midstream) *(continued)*

OUTCOME IDENTIFICATION AND PLANNING

The expected outcome to achieve is that an adequate amount of urine is obtained from the patient without contamination. Other outcomes include that the patient demonstrates an understanding of the need and process for specimen collection.

IMPLEMENTATION

ACTION	**RATIONALE**
1. Verify the prescribed intervention for a urine specimen collection in the patient's health record. Gather equipment.	Verifying the prescribed intervention is crucial for ensuring that the proper procedure is administered to the right patient. Assembling equipment provides for an organized approach to the task.
2. Perform hand hygiene and put on PPE, if indicated.	Hand hygiene and PPE prevent the transmission of microorganisms. PPE is required based on transmission precautions.
3. Identify the patient.	Identifying the patient ensures the right patient receives the intervention and helps prevent errors.
4. Explain the procedure to the patient. If the patient can perform the task without assistance after instruction, leave the container at the bedside with instructions to call the nurse as soon as a specimen is produced.	Explanation provides reassurance and promotes engagement. Timely transport of the specimen ensures accurate results.
5. Check the specimen label with the patient's identification bracelet. The label should include the patient's name and identification number, the time the specimen was collected, the route of collection, identification of the person obtaining the sample, and any other information required by facility policy.	Confirmation of patient identification information ensures the specimen is labeled correctly for the right patient.
6. Assemble equipment on the overbed table or other surface within reach.	Arranging items nearby is convenient, saves time, and avoids unnecessary stretching and twisting of muscles on the part of the nurse.
7. Have the patient perform hand hygiene, if performing self-collection.	Hand hygiene prevents the transmission of microorganisms.
8. Close the curtains around the bed and close the door to the room, if possible.	Closing the door or curtain provides for patient privacy.
9. Put on gloves. Assist the patient to the bathroom or onto the bedside commode or bedpan. Instruct the patient not to defecate or discard toilet paper into the urine (Figure 1).	Gloves reduce the transmission of microorganisms. Stool and/or toilet paper may contaminate the specimen.

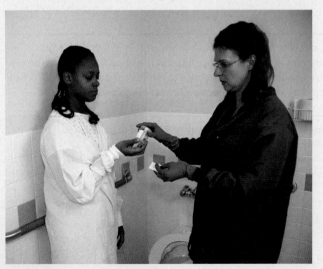

FIGURE 1. Instructing patient about urine collection procedure.

ACTION

10. Instruct the patient with female genitalia to separate the labia for cleaning of the area and during collection of urine. The patient should use the towelettes or wet washcloth to clean each side of the urinary meatus, then the center over the meatus, from front to back, using a new wipe or a clean area of the washcloth for each stroke. Instruct the patient with female genitalia to **keep the labia separated after cleaning and during collection** (MedlinePlus, 2021c) (Figure 2). Patients with male genitalia should use a towelette to clean the area around the meatus of the penis, wiping in a circular motion away from the urethral meatus. Instruct the uncircumcised patient to retract the foreskin before cleaning and during collection (MedlinePlus, 2021c) (Figure 3).

RATIONALE

Cleaning the perineal area or penis reduces the risk for contamination of the specimen. Separation of the labia avoids contamination by perineal skin and hair. Retraction of the foreskin avoids contamination by skin.

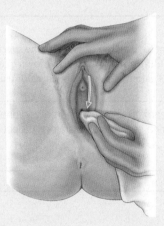

FIGURE 2. Cleaning female perineum. Separating labia and cleansing from front to back.

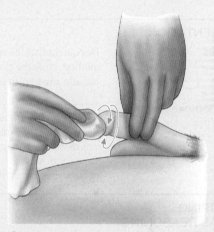

FIGURE 3. Cleaning male perineum. Wiping in a circular motion away from urethra.

11. **Do not let the container touch the perineal skin or hair during collection. Do not touch the inside of the container or the lid.** Have patient void a small amount of urine into the toilet, bedpan, or commode. The patient should then stop urinating briefly, and then continue voiding into the collection container. Collect the urine specimen (at least 3 to 5 mL) (Fischbach et al., 2022), and then instruct the patient to finish voiding in the toilet, bedpan, or commode. Instruct the uncircumcised male patient to replace the foreskin after collection.

Collecting a midstream specimen ensures that fresh urine is analyzed. Some urine may have collected in the urethra from the last void. By voiding a little before collecting the specimen, the specimen will contain only fresh urine.

12. Place the lid on the container. If necessary, transfer the specimen to appropriate containers/tubes for the specific test prescribed, according to facility policy.

Placing the lid on the container helps to keep the specimen clean and prevents spills.

13. Assist the patient from the bathroom, off the commode, or off the bedpan. Provide perineal care, if necessary.

Perineal care promotes patient comfort and hygiene.

14. Remove gloves and perform hand hygiene.

Removing gloves properly reduces the risk for infection transmission and contamination of other items. Hand hygiene reduces the transmission of microorganisms.

15. Place a label on the container per facility policy. Note the specimen collection method, according to facility policy. Place the container in a plastic, sealable biohazard bag.

Proper labeling ensures accurate communication of results. Packaging the specimen in a biohazard bag prevents the person transporting the container from coming in contact with urine.

(continued on page 1132)

Skill 18-4 ▶ Collecting a Urine Specimen (Clean Catch, Midstream) *(continued)*

ACTION	**RATIONALE**
16. Remove other PPE, if used. Perform hand hygiene.	Proper removal of PPE reduces the risk for infection transmission and contamination of other items. Hand hygiene reduces the transmission of microorganisms.
17. Transport the specimen to the laboratory as soon as possible. If unable to take the specimen to the laboratory immediately, refrigerate it (Fischbach et al., 2022).	If not refrigerated immediately, urine may act as a culture medium, allowing bacteria to multiply and skewing the results of testing. Refrigeration (up to 24 hours [Fischbach et al., 2022]) prevents the bacteria from multiplying.

EVALUATION

The expected outcomes have been met when an adequate amount of urine has been obtained from the patient without contamination, and the patient has demonstrated an understanding of the need and process for specimen collection.

DOCUMENTATION

Guidelines

Document that the specimen was collected and sent to the laboratory. Note the specimen collection method. Note the characteristics of the urine, including odor, amount (if known), color, and clarity. Include any significant patient assessments, such as patient reports of burning or pain on urination.

Sample Documentation

> <u>7/10/25</u> 2200 Patient instructed to collect midstream urine sample. Verbalized understanding of directions; 70 mL of cloudy, odorless, yellow urine sent to the laboratory. Patient denies pain or discomfort on urination.
>
> —*A. Blitz, RN*

DEVELOPING CLINICAL REASONING AND CLINICAL JUDGMENT

UNEXPECTED SITUATIONS AND ASSOCIATED INTERVENTIONS

- *Patient cannot provide a sufficient urine sample:* Offer the patient fluids to drink, although drinking too much fluid may dilute the urine, invalidating the test. The patient may return later in the day to supply a sample. Offer the patient assistance with the next void.
- *Patient missed voiding into the specimen container but did void into the collection receptacle in the toilet:* Do not use this urine as a sample for a culture; it could be heavily contaminated with bacteria and give a misleading result. Attempt to collect urine with the next void. Offer the patient assistance when trying to collect the sample.

SPECIAL CONSIDERATIONS

General Considerations

- For many urine tests, such as a urinalysis, drug testing, or diabetes testing, the specimen does not need to be sterile and does not need to be collected as a midstream specimen. However, in the case of urinalysis, if the specimen shows nitrates and white blood cells, a culture of a urine specimen may be prescribed as well.
- Because the first voiding of the day (early morning) contains the highest bacterial counts, collect this sample whenever possible (Fischbach et al., 2022).
- If possible, ensure the specimen is obtained before antibiotics are started (Fischbach et al., 2022).
- Urine specimens may also be obtained by direct urethral catheterization. Refer to Skills 12-7 and 12-8 for catheterization procedure.
- Urine specimens may also be obtained from urinary diversions. See the accompanying Skill Variation below.
- Urine specimens must never be obtained from a urine collection bag that is part of an indwelling urinary catheter drainage system (Fischbach et al., 2022). Refer to Skill 18-5 for the procedure to obtain a urine specimen from an indwelling urinary catheter.

Infant and Child Considerations

- The most reliable method to obtain a urine specimen for culture (associated with lower contamination rates) in neonates and young infants is to perform a suprapubic aspiration or transurethral catheterization (American Academy of Pediatrics [AAP], 2016; Cheek et al., 2015). Suprapubic aspiration is not within the scope of practice of registered nurses (May, 2018). Discuss sampling options with the health care team and the patient's parents. Suprapubic aspiration is painful; pain management during the procedure is important—topical anesthetic cream should be used when time permits, as well as age-appropriate distraction techniques (Cheek et al., 2015).
- Midstream collection can be accomplished with children older than age 2 years, provided the child is able to follow directions and engage in their care and with the nurse. Try having the child sit facing the back of the toilet, straddling the toilet seat. The nurse or parent can position themselves behind the child, holding the sterile container for urine collection.
- Urine should be obtained through urethral catheterization or suprapubic aspiration in ill-appearing febrile infants (AAP, 2016).
- Familiar terms, such as "pee-pee," "potty" or "tinkle," may be used with young children to ensure they understand what is being explained and to gain cooperation (Kyle & Carman, 2021, p. 712). Enlist the assistance of the patient's parents or significant others to identify appropriate terms.

Community-Based Care Considerations

- If the patient is to collect a specimen at home, ensure that the patient has a clear understanding of the collection procedure, understands the need to transport the specimen immediately to the laboratory, and has obtained the necessary equipment from their health care provider or laboratory. Reinforce that the patient cannot touch the inside of the collection container. Urine specimens must be refrigerated (up to 24 hours [Fischbach et al., 2022]) until they can be brought to the laboratory.

Skill Variation ▶ Obtaining a Urine Specimen From a Urinary Diversion

Urine specimens can be obtained from urinary diversions via several methods. Clean urine specimens can be obtained from a urinary diversion appliance into a clean container for a routine urinalysis (Williams, 2013). Specimens for culture should never be obtained directly from an existing urostomy pouch or drainage bag (Mahoney et al., 2013; WOCN, 2018). If a urine sample is needed for culture and sensitivity, most sources suggest that it should be obtained by sterile catheterization or clean catch drip collection (Mahoney et al., 2013; Williams, 2013; WOCN, 2018). However, results of at least one study suggest that collection from a clean urostomy pouch is also acceptable (Vaarala, 2018).

Equipment: Cleansing solution, based on facility policy; sterile gauze; sterile water or saline, or other cleansing solution for stoma site (povidone-iodine, chlorhexidine, soap and water), based on facility policy; double-lumen or straight catheter (16 Fr); sterile water-based lubricant if catheter not self-lubricated; sterile specimen container and urine collection tubes, based on facility policy; sterile and nonsterile gloves; new ostomy appliance; skin cleanser; disposable washcloth or washcloth and towel

1. Follow Steps 1 to 6 in Skill 18-4. Open the supplies, maintaining sterility.
2. Put on gloves. Remove ostomy appliance.
3. Remove gloves and perform hand hygiene.

4. Put on sterile gloves. Using a circular motion from the stoma opening outward, clean the stoma site with the sterile water, sterile saline, or other cleansing solution, based on facility policy. Blot the stoma with sterile gauze.

5. Place the open end of the urinary catheter into the specimen container. Lubricate the catheter with water-soluble lubricant. If using a straight catheter, gently insert the urinary catheter into the stoma site and advance no more than 2 to 3 inches (5 to 7.5 cm) (WOCN, 2018).
6. Hold the catheter in position until urine begins to drip. **If you meet resistance, rotate the catheter gently until it slides forward. Do not force the catheter. If you continue to meet resistance, do not force it any further.** If urine does not flow into the catheter, ask the patient to shift position and/or cough to mobilize urine (Williams, 2013).
7. Collect approximately 5 to 10 mL of urine before removing catheter. This may take 5 to 15 minutes (WOCN, 2018). Once the catheter is removed, cap the specimen container. Clean and dry the stoma and peristomal skin. Replace the ostomy appliance; refer to Skill 12-11. If necessary, transfer the specimen to appropriate containers/tubes for the specific test prescribed, according to facility policy.
8. Remove gloves and perform hand hygiene.

9. Continue with Steps 15 to 17 in Skill 18-4.
10. Alternatively, once the appliance is removed and the stoma cleansed, blot the stoma with sterile gauze. Discard the first few drops of urine by allowing urine to drip onto the sterile gauze (WOCN, 2018). Hold the sterile specimen cup under the stoma to collect urine. Collect approximately 5 to 10 mL of urine; collecting a sufficient amount may take 5 to 15 minutes (WOCN, 2018).

Skill 18-4 ▶ Collecting a Urine Specimen (Clean Catch, Midstream) *(continued)*

EVIDENCE FOR PRACTICE ▶

PRACTICE GUIDELINES: URINE SAMPLES AND URINARY DIVERSIONS

Wound Ostomy and Continence Nurses Society. (2018). *Catheterization of an ileal or colon conduit stoma: Best practice for clinicians.* https://www.ostomy.org/wp-content/uploads/2021/04/Catheterization-of-Urinary-Stoma-2018.pdf.

This best practice guideline was developed by a panel of certified ostomy nurses serving on the Wound, Ostomy and Continence Nurses (WOCN) Society's Clinical Practice Ostomy Committee. This guideline has been validated by the WOCN Society.

EVIDENCE FOR PRACTICE ▶

URINARY SAMPLE COLLECTION METHODS AND URINARY DIVERSIONS

Urine specimens can be obtained from urinary diversions via several methods, including catheterization, by dripping the urine directly from the stoma or from a fresh urostomy pouch after stoma care. Is the use of catheterization, which is an invasive procedure, necessary to ensure obtaining a reliable urine culture sample?

Related Evidence

Vaarala, M. H. (2018). Urinary sample collection methods in ileal conduit urinary diversion patients. A randomized controlled trial. *Journal of Wound, Ostomy, and Continence Nursing,* *45*(1), 59–62. https://doi.org/10.1097/WON.0000000000000397

The purpose of this randomized controlled trial was to compare bacteriologic urinalysis findings using three urinary sample collection methods in patients with ileal conduit urinary diversions. Patients who were age 18 years and older with an ileal conduit urinary diversion at a hospital clinic in Finland ($n = 36$) were randomized into two groups. Group A had a first urine sample collected by clean stoma catheterization, followed by urine sample collection by dripping urine from the stoma. Group B had the first urine sample collected by dripping urine from the stoma, followed by urine sample collection by clean stoma catheterization. Subsequently, all participants had a third urine sample collected from a factory-clean urostomy pouch immediately after approximately 20 mL of urine was present in the pouch. Each urine sample was evaluated by urine culture. The primary outcome measure was the incidence of uropathogenic bacteria in the urinary culture following the dripping urine from the stoma and urine from the urostomy pouch sample collection methods compared with the sample collection by clean stoma catheterization. Results indicated that uropathogenic bacteria were detected in the urinary culture in 16 of 36 samples (44%) collected by clean stoma catheterization; 15 of 36 samples (42%) collected by urine dripping directly from the stoma; and 13 of 35 samples (37%) collected from the clean urostomy pouch. Significant differences among the urine collection methods were not detected. Assuming catheterization as the most reliable method of sample collection, the sensitivity and specificity of the urine dripping from the stoma collection method were 81.3% and 90.0%, respectively. There were no significant differences in the incidence of uropathogenic bacteria when clean stoma catheterization was compared with urine dripping from the stoma and urostomy pouch methods. The researchers concluded that urine sample collection technique had a minor effect on the detection of potential uropathogenic bacteria. The researchers suggested that urinary samples collected by urine dripping from the stoma method or from a clean urostomy pouch would, in most cases, provide similar clinically significant uropathogenic bacteria findings compared with sample collection by clean stoma catheterization and could be considered as an alternative to collection of a urine sample by catheterization of the urinary stoma.

Relevance for Nursing Practice

Nurses have a responsibility to collaborate with members of the health care team to provide thoughtful person-centered interventions and care. Consideration of patient circumstances and needs should be part of planning treatment and care decisions to implement the least invasive interventions possible.

Skill 18-5 ▶ Obtaining a Urine Specimen From an Indwelling Urinary Catheter

Indwelling catheter drainage tubes have special sampling ports in the tubing for removal of urine for testing. Most sampling ports are needleless systems. However, some ports require the use of a needle or blunt cannula to access the sampling port. The drainage tubing below the access port may be bent back on itself or clamped so that urine collects near the port, unless contraindicated, based on the patient's condition. **Do not open the drainage system to obtain urine specimens, to avoid contamination of the system and bladder infection. Never take urine specimens from the catheter drainage bag because the urine is not fresh** (CDC, 2019d; Fischbach et al., 2022).

DELEGATION CONSIDERATIONS	Obtaining a urine specimen from an indwelling catheter may be delegated to assistive personnel (AP) as well as licensed practical/vocational nurses (LPN/LVNs). The decision to delegate must be based on careful analysis of the patient's needs and circumstances as well as the qualifications of the person to whom the task is being delegated. Refer to the Delegation Guidelines in Appendix A.
EQUIPMENT	• 10-mL sterile syringe • Blunt cannula, based on specific catheter in use • Alcohol or other antimicrobial wipe • Gloves • Additional PPE, as indicated • Sterile specimen container; urine collection tubes, based on facility policy • Biohazard bag • Appropriate label for specimen, based on facility policy and procedure
ASSESSMENT	After verifying the prescribed intervention for specimen collection, review the patient's health record for, or question the patient about, information about any medications they are taking, because medications may affect the results of the test. Assess the characteristics of the urine draining from the catheter. Inspect the catheter tubing to identify the type of sampling port.
ACTUAL OR POTENTIAL HEALTH PROBLEMS AND NEEDS	Many actual or potential health problems or issues may require the use of this skill as part of related interventions. An appropriate health problem or issue may include: • Impaired urination • Infection risk • Knowledge deficiency
OUTCOME IDENTIFICATION AND PLANNING	The expected outcome to achieve is that an adequate amount of urine is obtained without contamination or adverse effect. Other outcomes that may be appropriate include that the patient demonstrates an understanding of the need and process for specimen collection.

IMPLEMENTATION

ACTION	**RATIONALE**
1. Verify the prescribed intervention for a urine specimen collection in the patient's health record. Gather equipment.	Verifying the prescribed intervention is crucial for ensuring that the proper procedure is administered to the right patient. Assembling equipment provides for an organized approach to the task.
2. Perform hand hygiene and put on PPE, if indicated.	Hand hygiene and PPE prevent the transmission of microorganisms. PPE is required based on transmission precautions.
3. Identify the patient.	Identifying the patient ensures the right patient receives the intervention and helps prevent errors.
4. Explain the procedure to the patient.	Explanation provides reassurance and promotes engagement.

(*continued on page 1136*)

Skill 18-5 ▶ Obtaining a Urine Specimen From an Indwelling Urinary Catheter *(continued)*

ACTION	**RATIONALE**
5. Check the specimen label with the patient's identification bracelet. The label should include the patient's name and identification number, the time the specimen was collected, the route of collection, identification of person obtaining the sample, and any other information required by facility policy.	Confirmation of patient identification information ensures the specimen is labeled correctly for the right patient.
6. Assemble equipment on the overbed table or other surface within reach.	Arranging items nearby is convenient, saves time, and avoids unnecessary stretching and twisting of muscles on the part of the nurse.
7. Close the curtains around the bed and close the door to the room, if possible.	Closing the curtains or door provides for patient privacy.
8. Put on gloves.	Gloves reduce the transmission of microorganisms.
9. Clamp the catheter drainage tubing or bend it back on itself distal to the port, a minimum of 3 inches below the port (CDC, 2019d). If an insufficient amount of urine is present in the tubing, allow the tubing to remain clamped up to 30 minutes (Fischbach et al., 2022), to collect a sufficient amount of urine, unless contraindicated. Remove the lid from the specimen container, keeping the inside of the container and lid free from contamination.	Clamping the tubing ensures the collection of an adequate amount of fresh urine. Clamping for an extended period of time leads to overdistention of the bladder. Clamping may be contraindicated based on the patient's condition (e.g., after bladder surgery). The container needs to remain sterile so as not to contaminate the urine.
10. **Scrub the aspiration port vigorously with alcohol or other antimicrobial wipe and allow the port to air dry.**	Cleaning with alcohol or other antimicrobial deters entry of microorganisms when the needle punctures the port.
11. Attach the syringe to the needleless port. Alternatively, insert the blunt-tipped cannula into the port. Slowly aspirate enough urine for a specimen (at least 3 to 5 mL [Fischbach et al., 2022]; check facility requirements) (Figure 1). Remove the syringe from the port. **Unclamp the drainage tubing.**	Using a Luer-lock syringe or blunt-tipped cannula prevents a needlestick. Collecting urine from the port ensures that the specimen will contain fresh urine. Unclamping the catheter drainage tubing prevents overdistention of and injury to the patient's bladder.

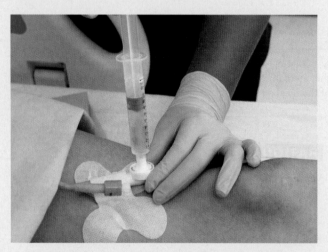

FIGURE 1. Attaching the syringe to the needleless aspiration port and slowly withdrawing urine specimen.

12. If a blunt-tipped cannula was used on the syringe, remove it from the syringe before emptying the urine from the syringe into the specimen cup. Place the cannula into a sharps collection container. **Slowly inject urine into the specimen container. Take care to avoid touching the syringe tip to any surface. Do not touch the edge or inside of the collection container.**	Forcing urine through the cannula breaks up cells and impedes accurate results of microscopic urinalysis. If the urine is injected quickly into the container, it may splash out of the container or into your eyes. Avoid touching the edge or inside of the container to avoid contamination.
13. Replace the lid on the container. If necessary, transfer the specimen to appropriate containers/tubes for the specific test prescribed, according to facility policy. Dispose of the syringe in a sharps collection container.	Proper disposal of equipment prevents injury and transmission of microorganisms. Safe disposal of sharps prevents accidental injury.

ACTION	RATIONALE
14. Remove your gloves and perform hand hygiene	Removing gloves properly reduces the risk for infection transmission and contamination of other items. Hand hygiene reduces the transmission of microorganisms.
15. Place a label on the container per facility policy. Note the specimen collection method, according to facility policy. Place the container in a plastic sealable biohazard bag.	Proper labeling ensures accurate communication of results. Packaging the specimen in a biohazard bag prevents the person transporting the container from coming in contact with the specimen.
16. Remove other PPE, if used. Perform hand hygiene.	Proper removal of PPE reduces the risk for infection transmission and contamination of other items. Hand hygiene reduces the transmission of microorganisms.
17. Transport the specimen to the laboratory as soon as possible. If unable to take the specimen to the laboratory immediately, refrigerate it (Fischbach et al., 2022).	If not refrigerated immediately, urine may act as a culture medium, allowing bacteria to multiply and skewing the results of testing. Refrigeration (up to 24 hours [Fischbach et al., 2022]) prevents the bacteria from multiplying.

EVALUATION

The expected outcomes have been met when an adequate amount of urine has been obtained without contamination or adverse effect, and the patient has demonstrated an understanding of the need and process for specimen collection.

DOCUMENTATION

Guidelines

Document the method used to obtain the specimen, the type of specimen sent, and characteristics of the urine. Note any significant patient assessments. Record urine volume on the intake and output record, if appropriate.

Sample Documentation

10/20/25 1515 Patient with indwelling urinary catheter in place. Urine noted to be dark yellow and cloudy. Patient's temperature 103°F, pulse 96, respirations 18, BP 118/64. Dr. Burning notified. Specimen for urine culture obtained from indwelling catheter and catheter removed per order. Patient due to void by 2115.

—B. Clapp, RN

DEVELOPING CLINICAL REASONING AND CLINICAL JUDGMENT

UNEXPECTED SITUATIONS AND ASSOCIATED INTERVENTIONS

- *No urine or insufficient amount noted in catheter tubing:* Clamp the tubing below the access port for up to 30 minutes, according to facility policy, unless contraindicated by patient condition.

SPECIAL CONSIDERATIONS

- Never obtain a urine specimen for culture from the urine collection bag that is part of an indwelling urinary catheter drainage system (CDC, 2019d; Fischbach et al., 2022).
- It is very important to remove the clamp from the drainage tubing as soon as the specimen is collected, unless there is a specific order to leave the tubing clamped, to prevent overdistention of the patient's bladder and injury.
- If possible, ensure the specimen is obtained before antibiotics are started (Fischbach et al., 2022).

(continued on page 1138)

Skill 18-5 ▶ Obtaining a Urine Specimen From an Indwelling Urinary Catheter *(continued)*

EVIDENCE FOR PRACTICE ▶

CATHETER-ASSOCIATED INFECTIONS
Resources and Guidelines
Centers for Disease Control and Prevention (CDC). (2015, October 16). *Healthcare-associated infections (HAI). Catheter-associated urinary tract infections (CAUTI).* https://www.cdc.gov/hai/ca_uti/uti.html

Centers for Disease Control and Prevention (CDC). (2017, February). *Catheter-associated urinary tract infections (CAUTI). Guidelines for prevention of catheter-associated urinary tract infections.* https://www.cdc.gov/infectioncontrol/guidelines/cauti/index.html

This site provides resources for health care providers and patients, including the CDC guidelines for prevention of catheter-associated infections. These guidelines recommend that alternatives to indwelling urethral catheterization should be considered in selected patients, when appropriate, such as the use of external catheters and intermittent catheterization. In addition, catheters should only be used for appropriate indications and should be removed as soon as they are no longer needed.

Skill 18-6 ▶ Testing Stool for Occult Blood

Fecal occult blood testing (FOBT) may be used to detect **occult blood** in the stool. It is used for initial/early screening for disorders such as cancer and for gastrointestinal (GI) bleeding in conditions such as ulcer disease, inflammatory bowel disorders, and intestinal polyps (MedlinePlus, 2020). Consecutive stool samples (three to six) should be collected from different stool samples to increase accuracy (Fischbach et al., 2022). FOBT may be performed within an institution, collected at the bedside, and sent to the laboratory for analysis. It may also be collected by the patient at home and delivered or mailed to the health care provider's office or to the laboratory for analysis.

The *guaiac fecal occult blood test* (gFOBT) is a chemical test that detects the enzyme peroxidase in hemoglobin molecules when blood is present in the stool sample. A positive gFOBT result indicates that abnormal bleeding is occurring somewhere in the digestive tract. Certain medications, such as a salicylate intake of more than 325 mg daily, other nonsteroidal anti-inflammatory drugs, steroids, iron preparations, and anticoagulants, also may lead to *false-positive* readings (Fischbach et al., 2022). The evidence for practice is conflicting regarding the impact of ingestion of certain foods and supplements before specimen collection on the accuracy of the test results (Doubeni, 2021; MedlinePlus, 2021). Foods and supplements that are suggested to have a possible effect on test results include red meat, cantaloupe, turnips, radishes, parsnips, horseradish, mushrooms, broccoli, cauliflower, apples, bananas, cantaloupe, and vitamin C–enriched foods and juices as well as vitamin C in excess of 250 mg/day (American Cancer Society, 2020; Colorectal Cancer Alliance, 2019a; Fischbach et al., 2022; MedlinePlus, 2021). Patients should consult with their health care providers and follow directions provided for the collection test kit provided.

The *fecal immunochemical test* (FIT) uses antibodies directed against human hemoglobin to detect blood in the stool. A positive FIT is more specific for bleeding in the lower GI tract (Fischbach et al., 2022). No drug or dietary restrictions are required for the FIT (American Cancer Society, 2020; Colorectal Cancer Alliance, 2019b).

The following are recommendations for the patient preparing for a fecal occult blood test (Fischbach et al., 2022):

- Avoid barium enemas for 72 hours before and during stool specimen collection.
- Do not collect samples during or until 3 days after a menstrual period.
- Do not collect samples while the patient has bleeding hemorrhoids or hematuria.

In clinical settings, these restrictions are usually not practical. Be sure to note the presence of any of the previously mentioned conditions in the clinical setting.

A positive result from either the gFOBT or the FIT requires follow-up testing, such as a sigmoidoscopy or colonoscopy (American Cancer Society, 2020).

DELEGATION CONSIDERATIONS	Obtaining a stool specimen for FOBT may be delegated to assistive personnel (AP) as well as to licensed practical/vocational nurses (LPN/LVNs). Developing the FOBT at the point of care is not delegated to AP. Developing the FOBT at the point of care may be delegated to LPN/LVNs. The decision to delegate must be based on careful analysis of the patient's needs and circumstances as well as the qualifications of the person to whom the task is being delegated. Refer to the Delegation Guidelines in Appendix A.
EQUIPMENT	• Gloves; other PPE as indicated • Wooden applicator • gFOBT: Wooden applicator, testing card, and developer (if processing is being done at point of care) • FIT: Applicator stick or brush, depending on collection kit in use • Bedpan, or plastic collection receptacle for commode or toilet • Biohazard bag • Appropriate label for specimen, based on facility policy and procedure
ASSESSMENT	Assess the patient's understanding of the collection procedure and their ability to engage in their care. Assess the patient for a history of GI bleeding. Review prescribed restrictions for medications and evaluate patient engagement with the required restrictions. Assess the patient for any blood in the perineal area, including hemorrhoids, menstruation, urinary tract infection, or vaginal or rectal tears. Blood may be from a source other than the GI tract.
ACTUAL OR POTENTIAL HEALTH PROBLEMS AND NEEDS	Many actual or potential health problems or issues may require the use of this skill as part of related interventions. An appropriate health problem or issue may include: • Knowledge deficiency • Anxiety
OUTCOME IDENTIFICATION AND PLANNING	The expected outcomes to achieve are that an uncontaminated stool sample is obtained following collection guidelines, and it is then transported to the laboratory within the recommended time frame. Other outcomes may include that the patient demonstrates accurate understanding of testing instructions and rationale for use.

IMPLEMENTATION

ACTION	**RATIONALE**
1. Verify the prescribed intervention for a stool specimen collection in the patient's health record. Gather equipment.	Verifying the prescribed intervention is crucial for ensuring that the proper procedure is administered to the right patient. Assembling equipment provides for an organized approach to the task.
2. Perform hand hygiene and put on PPE, if indicated.	Hand hygiene and PPE prevent the transmission of microorganisms. PPE is required based on transmission precautions.
3. Identify the patient.	Identifying the patient ensures the right patient receives the intervention and helps prevent errors.
4. Discuss with the patient the need for a stool sample. Explain the process by which the stool will be collected, either from a bedpan, commode, or plastic receptacle in the toilet.	Discussion and explanation help to allay some of the patient's anxiety and prepare them for what to expect.

(continued on page 1140)

Skill 18-6 ▶ Testing Stool for Occult Blood *(continued)*

ACTION	RATIONALE
5. If sending the specimen to the laboratory, check the specimen label with the patient identification bracelet. The label should include the patient's name and identification number, the time the specimen was collected, the route of collection, identification of the person obtaining the sample, and any other information required by facility policy.	Facilities may allow point-of-service testing (at the bedside or on unit), or the specimen may have to be sent to the laboratory for testing. Confirmation of patient identification information ensures the specimen is labeled correctly for the right patient.
6. Assemble equipment on the overbed table or other surface within reach.	Arranging items nearby is convenient, saves time, and avoids unnecessary stretching and twisting of muscles on the part of the nurse.
7. Close the curtains around the bed or close the door to the room, if possible.	Closing the door or curtain provides for patient privacy.
8. Place the plastic collection receptacle in the toilet, if applicable. Assist the patient to the bathroom, onto the bedside commode, or onto the bedpan. Instruct the patient not to urinate or discard toilet paper with the stool.	Proper collection into an appropriate receptacle for stool prevents inaccurate results. Urine or toilet paper can contaminate the specimen, interfering with accurate results.
9. After the patient defecates, assist the patient out of the bathroom or off the commode, or remove the bedpan. Perform hand hygiene and put on disposable gloves.	Hand hygiene deters the spread of microorganisms. Gloves protect the nurse from microorganisms in feces.

If Using gFOBT:

ACTION	RATIONALE
10. Open the flap on the sample side of the card. With the wooden applicator, apply a small amount of stool from the center of the bowel movement onto one window of the testing card. With the opposite end of the wooden applicator, obtain another sample of stool from another area and apply a small amount of stool onto the second window of the testing card (Figure 1).	Two separate areas of the same stool sample are tested to ensure accuracy. By using opposite ends of the wooden applicator, cross-contamination is avoided.

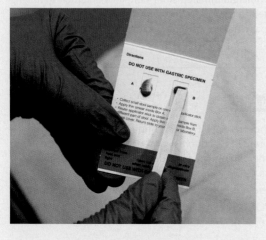

FIGURE 1. Using a wooden applicator to transfer stool specimen to window of testing card.

ACTION	RATIONALE
11. Close the flap over the stool samples.	Closing the flap prevents contamination of the samples.
12. If sending the stool to the laboratory, label the specimen card per facility policy. Place it in a sealable plastic biohazard bag and send it to the laboratory immediately.	Facilities may allow point-of-service testing (at bedside or on unit), or the specimen may have to be sent to the laboratory for testing. Correct labeling is necessary to ensure accurate results. Packaging the specimen in a biohazard bag prevents the person transporting the container from coming in contact with the specimen.

ACTION

13. If testing at the point of care, wait 3 to 5 minutes before developing. Open the flap on the opposite side of the card and place two drops of developer over each window and **wait the time stated in the manufacturer's instructions** (Figure 2).
14. Observe the card for any blue areas (Figure 3).

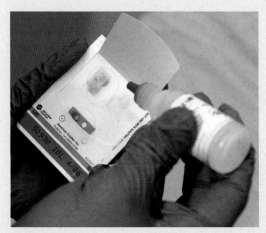

FIGURE 2. Applying developer to card windows.

If Using FIT:

15. Open the flap on the sample side of the card. With the applicator, brush, or sampling probe, apply a small amount of stool from the center of the bowel movement onto the top half of the window of the testing card. With the opposite end of the device, obtain another sample of stool from another area and apply a small amount of stool onto the bottom half of the window of the testing card.
16. Use the applicator to mix the samples and spread them over the entire window. Close the flap over the sample. Allow the card to dry.
17. If sending to the laboratory, label the specimen card per facility policy. Place it in a sealable plastic biohazard bag and send it to the laboratory immediately.

18. If testing at the point of care, open the collection card according to the manufacturer's instructions. Add three drops of developer to the center of the sample on the sample pad. Developer should flow through the test (T) line and through the control (C) line. Snap the test device closed.
19. Wait 5 minutes or the time specified by the manufacturer. Observe the card for a pink color on the test (T) line. The control (C) line must also turn pink within 5 minutes (Figure 4). If the control (C) line turns pink, read and communicate the result.

RATIONALE

If immediate testing is required, waiting 3 to 5 minutes before developing allows adequate time for the sample to penetrate the test paper and dry (Fischbach et al., 2022). The developer will react with any blood in the stool. Following the manufacturer's instructions promotes accuracy of results.

Any blue coloring on the card indicates a positive test result for blood.

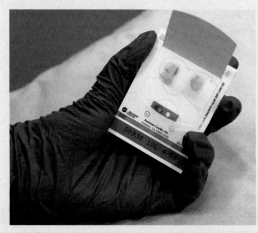

FIGURE 3. Observing windows on card for blue areas.

Two separate areas of the same stool sample are tested to ensure accuracy. By using opposite ends of the wooden applicator, cross-contamination is avoided.

Drying the samples stabilizes hemoglobin, if present.

Facilities may allow point-of-service testing (at bedside or on unit), or the specimen may have to be sent to the laboratory for testing. Correct labeling is necessary to ensure accurate results. Packaging the specimen in a biohazard bag prevents the person transporting the container from coming in contact with the specimen.

The developer will react with any blood in the stool. Following the manufacturer's instructions promotes accuracy of results.

The developer will react with any blood in the stool. Following the manufacturer's instructions promotes accuracy of results. Any pink color on the test (T) line indicates a positive result.

(continued on page 1142)

Skill 18-6 ▶ Testing Stool for Occult Blood *(continued)*

ACTION

RATIONALE

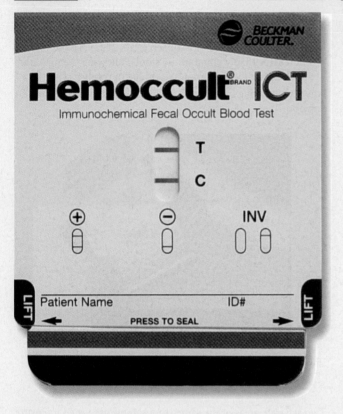

FIGURE 4. Observing for pink color on test (T) line and the control (C) line. (*Source:* Image courtesy of Beckman Coulter, Inc.)

20. After reading the results, discard the testing slide appropriately, according to facility policy. Remove your gloves and any other PPE, if used. Perform hand hygiene.

Proper removal of PPE reduces the risk for infection transmission and contamination of other items. Hand hygiene and proper disposal of equipment reduce the transmission of microorganisms.

EVALUATION

The expected outcomes have been met when an uncontaminated stool sample has been obtained following collection guidelines and transported to the laboratory within the recommended time frame, and the patient has demonstrated accurate understanding of testing instructions and rationale for use.

DOCUMENTATION

Guidelines

Document the method used to obtain the specimen and transport it to the laboratory. If testing is done by the nurse, document results and communication of results to the health care team. Document significant assessment findings and stool characteristics.

Sample Documentation

07/12/25 1040 Stool sample obtained from bowel movement. Labeled and sent to laboratory for occult blood testing. Stool noted to be semi-formed, dark brown, without evidence of gross blood.

—*K. Sanders, RN*

DEVELOPING CLINICAL REASONING AND CLINICAL JUDGMENT

UNEXPECTED SITUATIONS AND ASSOCIATED INTERVENTIONS

- *When developing a gFOBT, one window tests positive, whereas the second window tests negative:* This could indicate that the blood is from a source other than the GI tract. Document these results and notify the health care team.
- *When developing an FIT test, the control (C) line does not turn pink:* This is an invalid test; do not communicate the result. Repeat the test with a new collection card and test device (Beckman Coulter, 2015b).

SPECIAL CONSIDERATIONS

General Considerations

- *gFOBT* testing must be repeated with three to six different samples of stool (Fischbach et al., 2022).
- *FIT* sample collection is simpler, requiring only one to two different samples of stool (Bechtold et al., 2016).
- Positive *FIT* test results may appear before 5 minutes. To verify a negative result, wait the full 5 minutes after closing the test device. Do not interpret *FIT* results after 5 minutes (Beckman Coulter, 2015b).
- A specimen can be collected from an ostomy appliance. Apply a clean ostomy appliance and obtain a sample as soon as the patient passes stool into the appliance.
- Stool can be collected from the diaper of an infant or child, as long as the specimen is not contaminated with urine.

Community-Based Care Considerations

- Patients/caregivers are often instructed on how to collect stool specimens for occult blood at home and bring the samples to the office, clinic, or laboratory. Patients/caregivers should understand that it is important to follow instructions carefully to ensure validity of results. Any clean, dry container can be used to collect stool before contact with toilet bowl water. Patients are responsible only for obtaining a sample of stool and applying it to the collection card. Testing is done at the clinic, office, or laboratory.
- Some FIT collection kits use a sampling probe; the patient inserts the probe in the stool sample and inserts the probe in the collection device before returning for testing.
- Once the samples are collected, the collection devices can remain at room temperature until they are mailed or delivered to the testing location.

Skill 18-7 ▶ Collecting a Stool Specimen

A stool specimen may be prescribed to screen for pathogenic organisms, such as bacteria associated with enteric infection or ova and parasites; the presence of toxins indicating *Clostridioides difficile* infection; or for electrolytes, fat, and leukocytes. The nurse is responsible for obtaining the specimen according to facility procedure, labeling the specimen, and ensuring that the specimen is transported to the laboratory in a timely manner. The facility's policy and procedure manual or laboratory manual identifies specific information about the amount of stool needed, the time frame during which stool is to be collected, and the type of specimen container to use.

Usually, 1 inch (2.5 cm) of formed stool or 30 mL of liquid stool is sufficient (Fischbach et al., 2022). If portions of the stool include visible blood, mucus, or pus, include these with the specimen (Fischbach et al., 2022). Also be sure that the specimen is free of any barium or enema solution. Because a fresh specimen produces the most accurate results, send the specimen to the laboratory immediately. If this is not possible, the specimen should be either refrigerated or kept warm; contact the laboratory for instructions based on the type of testing (Fischbach et al., 2022). Do not refrigerate specimens for ova and parasites (Fischbach et al., 2022).

(continued on page 1144)

Skill 18-7 ▶ Collecting a Stool Specimen *(continued)*

DELEGATION CONSIDERATIONS	Obtaining a stool specimen may be delegated to assistive personnel (AP) as well as to licensed practical/vocational nurses (LPN/LVNs). The decision to delegate must be based on careful analysis of the patient's needs and circumstances as well as the qualifications of the person to whom the task is being delegated. Refer to the Delegation Guidelines in Appendix A.
EQUIPMENT	• Wooden applicators (2) • Clean specimen container (or container with preservatives for ova and parasites) • Biohazard bag • Gloves • Additional PPE, as indicated • Appropriate label for specimen, based on facility policy and procedure
ASSESSMENT	Assess the patient's understanding of the need for the test and the requirements of the test. Assess the patient's understanding of the collection procedure and their ability to engage in their care. Ask the patient when their last bowel movement was and check their health record for this information. Assess the characteristics of the stool.
ACTUAL OR POTENTIAL HEALTH PROBLEMS AND NEEDS	Many actual or potential health problems or issues may require the use of this skill as part of related interventions. An appropriate health problem or issue may include: • Knowledge deficiency • Diarrhea
OUTCOME IDENTIFICATION AND PLANNING	The expected outcome to achieve is that an uncontaminated specimen is obtained and sent to the laboratory promptly. Additional outcomes that may be appropriate include that the patient demonstrates an understanding of the need and process for specimen collection.

IMPLEMENTATION

ACTION	RATIONALE
1. Verify the prescribed intervention for a stool specimen collection in the patient's health record. Gather equipment.	Verifying the prescribed intervention is crucial for ensuring that the proper procedure is administered to the right patient. Assembling equipment provides for an organized approach to the task.
2. Perform hand hygiene and put on PPE, if indicated.	Hand hygiene and PPE prevent the transmission of microorganisms. PPE is required based on transmission precautions.
3. Identify the patient.	Identifying the patient ensures the right patient receives the intervention and helps prevent errors.
4. Discuss with the patient the need for a stool sample. Explain the process by which the stool will be collected, either from a bedpan, commode, or plastic receptacle in the toilet (Figure 1) to catch stool without urine. Instruct the patient to void first and not to discard toilet paper with stool. Tell the patient to call you as soon as a bowel movement is completed.	Discussion and explanation help to allay some of the patient's anxiety and prepare them for what to expect. The patient should void first because the laboratory study may be inaccurate if the stool contains urine. Placing a container in the toilet or bedside commode aids in obtaining a clean stool specimen uncontaminated by urine.

ACTION	RATIONALE
5. Check the specimen label with the patient's identification bracelet. The label should include the patient's name and identification number, the time the specimen was collected, the route of collection, identification of the person obtaining the sample, and any other information required by facility policy.	Confirmation of patient identification information ensures the specimen is labeled correctly for the right patient.
6. Assemble equipment on the overbed table or other surface within reach.	Arranging items nearby is convenient, saves time, and avoids unnecessary stretching and twisting of muscles on the part of the nurse.
7. After the patient has passed a stool, put on gloves. Use the wooden applicators to obtain a sample, free of blood or urine, and place it in the designated clean specimen container (Figure 2).	The container does not have to be sterile, because stool is not sterile. To ensure accurate results, the stool should be free of urine or menstrual blood.

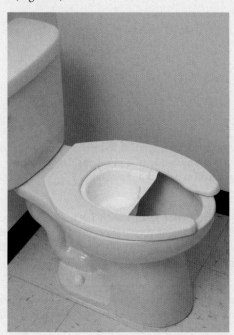

FIGURE 1. Plastic specimen collection receptacle in toilet to catch stool.

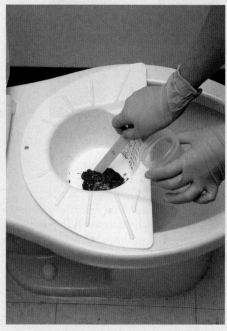

FIGURE 2. Transferring stool to specimen container.

8. Collect as much of the stool as possible to send to the laboratory.	Different tests and laboratories require different amounts of stool. Usually, 1 inch (2.5 cm) of formed stool or 30 mL of liquid stool is sufficient (Fischbach et al., 2022). If portions of the stool include visible blood, mucus, or pus, include these with the specimen (Fischbach et al., 2022). Collecting as much as possible helps to ensure that the laboratory has an adequate amount of specimen for testing.
9. Place the lid on the container. Dispose of used equipment per facility policy. Remove your gloves and perform hand hygiene.	Proper disposal of equipment reduces the transmission of microorganisms. Removing gloves properly reduces the risk for infection transmission and contamination of other items. Hand hygiene deters the spread of microorganisms.
10. Place a label on the container per facility policy. Place the container in a plastic, sealable biohazard bag (Figure 3).	Correct labeling is necessary to ensure accurate results. Packaging the specimen in a biohazard bag prevents the person transporting the container from coming in contact with stool.

(continued on page 1146)

Skill 18-7 ▶ Collecting a Stool Specimen *(continued)*

ACTION | **RATIONALE**

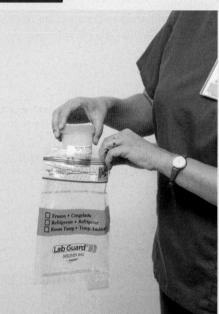

FIGURE 3. Placing specimen container in biohazard bag.

11. Remove other PPE, if used. Perform hand hygiene.

Proper removal of PPE reduces the risk for infection transmission and contamination of other items. Hand hygiene reduces the transmission of microorganisms.

12. Transport the specimen to the laboratory while the stool is still warm. If immediate transport is impossible, check with laboratory personnel or the policy manual to see whether refrigeration is contraindicated.

Most tests have better results with fresh stool. Different tests may require different preparation if the test is not immediately completed. Some tests will be compromised if the stool is refrigerated.

EVALUATION

The expected outcomes have been met when an uncontaminated specimen has been obtained and sent to the laboratory promptly, and the patient has demonstrated an understanding of the need and process for specimen collection.

DOCUMENTATION

Guidelines

Document the amount, color, and consistency of stool obtained, the time of collection, the specific test for which the specimen was collected, and transport to the laboratory.

Sample Documentation

> 7/12/25 2045 Large amount of pasty, green stool sent to laboratory for ova and parasite testing.
>
> —K. Sanders, RN

DEVELOPING CLINICAL REASONING AND CLINICAL JUDGMENT

UNEXPECTED SITUATIONS AND ASSOCIATED INTERVENTIONS

• *Patient is menstruating or has discarded toilet paper into the commode with stool:* Call the laboratory to discuss possible effects on test results. Not all tests will be affected by contaminants. The laboratory may accept the specimen even with the contaminant. Make a notation in the information submitted with specimen.

• *Specimen is inadvertently left on the counter instead of being sent to the laboratory:* Call the laboratory to discuss possible effects on test results. Not all tests will be affected by leaving the specimen on the counter for a period of time. The laboratory may accept the specimen even though it has been sitting out. Make sure that the time documented in the information submitted with the specimen accurately reflects the actual time the specimen was obtained.

SPECIAL CONSIDERATIONS

General Considerations

• Do not retrieve stool from the toilet for specimen use (Fischbach et al., 2022).
• At least three stool specimens collected on separate days are recommended for stool cultures related to potential bacterial infection (Fischbach et al., 2022).
• If possible, ensure specimens for culture are obtained before antibiotics are started, as therapy with antibiotics before specimen collection could affect results (Fischbach et al., 2022).
• If the patient is wearing an adult incontinence brief, the stool may be collected from the brief as long as it is not contaminated with urine.
• Barium procedures and laxatives should be avoided for 1 week before specimen collection (Fischbach et al., 2022).
• A specimen can be collected from an ostomy appliance. Apply a clean ostomy appliance and obtain a sample as soon as the patient passes stool into the appliance.
• If a timed stool test is prescribed, such as fecal fat, the entire amount of stool produced for 24 to 72 hours is sent to the laboratory. Be sure to follow instructions for storage while collection is ongoing.

Infant and Child Considerations

• Stool can be collected from the diaper of an infant or child, as long as the specimen is not contaminated with urine.

Community-Based Care Considerations

• Patients are often instructed on how to collect stool specimens at home and bring the samples to the office, clinic, or laboratory. Patients should understand that it is important to follow instructions carefully to ensure validity of results. Ensure the patient understands the proper procedure for sample storage before bringing it to the laboratory or office.

Skill 18-8 ▶ Obtaining a Capillary Blood Sample for Glucose Testing

Blood glucose monitoring provides information about how the body is controlling glucose metabolism. Controlling the patient's blood glucose levels is an important part of care for patients with many conditions, including diabetes, seizures, liver disease, pancreatitis, head injury, stroke, alcohol and drug intoxication, and sepsis and in patients taking corticosteroids or on enteral or parenteral feeding. Point-of-care testing (testing done at the bedside and samples are not sent to the laboratory) provides a convenient, rapid measurement of blood glucose. Patients with diabetes use this type of testing as an important part of disease management to monitor blood glucose and adjust lifestyle interventions and treatment (U.S. FDA, 2019). Blood samples are commonly obtained from the edges of the fingers for adults, but samples can be obtained from alternative sites, such as the palm of the hand, the forearm, upper arm, calf, or anterior thigh, depending on the time of testing and monitor used (U.S. FDA, 2019). Alternative site testing (AST) should not be performed at times when the blood glucose may be changing rapidly, as the results may be inaccurate (U.S. FDA, 2019). Avoid the fingertips because they are more sensitive. Rotate sites to prevent skin and tissue damage. **It is important to be familiar with and follow the manufacturer's guidelines and facility policy and procedure to ensure accurate results.** Blood glucose target levels are individualized for patients with diabetes, based on duration of diabetes, comorbid conditions, cardiovascular disease or diabetes complications, hypoglycemia unawareness, age/life expectancy, and individual patient considerations (ADA, n.d.). Normal fasting glucose for adults without diabetes is less than 99 mg/dL (NIDDK, 2016).

(continued on page 1148)

Skill 18-8 ▶ Obtaining a Capillary Blood Sample for Glucose Testing *(continued)*

DELEGATION CONSIDERATIONS	Obtaining a capillary blood sample for glucose testing may be delegated to assistive personnel (AP) as well as to licensed practical/vocational nurses (LPN/LVNs). The decision to delegate must be based on careful analysis of the patient's needs and circumstances as well as the qualifications of the person to whom the task is being delegated. Refer to the Delegation Guidelines in Appendix A.
EQUIPMENT	• Blood glucose meter • Sterile lancet • Cotton balls or gauze squares • Testing strips for meter • Nonsterile gloves • Additional PPE, as indicated • Skin cleanser and water or alcohol swab
ASSESSMENT	Assess the patient's history for indications necessitating the monitoring of blood glucose levels, such as high-carbohydrate feedings, history of diabetes mellitus, or corticosteroid therapy. Assess for signs and symptoms of hypoglycemia and hyperglycemia. In addition, assess the patient's knowledge about monitoring blood glucose. Inspect the area of the skin to be used for testing. Avoid bruised and open areas.
ACTUAL OR POTENTIAL HEALTH PROBLEMS AND NEEDS	Many actual or potential health problems or issues may require the use of this skill as part of related interventions. An appropriate health problem or issue may include: • Hyperglycemia risk • Knowledge deficiency • Anxiety
OUTCOME IDENTIFICATION AND PLANNING	The expected outcome to achieve is that the blood glucose level is measured accurately without adverse effect. In addition, the patient demonstrates an understanding of the need and process for specimen collection.

IMPLEMENTATION

ACTION	**RATIONALE**
1. Check the patient's health record or plan of care for the monitoring schedule. Additional testing may be indicated based on nursing judgment and the patient's condition.	This confirms scheduled times for checking blood glucose. Independent nursing judgment may lead to the decision to test more frequently, based on the patient's condition.
2. Gather equipment. Check the expiration date on the blood test strips.	This provides an organized approach to the task. Blood test strips that are past expiration date could cause inaccurate results and should not be used.
3. Perform hand hygiene and put on PPE, if indicated.	Hand hygiene and PPE prevent the transmission of microorganisms. PPE is required based on transmission precautions.
4. Identify the patient. Explain the procedure to the patient and instruct them about the need for monitoring blood glucose.	Identifying the patient ensures the right patient receives the intervention and helps prevent errors. Explanation helps to alleviate anxiety and facilitate engagement.
5. Close the curtains around the bed and close the door to the room, if possible.	Closing the curtain or door provides for patient privacy.
6. Turn on the monitor.	The monitor must be on for use.
7. Enter the patient's identification number or scan their identification bracelet, if required, according to facility policy.	Use of an identification number allows for electronic storage and accurate identification of patient data.

ACTION	RATIONALE
8. Put on gloves.	Gloves protect the nurse from exposure to blood or body fluids.
9. Prepare the **lancet** using aseptic technique.	Aseptic technique maintains sterility.
10. Remove the test strip from the vial. **Recap the container immediately.** Test strips also come individually wrapped. **Check that the code number for the strip matches the code number on the monitor screen.**	Immediate recapping protects strips from exposure to humidity, light, and discoloration. Matching code numbers on the strip and glucose monitor ensures that the machine is calibrated correctly.
11. Insert the strip into the meter according to directions for that specific device. Alternatively, the strip may be placed in the meter after collection of the sample on the test strip, depending on the meter in use.	A correctly inserted strip allows the meter to read the blood glucose level accurately.
12. **Have the patient wash their hands with skin cleanser and warm water and dry thoroughly. Alternatively, cleanse the skin with an alcohol swab. Allow the skin to dry completely.**	Washing with skin cleanser and water or alcohol cleanses the puncture site. Warm water also helps to cause vasodilation. Alcohol can interfere with accuracy of results if not completely dried.
13. Choose a skin site that is intact, warm, and free of calluses and edema (Van Leeuwen & Bladh, 2017).	Areas with lesions are not suitable for capillary sampling. Calluses, edema, and vasoconstriction (cool to palpation) interfere with the ability to obtain a blood sample.
14. Hold the lancet perpendicular to the skin and pierce the skin with the lancet (Figure 1).	Holding the lancet in the proper position facilitates proper skin penetration.
15. Encourage bleeding by lowering the patient's hand, making use of gravity. Lightly stroke their finger, if necessary, until a sufficient amount of blood has formed to cover the sample area on the strip, based on monitor requirements (check instructions for the monitor). If necessary, squeeze from the base of the finger (CDC, 2021d). Take care not to squeeze at the puncture site or to touch the puncture site or blood.	An appropriate-sized droplet facilitates accurate test results. Squeezing can cause injury to the patient and alter the test.
16. Gently touch a drop of blood to the test strip without smearing it (Figure 2). Depending on the meter in use, insert the strip into the meter after collection of the sample on the test strip.	Smearing blood on the strip may result in inaccurate test results.

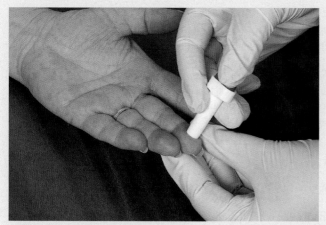

FIGURE 1. Piercing patient's finger with lancet.

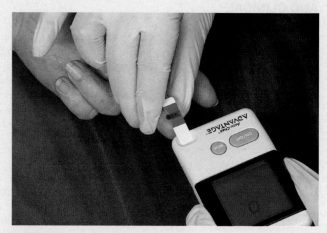

FIGURE 2. Applying blood to test strip.

17. Apply pressure to the puncture site with a cotton ball or dry gauze. **Do not use an alcohol wipe.**	Pressure causes hemostasis. Alcohol stings and may dry the skin.
18. Read blood glucose results and document the results in the EHR or other designated location, based on facility policy. Inform the patient of the test result.	Timing depends on the type of meter.

(continued on page 1150)

Skill 18-8 ▶ **Obtaining a Capillary Blood Sample for Glucose Testing** *(continued)*

ACTION	RATIONALE
19. Turn off the meter, remove the test strip, and dispose of supplies appropriately. Place the lancet in the sharps container.	Proper disposal prevents exposure to blood and accidental needlestick.
20. Remove your gloves and any other PPE, if used. Perform hand hygiene.	Proper removal of PPE reduces the risk for infection transmission and contamination of other items. Hand hygiene reduces the transmission of microorganisms.

EVALUATION

The expected outcomes have been achieved when the patient's blood glucose level has been measured accurately without adverse effect, and the patient has demonstrated an understanding of the need and process for testing.

DOCUMENTATION

Guidelines

Document blood glucose level in the patient's health record, according to facility policy. Document pertinent patient assessments, any intervention related to glucose level, and any patient teaching. Communicate abnormal results and/or significant assessments to the health care team.

Sample Documentation

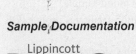

Practice documenting blood glucose testing in *Lippincott DocuCare*.

> 11/1/25 0800 Patient performed own fingerstick blood glucose test with minimal guidance. Verbalized rationale for fasting measurement and able to state symptoms of hypoglycemia. Patient's fingerstick blood glucose level 168. Four units regular Humulin insulin given per sliding scale, in addition to 10 units NPH Humulin insulin scheduled for 0800. Patient encouraged to review written guidelines for subcutaneous insulin administration; will review procedure and plan to have patient administer insulin at dinnertime. Patient verbalized an understanding.
>
> —B. Clapp, RN

DEVELOPING CLINICAL REASONING AND CLINICAL JUDGMENT

UNEXPECTED SITUATIONS AND ASSOCIATED INTERVENTIONS

- *Extremity is pale and cool to the touch:* Begin by warming the extremity. Have adult patients warm their hands by rubbing them together or washing them with warm water. Warm, moist compresses may also be used.
- *Blood glucose level results are above- or below-normal parameters:* Assess the patient for signs of hyperglycemia or hypoglycemia, respectively. Check the patient's health record for prescribed interventions, such as insulin dosage or glucose-containing carbohydrate administration (ADA, 2021). Notify the health care team of results, assessment data, and interventions.

SPECIAL CONSIDERATIONS

General Considerations

- If the selected site feels cool or appears pale, warm compresses can be applied for 3 to 5 minutes to dilate the capillaries.
- Sampling of blood from an alternative site other than fingertips may have limitations. Blood in the fingertips shows changes in glucose levels more quickly than blood in other parts of the body. This means that alternative site test results may differ from fingertip test results when glucose levels are changing rapidly (e.g., after a meal, taking insulin, or during or after exercise) because the results may be inaccurate. Caution patients to use a fingertip sample if it is less than 2 hours after eating, less than 2 hours after injecting rapid-acting insulin, during exercise or within 2 hours of exercise, when sick or under stress, when having symptoms of hypoglycemia, if unable to recognize symptoms of hypoglycemia, or if site results do not agree with the way the patient feels (U.S. FDA, 2019).

- Meters require calibration at least monthly or according to the manufacturer's recommendation, and when a new bottle of test strips is opened. The manufacturer's directions for calibration should be followed. After calibration, the meter is checked for accuracy by testing a control solution containing a known amount of glucose.
- Alternative testing sites, other than fingertips, should not be used to calibrate a continuous glucose monitor or for insulin dosing calculations (U.S. FDA, 2019).
- Inadequate sampling can cause errors in the results. It is very important to be aware of requirements for the specific monitor used.
- Continuous glucose monitoring (CGM) systems use sensors placed just below the skin to check glucose levels in tissue fluid. A transmitter sends information about glucose levels from the sensor to a wireless monitor. These devices provide real-time measurements of glucose levels every few minutes (NIDDK, 2017). These systems provide a way to see glucose trends and track patterns (NIDDK, 2017).
- Most CGM models require confirmation of a CGM reading with a fingerstick blood glucose test before taking insulin or treating hypoglycemia (NIDDK, 2017).

Infant and Child Considerations

- Heel sticks, using the outer aspect of the heel, may be used for infants. Warming the heel for 5 to 10 minutes before the sample is taken dilates the blood vessels in the area and aids in sampling (KarabiyikOğurlu et al., 2020; Vedder, 2021). This technique is not without controversy, as it is painful and can lead to scarring and infection, including infection of bone and cartilage, due to excessive depth of the puncture (Gorski et al., 2021; Vedder, 2021). Venipuncture by a skilled phlebotomist is suggested instead of heel lance methods due to the increased pain from the heel lance (Gorski et al., 2021). Automatic lancing devices are preferred over manual devices to control the depth of puncture and to reduce the risk of bone or cartilage infection (Gorski et al., 2021).

Older Adult Considerations

- Blood glucose meters are available with large digital readouts or audio components for patients with visual impairments (Williams, n.d.).

Community-Based Care Considerations

- Patients monitor blood glucose levels routinely at home. Provide education focusing on important elements of diabetes education to assist patients in managing their diabetes, including the signs, symptoms, and management of hypoglycemia and hyperglycemia; correct administration of oral hypoglycemic agents and/or insulin; fingerstick blood glucose monitoring; and the accurate use of fingerstick blood glucose monitoring equipment.
- Many different types of monitors are available. Assist patients to identify desirable features for individual use.

EVIDENCE FOR PRACTICE ▶

STANDARDS OF MEDICAL CARE IN DIABETES—2021

American Diabetes Association (ADA). (2021). Standards of medical care in diabetes—2021. *Diabetes Care, 44*(Suppl 1), S1–S232. https://care.diabetesjournals.org/content/44/Supplement_1

These standards of care provide clinicians, patients, researchers, payers, and other interested people with the components of diabetes care with general treatment goals and tools to evaluate the quality of care. The recommendations included are screening, diagnostic, and therapeutic actions that are known or believed to favorably affect health outcomes of patients with diabetes.

Skill 18-9 ▶ Using Venipuncture to Collect a Venous Blood Sample

Venipuncture involves piercing a vein with a needle to obtain a venous blood sample, which is collected in a syringe or tube or to initiate an intravenous access. The superficial veins of the arm in the antecubital fossa, which include the basilic, median cubital, and cephalic veins, are typically used for venipuncture for blood sampling (Figure 1) (Fischbach et al., 2022). However, venipuncture for blood sampling can be performed on a vein in the wrist, dorsal forearm, the dorsum of the hand, or another accessible location (Fischbach et al., 2022). When performing a venipuncture for blood sampling, remember the following:

- Do not use the inner wrist because of the high risk for damage to underlying structures.
- Avoid areas that are edematous, paralyzed, burned, scarred, or have a tattoo or are on the same side as a mastectomy, arteriovenous shunt, or graft.
- Avoid an extremity affected by a cerebrovascular accident, areas of infection, or areas with abnormal skin conditions.
- Do not draw blood from the same extremity being used for administration of intravenous medications, fluids, or blood transfusions. Some facilities will allow use of such sites as a "last resort," after the infusion has been held for a period of time. If necessary, choose a site below or distal to the infusion site (Fischbach et al., 2022; Gorski et al., 2021). Check facility policy and procedure.

Explanation and communication with patients about the need for venipuncture can reduce anxiety. It is important to carefully explain the information about the need for blood tests to ensure patient understanding.

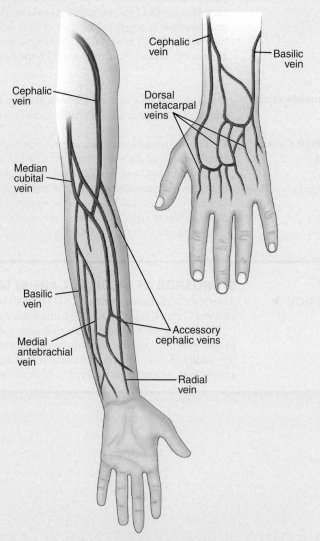

FIGURE 1. Blood vessels in the arm typically used for venipuncture.

DELEGATION GUIDELINES	The use of venipuncture to obtain a blood sample may be delegated to assistive personnel (AP) as well as to licensed practical/vocational nurses (LPN/LVNs). The decision to delegate must be based on careful analysis of the patient's needs and circumstances as well as the qualifications of the person to whom the task is being delegated. Refer to the Delegation Guidelines in Appendix A.

EQUIPMENT	• Tourniquet • Gloves • Additional PPE, as indicated • Antimicrobial wipes, such as chlorhexidine or alcohol • Sterile needle, gauge appropriate to the vein and sampling needs, using the smallest possible • Vacutainer needle adaptor • Blood collection tubes appropriate for prescribed tests • Appropriate label for specimen, based on facility policy and procedure • Waterproof protective pad • Prescribed local anesthetic cream, as indicated • Biohazard bag • Gauze pads (2 × 2) • Adhesive bandage

ASSESSMENT	Review the patient's health record for the blood specimens to be obtained. Ensure that the necessary computerized laboratory request has been completed. Assess the patient for any allergies, especially to the topical antimicrobial to be used for skin cleansing. Investigate for the presence of any conditions or use of medications that may prolong bleeding time, necessitating additional application of pressure to the puncture site. Ask the patient about any previous laboratory testing they may have had, including any problems, such as difficulty with venipuncture; fainting; or reports of dizziness, lightheadedness, or nausea. Assess the patient's anxiety level and understanding of the reasons for the blood test. Assess the need/patient preference for use of a prescribed local anesthetic cream (Fischbach et al., 2022). Assess the patency of the veins in both upper limbs and for circulation problems. Avoid areas that are edematous, burned, scarred, or paralyzed; have a tattoo, infectious or skin conditions, or hematoma present; are paralyzed; or are on the same side as a mastectomy or have an actual or planned dialysis access (Fischbach et al., 2022; Van Leeuwen & Bladh, 2017). Palpate the veins to assess the condition of the vessel; the vein should be straight, feel soft, cylindrical, and bounce when lightly pressed. Appropriate vessels will compress without rolling and have rapid rebound filling after compression. Avoid veins that are tender, sclerosed, thrombosed, fibrosed, or hard (Van Leeuwen & Bladh, 2017).

ACTUAL OR POTENTIAL HEALTH PROBLEMS AND NEEDS	Many actual or potential health problems or issues may require the use of this skill as part of related interventions. An appropriate health problem or issue may include: • Knowledge deficiency • Injury risk • Infection risk

OUTCOME IDENTIFICATION AND PLANNING	The expected outcome to achieve is that an uncontaminated specimen will be obtained without injury to the patient and sent to the laboratory promptly. In addition, the patient demonstrates an understanding of the need and process for specimen collection.

IMPLEMENTATION

ACTION	**RATIONALE**
1. Gather the necessary supplies. Check product expiration dates. Identify the prescribed laboratory tests and select the appropriate blood collection tubes.	Organization facilitates efficient performance of the procedure. Use of products that have not expired ensures proper functioning of equipment. Using correct bottles ensures accurate blood sampling.

(continued on page 1154)

Skill 18-9 ▶ Using Venipuncture to Collect a Venous Blood Sample *(continued)*

ACTION	RATIONALE
2. Perform hand hygiene and put on PPE, if indicated.	Hand hygiene and PPE prevent the transmission of microorganisms. PPE is required based on transmission precautions.
3. Identify the patient.	Identifying the patient ensures the right patient receives the intervention and helps prevent errors.
4. Explain the procedure to the patient. Allow them time to ask questions and verbalize concerns about the venipuncture procedure. Assess for the need/patient preference for the use of a prescribed local anesthetic cream.	Explanation provides reassurance and promotes engagement. Venipuncture is associated with pain; local anesthetic crease may be applied to the area before venipuncture (Fischbach et al., 2022.
5. Check the specimen label with the patient's identification bracelet. The label should include the patient's name and identification number, the time the specimen was collected, the route of collection, identification of the person obtaining the sample, and any other information required by facility policy. Depending on facility policy, specimen labels may be verified after obtaining blood samples, prior to application to blood sample tubes.	Verifying the patient's identity validates that the correct procedure is being done on the correct patient, and the specimen is accurately labeled.
6. Assemble equipment on the overbed table or other surface within reach.	Arranging items nearby is convenient, saves time, and avoids unnecessary stretching and twisting of muscles on the part of the nurse.
7. Close the curtains around the bed and close the door to the room, if possible.	Closing the door or curtain provides for patient privacy.
8. Provide for good light. Artificial light is recommended. Place a trash receptacle within easy reach.	Good lighting is necessary to perform the procedure properly. Having the trash receptacle within easy reach allows for safe disposal of contaminated materials.
9. Assist the patient to a comfortable position, either sitting or lying. If the patient is lying in bed, raise the bed to a comfortable working height (VHACEOSH, 2016).	Proper positioning allows easy access to the site and promotes patient comfort and safety. The proper bed height helps reduce back strain on the part of the nurse while performing the procedure.
10. Determine the patient's preferred site for the procedure based on their previous experience. Expose the arm, supporting it in an extended position on a firm surface, such as a tabletop. Position yourself on the same side as the site selected. Apply a tourniquet to the upper arm on the chosen side approximately 3 to 4 inches above the potential puncture site. Apply sufficient pressure to impede venous circulation but not arterial blood flow.	Eliciting the patient's preference promotes patient participation in their treatment and gives the nurse information that may aid in site selection. Positioning yourself close to the chosen site reduces back strain. Use of a tourniquet increases venous pressure to aid in vein identification. The tourniquet should remain in place no more than 60 seconds to prevent stasis and hemoconcentration (Gorski et al., 2021).
11. Put on gloves. Assess the veins using inspection and palpation to determine the best puncture site. Refer to the Assessment section above.	Gloves reduce transmission of microorganisms. Using the best site reduces the risk of injury to the patient. Observation and palpation allow for making distinction between other structures, such as tendons and arteries in the area, to avoid injury.
12. **Release the tourniquet. Check that the vein has decompressed.**	Releasing the tourniquet reduces the length of time the tourniquet is applied. The tourniquet should remain in place no more than 1 minute; prolonged tourniquet application causes stasis and hemoconcentration and alterations in test results (Fischbach et al., 2022). Thrombosed veins will remain firm and palpable and should not be used for venipuncture.
13. Attach the needle to the Vacutainer device. Place the first blood collection tube into the Vacutainer but not engaged in the puncture device in the Vacutainer.	The device is prepared for use to ensure efficiency with the task.

| ACTION | RATIONALE |

14. Use a single-use sterile applicator containing sterile antiseptic solution to **cleanse the patient's skin at the selected puncture site with the antiseptic solution identified in facility policy (Figure 2). Follow the manufacturer's directions for use to determine the product application process and dry times (Gorski et al., 2021). Allow the antiseptic to dry naturally; do not wipe, fan, or blow on the skin** (Gorski et al., 2021).

Cleaning the patient's skin reduces the risk for transmission of microorganisms. Allowing the skin to dry maximizes antimicrobial action and prevents contact of the substance with the needle on insertion, thereby reducing the sting associated with insertion. Allowing the area to thoroughly dry avoids the possibility of the solution causing hemolysis (Gorski et al., 2021).

15. Reapply the tourniquet approximately 3 to 4 inches above the identified puncture site (Figure 3). Apply sufficient pressure to impede venous circulation but not arterial blood flow. **After disinfection, do not palpate the venipuncture site. If repeated palpation is necessary, the antiseptic solution must be reapplied before venipuncture** (Gorski et al., 2021).

Use of a tourniquet increases venous pressure to aid in vein identification. The tourniquet should remain in place no more than 1 minute; prolonged tourniquet application causes stasis and hemoconcentration and alterations in test results (Fischbach et al., 2022).

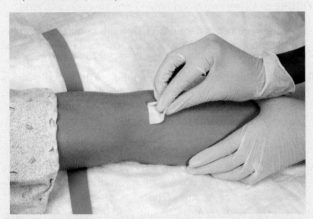

FIGURE 2. Cleaning the patient's skin at the venipuncture site.

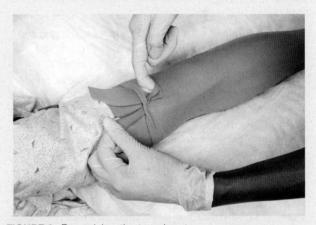

FIGURE 3. Reapplying the tourniquet.

16. Hold the patient's arm in a downward position with your nondominant hand. Align the needle and Vacutainer device with the chosen vein, holding the Vacutainer and needle in your dominant hand. Use the thumb or first finger of your nondominant hand to apply pressure and traction to the skin about 1 to 2 inches below the identified puncture site (Fischbach et al., 2022; Van Leeuwen & Bladh, 2017).

Applying pressure helps immobilize and anchor the vein. Taut skin at the entry site aids smooth needle entry; pressure on the distal end of the vein during the puncture decreases the possibility of rolling veins (Fischbach et al., 2022).

17. **Inform the patient that they are going to feel a pinch.** With the bevel of the needle up, insert the needle into the vein at a 15- to 30-degree angle to the skin (Van Leeuwen & Bladh, 2017) (Figure 4).

Warning the patient prevents a reaction related to surprise. Positioning the needle at the proper angle reduces the risk of puncturing through the vein.

18. Grasp the Vacutainer securely to stabilize it in the vein with your nondominant hand, and push the first collection tube into the puncture device in the Vacutainer, until the rubber stopper on the collection tube is punctured. You will feel the tube push into place on the puncture device. Blood will flow into the tube automatically (Figure 5).

The collection tube is a vacuum; negative pressure within the tube pulls blood into the tube.

19. **Remove the tourniquet as soon as blood flows adequately into the tube** (Gorski et al., 2021).

Tourniquet removal reduces venous pressure and restores venous return to help prevent venous stasis, bleeding, bruising, and inaccurate results (Fischbach et al., 2022; Van Leeuwen & Bladh, 2017).

(continued on page 1156)

Skill 18-9 ▶ Using Venipuncture to Collect a Venous Blood Sample *(continued)*

ACTION

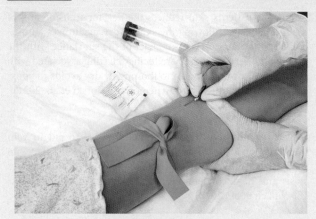

FIGURE 4. Inserting the needle at a 15-degree angle, with the bevel up.

20. Continue to hold the Vacutainer in place in the vein and continue to fill the required tubes, removing one and inserting another. Gently rotate each tube as you remove it.

21. After you have drawn all required blood samples, remove the last collection tube from the Vacutainer. **Place a gauze pad over the puncture site and slowly and gently remove the needle from the vein. Engage the needle guard. Do not apply pressure to the site until the needle has been fully removed.**

22. Apply gentle pressure to the puncture site for 2 to 3 minutes or until bleeding stops.

23. After bleeding stops, apply an adhesive bandage. Discard the Vacutainer and needle in the sharps container. Remove your gloves and perform hand hygiene.

24. Remove equipment and return the patient to a position of comfort. Raise the side rail and lower the bed.

25. Record the date and time the samples were obtained on the labels as well as the required information to identify the person obtaining the samples. Compare the specimen label with the patient identification bracelet, as required by facility policy. Depending on facility policy, specimen labels may be verified prior to obtaining blood samples (refer to Step 5). Apply labels to the specimens, according to facility policy. Place them in a biohazard bag.

26. Put on gloves. Check the venipuncture site to see if a hematoma has developed.

27. Remove your gloves and other PPE, if used. Perform hand hygiene.

28. Transport the specimen to the laboratory immediately. If immediate transport is not possible, check with laboratory personnel or the policy manual to see whether refrigeration is contraindicated.

RATIONALE

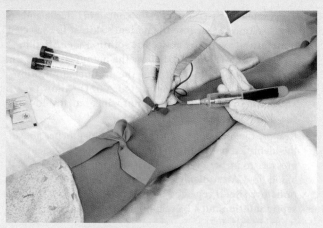

FIGURE 5. Observing blood flowing into the collection tube.

Filling the required tubes ensures that the sample is accurate. Gentle rotation helps to mix any additive in the tube with the blood sample.

Slow, gentle needle removal prevents injury to the vein. Releasing the vacuum before withdrawing the needle prevents injury to the vein and hematoma formation. Use of a needle guard prevents accidental needlestick injuries.

Applying pressure to the site after needle removal prevents injury, bleeding, and extravasation into the surrounding tissue, which can cause a hematoma.

The bandage protects the site and aids in applying pressure. Proper disposal of equipment reduces transmission of microorganisms. Removing gloves and performing hand hygiene reduce transmission of microorganisms.

Repositioning promotes patient comfort. Raising the rails promotes safety.

Proper labeling ensures accurate communication of results. Use of a biohazard bag prevents contact with blood and body fluids.

Gloves prevent contact with blood and body fluids. Development of a hematoma requires further intervention.

Proper removal of PPE reduces the risk for infection transmission and contamination of other items. Hand hygiene reduces the transmission of microorganisms.

Timely transport ensures accurate results.

EVALUATION

The expected outcomes have been met when an uncontaminated specimen has been obtained without injury to the patient and has been sent to the laboratory promptly, and the patient has demonstrated an understanding of the need and process for specimen collection.

DOCUMENTATION

Guidelines

Document any pertinent assessments; the laboratory specimens obtained; the date and time specimens were obtained; disposition of specimens; the amount of blood collected, if required; and any significant assessments or patient reactions.

Sample Documentation

6/10/25 0945 Blood specimen for CBC with differential obtained from right antecubital space. Approximately 8 mL of blood collected and sent to laboratory. No evidence of bleeding or hematoma at venipuncture site. Patient denied any reports of pain or feelings of lightheadedness.

—C. Lewis, RN

DEVELOPING CLINICAL REASONING AND CLINICAL JUDGMENT

UNEXPECTED SITUATIONS AND ASSOCIATED INTERVENTIONS

- *After applying the tourniquet, you have trouble finding a distended vein:* Have the patient make a fist, or try tapping the skin over the vein lightly several times. **To prevent venous stasis and reduce risk for inaccurate results, do not have the patient repeatedly clench their fist or pump their hand (Gorski et al., 2021), which may increase plasma potassium levels** (Fischbach et al., 2022). If unsuccessful, remove the tourniquet and try lowering the patient's arm to allow blood to pool in the veins. If necessary, apply warm compresses for about 10 minutes before reapplying the tourniquet.
- *Patient has large, distended, highly visible veins:* Perform venipuncture without a tourniquet to minimize the risk for hematoma (Fischbach et al., 2022).
- *Patient has a clotting disorder or is receiving anticoagulant therapy:* Maintain firm pressure on the venipuncture site for at least 5 minutes after withdrawing the needle to prevent hematoma formation.
- *Oozing or bleeding continues from the puncture site for more than a few minutes:* Elevate the area and apply a pressure dressing. If bleeding is excessive or persists for longer than 10 minutes, notify the health care team.
- *Hematoma develops at the venipuncture site:* Apply pressure until you are sure the bleeding has stopped (about 5 minutes). Notify the health care team. Document the size and appearance of the hematoma, notification of the health care team, and any prescribed interventions.
- *Patient reports feeling lightheaded and says they are going to faint:* Stop the venipuncture. If the patient is in bed, have them lie flat and elevate their feet. If the patient is in a chair, have them put their head between their knees. Encourage the patient to take slow, deep breaths. Call for assistance and stay with the patient. Obtain vital signs, if possible.

SPECIAL CONSIDERATIONS

General Considerations

- **Obtain only the volume of blood needed for accurate testing. Phlebotomy** (puncture of a vein to withdraw blood) contributes to anemia in newborns, pediatrics, and critically ill adult patients and hospital-acquired anemia in patients of all ages (Gorski et al., 2021). Consider interventions to conserve blood, including the use of small-volume blood collection tubes, point-of-care testing methods, avoidance of routine and/or unnecessary testing, and consolidation of all daily tests with one blood draw (Gorski et al., 2021).
- Perform venipuncture for phlebotomy on the opposite extremity of an infusion (Gorski et al., 2021). If phlebotomy must be performed on an extremity with infusing solutions, use a vein below or distal to the site of infusion (Gorski et al., 2021).
- In patients with a dialysis fistula or graft, or patients who have a planned dialysis fistula or graft, restrict venipuncture for blood sampling to the dorsum of the hand whenever possible (Gorski et al., 2021).

(*continued on page 1158*)

Skill 18-9 ▶ Using Venipuncture to Collect a Venous Blood Sample *(continued)*

- Be aware of the facility's policy regarding the order of collection of multiple tubes of blood to ensure accurate results.
- If the flow of blood into the collection tube or syringe is sluggish, leave the tourniquet in place longer, but always remove it before withdrawing the needle. Do not leave the tourniquet on for more than 1 minute (Fischbach et al., 2022).
- If necessary, use a blood pressure cuff inflated to a point between systolic and diastolic pressure values as an alternative to a tourniquet (Fischbach et al., 2022).
- Avoid collecting blood from edematous areas, arteriovenous shunts, an upper extremity on the same side as a previous lymph node dissection or mastectomy, infected sites, the same extremity as an intravenous infusion, and sites of previous hematomas or vascular injury.
- Avoid previous sites of venipuncture to reduce the potential for infection (Van Leeuwen & Bladh, 2017).
- Do not use veins in the lower extremities for venipuncture, because of an increased risk of thrombophlebitis. Some facilities allow collection from lower extremities as a prescribed intervention to collect blood from a leg or foot vein. Check your facility's policies.
- Apply warm compresses to the selected site 15 to 20 minutes before venipuncture to aid in distending veins that are difficult to locate.
- Consider the use of topical anesthetic creams to minimize discomfort and pain for the patient, based on facility policy. Allow 60 seconds after application for patients with light skin tones and 120 seconds for patients with dark skin tones before performing the venipuncture (Fischbach et al., 2022). Be familiar with the requirements and specifications for a particular product available for use. Application needs to occur sufficiently in advance to allow enough time to become effective.
- Use distraction, if appropriate. Distraction has been shown to be of benefit in reducing anxiety related to venipuncture, especially with children (Erdogan & Ozdemir, 2021; Kuo et al., 2018). Asking the patient to concentrate on relaxing and performing deep breathing may help them relax.

Infant and Child Considerations

- Use smaller-gauge needles with infants and children because their veins are smaller and more fragile.
- Consider automatically applying warm compresses to distend the small veins of infants and young children before attempting any venipuncture.
- Use butterfly needles, as appropriate, for obtaining blood from infants and small children.
- Heelsticks, using the outer aspect of the heel, may be used for infants. Warming the heel for 5 to 10 minutes before the sample is taken dilates the blood vessels in the area and aids in sampling (KarabiyikOğurlu et al., 2020; Vedder, 2021). This technique is not without controversy, as it is painful and can lead to scarring and infection, including infection of bone and cartilage, due to excessive depth of the puncture (Gorski et al., 2021; Vedder, 2021). Venipuncture by a skilled phlebotomist is suggested instead of heel lance methods due to the increased pain from the heel lance (Gorski et al., 2021). Automatic lancing devices are preferred over manual devices to control the depth of puncture and to reduce the risk of bone or cartilage infection (Gorski et al., 2021).
- Consider a combination of techniques including swaddling, breastfeeding, pacifiers, rocking, and/or administration of oral sucrose (24%) beginning 1 to 2 minutes before the venipuncture procedure for young infants to decrease the incidence of procedure-related pain (De Bernardo et al., 2018; Gorski et al., 2021).
- Consider using topical anesthetic creams or gels, refrigerant spray, or iontophoresis (application of electric current to carry ionized lidocaine through the skin) with infants and children, to decrease the incidence of procedure-related pain (Kyle & Carman, 2021). Apply the product for a sufficient time to reach maximal effectiveness.
- Consider the use of distraction to reduce anxiety and procedure-related pain (Erdogan & Ozdemir, 2021; Gorski et al., 2021; Kuo et al., 2018).

Older Adult Considerations

- Keep in mind that the veins of an older adult are fragile and may collapse easily. In addition, the skin is less elastic and may be more difficult to pull taut.
- The superficial veins of the hands of older adults are fragile, and venipuncture can cause a hematoma to form. Insert the needle for venipuncture at no more than a 30-degree angle unless using ultrasound guidance; use a 5- to 15-degree angle for veins of older adults (Gorski et al., 2021). In addition, these veins move due to the age-related loss of supportive muscle and connective tissue, making it difficult to enter the lumen of the vein.
- Consider performing venipuncture without a tourniquet for older adults to prevent rupture of capillaries (Fischbach et al., 2022).

EVIDENCE FOR PRACTICE ▶

RELIEF OF PAIN DURING BLOOD SPECIMEN COLLECTION IN PEDIATRIC PATIENTS

Needle insertion for venipuncture is painful, frightening, and distressful for children. What interventions can assist nurses to reduce the emotional and physical effects of painful procedures, such as venipuncture, in children?

Related Research

Erdogan, B., & Ozdemir, A. A. (2021). The effect of three different methods on venipuncture pain and anxiety in children: Distraction cards, virtual reality, and Buzzy® (randomized controlled trial). *Journal of Pediatric Nursing, 58,* e54–e62. https://doi.org/10.1016/j.pedn.2021.01.001

The purpose of this randomized-controlled study was to determine the effect of distraction cards, virtual reality, and Buzzy® methods on venipuncture pain and anxiety in children ages 7 to 12 years at a pediatric venipuncture unit of a university hospital in Turkey. Participants ($n = 142$) were randomized into four groups: the experimental groups ($n = 108$) received one of three interventions, and the control group received no intervention during venipuncture ($n = 34$). Participants in the distraction card group ($n = 35$) were asked several questions requiring them to focus on cards with hidden pictures and patterns just before during venipuncture. The participants in the virtual reality group ($n = 37$) engaged with a 3D dinosaur animation on a smartphone using virtual reality glasses and a headset. The Buzzy® intervention group received application of cold and vibration 60 seconds before the procedure on the venipuncture site, which was then moved to an area 3 cm above the site and continued during venipuncture. Participants' pain and anxiety levels were measured immediately after the venipuncture procedure, and a volunteer parent and the researcher observed the participants' behavior to measure pain and anxiety levels. Results indicated that all intervention groups had significantly lower pain and anxiety scores than the control group, with the Buzzy® group scoring the lowest mean on all measurements according to all raters (participant, parent, researcher). The researchers concluded that the Distraction Cards, virtual reality, and Buzzy® methods were all effective in reducing pain and anxiety related to venipuncture in children.

Relevance for Nursing Practice

Nurses are often responsible for obtaining blood samples from their patients, including children. Using the most efficient techniques can result in decreased pain and anxiety for both the children and their parents. This study suggests several methods of reducing pain associated with venipuncture and should be considered for use when caring for these young patients.

Skill 18-10 ▶ Obtaining a Venous Blood Specimen for Culture and Sensitivity

Normally bacteria-free blood is susceptible to infection through infusion lines as well as from thrombophlebitis, surgical drains, infected shunts, and bacterial endocarditis due to prosthetic heart-valve replacements. Bacteria may also move into the bloodstream through the lymphatic system from an infection of a specific body site when the person's immune system cannot contain the infection at its source, such as the bladder or kidneys, from a urinary tract infection. Patients with a compromised immune system are at higher risk for septicemia.

Blood cultures are performed to detect bacterial invasion (bacteremia) or fungi (fungemia) and the systemic spread of such an infection (septicemia) through the bloodstream. In this procedure, a venous blood sample is collected by venipuncture into two bottles (one set), one containing an anaerobic medium and the other an aerobic medium. The bottles are incubated, encouraging any organisms present in the sample to grow in the media. In acute febrile illness, two sets of cultures from different venipuncture sites are collected. In fever of unknown origin, two sets of cultures can

(continued on page 1160)

Skill 18-10 ▶ Obtaining a Venous Blood Specimen for Culture and Sensitivity *(continued)*

be drawn 45 to 60 minutes apart (Fischbach et al., 2022). If necessary, two more sets of samples can be drawn 24 to 48 hours later (Fischbach et al., 2022).

The main problem encountered with blood culture testing is that the specimen is easily contaminated with bacteria from the environment. Care must be taken to clean the skin at the venipuncture site properly to prevent contamination with skin flora, and aseptic technique must be used during the procedure. In addition, the access ports on the blood culture bottles must be properly cleaned before use.

Refer to Skill 18-9 for additional considerations related to venipuncture and blood sample collection.

DELEGATION GUIDELINES	The use of venipuncture to obtain a blood sample for blood culture may be delegated to assistive personnel (AP) in some settings as well as to licensed practical/vocational nurses (LPN/LVNs). The decision to delegate must be based on careful analysis of the patient's needs and circumstances as well as the qualifications of the person to whom the task is being delegated. Refer to the Delegation Guidelines in Appendix A.
EQUIPMENT	• Tourniquet • Gloves • Additional PPE, as indicated • Antimicrobial wipes, such as chlorhexidine or alcohol per facility policy, for cleaning skin and culture bottle tops • Vacutainer needle adaptor • Sterile butterfly needle, gauge appropriate to the vein and sampling needs, using the smallest possible, with extension tubing • Two blood culture collection bottles for each set being obtained: one anaerobic bottle and one aerobic bottle • Appropriate label for specimen, based on facility policy and procedure • Waterproof protective pad • Biohazard bag • Nonsterile gauze pads (2 × 2) • Sterile gauze pads (2 × 2) • Adhesive bandage
ASSESSMENT	Review the patient's health record for the number and type of blood cultures to be obtained. Ensure that the appropriate computer laboratory request has been completed. Assess the patient for signs and symptoms of infection, including vital signs, and note any antibiotic therapy being administered. Inspect any invasive monitoring insertion sites or incisions for indications of infection. Assess the patient for any allergies, especially related to the topical antimicrobial used for skin cleansing. Assess for the presence of any conditions or use of medications that may prolong bleeding time, necessitating additional application of pressure to the puncture site. Ask the patient about any previous laboratory testing they may have had, including any problems, such as difficulty with venipuncture; fainting; or reports of dizziness, lightheadedness, or nausea. Assess the patient's anxiety level and understanding about the reasons for the blood test. Assess the need/patient preference for use of a prescribed local anesthetic cream (Fischbach et al., 2022). Assess the patency of the veins in both upper limbs and for circulation problems. Avoid areas that are edematous, burned, scarred, or paralyzed; have a tattoo or hematoma present; are on the same side as a mastectomy; or have an actual or planned dialysis access or infectious or skin conditions present (Fischbach et al., 2022; Van Leeuwen & Bladh, 2017). Palpate the veins to assess the condition of the vessel; the vein should be straight, feel soft, cylindrical, and bounce when lightly pressed. Appropriate vessels will compress without rolling and have rapid rebound filling after compression. Avoid veins that are tender, sclerosed, thrombosed, fibrosed, or hard (Van Leeuwen & Bladh, 2017).

ACTUAL OR POTENTIAL HEALTH PROBLEMS AND NEEDS	Many actual or potential health problems or issues may require the use of this skill as part of related interventions. An appropriate health problem or issue may include: • Knowledge deficiency • Injury risk • Infection risk
OUTCOME IDENTIFICATION AND PLANNING	The expected outcome to achieve is that an uncontaminated specimen will be obtained without injury to the patient and sent to the laboratory promptly. In addition, the patient demonstrates an understanding of the need and process for specimen collection.

IMPLEMENTATION

ACTION	RATIONALE
1. Gather the necessary supplies. Check product expiration dates. Identify prescribed number of blood culture sets and select the appropriate blood collection bottles (at least one anaerobic and one aerobic bottle). **If tests are prescribed in addition to the blood cultures, collect the blood culture specimens before other specimens.**	Organization facilitates efficient performance of the procedure. Use of products that have not expired ensures proper functioning of equipment. Using correct tubes ensures accurate blood sampling.
2. Perform hand hygiene and put on PPE, if indicated.	Hand hygiene and PPE prevent the transmission of microorganisms. PPE is required based on transmission precautions.
3. Identify the patient.	Identifying the patient ensures the right patient receives the intervention and helps prevent errors.
4. Explain the procedure. Allow the patient time to ask questions and verbalize concerns about the venipuncture procedure. Assess for the need/patient preference for the use of a prescribed local anesthetic cream.	Explanation provides reassurance and promotes engagement. Venipuncture is associated with pain; local anesthetic crease may be applied to the area before venipuncture (Fischbach et al., 2022).
5. Check the specimen label with the patient's identification bracelet. The label should include the patient's name and identification number, the time the specimen was collected, the route of collection, identification of person obtaining the sample, and any other information required by facility policy. Depending on facility policy, specimen labels may be verified after obtaining blood samples, prior to application to blood sample tubes.	Verifying the patient's identity validates that the correct procedure is being done on the correct patient, and the specimen is accurately labeled.
6. Assemble equipment on the overbed table or other surface within reach.	Arranging items nearby is convenient, saves time, and avoids unnecessary stretching and twisting of muscles on the part of the nurse.
7. Close the curtains around the bed, and close the door to the room, if possible.	Closing the door or curtain provides for patient privacy.
8. Provide for good light. Artificial light is recommended. Place a trash receptacle within easy reach.	Good lighting is necessary to perform the procedure properly. Having the trash receptacle within easy reach allows for safe disposal of contaminated materials.
9. Assist the patient to a comfortable position, either sitting or lying. If the patient is lying in bed, raise the bed to a comfortable working height (VHACEOSH, 2016).	Proper positioning allows easy access to the site and promotes patient comfort and safety. The proper bed height helps reduce back strain on the part of the nurse while performing the procedure.

(continued on page 1162)

Skill 18-10 ▶ Obtaining a Venous Blood Specimen for Culture and Sensitivity *(continued)*

ACTION	RATIONALE
10. Determine the patient's preferred site for the procedure based on their previous experience. Expose their arm, supporting it in an extended position on a firm surface, such as a tabletop. Position yourself on the same side as the selected site. Apply a tourniquet to the upper arm on the chosen side approximately 3 to 4 inches above the potential puncture site (Figure 1). Apply sufficient pressure to impede venous circulation but not arterial blood flow.	Eliciting the patient's preference allows the patient to be involved in their treatment and gives the nurse information that may aid in site selection. Positioning yourself close to the chosen site reduces back strain. Use of a tourniquet increases venous pressure and distention to aid in vein identification. The tourniquet should remain in place no more than 1 minute; prolonged tourniquet application causes stasis and hemoconcentration and alterations in test results (Fischbach et al., 2022).

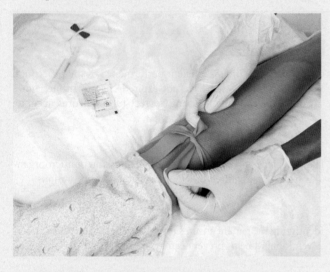

FIGURE 1. Applying the tourniquet.

ACTION	RATIONALE
11. Put on gloves. Assess the veins using inspection and palpation to determine the best puncture site. Refer to the Assessment section above.	Gloves reduce transmission of microorganisms. Using the best site reduces the risk of injury to the patient. Palpation allows for making a distinction between other structures, such as tendons and arteries in the area, to avoid injury.
12. **Release the tourniquet. Check that the vein has decompressed.**	Releasing the tourniquet reduces the length of time the tourniquet is applied. The tourniquet should remain in place no more than 1 minute; prolonged tourniquet application causes stasis and hemoconcentration and alterations in test results (Fischbach et al., 2022). Thrombosed veins will remain firm and palpable and should not be used for venipuncture.
13. Attach the butterfly needle extension tubing to the Vacutainer device.	The connection prepares the device for use.
14. Move collection bottles to a location close to the arm.	The bottles must be close enough to reach easily once venipuncture is successful.
15. Use a single-use sterile applicator containing sterile antiseptic solution to **cleanse the patient's skin at the selected puncture site with antiseptic solution identified in facility policy. Follow the manufacturer's directions for use to determine the product application process and dry times (Gorski et al., 2021). Allow the antiseptic to dry naturally; do not wipe, fan, or blow on the skin** (Gorski et al., 2021).	Cleaning the patient's skin reduces the risk for transmission of microorganisms. Allowing the skin to dry maximizes antimicrobial action and prevents contact of the substance with the needle on insertion, thereby reducing the sting associated with insertion. Allowing the area to thoroughly dry avoids the possibility of the solution causing hemolysis (Gorski et al., 2021).
16. Using a new antimicrobial swab, clean the stoppers of the culture bottles with the appropriate antimicrobial, per facility policy. Cover the bottle top with a sterile gauze square, based on facility policy.	Cleaning the bottle top reduces the risk for transmission of microorganisms into the bottle. Covering the top reduces risk of contamination.

ACTION

17. Reapply the tourniquet approximately 3 to 4 inches above the identified puncture site. Apply sufficient pressure to impede venous circulation but not arterial blood flow. **After disinfection, do not palpate the venipuncture site. If repeated palpation is necessary, the antiseptic solution must be reapplied before venipuncture** (Gorski et al., 2021).

18. Hold the patient's arm in a downward position with your nondominant hand. Use the thumb or first finger of your nondominant hand to apply pressure and traction to the skin about 1 to 2 inches below the identified puncture site (Fischbach et al., 2022; Van Leeuwen & Bladh, 2017). Align the butterfly needle with the chosen vein, holding the needle in your dominant hand (Figure 2).

19. **Inform the patient that they are going to feel a pinch.** With the bevel of the needle up, insert the needle into the vein at a 15- to 30-degree angle to the skin (Van Leeuwen & Bladh, 2017). You should see a flash of blood in the extension tubing close to the needle when the vein is entered (Figure 3).

RATIONALE

Use of a tourniquet increases venous pressure to aid in vein identification. The tourniquet should remain in place no more than 1 minute; prolonged tourniquet application causes stasis and hemoconcentration and alterations in test results (Fischbach et al., 2022).

Applying pressure helps immobilize and anchor the vein. Taut skin at the entry site aids smooth needle entry; pressure on the distal end of the vein during the puncture decreases the possibility of rolling veins (Fischbach et al., 2022).

Warning the patient prevents a reaction related to surprise. Positioning the needle at the proper angle reduces the risk of puncturing through the vein. A flash of blood indicates entrance into the vein.

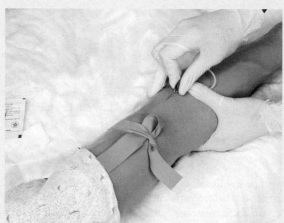

FIGURE 2. Aligning the butterfly needle with the chosen vein.

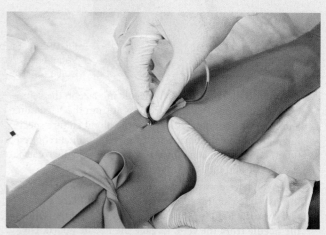

FIGURE 3. Inserting the needle with the bevel up at a 15- to 30-degree angle.

20. **Keeping the specimen bottle upright,** fill the aerobic bottle first (Fischbach et al., 2022; Laboratory Alliance of Central New York, 2017). Grasp the butterfly needle securely to stabilize it in the vein with your nondominant hand, and push the Vacutainer onto the first collection bottle (aerobic bottle), until the rubber stopper on the collection bottle is punctured (Figure 4). You will feel the bottle push into place on the puncture device. Blood will flow into the bottle automatically. Fill to the level indicated on the bottle; do not overfill (Fischbach et al., 2022).

21. **Remove the tourniquet as soon as blood flows adequately into the tube** (Gorski et al., 2021).

Specimen bottles should remain upright to prevent backflow of contents to the patient. The collection bottle is a vacuum; negative pressure within the bottle pulls blood into the bottle. Bottles should be filled as indicated to ensure an adequate sample; in adults, cultures should be 20 to 30 mL of blood (Fischbach et al., 2022).

Tourniquet removal reduces venous pressure and restores venous return to help prevent venous stasis, bleeding, bruising, and inaccurate results (Fischbach et al., 2022; Van Leeuwen & Bladh, 2017).

(continued on page 1164)

Skill 18-10 ▶ Obtaining a Venous Blood Specimen for Culture and Sensitivity *(continued)*

ACTION	RATIONALE

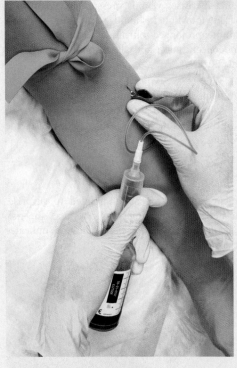

FIGURE 4. Stabilizing the butterfly needle and pushing the Vacutainer onto the aerobic collection bottle, keeping the bottle upright while filling.

22. Continue to hold the butterfly needle in place in the vein. Once the first bottle is filled, remove it from the Vacutainer and insert the second bottle. After the blood culture specimens are obtained, continue to fill any additional required tubes, removing one and inserting another. Gently rotate each bottle and tube as you remove it.

Filling the required bottles ensures that the sample is accurate. Gentle rotation helps to mix any additive in the tube with the blood sample.

23. After you have drawn all required blood samples, remove the last collection tube from the Vacutainer. **Place a gauze pad over the puncture site and slowly and gently remove the needle from the vein. Engage the needle guard. Do not apply pressure to the site until the needle has been fully removed.**

Slow, gentle needle removal prevents injury to the vein. Releasing the vacuum before withdrawing the needle prevents injury to the vein and hematoma formation. Use of a needle guard prevents accidental needlestick injuries.

24. Apply gentle pressure to the puncture site for 2 to 3 minutes or until bleeding stops.

Applying pressure to the site after needle removal prevents injury, bleeding, and extravasation into the surrounding tissue, which can cause a hematoma.

25. After bleeding stops, apply an adhesive bandage. Discard the Vacutainer and needle in a sharps container. Remove your gloves and perform hand hygiene.

The bandage protects the site and aids in applying pressure. Proper disposal of equipment reduces transmission of microorganisms. Removing gloves and performing hand hygiene reduce transmission of microorganisms.

26. Remove equipment and return the patient to a position of comfort. Raise the side rails and lower the bed.

Repositioning promotes patient comfort. Raising the rails promotes safety.

27. Record the date and time the samples were obtained on the labels as well as the required information to identify the person obtaining the samples. Compare the specimen label with the patient identification bracelet, as required by facility policy. Depending on facility policy, specimen labels may be verified prior to obtaining blood samples (refer to Step 5). Apply labels to the specimens, according to facility policy (Figure 5). Place them in a biohazard bag (Figure 6).

Proper labeling ensures accurate communication of results. Use of a biohazard bag prevents contact with blood and body fluids.

ACTION

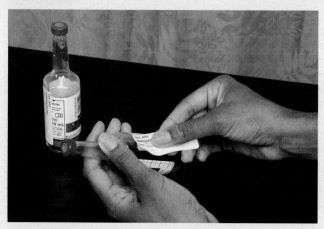

FIGURE 5. Placing a label on specimen container.

RATIONALE

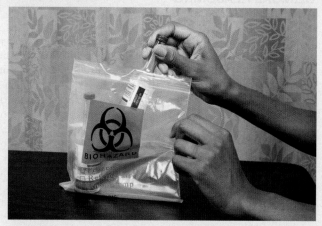

FIGURE 6. Placing specimen containers in biohazard bag.

28. Put on gloves. Check the venipuncture site to see if a hematoma has developed.

Gloves prevent contact with blood and body fluids. Development of a hematoma requires further intervention.

29. Remove gloves and other PPE, if used. Perform hand hygiene.

Proper removal of PPE reduces the risk for infection transmission and contamination of other items. Hand hygiene reduces the transmission of microorganisms.

30. Remove other PPE, if used. Perform hand hygiene.

Proper removal of PPE reduces the risk for infection transmission and contamination of other items. Hand hygiene reduces the transmission of microorganisms.

31. Transport the specimen to the laboratory immediately. If immediate transport is not possible, check with laboratory personnel or the policy manual to see whether refrigeration is contraindicated.

Timely transport ensures accurate results.

EVALUATION

The expected outcomes have been met when an uncontaminated specimen has been obtained without injury to the patient and sent to the laboratory promptly, and the patient has demonstrated an understanding of the need and process for specimen collection.

DOCUMENTATION

Guidelines

Document any pertinent assessments, the laboratory specimens obtained; the date and time specimens were obtained; disposition of specimens; the amount of blood collected, if required; and any significant assessments or patient reactions.

Sample Documentation

6/6/25 1710 Patient's temperature increased to 104.2°F. Patient very lethargic, pale, diaphoretic; with cool, clammy skin. Bradycardic with pulse rate of 56 beats/min and hypotensive with blood pressure of 90/50 mm Hg. Dr. Barrie notified. Blood cultures ×2 prescribed; drawn at left and right antecubital veins. No evidence of bleeding or hematoma at venipuncture sites.

—B. Pearson, RN

(continued on page 1166)

Skill 18-10 ▶ Obtaining a Venous Blood Specimen for Culture and Sensitivity *(continued)*

DEVELOPING CLINICAL REASONING AND CLINICAL JUDGMENT

UNEXPECTED SITUATIONS AND ASSOCIATED INTERVENTIONS

- *After applying the tourniquet, you have trouble finding a distended vein:* Have the patient make a fist, or try tapping the skin over the vein lightly several times. **To prevent venous stasis and reduce risk for inaccurate results, do not have the patient repeatedly clench their fist or pump their hand (Gorski et al., 2021), which may increase plasma potassium levels** (Fischbach et al., 2022). If unsuccessful, remove the tourniquet and try lowering the patient's arm to allow blood to pool in the veins. If necessary, apply warm compresses for about 10 minutes before reapplying the tourniquet.
- *Patient has large, distended, highly visible veins:* Perform venipuncture without a tourniquet to minimize the risk for hematoma (Fischbach et al., 2022).
- *Patient has a clotting disorder or is receiving anticoagulant therapy:* Maintain firm pressure on the venipuncture site for at least 5 minutes after withdrawing the needle to prevent hematoma formation.
- *Oozing or bleeding continues from the puncture site for more than a few minutes:* Elevate the area and apply a pressure dressing. If bleeding is excessive or persists for longer than 10 minutes, notify the health care team.
- *Hematoma develops at the venipuncture site:* Apply pressure until you are sure bleeding has stopped (about 5 minutes). Notify the health care team. Document the size and appearance of the hematoma, notification of the health care team, and any prescribed interventions.
- *Patient reports feeling lightheaded and says they are going to faint:* Stop the venipuncture. If the patient is in bed, have them lie flat and elevate their feet. If the patient is in a chair, have them put their head between their knees. Encourage the patient to take slow, deep breaths. Call for assistance and stay with the patient. Obtain vital signs, if possible.

SPECIAL CONSIDERATIONS

General Considerations

- Be aware that the size of the culture bottles may vary according to facility policy, but the sample dilution should always be 1:10.
- If possible, ensure the specimen is obtained before antibiotics are started (Fischbach et al., 2022).
- Draw blood from different peripheral venipuncture sites and document each site. This increases the likelihood of detecting a bloodstream infection and helps differentiate true bacteremia from a false-positive finding due to skin contamination. Peripheral sites are preferred (Fischbach et al., 2022; Gorski et al., 2021; Kyle & Carman, 2022).
- In the case of suspected catheter-related bloodstream infection, blood samples should be drawn from the central venous access device (CVAD). Remove and discard the used needleless connector prior to drawing the blood sample to reduce the risk of false-positive blood culture results. Do not collect a discard volume; send the initial blood volume aspirated from the CVAD for blood culture (Groski et al., 2021). Clearly document the site of collection.
- Avoid collecting blood from edematous areas, arteriovenous shunts, an upper extremity on the same side as a previous lymph node dissection or mastectomy, infected sites, the same extremity as an intravenous infusion, and sites of previous hematomas or vascular injury.
- Do not use veins in the lower extremities for venipuncture, because of an increased risk of thrombophlebitis. However, some facilities do allow collection from lower extremities as a prescribed intervention to collect blood from a leg or foot vein. Check your facility's policies.
- Apply warm compresses to the selected site 15 to 20 minutes before venipuncture to aid in distending veins that are difficult to locate.
- Consider the use of topical anesthetic creams to minimize discomfort and pain for the patient, based on facility policy. Allow 60 seconds after application for patients with light skin tones and 120 seconds for patients with dark skin tones before performing the venipuncture (Fischbach et al., 2022). Be familiar with requirements and specifications for a particular product available for use. Application needs to occur sufficiently in advance to allow enough time to become effective.
- Use distraction, if appropriate. Distraction has been shown to be of benefit in reducing anxiety related to venipuncture, especially with children (Erdogan & Ozdemir, 2021; Kuo et al., 2018). Asking the patient to concentrate on relaxing and performing deep breathing may help them relax.

- The application of molecular diagnostics techniques using identification of specific sequences of DNA and the development of automated instruments that can identify pathogens from a small amount of blood has made faster diagnosis of bloodstream infections and detection of antibiotic resistance possible (Peker et al., 2018).

Infant and Child Considerations

- Consider automatically applying warm compresses to distend the small veins of infants and young children before attempting any venipuncture.
- Heelsticks, using the outer aspect of the heel, may be used for infants. Warming the heel for 5 to 10 minutes before the sample is taken dilates the blood vessels in the area and aids in sampling (KarabiyikOğurlu et al., 2020; Vedder, 2021). This technique is not without controversy, as it is painful and can lead to scarring and infection, including infection of bone and cartilage, due to excessive depth of the puncture (Gorski et al., 2021; Vedder, 2021). Venipuncture by a skilled phlebotomist is suggested instead of heel lance methods due to the increased pain from the heel lance (Gorski et al., 2021). Automatic lancing devices are preferred over manual devices to control the depth of puncture and to reduce the risk of bone or cartilage infection (Gorski et al., 2021).
- For infants and small children, only 1 to 5 mL of blood can safely be drawn for culture; quantities <1 mL may be insufficient to detect bacterial organisms (Fischbach et al., 2022).
- Consider a combination of techniques including swaddling, breastfeeding, pacifiers, rocking, and/or administration of oral sucrose (24%) beginning 1 to 2 minutes before the venipuncture procedure for young infants, to decrease the incidence of procedure-related pain (De Bernardo et al., 2018; Gorski et al., 2021).
- Consider using topical anesthetic creams or gels, refrigerant spray, or iontophoresis (application of electric current to carry ionized lidocaine through the skin) with infants and children, to decrease the incidence of procedure-related pain ((Kyle & Carman, 2021). Apply the product for sufficient time to reach maximal effectiveness.
- Consider the use of distraction to reduce anxiety and procedure-related pain (Erdogan & Ozdemir, 2021; Gorski et al., 2021; Kuo et al., 2018).

Older Adult Considerations

- Keep in mind that the veins of an older adult are fragile and may collapse easily. In addition, the skin is less elastic and may be more difficult to pull taut.
- The superficial veins of the hands of older adults are fragile, and venipuncture can cause a hematoma to form. Insert the needle for venipuncture at no more than a 30-degree angle unless using ultrasound guidance; use a 5- to 15-degree angle for veins of older adults (Gorski et al., 2021). In addition, these veins move due to the age-related loss of supportive muscle and connective tissue, making it difficult to enter the lumen of the vein.
- Consider performing venipuncture without a tourniquet for older adults to prevent rupture of capillaries (Fischbach et al., 2022).

EVIDENCE FOR PRACTICE ▶

RELIEF OF PAIN DURING BLOOD SPECIMEN COLLECTION
Needle insertion for venipuncture is painful. What interventions can assist nurses to reduce the pain associated with venipuncture and arterial puncture?

Related Research
Erdogan, B., & Ozdemir, A. A. (2021). The effect of three different methods on venipuncture pain and anxiety in children: Distraction cards, virtual reality, and Buzzy® (randomized controlled trial). *Journal of Pediatric Nursing, 58*, e54–e62. https://doi.org/10.1016/j.pedn.2021.01.001
Refer to the details in the Evidence for Practice in Skill 18-9.

Skill 18-11 ▶ Obtaining an Arterial Blood Specimen for Blood Gas Analysis

Arterial blood gases (ABGs) are obtained to determine the adequacy of oxygenation and ventilation, to assess acid–base status, and to monitor the effectiveness of treatment (Fischbach et al., 2022). The most common site for sampling arterial blood is the radial artery (Hess et al., 2021). Other arteries may be used, but it may be a prescribed intervention to obtain the sample from another artery, based on facility policy.

Analysis of ABGs evaluates ventilation by measuring blood pH and the partial pressure of arterial oxygen (Pao_2) and partial pressure of arterial carbon dioxide ($Paco_2$). Blood pH measurement reveals the blood's acid–base balance. Pao_2 indicates the amount of oxygen that the lungs deliver to the blood, and $Paco_2$ indicates the lungs' capacity to eliminate carbon dioxide. ABG samples can also be analyzed for oxygen content and saturation and for bicarbonate values. Table 18-1 highlights the normal values for ABG. A respiratory technician or specially trained nurse can collect most ABG samples, but an advanced practice professional usually performs collection from the femoral artery, depending on facility policy. An Allen test should always be performed before using the radial artery to determine whether the ulnar artery delivers sufficient blood to the hand and fingers, in case there is damage to the radial artery during the blood sampling. A negative Allen test indicates the circulation from the ulnar artery is inadequate and a site other than the radial artery must be used (the opposite arm or another site) (Hess et al., 2021). Refer to the guidelines in this skill for performing an Allen test.

A blood sample for ABG testing may also be drawn from an arterial line. Refer to Skill 18-13.

Table 18-1 Arterial Blood Gas: Normal Values

PARAMETER	NORMAL VALUE
pH	7.35–7.45
$PaCO_2$	35–45 mm Hg
HCO_3	22–26 mEq/L
SaO_2	Oxygen saturation >95%
PaO_2	>80–100 mm Hg
Base excess or deficit	±2 mEq/L

DELEGATION CONSIDERATIONS

Obtaining an arterial blood specimen for blood gas analysis is not delegated to assistive personnel (AP). Depending on the state's nurse practice act and the organization's policies and procedures, obtaining an arterial blood specimen for blood gas analysis may be delegated to licensed practical/vocational nurses (LPN/LVNs). The decision to delegate must be based on careful analysis of the patient's needs and circumstances as well as the qualifications of the person to whom the task is being delegated. Refer to the Delegation Guidelines in Appendix A.

EQUIPMENT

- ABG kit, *or* heparinized (100 to 200 IU) self-filling 10-mL syringe with 22- to 23-gauge, 1-inch needle attached
- Airtight cap for hub of syringe
- 2 × 2 gauze pad
- Adhesive bandage
- Antimicrobial swab, such as chlorhexidine or alcohol, per facility policy
- Waterproof protective pad
- Prescribed local anesthetic cream, as indicated
- Biohazard bag
- Appropriate label for specimen, based on facility policy and procedure
- Cup or bag of ice and water
- Gloves
- Goggles or face shield
- Additional PPE, as indicated
- Rolled towel

ASSESSMENT

Review the patient's health record for information about the need for an ABG specimen. Ensure that the necessary computerized laboratory request has been completed. Assess the patient for any allergies, especially to the topical antimicrobial to be used for skin cleansing. Investigate for the presence of any conditions or use of medications that may prolong bleeding time, necessitating additional application of pressure to the puncture site. Assess the patient's cardiac status, including heart rate, blood pressure, and auscultation of heart sounds. Also assess the patient's respiratory status, including respiratory rate, excursion, lung sounds, and use of oxygen, including the amount being used, if prescribed. Ask the patient about any previous laboratory testing they may have had, including any problems, such as difficulty with venipuncture; fainting; or reports of dizziness, lightheadedness, or nausea. Assess the patient's anxiety level and understanding of the reasons for the blood test. Assess the need/patient preference for use of a prescribed local anesthetic (Fischbach et al., 2022).

Determine the adequacy of peripheral blood flow to the extremity to be used by performing the Allen test (detailed below). If the Allen test reveals little or no collateral circulation to the hand, do not perform an arterial stick to that artery. Assess the patient's radial pulse. If unable to palpate the radial pulse, consider using the other wrist. Assess the patient's understanding about the need for specimen collection.

ACTUAL OR POTENTIAL HEALTH PROBLEMS AND NEEDS

Many actual or potential health problems or issues may require the use of this skill as part of related interventions. An appropriate health problem or issue may include:
• Impaired gas exchange
• Injury risk
• Acute pain

OUTCOME IDENTIFICATION AND PLANNING

The expected outcome to achieve is that an uncontaminated specimen will be obtained without injury to the patient or damage to the artery and sent to the laboratory promptly. In addition, the patient demonstrates an understanding of the need and process for specimen collection.

IMPLEMENTATION

ACTION	RATIONALE
1. Gather the necessary supplies. Check product expiration dates. Check the patient's health record to identify the prescribed ABG analysis. Check the health record to make sure the patient has not been suctioned within the past 20 to 30 minutes. Check facility policy and/or procedure for guidelines on administering local anesthesia for arterial punctures. Administer the anesthetic and allow sufficient time for the full effect before beginning procedure.	Organization facilitates efficient performance of the procedure. Use of products that have not expired ensures proper functioning of the equipment. Checking the prescribed intervention and policy ensures that the proper procedure is initiated. Suctioning may change the oxygen saturation and is a temporary change not to be confused with baseline for the patient. Arterial puncture is a source of pain and discomfort. Intradermal injection of lidocaine around the puncture site has been shown to decrease the incidence and severity of localized pain when used before arterial puncture (American Association of Critical-Care Nurses [AACN], 2017; Hess et al., 2021).
2. Perform hand hygiene and put on PPE, if indicated.	Hand hygiene and PPE prevent the transmission of microorganisms. PPE is required based on transmission precautions.
3. Identify the patient.	Identifying the patient ensures the right patient receives the intervention and helps prevent errors.
4. Explain the procedure to the patient. Tell the patient you need to collect an arterial blood sample and the needlestick will cause some discomfort, but that they must remain still during the procedure.	Explanation facilitates engagement and provides reassurance for the patient.

(continued on page 1170)

Skill 18-11 ▶ Obtaining an Arterial Blood Specimen for Blood Gas Analysis *(continued)*

ACTION

5. Check the specimen label with the patient's identification bracelet. The label should include the patient's name and identification number, the time the specimen was collected, the route of collection, identification of the person obtaining the sample, the amount of oxygen the patient is receiving, the type of oxygen administration device, the patient's body temperature, and any other information required by facility policy. Depending on facility policy, specimen labels may be verified after obtaining blood samples, prior to application to blood sample tubes.

6. Assemble equipment on the overbed table or other surface within reach.

7. Close the curtains around the bed, and close the door to the room, if possible.

8. Provide for good light. Artificial light is recommended. Place a trash receptacle within easy reach.

9. If the patient is on bed rest, ask them to lie in a supine position, with their head slightly elevated and their arms at their sides. Ask an ambulatory patient to sit in a chair and support their arm securely on an armrest or a table. Place a waterproof pad under the site and a rolled towel under their wrist.

10. **Perform the Allen test (Figure 1) before obtaining a specimen from the radial artery.**

   a. Have the patient clench their fist to minimize blood flow into the hand.

   b. Using your index and middle fingers, press on the radial and ulnar arteries (Figure 1A). Hold this position for a few seconds.

   c. Without removing your fingers from the arteries, ask the patient to unclench their fist and hold their hand in a relaxed position (Figure 1B). The palm will be blanched because pressure from your fingers has impaired the normal blood flow.

   d. Release pressure on the ulnar artery (Figure 1C). If the hand becomes flushed, which indicates that blood is filling the vessels, it is safe to proceed with the radial artery puncture. This is considered a positive test. If the hand does not flush, perform the test on the other arm.

11. Put on gloves and goggles or a face shield. Locate the radial artery and lightly palpate it for a strong pulse.

12. Use a single-use sterile applicator containing sterile antiseptic solution to **cleanse the patient's skin at the selected puncture site with the antiseptic solution identified in facility policy. Follow the manufacturer's directions for use to determine the product application process and dry times (Gorski et al., 2021). Allow the antiseptic to dry naturally; do not wipe, fan, or blow on the skin** (Gorski et al., 2021). **After disinfection, do not palpate the venipuncture site. If repeated palpation is necessary, the antiseptic solution must be reapplied before venipuncture** (Gorski et al., 2021).

RATIONALE

Verifying the patient's identity validates that the correct procedure is being done on the correct patient, and the specimen is accurately labeled. Oxygen information and the patient's body temperature are required for accurate analysis.

Arranging items nearby is convenient, saves time, and avoids unnecessary stretching and twisting of muscles on the part of the nurse.

Closing the door or curtain provides for patient privacy.

Good lighting is necessary to perform the procedure properly. Having the trash receptacle in easy reach allows for safe disposal of contaminated materials.

Positioning the patient comfortably helps minimize anxiety. Using a rolled towel under their wrist provides for easy access to the insertion site.

Allen testing assesses patency of the ulnar and radial arteries (Hess et al., 2021).

Gloves and goggles (or face shield) prevent contact with blood and body fluids. If you push too hard during palpation, the radial artery will be obliterated and hard to palpate.

Cleaning the patient's skin reduces the risk for transmission of microorganisms. Allowing the skin to dry maximizes antimicrobial action and prevents contact of the substance with the needle on insertion, thereby reducing the sting associated with insertion. Allowing the area to thoroughly dry avoids the possibility of the solution causing hemolysis (Gorski et al., 2021). Palpation after cleansing contaminates the area.

ACTION	**RATIONALE**

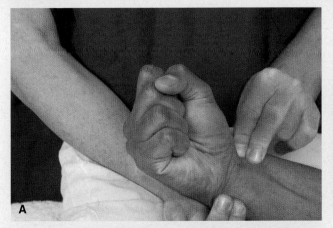

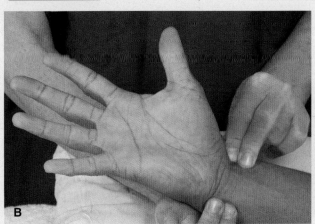

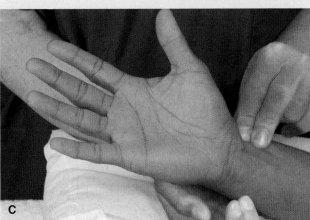

FIGURE 1. Performing Allen's test. **A.** Compressing the arteries with the patient's fist closed. **B.** Maintaining compression as patient unclenches fist. **C.** Compressing only the radial artery.

ACTION	**RATIONALE**
13. Stabilize the patient's hand with their wrist extended over the rolled towel, palm up. Palpate the artery above the puncture site with the index and middle fingers of your nondominant hand while holding the syringe over the puncture site with your dominant hand. **Do not directly touch the area to be punctured.**	Stabilizing the patient's hand and palpating the artery with one hand while holding the syringe in the other provides better access to the artery. Palpating the area to be punctured would contaminate the clean area.
14. Hold the needle bevel up at a 45-degree angle (Hess et al., 2021) at the site of maximal pulse impulse, with the shaft parallel to the path of the artery.	The proper angle of insertion ensures correct access to the artery. The artery is shallow and does not require a deeper angle to penetrate.
15. If local anesthetic was not used, **inform the patient that they are going to feel a pinch.** Puncture the skin and arterial wall in one motion. Watch for blood backflow in the syringe (Figure 2). Pulsating blood will flow into the syringe. Do not pull back on the plunger. Collect 2 to 3 mL (Hess et al., 2021).	Warning the patient prevents a reaction related to surprise. Positioning the needle at the proper angle reduces the risk of puncturing through the artery. The blood should enter the syringe automatically due to arterial pressure.
16. After collecting the sample, withdraw the syringe while your nondominant hand is beginning to place pressure proximal to the insertion site with the 2 × 2 gauze. **Press a gauze pad firmly over the puncture site until the bleeding stops—at least 5 minutes (Hess et al., 2021). If the patient is receiving anticoagulant therapy or has a blood dyscrasia, apply pressure for 10 to 15 minutes; if necessary, ask a coworker to hold the gauze pad in place while you prepare the sample for transport to the laboratory, but do not ask the patient to hold the pad.**	If insufficient pressure is applied, a large, painful hematoma may form, hindering future arterial puncture at the site.

(continued on page 1172)

Skill 18-11 ▶ Obtaining an Arterial Blood Specimen for Blood Gas Analysis *(continued)*

ACTION

RATIONALE

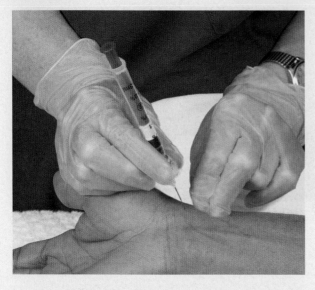

FIGURE 2. Observing blood backflow into syringe. (*Photo by B. Proud.*)

17. When the bleeding stops and the appropriate time has lapsed, apply a small adhesive bandage or small pressure dressing (fold a 2 × 2 gauze into fourths and firmly apply tape, stretching the skin tight).

Applying a dressing also prevents arterial hemorrhage and extravasation into the surrounding tissue, which can cause a hematoma.

18. Once the sample is obtained, check the syringe for air bubbles; remove excess air in the syringe by holding it upright and gently tapping it, allowing any air bubbles to reach the top of the syringe, and then expel the air (Hess et al., 2021).

Air bubbles can affect the laboratory values.

19. Engage the needle guard and remove the needle. Place the airtight cap on the syringe. Gently rotate the syringe. Do not shake it. Discard the needle in a sharps container. Remove your goggles and gloves and perform hand hygiene.

Engaging the needle guard prevents accidental needlestick injury. Using an airtight cap prevents the sample from leaking and keeps air out of the syringe, because blood will continue to absorb oxygen and will give a false reading if allowed to have contact with air. Rotating the syringe ensures proper mixing of heparin in the syringe with the sample; heparin prevents blood from clotting. Vigorous shaking may cause hemolysis. Removing goggles and gloves and performing hand hygiene reduce transmission of microorganisms.

20. Record date and time the sample was obtained on the label as well as the required information to identify the person obtaining the samples. Compare the specimen label with the patient identification bracelet, as required by facility policy. Depending on facility policy, the specimen label may be verified prior to obtaining blood samples (refer to Step 5). Apply labels to the specimens, according to facility policy. Place them in a biohazard bag. Insert the syringe into a cup or bag of ice water.

Labeling ensures the specimen is the correct one for the right patient. Packaging the specimen in a biohazard bag prevents the person transporting the samples from coming in contact with blood. Ice prevents the blood from degrading.

21. Remove equipment and return the patient to a position of comfort. Raise the side rail and lower the bed.

Repositioning promotes patient comfort. Raising the rails promotes safety.

22. Put on gloves. Check the puncture site for bleeding and to see if a hematoma has developed.

Gloves prevent contact with blood and body fluids. Continued bleeding or development of a hematoma requires further intervention.

23. Remove gloves and other PPE, if used. Perform hand hygiene.

Proper removal of PPE reduces the risk for infection transmission and contamination of other items. Hand hygiene reduces the transmission of microorganisms.

24. Transport the specimen to the laboratory immediately.

Timely transport ensures accurate results.

EVALUATION

The expected outcomes have been met when an uncontaminated specimen has been obtained without injury to the patient and sent to the laboratory promptly, and the patient has demonstrated an understanding of the need and process for specimen collection.

DOCUMENTATION

Guidelines

Document results of the Allen test, the time the sample was drawn, the arterial puncture site, the amount of time pressure was applied to the site to control bleeding, the type and amount of oxygen therapy the patient was receiving, pulse oximetry values, the respiratory rate and effort, the patient's other vital signs, and any other significant assessments or patient reactions.

Sample Documentation

9/22/25 1245 Allen's test positive at R radial artery. ABG obtained using R radial artery. Pressure applied to site for 5 minutes. Patient receiving 3 L/NC oxygen, pulse oximetry 94%, respirations even/unlabored, respiratory rate 18 breaths/min, oral temperature 98.9°F, patient denies dyspnea.

—C. Bausler, RN

DEVELOPING CLINICAL REASONING AND CLINICAL JUDGMENT

UNEXPECTED SITUATIONS AND ASSOCIATED INTERVENTIONS

- *While you are attempting to puncture the artery, the patient reports severe pain:* Using too much force may cause the needle to touch bone, causing the patient pain. Too much force may also result in advancing the needle through the opposite wall of the artery. If this happens, slowly pull the needle back a short distance and check to see if blood returns. If blood still fails to enter the syringe, withdraw the needle completely and restart the procedure.
- *You cannot obtain a specimen from the same site after two attempts:* Stop. Do not make more than two attempts from the same site. Probing the artery may injure it and the radial nerve.
- *After inserting the needle, you note that the syringe is filling sluggishly with dark red–purple blood:* If the patient is in critical condition, this may be arterial blood. But if the patient is awake and alert with a pulse oximeter reading within normal parameters, you have most likely obtained a venous sample. Discard the sample and redraw.
- *Patient is on anticoagulant therapy:* Expect to hold pressure on the puncture site for at least 10 minutes. If pressure is not held sufficiently long, a hematoma may form, place pressure on the artery, and decrease the flow of blood.
- *Blood was drawn without incident, but now, 2 hours later, the patient is reporting tingling in the fingers, and their hand is cool and pale:* Notify the health care team. An arterial thrombosis may have formed. If not treated, the thrombosis can lead to tissue necrosis on the extremity.
- *Puncture site continues to ooze:* If the site is not actively bleeding, consider placing a small pressure bandage on the insertion site. This will prevent the artery from continuing to ooze. Continually check the site for bleeding and assess the extremity to ensure that blood flow is adequate. The site should be monitored for several hours for bleeding (Fischbach et al., 2022).
- *Allen test is negative:* Try the other extremity. If the other extremity has a positive result (collateral circulation), use that extremity. If the Allen test is negative in both extremities, notify the health care team.

SPECIAL CONSIDERATIONS

General Considerations

- Be aware that use of a particular arterial site is contraindicated for the following reasons: absence of a palpable radial artery pulse, a negative Allen test indicating obstruction in the ulnar artery, cellulitis or infection in the area of the site, presence of an arteriovenous fistula or shunt, severe thrombocytopenia (platelet count 20,000/mm^3 or less, or based on facility policy), a prolonged prothrombin time or partial thromboplastin time, or an elevated international normalized ratio (Fischbach et al., 2022).

(continued on page 1174)

Skill 18-11 ▶ Obtaining an Arterial Blood Specimen for Blood Gas Analysis *(continued)*

- Anticipate possible adverse reaction and appropriate interventions: Some patients experience lightheadedness, nausea, or vasovagal syncope during arterial puncture (Fischbach et al., 2022).
- If the patient is receiving oxygen, wait 15 minutes after a change in type or mode of oxygen delivery or rate for specimen collection for ABG analysis (Fischbach et al., 2022). Indicate the amount and type of oxygen therapy the patient is receiving on the laboratory request. Also note the patient's current temperature, most recent hemoglobin level, and current respiratory rate. If the patient is receiving mechanical ventilation, note the fraction of inspired oxygen and tidal volume.
- If the patient is not receiving oxygen, indicate that they are breathing room air on the laboratory request for an ABG analysis.
- Specimens collected within 20 to 30 minutes of respiratory passage suctioning or other respiratory therapy will not be accurate (Van Leeuwen & Bladh, 2017).
- Consider obtaining an order for the use of a local anesthetic solution (1% lidocaine solution), gel, or cream to minimize discomfort and pain for the patient, based on facility policy (AACN, 2017; Fischbach et al., 2022). The use of 1% lidocaine without epinephrine injected intradermally around the artery puncture site has been shown to decrease the incidence of localized pain (AACN, 2017). Be familiar with the requirements and specifications for particular products available for use. Application needs to occur sufficiently far in advance to allow enough time to become effective, which may be contraindicated by the patient's condition. Consider such use of lidocaine carefully because it can delay the procedure. The patient may be allergic to the drug, or the resulting vasoconstriction may prevent successful puncture.
- Consider the use of topical anesthetic creams to minimize discomfort and pain for the patient, based on facility policy. Allow 60 seconds after application for patients with light skin tones and 120 seconds for patients with dark skin tones before performing the venipuncture (Fischbach et al., 2022). Be familiar with the requirements and specifications for a particular product available for use. Application needs to occur sufficiently in advance to allow enough time to become effective.
- If the femoral site is used for the procedure, apply pressure for a minimum of 10 minutes.
- Arterial lines may be used to obtain blood samples (refer to Skill 18-13). When sampling from arterial lines, record the amount of blood drawn for each sampling. Frequent sampling can result in a significant amount of blood being removed.
- Capillary blood gas samples may be used to estimate pH and PCO_2 in infants or other people when ABG analysis is indicated but arterial access is difficult (Hess et al., 2021).

Infant and Child Considerations

- Consider a combination of techniques including swaddling, breastfeeding, pacifiers, rocking, and/or administration of oral sucrose (24%) beginning 1 to 2 minutes before the venipuncture procedure for young infants to decrease the incidence of procedure-related pain (De Bernardo et al., 2018; Gorski et al., 2021).
- Consider using topical anesthetic creams or gels, refrigerant spray, or iontophoresis (application of electric current to carry ionized lidocaine through the skin) with infants and children, to decrease the incidence of procedure-related pain (Kyle & Carman, 2021). Apply the product for sufficient time to reach maximal effectiveness.
- Consider the use of distraction to reduce anxiety and procedure-related pain (Erdogan & Ozdemir, 2021; Gorski et al., 2021; Kuo et al., 2018).

EVIDENCE FOR PRACTICE ▶

RELIEF OF PAIN DURING BLOOD SPECIMEN COLLECTION

Needle insertion for venipuncture is painful. What interventions can assist nurses to reduce the pain associated with venipuncture and arterial puncture?

Related Research

Erdogan, B., & Ozdemir, A. A. (2021). The effect of three different methods on venipuncture pain and anxiety in children: Distraction cards, virtual reality, and Buzzy® (randomized controlled trial). *Journal of Pediatric Nursing, 58*, e54–e62. https://doi.org/10.1016/j.pedn.2021.01.001

Refer to the details in the Evidence for Practice in Skills 18-9.

Skill 18-12 ▶ Obtaining a Blood Sample From a Central Venous Access Device

Central venous (vascular) access devices (CVADs) provide access for many health care–related interventions, such as intravenous (IV) fluids, medications, hemodynamic monitoring, and blood sampling. (Refer to Skill 16-7 and Skill 16-8 in Chapter 16.) Obtaining a blood sample requires accessing the catheter and withdrawing the prescribed test samples using aseptic technique to avoid catheter-associated bloodstream infection (CABSI). Venous access device administration set entry points, end caps, and needleless connectors must be vigorously scrubbed and disinfected prior to each access to reduce the risk for introduction of microorganisms and prevent venous access device–related infection (Gorski et al., 2021). CVADs must be aspirated for a blood return prior to use to assess catheter function (Gorski et al., 2021). Flushing of the device before and after obtaining blood samples using 10 to 20 mL of preservative-free 0.9% sodium chloride solution is required (Gorski et al., 2021). CVADs should be locked with either a heparin solution (10 units/mL) or preservative-free 0.9% sodium chloride after each intermittent use, according to the directions for use for the specific CVAD and needleless connector (Gorski et al., 2021). If there is more than one lumen present, choose the appropriate CVAD lumen to use to obtain blood samples based on the largest lumen or the configuration of the lumen exit sites (refer to Step 12) (Gorski et al., 2021).

Nurses should evaluate the use of the discard method versus the push–pull (mixing) method for obtaining a sample from CVADs (Gorski et al., 2021; McBride et al., 2018). Closed blood sampling systems may also be used to reduce the risk of patient blood infections and health care–related anemia, and allow for return of any blood withdrawn for the purpose of clearing the catheter lumen (discard/waste) (Gorski et al., 2021). Refer to the policy and procedures and specific requirements for an individual facility.

The procedure below describes the discard method for obtaining blood samples from a CVAD. See the Special Considerations below for a brief description of the push–pull method.

DELEGATION CONSIDERATIONS	Obtaining a blood sample from a CVAD is not delegated to assistive personnel (AP) or licensed practical/vocational nurses (LPN/LVNs).
EQUIPMENT	• Gloves • Goggles or face shield • Additional PPE, as indicated • Vacutainer with needleless Luer adapter (or blunt cannula, for closed reservoir system) and appropriate blood collection tubes for prescribed tests • Two additional blood collection tubes, for discard blood volume • Prefilled commercially prepared syringes with 10-mL sterile normal saline for injection (minimum volume equal to twice the internal volume of the catheter system) (Gorski et al., 2021) • Prefilled commercially prepared syringe with heparin 10 units/mL in 10-mL (based on the manufacturer's directions for the use of the CVAD and needleless connector and facility policy) • Antimicrobial or chlorhexidine swabs, per facility policy • Waterproof protective pad • Passive disinfection caps (based on facility policy) or • Sterile cap for arterial catheter stopcock (based on facility policy) • Appropriate label for specimen, based on facility policy and procedure • Blank labels (2) • Biohazard bag • Bath blanket

(continued on page 1176)

Skill 18-12 ▶ Obtaining a Blood Sample From a Central Venous Access Device *(continued)*

ASSESSMENT

Review the patient's health record for the blood specimens to be obtained. Ensure that the necessary computerized laboratory requests have been completed. Assess the patency and functioning of the CVAD. Assess the CVAD site (refer to Skill 16-7 in Chapter 16). Assess the patient's understanding about the need for specimen collection.

ACTUAL OR POTENTIAL HEALTH PROBLEMS AND NEEDS

Many actual or potential health problems or issues may require the use of this skill as part of related interventions. An appropriate health problem or issue may include:
- Infection risk
- Knowledge deficiency
- Injury risk

OUTCOME IDENTIFICATION AND PLANNING

The expected outcome to achieve when obtaining a blood sample from a CVAD is that prescribed blood samples are obtained without compromise to the patency of the CVAD. In addition, the patient experiences minimal discomfort, remains free from infection, and verbalizes an understanding of the rationale for specimen collection.

IMPLEMENTATION

ACTION	RATIONALE
1. Verify the prescribed laboratory testing in the patient's health record and select the appropriate blood collection tubes. Consider the need to stop solutions and medications infusing through any of the lumens of the CVAD and wait the appropriate length of time before obtaining the blood samples.	Checking the prescribed intervention and policy ensures that the proper procedure is initiated. Using the correct blood collection tubes ensures accurate blood sampling. Stopping IV infusions prevents the presence of solutions contributing to inaccuracies in laboratory results. The length of time is associated with the internal volume of the specific CVAD (Gorski et al., 2021); refer as well to facility policy.
2. Gather all equipment. Check product expiration dates.	Assembling equipment provides for an organized approach to the task. Use of products that have not expired ensures proper functioning of the equipment.
3. Perform hand hygiene and put on PPE, if indicated.	Hand hygiene and PPE prevent the spread of microorganisms. PPE is required based on transmission precautions.
4. Identify the patient.	Identifying the patient ensures the right patient receives the intervention and helps prevent errors.
5. Close the curtains around the bed and close the door to the room, if possible. Explain the procedure to the patient.	This ensures the patient's privacy. Explanation relieves anxiety and facilitates engagement.
6. Assemble equipment on the overbed table or other surface within reach.	Arranging items nearby is convenient, saves time, and avoids unnecessary stretching and twisting of muscles on the part of the nurse.
7. Adjust the bed to a comfortable working height (VHACEOSH, 2016). Disconnect the infusion from the CVAD as necessary (refer to Chapter 16).	Having the bed at the proper height prevents back and muscle strain. Disconnection allows access to the device lumen for blood sampling.
8. Compare the specimen label with the patient identification bracelet. The label should include patient's name and identification number, the time the specimen was collected, the route of collection, identification of the person obtaining the sample, and any other information required by facility policy. Depending on facility policy, specimen labels may be verified after obtaining blood samples, prior to application to blood sample tubes.	Verifying the patient's identity validates that the correct procedure is being done on the correct patient, and the specimen is accurately labeled.
9. Use blank labels to label the two blood sample collection tubes to be used for the discard blood sample and the discard flush.	Labeling the discard tubes prevents accidental confusion with blood specimen tubes.

ACTION

10. Assist the patient to a comfortable position that provides easy access to the CVAD. Use the bath blanket to cover any exposed area other than the sampling site. Place a waterproof pad under the site.

11. Put on gloves and goggles or a face shield.

12. Locate the appropriate CVAD lumen to use to obtain blood samples based on the largest lumen or the configuration of the lumen exit sites; for catheters with a staggered lumen exit at the tip, the sample should be obtained from the lumen exiting at the point farthest away from the heart and above other lumen exits used for infusion (Gorski et al., 2021). Remove the passive disinfection cap or nonvented cap from the end of the lumen (Figure 1). If a nonvented cap was removed, use an antimicrobial swab to vigorously scrub the needleless connector or end cap. Allow it to air dry.

RATIONALE

Patient positioning and use of a bath blanket provide for comfort and warmth. The waterproof pad protects underlying surfaces.

Gloves and goggles (or face shield) prevent contact with blood and body fluids.

Use of the appropriate CVAD lumen reduces the risk for inaccuracies in results; refer also to the CVAD manufacturers' directions for use. Venous access device administration set entry points, end caps, and needleless connectors must be disinfected prior to each access to reduce the risk for introduction of microorganisms and prevent venous access device–related infection (Frimpong et al., 2015; Gorski et al., 2021; Harper, 2014; Loveday et al., 2014). Friction is needed to physically remove microorganisms from the top, sides, and threads of the needleless connector or end cap. Allow the antiseptic to dry completely following the manufacturer's directions for use (Gorski et al., 2021).

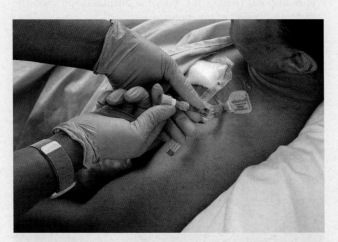

FIGURE 1. Removing the passive disinfection cap or nonvented cap from the end of the lumen.

13. **Prevent connection/disconnection reflux by using the appropriate sequence for flushing, clamping, and disconnecting determined by the type of needleless connector being used** (refer to Box 16-4 in Skill 16-5) (Gorski et al., 2021).

14. Insert the saline flush syringe into the needleless connector (Figure 2). Open the clamp on the lumen. Slowly inject the saline flush, noting any resistance or sluggishness, and slowly pull back on the syringe to aspirate for a positive blood return (Figure 3). If positive, instill the remaining solution over 1 minute or by using a pulsatile flushing technique of 10 short boluses of 1 mL interrupted by brief pauses; flush the line according to facility policy. Depending on facility policy, withdraw the volume of discard blood into syringe. Alternatively, the discard volume can be withdrawn using the blood sample tubes. Refer to Step 15.

Action of the positive pressure end cap is maintained with the appropriate sequence for flushing, clamping, and disconnecting determined by the type of needleless connector in use (Gorski et al., 2021).

Presence of a blood return upon aspiration and lack of resistance when flushing indicate patency of the VAD (Gorski et al., 2021). A pulsatile flushing technique of 10 short boluses of 1 mL interrupted by brief pauses may be more effective in removing solid deposits (e.g., fibrin, drug precipitate, intraluminal bacteria) (Gorski et al., 2021). A sufficient amount of discard volume needs to be withdrawn before obtaining the blood sample to be tested in the laboratory. This sample is discarded because it is diluted with flush solution, possibly leading to inaccurate test results. If an insufficient amount of discard volume is withdrawn, the specimen may be diluted and contaminated with flush solution. If an excessive amount of discard volume is withdrawn, the patient may experience an iatrogenic (treatment-induced) blood loss. The wide variation in discard volumes depends on the internal volume of the CVAD, saline flushing prior to drawing the discard volume, and the specific laboratory tests (Gorski et al., 2021).

(continued on page 1178)

Skill 18-12 ▶ Obtaining a Blood Sample From a Central Venous Access Device *(continued)*

ACTION

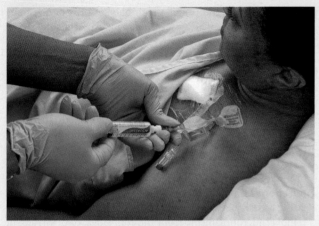

FIGURE 2. Inserting the flush syringe into the needleless connector.

15. Remove the syringe and dispose of it appropriately if used to collect the discard blood volume, according to facility policy.

16. Use an antimicrobial swab to vigorously scrub the needleless connector or end cap and allow it to dry. If a needleless Luer adapter is not part of the Vacutainer, attach a needleless Luer adapter to the Vacutainer. Connect the needleless adapter of the Vacutainer to the needleless connector or end cap on the CVAD lumen (Figure 4). Insert the labeled blood sample tube for the discard sample into the Vacutainer (Figure 5). Follow facility policy for the volume of discard blood to collect (2 to 25 mL) (Gorski et al., 2021).

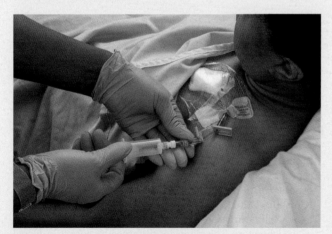

FIGURE 4. Connecting the needleless adapter of the Vacutainer to the connector or end cap on the CVAD lumen.

17. Remove the discard syringe and dispose of it appropriately, according to facility policy.

18. Insert each blood sample collection tube into the Vacutainer for each additional sample required. Gently rotate each tube as you remove it.

RATIONALE

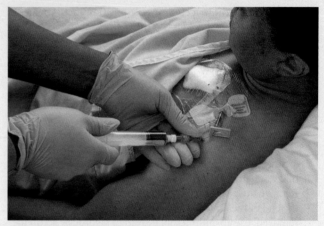

FIGURE 3. Pulling back on the syringe to aspirate for positive blood return.

Proper disposal reduces the risk of accidental blood exposure and transmission of microorganisms.

A sufficient amount of discard volume needs to be withdrawn before obtaining the blood sample to be tested in the laboratory. This sample is discarded because it is diluted with flush solution, possibly leading to inaccurate test results. If an insufficient amount of discard volume is withdrawn, the specimen may be diluted and contaminated with flush solution. If an excessive amount of discard volume is withdrawn, the patient may experience an iatrogenic (treatment-induced) blood loss. The wide variation in discard volumes depends on the internal volume of the CVAD, saline flushing prior to drawing the discard volume, and the specific laboratory tests (Gorski et al., 2021).

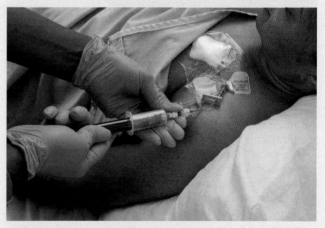

FIGURE 5. Inserting the blood sample tube to collect discard blood volume.

Proper disposal reduces the risk of accidental blood exposure and transmission of microorganisms.

The Vacutainer is a nonvented system, preventing backflow of patient blood. Filling the required tubes ensures that the sample is accurate. Gentle rotation helps to mix any additive in the tube with the blood sample.

ACTION

19. After obtaining the final blood sample, remove the Vacutainer.

20. Flush the lumen: Use an antimicrobial swab to vigorously scrub the needleless connector or end cap and allow it to dry. **Prevent connection/disconnection reflux by using the appropriate sequence for flushing, clamping, and disconnecting determined by the type of needleless connector being used** (see Box 16-4 in Skill 16-5) (Gorski et al., 2021). Insert the saline flush syringe into the needleless connector. Slowly inject the saline flush, noting any resistance or sluggishness, and slowly pull back on the syringe to aspirate for a positive blood return. If positive, instill the remaining solution over 1 minute or by using a pulsatile flushing technique of 10 short boluses of 1 mL interrupted by brief pauses; flush the line according to facility policy. Remove the syringe.

21. Use an antimicrobial swab to vigorously disinfect the connection surface and sides of each access site and allow them to dry. If the lumen is being used for infusion, reconnect the infusion. If the lumen is not in use, clamp the lumen and attach a passive disinfection cap.

22. Remove your face shield and gloves and perform hand hygiene. Record the date and time the samples were obtained on the labels as well as the required information to identify the person obtaining the samples. Compare the specimen label with the patient identification bracelet, as required by facility policy. Depending on facility policy, specimen labels may be verified prior to obtaining blood samples (refer to Step 8). Apply labels to the specimens, according to facility policy. Place them in a biohazard bag.

23. Return the patient to a comfortable position. Lower the bed height, if necessary, and adjust the head of the bed to a comfortable position.

24. Remove additional PPE, if used. Perform hand hygiene. Transport specimens to the laboratory immediately.

RATIONALE

The device is no longer needed.

Flushing maintains patency of the IV line. Venous access device administration set entry points, end caps, and needleless connectors must be disinfected prior to each access to reduce the risk for introduction of microorganisms and prevent venous access device–related infection (Frimpong et al., 2015; Gorski et al., 2021; Harper, 2014; Loveday et al., 2014). Friction is needed to physically remove microorganisms from the top, sides, and threads of the needleless connector or end cap. Allow the antiseptic to dry completely following the manufacturer's directions for use (Gorski et al., 2021). Action of the positive pressure end cap is maintained with the appropriate sequence for flushing, clamping, and disconnecting determined by the type of needleless connector in use (Gorski et al., 2021). The presence of a blood return upon aspiration and lack of resistance when flushing indicate patency of the VAD (Gorski et al., 2021). A pulsatile flushing technique of 10 short boluses of 1 mL interrupted by brief pauses may be more effective in removing solid deposits (e.g., fibrin, drug precipitate, intraluminal bacteria) (Gorski et al., 2021).

Venous access device administration set entry points, end caps, and needleless connectors must be vigorously scrubbed and disinfected prior to each access to reduce the risk for introduction of microorganisms and prevent venous access device–related infection (Frimpong et al., 2015; Gorski et al., 2021; Harper, 2014; Loveday et al., 2014). Friction is needed to physically remove microorganisms from the top, sides, and threads of the needleless connector or end cap. Allow the antiseptic to dry completely to ensure complete effectiveness. Clamping the lumen when not in use prevents accidental introduction of air into the lumen and loss of blood. Passive disinfection caps contain an antiseptic-impregnated sponge that dispenses the antiseptic over the connector's top and threads and protects the hub from contamination by touch or airborne sources (Gorski et al., 2021; Stango et al., 2014).

Proper removal of PPE and hand hygiene reduce the risk for infection transmission and contamination of other items. Proper labeling ensures accurate communication of results. Use of a biohazard bag prevents contact with blood and body fluids.

Repositioning promotes patient comfort.
Lowering the bed promotes patient safety.

Proper removal of PPE reduces the risk for infection transmission and contamination of other items. Hand hygiene prevents transmission of microorganisms. Specimens must be processed in a timely manner to ensure accuracy.

(*continued on page 1180*)

Skill 18-12 ▶ Obtaining a Blood Sample From a Central Venous Access Device *(continued)*

EVALUATION

The expected outcomes have been met when the blood samples have been obtained without compromise to the patency of the CVAD, and the patient has experienced minimal discomfort, remained free from infection, and verbalized an understanding of the rationale for and the steps of the procedure.

DOCUMENTATION

Guidelines

Document any pertinent assessments; the laboratory specimens obtained; the date and time specimens were obtained; the disposition of the specimens; the amount of blood collected and discarded, if required; and any significant assessments or patient reactions.

Sample Documentation

> 10/20/25 0230 Blood specimens for repeat PT/PTT, CBC, and BMP obtained via left subclavian multilumen CVAD after discarding 10 mL of blood. Catheter flushed, per policy; specimens sent to the laboratory.
>
> —R. Chin, RN

DEVELOPING CLINICAL REASONING AND CLINICAL JUDGMENT

UNEXPECTED SITUATIONS AND ASSOCIATED INTERVENTIONS

- *Blood flow from the lumen stops after beginning collection of blood:* Remove the blood specimen tube; the tube may have lost vacuum or be defective. Reattempt collection with a new tube; the tube may have lost vacuum or be defective.
- *Blood flow from the lumen stops after beginning collection of blood:* The exit site of the CVAD lumen may be lodged against the wall of the blood vessel; ask the patient to raise their arm on the side of the CVAD and/or ask the patient to cough. These actions may be sufficient to move the lumen away from the blood vessel wall and allow for blood flow.

SPECIAL CONSIDERATIONS

General Considerations

- Sampling from a CVAD is associated with some risks, including increased hub manipulation and the potential for intraluminal contamination, alterations in patency of the CVAD, and errors in lab values associated with adhesion of medications infused through the CVAD to the surface of the lumens (Gorski et al., 2021).
- Obtain blood samples for evaluation of drug levels from a lumen not used for administration of the drug being monitored, if possible (Gorski et al., 2021).
- Obtain only the volume of blood needed for accurate testing. Excessive blood sampling contributes to anemia in newborns, pediatrics, and critically ill adult patients and hospital-acquired anemia in patients of all ages (Gorski et al., 2021). Consider interventions to conserve blood, including the use of small-volume blood collection tubes, point-of-care testing methods, and avoidance of routine and/or unnecessary testing (Gorski et al., 2021).
- Be aware of the facility's policy regarding the order of collection of multiple tubes of blood to ensure accurate results.
- Blood cultures obtained from CVADs: Check facility policy for the need to change the needleless connector prior to obtaining blood for blood cultures.
- Blood cultures obtained from CVADs: At the first fever, obtain one peripheral set of blood cultures and one set from each lumen of the CVAD, with no blood discarded (Fischbach et al., 2022; Gorski et al., 2021). Subsequent cultures should be obtained from the CVAD only.
- Do not routinely use CVADs infusing parenteral nutrition for blood sampling to avoid increasing the risk for catheter-associated blood stream infections (Gorski et al., 2021).
- Do not reinfuse the discard sample in a disconnected syringe due to the risk of contamination and blood clot formation (Gorski et al., 2021).
- A closed-loop blood collection system may be used to allow return of any blood withdrawn for the purpose of clearing the catheter lumen (discard volume) (Gorski et al., 2021).

- The push–pull method can be used to reduce the amount of wasted blood and reduce hub manipulation (Gorski et al., 2021). Evidence suggests the use of 4 to 6 mL of blood withdrawn into the syringe and flushed back into the catheter lumen without disconnecting the syringe; the aspiration/return or push–pull cycles are repeated for a total of four cycles (Gorski et al., 2021).

EVIDENCE FOR PRACTICE ▶

BLOOD SAMPLING VIA A CVAD
Related Guideline
Infusion Nurses Society (INS) Standards of Practice
Gorski, L. A., Hadaway, L., Hagle, M. E., Broadhurst, D., Clare, S., Kleidon, T., Meyer, B. M., Nickel, B., Rowley, S., Sharpe, E., & Alexander, M. Infusion Nurses Society. (2021). Infusion therapy. Standards of practice, 8th edition. *Journal of Infusion Nursing, 44*(Suppl 1), S1–S224. doi: 10.1097/NAN.0000000000000396.

 The Infusion Nurses Society is recognized as the global authority in infusion therapy. The *Infusion Nursing Standards of Practice* is an evidence-based document, providing guidelines for nurses related to infusion therapy for use in all patient settings and addressing all patient populations. Specific guidance is provided for blood sampling via a CVAD.

EVIDENCE FOR PRACTICE ▶

BLOOD SAMPLING VIA A CENTRAL VENOUS ACCESS DEVICE AND PEDIATRIC INTENSIVE CARE
Blood sampling is a major source of blood loss in the pediatric intensive care unit (PICU) (Gorski et al., 2021; McBride et al., 2018). The push–pull method has been suggested for central venous access device (CVAD) sampling to reduce sampling-related blood loss and resulting anemia. Can this method be used safely and reliably?

Related Evidence
McBride, C., Miller-Hoover, S., & Proudfoot, J. A. (2018). A standard push-pull protocol for waste-free sampling in the PICU. *Journal of Infusion Nursing, 41*(3), 189–197. doi: 10.1097/NAN.0000000000000279.

 The purpose of this evidence-based practice project was to standardize a push–pull protocol for the majority of laboratory tests and CVADs and to determine if the protocol could be safely and reliably used as a routine sampling method in the PICU setting. A standard push–pull protocol for the PICU was developed, based on a review of protocols in the literature. Participants ($n = 37$) were a convenience sample of intermediate-acuity and high-acuity pediatric patients on trauma, organ transplant, and medical/surgical/cardiovascular intensive care units at a quaternary children's hospital. Participants had a variety of types of CVADs and prescribed laboratory tests ($n = 88$ total draws). Nurses on the units were educated about the project and trained in using the push–pull protocol, blood sampling instructions, and trouble-shooting tips for inadequate blood return. Samples using the push–pull method were collected over a 4-month period. A within-subject design was used, with laboratory values from push–pull samples compared to the patient's preceding and following laboratory values drawn according to standard practice (discard method). No significant differences were found in the means within each subject between the two methods ($p > 0.5$). No increase in catheter occlusions or infections were associated with the project. The researchers suggested that the protocol can be used safely and reliably as a standard waste-free sampling method in the PICU.

Relevance for Nursing Practice
Nurses have a responsibility to collaborate with members of the health care team to provide thoughtful person-centered interventions and care. Consideration of patient circumstances and needs should be part of planning treatment and care decisions to protect patients from the negative impact of blood loss and anemia.

Skill 18-13 ▶ Obtaining an Arterial Blood Sample From an Arterial Catheter

Obtaining an arterial blood sample requires percutaneous puncture of the radial (most common), brachial, or femoral artery. However, an arterial blood sample can also be obtained from an arterial catheter. Arterial catheters are used for hemodynamic monitoring (including measuring arterial pressures, continuous monitoring of blood pressure) and obtaining arterial blood samples without having to perform repeated arterial punctures, such as for blood gas analysis (Burns & Delgado, 2019; Hinkle et al., 2022). A pressure monitoring system (Figure 1) transmits pressures from the intravascular space or cardiac chambers through a catheter and fluid-filled tubing to a pressure transducer, which converts the physiologic signal from the patient to a pressure tracing and digital value. Patency of the system and prevention of backflow of blood through the catheter and tubing is maintained by using a continuous flush solution under pressure (Burns & Delgado, 2019; Morton & Fontaine, 2018).

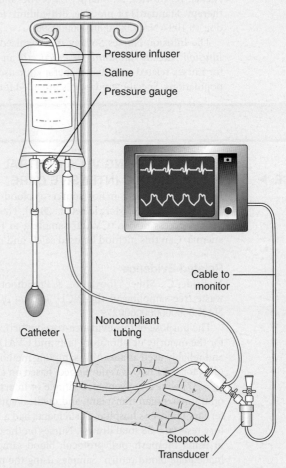

FIGURE 1. Pressure monitoring system. (*Source:* From Morton, P. G., & Fontaine, D. K. [2018]. *Essentials of critical care nursing. A holistic approach* [11th ed.]. Wolters Kluwer.)

The procedure below describes obtaining a sample from a closed reservoir system (Figure 2); a closed-loop system should be used when drawing from an existing arterial catheter to reduce health care–acquired anemia and intraluminal contamination and catheter-associated bloodstream infection (CABSI) compared to an open, stopcock system (Gorski et al., 2021).

| **DELEGATION CONSIDERATIONS** | Obtaining an arterial blood sample from an arterial catheter is not delegated to assistive personnel (AP) or licensed practical/vocational nurses (LPN/LVNs). |

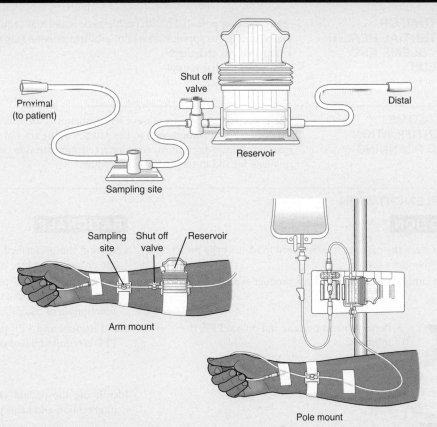

FIGURE 2. Closed blood collection/withdrawal system. (*Source:* Burns, S. M., & Delgado, S. A. (2019). *AACN Essentials of Critical Care Nursing* (4th ed.). McGraw Hill Education. Permission obtained from Edwards Lifesciences LLC, Irvine, CA.)

EQUIPMENT	• Arterial blood gas (ABG) kit heparinized (100 to 200 IU) self-filling 10-mL syringe with 22- to 23-gauge, 1-inch needle attached, rubber cap for ABG syringe hub, and ice-filled plastic bag or cup, if ABG is prescribed • Gloves • Goggles or face shield • Additional PPE, as indicated • Vacutainer with blunt cannula for closed reservoir system and appropriate blood collection tubes for prescribed tests • Two additional blood collection tubes, for discard blood volume • Antimicrobial swab, such as chlorhexidine or alcohol, per facility policy • Waterproof protective pad • Passive disinfection caps (based on facility policy) or • Sterile cap for arterial catheter stopcock (based on facility policy) • Appropriate label for specimen, based on facility policy and procedure • Blank labels (2) • Biohazard bag • Bath blanket
ASSESSMENT	Review the patient's health record and plan of care for information about their need for an arterial blood sample. Ensure that the necessary computerized laboratory request has been completed. Assess the patient's cardiac status, including heart rate, blood pressure, and auscultation of heart sounds. Also assess the patient's respiratory status, including respiratory rate, excursion, lung sounds, and use of oxygen, if prescribed. Check the patency and functioning of the arterial catheter. Assess the patient's understanding of the need for specimen collection.

(*continued on page 1184*)

Skill 18-13 ▶ Obtaining an Arterial Blood Sample From an Arterial Catheter *(continued)*

ACTUAL OR POTENTIAL HEALTH PROBLEMS AND NEEDS	Many actual or potential health problems or issues may require the use of this skill as part of related interventions. An appropriate health problem or issue may include: • Impaired gas exchange • Impaired cardiac output • Fluid imbalance
OUTCOME IDENTIFICATION AND PLANNING	The expected outcome to achieve when obtaining an arterial blood sample is that a specimen is obtained without compromise to the patency of the arterial catheter. In addition, the patient experiences minimal discomfort, remains free from infection, and verbalizes an understanding of the rationale for and the steps of the procedure.

IMPLEMENTATION

ACTION	RATIONALE
1. Check the patient's health record to identify the prescribed laboratory testing.	Checking the prescribed intervention and policy ensures that the proper procedure is initiated.
2. Gather all equipment. Check product expiration dates.	Assembling equipment provides for an organized approach to the task. Use of products that have not expired ensures proper functioning of equipment.
3. Perform hand hygiene and put on PPE, if indicated.	Hand hygiene and PPE prevent the spread of microorganisms. PPE is required based on transmission precautions.
4. Identify the patient.	Identifying the patient ensures the right patient receives the intervention and helps prevent errors.
5. Close the curtains around the bed and close the door to the room, if possible. Explain the procedure to the patient.	This ensures the patient's privacy. Explanation relieves anxiety and facilitates engagement.
6. Assemble equipment on the overbed table or other surface within reach.	Arranging items nearby is convenient, saves time, and avoids unnecessary stretching and twisting of muscles on the part of the nurse.
7. Adjust the bed to a comfortable working height (VHACEOSH, 2016).	Having the bed at the proper height prevents back and muscle strain.
8. Compare the specimen label with the patient identification bracelet. The label should include the patient's name and identification number, the time the specimen was collected, the route of collection, identification of the person obtaining the sample, and any other information required by facility policy. Depending on facility policy, specimen labels may be verified after obtaining blood samples, prior to application to blood sample tubes.	Verifying the patient's identity validates that the correct procedure is being done on the correct patient, and the specimen is accurately labeled.
9. Use blank labels to label the two blood sample collection tubes to be used for the discard blood sample and the discard flush.	Labeling the discard tubes prevents accidental confusion with blood specimen tubes.
10. Assist the patient to a comfortable position that provides easy access to the sampling site. Use the bath blanket to cover any exposed area other than the sampling site. Place a waterproof pad under the site.	Patient positioning and use of a bath blanket provide for comfort and warmth. The waterproof pad protects underlying surfaces.
11. Put on gloves and goggles or a face shield.	Gloves and goggles (or face shield) prevent contact with blood and body fluids.

ACTION	**RATIONALE**
12. Temporarily silence the arterial pressure monitor alarms.	The integrity of the system is being altered, which will cause the system to sound an alarm. Facility policy may require the alarm be left on.
13. Locate the closed-system reservoir and blood-sampling site. Use an antimicrobial swab to vigorously scrub the sampling site (Figure 2). Allow it to air dry.	Arterial access device administration set entry points, end caps, and needleless connectors must be disinfected prior to each access to reduce the risk for introduction of microorganisms and prevent access device–related infection (Frimpong et al., 2015; Gorski et al., 2021; Harper, 2014; Loveday et al., 2014). Friction is needed to physically remove microorganisms from the top, sides, and threads of the needleless connector or end cap. Allow the antiseptic to dry completely following the manufacturer's directions for use (Gorski et al., 2021).
14. Holding the reservoir upright, grasp the flexures and slowly fill it with blood over a 3- to 5-second period (Figure 2). If you feel resistance, reposition the patient's extremity and check the catheter site for obvious problems (e.g., kinking of the tubing). Then continue with blood withdrawal.	Filling the reservoir pulls the saline from the monitoring line, so the blood sample is not diluted by the fluid in the line.
15. Turn off the shut-off valve to the reservoir by turning the handle perpendicular to the tubing (Figure 2).	This prevents flow of fluid from the reservoir into the blood samples and allows blood from the patient to be drawn through the sampling port.
16. Insert the Vacutainer into the sampling site (see Figure 2). Insert the blood sample tubes into the Vacutainer. If coagulation tests have been prescribed, collect those sample tubes last. After obtaining the final blood sample, grasp the Vacutainer near the sampling site and remove the Vacutainer.	Inserting the Vacutainer or syringe into the sampling port allows blood to be drawn into blood sample tubes. The Vacutainer is a nonvented system, preventing backflow of patient blood. Obtaining coagulation samples last prevents dilution from the flush device.
17. After removal of the Vacutainer, turn the one-way valve to its original position, parallel to the tubing. Push down evenly on the reservoir (see Figure 2) plunger until the flexures lock in place in the fully closed position and all fluid has been reinfused. The fluid should be reinfused over a 3- to 5-second period. Activate the flush release.	Reinfusion of "waste" blood reduces hospital-acquired anemia, intraluminal contamination, and catheter-associated blood stream infection (Gorski et al., 2021). In-line flushing clears the sampling port and flush line to maintain the integrity of the system and prevent clotting and infection.
18. Use an antimicrobial swab to vigorously scrub the sampling site.	Arterial access device administration set entry points, end caps, and needleless connectors must be disinfected prior to each access to reduce the risk for introduction of microorganisms and prevent access device–related infection (Frimpong et al., 2015; Gorski et al., 2021; Harper, 2014; Loveday et al., 2014). Friction is needed to physically remove microorganisms from the top, sides, and threads of the needleless connector or end cap. Allow the antiseptic to dry completely, following the manufacturer's directions for use (Gorski et al., 2021).
19. Remove your gloves and goggles/face shield and perform hand hygiene. Check the monitor for return of the arterial waveform and pressure reading. Reactivate the monitor alarms. Record the date and time the samples were obtained on the labels as well as the required information to identify the person obtaining the samples. If arterial blood gas (ABG) was collected, record the oxygen flow rate (or room air) on the label. Apply the labels to the specimens, according to facility policy. Place them in biohazard bags; place the ABG sample in a bag with ice.	Proper removal of PPE and hand hygiene reduce the risk for infection transmission and contamination of other items. Confirmation of the return of arterial waveform and pressure readings ensures proper functioning and integrity of the system. Reactivating the alarm system ensures proper functioning. Proper labeling prevents error. Recording the oxygen flow rate ensures accurate interpretation of the results of the ABG. Use of a biohazard bag prevents contact with blood and body fluids. Ice maintains the integrity of the sample.

(continued on page 1186)

Skill 18-13 ▶ Obtaining an Arterial Blood Sample From an Arterial Catheter *(continued)*

ACTION	RATIONALE
20. Return the patient to a comfortable position. Lower the bed height, if necessary, and adjust the head of the bed to a comfortable position.	Repositioning promotes patient comfort. Lowering the bed promotes patient safety.
21. Remove additional PPE, if used. Perform hand hygiene. Send specimens to the laboratory immediately.	Proper removal of PPE reduces the risk for infection transmission and contamination of other items. Hand hygiene prevents transmission of microorganisms. Specimens must be processed in a timely manner to ensure accuracy.

EVALUATION

The expected outcomes have been met when an arterial specimen has been obtained without compromise to the patency of the arterial catheter, and the patient has experienced minimal discomfort, remained free from infection, and verbalized an understanding of the rationale for and the steps of the procedure.

DOCUMENTATION

Guidelines

Document any pertinent assessments, the laboratory specimens obtained, the date and time specimens were obtained, and the disposition of the specimens.

Sample Documentation

> <u>10/20/25</u> 0230 Continuous heparin IV infusion at 900 units/hr via left subclavian central catheter. Blood specimens for repeat PT/PTT, CBC, and BMP obtained via right radial arterial catheter, per order. Catheter flushed, per policy; specimens sent to the laboratory.
>
> —*R. Chin, RN*

DEVELOPING CLINICAL REASONING AND CLINICAL JUDGMENT

UNEXPECTED SITUATIONS AND ASSOCIATED INTERVENTIONS

• *After obtaining the specimen and reactivating the arterial pressure monitoring system, no waveform is noted:* Check the stopcock to make sure that it is open to the patient and recheck all connections and components of the system to ensure proper setup. If necessary, rebalance the transducer or replace the system, as necessary. If problem persists, suspect a clotted catheter tip. Follow facility policy to troubleshoot a potentially clotted arterial catheter and notify the health care team.

SPECIAL CONSIDERATIONS

• If the patient is receiving oxygen, wait 15 minutes after a change in type or mode of oxygen delivery or rate for specimen collection for ABG analysis (Fischbach et al., 2022). Indicate the amount and type of oxygen therapy the patient is receiving on the laboratory request. Also note the patient's current temperature, most recent hemoglobin level, and current respiratory rate. If the patient is receiving mechanical ventilation, note the fraction of inspired oxygen and tidal volume.

• If the patient is not receiving oxygen, indicate that they are breathing room air on the laboratory request for an ABG analysis.

EVIDENCE FOR PRACTICE ▶

BLOOD SAMPLING VIA A CENTRAL VENOUS ACCESS DEVICE
Related Guideline
Infusion Nurses Society (INS) Standards of Practice
Gorski, L. A., Hadaway, L., Hagle, M. E., Broadhurst, D., Clare, S., Kleidon, T., Meyer, B, M., Nickel, B., Rowley, S., Sharpe, E., & Alexander, M. Infusion Nurses Society. (2021). Infusion therapy. Standards of practice, 8th edition. *Journal of Infusion Nursing, 44*(Suppl 1), S1–S224. doi: 10.1097/NAN.0000000000000396.

The Infusion Nurses Society is recognized as the global authority in infusion therapy. The *Infusion Nursing Standards of Practice* is an evidence-based document, providing guidelines for nurses related to infusion therapy for use in all patient settings and addressing all patient populations. Specific guidance is provided for use of closed-loop systems as these systems return the blood to the patient and reduce blood loss associated with blood sampling.

Enhance Your Understanding

Focusing on Patient Care: Developing Clinical Reasoning and Clinical Judgment

Consider the case scenarios at the beginning of the chapter as you answer the following questions to enhance your understanding and apply what you have learned.

QUESTIONS

1. The nurse explained to Mr. Conklin the procedure for obtaining the required urine specimens. Unfortunately, it becomes clear that the patient is too confused at this time to follow the directions and obtain the specimen by himself. How would you handle this situation? How would you successfully obtain an uncontaminated specimen from a patient who is unable to engage in their care?

2. Huana Yon's health care provider provides pre- and postappointment education and information for the patients in the practice. Part of the nurse's responsibilities when contacting patients before their scheduled visit is to provide information related to anticipated laboratory tests and any necessary patient preparation. What information would you include if you were calling this patient before their visit in relation to collecting a stool specimen for occult blood? What medications or other habits would you question them about? What information would you give them to prepare for the test?

3. The nurse assigned to Mrs. Yeletsky questions them about their blood glucose testing at home. Mrs. Yeletsky states, "I never really figured out how to work the machine they gave me the last time I saw the doctor. The buttons are too small, and I can't see the writing on the screen very well. Besides, I'm only a little diabetic." What additional information would you want to obtain from this patient? How would you address their possible lack of understanding regarding diabetes? What interventions could you attempt to aid them in managing their blood glucose levels? What other aspects of their health habits would you want to assess?

You can find suggested answers after the Bibliography at the end of this chapter.

Integrated Case Study Connection

The case studies in the back of the book focus on integrating concepts. Refer to the following case studies to enhance your understanding of the concepts and skills in this chapter.

- Basic Case Studies: Joe LeRoy, page 1203; Tula Stillwater, page 1207.
- Intermediate Case Studies: Victoria Holly, page 1211.
- Advanced Case Studies: Cole McKean, page 1225.

Bibliography

American Academy of Pediatrics (AAP). (2016). Reaffirmation of AAP Clinical Practice Guideline: The diagnosis and management of the initial urinary tract infection in febrile infants and children 2 to 24 months of age. *Pediatrics, 138*(6), e20163026. https://doi.org/10.1542/peds.2016-3026

American Association for Clinical Chemistry (AACC). (2020, November 12). *Lab Tests Online®. Proper self-collection of nasal swabs critical for accurate COVID-19 testing.* https://labtestsonline.org/news/proper-self-collection-nasal-swabs-critical-accurate-covid-19-testing

American Association for Clinical Chemistry (AACC). (2021a, August 27). *Lab Tests Online®. Fecal immunochemical test.* https://labtestsonline.org/tests/fecal-immunochemical-test-and-fecal-occult-blood-test

American Association for Clinical Chemistry (AACC). (2021b, October 1). *Lab Tests Online®. Fecal immunochemical test.* https://labtestsonline.org/tests/fecal-occult-blood-test

American Association of Critical-Care Nurses (AACN). (2016, August 1). Prevention of CAUTI in adults. https://www.aacn.org/clinical-resources/practice-alerts/prevention-of-cauti-in-adults

American Association of Critical-Care Nurses (AACN). (2017). In D. L. Wiegand (Ed.). *AACN procedure manual for high acuity, progressive, and critical care* (7th ed.). Elsevier.

American Cancer Society (ACS). (2020). *Colorectal cancer screening tests.* https://www.cancer.org/cancer/colon-rectal-cancer/detection-diagnosis-staging/screening-tests-used.html

American Diabetes Association (ADA). (n.d.). *The big picture: Checking your blood sugar.* https://www.diabetes.org/healthy-living/medication-treatments/blood-glucose-testing-and-control/checking-your-blood-sugar

American Diabetes Association (ADA). (2021). Standards of medical care in diabetes—2021. *Diabetes Care, 44*(Suppl 1), S1–S232. https://care.diabetesjournals.org/content/44/Supplement_1

Bauldoff, G., Gubrud, P., & Carno, M. A. (2020). *LeMone and Burke's Medical-surgical nursing: Clinical reasoning in patient care* (7th ed.). Pearson.

Bechtold, M. L., Ashraf, I., & Nguyen, D. L. (2016). A clinician's guide to fecal occult blood testing for colorectal cancer. *Southern Medical Journal, 109*(4), 248–255. https://doi.org/10.14423/SMJ.0000000000000449

Beckman Coulter. (2013). *Hemoccult®: Screening test for fecal occult blood.* https://www.beckmancoulter.com/download/file/wsr-158620/462403EC?type=pdf

Beckman Coulter. (2015a, March). *Hemoccult® ICT: Immunochemical fecal occult blood test (FIT). Patient sample collection instructions.* https://www.beckmancoulter.com/download/file/wsr-118305/395887PM?type=pdf

Beckman Coulter. (2015b). *Hemoccult® ICT: Product instructions.* https://www.beckmancoulter.com/download/file/wsr-116763/395069FJ?type=pdf

Burns, S. M., & Delgado, S. A. (2019). *AACN essentials of critical care nursing* (4th ed.). McGraw Hill Education.

Centers for Disease Control and Prevention (CDC). (n.d.). *Influenza specimen collection.* Retrieved October 26, 2021, https://www.cdc.gov/flu/pdf/professionals/flu-specimen-collection-poster.pdf

Centers for Disease Control and Prevention (CDC). (2011, January 17). *Healthcare-associated infections (HAIs). Staphylococcus aureus in healthcare settings.* https://www.cdc.gov/hai/organisms/staph.html

Centers for Disease Control and Prevention (CDC). (2019a, November 18). *Pertussis (whooping cough). Specimen collection. Pertussis testing video: Collecting a nasopharyngeal swab clinical specimen.* https://www.cdc.gov/pertussis/clinical/diagnostic-testing/specimen-collection.html

Centers for Disease Control and Prevention (CDC). (2019b, February 28). *Methicillin-resistant Staphylococcus aureus (MRSA): Healthcare settings.* https://www.cdc.gov/mrsa/healthcare/index.html?CDC_AA_refVal=https%3A%2F%2Fwww.cdc.gov%2Fmrsa%2Fhealthcare%2Fclinicians%2Fprecautions.html

Centers for Disease Control and Prevention (CDC). (2019c). How to collect an anterior nasal swab specimen for COVID-19 testing. https://www.cdc.gov/coronavirus/2019-ncov/testing/How-To-Collect-Anterior-Nasal-Specimen-for-COVID-19.pdf

Centers for Disease Control and Prevention (CDC). (2019d, May 9). *Healthcare-associated infections (HAI). Patients with indwelling urinary catheter. Strategize initiatives you can incorporate into your program.* https://www.cdc.gov/hai/prevent/cauti/indwelling/strategize.html

Centers for Disease Control and Prevention (CDC). (2019e, October 25). *Interim guidelines for collecting and handling of clinical specimens for COVID-19 testing.* https://www.cdc.gov/coronavirus/2019-ncov/lab/guidelines-clinical-specimens.html

Centers for Disease Control and Prevention (CDC). (2021, August 10). *Monitoring your blood sugar.* https://www.cdc.gov/diabetes/managing/managing-blood-sugar/bloodglucosemonitoring.html

Centers for Disease Control and Prevention (CDC). (2021a). *Core curriculum on tuberculosis: What the clinician should know* (7th ed.). https://www.cdc.gov/tb/education/corecurr/pdf/CoreCurriculumTB-508.pdf

Centers for Disease Control and Prevention (CDC). (2021b, February 8). *Colorectal (colon) cancer. Colorectal cancer screening tests.* https://www.cdc.gov/cancer/colorectal/basic_info/screening/tests.htm

Centers for Disease Control and Prevention (CDC). (2021c, October 25). *Tuberculosis (TB).* https://www.cdc.gov/tb/default.htm

Centers for Disease Control and Prevention (CDC). (2021d, August 10). *Monitoring your blood sugar.* https://www.cdc.gov/diabetes/managing/managing-blood-sugar/bloodglucosemonitoring.html

Cheek, J. A., Craig, S. S., Seith, R. W., & West, A. (2015). Urine collection in young children. *Emergency Medicine Australasia, 27*(4), 348–350. https://doi.org/10.1111/1742-6723.12442

Collins, L. (2019). Diagnosis and management of a urinary tract infection. *British Journal of Nursing, 28*(2), 84–88. https://doi.org/10.12968/bjon.2019.28.2.84

Colorectal Cancer Alliance. (2019a). *Guaiac fecal occult blood test.* https://www.ccalliance.org/screening-prevention/screening-methods/guaiac-fecal-occult-blood-test

Colorectal Cancer Alliance. (2019b). *Fecal immunochemical test.* https://www.ccalliance.org/screening-prevention/screening-methods/fecal-immunochemical-test

Davis, C. (2019). Catheter-associated urinary tract infection: Signs, diagnosis, prevention. *British Journal of Nursing, 28*(2), 96–100. https://doi.org/10.12968/bjon.2019.28.2.96

De Bernardo, G., Riccitelli, M., Sordino, D., Giordano, M., Piccolo, S., Buonocore, G., & Perrone, S. (2018). Oral 24% sucrose associated with non-nutritive sucking for pain control in healthy term newborns receiving venipuncture beyond the first week of life. *Journal of Pain Research, 12,* 299–305. https://doi.org/10.2147/JPR.S184504

Doubeni, C. (2021, October 25). UpToDate®. *Tests for screening for colorectal cancer.* Wolters Kluwer. https://www.uptodate.com/contents/tests-for-screening-for-colorectal-cancer

Ehrhardt, B. S., Givens, K. E. A., & Lee, R. C. (2018). Making it stick: Developing and testing the Difficult Intravenous Access (DIVA) Tool. *American Journal of Nursing, 118*(7), 56–62. https://doi.org/10.1097/01.NAJ.0000541440.91369.00

Eliopoulos, C. (2018). *Gerontological nursing* (9th ed.). Wolters Kluwer.

Erdogan, B., & Ozdemir, A. A. (2021). The effect of three different methods on venipuncture pain and anxiety in children: Distraction cards, virtual reality, and Buzzy® (randomized controlled trial). *Journal of Pediatric Nursing, 58,* e54–e62. https://doi.org/10.1016/j.pedn.2021.01.001

Erzincanli, S., & Kasar, K. S. (2021). Effect of hand massage on pain, anxiety, and vital signs in patients before venipuncture procedure: A randomized controlled trial. *Pain Management Nursing, 22,* 356–360. https://doi.org/10.1016/j.pmn.2020.12.005

Fischbach, F. T., Fischbach, M. A., & Stout, K. (2022). *Fischbach's a manual of laboratory and diagnostic tests* (11th ed.). Wolters Kluwer.

Frimpong, A., Caguioa, J., & Octavo, G. (2015). Promoting safe IV management in practice using H.A.N.D.S. *British Journal of Nursing (IV Therapy Supplement), 24*(2), S18–S23. DOI: 10.12968/bjon.2015.24.Sup2.S18

Gorski, L. A., Hadaway, L., Hagle, M. E., Broadhurst, D., Clare, S., Kleidon, T., Meyer, B. M., Nickel, B., Rowley, S., Sharpe, E., & Alexander, M., Infusion Nurses Society. (2021). Infusion therapy. Standards of practice, 8th edition. *Journal of Infusion Nursing, 44*(Suppl 1), S1–S224. https://doi.org/10.1097/NAN.0000000000000396

Harper, D. (2014). I.V. Rounds. Infusion therapy: Much more than a simple task. *Nursing, 44*(7), 66–67. DOI: 10.1097/01.NURSE.0000446643.87747.1f

Hess, D. R., MacIntyre, N. R., Galvin, W. F., & Mishoe, S. C. (2021). *Respiratory care: Principles and practice* (4th ed.). Jones & Bartlett Learning.

Higgins, T. S., Wu, S. W., & Ting, J. Y. (2020). SARS-CoV-2 nasopharyngeal swab testing—False-negative results from a pervasive anatomical misconception. *JAMA Otolaryngology—Head and Neck Surgery, 146*(11), 993–994. https://doi.org/10.1001/jamaoto.2020.2946

Hill, S., & Moore, S. (2018). Arterial blood gas sampling: Using a safety and pre-heparinised syringe. *British Journal of Nursing, 27*(14), S20–S26. https://doi.org/10.12968/bjon.2018.27.14.S20

Hinkle, J. L., Cheever, K. H., & Overbaugh, K. (2022). *Brunner & Suddarth's Textbook of medical-surgical nursing* (15th ed.). Wolters Kluwer.

International Council of Nurses (ICN). (2019). *Nursing diagnosis and outcome statements.* https://www.icn.ch/sites/default/files/inline-files/ICNP2019-DC.pdf

Jarvis, C. (2016). *Physical examination and health assessment* (7th ed.). Elsevier.

Jarvis, C., & Eckhardt, A. (2020). *Physical examination & health assessment* (8th ed.). Elsevier.

Jensen, S. (2019). *Nursing health assessment. A best practice approach* (3rd ed.). Wolters Kluwer.

The Joint Commission. (2021). *National patient safety goals.* https://www.jointcommission.org/standards/national-patient-safety-goals/

KarabiyikOğurlu, Ö., TuralBüyük, E., & Yildizlar, O. (2020). The effect of warm compression applied before heel lance on pain level, comfort level and procedure time in healthy term newborns: A randomized clinical trial. *Journal of Midwifery & Reproductive Health, 8*(3), 1–8. https://doi.org/10.22038/jmrh.2020.41747.1475

Karch, A. M. (2020). *Focus on nursing pharmacology* (8th ed.). Wolters Kluwer.

Knapp, R. (Clinical Ed.). (2020). *Hemodynamic monitoring made incredibly visual* (4th ed.). Wolters Kluwer.

Kuo, H. C., Pan, H. H., Creedy, D. K., & Tsao, Y. (2018). Distraction-based interventions for children undergoing venipuncture procedures: A randomized controlled study. *Clinical Nursing Research, 27*(4), 467–482. https://doi.org/10.1177/1054773816686262

Kyle, T., & Carman, S. (2021). *Essentials of pediatric nursing* (4th ed.). Wolters Kluwer.

Laboratory Alliance of Central New York, LLC. (2017, November 24). *Collection and inoculation of blood specimens for routine culture (Bacterial, T.B. or fungus).* https://www.laboratoryalliance.com/healthcare-providers/laboratory-services/specimen-collection-documents/collection-and-inoculation-of-blood-specimens-for-routine-culture-bacterial-t-b-or-fungus

Loveday, H. P., Wilson, J. A., Pratt, R. J., et al. (2014). Epic3: National evidence-based guidelines for preventing healthcare-associated infections in NHS hospitals in England. *Journal of Hospital Infection, 86*(1), S1–S70. DOI: 10.1016/S0195-6701(13)60012-2

Mahoney, M., Baxter, K., Burgess, J., Bauer, C., Downey, C., Mantel, J., Perkins, J., Rice, M., Salvadalena, G., Schafer, V., Sheppard, S. (2013). Procedure for obtaining a urine sample from a urostomy, ileal conduit, and colon conduit. A best practice guideline for clinicians. *Journal of Wound, Ostomy and Continence Nursing, 40*(3), 277–279. https://doi.org/10.1097/WON.0b013e31828f1a47

Mark, M. E., LoSavio, P., Husain, I., Papagiannopoulos, P., Batra, P. S., & Tajudeen, B. A. (2020). Effect of implementing simulation education on health care worker comfort with nasopharyngeal swabbing for COVID-19. *Otolaryngology-Head and Neck Surgery, 163*(2), 271–274. https://doi.org/10.1177/0194599820933168

Marty, F. M., Chen, K., & Verrill, K. A. (2020, April 17). How to obtain a nasopharyngeal swab specimen. *The New England Journal of Medicine*. [Online]. https://www.nejm.org/doi/full/10.1056/nejmvcm2010260

May, O. W. (2018). Urine collection methods in children: Which is the best? *Nursing Clinics of North America, 53*(2), 137–143. https://doi.org/10.1016/j.cnur.2018.01.001

McBride, C., Miller-Hoover, S., & Proudfoot, J. A. (2018). A standard push-pull protocol for waste-free sampling in the PICU. *Journal of Infusion Nursing, 41*(3), 189–197. https://doi.org/10.1097/NAN.0000000000000279

McLaughlin, M. A. (Ed.). (2020). *Cardiovascular care made incredibly easy* (4th ed.). Wolters Kluwer.

MedlinePlus. (2020). Fecal occult blood test (FOBT). U.S. National Library of Medicine. https://medlineplus.gov/lab-tests/fecal-occult-blood-test-fobt/

MedlinePlus. (2021a, September 16). Nasal swab. U.S. National Library of Medicine. https://medlineplus.gov/lab-tests/nasal-swab/

MedlinePlus. (2021b, October 8). Nasopharyngeal culture. U.S. National Library of Medicine. https://medlineplus.gov/ency/article/003747.htm

MedlinePlus. (2021c, October 8). *Clean catch urine sample*. U.S. National Library of Medicine. https://medlineplus.gov/ency/article/007487.htm

MedlinePlus. (2021d). *Stool guaiac test*. U.S. National Library of Medicine. https://medlineplus.gov/ency/article/003393.htm

Morton, P. G., & Fontaine, D. K. (2018). *Critical care nursing. A holistic approach* (11th ed.). Wolters Kluwer.

National Institute of Diabetes and Digestive and Kidney Diseases (NIDDK). (2016, December). Diabetes tests & diagnosis. https://www.niddk.nih.gov/health-information/diabetes/overview/tests-diagnosis

National Institute of Diabetes and Digestive and Kidney Diseases (NIDDK). (2017, June). Continuous glucose monitoring. https://www.niddk.nih.gov/health-information/diabetes/overview/managing-diabetes/continuous-glucose-monitoring

Norris, T. L. (2020). *Porth's essentials of pathophysiology* (5th ed.). Wolters Kluwer.

Novotne, T. A., & Kaseb, H. O. (2013). The changing face of *Clostridium difficile* in critical care. *Nursing2013 Critical Care, 8*(3), 26–34.

Peker, N., Couto, N., Sinha, B., & Rossen, J. W. (2018). Diagnosis of bloodstream infections from positive blood cultures and directly from blood samples: Recent developments in molecular approaches. *Clinical Microbiology and Infection, 24*(9), 944–955. https://doi.org/10.1016/j.cmi.2018.05.007

Problem-based care plans. (2022). In Lippincott Advisor. Wolters Kluwer. https://advisor.lww.com/lna/home.do

Silbert-Flagg, J., & Pillitteri, A. (2018). *Maternal and child health nursing* (8th ed.). Wolters Kluwer.

Stango, C., Runyan, D., Stern, J., Macri, I., & Vacca, M. (2014). A successful approach to reducing bloodstream infections based on a disinfection device for intravenous needleless connector hubs. *Journal of Infusion Nursing, 37*(6), 462–465. DOI: 10.1097/NAN.0000000000000075

Taylor, C., Lynn, P., & Bartlett, J. (2023). *Fundamentals of nursing: The art and science of person-centered care* (10th ed.). Wolters Kluwer.

U.S. Food & Drug Administration (FDA). (2019, April 4). *Blood glucose monitoring devices*. https://www.fda.gov/medical-devices/in-vitro-diagnostics/blood-glucose-monitoring-devices

U.S. National Library of Medicine, National Institutes of Health, MedlinePlus. (2017). *Nasopharyngeal culture*. https://medlineplus.gov/ency/article/003747.htm

U.S. Preventive Services Task Force. (2021, May 18). *Final recommendation statement. Colorectal cancer: Screening*. https://www.uspreventiveservicestaskforce.org/uspstf/document/RecommendationStatementFinal/colorectal-cancer-screening#tab

Vaarala, M. H. (2018). Urinary sample collection methods in ileal conduit urinary diversion patients. A randomized controlled trial. *Journal of Wound, Sotomy, and Continence Nursing, 45*(1), 59–62. https://doi.org/10.1097/WON.0000000000000397

Van Leeuwen, A. M., & Bladh, M. L. (2017). *Davis's comprehensive handbook of laboratory & diagnostic tests with nursing implications* (7th ed.). F.A. Davis Company.

Vedder, T, G. (2021, January 14). Heel sticks. Medscape. https://emedicine.medscape.com/article/1413486-overview

VHA Center for Engineering & Occupational Safety and Health (CEOSH). (2016). *Safe patient handling and mobility guidebook*. http://www.tnpatientsafety.com/pubfiles/Initiatives/workplace-violence/sphm-pdf.pdf Williams, A. S. (n.d.). Monitoring your diabetes. American Federation for the Blind. https://www.afb.org/blindness-and-low-vision/eye-conditions/diabetes-and-vision-loss-guide-caring-yourself-when-you-2

Williams, J. (2013). Stoma care: Obtaining a urine specimen from a urostomy. *Gastrointestinal Nursing, 10*(5), 11–12. https://doi.org/10.12968/gasn.2012.10.5.11

World Health Organization (WHO). (2010). *WHO guidelines on drawing blood: Best practices in phlebotomy*. http://www.euro.who.int/__data/assets/pdf_file/0005/268790/WHO-guidelines-on-drawing-blood-best-practices-in-phlebotomy-Eng.pdf?ua-1

Wound Ostomy and Continence Nurses Society (WOCN). (2018). *Catheterization of an ileal or colon conduit stoma: Best practice for clinicians*. https://www.ostomy.org/wp-content/uploads/2018/11/Catheterization-of-Urinary-Stoma-2018.pdf

SUGGESTED ANSWERS FOR FOCUSING ON PATIENT CARE: DEVELOPING CLINICAL REASONING AND CLINICAL JUDGMENT

1. Obtaining a urine specimen is a priority in Mr. Conklin's care. Results will help determine the underlying cause of their symptoms and direct treatment. As a result, you will have to take a more involved role in the collection. You will have to obtain the specimen. Continue to reinforce the need for the urine specimen. Gather the necessary supplies and place them in the patient's room or bathroom. Plan to obtain the specimen the next time Mr. Conklin has to void. Share the plan with other caregivers. When the patient communicates their need to void, put on nonsterile gloves. Assist them to the bathroom. Explain again the need and rationale for the urine specimen. Explain that you are going to clean their penis to get the specimen. Clean their penis according to the guidelines in the procedure. Ask Mr. Conklin to void into the toilet; be ready to place the specimen cup in the stream of urine to obtain a sample. Put the lid on the specimen container. After assisting the patient with the rest of their toileting needs, clean the outside of the container, if urine contacted the outside during sampling. Label the sample and transport it to the laboratory.

2. Explain the reason for the test and the procedure for stool collection. Ask about any hematuria, bleeding hemorrhoids, or recent nose or throat bleeding. These situations would require the test to be postponed. Question Ms. Yon regarding medications she use, including certain medications, such as a salicylate intake of more than 325 mg daily, steroids, iron preparations, and anticoagulants, that may lead to false-positive readings, and use of vitamin C, as this may lead to false-negative results. Ask about the use of laxatives, enemas, or suppositories for 3 days before testing. Ms. Yon should understand that they should collect the specimen the morning of her appointment and know how to handle the specimen once she has obtained it.

3. Assess Mrs. Yeletsky's knowledge regarding her understanding of what diabetes is, its effects on the body, possible complications, dietary guidelines, medications prescribed to treat their diabetes, activity level/habits, and personal hygiene, particularly foot care. You should incorporate education regarding diabetes, including simple explanations of the definition of diabetes, normal blood glucose ranges, effect of insulin and exercise, effect of food and stress, and basic treatment approaches. A referral to the diabetic clinical specialist, if available, would be appropriate, as well as a referral for outpatient follow-up. Review the patient's understanding of blood glucose monitoring and the use of the blood glucose monitor. Investigate alternative blood glucose monitors; models are available to aid people with impaired vision. Explore the support the patient has available and the possibility of a significant other assisting with their diabetes management, if appropriate.

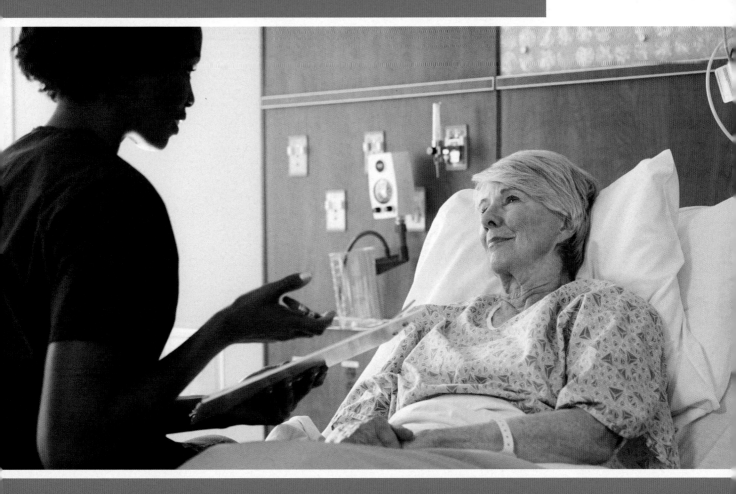

Integrated Case Studies

These case studies are designed to focus on integrating concepts. They are not meant to be all-inclusive. The Developing Clinical Reasoning and Clinical Judgment questions should guide your discussions of related issues. The discussion within the Integrated Nursing Care section represents possible nursing care solutions to problems; you may find other solutions that are equally acceptable.

PART 1

Basic Case Studies

Nursing Concepts

- Advocacy
- Assessment
- Clinical Decision Making/Clinical Judgment
- Collaboration/Teamwork and Collaboration
- Comfort
- Communication
- Elimination
- Functional Ability
- Infection
- Mobility
- Nutrition
- Oxygenation/Gas Exchange
- Safety
- Teaching and Learning/Patient Education
- Tissue Integrity

Case Study

Abigail Cantonelli

Abigail Cantonelli, age 80, injured her left knee and wrist when she fell on an icy sidewalk. She has been on your orthopedic and neurologic unit for several days. She has a history of cardiomyopathy, for which she receives furosemide. Her vital signs are stable and she rates her pain as aching, intermittent, and a 2 on a scale of 1 to 10 (10 = worst pain). Because Mrs. Cantonelli has an increased risk of falling, she has been prescribed physical therapy and cane-walking instructions before discharge. Although the physical therapy staff has already initiated the cane-walking instructions, you will need to ambulate Mrs. Cantonelli with her cane during your shift. While you are ambulating down the hall, she says, "Oh, dear! I feel dizzy." She begins to lose her balance and fall toward you.

continued

Abigail Cantonelli (continued)

Prescribed Interventions

Physical therapy for cane-walking instruction
Ambulate every shift with cane assistance
Furosemide 20 mg PO every morning

Potassium chloride 10 mEq PO every day
Naproxen 275 mg PO q6–8h prn pain

Developing Clinical Reasoning and Clinical Judgment

- Identify Mrs. Cantonelli's risk factors for falling.

- Considering these risk factors, what special assessments and precautions should you implement before assisting her to ambulate or while assisting her with ambulation?

- Describe the actions you would implement when Mrs. Cantonelli begins to fall.

Suggested Responses for Integrated Nursing Care

- Falls are the leading cause of unintentional injury death in people aged 65 years and older (CDC, 2018). Because of Mrs. Cantonelli's age, history of falls, and impaired mobility, she continues to be at risk for falls. Her weakness and pain from her injuries also contribute to this risk. In addition, she is taking furosemide, a diuretic. This medication contributes to an increased risk for falling and subsequent injury (Kapas, 2021). Implement fall-prevention interventions (refer to Chapter 4).

- Before ambulating Mrs. Cantonelli, implement several assessments and precautions to prevent orthostatic hypotension. Assess for orthostatic hypotension (refer to Chapter 2). Have her sit on the side of the bed for a few minutes and make sure she does not feel dizzy, weak, or lightheaded (refer to Chapter 9). Because she has a history of cardiomyopathy, assess for shortness of breath and chest pain. If she cannot tolerate sitting up on the side of the bed without having these symptoms, then she will not tolerate standing up or ambulating. Assess her pain level immediately before ambulation (Chapter 10). If you have to medicate her for pain, then wait until the pain medicine has had time to take effect before ambulating. Because she is weaker on her left side, assess strength on her right side to ensure she will be able to support her weight with the cane (refer to Chapter 9). If she has difficulty

maintaining her balance, apply a safety belt (gait belt) before she begins to ambulate with the cane (some institutions require the use of a safety belt).

- While Mrs. Cantonelli is ambulating with her cane, observe her closely. Assess her technique with the cane. Observe for symptoms such as dizziness, chest pain, and shortness of breath. As she continues ambulating, evaluate how she tolerates this activity (Chapter 9). Before she is discharged from the hospital, assess her self-confidence as well as her overall ability to use the cane.

- If Mrs. Cantonelli begins to fall, it is important to protect her while also protecting yourself. If you feel her start to fall, maintain a wide base of support, grasp the safety/gait belt firmly and slowly guide her down toward the floor, supporting her on your thigh and large quadriceps muscle and protecting her head (Wintersgill, 2019) (refer to Chapter 9). Assess her orientation and stay with her while waiting for help from another health care provider. Take her vital signs to determine if there is a change from baseline. Thoroughly explore other factors that may have contributed to her fall, and plan interventions that will prevent future falls. If Mrs. Cantonelli continues to have problems with falling or difficulty using the cane, consider having her use a walker.

Case Study

Tiffany Jones

Tiffany Jones, age 17, is scheduled to undergo an ovarian cyst biopsy under local anesthesia. She has been NPO since midnight. Her ID bracelet is on and her consent form is signed. Her mother is in the waiting room. You are to provide Tiffany's immediate preoperative care. You place an IV in her left hand without difficulty. The next procedure is to insert an indwelling urinary (Foley) catheter. You set up the sterile field between her legs. As you clean the urinary meatus, Tiffany keeps drawing her legs closer together. When you remind her, she opens her legs and says, "Sorry, I didn't mean to move." As you insert the catheter into the urethra, Tiffany is startled and slams her knees together. When she opens her knees, the catheter appears to be inserted, but no urine is flowing.

Prescribed Interventions

Intravenous fluids: D5 ½ NSS at 50 mL/hr

Foley catheter to straight drainage

Developing Clinical Reasoning and Clinical Judgment

- Where might the urinary catheter be positioned, and should you advance the catheter further?

- Identify issues of concern to patients before surgery.

- How do you determine whether the catheter and the sterile field are still sterile?

- Describe methods of responding to Tiffany's nervousness.

- How could you have set up a more stable sterile field?

continued

Tiffany Jones (continued)

Suggested Responses for Integrated Nursing Care

- The female urethra is short, only about 1.6 inches (4 cm) long (Norris, 2020). If the catheter is advanced that far and no urine is flowing, the catheter may be in the vagina. Do not remove the catheter; it will serve as a guide to locate the urethral opening, which is just above the vagina (refer to Chapter 12). You would not advance the catheter further even if it were in the urethra, because when Tiffany closed her legs, the catheter probably came into contact with her skin and is no longer sterile. Advancing a nonsterile catheter into the urethra would increase her risk for developing a urinary tract infection. Because you are not certain whether her legs touched the sterile field, the sterile field is also no longer considered sterile (refer to Chapters 1 and 12).

- You will need to obtain another complete catheter insertion kit. Cover Tiffany and verify that she understands your plans. As you set up the new kit, place it on the bedside table, not between her legs, to prevent accidental contamination (refer to Chapter 12).

- Teenagers are generally uncomfortable with urinary catheterization because in this procedure, the nurse must look at and touch a very private area. Such an invasion of privacy is traumatic at an age when girls are easily embarrassed. Teenage girls may have "nervous legs": As you touch their inner thighs or labia, the knees slam shut almost involuntarily. Have a second nurse, caregiver, or a relative attend to the teenager. The nurse or relative can distract and soothe the teen, minimizing the unpleasantness of the experience, and can also keep a "reminder" hand on Tiffany's open knee to help you maintain sterility.

- As with most preoperative patients, Tiffany has several reasons to feel nervous. She is facing surgery, an unknown and anxiety-producing experience. The preoperative procedures, such as IV insertion and urinary catheterization, are unpleasant and uncomfortable. You can implement several strategies to reduce preoperative patients' anxiety. Have a familiar person stay with the patient. Tell the patient your name. Clearly explain procedures and provide instructions to the patient before you begin. Instructions should include the rationale and the length of time the procedure will take. For urinary catheterization, the patient may also want to know how long they will have the catheter in place. Emphasize to the patient that it is all right to ask questions. Describe how the procedure will feel to the patient—for example, "when I clean you, it will feel cold and wet." Keep your voice calm and very matter-of-fact throughout the procedure (refer to Chapters 6 and 12).

Case Study

James White

James White, a patient with an exacerbation of chronic obstructive pulmonary disease (COPD), is on your medical-surgical unit. You need to obtain his vital signs and give him a bath. His vital signs at 0800 were as follows: temperature, 98.4°F; pulse, 86 beats/min and regular; respirations, 18 breaths/min; blood pressure, 130/68 mm Hg. The physical therapist who is working with this patient on conditioning therapy has just brought him back from his exercises. You notice that his breathing is labored, with audible expiratory wheezes. While you are obtaining his oral temperature and vital signs, you continue to hear audible expiratory wheezing. His vital signs now are as follows: temperature, 96.8°F; pulse, 106 beats/min and irregular; respirations, 26 breaths/min; blood pressure, 140/74 mm Hg.

Prescribed Interventions

Daily physical therapy for conditioning

Oxygen at 2 L via nasal prongs prn for pulse oximetry <90%

Vital signs q4h

Oxygen saturation levels via pulse oximeter every shift and prn

continued

Developing Clinical Reasoning and Clinical Judgment

- Did you take the second set of vital signs at the most appropriate time? Why or why not?

- How has Mr. White's physical activity affected the accuracy of his vital signs?

- Describe the timing and type of bath you think Mr. White requires and the degree of assistance he will need. Explain your rationale.

- What would be your course of action in response to his labored breathing?

Suggested Responses for Integrated Nursing Care

- Always compare vital signs with the baseline before making further clinical decisions (refer to Chapter 2). As you compare the previous vital signs with the ones you just obtained, you notice that Mr. White's pulse rate, respiratory rate, and blood pressure are elevated. Your assessment of his pulse also indicates that his pulse is now irregular. Mr. White has just experienced a significant increase in activity; waiting until he has recovered from the exertion would be more appropriate in order to obtain a resting set of vital signs.

- What does the very low temperature indicate? Remember, you continued to hear Mr. White's heavy breathing while obtaining the remainder of the vital signs. Mr. White could not keep his lips pursed in a seal around the thermometer, and this often gives an inaccurate temperature (refer to Chapter 2). Mouth breathing and respiratory distress are contraindications for obtaining an oral temperature. As a nurse, you are responsible for determining the most appropriate site to obtain the temperature (refer to Chapter 2).

- Does Mr. White's elevated respiratory rate and noisy breathing indicate respiratory distress or a need for

oxygen? Obtain an oxygen saturation level via pulse oximetry (refer to Chapter 14). If the oxygen saturation level is satisfactory for Mr. White, then you can be confident that his body is compensating for the increased oxygen demand. Allow him to rest, with the head of his bed elevated, and retake his vital signs in 15 to 30 minutes. Take vital signs as often as the patient's condition warrants. If Mr. White's oxygen saturation and vital signs continue to deviate from baseline after a rest period, obtain additional information through a more focused respiratory assessment and notify the health care provider (refer to Chapters 2, 3, and 14).

- A bath represents another increase in activity. Mr. White needs time to recover from the physical therapy exercises before attempting the bath. He should be able to sit in a chair and, in fact, will breathe more comfortably sitting up than lying down. Having him lie flat could make him decompensate (deterioration in respiratory function), so you should not perform occupied bed-making (refer to Chapter 7). If encouraged to sit up, he will probably be able to complete much of his bath by himself.

UNIT III Integrated Case Studies

Case Study

Naomi Bell

Naomi Bell, age 90, was admitted to the hospital yesterday after experiencing chest pain. She wears a hearing aid in her left ear. In the report you were told that she is "confused" and "doesn't answer questions appropriately." Her vital signs overnight were as follows: temperature, 98.0°F; pulse, 62 beats/min; respirations, 18 breaths/min; blood pressure, 132/86 mm Hg. She is due for her morning medications. As you give Mrs. Bell her medications and state their purpose, she points to the digoxin and says, "Honey, I don't take that pill."

Prescribed Interventions

Digoxin 0.125 mg PO every morning
Enteric-coated aspirin 81 mg PO every day
Furosemide 20 mg PO every morning

Famotidine 20 mg PO BID
Potassium chloride 10 mEq PO every morning
Captopril 50 mg PO TID

Developing Clinical Reasoning and Clinical Judgment

• How would you respond to Mrs. Bell's statement, "Honey, I don't take that pill"?

• Describe factors that can contribute to inappropriate answers, and identify nursing actions to diminish these factors.

• Suggest ways in which you can confirm that you are giving Mrs. Bell the correct medications.

• How would you determine Mrs. Bell's level of confusion, if any?

• Identify the medications that require assessment before administration.

Suggested Responses for Integrated Nursing Care

- When patients question you regarding their medications, listen to them. Questions like this should send a "red flag" to the nurse. Often, patients are familiar with what they normally take and can alert you that this may not be the right medication. Do not insist that Mrs. Bell take the digoxin until you confirm the accuracy of the prescribed intervention. In this case, it could be that Mrs. Bell just did not hear what you said. Always confirm what patients say to you by restating it back to them. It could also be that she is more familiar with the trade name for this drug or the medication may look different from the medication she uses at home.

- You should use multiple safety checks to give medications safely (refer to Chapter 5). Some measures include researching the drug before administration and double-checking all of the "rights." Compare the electronic medication administration record with the original prescribed intervention in the health record. If the prescribed intervention still remains unclear to you, call the prescriber to clarify it (refer to Chapter 5).

- Some medications require assessment before you administer them to the patient. In this case, Mrs. Bell takes four medications that will require assessment before administration. Digoxin, furosemide, and captopril will affect pulse and blood pressure and these vital signs should be assessed prior to administration (refer to Chapter 2). In addition, laboratory test results should be available on potassium and digoxin levels. If Mrs. Bell has a low pulse rate, low blood pressure, or a toxic laboratory value, you will not administer these medications and will notify the health care provider (refer to Chapter 5).

- Sometimes, older patients become confused in unfamiliar settings—in this case—the hospital. However, do not assume this is always the case. The nurse who gave you the report may have assumed that Mrs. Bell's inappropriate answers were due to confusion, when in fact they may be related to Mrs. Bell's hearing problem. When patients with a hearing impairment are in an unfamiliar setting, such as a hospital admission, encourage them to wear their hearing aids and help them check their batteries to ensure they are working. If you are still unclear whether Mrs. Bell is confused, perform a standard mental status examination used by your institution (refer to Chapter 3). This will establish a baseline assessment of her mental status that you can use to individualize her nursing care plan.

- If you determine Mrs. Bell is confused, assess the source of confusion. Given Mrs. Bell's cardiac condition, assess her respiratory status and oxygen saturation level via pulse oximetry to determine whether she is experiencing hypoxia or ischemia (refer to Chapters 2, 3, and 14). If the cause is physiologic, notify the health care team immediately. Another source contributing to confusion could be isolation caused by hearing loss. One way to reduce possible confusion for Mrs. Bell is to improve communication. Ensure that her hearing aid battery is operating and that the unit is placed correctly. Other ways to improve communication include talking to her at eye level, facing her directly when speaking, or even speaking into her unaffected ear. If Mrs. Bell's vision is better than her hearing, you can also give her pertinent information in writing.

Case Study

John Willis

You are a nursing student in your first semester of nursing school. Your assigned patient has been discharged before your arrival. Your instructor provides you with the name of another patient to care for, based on the recommendation of the staff. Before you can review the information about the patient with your instructor, she is called to consult with another student and a physician about an emergent patient situation. You read the clinical pathway for John Willis and find that he has methicillin-resistant *Staphylococcus aureus* (MRSA) in his sputum and suspected pulmonary tuberculosis (TB). You remember reviewing these topics in class and in the learning resource center. Because your instructor is still occupied with the patient emergency,

continued

you decide to begin caring for your new patient, instead of wasting time waiting to review the information with her. When you go to your patient's room, you see the isolation cart containing the transmission-based precaution supplies outside the room, with the hospital's policy and procedure posted for precautions to use for TB and MRSA. You see there are individual masks in plastic bags with different people's names on them, as well as masks with protective eye shields. You recall something from class about wearing a specially fitted mask when implementing these precautions, but realize you do not remember as much as you thought you did. You are unsure of exactly what you need to do. You find the staff nurse assigned to the patient in another patient's room, interrupt his conversation, and say, "I don't have a mask to care for my patient." The nurse sharply responds, "Just go get started. I'm in the middle of something." You consider just going in and introducing yourself and checking on the patient's status. Should you "borrow" a mask from one of the bags? You think it is your duty to care for this patient, but think you may need more information to be safe.

Prescribed Interventions

Airborne precautions
Contact precautions

Sputum specimen for culture and sensitivity and acid-fast bacillus (AFB)
Vital signs every shift

Developing Clinical Reasoning and Clinical Judgment

- Compare the mode of transmission for TB and MRSA.

- Describe another way in which you could have approached this situation.

- What may have led to the nurse's abrupt and sharp response?

- What are the potential consequences of a lack of use of appropriate transmission-based precautions?

- Identify the appropriate protective equipment needed to care for a patient with TB and a patient with MRSA.

continued

Suggested Responses for Integrated Nursing Care

- Pulmonary TB transmission occurs through the air from one person to another. MRSA transmission can occur through direct contact with contaminated blood or body fluids. MRSA can be spread by direct or indirect contact. In this case, MRSA could be transmitted indirectly by coming into contact with items used to care for the patient, such as blood pressure cuffs or linen, or contact with contaminated surfaces in the room.

- Facilities require the use of appropriate personal protective equipment (PPE), including gowns, gloves, and masks, when caring for patients with TB and MRSA. Unique to the Airborne Precautions needed for TB is the use of specially fitted masks, either a high-efficiency particulate air (HEPA) filter respirator or N95 respirator mask certified by NIOSH to prevent the inspiration of airborne microorganisms (refer to Chapter 1). N95 respirators require fit-testing to ensure the mask is on correctly and adjusted to fit properly. If a fit-tested mask is required by your facility, you would either need to be fit-tested for a mask (often done by Employee Health) or reassigned to another patient. In addition, to protect yourself whenever there is the potential for contamination to your eyes, such as coughing, you should wear goggles or a mask with a face shield. Institutions vary greatly in their supplies. If you do not take the appropriate transmission-based precautions, you put yourself at risk for exposure to disease; in this case, TB and MRSA. In addition, entering other patients' rooms results in the potential for transmission of microorganisms and infection (refer to Chapter 1). It is always your responsibility, even as a student, to follow the policies and procedures of the facility where you are placed for clinical experiences.

- Hospitals are stressful places. Understanding when and how to communicate with others is an invaluable set of skills. Waiting for the nurse to complete a conversation and task before asking for guidance would have been the ideal situation. Nurses have to prioritize the care they provide. Asking, "Do you have a moment to review something with me?" is a good way to ensure getting the time and attention you need. Because there was no emergency to obtain the vital signs and sputum specimen, they can wait until you are sure you can provide safe care.

- You were right to question the appropriateness of caring for this patient and in thinking you may need more information to be safe. In this situation, waiting to review the patient information with your instructor is the ideal solution. Your instructor did not have all the information about the patient before being called away to an emergency. She would not have assigned this patient to you after reviewing his diagnosis, realizing that you would need a specially fitted mask to care for the patient. While waiting for your instructor, you should obtain as much information as possible. Background research and knowledge are powerful tools. Examples of resources you can access include the hospital policies and procedure files, the infection control manual, the infection control nurse, and experienced staff members, provided they are able to take time out from their patient care responsibilities. Then, when your instructor is available, you can share this information with them to plan your care for that day.

Case Study

Claudia Tran

Claudia Tran, age 84, has been on your skilled nursing unit following a cerebral vascular accident (CVA). Her neurologic checks and vital signs are unchanged from her baseline admission. Her CVA has impaired her ability to chew and swallow and she is receiving weekly vitamin B_{12} injections for pernicious anemia. She has left-sided weakness, with flaccidity of her left hand. Ms. Tran is emaciated and her skin is very fragile. She has reddened areas on her coccyx, heels, left hip, and elbows. Over the past week, Ms. Tran has become increasingly confused and incontinent. She has a gastric tube for feedings, which she receives every 8 hours. Ms. Tran constantly

continued

Claudia Tran (continued)

pulls at her feeding tube and has had to have it reinserted today after pulling it out. Because of this, a soft wrist restraint has been prescribed for the next 4 hours.

Prescribed Interventions

Soft wrist restraint for safety for the next 4 hours (end at 1330), then reevaluate

Vitamin B_{12} injection 1,000 mcg IM weekly

Gastric tube feedings—FiberSOURCE HN 320 mL q8h

Physical therapy daily, passive and active range of motion (ROM) as tolerated

Developing Clinical Reasoning and Clinical Judgment

- Considering Ms. Tran's condition, what special safety measures should be implemented related to the use of the wrist restraint?

- What are the risks of falling for this patient?

- Identify the risks associated with gastric tube feeding for this patient.

- Identify risk factors and preventive measures to maintain the integrity of Ms. Tran's skin.

- Identify appropriate sites and administration considerations related to the vitamin B_{12} injections prescribed for Ms. Tran.

Suggested Responses for Integrated Nursing Care

- Restraints are used only as a last resort after all other measures have failed. Implement alternatives to the use of restraints (refer to Chapter 4). Other measures could include placing her bed in a low position, having a family member sit with her, and placing her in a room near the nurses' station. Only use restraints as prescribed by the health care provider, and follow facility guidelines to protect the patient. Because Ms. Tran already has alterations in the integrity of her skin, pad the restraints and make sure they are the correct size. An additional safety measure would be performing frequent neurovascular checks to the extremity, including checking warmth, sensation, and capillary refill. Restraints are released at specified

frequencies. This will improve the circulation to her extremities, reduce the chance of skin breakdown, and give you an opportunity to assess the site. Ms. Tran has left-sided weakness; therefore, applying a restraint on her flaccid arm could cause harm and is not needed (refer to Chapter 4).

- Ms. Tran has many factors that increase her risk for alterations in skin integrity, including decreased mobility, malnutrition, altered mental status, advanced age, incontinence, and positioning for tube feedings. A multifaceted approach is necessary to reduce her risk and prevent further alterations in her skin integrity (refer to Chapter 8). It is essential to develop a schedule for repositioning (refer to Chapter 9). Ms. Tran could

continued

benefit from a special type of mattress, such as one with a pressure-reducing surface. Implementing a physical therapy program of active and passive ROM exercises would be helpful. Arrange for a nutritional consult to ensure that she will receive adequate protein, as well as other vitamins and minerals essential to maintain skin integrity.

- What complications could result from the combination of decreased mobility and incontinence? A noninvasive way to reduce the chance of recurrent incontinence is to offer Ms. Tran a bedpan at regular intervals. Frequent skin care and use of a skin protectant/barrier to prevent damage from excessive moisture is an important part of her nursing care (refer to Chapter 7).
- Because Ms. Tran is older, confused, and in a restraint, her risk for falling is high. Keep her bed in a low position at all times and make sure her call light is within reach. Frequently check on patients such as Ms. Tran to decrease isolation, provide reorientation, and assess for patient needs (refer to Chapter 4).
- Ms. Tran is receiving tube feedings to meet her nutritional needs. Monitoring patient tolerance of enteral nutrition (EN) is part of the nursing care for patients receiving this nutritional intervention. Nursing actions that contribute to successful enteral tube feedings focus on monitoring patient tolerance of EN, patient safety, and monitoring for complications. Patient tolerance of the volume and type of formula must be monitored daily (Boullata et al., 2017; McClave, Taylor et al., 2018). Criteria to consider when evaluating patient feeding tolerance include the absence of nausea, vomiting, diarrhea and constipation, abdominal pain and feelings of fullness, and distention. In addition, the patient should have bowel sounds present within normal limits and achieve the target goal for administration of the EN. Ms. Tran is at increased risk for reflux, aspiration, and pneumonia. Make sure the patient is as upright as possible during feeding. Keep the head of the bed elevated at 30 to 45 degrees at all times during administration of enteral feedings and for 1 hour afterward to prevent these complications, unless contraindicated (McClave, Taylor et al., 2016; Roveron et al., 2018). Patients for whom semirecumbent position is contraindicated or who cannot tolerate a semi-Fowler position should be placed in reverse- or anti-Trendelenburg position (Boullata et al., 2017; Roveron et al., 2018) (refer to Chapter 11).
- When giving Ms. Tran vitamin B_{12} injections, use larger muscles and rotate sites. Implement the rotation schedule for this injection in her care plan. This is particularly important because Ms. Tran is emaciated and does not have good muscle mass. Avoid areas that are reddened or have palpable nodules and scars. Because vitamin B_{12} injections can be irritating, inject the medication using the Z-track method to minimize pain, trauma, and discomfort (refer to Chapter 5) (Taylor et al., 2023).

Case Study

Joe LeRoy

Joe LeRoy, age 60, was brought in by his daughter and admitted to your small rural hospital. He has had the stomach flu at home for several days and is suffering from dehydration. He has right-sided hemiplegia due to a cerebral vascular accident (CVA) 3 years ago. Mr. LeRoy has remained in bed during his hospital stay due to extreme weakness and fatigue.

You received the report from the previous nurses related to your five patients. From the report, you note that Mr. LeRoy continues to have frequent liquid stools (averaging about three or four times per shift). The doctor has requested a stool sample for culture and sensitivity. When entering your patient's room, you notice his sheets are very dirty and he has a strong body odor.

Prescribed Interventions

Intravenous fluids: D5 ½ NSS at 125 mL/hr

Stool sample for culture and sensitivity

Vital signs every shift

continued

Joe LeRoy (continued)

Developing Clinical Reasoning and Clinical Judgment

- Develop your priorities and rationales for the following nursing care for Mr. LeRoy:
  - Considerations when collecting the stool sample
  - Changing his sheets
  - Completing the initial nursing assessment

- Are there any assessments that you would want to pay particular attention to during your nursing care?
  - Obtaining vital signs
  - Collecting the sample
  - Giving a bath

- Describe how your attitude and nonverbal behavior could affect Mr. LeRoy's hospital experience.

Suggested Responses for Integrated Nursing Care

- Prioritizing care is sometimes a difficult, but important skill for all nurses. Determine whether Mr. LeRoy can provide his own personal care, although this is unlikely due to his hemiplegia and weakness. If you need to assist him with his personal care, determine the needs of your other patients before beginning this care (refer to Chapter 7). Before leaving Mr. LeRoy, let him know your plan and the time he can expect to have assistance with his bath. Another alternative is to delegate the bath and changing of bed linens to assistive personnel (AP) (refer to Chapter 7). During your initial assessment of Mr. LeRoy, cover any very obviously dirty areas of his sheets with a blue waterproof pad or a clean sheet. You could also offer him a wet, warm washcloth and a dry towel for initial cleaning while you are completing the nursing assessment. You should also inform Mr. LeRoy of the need for a stool specimen (refer to Chapter 18).

- If an AP is not available, return to his room after completing your other patient assessments. First, obtain the warm stool sample, give the bath, and then change his linens (refer to Chapter 7). This sequence saves time and energy for both the nurse and the patient, because the linens may become soiled when providing a bed bath or assisting a patient on a bedpan.

- While wearing gloves, collect and send the stool specimen promptly to the laboratory. Specimens should be sent while still warm, because the microorganisms present at body temperature may die when

the specimen temperature changes, and this would produce a false-negative result (refer to Chapter 18).

- Measurement of Mr. LeRoy's vital signs will provide insight into his fluid and electrolyte status, which may be altered related to complications from the flu, including dehydration and diarrhea. Mr. LeRoy's age and underlying chronic health condition impacts his ability to maintain homeostasis. Measurement of vital signs should be implemented based on the nurse's judgment of this patient's situation (refer to Chapter 2). During your assessment, pay particular attention to Mr. LeRoy's skin. Mr. LeRoy is at risk for alterations in skin integrity and pressure injury due to his age, diarrhea, altered nutrition, and immobility (refer to Chapters 3 and 8). Assist Mr. LeRoy to turn over so that you can inspect his back and bony prominences, the most likely areas for alterations in skin integrity. Institute nursing interventions to prevent pressure injury. If you notice any skin breakdown, institute appropriate nursing interventions, based on facility policy, and notify the health care team (refer to Chapters 7 and 8).

- A nurse's nonverbal behavior can have a dramatic impact on a patient's health care experience. Projecting a positive attitude and providing nonjudgmental care help a patient cope with hospitalization. You may be offended by Mr. LeRoy's body odor and the smell of his stool, but as a nurse, you need to learn strategies to manage strong odors and make sure that your facial expressions or body language do not convey discomfort or disgust.

continued

Case Study

Kate Townsend

Kate Townsend, a 70-year-old patient with chronic obstructive pulmonary disease (COPD), has just returned to your medical-surgical unit from surgery for repair of a bowel obstruction and lysis of intestinal adhesions. She has a midline abdominal transverse incision secured with sutures and covered with a dry sterile dressing. She has a right peripheral IV with D5 ½ NSS at 75 mL/hr. She has a history of long-term steroid use for her COPD. She has a nasogastric (NG) tube in her right naris, which is clamped at this time. The health care provider prescribes oxygen 2 L/min via nasal cannula. The patient's primary nurse asks you to place the patient on oxygen. When you attempt to place the cannula in the patient's naris with the NG tube, you think it is uncomfortable and a little odd. For comfort, you consider placing a simple oxygen mask on Mrs. Townsend instead. Her vital signs are as follows: temperature, 99.6°F; pulse, 76 beats/min; respirations, 24 breaths/min; blood pressure, 110/70 mm Hg; oxygen saturation (O$_2$ 2 L/min), 92%.

Prescribed Interventions

NG tube to low intermittent suction

Cough and deep breathe/incentive spirometry every hour while awake

Morphine sulfate 1 to 2 mg IV q4h prn pain

Oxygen 2 L/min via nasal cannula

Intravenous fluid: D5 ½ NSS at 75 mL/hr

Developing Clinical Reasoning and Clinical Judgment

- What is the difference between oxygen given by nasal cannula and that given via a simple oxygen mask?

- What comfort measures would you want to provide for Mrs. Townsend?

- What do you need to consider in changing to a simple oxygen mask for delivery of the oxygen?

- Develop a discharge plan for Mrs. Townsend.

- Considering Mrs. Townsend's chronic lung disease, what complications can occur postoperatively, and what nursing interventions could decrease these complications?

continued

Suggested Responses for Integrated Nursing Care

- Several delivery systems exist to provide oxygen to patients, and they deliver varying amounts of oxygen. Oxygen delivered via a nasal cannula set at 2 L/min would deliver about 28% oxygen, whereas oxygen delivered in a simple mask could deliver 40% to 60% oxygen, depending on the flow meter setting (refer to Chapter 14). Oxygen is considered a medicine, so it is not an independent nursing intervention outside of emergency circumstances but a prescribed intervention. The oxygen concentration and delivery system are adjusted according to a prescribed intervention or parameters from a physician or other advanced practice professional.

- When changing Mrs. Townsend for comfort reasons from the nasal cannula to the mask, you could increase the delivery of oxygen anywhere from 12% to 32%; a change in delivery method may have significant implications. Although it is not entirely comfortable to have an NG tube, much less another tube in the naris, it is not unusual for this to occur. Both will fit with some manipulation by the nurse. Oxygen is considered a medicine, so it is not an independent nursing intervention outside of emergency circumstances but a prescribed intervention. The oxygen concentration and delivery system are adjusted according to a prescribed intervention or parameters from a physician or other advanced practice professional.

- Patients with chronic lung disease are at increased risk after surgery for pulmonary complications, including atelectasis and pneumonia. General anesthesia alters all of the muscles involved in breathing and clearing the airway. COPD is a restrictive lung disease, meaning that the patient's lungs lose their elasticity and become less compliant. For Mrs. Townsend, this combination of underlying disease and the effects of surgery results in a decreased ability to mobilize secretions, which could lead to atelectasis and possibly pneumonia. Mrs. Townsend may be experiencing atelectasis, indicated by her temperature of 99.6°F. Other signs of atelectasis would be decreased breath sounds and/or crackles in the lung bases, shortness of breath, increased respiratory rate, and decreased oxygen saturation of pulse oximetry (refer to Chapters 3, 6, and 14). Without nursing intervention, atelectasis could lead to pneumonia. Measures to facilitate lung expansion and mobilization of secretions will minimize atelectasis. These nursing measures include elevation of the head of her bed, deep-breathing and coughing exercises, adequate pain control, and early ambulation (refer to Chapters 6, 10, and 14).

- Long-term steroid use can make the skin very fragile, increase the potential for alterations in skin integrity, and delay wound healing. To prevent this, observe the skin under her NG tube and oxygen cannula tubing. The pressure of the tubes on her face and behind her ears could cause a break in skin integrity. Secure the nasogastric tube with a commercial securement device (Schroeder & Sitzer, 2019). You may need to protect the skin under the cannula tubing with a hydrocolloid dressing (refer to Chapter 8), especially if the skin becomes reddened. There are many commercial products to hold oxygen nasal cannulas which may also increase her comfort.

- Discharge plans for Mrs. Townsend would need to address both her underlying lung disease as well as her recent intestinal surgery. Patient education should focus on measures that enable Mrs. Townsend to improve her lung compliance and increase her oxygenation. Deep breathing, coughing, and a daily activity schedule are imperative (refer to Chapter 6). Due to her prolonged use of steroids, she may also experience delayed wound healing at her incision site. Patient education should address optimal nutrition and prevention of infection. Before discharge, validate Mrs. Townsend's knowledge of measures to prevent pulmonary and wound complications.

Case Study

Tula Stillwater

Tula Stillwater is 36 years old and has had diabetes since age 26. Ms. Stillwater weighs 218 lb, is gravida 1 para 1, and delivered a 9 lb, 8 oz boy via cesarean section 3 days ago, resulting in a transverse abdominal incision with staples. She reports tenderness on the right side of the incision, but acute pain on the left side of the incision. Her 0800 vital signs are as follows: temperature, 101.6°F; pulse, 76 beats/min; respirations, 18 breaths/min; blood pressure, 134/78 mm Hg. Her blood glucose before breakfast is 185 mg/dL; her blood glucose on previous days had ranged from 90 to 124 mg/dL.

On initial assessment, you note the dressing is intact on her incision. The staples are intact in the incision; the incision is well approximated and without erythema on the right side. However, the left side of the incision is pulling apart and is edematous and warm to the touch, with a scant amount of purulent drainage.

Prescribed Interventions

Vital signs q4h

Fingerstick blood glucose before meals and at bedtime

Regular insulin per sliding scale

Prescribed interventions:
- Remove staples before discharge.
- Discharge on third day, if stable.

Developing Clinical Reasoning and Clinical Judgment

- What is your interpretation of her vital signs? Who should be notified and when?

- How would you determine whether Ms. Stillwater meets the criteria for discharge?

- What is the relationship between Ms. Stillwater's diabetes and her postsurgical condition?

- What factors affect her staple removal?

- How should you respond to her fingerstick blood glucose level?

- What nursing interventions do you foresee performing?

- Describe the timing and the technique for administering her insulin.

continued

Suggested Responses for Integrated Nursing Care

- Ms. Stillwater's vital signs and other symptoms should alert you to a potential complication. She may have an infection related to her incision, as evidenced by her increased temperature and her subjective report of acute pain at the incision. Her blood pressure could be a result of her pain, but you should compare it with her baseline and continue to monitor it. You assessed the incision carefully for signs of infection (refer to Chapter 8). Notify her health care team immediately of this potential complication.

- Wound healing may be impaired in people with diabetes, so any patient with diabetes requires vigilant wound assessment. In addition, the stress of surgery usually results in increased blood glucose levels. Ms. Stillwater's fingerstick blood sugar is elevated from her baseline, another symptom of a possible infection. When you see a dramatic increase in blood glucose in a patient with diabetes, consider the possible causes.

- Despite the urgency of this new complication of wound infection, Ms. Stillwater should receive her insulin and breakfast as she usually would. Administer her insulin in a subcutaneous site; she can help you identify the site where she should receive her insulin. Patients who are accustomed to managing their diabetes at home will have preferences when in the hospital, and you should honor these preferences when possible (refer to Chapter 5).

- Many patients who have had cesarean sections are discharged on the third day. One of the expected outcomes for discharge would include being free of infection. Ms. Stillwater is not free of infection; she has pain at her incision site, a fever, incision assessment findings indicating alterations in healing, and an elevated fingerstick blood sugar. When you notify the health care team of these symptoms, a complete blood count (Chapter 18), a wound culture (Chapter 8), incision site care (Chapter 8), and cancellation of the discharge are prescribed.

- Given the delayed discharge and impaired wound healing, you would not want to remove the staples from this incision because removing the staples at this time could place Ms. Stillwater at risk for dehiscence (Chapter 8). Another factor affecting the risk for dehiscence and impaired wound healing is Ms. Stillwater's increased subcutaneous fat.

- Did you foresee obtaining a complete blood count and a wound culture and performing incision site care? Did you also anticipate that this patient should not be discharged nor have her staples removed? In addition, although her physiologic care is very important, you will also need to relieve anxiety related to this infection and acknowledge her disappointment and potential concerns regarding the care of her son, since she cannot go home today.

PART 2

Intermediate Case Studies

Nursing Concepts

- Advocacy
- Assessment
- Clinical Decision Making/Clinical Judgment
- Collaboration/Teamwork and Collaboration
- Comfort
- Communication
- Elimination
- Fluids and Electrolytes
- Functional Ability
- Infection
- Mobility
- Nutrition
- Oxygenation/Gas Exchange
- Perfusion
- Safety
- Teaching and Learning/Patient Education
- Thermoregulation
- Tissue Integrity

Case Study

Olivia Greenbaum

Olivia Greenbaum is a 9-month-old infant admitted to the hospital with respiratory syncytial virus (RSV). She was born prematurely at 30 weeks' gestation. Her complications at birth included respiratory distress syndrome (RDS), suspected sepsis, and formula intolerance. She was discharged home after 8 weeks on soy-based formula. This is her first hospitalization since her birth. Olivia is Mr. and Mrs. Greenbaum's only child, and they are very anxious. Mrs. Greenbaum is her primary caregiver.

Olivia is receiving supplemental humidified oxygen administered via oxygen tent at 40%. She is very fussy and is not tolerating separation

continued

from her mother well. She has a peripheral IV inserted in her right hand with D5 ¼ NSS with 10 mEq of potassium chloride infusing at 20 mL/hr. It is covered with a sock puppet. She is wearing a T-shirt and a disposable diaper. She is quite active within the crib. Her previous vital signs were as follows: temperature, 36.4°C (97.5°F); pulse, 84 beats/min; respirations, 38 breaths/min; blood pressure, 94/58 mm Hg.

Mrs. Greenbaum spent the night and is currently sleeping in the recliner in Olivia's room. You enter the room and observe Olivia sleeping. She is pale with circumoral cyanosis. Her respiratory rate is 40 breaths/min with an audible expiratory wheeze. Her heart rate on the monitor is 86 beats/min; her pulse rate on the pulse oximeter is 62 beats/min. The pulse oximeter is currently showing an oxygen saturation level of 68%.

Prescribed Interventions

Vital signs q4h

Encourage coughing

Oxygen via tent at 40%

Continuous pulse oximetry when quiet; may obtain every hour intermittent pulse oximeter readings when active

Maintain O_2 saturation 93% to 97%. Adjust O_2 in increments of 2% up to a max of 50%

Isomil 6 to 8 oz every 4 hours when awake

Intravenous fluids: D5 ¼ NSS with 10 mEq potassium chloride at 20 mL/hr

Heart rate/resp. monitor

Developing Clinical Reasoning and Clinical Judgment

- What is your first priority after observing Olivia sleeping?

- Identify factors that affect the accuracy of the oxygen saturation reading.

- Should you increase the oxygen being administered?

- How frequently should Olivia's IV site be assessed? What is the function of the sock puppet?

- What is your interpretation of her vital signs and oxygen saturation?

- How do you encourage coughing in a 9-month-old infant?

- Give examples of how to manage thermoregulation within an oxygen tent.

continued

Suggested Responses for Integrated Nursing Care

- Your first priority is to establish whether Olivia is hypoxic. You noted a rapid respiratory rate and circumoral cyanosis, both potential symptoms of hypoxia. The pulse oximeter heart rate does not match the cardiac monitor heart rate. Gently, without disturbing Olivia, you remove and replace the pulse oximeter.

- Your preliminary assessment is that the pulse oximeter is not accurately assessing her oxygenation. You are able to hold the probe to her toe and get a reading of 95%. Olivia begins to wake up. Take her apical heart rate, which is the most reliable site for infants and small children (see Chapter 2). Compare her apical pulse rate with the heart rate on the pulse oximeter as well as the heart rate on the cardiac monitor. Nurses must always verify that the equipment is accurately reflecting the patient's status. Next, you take her temperature, which is 97.1°F (36.2°C). The humidified oxygen is also cooling Olivia, making her hands, feet, and lips appear cold, blue, and dusky (refer to Chapter 14).

- Once Olivia is awake, she will not tolerate having the pulse oximeter probe on her toe and will keep pulling it off. You will need to check the oxygen saturation intermittently, as well as a more focused respiratory assessment (refer to Chapters 2 and 3). Your next priority is to warm her up. When children become chilled, they have increased energy expenditure. When infants are stressed beyond aerobic metabolism, they use anaerobic metabolism. This produces lactic acid, which increases the acidity of the blood,

exacerbating respiratory distress. Urge her parents to bring in more clothes and to layer clothing to keep Olivia thermoregulated within the humidified tent. You do not need to increase the oxygen level; what at first looked like hypoxia is in fact hypothermia!

- The accuracy of a pulse oximetry reading is affected by several factors, including patient perfusion and peripheral vasoconstriction. Other factors that prevent the detection of oxygen saturation may be as simple as nail polish or artificial nails (see Chapter 14).

- Encouraging coughing in an infant is accomplished either through crying or laughing. Crying and laughing require deep breaths and will cause a patient to cough, thus promoting airway clearance. If the infant is periodically crying vigorously, that is sufficient. You can try tickling or playing peekaboo to get a 9 month old to laugh.

- Check this patient's IV site every hour to ensure there are no signs of infiltration (Chapter 16). The sock puppet is one way to disguise the IV site dressing while leaving it accessible for examination. If a young child can see the IV site dressing, they will often persist in trying to remove the tape and dressing despite all your efforts. If you cover the site, the child will not remember it is there. Piaget's theory of cognitive development includes the concept of object permanence. At 9 months old, a child cannot imagine what they cannot see—in other words, what is out of sight is out of mind. Other alternative to restraints may also be appropriate (refer to Chapter 4).

Case Study

Victoria Holly

Victoria Holly, age 68, is newly admitted to the hospital due to anemia and severe dehydration. They have been prescribed an IV of D5 ½ NSS infusing into the right hand to address the dehydration. Mrs. Holly has a second IV access in her left arm to be used for blood administration only. She recently received 2 units of packed red blood cells in response to the anemia. There are prescribed interventions to draw a complete blood count (CBC) and a complete metabolic profile (CMP). Mrs. Holly also has an ileostomy, which she has managed for several years on her own. Upon your initial nursing assessment of Mrs. Holly, you find her vital signs are as follows: temperature, 97.2°F; pulse, 96 beats/min; respirations, 18 breaths/min; blood pressure, 88/50 mm Hg. Her skin is "tenting" and you are having difficulty palpating her peripheral pulses. Her lips are dry and cracked. The skin around her stoma site is bright red and open in areas. You notice that her ostomy pouch was cut much larger than the stoma site. She reports she is very tired and "lacks energy." Her family informs you that she has always been a very independent person but in the last couple of months she just "hasn't been herself."

continued

Prescribed Interventions

Intravenous fluids: D5 ½ NSS IV at 125 mL/hr
Strict I&O

Daily weights
CBC and CMP stat

Developing Clinical Reasoning and Clinical Judgment

- Identify the equipment needed and appropriate sites to consider to obtain the blood samples.

- What is alarming about the assessment of her ileostomy? Identify possible explanations for the stoma's condition.

- Describe how you would assess Mrs. Holly's peripheral circulation.

- What are measurable physical parameters you can use to determine whether the fluid replacement therapy and blood administration have had a therapeutic effect?

- What concerns you about Mrs. Holly's present condition in relationship to performing her activities of daily living (ADLs) independently?

- Develop a discharge teaching plan for Mrs. Holly related to ostomy care.

Suggested Responses for Integrated Nursing Care

- You cannot obtain the specimen from above the IV in her right hand because the specimen will be diluted with the D5 ½ NSS solution and, thus, will be inaccurate. It is not considered best practice to draw laboratory specimens from an IV site unless absolutely necessary, according to facility policy. Also, you cannot draw blood specimens from a dedicated IV access such as the one Mrs. Holly has for blood administration. Collect Mrs. Holly's laboratory work from her left arm via venipuncture, avoiding the right arm due to the IV infusion (Chapter 18).

- When a patient has no peripheral pulses, you must investigate further (refer to Chapters 2 and 3). Never ignore the absence of pulses, as this could signal a life-threatening condition. Have another nurse check the pulses, or use a Doppler. Upon checking Mrs. Holly's pulses with a Doppler device, you were able to hear them and marked them with an "x" to facilitate future assessments. In your initial assessment, you

were not surprised that Mrs. Holly's pulses were non-palpable, as she has a very low circulating volume.

- Mrs. Holly's vital signs are disconcerting because her blood pressure is low. Because of her hypotension, ADLs may unduly tax her. Until you see a positive change in her vital signs, provide assistance with her ADLs (see Chapter 7). In addition, Mrs. Holly has an IV in each arm. It may be difficult for her to care for the ostomy and perform personal care when one or both of the access sites are used for infusions.

- Mrs. Holly's ileostomy site is very red and excoriated. You are alarmed, as this could place her at risk for infection. Do not assume that a health care provider has seen the excoriation around the ostomy site. If the patient came into the hospital with more pressing matters, such as decreased blood pressure, the health care provider may not have observed the ileostomy. Notify the health care team. Mrs. Holly may lack knowledge about the appropriate method for sizing

continued

and cutting her ostomy appliance. You suspect that she may be cutting the faceplate in such a way as to leave her skin exposed to the liquid stool, which is then causing the excoriation (see Chapter 13).

- One therapeutic outcome to anticipate with Mrs. Holly would be an increase in blood pressure. Other outcomes include palpable peripheral pulses and normal skin turgor. Subjectively, Mrs. Holly should report that her energy has increased. Her family may also comment that she is becoming more "like herself." Sometimes health care workers make judgments about older adults, thinking that they are always tired. Since health care workers are often unfamiliar with their patients' normal conditions, comments made by family members can often be very helpful in determining progress. This is especially true if your patient cannot communicate. Objectively, one outcome would be that Mrs. Holly becomes more active in her own care.

- One area you should investigate is Mrs. Holly's ability to care for the ostomy before she came to the hospital. It is possible that her skin around the stoma site has looked like this for some time. Before her hospital discharge, evaluate her knowledge through return demonstration to ensure that she can care for the stoma and can identify possible family resources. She may benefit from a home health referral to ensure she is caring for her stoma properly.

Case Study

Tula Stillwater

It is now day 5 in the hospital for Ms. Stillwater (refer to related Case Study in the Basic Case Studies section on p. 1207). Ms. Stillwater has developed a staphylococcal infection in her cesarean section incision. This is the second time you have cared for this patient. You are familiar with her diabetic status, baseline vital signs, and routine postpartum care. She is currently receiving an IV antibiotic. Her vital signs are as follows: temperature, 99.2°F; pulse, 74 beats/min; respirations, 18 breaths/min; blood pressure, 130/80 mm Hg. Her fingerstick blood glucose before breakfast is 120 mg/dL.

You learned in the report that her incision is intact and healing on the right side, but the far left side of her incision is being treated with a calcium alginate wound dressing. The open part of the incision is approximately 1 inch long, 0.5 inch wide, and 1 inch deep. This part of her incision is draining copious amounts of foul-smelling, yellow-to-green purulent drainage. The incision is very painful. Ms. Stillwater reports her pain as a constant, stabbing and burning pain at a 6 on a scale of 1 to 10 (10 = worst) before her pain medication is administered.

Ms. Stillwater's 5-day-old boy is now bottle-feeding regularly. He is taking 3 oz of Similac with Iron every 4 hours. Ms. Stillwater is eager to assume the majority of his care.

Prescribed Interventions

Medication or saline lock; flush every shift and prn
Vancomycin 1.0 g IV q12h
Sterile dressing change with calcium alginate wound dressing; pack loosely, change when outer dressing is saturated with drainage. Irrigate wound with normal saline before removing dressing
Irrigate wound with NSS with dressing change

Fingerstick blood glucose before meals and at bedtime
Humalog insulin per sliding scale
Vital signs q4h
Ibuprofen 600 mg po q4–6h prn pain
Hydrocodone 5 mg and acetaminophen 325 mg po q4–6h prn pain unrelieved by ibuprofen

continued

Developing Clinical Reasoning and Clinical Judgment

- How will you plan the dressing change for Ms. Stillwater and what equipment will you need?

- What techniques can you show Ms. Stillwater to improve her mobility and ability to hold and care for her infant?

- Describe your assessment and interventions for this wound.

- Identify factors that will promote wound healing in Ms. Stillwater.

- How will you organize your nursing care to provide uninterrupted time for Ms. Stillwater to care for her 5-day-old son?

- Describe the procedure you will use to administer the IV antibiotic.

Suggested Responses for Integrated Nursing Care

- Ms. Stillwater's dressing change will be stressful and uncomfortable (Chapter 8). To manage the pain, perform the dressing change after she has taken her pain medication and you have allowed enough time for it to be effective. Consider nonpharmacologic interventions to help increase comfort and decrease pain (Chapter 10). Given her diabetic status, allow her to eat her breakfast and receive her insulin before you begin her dressing change. Ms. Stillwater's focus is probably on her son. Encourage her to give him his morning bottle and to be satisfied that he is comfortable before you begin the dressing change.

- Review Chapter 8 to develop the list of equipment you will need for the dressing change. You will need to set up a sterile field and maintain the sterility during the dressing change (Chapter 1). Ms. Stillwater can be positioned supine and rotated slightly to her left to promote drainage of the wound during irrigation.

- Make sure your assessment of the wound includes the size, the presence of granulation tissue, a description of the drainage, wound color, the presence of edema and erythema, and temperature (see Chapter 8). Note the condition of the skin at the wound edges as well as the surrounding skin, including the location of the dressing tape. Look for changes in the condition of the wound and note how Ms. Stillwater is tolerating the dressing change. If she will be taught to care for this wound and perform the dressing changes at home, instruction and return

demonstration would become part of her discharge planning.

- For Ms. Stillwater's wound to heal, the infection must be resolved, and the wound edges will need to become approximated. To optimize wound healing, Ms. Stillwater will need a diet high in protein, calories, and minerals. Collaborate with the health care team to obtain a nutritional consultation.

- The care of her infant son is a priority for Ms. Stillwater. Cluster your nursing care, such as wound dressing changes, vital signs, and medication administration, to allow her sufficient time to provide care for her son.

- Make sure Ms. Stillwater knows how to use a splint, such as a pillow or folded blanket, across her abdomen to give support to her abdominal musculature when moving or coughing (see Chapter 6). Spending time in a comfortable chair may be preferable to getting in and out of bed. Assess that Ms. Stillwater is using the "football hold" to feed and comfort her son. The advantage of this position is that the infant does not rest on the mother's abdomen. Ms. Stillwater should have several pillows available to provide support for her arms when holding her infant.

- To give the IV antibiotic, assess the IV site for patency (Chapter 16), flush the IV per facility policy prior to administration, administer the antibiotics according to the facility and/or manufacturer's guidelines, and then flush the medication or saline lock after the antibiotic is infused (see Chapter 5).

Case Study

Jason Brown

Jason Brown is a 21-year-old college football player. It is the second postop day following surgical repair of a fracture of his right tibia and fibula. He has sutures over the anterior knee and lateral malleolus and a posterior splint on the right leg. He continues to report considerable pain. His vital signs at midnight were as follows: temperature, 98.3°F; pulse, 58 beats/min; respirations, 12 breaths/min; blood pressure 118/70 mm Hg. He reported his incisional pain as sharp, stabbing, and a 3 on a scale of 1 to 10 (10 = worst) at about 10 PM. He has a peripheral IV in his left forearm infusing D5 ½ NSS at a rate of 20 mL/hr. He is using a patient-controlled anesthesia (PCA) pump for pain relief. The nursing care for the morning includes routine AM care, cast care, and a trip to physical therapy (PT). Shortly after morning report, the unit secretary catches you and says, "Jason says he needs a nurse. He is in terrible pain."

You enter the room. Jason is pale and diaphoretic. His sheets are damp with some wet spots. He says, "My leg hurts. It really hurts." You ask him to rate his pain, and he answers, "At least an 8. I've been pushing my pain pump but I'm still in pain." His IV site looks okay. You say, "I'm going to find out why it is hurting. I need to get your vital signs first." His vital signs now are as follows: temperature, 98.9°F; pulse, 72 beats/min; respirations, 20 breaths/min; blood pressure, 124/78 mm Hg.

Prescribed Interventions

Vital signs q4h

Intravenous fluids: D5 ½ NSS at 20 mL/hr

PCA—morphine sulfate 1 mg/mL, 1 mg q6min; lockout max 10 mg in 1 hr

Zolpidem 5 mg prn at bedtime for sleep

PT for weight bearing, as tolerated

Developing Clinical Reasoning and Clinical Judgment

- What is the significance of the changes in Jason's vital signs?

- How do you assess the following:
  - Infection versus inflammation?
  - Neurovascular compromise?
  - IV patency?

- What interventions for Jason's pain must occur immediately before administering nursing care and PT?

continued

Suggested Responses for Integrated Nursing Care

- Always compare vital signs with a baseline and the previous vital signs (see Chapter 2). While Jason's temperature is elevated slightly, it has not increased dramatically, as it would be with an infection. His respiratory rate and pulse rate were quite low at midnight. Since he is a young, healthy athlete, his resting pulse rate may be lower than what is often considered as the norm. You notice that his resting pulse rates on the night shift have been running from 56 to 60 beats/min. Another factor contributing to his decreased pulse rate may be the effect of the zolpidem that he took at 2200 to help him sleep. Therefore, while his morning respiratory rate and pulse rate are still within normal range, they represent a significant increase from his resting baseline. These are objective assessments that correlate with his identification of increased pain.

- One reason for an increase in pain with any postsurgical patient is the possibility of infection. Quickly assess all surgical incision sites and observe for redness, swelling, or a foul odor (Chapter 8). Due to short hospital stays, signs and symptoms of infection do not usually appear until after the patient is discharged. The assessment of the surgical site should also include checking for bleeding. Hemorrhage in the postoperative period is always a potential complication (see Chapter 6).

- In addition to infection, Jason is at risk for neurovascular compromise because of the trauma to his right leg as well as from the splint and dressing. Assess for neurovascular compromise and perform cast care (refer to Chapters 3 and 9). Jason's fracture has been placed in a splint rather than a cast, which is a more current surgical practice, but nurses still refer to the care of the affected extremity as "cast care." Determine whether there are any signs of compartment

syndrome (refer to Chapters 3 and 9). You need no additional equipment for this assessment, and it should take very little time; do this immediately.

- Upon assessment, you find that Jason's foot and leg are pink and warm with 2+ pulses, no edema, full sensation, motion, and capillary refill measuring less than 3 seconds. The incision sites show no redness, swelling, drainage, or foul odor, and no bleeding is evident.

- Another possible reason for his pain is that his IV may no longer be patent and, therefore, he would not be receiving any pain medication. You remember the wet spots on the bed as you begin systematically checking each of the IV administration-set connections. Your assessment of the IV site shows no swelling, and he reports no pain at the site. Your next check should be from the IV site to the IV tubing. You find that the connection of the IV tubing to the IV insertion catheter is loose and leaking. Determine whether the IV site is still patent (see Chapter 16). If the IV is still patent, replace the IV tubing (see Chapter 16). Check the medication in the PCA pump to ensure it is the correct medication. You will be required to check the PCA history to determine the amount of medication used as well as the amount remaining every 4 hours or according to facility policy (see Chapter 10).

- Contact the health care provider to explain that the PCA pain medication was infusing onto the bed linens, and obtain a prescribed intervention for an appropriate bolus dose so that Jason can obtain immediate pain relief. After 30 minutes, obtain another set of vital signs and perform a pain assessment. Document the evaluation of your interventions. Jason's pain will need to be controlled before initiating additional nursing care. Coordinating with PT to reschedule his therapy until his pain is controlled is a nursing responsibility.

Case Study

Kent Clark

Kent Clark, age 29, was admitted 24 hours ago for observation related to a suspected closed head injury following a motor vehicle accident (MVA). Mr. Clark's baseline vital signs are stable. He has a cervical collar and is scheduled to undergo an MRI to determine if he has a cervical spine injury. The health care provider has asked you to reduce his activity until cervical spinal injuries are ruled out.

Currently, Mr. Clark is awake, alert, and oriented (to person, place, and time); his pupils are equally round and reactive to light and accommodation (PERRLA). He moves all four extremities bilaterally. His head is elevated 30 degrees to minimize increased intracranial pressure (ICP) and edema. A peripheral IV in his right arm is infusing D5 ½ NSS at 40 mL/hr.

Just before you are scheduled to take him to Special Procedures for the MRI, Mr. Clark becomes restless and anxious. During the neuro check, you notice that his right pupil is sluggish. Although he denies pain, he says, "I don't care what the doctors say. I am not going to stay in this bed any longer!" When you call the health care provider, they prescribe lorazepam 0.5 mg IV push. However, as you give the IV push medication to Mr. Clark, you notice a cloudy substance forming in the IV line and the patient reports a slight burning at his IV insertion site.

Prescribed Interventions

Bed rest
Intravenous fluids: D5 ½ NSS at 40 mL/hr
HOB elevated 30 degrees

Neurologic checks q2h
Lorazepam 0.5 mg IV push now × one dose
Cervical collar

Developing Clinical Reasoning and Clinical Judgment

• What clinical symptoms alert you that Mr. Clark's condition is changing? What additional assessments will you do?

• Identify the source of the pain at the IV insertion site and the cloudy substance in the IV tubing.

• Describe special positioning and transfer techniques to be followed for Mr. Clark.

• What could you have done to prevent these complications, and how will you intervene now?

• How will you handle Mr. Clark's anger and maintain reduced activity?

continued

Suggested Responses for Integrated Nursing Care

- In a patient with a closed head injury, bleeding or swelling may occur within the confines of the skull, leading to increased ICP. This increased ICP could cause extensive brain damage. Mr. Clark became increasingly restless and anxious, which could be a subtle sign of increased ICP. Even slow bleeding inside the cranium can cause changes. When you observe a change, immediately perform a neurologic assessment to determine if there are further neurologic alterations (refer to Chapters 3 and 17). When Mr. Clark became restless, you noticed that his right pupil was more sluggish to light than the left, which is another sign of increased ICP. Complete neurologic checks as often as his condition warrants, and immediately report subtle changes in neurologic checks to the health care team. Meticulous documentation of baseline neurologic checks and subsequent assessments is important to detect subtle neurologic changes (Chapters 3 and 17).

- Cervical spinal injuries can vary in severity, and even hairline fractures can become unstable if the patient is not positioned and transferred correctly. Mr. Clark has a cervical collar and the health care provider has asked you to minimize his movement (refer to Chapter 17). If you need to turn Mr. Clark, keep his head lowered and then turn him as a unit without flexing or turning his neck. Obtain help from additional staff so that you can stabilize his head, neck, and torso in straight alignment while he is being turned. When Mr. Clark is transferred from the bed to a stretcher, use a friction-reducing sheet or lateral transfer device to move him gently and carefully as a unit (refer to Chapter 9). Even though he has a cervical collar, do not assume that it is safe for him to sit up further in the bed or get up and move around.

- Mr. Clark is angry and wants to get out of bed. For Mr. Clark, careful pharmacologic sedation may be a good option. The health care provider has prescribed lorazepam to reduce his agitation and anxiety. Another possible intervention is to help Mr. Clark feel more in control of his environment. This could be as simple as having a family member stay with him, and frequently checking his needs. Restraints would be the least desirable option for him. At this time, placing restraints on him could increase his agitation and make him feel more trapped, and this could increase his ICP; alternatives to restraints should be implemented (refer to Chapter 4).

- Pain at the IV site could mean that the IV is not patent. Carefully observe the IV site for any signs of phlebitis or infiltration before and while giving the IV push (refer to Chapers 5 and 16). If you determine that Mr. Clark's IV has a good blood return and is not infiltrated, the burning sensation at his IV site may be related to the administration of the lorazepam IV. Medications given by intravenous (IV) bolus can be irritating. Give the medication and the flush that follows at a slower rate. If not contraindicated, some medications can also be diluted, based on facility policy and/or as prescribed.

- The most probable cause for the cloudy appearance in Mr. Clark's IV line is precipitation of the drug due to chemical incompatibility of the lorazepam and the IV fluid of D5 ½ NSS. When giving any medication through an IV line, you must know whether the drug and IV solution are chemically compatible (refer to Chapter 5). When IV drugs are not compatible, a reaction immediately occurs that may or may not be visible to the eye, but nevertheless can be dangerous. To prevent this, flush the IV line before and after medication administration per facility policy. Since a precipitate has already formed, clamp the tubing off using the clamp closest to Mr. Clark and make sure that the cloudy substance does not reach him (see Chapter 5). Some facilities require discontinuing the IV and restarting another IV with new IV tubing; other hospitals require changing only the IV tubing. If signs of incompatibility occur, notify the health care team and continue to assess Mr. Clark's need for further medication.

Case Study

Lucille Howard

Lucille Howard, age 78, is in the hospital for a severe urinary tract infection (UTI). She has a history of urinary retention and UTIs. She is overweight, has a history of heart failure, and is allergic to many medications, including several antibiotics. Twenty-four hours ago she had severe nausea and vomiting and was prescribed nothing by mouth (NPO). She has an IV catheter inserted in her left arm, infusing D5 ½ NSS at 75 mL/hr. While caring for Ms. Howard, you notice that she begins to have some coarse audible breath sounds and difficulty breathing. She reports pain in her abdomen.

Prescribed Interventions

Intravenous fluids: D5 ½ NSS at 75 mL/hr

Ciprofloxacin 200 mg IV q12h

NPO

Strict I&O

Developing Clinical Reasoning and Clinical Judgment

• What are possible causes of Ms. Howard's current symptoms?

• How would you identify the source of her current symptoms?

• What actions will you take?

Suggested Responses for Integrated Nursing Care

• There are several potential causes for Ms. Howard's symptoms. In light of her drug sensitivities, she may be allergic to the ciprofloxacin. Allergic responses can include difficulty breathing as well as itching and a rash. Another source of her symptoms could be related to her heart problems. People with heart problems can easily become overloaded with fluid. Symptoms of fluid overload, a common problem for patients with heart failure, include crackles in the lungs, abnormal heart sounds, and possibly edema.

• To determine the cause of Ms. Howard's symptoms, you need to perform several assessments. First, obtain vital signs (refer to Chapter 2), auscultate her heart and lung sounds and palpate her abdomen (refer to Chapter 3). Assess for edema. Also assess for a rash on her skin, and ask her if she has any

itching. Review her voiding history and volume of urine per episode of voiding.

• If her heart and lung sounds are normal, but her abdominal discomfort persists, she may have to urinate. Review the method she has been using to void. Ms. Howard is overweight and positioning on a bedpan may be difficult and is not conducive to emptying of her bladder. Arrange for and encourage her to get out of bed to void; use of a bedside commode is probably the best intervention, as she is experiencing some difficulty breathing and probably has decreased energy related to her acute illness (refer to Chapter 12). Consider checking postvoid residual to confirm she is emptying her bladder (refer to Chapter 12). Consult a safe patient handling algorithm to help you make decisions about safe patient handling and movement (refer

continued

Lucille Howard (continued)

to Chapter 9). Utilize appropriate transfer devices and the assistance of others when assisting Ms. Howard out of bed.

- If Ms. Howard seems to be emptying her bladder and the postvoid bladder scans reveal minimal retention, her discomfort could be related to the UTI. Collaborate with the health care provider regarding appropriate analgesia.

- You should also review the patient's intake and output, for the most recent hours and for the last 24 hours (refer to Chapter 16). Currently, Ms. Howard is getting 75 mL/hr of IV fluid. She should be voiding an average of at least 30 mL/hr, the least amount of urine you would expect to see in an hour (30 mL). You could weigh the patient and compare today's weight with her admission weight (refer to Chapter 3). The record of a patient's daily weight may more

accurately depict fluid balance status, due to possible numerous sources of inaccuracies in fluid intake and output measurement. Weigh the patient at the same time every day. If Ms. Howard's input is higher than her output, she is at risk for overload. New or worsening edema or significantly increased body weight in 24 hours indicates an accumulation of fluid related to fluid overload or worsening heart failure.

- If Ms. Howard is having an allergic reaction, hold any dose of the ciprofloxacin that may be due, follow anaphylaxis protocol, and notify the health care team. If she is beginning to have problems with fluid overload due to her heart problems, reduce the IV rate to a keep open rate (20 to 40 mL/hr), and consult with the health care team regarding further intervention. Continue to monitor Ms. Howard until you are certain she is stabilized and her symptoms have resolved.

Case Study

Janice Romero

Janice Romero, age 24, has recently been diagnosed with acute lymphocytic leukemia (ALL). To provide long-term venous access, she is having an implanted port placed. She had a 21-gauge peripheral IV inserted in her right arm prior to surgery. After her port was placed, Mrs. Romero's health care provider prescribed two units of packed red blood cells (PRBCs). You note a prescribed intervention for the use of a blood warmer for the transfusions. When you talk to Mrs. Romero about the blood transfusion, she tells you that the last time she received blood she had chills and fever during the transfusion.

Prescribed Interventions

Two units PRBCs via blood warmer stat

Intravenous fluids: D5 ½ NSS at 50 mL/hr

Developing Clinical Reasoning and Clinical Judgment

- Identify the site you will use to administer blood to Mrs. Romero. Why did you choose this site?

- Describe the technique you will use to administer blood to Mrs. Romero.

continued

- Identify the purposes for warming blood, and describe the safest way to warm blood.

- Considering Mrs. Romero's history and diagnosis, describe the precautions you will implement before giving her blood.

Suggested Responses for Integrated Nursing Care

- Before Mrs. Romero can receive blood, you must select an appropriate site (see Chapter 16). Site selection depends on the gauge of the IV and the fluid infusing in the IV. Use a 20- to 24-gauge PIVC based on vein size for blood transfusion; a large-gauge PIVC is recommended when rapid transfusion is required. Since dextrose will cause hemolysis, blood can be administered only with normal saline. For these two reasons, the optimal site for blood administration is her implanted port (Chapter 16). Before you give her blood through the port, be certain that the port is not dedicated for other infusions, such as chemo.

- Since the implanted port is new, check the patient's health record for indications that the port has been approved for use; confirmation of location of the tip of the port catheter either by postprocedure chest radiograph or by technology used during the placement procedure is required prior to use and should be documented in the patient's health record. Maintain sterile technique when accessing the port and wear a mask (see Chapter 16). Ensure that the port is patent prior to use. Check the port for patency and blood return per facility policy. Infuse the normal saline slowly while you observe the implanted port site for signs of swelling and pain. If the port shows any

sign of infiltration, notify the health care provider and choose another site to give her blood.

- Some patients may need to have their blood warmed before it is administered. This includes patients who are at risk for cardiac arrhythmias, patients with unusual immune responses, as well as neonatal and pediatric patients. A health care provider must prescribe warming of blood products during transfusion. Various devices exist to warm blood. Whenever you need to warm blood, always use a blood warmer approved by your facility. Do not use the microwave to warm any blood product.

- Mrs. Romero's history of chills and fever are signs of a possible transfusion reaction; thus, she is at increased risk for a transfusion reaction. Ensure that she has a signed consent form and that she fully understands her need for the blood. The health care provider should be aware of this history of a transfusion reaction. Stay with the patient for at least 15 minutes at the beginning of the transfusion. Assess the patient at least every 30 minutes for adverse reactions (Gorski et al., 2021). Continue to monitor her vital signs frequently per hospital policy (see Chapters 2 and 16). When you leave her room, make sure her call light is available, and instruct her to contact you if she has any symptoms.

Case Study

Gwen Galloway

Mrs. Galloway, age 64, had a left-sided mastectomy and is now receiving follow-up chemotherapy for recurrent breast cancer with axillary node involvement at the outpatient oncology center. She reports intermittent pain and soreness on her left side and under her left arm. She has a central venous access device (CVAD) (double-lumen Hickman catheter) inserted in the right side of her chest. Recent laboratory work shows a low white blood cell count of 1,800/mm^3 and a low platelet count of 39,000/mm^3. She also bleeds and bruises very easily. You have to obtain vital signs and draw a complete blood count (CBC). The dressing on her CVAD must be changed.

continued

Gwen Galloway (continued)

Prescribed Interventions

Vital signs on arrival

CBC on arrival

Acetaminophen 650 mg po q6h prn pain

Change central line dressing q week

Developing Clinical Reasoning and Clinical Judgment

- What special precautions should you take while obtaining Mrs. Galloway's vital signs?

- Explain why some sites would be contraindicated when taking Mrs. Galloway's temperature.

- Identify your interventions when changing Mrs. Galloway's central line dressing and the rationale for these interventions.

- Describe the special precautions you would take when drawing blood from Mrs. Galloway. Identify the site where you would draw the blood.

Suggested Responses for Integrated Nursing Care

- To individualize care, always assess your patient's condition and special needs. When a patient undergoes a mastectomy, they will often have lymph nodes removed from the affected side. Taking a blood pressure reading in the affected arm could interfere with circulation and harm the extremity (see Chapter 2). In Mrs. Galloway's case, her affected side is on the left, so take her blood pressure on the right side.

- Mrs. Galloway has a low platelet count, which places her at risk for bleeding. In addition, her low white blood cell count places her at risk for infection and other complications. Therefore, taking a rectal temperature would be contraindicated for Mrs. Galloway. It would also be contraindicated to take a left-sided axillary temperature on Mrs. Galloway because she is still having some discomfort due to her recent mastectomy (see Chapter 2).

- Given Mrs. Galloway's risk for bleeding, would a peripheral venipuncture be the best choice to obtain the prescribed CBC? Due to the risk for prolonged

bleeding, her central line may provide the best access for a blood specimen (Chapter 18). Determine whether her health care provider has restricted her central line for chemotherapy. If her central line is dedicated to chemotherapy only, obtain a blood specimen via venipuncture (Chapter 18). If you needed to do a venipuncture, using Mrs. Galloway's left side would be contraindicated due to the mastectomy. You will need to apply pressure to the site for a longer period of time because of her increased risk for bleeding.

- When changing Mrs. Galloway's central line dressing, use sterile technique due to her increased risk for infection (Chapter 1). Maintain sterile technique when changing the CVAD dressing and wear a mask (see Chapter 16). Ensure that the CVAD is patent prior to use. Check the CVAD for patency and blood return per facility policy (Chapter 16). To prevent bleeding and bruising at the central line site, do not move or pull on the catheter as you are manipulating the central line dressing.

Case Study

George Patel

George Patel, age 64, was admitted to your floor 3 days ago following surgical insertion of a tracheostomy tube. His diagnosis prior to surgery was acute upper airway obstruction. He has a medication (saline) lock. Currently, he is receiving oxygen via his tracheostomy at 40%. His pulse oximetry readings have been consistently running in the low 90s. He quickly becomes short of breath when his oxygen is interrupted during suctioning. During your shift, you will have to suction Mr. Patel as needed and provide routine tracheostomy care. You will also need to transport him with portable oxygen to radiology for his chest x-ray (AP and lateral).

Prescribed Interventions

Morphine sulfate 1 to 4 mg IV q3h prn for pain

AP and lateral chest x-ray

Pulse oximetry every shift and prn

Oxygen via trach Venturi mask at 40%

Tracheostomy care every shift and prn

Medication or saline lock, flush every shift

Tracheal suctioning prn

Developing Clinical Reasoning and Clinical Judgment

- How would you determine when Mr. Patel needs to be suctioned?

- How would you determine when Mr. Patel needs to have tracheostomy care?

- Describe expected outcomes when suctioning and providing tracheostomy care.

- When transporting Mr. Patel to the radiology department, what interventions should you implement to ensure his safety?

Suggested Responses for Integrated Nursing Care

- To evaluate the need for suctioning, first assess Mr. Patel's respiratory status (refer to Chapters 3 and 14). Examine his oxygen saturation and compare it with his baseline (Chapter 14). If his oxygen saturation is decreased from his baseline, this may be an indication that he needs to be suctioned. Observe his respirations to determine if they are more labored than usual (refer to Chapters 2 and 3). Listen to his lung sounds for crackles or wheezes. Also, listen around his tracheostomy for gurgling. Does he have

a productive cough? All of these signs and symptoms are indications that he needs to be suctioned.

- To assess the need for tracheostomy care (see Chapter 14), closely examine his tracheostomy as well as the tracheostomy holder/ties and precut gauze dressing. If it appears wet or moist, tracheostomy care would be indicated. If his tracheostomy dressing appears dry and intact, you may want to wait until later in your shift to do tracheostomy care. Suctioning and subsequent coughing will often soil the tracheostomy

continued

George Patel (continued)

dressings, so wait until after suctioning to change the trachcostomy dressing.

- Your expected outcomes when suctioning a tracheostomy include minimizing hypoxia, discomfort, and fatigue. Hypoxia may be reduced by hyperoxygenating the patient before suctioning according to facility policy. When you suction Mr. Patel (using sterile technique), limit the length of suction time to 10 to 15 seconds and allow him to rest before suctioning him again (see Chapters 1 and 14). During tracheostomy care or repeat suctioning, quickly replace his oxygen source and limit the time his oxygen is interrupted. Since Mr. Patel has a new tracheostomy, it is very likely he will need to be premedicated with morphine for pain. Morphine may depress respirations, so continually assess Mr. Patel's respiratory status after administering the pain medication. In addition, adequate rest periods are needed to minimize fatigue from suctioning. Mr. Patel may require a rest period between suctioning the tracheostomy and his tracheostomy care.

- Important interventions when transporting Mr. Patel focus on providing adequate oxygenation. First, assess Mr. Patel's oxygen saturation and respiratory status prior to transport (Chapters 2 and 3). If indicated, suction Mr. Patel before he leaves his room. You must also check that the portable oxygen tank is full and the label says "oxygen." Before turning off his wall oxygen, make sure the portable oxygen tank is working properly and that the equipment is ready. This avoids interruption of the oxygen supply while placing him on the portable oxygen.

Advanced Case Studies

Nursing Concepts

- Advocacy
- Assessment
- Clinical Decision Making/Clinical Judgment
- Collaboration/Teamwork and Collaboration
- Comfort
- Communication
- Elimination
- Fluids and Electrolytes
- Functional Ability
- Infection
- Inflammation
- Mobility
- Nutrition
- Oxygenation/Gas Exchange
- Perfusion
- Professionalism/Professional Behaviors
- Safety
- Teaching and Learning/Patient Education
- Thermoregulation
- Tissue Integrity

Case Study

Cole McKean

Cole McKean is a 4-year-old boy in the pediatric intensive care unit (PICU). He weighs 22 kg. He was admitted 3 days ago after nearly drowning in a neighbor's pool. He was submerged for 5 to 10 minutes. The neighbor initiated CPR and the rescue team had a heart rate established within 10 minutes of their arrival. The aspirated pool water caused a severe inflammatory response resulting in pulmonary edema. Cole is intubated with an endotracheal tube (ETT) and is on a mechanical ventilator. Throughout the past 2 days, he has been producing copious bronchial secretions and has required suctioning

continued

Cole McKean (continued)

about every 2 hours. Today, his breath sounds are clearer and he requires less frequent suctioning. He is being weaned off oxygen. The care plan for today includes possible extubation. An arterial line is in place in his left radial artery, infusing NSS at 2 to 3 mL/hr. A peripherally inserted central catheter (PICC) line with an infusion of D5 ½ NSS at 75 mL/hr is inserted into his right arm. His heart rate, respiratory rate, and arterial waveform are being monitored. The pulse oximeter sensor is applied to his right toe. He has an indwelling urinary catheter to gravity drainage and a nasogastric tube in place and set to low intermittent suction. Cole is receiving sedation but is opening his eyes at times and moving his extremities. He is becoming more active.

Suddenly, the alarm goes off on the ventilator. You look at Cole. His eyes are open and he is making crying sounds. You know when a child is properly intubated they cannot make sounds. You notice that his oxygen saturation level has dropped to 81% and his color is dusky. He is breathing on his own around the tube and his abdomen is rounded. You and the pediatric intensivist assess Cole's respiratory status and oxygenation and decide to remove the ETT and begin oxygen at 40% via face mask. When you place Cole on the face mask, his oxygen saturation returns to the mid-90s. The health care provider says, "This little fellow was ready to get rid of his tube." She prescribes a follow-up arterial blood gas (ABG) to be drawn in 15 minutes.

Prescribed Interventions

Continuous pulse oximetry

Foley to gravity

Maintain O_2 saturation 92% to 98%

I&O

Oxygen 40% via face mask

Nasogastric tube to low intermittent suction

Vital signs q1h

Neurologic checks q1h

Intravenous fluids: D5 ½ NS at 75 mL/hr

Endotracheal suctioning prn

Arterial line: NSS 2 to 3 mL/hr

Developing Clinical Reasoning and Clinical Judgment

• Describe your initial actions in response to a possible extubation.

• Develop a care plan that will allow Cole rest and sleep periods, but also allow hourly assessments.

• How can the technique of drawing ABGs be adapted for a pediatric patient?

• Identify the nursing skills involved in monitoring Cole's respiratory status.

• How will Cole's response be evaluated now that he is on an oxygen mask?

continued

Suggested Responses for Integrated Nursing Care

- When a patient is intubated, the patency of this airway is a critical priority. When you hear Cole cry, you must determine if his ETT is in the proper place (refer to Chapter 14). Listen with your stethoscope over the lung fields and abdomen. If you do not hear ventilator-induced breath sounds over the lung fields, then the ETT is not in place. Because a child's neck is so short, it is not difficult to displace a tracheal tube into the esophagus. If this occurs, you may hear ventilator-cycled sounds in the abdomen. Signs that an ETT is not in the correct position include unstable oxygen saturation levels, cyanosis, and abdominal distention. In Cole's situation, you determine that the ETT is no longer in the lungs. All patients on mechanical ventilation must have an Ambu bag and a mask of the correct size at the bedside. Cole did not require mask-bag respirations at this time, but he has the potential for this need.

- When you are evaluating Cole's response, the ABG results will guide clinical decision making regarding oxygen delivery. In Cole's case, 10 to 15 minutes after changing to the 40% oxygen mask, you draw an ABG (see Chapter 18). The results come back as follows: Pao_2, 82 mm Hg; $Paco_2$, 46 mm Hg; pH, 7.34; Hco_3, 20 mEq/L. This ABG shows that Cole's oxygen level is acceptable and there is no indication to support immediate reintubation. Continue to assess Cole's respiratory status and oxygenation (see Chapters 3 and 14) and obtain ABGs periodically, as prescribed, to evaluate Cole's response to treatment.

- Monitor and assess Cole's respiratory status: observe his work of breathing, count his respiratory rate, observe his color, and auscultate breath sounds (refer to Chapters 2, 3, and 14). If he shows no significant respiratory distress and has a stable respiratory rate and clear breath sounds, he is responding well to the change in his oxygen source. In addition, continuously monitor the oxygen saturation level via pulse oximetry. Immediately report any increases or decreases in oxygen saturation to the health care provider.

- Because children have a small total blood volume, the blood drawn back in the arterial line is usually not discarded but returned to the patient after the laboratory sample is drawn. Smaller volumes of blood are sent to the laboratory in pediatric specimen tubes. The setup for a pediatric arterial line delivers a smaller volume of fluid when the inline flushing device is activated (see Chapter 18).

- When a patient, especially a child, is critically ill, cluster your hands-on care so that the patient will have a significant amount of time to sleep and rest between interventions. One of the initial assessments a nurse makes in an intensive care setting is to determine that each of the monitoring devices is accurately displaying the patient's status (see Chapters 14 and 15). After you determine that the monitors accurately reflect the patient's vital signs, obtaining alternating sets of vital signs from the patient and from the monitor may be permitted, according to hospital policy (refer to Chapter 2). Consider interventions to decrease discomfort and increase patient comfort (Chapter 10). Maintain a quiet environment (Chapter 10). Because of the noise and activity of the intensive care unit, many infant and child intensive care units dim the lights at night to create day/night cycles for the children.

Case Study

Damian Wallace

Damian Wallace, age 19, was admitted to the emergency department approximately 4 hours ago with a stab wound to the chest that he received in a knife fight while intoxicated. You are asked to care for Damian while his nurse attends to a new emergency. She gives you the following report: He was admitted in respiratory distress and bleeding from the stab wound. His wound is on the right side at the sixth intercostal space and is approximately 1 inch in length, sutured, and intact. The chest x-ray confirmed a right hemothorax and, as a result, the emergency department physician inserted a chest tube. The chest tube is connected to a disposable drainage system and placed to suction at -20 cm H_2O. The chest tube is draining a small amount of dark-red blood. There has not been any new drainage for the past 2 hours.

continued

Damian Wallace (continued)

Damian's most recent vital signs were as follows: temperature, 98.4°F; pulse, 88 beats/min; respirations, 24 breaths/min; blood pressure, 112/74 mm Hg. He is receiving oxygen via face mask at 30% and is on continuous pulse oximetry. The oxygen saturation level is currently 96%. He says he feels short of breath. He does not have labored breathing and is not using accessory muscles. He reports pain at the chest tube insertion site and stab wound site. He has a patent IV infusing in his left forearm. His laboratory work reported a blood alcohol level of 0.12. The nurse giving report says, "Good luck—He says he's in pain, but I think he already drank his pain medication from a bottle."

Damian turns on his call light. When you approach him, you notice his breathing is labored with subclavicular retractions. The pulse oximeter reads 95%. Damian says, "This thing in my side really hurts."

You take another set of vital signs: temperature, 98.6°F; pulse, 90 beats/min; respirations, 37 breaths/min; blood pressure, 118/78 mm Hg. You find the breath sounds are diminished on the right. The chest drainage tubing is in the bed without a dependent loop, and Damian has been lying on a segment of the tubing. You ask him to describe his pain and rate it on a scale of 1 to 10 (10 = worst), and he says, "Really bad, sharp, about a 5, like I'm being stabbed again!" You ask if the medicine he got earlier helped with the pain, and he replies, "it didn't help one bit!" When you review the eMAR, you find that Damian has been prescribed ketorolac 30 mg IV, which was given 3 hours ago, and hydrocodone 5 mg and acetaminophen 325 mg po for pain unrelieved by ketorolac, which has not been administered. You find his nurse and ask if pain medication was administered. The nurse responds, "Are you kidding? If he's tough enough to drink and fight, he's tough enough for a little chest tube. If the anti-inflammatory doesn't help, he doesn't deserve anything stronger."

Prescribed Interventions

Chest tube with drainage system to suction at −20 cm H_2O

Intravenous fluids: NSS at 100 mL/hr

Oxygen at 30% via face mask

Ketorolac 30 mg IV q6h prn pain

Hydrocodone 5 mg and acetaminophen 325 mg po q4–6h prn pain unrelieved by ketorolac

Continuous pulse oximetry

Developing Clinical Reasoning and Clinical Judgment

• Which of Damian's needs is your first priority? Describe your assessments related to your first priority.

• How would you troubleshoot his chest tube drainage system? What could be the source of his respiratory distress?

continued

- Describe the purpose of a chest tube drainage system for a hemothorax.

- Discuss valid reasons a nurse might not give a pain medication when there is a prn order.

- Discuss prejudices nurses may have that may prohibit adequate pain management.

Suggested Responses for Integrated Nursing Care

- Your first priority is Damian's increased respiratory distress (refer to Chapters 2 and 3). Although the change in oxygen saturation levels is very small, this is only because Damian's body is compensating for it now. Damian's work of breathing has dramatically changed, signaling a change in his respiratory status. Your preliminary assessment showed a respiratory rate of 37 breaths/min, up significantly from his earlier respiratory rate of 24. When you inspected the chest, you found subclavicular retractions; this indicates that Damian is using his intercostal muscles to breathe. When you auscultated breath sounds, you found decreased air movement on the right, indicating a hemothorax.

- In a hemothorax, blood collects in the pleural space and compresses a lung. The purpose of the chest tube is to evacuate the blood and allow the lung to expand fully (Chapter 14). In Damian's case, the stab wound created a puncture in the pleura, allowing blood to accumulate within the pleural space. It is important to evaluate the right lung on a routine basis to make sure the blood in the pleural space has been removed so that the lung can reexpand (refer to Chapter 3). Any change in respiratory status may indicate a problem with the chest tube drainage system.

- As you noted in this case, Damian has had a change in his respiratory status. Since you have completed his assessment, now begin inspecting the equipment. As with any equipment check, begin inspection at the patient and move to the equipment. Start your inspection at the insertion site of the chest tube (refer to Chapter 14). Observe the dressing to ensure it is occlusive and inspect the tubing for leaks, kinks, and dependent loops. Compare the amount of recent drainage in the drainage system, with the volume of old drainage, and check the amount of suction (see Chapter 14). In this case, Damian has been lying on his tubing, which would prevent it from draining

properly. When you reposition Damian's tubing, approximately 60 mL of dark old blood flows into the drainage set. His respiratory status improves quickly. Thus, this accumulated blood in the pleural space was the source of his respiratory distress.

- There are several situations in which giving an opioid analgesic may be contraindicated. During a life-saving procedure, pain is not always a priority. In this case, Damian did not receive pain medication before the insertion of his chest tube, because he was at risk for respiratory arrest. Opioids may also be contraindicated when it is critical to assess mental status, because the opioid might mask neurologic changes. Opioid analgesics also are associated with the adverse effects of respiratory depression and vital sign changes. Patients sometimes do not receive the prescribed pain medication because the nurse is worried about these adverse effects (refer to Chapter 10). Because of this, controversy exists as to whether the benefit of pain control outweighs the risk of adverse drug reactions. Many hospitals have committees that can assist with these ethical decisions. Collaboration among nurses, doctors, and pharmacists can result in optimal pain control with minimal adverse effects. Speak with the health care provider before independently deciding to withhold pain medication to prevent adverse drug reactions.

- Another reason nurses may withhold medication is their own preconception of the patient's pain and their own prejudices. Some nurses are not even aware that they have these feelings. As a nursing student, you need to understand how you will respond to patients, and you need to explore your own beliefs and prejudices. The accepted standard in nursing is that a patient defines their own pain and that it is the nurse's responsibility to manage it properly. Guidelines for pain management have been written by State Boards of Nursing, the U.S. Department of Health and Human Services, the World Health Organization, as well as other professional organizations.

Case Study

Robert Espinoza

Robert Espinoza, age 44, has just had exploratory abdominal surgery. The postanesthesia recovery room (PACU) nurse calls at 1410 to provide report for Mr. Espinoza and tells you that he has a peripheral IV inserted in his right arm, infusing NSS at 50 mL/hr. He has a midline abdominal dressing that is dry and intact with two Jackson–Pratt (JP) drains in place. He also has a nasogastric (NG) tube and an indwelling urinary catheter to gravity drainage. The nurse reports that his NG tube has been checked for placement and has been draining moderate amounts of yellow-green contents. His vital signs in the PACU are as follows: temperature, 98.0°F; pulse, 86 beats/min; respirations, 16 breaths/min; blood pressure, 134/80 mm Hg. At 1400, he received 4 mg morphine sulfate IV for sharp incisional pain reported as 8 on a scale of 1 to 10 (10 = worst).

At 1500, you receive Mr. Espinoza on your medical-surgical unit via stretcher by a hospital transporter. The NG tube tape that secured the NG to his nose is no longer in place. You also notice that the urinary drainage bag lying on top of his legs has a small amount of amber urine in the reservoir. While you are in his room, Mr. Espinoza says, "Hey, it feels like there's something wet under my back." His vital signs on arrival are as follows: temperature, 98.0°F; pulse, 130 beats/min; respirations, 18 breaths/min; and blood pressure, 100/68 mm Hg. His respirations are regular and unlabored and his skin color is pink. He now rates his pain as dull and 2 on a scale of 1 to 10 (10 = worst). Mr. Espinoza's family is anxiously waiting in the waiting room on your unit.

Prescribed Interventions

Indwelling urinary catheter to gravity × 24 hours; discontinue at 0800 on 8/24

Routine JP drain care

Strict I&O

Routine postoperative vital signs

NG tube to intermittent suction; 30 mL NSS flush q4h

Intravenous fluids: NSS at 50 mL/hr

Morphine sulfate 3 mg IV q4h prn for pain

Developing Clinical Reasoning and Clinical Judgment

- Considering Mr. Espinoza's immediate postoperative status, describe how you would transfer him from the stretcher to his bed.

- Prioritize, with rationales, your assessments and nursing care for Mr. Espinoza in the following areas:
  - Immediate assessments and interventions
  - Assessment and management of tubes
  - Pain management and comfort level
  - Care of his family

continued

Suggested Responses for Integrated Nursing Care

- When transferring Mr. Espinoza to his bed, consider the following factors: minimizing his pain level, protecting his incision, and protecting the patency of his tubes. Excessive strain from moving can cause disruption and bleeding to his abdominal incision. Per facility policy, carefully transfer him, utilizing appropriate transfer devices and the assistance of others (refer to Chapter 9). Consult a safe patient-handling algorithm to help you make decisions about safe patient handling and movement (see Chapter 9). During transfer, be careful not to disrupt his tubes or dressings. Once Mr. Espinoza is in his bed, place his urinary drainage bag on the bed frame so that it hangs below the level of his bladder. This position will allow the urine to drain by gravity and decrease the possibility of a urinary tract infection (see Chapter 12).

- Because Mr. Espinoza is a new postoperative patient, your first priority is to perform an assessment based on the airway, breathing, and circulation (ABC) criteria. Assess his respiratory status (refer to Chapters 2 and 3). Compare his vital signs on arrival with his baseline vital signs. Mr. Espinoza's respiratory rate has not changed significantly from his baseline. If not contraindicated, elevate his head to facilitate deep breathing and continue to assess his airway and respiratory status (see Chapter 6).

- Circulation is the next immediate priority. In Mr. Espinoza's case, his blood pressure has decreased and his heart rate has increased from his baseline in the PACU. Both of these changes could indicate decreased blood volume related to bleeding. Therefore, assess Mr. Espinoza's abdominal dressing to evaluate if it is dry and intact (refer to Chapters 6 and 8). Never assume that an incision is dry just because you cannot see any blood on top of the dressing. If the abdominal dressing is covered by foam tape, blood underneath the tape may not be easily visualized. Look under the patient to see if blood has trickled underneath the dressing. Mr. Espinoza said that he felt something "wet" under his back, and when turning him, you discover that there is a large puddle of bright-red blood underneath him that is caused by acute bleeding from his abdominal incision. Do not remove the abdominal dressing. You may, however, reinforce the dressing per prescribed intervention or facility policy.

- Identify all other possible sources of bleeding. When you assess the JP drains, note the color, amount, and consistency of blood (refer to Chapter 8). Assess his abdomen for signs of internal bleeding, such as abdominal distention. Also check for decreased urine output, another sign indicating a possible decrease in blood volume. A urine output of less than 30 mL/hr may be a sign of hypovolemic shock. Although Mr. Espinoza is bleeding and has signs of decreased blood volume, he is not yet in hypovolemic shock. If Mr. Espinoza's blood pressure continues to drop, elevate his feet to increase venous return. Report all indications of internal and/or external bleeding and other assessment findings to the health care provider (refer to Chapter 6). Acute postoperative bleeding may require surgical repair.

- Your next priority is to ensure that all of his tubes are intact and working properly. One of the first tubes you want to assess for patency is his IV, particularly because he may be returning to surgery (refer to Chapter 16). The next tubes you want to examine are the JP drains. To maintain suction, a JP drain must be less than half full. Assess the color and other characteristics of the JP drainage (see Chapter 8). Next, assess his NG tube (refer to Chapter 13). Mr. Espinoza's NG tube tape is not secure, so you cannot assume that the tube is still in his stomach. Check the NG for placement; assess the pH and amount of the return; measure the length of the exposed tube and compare it with the length documented at the time of insertion; collaborate with the health care team to determine if a radiograph is necessary to confirm placement; once correct placement is verified, place the NG to intermittent suction (refer to Chapter 13). Next, evaluate his urinary catheter to determine if it is draining properly (refer to Chapter 12).

- The next priority is to monitor Mr. Espinoza's pain level (refer to Chapter 10). If he is in acute pain, immediately consider incisional disruption. Because Mr. Espinoza is bleeding, you may need to give small increments as opposed to large amounts of morphine (refer to Chapter 5) to prevent a further drop in his blood pressure; consult with the health care team in light of the assessment findings and changes from baseline. In addition to his physical comfort, attend to potential anxiety about returning to the operating room. Maintain a calm voice and demeanor when caring for Mr. Espinoza.

- Notify the health care team of all assessment findings.

- Do not forget Mr. Espinoza's family, who are anxious to see him. It is helpful to send another staff nurse to keep them updated while you are busy in his room. When his condition stabilizes and before the family visits him, tell them about the tubes that they will see, including the reason for and function of each of the tubes. Be flexible when allowing the family to come in and visit Mr. Espinoza.

Case Study

George Patel, Gwen Galloway, Claudia Tran, and James White

This is your first week as an RN in a small rural hospital. You work the night shift on a medical-surgical unit. Tonight your only assistive personnel (AP) and a staff nurse have called in sick, which makes the unit short-staffed. You have notified the night supervisor that you need help, and they send an AP from another floor to assist you. The AP tells you they can send another nurse in about an hour, and instructs you to take care of the priority cases until that time.

You have six relatively uncomplicated patients; caring for them involves checking their vital signs and giving medications. You instruct the aide to obtain vital signs for these patients and report the results back to you. A quick review of the medications reveals nothing that is urgent; you can wait and have the second nurse administer the medications when they arrive. You have four other patients with more complicated issues, who require additional assessments and urgent care:

- *George Patel, a 64-year-old patient with a tracheostomy, has gurgling sounds coming from his tracheostomy and a frequent, nonproductive cough. His oxygen saturation level via pulse oximetry is 88%. Prescribed interventions include suctioning his tracheostomy prn.*

- *Gwen Galloway had been receiving chemotherapy and has now come back to the hospital with gastroenteritis. When you arrive on your shift, she is experiencing bouts of nausea and vomiting.*

- *Claudia Tran, an 84-year-old patient from a skilled nursing unit, is post-CVA. She has a stage III pressure injury on her coccyx and a stage I pressure injury on her left hip. She needs to be turned every 30 minutes because of rapidly developing erythema on bony prominences. She is confused and has fallen the past two nights when left unattended, even with implementation of fall precautions. Her family is visiting her now but plans to leave in 30 minutes.*

- *James White has COPD. The AP reports that the blood pressure from the automatic cuff is 168/100 mm Hg; his baseline is usually 130/70 mm Hg. The AP also reports that he is complaining of a severe headache, but has no other complaints.*

Developing Clinical Reasoning and Clinical Judgment

- Identify the order in which you would provide care to these patients. Explain your rationales as well as your interventions.

Suggested Responses for Integrated Nursing Care

- Mr. Patel is having difficulty with airway clearance and oxygenation, so he will be your first priority. Nursing priorities follow the ABCs: airway, breathing, and circulation. He will require prompt tracheal suctioning and further evaluation of his respiratory status (see Chapters 3 and 14).

continued

- Next, address the dramatic change in vital signs that Mr. White is experiencing. Mr. White is at risk for adverse effects if his blood pressure continues to stay elevated and is not controlled. Before planning any other interventions, verify the blood pressure by taking it yourself with a manual cuff (see Chapter 2). Initial nursing assessment includes assessing the accuracy of the equipment as well as the accuracy of the information reported to you by assistive personnel. The blood pressure you obtain is 190/110 mm Hg. Check for prescribed interventions regarding possible prn blood pressure medication to administer. Call the health care provider right away and notify them of the change in Mr. White's status.

- You know that Ms. Tran is at high risk for falls if left unattended, and she may injure herself seriously if this occurs. Reducing her risk for injury is your next priority (see Chapter 4). In Ms. Tran's case, you could ask a family member to stay the night, or at least until you get more help on the unit. Many families are willing to help if you make them aware of such situations. If the family leaves, ask the AP to make sure the bed is in a low position, and stay with Ms. Tran until you get further help. You can delegate Ms. Tran's positioning schedule to the aide.

- Despite the obvious distress of vomiting, this is not a life-threatening situation for Mrs. Galloway. Therefore, her condition is a lower priority than that of the other three patients. Mrs. Galloway requires comfort. Check if an antiemetic medication has been prescribed; if not, call the health care provider and obtain a prescription. Other interventions you can perform until her medication takes effect are lowering the lights, applying a cool cloth to the neck, decreasing noises, removing substances that may have a strong odor (e.g., food and vomitus), and keeping her head elevated.

- When prioritizing and delegating care, here are some questions that might help guide your decision-making process:
  - Is the situation life threatening?
  - How rapidly could this patient's condition deteriorate?
  - How quickly can you remedy the problem?
  - Who can provide assistance?

- Whenever a patient's airway, breathing, or circulation is jeopardized, this is a life-threatening emergency. Base your priorities on the ABC criteria. Mr. Patel is your first priority because his airway and oxygenation are a problem. When a patient's condition has the potential to deteriorate rapidly, this is also a priority. In Mr. White's case, because of the spike in his blood pressure, he has the potential for adverse effects. Preventing potential life-threatening effects requires immediate action. When two patients have problems of similar urgency, such as oxygenation, respond to the problem that you can remedy the quickest. Sometimes when you have many activities to accomplish in a short period of time, it is difficult to take time to seek additional help. Many hospitals will have night supervisors to assist you with problem solving. In addition, health care providers are available by phone or in the hospital. Assistive personnel (AP) are sometimes available to assist with noncritical tasks. A nursing skill to develop is prioritization of nursing care and delegation of appropriate tasks and care.

Case Study References

Boullata, J. I., Carrera, A. L., Harvey, L., Escuro, A. A., Hudson, L., Mays, A., McGinnis, C., Wessel, J. J., Bajpai, S., Beebe, M. L., Kinn, T. J., Klang, M. G., Lord, L., Martin, K., Pompeii-Wolfe, C., Sullivan, J., Wood, A., Malone, A., & Guenter, P., & ASPEN Safe Practices for Enteral Nutrition Therapy; American Society for Parenteral and Enteral Nutrition. (2017). ASPEN safe practices for enteral nutrition therapy. *Journal of Parenteral and Enteral Nutrition, 41*(1), 15–103. https://doi.org/10.1177/0148607116673053

Centers for Disease Control and Prevention (CDC). (n.d.). *Sequence for putting on personal protective equipment and how to safely remove personal protective equipment.* [Poster]. https://www.cdc.gov/hai/pdfs/ppe/PPE-Sequence.pdf

Centers for Disease Control and Prevention (CDC). (2018, May 17). Deaths from falls among persons aged ≥ 65 years – United States, 2007–2016. *Morbidity and Mortality Weekly Report (MMWR), 67*(18), 509–514. https://www.cdc.gov/mmwr/volumes/67/wr/mm6718a1.htm

Centers for Disease Control and Prevention (CDC). (2019a). *Hand hygiene in healthcare settings.* https://www.cdc.gov/handhygiene/index.html

Centers for Disease Control and Prevention (CDC). (2019b). *Guideline for isolation precautions: Preventing transmission of infectious agents in healthcare settings.* https://www.cdc.gov/infectioncontrol/guidelines/isolation/index.html

Gorski, L. A., Hadaway, L., Hagle, M. E., Broadhurst, D., Clare, S., Kleidon, T., Meyer, B. M., Nickel, B., Rowley, S., Sharpe, E., & Alexander, M. (2021). Infusion therapy standards of practice, 8th edition. *Journal of Infusion Nursing, 44*(Suppl 1), S1–S224. https://doi.org/10.1097/NAN.0000000000000396

The Joint Commission. (2022). *National patient safety goals. Hospital: 2022 National patient safety goals.* https://www.jointcommission.org/standards/national-patient-safety-goals/hospital-national-patient-safety-goals/

Kapas, S. (2014, February 12). Preventing falls in older people. *The Pharmaceutical Journal, 293*(7834). [Online]. https://pharmaceutical-journal.com/article/ld/preventing-falls-in-older-people

McClave, S. A., DiBaise, J. K., Mullin, G. E., & Martindale, R. G. (2016). ACG clinical guideline: Nutrition therapy in the adult hospitalized patient. *The American Journal of Gastroenterology, 111*(3), 315–334. https://doi.org/10.1038/ajg.2016.28

Norris, T. L. (2020). *Porth's essentials of pathophysiology* (5th ed.). Wolters Kluwer.

Roveron, G., Antonini, M., Barbierato, M., Calandrino, V., Canese, G., Chiurazzi, L. F., Coniglio, G., Gentini, G., Marchetti, M., Minucci, A., Nembrini, L., Neri, V., Trovato, P., & Ferrara, F. (2018). Clinical practice guidelines for the nursing management of percutaneous endoscopic gastrostomy and jejunostomy (PEG/PEJ) in adult patients. *Journal of Wound, Ostomy, and Continence Nursing, 45*(4), 326–334. https://doi.org/10.1097/WON.0000000000000442

Schroeder, J., & Sitzer, V. (2019). Nursing care guidelines for reducing hospital-acquired nasogastric tube-related pressure injuries. *Critical Care Nurse, 39*(6), 54–63.

Taylor, S. J., Allan, K., Clemente, R., Marsh, A., & Toher, D. (2018). Feeding tube securement in critical illness: Implications for safety. *British Journal of Nursing, 27*(18), 1036–1041.

Taylor, C. R., Lynn, P. B., & Bartlett, J. L. (2023). *Fundamentals of nursing: The art and science of person-centered care* (10th ed.). Wolters Kluwer.

Wintersgill, W. (2019). Gait belts 101: A tool for patient and nurse safety. *American Nurse Today, 14*(5), 31–34.

INTRODUCTION

Delegation is the process for a nurse to direct another person to perform nursing tasks and activities (American Nurses Association [ANA] & National Council of State Boards of Nursing [NCSBN], 2019). Delegation involves the transfer of responsibility for the performance of an activity to another individual while retaining accountability for the outcome. Used appropriately, delegation can result in safe and effective nursing care and contribute to improved patient care outcomes (Barrow & Sharma, 2021). Delegation allows the registered nurse (RN) to attend to more complex patient care needs, develops the skills of assistive personnel, and promotes cost containment for the health care organization (ANA & NCSBN, 2019). The decision to delegate is based upon the RN's judgment concerning the condition of the patient, the competence of all members of the nursing team, and the degree of supervision that will be required of the RN if a task is delegated (ANA & NCSBN, 2019).

In delegating, the RN must ensure appropriate assessment, planning, implementation, and evaluation. Decision making about delegation is a continuous process. These guidelines provide a quick reference for the delegation decision-making information found in each skill.

DELEGATION CRITERIA

Criteria to be considered by the RN when deciding to delegate care activities (ANA & NCSBN, 2019) include:

1. The State Nursing Practice Act must permit delegation and outline the authorized task(s) to be delegated or authorize the RN to decide delegation.
2. The person delegating has the appropriate qualifications: appropriate education, skills, and experience as well as current competency.
3. The person receiving the delegation must have the appropriate qualifications: appropriate education, training, skills, and experience as well as evidence of current competency.

In addition, according to the ANA and NCSBN (2019), the delegated task(s) must not involve critical decision making or nursing judgment.

DELEGATION PROCESS

Delegation is a multistep, continuous process.

1. The RN must be fully aware of the parameters for delegation as outlined in their state's Nurse Practice Act as well as the employing organization's policies and procedures regarding delegation (Daley, 2013).
2. The RN must assess the situation, identifying the needs of the patient, considering the circumstances and setting, as well as the competence of the person to whom the task is being delegated (delegatee). The RN may proceed with delegation if patient needs, circumstances, and available resources indicate patient safety will be maintained with delegated care.
3. The RN plans for and clearly communicates the specific task(s) to be delegated. The RN may proceed with delegation if the nature of the task, competence of the person receiving the delegation, and patient implications indicate patient safety will be maintained with delegated care.
4. The RN maintains overall accountability for the patient. The delegatee bears the responsibility for the delegated activity, skill, or procedure (ANA & NCSBN, 2019). The RN may proceed with delegation if the RN and person receiving the delegation accept the accountability for their respective roles in the delegated patient care.
5. The RN supervises performance of the delegated task(s), providing directions and clear expectations of how the task(s) is to be performed. The RN monitors performance, intervenes if necessary, and ensures the appropriate documentation.
6. The RN must evaluate the entire delegation process, evaluating the patient, the performance of the task(s), and obtain and provide feedback.
7. The RN must reassess and adjust the overall plan of care, as needed.

FIVE RIGHTS OF DELEGATION

The Five Rights of Delegation provide a resource to facilitate decisions about delegation. The ANA and NCSBN (2019) identify the Five Rights of Delegation as follows:

- **Right Task:** One that falls within the delegatee's job description or is included as part of the established written policies and procedures of the practice setting.
- **Right Circumstances:** The health condition of the patient must be stable. Changes in the patient's condition require the delegatee to communicate this to the RN, and the RN must reassess the situation and the appropriateness of the delegation.
- **Right Person:** The delegatee possesses the appropriate skills and knowledge to perform the activity.

- **Right Direction/Communication:** Each delegation situation should be specific to the patient, the licensed nurse, and the delegatee. A clear, concise description of the task, including its objective, limits, and expectations should be provided.
- **Right Supervision/Evaluation:** This includes appropriate monitoring, evaluation, intervention, as needed, and feedback.

"DO-NOT-DELEGATE" CARE

Nursing care or tasks that should never be delegated except to another RN include:

- Initial and ongoing nursing assessment of the patient and their nursing care needs
- Determination of the nursing diagnosis, nursing care plan, evaluation of the patient's progress in relation to the care plan, and evaluation of the nursing care delivered to the patient
- Supervision and education of nursing personnel; patient teaching that requires an assessment of the patient and their education needs
- Any other nursing interventions that require professional nursing knowledge, judgment, and/or skill

DELEGATION DECISION TREE

Using skills, knowledge, and professional judgment, the RN determines appropriate nursing practice based on the state practice act and professional scope of practice, the standards and code of ethics, and the organization's policies and procedures related to delegation (ANA & NCSBN, 2019).

The Decision Tree for Delegation by Registered Nurses distributed by the American Nurses Association and the National Council of State Boards of Nursing can assist nurses with delegation decisions. The Decision Tree for Delegation can be found at https://www.ncsbn.org/Delegation_joint_statement_NCSBN-ANA.pdf

References and Resources

American Nurses Association (ANA) and National Council of State Boards of Nursing (NCSBN). (2019). *National guidelines for nursing delegation.* https://www.nursingworld.org/~4962ca/globalassets/practiceandpolicy/nursing-excellence/ana-position-statements/nursing-practice/ana-ncsbn-joint-statement-on-delegation.pdf

Barrow, J. M., & Sharma, S. (2021, July 26). *Five rights of nursing delegation.* StatPearls [Internet]. https://www.ncbi.nlm.nih.gov/books/NBK519519/

Daley, K. (2013). Helping nurses strengthen their delegation skills. *American Nurse Today, 8*(3), 18.

National Council of State Boards of Nursing (NCSBN). (2016). National guidelines for nursing delegation. *Journal of Nursing Regulation, 7*(1), 5–12. https://www.ncsbn.org/NCSBN_Delegation_Guidelines.pdf

National Council of State Boards of Nursing (NCSBN). (2021). *Delegation.* https://www.ncsbn.org/1625.htm

Note: Page number followed by b, f, and t indicates text in box, figure, and table respectively.